evolve

∴ To access your Student Resources, visit the Web address below:

http://evolve.elsevier.com/Pellerito/driver

Evolve Student Learning Resources for Pellerito: Driver Rehabilitation and Community Mobility: Principles and Practice offers the following features

- **WebLinks**
  Links to organizations and other helpful websites.

- **References**
  Links to Medline abstracts.

- **Crossword Puzzles**
  Vocabulary-building exercises.

- **Additional Readings**
  List of additional references for research.

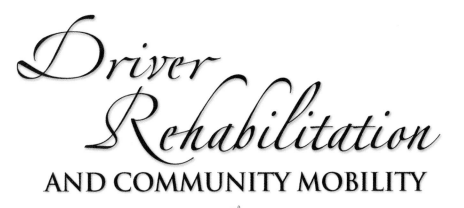

Driver Rehabilitation

AND COMMUNITY MOBILITY

Principles and Practice

Driver *Rehabilitation*

AND COMMUNITY MOBILITY

PRINCIPLES AND PRACTICE

JOSEPH MICHAEL PELLERITO, JR., MS, OTR

ASSOCIATE PROFESSOR AND ACADEMIC PROGRAM DIRECTOR

OCCUPATIONAL THERAPY PROGRAM

EUGENE APPLEBAUM COLLEGE OF
PHARMACY AND HEALTH SCIENCES

WAYNE STATE UNIVERSITY

DETROIT, MICHIGAN

WITH 48 CONTRIBUTING AUTHORS

FOREWORD BY
WILLIAM CLAY FORD, JR.

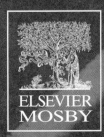

ELSEVIER
MOSBY

ELSEVIER
MOSBY

11830 Westline Industrial Drive
St. Louis, Missouri 63146

Driver Rehabilitation and Community Mobility   ISBN 0-323-02937-X
Copyright © 2006, Mosby, Inc.

NOTICE

Knowledge and best practice in this field are constantly changing. As new research and experience broaden our knowledge, changes in practice, treatment and drug therapy may become necessary or appropriate. Readers are advised to check the most current information provided (i) on procedures featured or (ii) by the manufacturer of each product to be administered, to verify the recommended dose or formula, the method and duration of administration, and contraindications. It is the responsibility of the practitioner, relying on their own experience and knowledge of the patient, to make diagnoses, to determine dosages and the best treatment for each individual patient, and to take all appropriate safety precautions. To the fullest extent of the law, neither the Publisher nor the Editors assumes any liability for any injury and/or damage to persons or property arising out or related to any use of the material contained in this book.
Neither the Publisher nor the Editors assume any responsibility for any loss or injury and/or damage to persons or property arising out of or related to any use of the material contained in this book. It is the responsibility of the treating practitioner, relying on independent expertise and knowledge of the patient, to determine the best treatment and method of application for the patient.

International Standard Book Number 0-323-02937-X

Publishing Director: Linda Duncan
Editor: Kathy Falk
Developmental Editor: Melissa Kuster Deutsch
Publishing Services Manager: Pat Joiner
Project Manager: David Stein
Designer: Jyotika Shroff

Printed in the United States of America

Last digit is the print number: 9 8 7 6 5 4 3 2 1

REVIEWERS

Karmen M. Brown, MPH, OTR, FMOTA
Director, Fieldwork Education & Assistant
   Professor
Occupational Therapy Program
Eugene Applebaum College of Pharmacy and
   Health Sciences
Wayne State University
Detroit, Michigan

Randall L. Commissaris, Ph.D.
Associate Professor
Department of Pharmaceutical Sciences
Eugene Applebaum College of Pharmacy and
   Health Sciences
Wayne State University
Detroit, Michigan

Gerry E. Conti, MS, OTR
Assistant Professor
Occupational Therapy Program
Eugene Applebaum College of Pharmacy and
   Health Sciences
Wayne State University
Detroit, Michigan

Tapan K. Datta, PhD, PE
Professor
Department of Civil and Environmental
   Engineering
Wayne State University
Detroit, Michigan

Maggie Katz, BA, MBA
Director of Development
Eugene Applebaum College of Pharmacy and
   Health Sciences
Wayne State University
Detroit, Michigan

Catherine L. Lysack, PhD, OT(C)
Associate Professor
Institute of Gerontology and the Occupational
   Therapy Program
Wayne State University
Detroit, Michigan

Linda McQuistion, PhD, PE, CPE
Rehabilitation Engineer
Rehabilitation Technology Support Unit
Ohio Rehabilitation Services Commission
Canton, Ohio

Regina Parnell, MS, OTR
Senior Lecturer
Occupational Therapy Program
Eugene Applebaum College of Pharmacy and
   Health Sciences
Wayne State University
Detroit, Michigan

Fredrick D. Pociask, PhD, PT, OCS
Assistant Professor
Physical Therapy Program
Wayne State University
Detroit, Michigan

Wynefred Schumann, MS, FAASCU
Assistant Dean Student & Alumni Affairs (Retired)
Associate Professor
Department of Pharmacy Practice
Eugene Applebaum College of Pharmacy and
   Health Sciences
Wayne State University
Detroit, Michigan

Stacey L. Schepens, BS, OTR
Occupational Therapist and Graduate Research
Assistant
Occupational Therapy Program
Eugene Applebaum College of Pharmacy and
Health Sciences
Wayne State University
Detroit, Michigan

Suzanne B. Siegel, MFA, BA
Kalamazoo, Michigan

Susan Ann Talley, PT, MA, DPT
Director and Academic Coordinator of Clinical
Education
Physical Therapy Program
Eugene Applebaum College of Pharmacy and
Health Sciences
Wayne State University
Detroit, Michigan

Mary Warren, MS, OTR/L
Assistant Professor, Occupational Therapy
Director Graduate Certificate in Low Vision
Rehabilitation
University of Alabama at Birmingham
Birmingham, Alabama

CONTRIBUTORS

Beth E. Anderson, OTR/L, CDRS
Certified Driver Rehabilitation Specialist
Rehab Results Group
DeKalb Medical Center
Decatur, Georgia

Patrick T. Baker, MHS, OTR/L, CLVT, CDRS
Geriatric Clinical Specialist
The Cleveland Clinic Foundation
Cleveland, Ohio

Lori Benner, MPA, OTR/L, CDRS
Manager Ortho/General Medical
    Therapy Services Team
Drivers Evaluation and Training
Hershey, Pennsylvania

Carol A. Blanc, OTR/L, CDRS, BS
Senior Occupational Therapist, Certified Driver
    Rehabilitation Specialist
Occupational Therapy, Adapted Driving Program
Banner Good Samaritan Rehabilitation Institute
Phoenix, Arizona

Kevin Borsay, MS, EE
Archive Design Studio
Detroit, Michigan

Jerry Bouman, BA, CDRS
Program Manager
Driver Rehabilitation Program
Mary Free Bed Rehabilitation Hospital
Grand Rapids, Michigan

Bethany Broadwell, BA
Disabilities Issues Journalist
West Bloomfield, Michigan

Renee Coleman Bryer, PhD
Assistant Professor
Department of Physical Medicine and Rehabilitation
Wayne State University
Clinical Neuropsychologist
Department of Rehabilitation Psychology and
    Neuropsychology
Rehabilitation Institute of Michigan
Detroit, Michigan

Cynthia J. Burt, OTR, CDRS
Senior Therapist
Rehabilitation Institute of Michigan
Detroit, Michigan

Tapan K. Datta, PhD, PE
Professor
Department of Civil and Environmental
    Engineering
Wayne State University
Detroit, Michigan

Elin Schold Davis, OTR, CDRS
Senior Occupational Therapist
Sister Kenny Rehabilitation Institute
Minneapolis, Minnesota
Coordinator, AOTA Older Driver Initiative
American Occupational Therapy Association
Bethesda, Maryland

Marilyn Di Stefano, BAppSc (Occ Ther), GradDipErg, AccOT, Associate Fellow ACRS
Senior Lecturer, Co-ordinator
Postgraduate Occupational Health and Safety
  Programs
Joint Course Co-ordinator: Driver Education and
  Rehabilitation
Occupational Therapy
La Trobe University
Buncoora, Victoria, Australia
Convenor, National Advisory Group: Driving, OT
  Australia
Australian Occupational Therapy Association
Melbourne, Victoria, Australia
Associate Fellow,
Australasian College of Road Safety
Mawson, Australian Capital Territory, Australia

David W. Eby, PhD
Research Associate Professor
University of Michigan Transportation Research
  Institute
Ann Arbor, Michigan

R. Darin Ellis, PhD
Associate Professor
Department of Industrial and Manufacturing
  Engineering
Wayne State University
Detroit, Michigan

Richard J. Genik II, PhD
Assistant Professor
Psychiatry and Behavioral Neurosciences
Emergent Technology Research Division
Deputy Director for Technology Integration and
  Planning
Department of Psychiatry and Behavioral
  Neurosciences
Wayne State University School of Medicine
Detroit, Michigan

Christopher C. Green, MD, PhD
Executive Director
Emergent Technology Research Division
Assistant Professor
Department of Psychiatry and Behavioral
  Neurosciences, and Diagnostic Radiology
Fellow, Clinical Neuroimaging
Diagnostic Radiology
Wayne State University School of Medicine
Detroit, Michigan

Elizabeth L. Green, OTR/L, CDRS
Director
Occupational Therapy Program
Frye Regional Medical Center
Hickory, North Carolina

Robin A. Hanks, PhD, ABCN-ABPP
Assistant Professor
Department of Physical Medicine and
  Rehabilitation
Wayne State University
Chief of Rehabilitation Psychology and
  Neuropsychology
Department of Rehabilitation Psychology and
  Neuropsychology
Rehabilitation Institute of Michigan
Detroit, Michigan

Ann B. Havard, LOTR, CDRS, ATP
Driver Rehabilitation Program Manager
Center for Biomedical Engineering and
  Rehabilitation Science
Louisiana Tech University
Ruston, Louisiana

Li Hsieh, PhD
Assistant Professor
Department of Audiology & Speech-Language
  Pathology
Wayne State University
Detroit, Michigan

Charles P. Huss, MA
ACVREP Certified Orientation & Rehabilitation
  Specialist
Life Skills Training Unit—Blind & Visually
  Impaired Services
West Virginia Rehabilitation Center
Institute, West Virginia

Charles K. Hyde, PhD
Professor
Department of History
Wayne State University
Detroit, Michigan

Deena Garrison Jones, OTL, CDRS
Founder, President
Boundless Mobility
Waynesboro, Virginia

Thomas D. Kalina, MS, OTR/L, CDRS
Adapted Driving Supervisor
Adapted Driving Program
Bryn Mawr Rehabilitation Hospital
Malvern, Pennsylvania

Annette Lavezza, OTR/L, CDRS
Senior Occupational Therapist
Johns Hopkins Driving Program
Lutherville, Maryland

Catherine L. Lysack, PhD, OT(C)
Associate Professor
Institute of Gerontology and Occupational Therapy
    Program
Wayne State University
Detroit, Michigan

**Wendy Macdonald, PhD, DipPsych, BSc (Hons),
FSIA, MAPS, MHFESA, MHFES**
Associate Professor
Centre for Ergonomics and Human Factors,
    Faculty of Health Sciences
La Trobe University
Melbourne, Victoria, Australia

Miriam Ashley Manary, MSE
Senior Engineering Research Associate
Biosciences Division
University of Michigan Transportation Research
    Institute
Ann Arbor, Michigan

Susan L. Martin, OTR/L, DRS
Occupational Therapist, Driver Rehabilitation
    Specialist
Physical Medicine and Rehabilitation
Johns Hopkins Driving Program
Baltimore, Maryland

Chris Maurer, MPT, ATP
Physical Therapist
Assistive Technology Center
Atlanta, Georgia

Linda McQuistion, PhD, PE, CPE
Rehabilitation Engineer
Rehabilitation Technology Support Unit
Ohio Rehabilitation Services Commission
Canton, Ohio

Lisa J. Molnar, MHSA
Senior Research Associate
Social and Behavioral Analysis
University of Michigan Transportation Research
    Institute
Ann Arbor, Michigan

Karen Monaco, OTR, CDRS
President
Monaco's Therapy on Wheels, Inc.
Augusta, Georgia

Mark Nickita, AIA
Archive Design Studio
Detroit, Michigan

Susan Popek-Boeve, CTRS, ATRIC
Senior Therapeutic Recreation Specialist
Adult Neuro Outpatient and Campus Inpatient
Rehabilitation Institute of Michigan
Detroit, Michigan

Lisa J. Rapport, PhD
Associate Professor
Department of Psychology
Wayne State University
Detroit, Michigan

Susan Redepenning, OTR/L, CDRS
Occupational Therapist
Occupational Therapy Solutions, Inc.
Minneapolis, Minnesota

Dana L. Roeling, MEd
Executive Director
National Mobility Equipment Dealers Association
Tampa, Florida

Lawrence W. Schneider, PhD
Research Professor
Biosciences Division
University of Michigan Transportation Research
    Institute
Ann Arbor, Michigan

Janie B. Scott, MA, OTR/L, FAOTA
Occupational Therapy Consultant
Columbia, Maryland

Michael K. Shipp, MEd, CDRS
Associate Director for Rehabilitation Services
Center for Biomedical Engineering and
    Rehabilitation Science
Louisiana Tech University
Assistant Director for Rehabilitation Services
Ruston, Louisiana

Franklin Stein, PhD, OTR, FAOTA
Professor Emeritus
Occupational Therapy
University of South Dakota
Vermillion, South Dakota
Editor, Occupational Therapy International

Erica B. Stern, PhD, OTR/L, FAOTA
Associate Professor
Program in Occupational Therapy
University of Minnesota
Minneapolis, Minnesota

Chad Strowmatt, LOT, CDRS
Strowmatt Rehabilitation Services, Inc.
Houston, Texas
President
Association for Driver Rehabilitation Specialists
Ruston, Louisiana

Gary Leonard Talbot, BSME
Lake Buena Vista, Florida

Renee Tyree, PharmD, CDRS
Certified Driver Rehabilitation Specialist
Ability Driver Rehabilitation Services
Tucson, Arizona

Carol J. Wheatley, OTR/L, CDRS
Occupational Therapist, Driver Rehabilitation
  Specialist
Rehabilitation Technology Services
Workforce and Technology Center
Maryland Division of Rehabilitation Services
Baltimore, Maryland

This book is dedicated to my wife, Laura;
my anchor, compass, and inspiration.

To my children, Lillian Alexandra and Joseph III;
my precious, enduring, and living legacy;
they are grace and beauty,
and all that I aspire to be.

To the people with disabilities, aging-related concerns, and their caregivers who
I have had the privilege to serve, over the past 25 years.

To my mother;
she has taught me the meaning of optimism, courage, and perseverance.

And to my father (In memorium);
he thought cars were a pain in his derrière.

FOREWORD

Mobility speaks volumes in today's world. Its definitions are as rich and varied as the contexts of people's lives. We take mobility as our birthright. Bikes and cars mark rites of passages as children grow into adulthood and experience the freedom and independence to push the boundaries of their known worlds. The open road is our metaphor for limitless possibilities and the freedom to explore what lies beyond the horizon. We have mastered the open road, we have been to the moon and back, we have only to choose the vehicle that will take us.

My great-grandfather, Henry Ford, founded Ford Motor Company at a time when mobility was not assumed or taken for granted. It was his dream to make mobility available to the average working man. His Model T, a car for the multitude, put the world on wheels, and the world has been defining and redefining *mobility* ever since. One such redefinition was born of Henry Ford's friendship with the Wright Brothers and his interest in flight. His support of civil and commercial aviation advanced private investment and public confidence in, and national acceptance of, the viability of a new mode of transport and travel.

Our passion at Ford to make mobility available to *all* our customers continues today. Because we recognize the needs of a population that does not take movement for granted, the Ford Mobility Motoring program was created to assist customers with disabilities to adapt the vehicle of their choice to their special needs. Vehicles are customized to fit an individual's particular driving requirements as he or she works in concert with our dealers and adaptive equipment suppliers to obtain the best fit possible between driver and vehicle.

I am particularly grateful to Joseph M. Pellerito, Jr. for the contribution he is making to exploring the challenges of mobility for the disabled, their caregivers, and aging drivers in his latest work, *Driver Rehabilitation and Community Mobility: Principles and Practice*. Thanks to the work of experts like Professor Pellerito and his colleagues in the field of occupational therapy, and other professionals in medical and engineering disciplines, evidence-based data are creating an increasingly scientific approach to solving the problems of adaptive motoring. As a leader in this special-market industry, Ford intends to keep the momentum going.

Professor Pellerito also studies the mobility issue for people who do not drive but rely on community-provided mobility. He explores alternate sources of transportation that enable nondrivers to remain connected to their communities, needed services, and each other. In the context of an aging population of baby boomers, increased lifetime expectancies, and an increased emphasis on quality of life, the research set before us is timely and compelling.

As we improve the mobility of customers who are disabled and challenged by conventional driving skills and vehicles, we are enabling all our customers to enjoy a birthright of autonomy and freedom of movement. When we make a positive difference in the lives of one community, we are helping to make a positive difference—and building a better world—for everyone.

William Clay Ford, Jr.
Chairman and CEO
Ford Motor Company
Dearborn, Michigan

PREFACE

Working with people with disabilities, the elderly, and their caregivers within the context of driver rehabilitation and community mobility has been a practice area of great interest and importance to me throughout most of my professional career. My interest was cultivated during the many years of adult physical medicine and rehabilitation services (i.e., occupational therapy services) I was involved in providing along with my colleagues at Rehabilitation Institute of Michigan (RIM) in the Detroit Medical Center (DMC) in Detroit, Michigan. It was early in my career when I first began to notice that my clients would consistently identify their desire to return to driving as a primary goal that often superseded other team-supported goals, such as those related to achieving higher levels of independence when performing basic activities of daily living (ADL).

Driving provided my clients with more than the means to move from place to place; driving provided them with the means to preserve critical links to their communities and to the personal and professional ties or relationship networks that are necessary for a robust and vital social life. Irrespective of age, obtaining and keeping a driver's license is much more than what the law defines as a privilege; it is a universal symbol of autonomy and independence.

Clients more often than not were highly motivated to successfully return to driving, especially while overcoming the challenges associated with serious injuries, illnesses, and/or the aging process. Driving was their primary mode for community mobility and appeared to empower them in numerous ways. First, driving enabled them to reconnect with their primary (e.g., family, neighborhood) and secondary (e.g., friends, associates) group members, return to their preillness/preinjury roles and responsibilities, and participate in meaningful activities within their personal and professional communities. Conversely, I also witnessed the negative effects that driving cessation had on my clients young and old. Most of them lived in an urban setting, were no longer able to drive, and could not access dependable alternative transportation (e.g., mass transit, public transportation, an available family member or friend willing to drive them around town, or private transportation). More often than not driving cessation resulted in my clients reporting that they had increased feelings of isolation, loneliness, and depression; weakened personal and professional ties (i.e., networks) because of diminished contact with others; declining health; reduced community participation; and marginalized quality of life. These revelations motivated me to begin developing and honing my professional skills in the areas of driver rehabilitation and community mobility.

It was a combination of experiences that motivated me to begin examining driver rehabilitation more closely. Community mobility would also become an important area to address (e.g., alternative transportation and driving cessation) for those clients who were unable to return to driving because they could not afford an adapted vehicle or because of any number of other factors that precluded them from procuring a motor vehicle. Not enough research was focused on driver rehabilitation and there was a paucity of research on community mobility and driving cessation.

Why Community Mobility?

Driver rehabilitation services should include addressing *community mobility* because not everyone can safely drive a motor vehicle. Managing the effects of driving cessation and educating clients about alternative transportation options are critical services that driver rehabilitation specialists should provide for their clients and their clients' caregivers.

Professional Credentials

It remains unclear as to the "optimal" credentials and experience DRSs should possess. Occupational therapists and driver educators possess skills, knowledge, experience, and perspectives that are complementary. Clients and their caregivers are best served when occupational therapists and driver educators work together to provide driver rehabilitation and community mobility services that are client-focused and evidence-based.

Professional organizations including the AOTA, ADED, NHTSA, and NMEDA are working together to help ensure that the public is best served by exploring ways to expand the capacity for meeting the increased demand for DRSs, providing shared oversight of the credentialing processes for individuals wanting to develop an expertise in this rapidly evolving field, and facilitating research that will provide evidence to support or refute current evaluation and intervention practices. This book is another valuable tool that will help facilitate both the growth and development of individual practitioners and driver rehabilitation and community mobility as a respected profession that spans the globe.

The Book

It was a privilege to have had the opportunity to fulfill the role of editor and author for this unique and dynamic textbook and supplemental CD-ROM. I am honored to introduce the world's first book that offers a comprehensive overview of driver rehabilitation and community mobility for people with disabilities, the elderly, and their caregivers. It presents historical and global perspectives that link sound theoretical principles with the application of knowledge that drives innovative and evidence-based practice. The book comprises 26 chapters and 9 appendices that were written by leading experts who work within the rapidly evolving field of driver rehabilitation and community mobility. Their collective wisdom and years of experience have been instrumental in helping to ensure that this book reflects the belief that efficacious and evidence-based practice should be founded on sound research that supports professional judgment, reasoning, and experience.

In addition to the book's chapters and appendices, an Adapted Driving Decision Guide is on the supplemental CD-ROM. The guide features a dynamic algorithm (i.e., a series of questions) pertaining to a client's adapted driving needs. The client's physical and cognitive status, currently used mobility equipment, ability to access a vehicle, optimal vehicle type, and potential adapted driving controls or aids are examined. The client and the DRS can explore rich content and images reflecting recommendations for potential solutions that address optimal transfer techniques, best vehicle type, options for stowing a mobility aid, and suggested adapted driving controls. Presenting the guide in electronic format on CD-ROM will enable service providers, teachers, and students alike to use it as a tool that readily augments the book's rich content. As the professional or student moves through the guide with an actual or hypothetical client, topic areas can be explored reflecting key considerations and potential solutions to meet driver rehabilitation and community mobility needs.

Primary Aims

The primary aims of this book are to advance the health, safety, and well-being of society through the preparation of highly skilled DRSs and, through evidence-based content, to help them to discover, evaluate, and implement new knowledge related to driver rehabilitation and community mobility. This book will contribute to ensuring that clinicians, researchers, practitioners, teachers, and students achieve these aims by:

- Educating and preparing learners to become practitioners who function effectively and efficiently in a rapidly changing, culturally diverse, and multidisciplinary health care environment
- Promoting research directed toward generating new knowledge and understanding of driver rehabilitation and community mobility services, while improving DRS practice and interventions
- Developing researchers and scientists to create new knowledge and understanding that will enhance driver evaluation and rehabilitation
- Developing new and strengthening existing collaborative relationships with healthcare providers, private sector industries, academia, consumer groups, and other organizations that enrich learning, support current research, and improve the design and delivery of driver rehabilitation and community mobility services
- Disseminating new knowledge and understanding to occupational therapists working as DRSs, occupational therapy generalists, professionals working within the health care industry, other DRSs, and organizations committed to improving life conditions related to community mobility for clients and their families
- Disseminating knowledge about disability and rehabilitation to promote overall health, safety, and well-being, as it relates to the urban, rural, and global driver rehabilitation and community mobility
- Influencing policy to improve individual access to safe and reliable transportation

Evidence-Based Practice

This book examines driver rehabilitation and community mobility through the lens of the helping professions and, whenever possible, from an evidence-based perspective. However, much of what is considered acceptable practice today is not necessarily grounded in research, but is founded instead on clinical and on-road experience of DRSs. Specialists have always been willing to share their successes, challenges, and even failures with others who are involved in driver rehabilitation, and professional networking may be the DRS's most valuable asset. More recently, specialists have begun to explore community mobility issues (alternative transportation and driving cessation), especially for those individuals who are no longer able to drive. The result of the informal and formal collaboration is a kind of cumulative knowledge that has developed over time and that has filled a critical void (i.e., the immediate needs of clients and caregivers) while valid research that could be translated into evidence-based practice was just beginning to inform practice. This is not to diminish the value that experience, imagination, and creativity play in guiding and informing practitioners and researchers in the pursuit of efficacious driver rehabilitation and community mobility practice. Nevertheless, thoughtful examination of the existing standards of practice in order to support or refute the evaluation and intervention methods employed by contemporary DRSs is warranted. What better place to capture and compile their collective wisdom, experience, research, and vision than in a comprehensive book?

The Contributors

Contributors with diverse backgrounds (e.g., credentials, work settings, roles, and experiences) were invited to participate in this project to emphasize the importance of the team approach—one that values and respects a client-centered orientation. In this text, the contributors and I aim to make a valuable contribution to the identification, explication, and application of knowledge about driver rehabilitation and community mobility. Within this focus, I have strived to present a range of topics that will speak to driver rehabilitation and community mobility for people with disabilities, the elderly, and their caregivers across the lifespan. The topics presented in this textbook under the broad heading of driver rehabilitation and community mobility examine the impact mobility has on what people can do within the context of daily occupations (i.e., meaningful activities), roles, habits, and community participation leading to a full and robust social life. The term "participation" as used in this text is congruent with its use in the World Health Organization's (WHO) International Classification for Functioning, Disability, and Health, also known as the ICF, because it acknowledges that participation is enhanced when individuals are empowered by removing social barriers and providing social supports.

My Cultural Perspective

How society views and values mobility is fashioned by its culture and is influenced by an individual's gender, habits, roles, ethnicity, race, age, economic status, geographic location, and political affiliation. My cultural perspective (and that of the book's contributors) is fundamentally that from developed, western, and industrialized countries. There are a constellation of issues pertaining to driver rehabilitation and community mobility that are universal, and much of the content that is presented can be effectively applied in order to improve driver rehabilitation and community mobility service delivery, irrespective of geographic location or socioeconomic or geopolitical status. In urban, suburban, and rural settings around the world people must rely on safe, reliable, and accessible transportation. I am not asserting that this book is some kind of panacea for mobility issues; instead, I believe that our collective effort will help to improve the quality of services and research centering on driver rehabilitation and community mobility for people with disabilities, the elderly, and their caregivers on both macro (i.e., global) and micro (i.e., individuals, small groups, and towns) levels.

Many of the contributors that participated in writing portions of this textbook are from the United States; however, others are from countries such as Australia and Canada. Their perspectives have added greatly to the depth and breadth of the content presented here and will help to further the global effort to understand and improve evaluation and intervention strategies that aim to address driver rehabilitation and community mobility. We have much to learn from one another and are strengthened by the professional collaboration that can occur with ease over great distances thanks to computing and information technology, the Internet, the World Wide Web (WWW), and people who are willing and able to use technology for electronic collaboration.

Topic Selection

There are additional topics that I wanted to include or present in greater detail in this textbook but did not because of time and space constraints: For example, leading-edge strategies for driver education along gender, age, or ethnic (i.e., people who speak English as a second language) lines; problems associated with driving while under the influence of drugs or alcohol or both; and driving and community mobility within developing countries. Although these topics are outside my own professional experience and expertise, I acknowledge their importance and take some comfort in knowing that they are being addressed elsewhere by other researchers and practitioners interested in driver rehabilitation and community mobility.

Driver rehabilitation and community mobility cannot be neatly presented in a concrete or "linear" fashion. Nor can the clinical reasoning that is driven by an understanding of the available evidence in the professional literature and tempered by real-world experience be presented as a static bundle of neatly organized concepts. The issues, perspectives, and constructions of reality vary from person to person and are influenced by the role or roles each of us assumes (e.g., client, caregiver, DRS, mobility equipment dealer, academic). The contributors provided dynamic content that reflects their unique perspectives and respective areas of expertise. We attempted to include viewpoints from the entire team of professionals, which included the client (i.e., the center of the team) and his or her caregivers. We examined driver rehabilitation and community mobility activities that range from topics and issues that appear to be universal (i.e., understood on a global level) to the unique and even idiosyncratic personal needs that clients and caregivers may present. For example, we explored driver rehabilitation and community mobility within the larger context of a worldwide car culture in which driving is viewed by most people as much more than a privilege but, in fact, a rite of passage. We also discovered that driving and community mobility play a critical role in fostering a robust social life for people throughout the world, examined the negative effects of driving cessation, and have identified the need for an evidence-based approach to driver rehabilitation and community mobility services.

How this Book Is Organized

The 26 chapters in this book are organized into seven main parts. Additionally, nine appendices, a glossary of terms, an index, and a supplemental CD-ROM featuring the Adapted Driving Decision Guide have been provided to augment the book's rich chapter content. Part I includes chapters 1 through 4 and provides an introduction (Chapter 1), an historical perspective of driving (Chapter 2), the role driving plays in American culture (Chapter 3), and an introduction of the driver rehabilitation team (Chapter 4).

Part II includes Chapters 5 through 10. In this section, methods of measuring driving potential before taking a client on the road are described in great detail. These include introducing the reader to the Adapted Driving Decision Guide that is a tool for facilitating discussion between the driver rehabilitation specialist, the client, and his or her caregivers about potential adapted driving solutions (Chapter 5); examining the driver rehabilitation and community mobility clinical evaluation (Chapter 6); exploring how neuropsychologists help predict a client's readiness to drive after an injury, illness, or the aging process (Chapter 7); reviewing how medications can effect drivers and driving outcomes (Chapter 8); discovering the impact of positioning and mobility devices on driving and community mobility (Chapter 9); and determining how simulators are bridging the gap between the clinical and on-road driving evaluations (Chapter 10).

Part III includes Chapters 11 through 13 and contains information on the steps involved in performing an on-road driver evaluation. These include how DRSs prepare for the on-road evaluation by identifying the optimal vehicle type and setting-up the adaptive driving equipment before taking a client on the road (Chapter 11). A comprehensive on-road driver evaluation with considerations related to vision, hearing, orthopedic, neurological, and psychosocial conditions and impairments is provided as well (Chapter 12). On-road driver rehabilitation and training are also covered (Chapter 13).

Part IV includes Chapters 14 and 15 and presents content on how to document the clinical and on-road evaluations (Chapter 14) as well as how to secure funding for driver rehabilitation and community mobility products and services (Chapter 15).

Part V explores the environmental factors that impact drivers, passengers, and pedestrians. These factors include how principles of universal design are impacting the design and ultimate functionality of vehicles today and in the future (Chapter 16); how wheelchairs, wheelchair tiedowns, and occupant restraints influence safety and crash protection for drivers and passengers (Chapter 17); the various types of In-vehicle Intelligent Transport Systems and how IITS design influences driving task demands (Chapter 18); how designing the external environment can impact traffic safety for drivers, passengers, and pedestrians (Chapter 19); the role driving and community mobility play while individuals pursue sports, recreation, and leisure interests (Chapter 20); the negative consequences that are often associated with driving cessation and some unique tools to address issues pertaining to alternative transportation (Chapter 21); and the impact that sound urban planning and reliable alternative transportation have on communities and individuals (Chapter 22).

Part VI examines the important role that professional ethics plays (Chapter 23), research that supports evidence-based driver rehabilitation (Chapter 24), and next-generation neuroimaging that enables researchers to watch people think in order to understand deficits and improve driving performance (Chapter 25).

Part VII, consisting of Chapter 26, delves into program development in a rapidly evolving field. Numerous appendices follow Section VII and offer a plethora of information for the DRS, student, academic (i.e., teacher, researcher, or both), healthcare worker, entrepreneur, client, caregiver, and others who share an interest in driver rehabilitation and community mobility.

Joseph M. Pellerito, Jr.

ACKNOWLEDGMENTS

Driver Rehabilitation and Community Mobility: Principles and Practice is the first comprehensive textbook on the topic of driver rehabilitation and community mobility published in the Unites States. It was constructed chiefly due to the valuable contributions of 50 contributors and 14 reviewers who brought diverse professional perspectives to this project from academe, the private business and corporate sectors, healthcare, and the automotive industry. The book's dynamic content reflects their dedication to excellence and willingness to share their unique insight and knowledge gained over years of experience in a rapidly changing field. I want to extend my heartfelt thanks to them for making this project possible and a success.

Heartfelt thanks to William Clay Ford, Jr., Chairman of the Board and Chief Executive Officer of Ford Motor Company, for writing the captivating forward to this book. His vision and leadership have continued a proud and distinct legacy that his great grandfather, Henry Ford, started more than a century ago in a small factory just outside of Detroit, Michigan. I am thrilled for many reasons that he agreed to be a part of this project and cannot possibly list each of them here. However, I would like to convey that I hold a deep respect for him as a corporate leader and as a human being. He presents an industrious and inspiring vision for tomorrow that requires dedication to the notion of enhancing the safety, well-being, and quality of life for the talented men and women ultimately responsible for producing motor vehicles; the safety and well-being of consumers and other roadway users; and the health and wellness of the planet's natural resources for future generations.

I would be remiss if I did not recognize the contributions that were made indirectly to this project by the contributors' family members. Encouragement, sacrifices, and accommodations enabled the contributors to complete the constellation of tasks involved in completing this book project. I would also like to extend my thanks to my colleagues at Wayne State University in the Occupational Therapy Program: Karmen Brown, Gerry Conti, Rosanne Di Zazzo-Miller, Doreen Head, Catherine Lysack, Regina Parnell, and Tamra Samuels. Their encouragement and willingness to help out in so many thoughtful ways made a significant difference, especially during the last few weeks of the project that included last minute editing and the proverbial tying-up of a thousand and one loose ends. I would also like to acknowledge my friends and colleagues at the American Occupational Therapy Association (AOTA), the Association for Driver Rehabilitation Specialists (ADED), the National Highway Traffic Safety Administration (NHTSA), the National Mobility Equipment Dealers Association (NMEDA), Rehabilitation Institute of Michigan (RIM), University of Michigan Transportation Research Institute (UMTRI), and iCan! Inc. for their support and commitment to fostering a worldwide culture that respects and values the importance of driving and alternative community mobility for people with disabilities, aging-related concerns, or both.

The *Adapted Driving Decision Guide's* content (introduced in Chapter 6 and presented in its entirety on the supplemental CD-ROM) was greatly enhanced thanks to Cynthia Burt and Jerry Bauman. Fredrick Pociask's creativity, attention to detail, and expertise in instructional design guided the development of the CD-ROM version of the *Adapted Driving Decision Guide*. Dennis Anson's book *Alternative Computer Access: A Guide to Selection* (1997) was the original inspiration for creating the guide. The electronic version of the guide also was improved by the generosity of the professionals who freely shared their knowledge or permitted me to include a number of previously published reports including Clair Wang at the American Medical Association (AMA); David Eby and Lisa Molnar at the University of Michigan Transportation Research Institute (UMTRI); Dana Roeling at the National Mobility Equipment Dealers Association (NMEDA); Linda McQuistion and Chad Strowmatt at the Association for Driver Rehabilitation Specialists (ADED); Essie Wagner at the National Highway Traffic Safety Association (NHTSA), Maureen Peterson and Elin Schold Davis at the American Occupational Therapy Association (AOTA), and my colleagues who sit with me on the AOTA's Elder Driver Advisory Panel: Elin Schold

Davis, Dennis McCarthy, Susan Redepenning, Carol Wheatley, Linda Hunt, Wendy Stav, and Susan Pierce.

Everyone who contributed to this project cannot be named; however, I would like to acknowledge the colleagues and friends with whom I discussed the rationale for a comprehensive textbook that examines driver rehabilitation and alternative community mobility, or helped in some other meaningful way, perhaps in the distant past or more recently: Daniel Smingel, David Herbst, Pamela Morenzetti, Laura Pellerito, Cindi Burt, Catherine Lysack, Kenny Rudolph, James Fielding III, Heather Dillaway, Susan Esdaile, Bud Rizer, Damon Page, Jeff Finn, James Cole, Larry Zatkoff, Ken Pelon, Dale Bills, Tom Stowers, Frank Stein, Doreen Head, Regina Parnell, Louis Amundson, Eileen Andreassi, Karmen Brown, Gerry Conti, Clarence Dorey, Eberhard Mammen, Heidi Van Arnem (In memoriam), Burl Von All-men, Robert Raleigh, John Rybicki, Doug Cordier, Beverly Maiers, Rosanne DiZazzo Miller, Cheryl Davidge, Doug Mitchell, Mary Sullivan, John Bibbler, Donald Bouma, Patti DeBear, Lisa Pellerito, Paul Pellerito, Christopher Pellerito, and Lynn Ann Pellerito.

The knowledgeable, highly competent, and supportive team at Elsevier-Mosby publishing has my utmost respect and gratitude for their professionalism, accessibility, and willingness to assist me in addressing the plethora of issues and challenges that would inevitably arise throughout the course of this project: Kathy Falk, Melissa Kuster Deutsch, and David Stein. Finally, the professionals who generously gave of their time and intellect to review chapter content and provide constructive feedback, which was especially helpful because it made the editing task manageable and improved the overall quality of the book's content.

ABOUT THE EDITOR

Joseph M. Pellerito, Jr. was born in 1961 in Detroit, Michigan, and grew up in and around the Motor City. He graduated from Western Michigan University's Honor's College in 1984 with a Baccalaureate of Science (BS) degree in Occupational Therapy (OT), completed a Master of Science (MS) degree in Rehabilitation Technology at Johns Hopkins University in 1994, and is currently working to complete a PhD degree at Wayne State University (WSU) in Detroit, Michigan.

Professor Pellerito worked in the Detroit Medical Center (DMC) at the Rehabilitation Institute of Michigan (RIM) from 1984-1999. At the time of his departure from RIM, he was fulfilling multiple roles that included directing the OT, physical therapy (PT), and therapeutic recreation (TR) professional practices, as well as managing the DMC Nursing Centers' Therapy Staff, assistive technology laboratory, home and job site environmental evaluation services, and the driver rehabilitation program.

Professor Pellerito is an Associate Professor and Academic Program Director of the Occupational Therapy Program in the Eugene Applebaum College of Pharmacy and Health Sciences at WSU in Detroit, Michigan.

He possesses a passion for teaching, conducting research, and performing service work that focuses on empowering the underserved by conducting assistive technology evaluations and providing training in the use of leading-edge products. He has lectured nationally and internationally on various topics including driver rehabilitation and alternative community mobility, alternative computer access, electronic aids to daily living, home and jobsite environmental evaluations, and the impact that technology has on society generally and individuals specifically.

In 2002, Professor Pellerito founded Pellerito + Associates, LLC, a company committed to improving quality of life, enhancing self-reliance, and optimizing the health, safety, and well-being of people with disabilities, the elderly, and their caregivers by providing safe, functional, and affordable assistive technology services and products. He is preparing to launch a non-profit company called AbilityMart (www.abilitymart.com) that will specialize in adaptive devices and assistive technology products that are designed to help facilitate a client's participation in meaningful activities at home, work, school, and other contexts where life happens.

CONTENTS

PROFESSIONAL ETHICS, CONTINUING COMPETENCE, AND ORGANIZATIONS, 599

EDUCATIONAL MATERIALS, COMMUNITY MOBILITY, AND DRIVING CESSATION, 623

INTRODUCTION: AN HISTORICAL PERSPECTIVE ON DRIVING AND THE DRIVER REHABILITATION TEAM

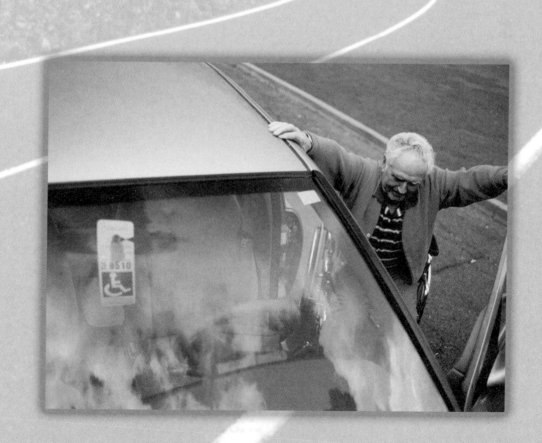

Chapter 1

INTRODUCTION TO DRIVER REHABILITATION AND COMMUNITY MOBILITY

Wendy Macdonald • Joseph M. Pellerito, Jr. • Marilyn Di Stefano

KEY TERMS

- Driver rehabilitation specialist (DRS)
- Community mobility
- Instrumental activities of daily living (IADL)
- International classification of functioning, disability, and health (ICF)
- Risk
- Competencies
- Attentional resources
- Operational behavior
- Tactical behavior
- Strategic behavior

CHAPTER OBJECTIVES

After completing this chapter, the reader will be able to do the following:

- Describe the different conceptual framework models that driver rehabilitation specialists use.
- Explain the importance of the International Classification of Functioning, Disability, and Health on the field of driver rehabilitation.
- Explain the role that driver strategies and driving tactics may play in optimizing driver, passenger, and pedestrian safety.

DRIVER REHABILITATION AND COMMUNITY MOBILITY SERVICES

One of the most important "rites of passage" for young people in economically developed countries throughout the world is passing a test to earn a driver's license. In such countries people of all ages living in urban and rural areas are highly dependent on the automobile to meet their travel and community mobility needs.[1-3] Driving is an important symbol of adult autonomy and independence. It provides a sense of personal competence and enables access to essential services and meaningful social interactions, and for older people it can support their ability to "age in place" in familiar surroundings.[2] The independent community mobility afforded by driving also influences the roles people assume,[4] the formation and maintenance of primary and secondary group ties, the daily operation of households and businesses, the pursuit of meaningful activities in a variety of social settings,[5-8] and the construction of positive self-concepts and high self-esteem more generally.[6,9-12] Overall, driving and its associated car culture influence the ways in which we interact with others, perceive the world and ourselves, and imagine how others perceive us.[13]

Most drivers with functional impairments—whether because of accidental injury, illness, aging-related changes, or some other cause—have similar needs to drive and to maintain their community mobility as those of the general population. However, in attempting to meet these needs, they often experience unique challenges. The professional services of driver rehabilitation specialists can be invaluable in helping people

3

with physical and/or cognitive limitations to maintain their community mobility and in protecting the safety of the individual driver and the public at large.

FORMATION OF THE ASSOCIATION FOR DRIVER EDUCATORS OF THE DISABLED

During the 1940s and 1950s hospitals and privately owned businesses had historically experienced difficulty finding individuals to provide driver rehabilitation services for their clients who were unable to drive or access the community by some other means because of physical, mental, and/or psychological disabilities. The Association for Driver Educators of the Disabled (ADED) was formed by a small group of people in response to a growing need for professionals interested in sharing ideas about "best practices" and in developing formal and informal channels of communication. The first organizational meeting was held in Detroit, Michigan during a 2-day period in August 1977. The emerging field of driver rehabilitation was continuing to evolve during the latter half of the twentieth century as rapidly as the automotive industry itself. These pioneering professionals soon recognized the need to develop a certification process sponsored and administered by the ADED, the fledgling professional association that was working to build a foundation for future practitioners. Professionals who successfully passed the rigorous examination were (and still are) granted the coveted credential of Certified Driver Rehabilitation Specialist (CDRS).

ADED's membership, and those members who have been granted the CDRS credential in particular, comprises a diverse group of professionals who have education, training, and experience in rehabilitation, education, and/or some other related field. Most CDRSs have a background in occupational therapy (OT); however, CDRSs may also be driver educators, physical therapists, pharmacists, and/or owners of commercial driving schools, to name a few. (See Appendix K for more information on the history of ADED.)

THE OCCUPATIONAL THERAPIST AS DRIVER REHABILITATION SPECIALIST

The education and training of occupational therapists provide them with an ideal basis on which to develop the skills required to provide driver rehabilitation and community mobility services. Occupational therapists have expertise in assessing the individual's holistic status (i.e., mind, body, and spirit), including an understanding of how medical conditions and impairments can impede driver readiness. The occupational therapist working as a *driver rehabilitation specialist* (DRS) is

therefore often recognized as possessing an ideal professional background to perform predriving or clinical driver rehabilitation evaluations. Some models of practice team an occupational therapist with another member of the driver rehabilitation team who may lack clinical training but possesses highly developed insight developed during years of experience. For example a driver educator who has worked to provide driver rehabilitation services to people with disabilities and elderly persons can make a valuable contribution even though he or she may not have had any formal education concerning the disabling medical conditions often presented by clients seeking services.

DRIVER REHABILITATION SPECIALIST CREDENTIALS

Becoming a CDRS requires a DRS to pass an examination and to submit a series of reflective reports on their professional practice experiences. However, this is still a voluntary process that DRSs may or may not undertake. To complicate matters further, the American Occupational Therapy Association (AOTA) is currently working to develop its own certification programs in driver rehabilitation and community mobility—a process that is an entirely separate process from the ADED credentialing route. In recognition of these differences and to simplify the presentation, the phrase *driver rehabilitation specialist* (or DRS) will be used throughout this book. This and other pertinent issues affecting the evolution of the driver rehabilitation field of practice will be examined, where relevant, throughout the book. See Chapter 23 for more information on legal and professional ethics in driver rehabilitation.

SERVICE DELIVERY MODELS IN DRIVER REHABILITATION

The service delivery models presented in this chapter and in Chapters 4 and 26 and Appendix C reflect current standards of practice in the United States. However, these brief descriptions should not be considered exhaustive; they do not include all of the programmatic variations offered throughout the United States or in other places around the world. Irrespective of the service delivery model that is being examined, driver rehabilitation programs are most likely to employ occupational therapists to provide driver rehabilitation (and more recently community mobility) services to people with specific disabilities, the elderly population, and/or their caregivers. *Community mobility* has recently been acknowledged as a key component addressed by the comprehensive driver evaluation that all DRSs, irrespective of their professional training and experience, should undertake. Box 1-1 provides a brief description of community mobility.

The following sections outline three common service delivery models wherein DRSs provide driver rehabilitation services.

Programs Offering Clinical Evaluations Only

Programs that conduct only clinical evaluations provide key information that can be used by the driver rehabilitation team members (e.g., physiatrist, family physician, driver educator, case manager, and occupational therapist specializing in driver rehabilitation services) in determining how best to address return-to-driving and/or community mobility issues. Additionally, clinical evaluations can help to identify clients who are at risk, and they provide concrete data to support decisions to discontinue the evaluation process before the client has received an on-road evaluation. For example during a clinical evaluation a client may report that he or she has experienced grand mal seizures only 1 week previously, which is a clear indication that driving would be inadvisable, warranting interruption of the evaluation process at that point. This is a serious decision that requires the collection and thorough analysis of valid assessment data and that is then based on communication with and the concurrence of other members of the driver rehabilitation team. The client, and perhaps also his or her caregivers, needs a clear and concise explanation of why his or her driving should cease. However, it is important to note that discovery of such a clear-cut contraindication during the clinical evaluation is not a common occurrence. Most clients require a behind-the-wheel evaluation because on-road driving behavior is the best indicator of that individual's ability to drive safely, and obviously this key evaluation variable cannot be tested indoors in a clinical setting while the client and DRS are sitting at a table. In normal circumstances, therefore, it is important that any DRSs who provide solely clinical evaluations should work in coordination with an established driver rehabilitation program, which can augment the clinical evaluation with an on-road evaluation.

Programs Offering Clinical Evaluations and Simulator Assessments

Some programs offer driving simulator assessment within their evaluation and training services. There are various possible advantages of using a driving simulator, including the capability to assess the following: client responses to challenging stimuli, including animate and inanimate obstacles; how they cope during variable inclement and clement weather conditions; their topographic orientation in familiar and unfamiliar environments; and night driving performance. Simulators also enable the client to drive while using adapted driving aids that may be unfamiliar to him or her, to navigate virtual communities and develop strategies for topographic orientation, and to work to improve executive functions, such as problem solving in a low-risk, virtual environment before tackling these tasks in the real world. Simulators may also bridge the gap between clinical and on-road evaluations by providing a tangible way for clients to practice driving skills after narrowly failing a clinical or on-road evaluation. In the past clients were

---

BOX 1-1	A Brief Description of Community Mobility

COMMUNITY MOBILITY
Depending on a person's age and health status, community mobility is most often accomplished by one or more of the following:
1. Walking
2. Using a wheeled mobility device that requires the initiation of movement by one's own volition, such as a manual wheelchair, bicycle, skateboard, roller blades/roller skates, or child's "manual" scooter
3. Using a powered or power-assisted wheeled mobility device such as a power wheelchair, Segway, manual wheelchair with power assist, or adult's scooter
4. Using public and private transportation such as a bus, train, taxi, mass transit, or streetcar (i.e., trolley), and getting a ride from a friend or family member
5. Driving a motor vehicle such as a car, van, SUV, or truck with or without structural modifications to the vehicle, adapted driving equipment, or both

Historically, DRSs have focused on assisting people with disabilities and/or aging-related concerns to access stock or modified vehicles, stow and secure mobility aids as needed, and drive with or without adapted driving aids, as well as achieve an optimal level of safety and comfort when riding as passengers in motor vehicles. Programs today, however, must also provide services that focus on alternative community mobility including helping clients plan for, and contend with, driving cessation. DRSs have an ethical responsibility to assist clients and caregivers in effectively identifying and using cost-effective and dependable alternatives to driving that enable alternative community mobility in areas where clients engage in meaningful activities and relationships.

told to return to the facility for a follow-up evaluation at some point in the future (e.g., 3 to 6 months later) without being given instructions on how to remediate skills necessary for improving their chances of passing the comprehensive driver rehabilitation evaluations (i.e., clinical and on-road evaluations) that can lead to safe and independent driving. See Chapter 10 for more information on driving simulators.

Programs Offering Comprehensive Driver Rehabilitation Evaluations and More

Inclusion of clinical and on-road evaluations ensures that clients are provided with a comprehensive driver evaluation. After the comprehensive evaluation has been completed, additional services should include driver training and/or addressing alternative community mobility as a critical IADL. Alternative community mobility may include, but is certainly not limited to, assisting clients and their caregivers with identifying viable and safe alternatives to driving, or riding as a passenger in, motor vehicles. Irrespective of whether or not a client relies upon an ambulation aid, wheeled mobility device, private or public transportation service, friend or family member, or any number of other community mobility options, he or she will also need support to carry out the IADL tasks that are often performed while traveling about in the community. IADL, within the context of community mobility, therefore is another key service area that occupational therapists specializing in driver rehabilitation services should address in order to provide a full continuum of services to their clients and caregivers.

CONCEPTUAL FRAMEWORKS SUPPORTING DRIVER REHABILITATION AND COMMUNITY MOBILITY SERVICES

The conceptual frameworks that are used by rehabilitation professionals play a key role in underpinning their evaluation procedures and guiding their observations, decisions, and intervention processes.[14] In this section a selection of conceptual and theoretical frameworks that are most relevant to the activities of DRSs is examined.

Occupational therapists and occupational therapy assistants have historically drawn from a rich tapestry of theoretical and conceptual frameworks that have originated within and outside the OT professional literature. Models of human activity or occupation that identify driving as one of the most important IADLs can be instructive in guiding DRSs in providing driver rehabilitation evaluation and training services. These models

can also support our understanding of an individual's driving behavior in relation to the physical environment within which driving occurs and in relation to its broader social and environmental contexts.

THE MODEL OF HUMAN OCCUPATION

The Model of Human Occupation (MOHO) has been undergoing development since the 1980s and continues to be refined.[15] Key components of the MOHO framework include the following constructs:
- Volition: The thoughts, feelings, and motivations related to particular activities.
- Habituation: Behavioral routines and patterns.
- Performance capacity: Influenced by physical and mental abilities and by subjective experiences.
- Environmental influences, physical and social, that affect performance.

The application of the MOHO to a nonexhaustive list of factors that may influence driving performance is presented in Table 1-1. This framework highlights issues that may need to be considered when an individual's driving and community mobility needs and abilities are evaluated.

THE PERSON–ENVIRONMENT–OCCUPATION MODEL

The Person–Environment–Occupation (PEO) model is similar to the MOHO in many of its basic assumptions, definitions, and key concepts. It highlights transactional interrelationships between the person, environment, and occupation (i.e., elements that influence human performance).[17] The PEO model depicts these three elements as linked in "transactional relationships" that result in occupational performance. These elements are purported to change over time and space, consistent with the notion that occupational performance occurs within a developmental framework with changes during the lifespan. The quality of fit between the model's elements is measured in terms of the quality of occupational performance and the person's associated experience.

CANADIAN MODEL OF OCCUPATIONAL PERFORMANCE

The Canadian Model of Occupational Performance (CMOP)[18] is another conceptual framework used by DRSs and is similar in many ways to the PEO model. In relation to driving performance, the CMOP emphasizes interactional issues and performance factors relevant to a person's age and lifestyle.[19]

Models such as the PEO and the CMOP support OT practice by facilitating a broad view of the various

Table 1-1   Use of the Model of Human Occupations (MOHO) to Identify Some of the Factors and Issues that May Be Relevant in Driver Rehabilitation

Some MOHO Constructs	Examples Related to Driving and Maintenance of Community Mobility
VOLITION Personal causation	Role of self in relation to road safety; insight into own driving abilities.
Values	Beliefs and associated values concerning driving, risk taking while driving, and personal responsibility for safety.
Interests	Interest in driving and associated satisfaction or pleasure derived from it, including perceived benefits of interacting with peers.
HABITUATION Habits	Habitual behavior patterns are likely to influence why, how, when, and where an individual drives or accesses alternative transportation to maintain community mobility.
Roles	Life roles may be associated with driving tasks (e.g., among older couples the husband may be the primary or sole driver). Some worker roles involve a substantial amount of driving.
PERFORMANCE CAPACITY Body function	Impaired cognition or physical capacities caused by an injury, illness, or the aging process can negatively affect IADL such as driving and community mobility. For example, navigating while driving may be difficult or impossible for an individual alone in the vehicle. Cognitive and physical limitations may also affect the person's ability to use primary or secondary vehicle controls.
ENVIRONMENT Physical	Vehicle components may impede performance (e.g., door openings may restrict ingress/ egress; seat design may not provide sufficient postural support; and primary or secondary vehicle controls may not be adaptable for the user).
Social	Interactions with passengers may support or hinder driving performance. Family or peer group associations may positively or negatively influence client decisions (e.g., when/where to drive) that affect the degree of exposure to risk.

factors that together determine an individual's performance and well-being in a specific situation.[19] For example a teenager with a disability who is learning to drive for the first time will probably be contending with different issues from those faced by a much older person who is attempting to return to driving after a stroke. Such differences need to be considered by DRSs in their approach to evaluation and intervention.

THE OCCUPATIONAL ADAPTATION MODEL

Central to this model is the notion that humans learn to adapt to the demands of their activities within a particular environment.[20,21] The model's key assumptions include the following:

• Demands are internal and external to the individual and are most usefully viewed within a person-occupational-environment context.

• Dysfunction occurs when a person's adaptive capacity cannot match performance demands, creating a need for the person to change his or her adaptive processes.
• The process of adaptation involves stages that reflect planning, evaluating, and integrating responses to internal and/or external stimuli.
• At any stage of the lifespan, life events and/or disabling conditions can impede an individual's ability to adapt.
• A person's adaptive skills will ultimately determine the success of his or her occupational performance.

Within this framework the central emphasis on adaptation is clearly applicable to the work of DRSs. Conceptually it supports the promotion of a wide range of remediation strategies to overcome functional limitations and maintain optimal activity performance and community participation.

A centrally important feature of all of the aforementioned OT models is their client-centered approach to evaluation and intervention. Each of these conceptual frameworks also suggests that a range of environmental, social, and individual factors influence performance. Identification and implementation of effective driver rehabilitation and community mobility services require a thorough understanding of these factors and how they may interact in affecting different individuals.

WORLD HEALTH ORGANIZATION INTERNATIONAL CLASSIFICATION OF FUNCTIONING, DISABILITY, AND HEALTH

The World Health Organization (WHO) has developed a different type of framework to foster greater consistency in the categorization of functioning, disability, health, and well-being: the *International Classification of Functioning, Disability, and Health* (ICF). The ICF provides a standard lexicon (i.e., universal vocabulary) for describing interrelationships between health, disability, functioning, and other related issues such as driving. More disease-orientated classification systems have tended to link impairment directly to activity limitations without consideration of social or environmental factors.[22] In contrast the ICF takes a broader systems approach, documenting characteristics of individuals, their activities, and the context of their occupational engagement.

The full version of the ICF has two parts: (1) Part 1: Functioning and Disability and (2) Part 2: Contextual Factors. Part 1 is subdivided into "Body Functions and Structures" and "Activities and Participation," and Part 2 is subdivided into "Environmental Factors" and "Personal Factors." Table 1-2 shows how the ICF can be used to describe someone's status after he or she has experienced a complete spinal cord injury. This hypo-

thetical individual has been evaluated for driving, with special consideration given to driving-related issues that may affect his or her possible return to work as a sales representative. It should be noted that each cell within the "constructs" row of Table 1-2 would be coded and that this information could be part of a database containing information on all of the individuals who received driver rehabilitation and community mobility services within participating driver rehabilitation and community mobility programs.

Although personal factors are included in the ICF framework, detailed operational definitions are not provided. Driving is a specific activity within the subsection mobility (i.e., moving around using transportation), and this in turn is a section within the higher-level activities and participation classification. Various subcategories of driving are also included in the ICF, such as driving motorized vehicles, human-powered transportation (e.g., bicycles and rowboats), and animal-powered vehicles (e.g., horse-drawn carts).[23] The simplified example in Table 1-2 illustrates how the ICF classification system may help DRSs to describe more consistently the nature and extent of client problems and related factors.

Because the ICF is applicable to everyone, not just to people with disabilities, it has many potential uses, including application across research, education, health care, insurance, policy, clinical, and statistical domains. It is anticipated that wider application of the ICF will encourage improved communication between researchers and the establishment of larger data sets at national and international levels, which would facilitate comparative data analyses at a global level.[23,24] Such developments would be useful in research on relationships between disability, health, and wellness on the one hand and driving and community mobility on the other.

Research is underway to investigate the opportunities and challenges the ICF presents in particular for the OT profession.[25] It has engendered considerable debate,[26] and its implications for professional practice have not yet been fully developed.[27,28] Further details are available from the WHO web site (*www.who.int/classification/icf*).

RISK MANAGEMENT FRAMEWORKS

DRIVING AS A HAZARDOUS ACTIVITY

Driving a vehicle in ordinary traffic is an inherently hazardous activity for drivers, passengers, and pedestrians alike. There is an expectation that drivers will maintain an appropriate distance from each other and from inanimate objects and pedestrians. Vehicles that are traveling at high speeds in close proximity to each other and

Table 1-2 **Classification of an Individual with a Complete Spinal Cord Injury Who Wishes to Return to Work-Related Driving as a Sales Representative**

	Part 1: Functioning and Disability		Part 2: Contextual Factors	
Components	Body functions, structures, and impairments	Activities and participation	Environmental factors	Personal factors
Domains	Body functions Body structures	Life areas (e.g., communication, mobility, self-care, domestic life, and interpersonal)	External influences on functioning and disability	Internal influences on functioning and disability
Constructs	Physiologic and anatomical changes to the spinal cord: client suffers a spinal cord injury with resultant major impairments.	Mobility (i.e., driving). Client is unable to drive a standard vehicle but able to drive a vehicle with modified primary and secondary vehicle controls and transfer assist (e.g., electromechanical lift) and mobility aid stowing device.	Standard fleet vehicles do not have the required modifications and equipment. The employer is reluctant to modify a fleet vehicle.	The client is motivated to pursue driver rehabilitation and to seek alternative funding to secure the necessary vehicle type and/or modifications.

to other road users present the potential for disaster because the large amount of kinetic energy that is dissipated in the event of a collision between two or more objects can easily cause injury or death. In economically developed countries driving is one of the most dangerous activities routinely undertaken by a high proportion of the population. Perhaps the only comparable activity that has a higher associated risk of injury or death is that of being a pedestrian versus a driver or passenger in a vehicle. The risk of being severely injured or killed is significantly greater for pedestrians because they are without any protection unlike vehicle occupants, who in the event of a crash gain significant protection from their own vehicle's safety infrastructure (e.g., crumple zones, seat belts, and airbags), especially if the vehicle is designed to be highly crashworthy.

VARIATION IN CRASH RISK BY AGE GROUP

The population demographics of economically developed countries indicate that within the next few decades there will be a substantial increase in the proportion of drivers in older age groups. The increase will be particularly marked for women drivers because in earlier decades it was much less common for women to drive compared with the contemporary situation.

Calculated risk levels per unit distance driven, such as those shown in Figure 1-1, support the view that older drivers have a substantially higher crash risk than their younger counterparts. However, these figures do not take into account the frailty bias (i.e., older drivers' greater vulnerability to injury), which means that the collisions in which they are involved are more likely to be officially recorded as injury-related accidents and more often result in fatalities.[29] There is also evidence that individuals who drive less tend to have a higher crash risk,[30] and on this basis some have argued that because older people typically drive less than their younger counterparts, calculation of their crash risk should control for this factor.[31] However, the general consensus of opinion among road safety researchers is that crash risk *does* increase with increasing age beyond approximately 75 to 80 years of age, although not to the extent depicted in Figure 1-1.[32] Empirical data on older drivers' performance under test conditions support such a view.

ELEVATION IN CRASH RISK RELATED TO COMMON MEDICAL CONDITIONS

There have been several major reviews of empirical evidence of relationships between diagnosed medical

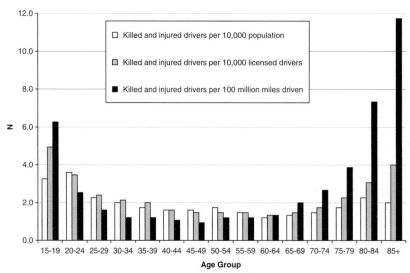

Figure 1-1   Variation in numbers of U.S. driver fatalities and injuries by age for three sets of data: per head of population, per number of licensed drivers, and per distance driven (FARS 1997). (From Hu P, Jones D, Reuscher T, et al: *Projecting fatalities in crashes involving older drivers,* Report for the National Highway Traffic Safety Administration, Oak Ridge National Laboratory, Tennessee, 2000, ONRL.)

conditions and crash risk.[33-35] There is a paucity of research related to some medical conditions, and interpretation of available evidence is difficult because of variable and often poor quality of available information and inconsistencies in diagnostic criteria. For example the review by Charlton et al[35] highlighted a range of methodological shortcomings and the need for large and well-controlled, population-based studies. Nevertheless they noted from the available evidence that people diagnosed with any of the following eight conditions had a relative risk at least double that of people in control groups: dementia, epilepsy, multiple sclerosis, psychiatric disorders (grouped into one category), schizophrenia, sleep apnea, alcohol abuse, and cataracts.

Review of this literature is beyond the scope of this book; however, it is important that DRSs maintain a keen awareness of the issues that may arise because of needs that are often associated with a variety of medical conditions. For this purpose the *Physician's Guide to Assessing and Counseling Older Drivers*, developed by the American Medical Association (AMA) in cooperation with the National Highway Traffic Safety Administration (NHTSA), may be helpful.[33] Part of this guide has been included in this book's Appendixes A, B, F, H, and I, and the entire document is available in PDF format in this book's supplemental CD: *The Adapted Driving Decision Guide.*

It also is important to remember that some medical conditions affect not only driving but also people's ability to use alternative forms of transportation as a means for community mobility. Research such as that summarized in the Organization for Economic

Cooperative Development (OECD) report, *Aging and Transport: Mobility Needs and Safety Issues*, reveals that because most people experience increasing difficulties with walking community distances as they age, they are likely to be capable of driving safely for longer than they are able to use alternative transportation methods.[36] This kind of research highlights the need for DRSs to see their clients holistically and to focus on more than just their medical diagnoses to determine the overall impact of functional impairments on driving and community mobility.[23]

BALANCING INJURY RISK AND A CLIENT'S DESIRE TO DRIVE

The need to manage road injury risks is only one of several important goals for DRSs. In many cases a primary goal is to help clients achieve or maintain a satisfactory level of community mobility, and to achieve this it can be important to maintain driving as an IADL. For example it has been found that older people who become unable to drive typically experience diminished community mobility, often associated with increased depression and related illnesses.[37,38] Fonda et al[39] found that Americans aged ≥70 years who stopped driving were at greater risk of depression than those who just restricted their normal driving patterns, as well as those whose driving was reportedly unmodified. Issues related to driving cessation and community mobility are discussed further in Chapters 7, 21, and 22.

Because the loss of a driver's license can negatively affect a client's health and well-being, it is essential that the evaluation procedures used to assess driving-related capacities and on-road performance are reliable and that they use realistic, evidence-based performance criteria. However, the need to maintain clients' community mobility must be balanced against the need to maintain his or her safety and the safety of passengers and pedestrians within the wider community. From a safety standpoint the process of evaluating functionally impaired drivers should reliably screen (i.e., filter out) those individuals whose driving performance would present an unacceptable risk to the drivers themselves, prospective passengers, pedestrians, and public and private property (e.g., buildings, fences, landscape, and signage). Balancing issues that are often in mutual opposition is a key concern of licensing authorities and DRSs.

Antrim and Engum[40] state that:

> Necessary in striking this balance is the rehabilitation professional who seeks to increase the patient's activities and independence while also, at times, acting as the patient's advocate. However, acting to maximize independence, however well intentioned, without utilizing the reliable, valid and relatively comprehensive evaluation tools now available will unnecessarily result in increased professional liability exposure. (p. 19)

For more information on driver evaluation procedures and related evaluation criteria, see Chapters 7 and 14. For more information covering legal and ethical issues, see Chapter 24.

MANAGING DRIVER CRASH RISK WITHIN A SYSTEMS FRAMEWORK

As previously outlined in this chapter the work of DRSs can usefully be conceptualized within a broad systems framework. Within the domain of road safety, risk management experts—particularly human factors professionals—also view their roles within the kind of systems framework that is depicted in Figure 1-2. This figure shows that the behavior of individual drivers occurs within a broad system of interacting factors that encompass task demands, the immediate environment, and the broader sociolegal context. It highlights some of the wide variety of potential risk management strategies that are meant to target and ameliorate the potentially destructive effects of the primary factors that influence injury risk.

Within this systems framework, measures to promote safer driving performance as a means of managing injury risk represent only one of many potential approaches to managing the system risks. Other approaches to risk management include those that address the need for safer designs of vehicles and for safer design and maintenance of the physical road traffic environment, including road signs, traffic signals, and so on. See Chapter 19 for more information on designing the external environment for traffic safety.

It is important to recognize the general nature of risk in the context of driving and the factors that influence an individual driver's risk level. In general terms *risk* is usually defined as the product of the probability of a particular negative consequence multiplied by the severity of that consequence. Within the road traffic system the negative consequences of primary concern to system risk managers are personal injuries or deaths resulting from collisions between road users and a broad range of associated and subsequent financial and personal costs.

Risk management strategies vary in their objectives: to minimize the probability of a crash occurring (i.e., crash prevention) or to minimize injury severity if there *is* a crash. In the present context our primary focus is

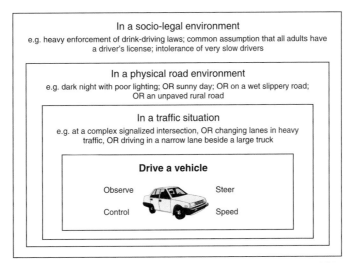

Figure 1-2 The road traffic system depicting the individual driver as one component within a complex system of interacting factors.

on strategies that entail modification of a client's behavior (when behavior includes but is not confined to driving performance) in ways that may influence one or another of these objectives. Strategies to reduce injury severity that are within the control of individual drivers include the use of a seat belt and use of a vehicle with good crash protection characteristics. The most important driving-related strategy to reduce injury severity is avoidance of excessive speed because this reduces the amount of potentially harmful energy that will be dissipated in the event of a crash. This strategy also promotes crash prevention because lower speeds provide all drivers with more time to process information—an advantage that is particularly important in the case of drivers whose information processing speed is reduced (e.g., many older drivers). Other strategies to reduce the probability of being involved in a crash include planning trips to avoid driving at times and in environments where traffic will be particularly heavy or where the driving task is likely to be particu-

larly difficult for that individual. Examples of such strategies are shown at priority level 4 of Table 1-3.

Table 1-3 prioritizes different types of risk control measures according to their relative effectiveness based on the standard risk management Hierarchy of Hazard and Risk Control Measures.[41] This general hierarchy is widely accepted by safety professionals and is incorporated within many standards governing occupational safety throughout the world.[42] Contrary to popular belief, measures to improve driver behavior are at the lowest and least effective level of the hierarchy, priority 4. The hierarchy specifies that measures to control hazards (including hazardous behavior) and risk factors should assign the highest priority to the elimination or reduction of potentially injurious energy sources (e.g., heavy vehicles traveling at high speeds). The next highest priority should be given to engineering control strategies, such as redesigning traffic signals to achieve safer control of vehicle movements at intersections, designing vehicles to improve their crash worthiness,

Table 1-3   Hierarchy of Hazard and Risk Control Measures (based on ILO-OSH, 2001)

Levels of the Risk Control Hierarchy	Examples of Road Injury Risk Control Measures in Context of Driver Rehabilitation
Priority 1: Eliminate the hazard or risk	DRSs can do little to eliminate the hazard because this stems from vehicles traveling at significant speeds in close proximity to each other. They may encourage clients to minimize their exposure to hazard (i.e., their use of roadways as a driver and pedestrian). However, such a strategy will often conflict with mobility needs unless, for example, a client can live in a vehicle-free residential community with infrastructure that supports aging in place.
Priority 2: Control the hazard/risk at source using engineering or organizational measures	Safe design of the road system, including the road environment and vehicles (e.g., with airbags), is a key requirement. At individual driver level, using a vehicle rated as highly crashworthy,* including use of its seatbelt, falls into this category.
Priority 3: Minimize the hazard/risk by specifying safe procedural requirements and administrative control measures	Examples at a system management level include the driver licensing and testing system, road traffic laws more generally, and police enforcement of such laws. By definition there are no equivalent strategies at the individual driver level.
Priority 4: Where some hazards/risks remain, take measures to ensure that people take appropriate protective measures at an individual level	A system-level measure would be public information campaigns intended to influence driver behavior. At the individual level possible strategies include route planning to maximize use of controlled rather than uncontrolled intersections, avoidance of driving at night or in heavy traffic or on high-speed roads *except* high-standard freeways (dual carriageway, no intersections), and in some circumstances specialist driver training.

*Information on vehicle safety is available from the National Highway Traffic Safety Administration, at http://www.nhtsa.dot.gov/.
DRS, Driver rehabilitation specialist.

and designing the roadside environment to minimize the occurrence of rigid objects such as large posts that have the potential to cause severe damage if struck by a vehicle. Strategies to modify the driver's behavior are at the lowest and least effective level in this hierarchy, falling within the category of administrative or procedural controls. Despite these findings DRSs who are not involved in traffic safety research typically see measures to improve driving behavior as centrally important to maintaining road safety. It is important that DRSs understand the levels of risk management and control in relation to road safety, and give some consideration to the role of higher-order risk management strategies after considering a client's particular situation and needs.

MODIFICATION OF DRIVER BEHAVIOR TO REDUCE RISK EXPOSURE

At system management level common risk management strategies that target driver behavior include licensing procedures and enforcement of traffic laws that are intended to regulate driving performance. The work of DRSs is often closely linked to that of driver educators, and their role may even be incorporated within road safety legislation, as is the case for occupational therapists with specialist training in driver rehabilitation in Victoria, Australia.

Within a DRS's role there is usually considerable scope to promote a wide variety of methods for reducing clients' exposure to risk. DRSs may assist their clients to develop and implement strategies to decrease their quantity of exposure to risk, for example by fostering client decisions that result in less frequent and/or shorter trips. Risk can also be reduced by changing the quality of exposure, for example by a driver planning trips and routes that minimize the proportion of time during which he or she will be driving in higher-risk situations (e.g., night driving, inclement weather, or under other circumstances or in environments in which driving may be excessively demanding). See Appendix G for more information on making driving-related decisions, including voluntary driving cessation.

MODIFYING THE DRIVER'S BEHAVIOR TO IMPROVE ON-ROAD DRIVING PERFORMANCE

DRSs should also help functionally impaired drivers to develop strategies that foster self-management of on-road driving behavior to reduce its riskiness (i.e., to drive more safely). Strategies that focus on improving driver behavior include driver training, which is commonly seen by people without expertise in road safety as an important means of promoting road safety. Unfortunately research evidence on the effects of defensive or advanced driver training on subsequent driver risk levels does not support this view. There is a large body of evidence that does *not* show that more highly trained drivers tend to be safer drivers or that completion of a particular type of driver training program is more likely to result in a lower crash risk.[43]

However, there are various situations in which driver rehabilitation and community mobility professionals need to use training techniques to help their clients acquire the necessary knowledge and skills to use adaptive driving aids identified by the DRS as medically necessary. In the case of older drivers there may be some benefit gained by providing training that focuses on updating the client's knowledge and understanding of laws that pertain to driving and his or her "road craft" (i.e., driving tactics people adopt in various common situations), such as roundabouts, making a left turn at an intersection, and merging onto a freeway.

Perhaps most importantly there is a need to help drivers to adopt a range of strategies and driving tactics that will at least partially compensate for their impairments and help to minimize the risk of injury that is associated with their driving performance. To clarify the role that driver strategies and driving tactics may play in optimizing driver, passenger, and pedestrian safety, the remainder of this chapter provides detailed analyses of the driving task within several different frameworks.

MODELS OF THE DRIVING TASK

DRSs are concerned with assisting people to attain or retain skills that are necessary for driving competence. This process involves evaluating driving-related capacities and driving performance to determine whether the driver is able to perform at an adequately competent level and likely to do so in practice. It is therefore important to understand the nature of the driving task and of driving *competencies.*

Driving can be analyzed from a variety of perspectives. As described previously in this chapter, there are several descriptive frameworks that can be useful in understanding the complexities of driving performance and the wide range of factors that may affect it. The WHO's ICF also provides a useful means of describing and categorizing functional impairments.

However, because driving a vehicle is a highly complex activity with associated risk of severe injury or death, it is essential that the expertise of DRSs is founded on a theory-based model of practice that has been empirically evaluated to support critical thinking and valid decision making during driver evaluation and training. Such theory-based models have been developed by cognitive ergonomists and neuropsychologists, drawing on evidence from psychological and behavioral sciences research.[44,45] Theory-based models support a more detailed understanding of the processes underlying driver abilities, performance, and behavior; they also play a key role in defining the requirements for a valid assessment of driver capacities and performance. For more information, please see below and also Chapters 6, 7, and 12.

THE HUMAN AS A PROCESSOR OF INFORMATION

Within the research literature that focuses on driver rehabilitation and alternatives to driving that enable community mobility, theoretical models often depict driving as an information-processing activity that falls within this framework (see Proctor and Van Zandt[46] and Wickens and Hollands[47] for accounts of human information–processing capacities, limitations, and system characteristics). Such models conceptualize the activity of driving and related driver competencies within broad categories related to information intake, central decision making and response selection, and action or response execution.

Figure 1-3 depicts a generic view of information processing, starting on the left with the flow of information from the environment to the driver's sensory organs. Only some of this information progresses beyond sensory memory stores to be perceived (entailing some initial interpretation) and still less goes on to enter fully into conscious awareness, the central, cognitive stage of the human information–processing system.

For driving, visual information is clearly the most important type of sensory input, which is why effective visual sensory functioning is an important requirement for competent driving performance. Despite this it should be noted that some aspects of visual functioning are more important for safe driving than are others; for example dynamic visual acuity appears to be more important than the static acuity that is most commonly measured.[48] To ensure that evaluation of visual functioning as part of driver evaluation is valid for the intended purpose, it should focus on those aspects that have been shown to be most important for safe driving. Processing at the perceptual stage is critical for safety. It entails identification and interpretation of information about the road traffic environment, which sustains the driver's awareness of the current situation and supports ongoing cognitive predictions of the immediate future to provide a basis for vehicle-control actions.

The selection of information in the environment for initial processing and the interpretation of this information are influenced by the driver's preexisting knowledge and skills, as depicted in Figure 1-3. Note also that information selection and interpretation can be influenced (perhaps less directly) by the driver's preexisting attitudes and specific motives. Key visual sensory and perceptual requirements are discussed in Chapters 6, 12, 13, and 21.

A centrally important feature of human information processing is the role of *attentional resources*, depicted at the top of Figure 1-3. In this figure arrows show that some attention is required at all stages of information processing, with the requirement for attention being minimal at the information-intake stage and maximal at the central, cognitive stage of conscious awareness. Because of its high demand for attention and because attentional resources are finite, this central stage often

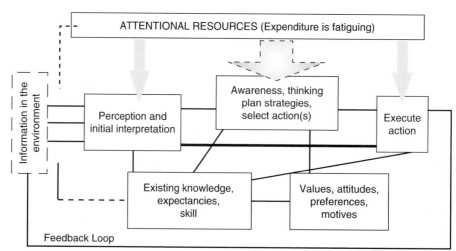

Figure 1-3 A generic depiction of how people "process" information during activities such as driving. (From Macdonald W: *Human error: causes and countermeasures,* Proceedings of the Safety in Action Conference 2004, Safety Institute of Australia, Victorian Division, 2004.)

acts as a bottleneck in the processing system. Closely tied to this resource limitation is the existence of a maximum rate at which humans can process information.

Because of these attentional and information-processing limitations that characterize all of us, it is important that drivers are able to allocate their available attentional resources optimally between different environmental sources of sensory input and between different stages of the information-processing system (e.g., intake of environmental information and decision making related to vehicle control and driving tactics). Common problems leading to the deterioration in the quality of many older drivers' performance include a decrease in their overall attentional capacity, slowing of their information-processing rate, and suboptimal allocation of available attentional resources. Such problems may also be key factors leading to poorer driving performance among people with some medical conditions.

The large arrow in Figure 1-3 that connects perception and initial interpretation directly to execute action, thus bypassing conscious awareness, which is the stage most demanding of attentional resources, indicates another important feature of the human information–processing system. This bypass arrow depicts the fact that for experienced drivers, a substantial proportion of vehicle control activity is completely routine; as such, it demands little if any attention and occurs more or less automatically in response to specific, routinely occurring patterns of perceived information—based of course on a large amount of previous practice. For example each element in the sequence of actions entailed in steering a car around a curve occurs largely automatically in response to the preceding element. This chain of actions incorporates intermittent intake of visual information from the environment to support fine-tuning of control movements. Such visuomotor programs represent some of the basic building blocks of driving skill. However, persons whose motor control is impaired by injury may need to consciously attend to controlling movement of their limbs, which will reduce the amount of spare attentional capacity that they have available for allocation to other aspects of the driving task.

Largely automatic (more properly termed automatized) linkages between driving performance elements exist also at the perceptual stage. When a specific pattern of incoming information finds an immediate match with a preexisting template in memory (the template being based on past experience [i.e., perceptual practice]), the incoming information can be interpreted with minimal if any requirement for attention. For example the majority of drivers would immediately slow down and stop at a red light without much conscious effort being used to interpret the signal. This is sometimes called recognition-primed decision making.

A key characteristic of fully developed competence in experienced drivers is their memory representation of the traffic system, which is organized as schemata related to particular topics, or internal mental models representing the dynamic functioning of systems, such as the behavior of road users. These organized knowledge systems support all aspects of expert driver performance.

DESCRIPTIVE MODELS

In addition to the OT models discussed earlier, some other models play a useful role in conceptualizing driver performance at a more detailed level, two of which are described below. First the skills-rules-knowledge (SRK) hierarchy provides a detailed description of different performance levels that build on the theoretical model of the human as an information processor outlined above. Second a hierarchical model has been developed that is specific to driving. It focuses at the higher stages of the SRK model and provides a broader view of driver behavior that encompasses individual lifestyle and nondriving strategies to reduce exposure to risk as a driver, as well as lower-order strategies and tactics relevant to on-road driving performance.

The Skills-Rules-Knowledge Hierarchy

The extent to which performance is automatized, as opposed to requiring full attention, is central to what is commonly known as the SRK hierarchy.[49,50] This model is not specific to driving but has been widely applied to this activity. Building on information-processing theory and related evidence, it categorizes elements of human performance as one the following:

- Skill-based: Meaning that performance occurs with little or no attention
- Rule-based: Meaning that performance demands some attention to identify the routinely applicable "rule" that determines the required response to perceived information
- Knowledge-based: Meaning that full attention is required to interpret and evaluate the situation and to decide appropriate actions

Skill-based performance can entail the execution of automatized programs that comprise a series of perceptual and motor performance elements, operating as described in the previous section. Performance at skill- and rule-based levels is also demonstrated by the routine perception and interpretation of incoming information by experienced drivers in highly familiar road environments, where preexisting cognitive schemata or mental models heavily influence their perception and interpretation of incoming information. The cognitive schemata of experienced drivers, which encapsulate a vast amount of organized, highly detailed knowledge of system operation, make it possible for a driver's behavior in familiar circumstances to be so automatized that "one is able, for example, to drive practically without conscious control from home to work."[51] Therefore "... (experienced) drivers are, most of the time, driving quite routinely, according to their learned habits and using simple cues in the traffic environment."[51]

No matter how familiar the environment, the presence and activities of other road users are always to some degree unpredictable, so that driving is never without some degree of attentional demand. This demand can be very high when much of driving performance is at a knowledge-based level. This occurs when, for example, the driver is in an unfamiliar area and therefore must pay a lot of attention to the subtask of navigation; if the vehicle being driven is an unfamiliar one, the attentional demands will be even greater. Rule-based performance is intermediate in attentional requirements; people following learned procedures in fairly routine situations typify this level. Driving maneuvers such as changing lanes on a freeway are generally performed at this level.

This SRK framework has been particularly useful to identify the different types of errors that characterize skill-, rule-, and knowledge-based performances because different types of risk-management strategies are demanded by different error types.[52-55] When performance is largely automatized, errors typically involve misdirection of attention leading to lapses (accidental omissions at any stage of information processing [e.g., failure to notice a pedestrian about to step into the road]) or slips (errors in execution of the intended response [e.g., accidentally crunching a gear change in a manually controlled car]).

The majority of errors made by people performing at a skill-based or rule-based level are slips or lapses, typically caused by distractions or other nonroutine intrusions that can disrupt the routine execution of automatized perceptual and motor performance units. For example an interesting conversation with a passenger may cause even a highly experienced driver to fail to notice (a lapse) that a car behind has commenced an overtaking maneuver. If the driver should then decide to change lanes in the direction of the overtaking vehicle and fails to check that the adjacent lane is clear (a slip—omission of effective checking via rearview mirror or head turn), there may well be a near miss or even a crash.

Errors that occur during knowledge-based performance are termed mistakes, unless they result from a deliberate decision to do something wrong (e.g., deliberately driving faster than the legal speed limit), in which case they are termed violations. Nondeliberate mistakes are typically the result of inadequate information, whether because of a failure of the road traffic authorities to provide adequate signage, for example,

or because of the driver's inadequate understanding of something such as the meaning of a road sign or law. Among older drivers in particular, mistakes are more likely in complex situations where there is significant time pressure, such as at a complex intersection where a driver wanting to complete a turning maneuver has to select a safe gap in multiple streams of opposing traffic. In such situations mistakes are likely because the demands of the driving task simply exceed the driver's capacity to attend to and make decisions about all of the necessary information in the available time.

Fully skill-based performance cannot be enhanced by giving more attention to it than is demanded by the task; in fact the reverse may well be true. It follows that admonishing drivers always to pay attention is not a good strategy for managing road safety because much of normal driving performance is at least partially automatized. Expenditure of attentional resources also entails effort; therefore paying attention has a cost—it is fatiguing, just as the expenditure of physical effort is fatiguing, which can increase the risk of errors.

Drivers must necessarily pay more attention when the driving task is objectively more difficult (requiring greater concentration and/or a faster processing rate) and when their competence level is relatively low so that their performance is less automatized. A highly skilled driver who is performing a routine task that proceeds in accordance with his or her expectancies—for example driving along a very familiar route—will need to expend a relatively small amount of attentional resources because the performance will be automatized to the maximum extent possible for that particular set of task conditions (determined by the predictability of vehicle, road, and traffic conditions). In contrast a novice performing the same task would have to pay considerably more attention, as would an experienced driver for whom that particular road environment was unfamiliar.

The total amount of attention invested in performance and the effectiveness of its allocation to different component behaviors can vary considerably within the same driver over time, depending on variables such as driving experience, age, fatigue, stress, and state of health. Demand for attention can also vary with the particular performance strategy adopted. Drivers who have a realistic understanding of their own performance capacities and limitations in relation to the demands of different driving maneuvers and situations may be able to plan trips to compensate, at least partially, for their impairments. For example they may minimize their number of overtaking and lane-changing maneuvers and try to maximize their use of signalized intersections rather than ones that require them to select gaps in heavy traffic flows.

A Hierarchical Model Specific to Driving: the Gadget Matrix

The Gadget Matrix is the latest of several models specific to driving that have been developed. These have some similarity to the SRK hierarchy but differ in that they are not directly linked to the human information-processing model. For example Michon[57] described driving performance and behavior in terms of three hierarchical levels: operational, tactical, and strategic. *Operational behavior* is concerned with routine vehicle maneuvering at the level of vehicle control operations; thus it is generally at the skill-based level (in SRK terms) except for novice drivers. *Tactical behavior* is that involved in applying road rules and adapting to the demands of the immediate road and traffic conditions, including performance of maneuvers such as turning, overtaking, and parking; it may be performed at various levels of automatization, but much of it is at the rule-based level for most drivers. *Strategic behavior* considers the goals and more general driving context, including decisions about whether to drive under particular conditions and route planning; it is most commonly at the knowledge-based level.

The early Michon framework has been developed into a form known as the Gadget Matrix to support improved programs of young driver education.[58] The Gadget Matrix has added a fourth level in the hierarchy above Michon's strategic level. This highest level is concerned with broader goals for life and skills for living and includes drivers' knowledge of and control over how their own life goals and personal characteristics may affect their driving behavior. Relevant here are issues such as an individual's specific lifestyle or work requirements, perceived group norms, personal values, attitudes and motives concerning driving-related issues, level of self-control and related personality characteristics, and so on.

DRIVER COMPETENCIES AND BEHAVIORS: A REHABILITATION FRAMEWORK

Terminology and concepts from the aforementioned models have been used to formulate a framework suitable for use by driver rehabilitation professionals, incorporating categories of driver competencies and underlying capacities and attributes. This framework builds on previous work by Macdonald,[59] Evans and Macdonald,[60] Macdonald,[61] AustRoads,[62] and Macdonald and Scott.[63] The Gadget Matrix[58] has also been considered. This framework is hierarchical, specifying driver competencies and attributes within the following categories: driving-specific competencies and prerequisite driver characteristics.

DRIVING-SPECIFIC COMPETENCIES

- *General driver strategies:* Their aim is to optimize the balance between an individual's exposure to injury risk and his or her community mobility, as well as maximizing personal ability to drive safely.
- *On-road driving tactics:* Their aim is to achieve overall goals of the trip while also optimizing the balance between driving task demands and individual ability to drive safely and in compliance with road laws.
- *Control of vehicle operations:* Their aim is appropriate execution of the performance elements involved in basic vehicle control operations and maneuvers (incorporates execution of level 2 tactics).

PREREQUISITE DRIVER CHARACTERISTICS

Prerequisite driver characteristics consist of the driver's general capacities and personal attributes that are necessary for competent driving performance. This framework is shown in Box 1-2. Note that the two lowest levels of the hierarchy, control of vehicle operations and prerequisite driver characteristics, are subdivided within the main information-processing stages of perception, cognition, and motor responses. This division is not appropriate at tactical and strategic levels because driving performance and behavior at these two higher levels are primarily concerned with planning, decision making, and response selection.

Table 1-4 tabulates driver competencies within the four hierarchical levels of the Gadget Matrix, listing typical risk factors for each level within the hierarchy, separately for the two groups of drivers known to be at highest risk. These groups are those with the least experience as drivers and those with a significant degree of cognitive impairment, including people without a particular medical diagnosis but whose cognitive functioning is significantly impaired because of more general, aging-related changes.

Particularly at the higher hierarchical levels concerning goals, strategies, and driving tactics, these frameworks are intended to support a comprehensive, systems-based approach to driver evaluation and to the identification of a wide range of methods by which drivers may be (re)habilitated and their community mobility optimized, while maintaining an adequate level of road safety. A disability may affect only one of the basic capacities that underlie driver competence (e.g., some aspect of physical coordination or vision), or it may affect several specific capacities (e.g., vision, short-term memory, and the ability to allocate attention appropriately). See Chapters 5, 6, 11, 12, and 13 for additional information on issues relating to how particular types of functional impairments are addressed.

BOX 1-2	**Categories of Driver Competencies and Underlying Capacities and Attributes: A Framework to Support Driver Rehabilitation**

A. DRIVING-SPECIFIC COMPETENCIES

1. GENERAL STRATEGIES to optimize balance between risk exposure and mobility:

Consider alternative transport modes or alternatives to travel—drive only when optimal

Buy, and maintain well, a vehicle that provides good crash protection (and without "aggressive" design features likely to maximize damage to other vehicles or pedestrians)

Maximize personal abilities to drive safely (e.g., minimize fatigue, comply with prescribed drug regimen, use prescribed lenses, more generally apply knowledge and insight concerning own impairments to minimize their functional effects; and maintain good knowledge of current road laws)

Plan trips and specific routes for safest times and in safest circumstances (e.g., avoid night driving, peak traffic, passengers who may be a distraction, and highly demanding situations or maneuvers)

2. DRIVING TACTICS to optimize balance between task demands and own abilities; more generally, to maximize safety:

Minimize numbers of difficult maneuvers (e.g., overtaking, turning across opposing traffic streams, and lane-changing at high speed in heavy traffic)

Manage passenger behavior and any social pressures

If any impairment to attentional capacity or information processing rate, drive at a reasonably slow speed (provided that this does not impair the progress of other vehicles)

Use appropriate seat belt or other restraint system

3. CONTROL OF VEHICLE OPERATIONS (incorporates *execution* of above tactics):

Perceptual-Cognitive Operations

Accurate schemata, mental models, and expectancies concerning road traffic system operations and behavior of other drivers—supporting more automatized perceptual/cognitive performance

Maintain efficient visual searching/scanning of the environment (using vehicle headlights as required)

Based on mental models and expectancies, "read" traffic situations, maintain high situation awareness

Within the broader context of situation awareness, identify "hazards" (specific, higher-risk situations) in good time

Based on situation awareness and perception of specific hazards, together with personal "calibration," select appropriate driving responses

Allocate attentional resources in accord with driving task demands, sustaining vigilance as required

Motor Control Operations

Change speed or lateral position smoothly

Maintain safety margins by appropriate
- Speed for conditions
- Lateral and anterior/posterior position within lane or carriageway
- Position in relation to stationary objects/vehicles

Control vehicle smoothly and accurately during low-speed maneuvers

Use secondary controls (e.g., vehicle horn and turn indicators) as required.

B. PREREQUISITE DRIVER CHARACTERISTICS: CAPACITIES AND ATTRIBUTES

Sensory and Perceptual Capacities

Adequate vision (especially visual fields, dynamic acuity, contrast sensitivity)

Adequate proprioception, kinesthesia, cutaneous sensation

Visuospatial perception (including visual search) and related capacities (e.g., visualization of missing information) underlying ability to predict trajectories and arrival times of moving objects

Cognitive Capacities and Overall Executive Function

Level of insight regarding own functional abilities and impairments (i.e., accuracy of "self-calibration" as a driver)

Level of self-control in relation to and implementing higher-order strategies and tactics, including planning, organizing, and adapting knowledge to current and projected future situations

Information-processing capacity and rate, choice reaction time, working memory capacity

Level of attentional resources and attentional control:
To divide attention between concurrent task components, maintain focus, and resist distractions
To sustain concentration for extended periods

Physical Capacities and Psychomotor Coordination

Physical strength and endurance

Postural stability and flexibility (especially head-neck)

Range of motion

Coordination (e.g., simple tracking and motor control skills)

Gross mobility, seated balance

Table 1-4 Key Driver Competencies and Examples of Associated Risk Factors of Two Categories of High-Risk Drivers, Categorized Within the Four Hierarchical Levels of the European Union Model of Driver Behavior Known as the Gadget Matrix

Hierarchical Level	Key Driver Competencies	Examples of Risk Factors	
		Inexperienced Drivers	Cognitively Impaired Drivers
1. General goals for life and skills for living	Knowledge and insight concerning how life goals and personal tendencies affect driving behavior Personal values Lifestyle/life situation Group norms Motives Self-control and related personal characteristics Awareness of: Own risk-taking behavioral tendencies Own ability for impulse control	Tendencies: To accept risks For sensation-seeking To accept peer-group norms To comply with risky social pressures To use alcohol, recreational drugs To push boundaries in relation to authority figures (e.g., breaking the law by speeding)	Absence of satisfactory alternative means of maintaining community mobility and inadequate support to do so Lack of awareness of the nature and extent of own functional impairments Unwillingness or inability to make lifestyle changes to compensate for functional impairments
2. Driving-specific goals and strategies	Knowledge of the need to: Assess possible effects of trip goals on driving performance Plan and choose routes to avoid excessively difficult conditions Allow sufficient time for trip, considering likely conditions Avoid and/or manage any social pressures while driving Awareness of own: Personal planning skills Typical driving-related motives	Driving in impaired state (e.g., because of mood, fatigue, alcohol/drugs) Risky trip purpose: recreation Risky road environment: night driving, high speed, rural roads Risky social context: own-age peers Risky personal motives: sensation seeking, etc. Driving to enhance self-image (e.g., by law breaking)	Impaired condition because of illness/disability, prescription medications, or fatigue Inadequate insight regarding the impact of impairment on own driving performance Unnecessary trips, poor trip planning Inadequate knowledge of strategies to reduce quantity or quality of exposure to risk Inability to change behavioral patterns (e.g., continues to tow a trailer/caravan despite reduced driving skills)
3. Mastery of traffic situations	Awareness of and ability to implement safe driving tactics regarding Application of traffic rules Lateral position on road Vehicle speed Importance of adequate safety margins Communication with other road users Understanding of own inadequacies as a driver	Inaccurate or incomplete expectancies because of underdeveloped mental models Overestimation of own driving skill level Risky driving style (e.g., excessive levels of speed, lane-changing, and overtaking) Inadequate safety margins Risky road environments (e.g., night, rural roads, unfamiliar areas) Inadequate modification of driving tactics (e.g., by driving more slowly) to compensate for own skill deficiencies	Inadequate maintenance of knowledge regarding road law, traffic control devices, etc. Excessively long or fatiguing trips Highly demanding driving task: heavy, fast-moving traffic, complex intersections, towing, and other situations Inadequate modification of driving tactics (e.g., by avoiding lane changing, difficult maneuvers) to compensate for own impairments Failure to compensate for slower reaction/movement times Lack of insight into poor driver habits (e.g., failing to apply indicators) or extreme compensatory behaviors (e.g., driving 40 km/hr in 70 km/hr zone)

Continued

Table 1-4   **Key Driver Competencies and Examples of Associated Risk Factors of Two Categories of High-Risk Drivers, Categorized Within the Four Hierarchical Levels of the European Union Model of Driver Behavior Known as the Gadget Matrix—cont'd**

Hierarchical Level	Key Driver Competencies	Examples of Risk Factors	
		Inexperienced Drivers	Cognitively Impaired Drivers
4. Vehicle maneuvers	See table 4, Level 3 Competencies and Level 4 Prerequisite Driver Characteristics	Unfamiliar vehicle or driving conditions Incomplete development of all aspects of driving skill and consequent overloading of information-processing capacity under highly demanding driving task conditions	Unfamiliar vehicle or driving conditions Cognitive decrements affecting information processing (slow rate, limited resources) or attention allocation abilities, in combination with driving conditions that demand high levels of these abilities (e.g., fast, complex traffic flows and in-vehicle distractions) Health conditions that create an increased demand for attentional control (e.g., because of pain or use of some adaptive equipment)

SUMMARY

Driver rehabilitation specialists can provide invaluable assistance to people with specific disabilities and more general functional impairments. DRSs use strategies that are adapted to the unique characteristics and circumstances of their individual clients in accord with conceptual models of human occupation. Such models share a client-centered approach to evaluation and intervention, and they all highlight the need for DRSs to take account of a variety of environmental, social, activity-specific, and individual factors. Identification and implementation of the most effective service strategies for each individual client require a thorough understanding of these factors and their potential impacts.

Because of the inherently hazardous nature of driving a motor vehicle in traffic on our roads, DRSs help clients to balance their community mobility goals against the need to minimize injury risk for themselves and other road users. Achievement of this balance is often difficult; it requires DRSs to be familiar with a wide range of potential risk management strategies, some of which target crash prevention, whereas others target harm minimization in the event of a crash. Risk reduction can be achieved by helping clients to reduce their exposure to risk, as well as by helping them to drive in ways that will reduce risk. An important principle to follow is the hierarchy of control, which is based on evidence of the relative effectiveness of different types of risk control measure.

For most DRSs an essential part of their work is the evaluation of clients' functional abilities and limitations in relation to driving task demands. The results of these evaluations also provide the basis for helping clients to identify and implement a customized set of driving strategies and tactics that will at least partially compensate for their impairments. It is essential that the evaluation procedures used for this purpose are reliable and that they use realistic, evidence-based performance criteria. Therefore it is important for DRSs to have an expert understanding of driving task demands and related driver competencies founded on a theory-based model of practice that has been empirically evaluated.

To facilitate this, key concepts and empirical data from several theoretical models are used in this chapter to formulate a conceptual framework suitable for use by driver rehabilitation professionals. This hierarchical framework specifies driver competencies and underlying capacities and attributes within a number of different categories and supports analysis of a comprehensive range of impairments. On this basis key driver competencies and associated common risk factors are identified.

REFERENCES

1. Hensher D, Alsnih R: The mobility and accessibility expectations of seniors in an aging population, *Transportation Research Part A Policy and Practice* 37:903-916, 2003.

2. US Department of Transportation: *Safe mobility for a maturing society: challenges and opportunities*, Washington, DC, 2003, US Department of Transportation.

3. Molnar LJ, Eby DW, Miller LL: *Promising approaches to enhancing elderly mobility, Report No. UMTRI-2003-14*, Ann Arbor, MI, 2003, University of Michigan Transportation Institute.

4. Enterlante TM, Kerm JM: Wives' reported role changes following a husband's stroke: a pilot study, *Rehabilitation Nurs* 20(3):155-160, 1995.

5. Zropf R: *Occupational therapy driver assessment and training course manual*, Sydney, 1988, Cumberland College of Health Sciences, University of Sydney.

6. Carr DB: Assessing older drivers for physical and cognitive impairment, *Geriatrics* 48:46-48, 51, 1993.

7. Victor C: *Old age in modern society*, ed 2, London, 1994, Chapman and Hall.

8. Johnson JE: Rural elders and the decision to stop driving, *J Comm Health Nurs* 12(3): 131-138, 1995.

9. Stubbins J: *Social and psychological aspects of disability: a handbook for practitioners*, Baltimore, 1977, University Park.

10. Gillens L: Yielding to age: when the elderly can no longer drive, *J Gerontologic Nurs* 16(11):12-15, 1990.

11. Kalz RT, et al: Driving safety after brain damage: follow up of 22 patients with matched controls, *Arch Phys Med Rehab* 71:133-137, 1990.

12. Galski T, Bruno RL, Ehle HT: Driving after cerebral damage: a model with implications for evaluation, *Am J Occ Ther* 46:324-331, 1992.

13. Vidich AJ, Lyman SM: Qualitative methods: their history in sociology and anthropology. In Denzin NK, Lincoln YS, editors: *Handbook of qualitative research*, Thousand Oaks, CA, 1994, Sage Schegloff.

14. McColl MA, Pollock N, Law M, et al: *Theoretical basis of occupational therapy*, ed 2, Thorofare, NJ, 2003, Slack.

15. Kielhofner G: *A model of human occupation: theory and application*, Baltimore, 1985, Williams and Wilkins.

16. Kielhofner G: *A model of human occupation: theory and application*, ed 3, Baltimore, 2002, Williams and Wilkins.

17. Law M, Cooper BA, Strong S, et al: The person-environment-occupation model: a transactive approach to occupational performance, *Can J Occup Ther* 63:9-23, 1996.

18. Canadian Association of Occupational Therapists: *Enabling occupation: an occupational therapy perspective*, Ottawa, 1997, CAOT Publications ACE.

19. Strong S, Rigby P, Stewart C, et al: Application of the person-environment-occupation model: a practical tool, *Can J Occup Ther* 66:122-133, 1999.

20. Crepeau EB, Cohn ES, Boyt Schell BA, editors: *Willard and Spackman's occupational therapy*, Philadelphia, 2003, Lippincott Williams & Wilkins.

21. Schultz S, Schkade JK: Occupational adaptation. In Crepeau EB, Cohn ES, Boyt Schell BA, editors: *Willard and Spackman's occupational therapy*, Philadelphia, 2003, Lippincott Williams & Wilkins, pp 220-227.

22. Pfeiffer D: The devils are in the details: the ICIDH2 and the disability movement, *Disabil Soc* 15:1079-1082, 2000.

23. World Health Organization: *ICF International Classification of Functioning, Disability and Health*, Geneva, 2001, World Health Organization.

24. Law M, Baum BM, Dunn W: *Measuring occupational performance: supporting best practice in occupational therapy*, Thorofare, NJ, 2001, Slack.

25. Chard G: International Classification of Functioning, Disability and Health, *Br J Occup Ther* 67:1, 2004.

26. Bury M: A comment on the ICIDH2, *Disabil Soc* 15:1073-1077, 2000.

27. Dahl TH: International Classification of Functioning, Disability and Health: an introduction and discussion of its potential impact on rehabilitation services and research, *J Rehabil Med* 34:201-204, 2002.

28. Jette AM, Haley SM, Kooyoomjian JT: Are the ICF activity and participation dimensions distinct? *J Rehabil Med* 35:145-149, 2003.

29. Evans L: *Traffic safety and the driver*, New York, 1991, Van Nostrand Reinhold.

30. Janke MK: Accidents, mileage, and the exaggeration of risk, *Accident Analysis Prevention* 23:183-188, 1991.

31. Hakamies-Blomqvist L: *Ageing Europe: the challenges and opportunities for transport safety*, European Transport Safety Council, Rue du Cornet 34, B-1040, Brussels, 2003. Available at: *http://www.liikenneturva.fi/englanti/ikaluokat/iakkaat/AgeingEurope.pdf* Accessed May 2004.

32. Hu P, Jones D, Reuscher T, et al: *Projecting fatalities in crashes involving older drivers*, Report for the National Highway Traffic Safety Administration, Oak Ridge National Laboratory, Tennessee, 2000, ONRL.

33. American Medical Association and National Highway Traffic Safety Administration: *Physician's guide to assessing and counseling older drivers*, 2003. Available at: *http://www.ama-assn.org/ama/pub/category/10791.html*. Accessed September 2, 2003.

34. Austroads: *Assessing fitness to drive: for commercial and private vehicle drivers: medical standards for licensing and clinical management guidelines*, ed 3, Sydney, 2003, Austroads Incorporated.

35. Charlton J, Koppel S, O'Hare M, et al: *Influence of chronic illness on crash involvement of motor vehicle drivers* (Literature review No. 213), Melbourne, 2004, Monash University Accident Research Centre.

36. Organization for Economic Co-operative Development: *Aging and transport: mobility needs and transport issues; OECD Report*, Geneva, 2001, Organization for Economic Co-operative Development.

37. Marottoli RA, Mendes de Leon C, Glass T, et al: Driving cessation and increased depressive symptoms: prospective evidence from the New Haven EPESE, *J Am Geriatr Soc* 45:202-206, 1997.

38. Harris A: Transport research among non-driving older people, *ARRB/REAAA Conference Proceedings*, Cairns, May 2003.

39. Fonda SJ, Wallace RB, Herzog AR: Changes in driving patterns and worsening depressive symptoms among older adults, *J Gerontol Series B Psychologic Sci Social Sci* 56:S343-S351, 2001.

40. Antrim JM, Engum ES: The driving dilemma and the law: patients' striving for independence versus public safety, *Cognitive Rehabil* March/April:15-19, 1989.

41. International Labour Organization (ILO-OSH): *Guidelines on occupational safety and health management systems*, Geneva, 2001, International Labour Office.

42. Standards Australia International (SAI): *Occupational health and safety management systems. General guidelines on principles, systems and supporting techniques*, Australian Standard AS/NZS 4804:2001, ed 2, Sydney, 2001, Standards Australia International.

43. Christie R: *The effectiveness of driver training: a review of the literature* (Literature review No. 01/03), Melbourne, 2001, Royal Automobile Club of Victoria.

44. Ranney TA: Models of driving behaviour: a review of their evolution, *Accident Analysis Prevention* 26:733-750, 1994.

45. Rothengatter T: Psychological aspects of road user behaviour, *Applied Psychol Internat Rev* 46:223-234, 1997.

46. Proctor RW, Van Zandt T: *Human factors in simple and complex systems*, Boston, 1994, Allyn and Bacon.

47. Wickens CD, Hollands JG: *Engineering psychology and human performance*, ed 3, Upper Saddle River, NJ, 2000, Prentice Hall.

48. Messinger-Rapport BJ: *Assessment and counseling of older drivers: a guide for primary care physicians: primary care*, 2003. http://articles.findarticles.

com/p/articles/mi_m2578/is_12_58/ai_11236 Retrieved May 2004.

49. Rasmussen J, Jensen A: Mental procedures in real-life tasks: a case-study of electronic trouble shooting, *Ergonomics* 17:293-307, 1974.

50. Rasmussen J, Pejtersen A, Goodstein LP: *Cognitive systems engineering*, New York, 1994, Wiley.

51. Summala H: Modeling driver behavior: a pessimistic prediction? In Evans L, Schwing R, editors: *Human behavior and traffic safety*, New York, 1985, Plenum Press.

52. Hale AR, Glendon AI: *Individual behaviour in the control of danger*, Amsterdam, 1987, Elsevier.

53. Reason JT: *Human error*, Cambridge, 1990, Cambridge University Press.

54. Park K: Human error. In Salvendy G, ed. *Handbook of human factors and ergonomics*, New York, 1997, John Wiley & Son.

55. Macdonald WA: *Human error: causes and countermeasures*, Proceedings of the Safety in Action Conference 2004, Melbourne, Australia, 2004.

56. Reference deleted in pages.

57. Michon JA: Dealing with danger: summary of a workshop in the Traffic Research Centre. In van Zomeren AH, Brouwer WH, Minderhoud JK, editors: *Acquired brain damage and driving: a review*, vol 68, pp 697-705, The Netherlands, 1979, State University Groningen.

58. Hatakka M, Keskinen E, Gregersen NP, et al: Theories and aims of educational and training measures. In Siegrist SE, editor: *Driver training, testing and licensing—towards theory-based management of young drivers' injury risk in road traffic*, Berne, Switzerland, 1999, Human Research Department, Swiss Council for Accident Prevention, pp 13-44.

59. Macdonald WA: *Novice driver competencies*, Unpublished report to the Austroads Novice Car Driver Competencies Specification Project, Australia, 1994, National Association of Australian State Road Authorities.

60. Evans T, Macdonald W: The nature of novice drivers' situation awareness: an exploratory study. Proceedings of the *2002 Road Safety Research, Policing and Education Conference*, Adelaide, 2002, Causal Productions.

61. Macdonald W: *Driving competencies for learner drivers* (No. RUB 97/98-13), Melbourne, Victoria, 1998, VicRoads.

62. Austroads: *Novice car driver competency specification*. Report AP-121/95. Haymarket, NSW, Australia, 1995, Austroads.

63. Macdonald WA, Scott T: *Disabled driver test procedures*, Canberra, 1993, Federal Office of Road Safety.

Chapter 2

DRIVING AND COMMUNITY MOBILITY: AN HISTORICAL PERSPECTIVE

KEY TERMS

- Mass transit
- Mass automobility
- Interstate Highway Act of 1956

CHAPTER OBJECTIVES

After completing this chapter, the reader will be able to do the following:

- Understand how technological changes shaped transportation.
- Understand how the automobile has come to be the predominant form of transportation for most Americans and other people residing in industrialized countries around the world.
- Understand that the reliance on transportation creates a need for those who are elderly or have disabilities or other mobility issues to adapt automobiles to their needs.
- Understand the role that occupational therapists and driver educators played in creating the field of driver rehabilitation.

SECTION I

History of the Automobile

Charles K. Hyde

The automobile is the predominant form of transportation for virtually all Americans and other people residing in Western, industrialized countries around the world today. To be sure *mass transit* choices (i.e., subways, commuter railroads, buses, and trolleys) are important in a handful of large cities in North America, and Americans prefer airplanes for long-distance travel of more than 500 miles. The young, elderly, people with disabilities, and the poor are the main users of bus transportation but not by choice. Bicycles are most commonly used by children and youth not of driving age and by adults for recreation. Walking or riding a wheeled mobility device more than a few blocks is alien to most Americans. Today most Americans spend large parts of their lives in automobiles on the streets, roads, expressways, and parking lots that dominate the "built environment" of urban and suburban America. The automobile permeates everyday life in ways that are not often recognized. The driver's license, for example, has become the only easily accepted form of identification for adults. This dominant role for the automobile has developed in a little more than 100 years. In 1900 there were about 8000 motor vehicles registered in the United States. By 1929 that number had jumped to 26.5 million and in 2001 reached the astonishing figure of slightly under 230 million vehicles on U.S. roads and highways.[1]

STEAM, ELECTRIC, HYBRID, AND INTERNAL COMBUSTION ENGINES

In recent years there has been a growing interest in automobiles powered by electric motors or by various hybrid engines. These alternative designs are still viewed as technical oddities, not likely to be practical (i.e., economical) anytime soon. With few exceptions internal combustion engines burning some type of gasoline, diesel fuel, propane, or natural gas power automobiles and trucks; this has not always been the case. During the first two decades of the twentieth century automobiles powered by steam engines and electric motors were popular alternatives to automobiles with internal combustion engines. In 1900 the production of 4192 automobiles in the United States consisted of 1681 steam-powered vehicles, 1575 powered by electric motors, and only 936 with gasoline engines.

Five years later gasoline cars dominated sales of new vehicles, but steam and electric cars were manufactured until the late 1920s, each holding onto a group of loyal customers. The ascendancy of the internal combustion automobile and the simultaneous decline of the steamers and electrics is an important subplot in the story of the automobile's adoption in the United States.[2]

More than a dozen Americans invented steam-powered road vehicles during the period of 1860 to 1900, including several inventors who went on to manufacture gasoline cars. Ransom E. Olds made two operational steam-powered vehicles in Lansing, Michigan in the 1890s. The first steam vehicles produced in quantity for sale to the public took place around Boston in 1898, when George Whitney and the Stanley brothers (Francis E. and Freelan O.) developed successful models. The Locomobile Company of Bridgeport, Connecticut made 5000 steamers in the brief period of 1900 to 1903. The White brothers of Cleveland, Ohio, manufacturers of sewing machines, began making steam cars in 1901 and continued to sell them until 1910, when the company converted to gasoline automobiles. The Stanley Steamer Company made steamers until 1925 and was the last company to do so. Early technical improvements speeded the adoption of steamers. Initially the driver needed 20 minutes to get up a head of steam, but "flash" boilers reduced that time to 2 minutes. However, the steam-powered car had several drawbacks that led to its demise. Steamers required a good supply of soft water and burned as much fuel (kerosene or gasoline) as automobiles powered by internal combustion engines. The most important disadvantage of steam-powered vehicles was the low power-to-weight ratio for the engine.[3]

Automobiles powered by electric motors, with storage batteries providing the current, enjoyed even more success than steam-powered cars in the early twentieth century. William Morrison of Des Moines, Iowa drove the first electric car in the United States in 1891. Commercial production for the market started in Philadelphia, Pennsylvania in 1894 when Henry Morris and Pedro G. Salom offered the "Electrobat" to the public.[1] The Pope Manufacturing Company of Hartford, Connecticut, the highly successful manufacturer of the Columbia bicycle, introduced the Columbia electric car in May 1897. Pope Manufacturing also experimented with gasoline cars but initially concentrated on electrics. In 1898 and

1899 the Pope factory shipped 540 cars, and 500 of these were electrics. Other earlier electric car pioneers in the United States included Andrew Lawrence Riker, who commercially produced electrics starting in 1897. One year later Elmer Ambrose Sperry built six electric automobiles in Cleveland, Ohio, which soon became a center for electric car manufacturing. Even the Studebaker Corporation, makers of wagons and carriages since the Civil War, briefly offered electric cars in 1902 before moving to gasoline cars.[4]

Electric cars had many inherent advantages over their steam- and gasoline-powered competitors. They were quiet, clean, smokeless, and easy to operate, especially on paved roads. Women preferred them because there was no need to "get up steam" or to hand-crank the engine to start it. However, electric cars did have disadvantages compared with steamers and gasoline cars. They typically did not have the power to climb steep hills or to pull themselves out of deep ruts or mud. More importantly they had a short operating range, usually between 50 and 80 miles, between recharging the batteries.[2] Sharp regional differences in the pattern of early automobile ownership reflect the advantages and disadvantages of electrics. Registration of automobiles in the state of New York by source of power in May 1903 was as follows: steam engines (53%), gasoline engines (27%), and electric motors (20%). In early 1901 cars registered in the city of Chicago presented a markedly different pattern, with electrics accounting for 60% of the total, steam cars a distant second at 24%, and gasoline cars making up a mere 16% of the total. Chicago car owners probably used their vehicles mainly on well-paved streets on flat terrain within the city, whereas in New York car owners traveled greater distances on rougher roads over hilly terrain.[4]

Electric-powered taxicabs and city delivery vehicles enjoyed a brief stretch of popularity in the early twentieth century. In 1902 the Columbia Automobile Company and the Electric Vehicle Company merged to form a manufacturing giant that hoped to sell tens of thousands of electric taxicabs for use in cities like New York, Philadelphia, and Chicago. The firm produced about 2000 cabs in 1902 to 1903, but these proved impractical. In normal use the entire set of batteries (1200 pounds) had to be replaced after every trip. A second generation of electrics for personal use emerged with the introduction of the Detroit Electric by the Anderson Carriage Manufacturing Company in 1907. Anderson quickly increased production to 1600 electrics by 1910. The company became the Anderson Electric Car Company in 1911. The firm went into receivership in 1927 but only survived until 1940 as the last manufacturer of electric cars in the United States. By then some 50,000 electric cars had been made in the United States, and Anderson accounted for more than 25% of the total. The rapid demise of the electric automobile in the first decade of the twentieth century was precipitous. As early as 1904, when American automobile output was 21,693 units, electrics made up <7% of the total. In 1909 Americans bought 82,000 gasoline-engine cars but only 4000 electrics, <5% of the total. The New York Automobile Show of 1925 was the first show where all of the vehicles displayed were gasoline powered.[4]

GASOLINE-POWERED VEHICLES DOMINATE THE MARKET

The gasoline-powered car came to dominate the automobile market because it became more reliable, more comfortable, and less expensive over time. Brothers Charles and Frank Duryea invented the first American gasoline-powered car in Springfield, Massachusetts in 1893 and first manufactured them for general sale in 1896. Early gasoline automobile inventors emerged in many midwestern cities, including Cleveland, Indianapolis, and Detroit. The focus of the industry shifted to Michigan with the success of the Olds Motor Works (1899) and the Ford Motor Company (1903), among others. The discovery of huge oil deposits at Spindletop, near Beaumont, Texas in 1901 and subsequent discoveries in Oklahoma flooded the market with cheap gasoline, making the gasoline automobile even more appealing.[5]

Whereas the basic technologies used in steam and electric vehicles changed little after 1905, gasoline automobiles improved noticeably. Early automobiles, such as the "curved-dash Olds" of 1901, were called horseless carriages and looked the part. They looked like a horse-drawn buggy except that a tiller replaced reins as the steering device, while the engine and gas tank were located under the driver's seat. Between 1905 and 1910 the "buggy-type" car disappeared, and the new designs increasingly looked like modern automobiles. The engine, which had grown in size and power, moved under a separate hood well in front of the driver, who controlled the front wheels with a steering wheel. The underpowered car, the bane of early automobile owners, was disappearing. The 1901 Olds runabout had a 5-horsepower engine and weighed 900 pounds, whereas the 1908 Model T Ford had a 20-horsepower engine and weighed 1200 pounds. The H-slot slide-gear transmission, with three forward gears and one reverse, was nearly standard in the industry by 1910. The extensive use of strong, lightweight vanadium steel in cars, pioneered by the Ford Motor Company, reduced weight and improved mechanical reliability.[2]

MAKING CARS MORE AFFORDABLE AND RELIABLE

Before the Model T Ford of 1908 potential car buyers faced difficult choices. Several large, heavy, and reasonably reliable cars were available for purchase but typically cost between $2000 and $4000, well outside the reach of most buyers. Nameplates such as Packard, Pierce, Peerless, Thomas, and Locomobile were available in this price range. Most early automobile owners were moderately wealthy white men. There were also a variety of "buggy-type" cars, also called "runabouts," that would seat two passengers only and were available for <$1000. A 1907 Brush Runabout sold for a mere $500. These cheaper cars unfortunately were usually not reliable.

The Model T Ford changed the face of the automobile market because it was a reliable car that became more and more affordable over time. Henry Ford priced the Model T runabout at $825 in 1908 but in 1910 dropped the price to $680. He followed with additional price reductions, and in August 1916 Ford announced a price of $345 for the runabout. Ford's sales, a robust 34,528 cars in 1910 to 1911, skyrocketed to 730,041 units in 1916 to 1917. James Flink described the mass production of cars as the logical prerequisite for "mass automobility" in the United States in the twentieth century. Henry Ford made it happen by making the Model T affordable for most Americans— the middle class, farmers, and factory workers. Vehicle registrations in the United States jumped from 468,000 in 1910 to 9,239,000 in 1920 and then reached 26,532,000 a decade later.[2] The introduction of installment purchasing of automobiles also made them more affordable. Starting in 1916 the Guarantee Securities Corporation of New York financed sales for most vehicle brands. General Motors introduced the General Motors Acceptance Corporation (GMAC) in 1919 to encourage sales by offering consumers the opportunity to make payments over a predetermined amount of time versus being required to make a one-time payment up front. As early as 1922 73% of new car purchases were made with time payments.[3]

GASOLINE-POWERED AUTOMOBILES AND TECHNICAL IMPROVEMENTS

Technical improvements to the gasoline automobile in the 1910s and 1920s guaranteed a complete victory over the steam and electric alternatives. Perhaps the most important improvement was the development of the electric self-starter by Charles Kettering of General Motors in 1911. He installed his system on 1912 Cadillacs, and the hand crank quickly went out of existence. By 1916 virtually all of the new cars (98%) came equipped with electric starters. Cranking by hand required strength and skill but was also dangerous. If an engine backfired the result was often a broken arm or wrist. The electric starter opened automobile use to women and to some men of smaller stature as well. The automobile industry also moved the steering wheel from the right side of the car to the left side. Initially when roads were unpaved and the driver had to watch the shoulder of the road for ditches, having the wheel on the right made some sense. With the coming of better roads, a greater volume of traffic, and the need to avoid oncoming cars, left-side steering was needed. In 1910 only 2% of new automobiles sold in the United States had the steering wheel on the left side, but in 1916 some 98% did.[5]

IMPROVED SAFETY AND COMFORT

Cars also became more comfortable during the first decade of the twentieth century. The use of shock absorbers and improved springs helped to improve comfort, along with the introduction of pneumatic tires that replaced solid rubber tires. Improved wheel rims also made changing tires easier, an important advance during a period when tires routinely lasted for only ≤1000 miles. After Prest-O-Lite introduced reliable acetylene lamps in 1904, night driving became practical.[2]

During the first two decades of the twentieth century, virtually all of the new cars were open, with no solid roof or permanent windows enclosing the vehicle's occupants. In northern parts of the United States, the open car was used only part of the year and would spend many months in a garage or under a tarp. When hardy auto enthusiasts used their cars in the winter, they required special clothing (i.e., warm and waterproof) to drive. In 1912 the Edward G. Budd Manufacturing Company of Philadelphia introduced the all-steel automobile body, still an open vehicle type, but it quickly became popular, in part because of its strength and durability. Budd designed the first all-steel closed-body car for the Dodge Brothers in 1923, and the closed body (many using a composite design of steel and wood) became the industry standard. In 1919 only 10% of new cars had closed bodies, but by 1927 >82% of new cars were enclosed. The closed body allowed for year-round use of the vehicle and made it more attractive to men and women alike who did not want to wear special clothing just to drive their automobile.[3]

A series of additional technical improvements made driving more pleasant and made cars more reliable and safer. In the early 1920s Charles Kettering discovered that adding tetraethyl lead to gasoline reduced engine knock, making driving more pleasant. DuPont also developed more effective antifreeze mixtures, which helped control overheating. Improved gasoline and better engine designs also reduced engine vibrations. The brand-new Chrysler Six, introduced in January 1924, incorporated the latest in automotive technology. It featured a high-compression engine, which further increased the power-to-weight ratio, low-pressure "balloon" tires, and four-wheel hydraulic brakes, developed by Malcolm Lougheed (Lockheed) in the early 1920s. His brakes were first used on the 1922 Duisenberg, a luxury car. Chrysler's engineers improved Lockheed's design, and the 1924 Chrysler Six was the first American car produced in large quantities to have these improved brakes as standard equipment. Earlier cars had mechanical braking systems often installed on only two wheels.[3]

Mechanical refinements and improvements in comfort and safety continued through World War II but were seldom revolutionary or radical. Shatter-resistant laminated glass windshields were first used on the 1926 Rickenbacker and Stutz models, but the 1927 Model A Ford was the first mass-produced car to use these "safety" windshields.[6] The late 1920s witnessed the invention of the mechanical fuel pump, the downdraft carburetor, which increased engine power, and the automatic choke. For his 1932 models Henry Ford introduced a V-8 engine costing so little that it could be used in low-priced cars like the Ford. This was the beginning of an American automotive "horsepower race" that continued well into the 1970s. A typical American automobile engine in the 1920s developed about 20 horsepower, but by 1950 this average had jumped to 100 horsepower.[3] More powerful engines meant greater speed and therefore the need for better brakes to stop the vehicle. In 1930 Cadillac offered a V-16 engine rated at 165 horsepower and a power brake system run off the manifold vacuum. Power brakes spread in popularity during the 1930s as cars became heavier and engines more powerful.[7]

Shifting gears manually had always been a challenge for all but the most highly skilled drivers. Automotive engineers gradually introduced technical improvements to make shifting easier. The 1928 Cadillac, for example, incorporated an industry "first"—a synchromesh transmission, which eliminated the need to "double-clutch" to avoid grinding the gears.

The automatic transmission was perhaps the most important technical breakthrough because it made driving less complicated. The first fully automatic transmission was the 1940 Oldsmobile "Hydra-Matic

Drive," followed quickly by the "Fluid Drive," which was introduced in the 1941 Chrysler Corporation models.[3]

IMPROVED ROADS AND HIGHWAYS

The widespread acceptance of the automobile in the 1920s and after depended on the development of better roads and highways. The condition of roads in the United States at the turn of the century was appalling by today's standards. According to one estimate, in 1904 only 7% of U.S. highways were "improved," meaning that it had a surface other than dirt. Of the nearly 154,000 miles of "improved" roads, two-thirds of the mileage had gravel surfaces and another one-quarter was surfaced with water-bound macadam, which consisted of small stones. A mere 141 miles were surfaced with brick or asphalt. Most were impassible much of the year because of deep ruts, potholes, and mud. Ironically the first agitation for improved roads came from bicyclists in the late nineteenth century. The League of American Wheelmen, established in 1880, and the National League for Good Roads, founded in 1892, became the two major groups to lobby their state legislatures and the federal government for better roads. In 1893 Congress created an Office of Road Inquiry within the Department of Agriculture, but its purpose was purely educational.[8]

Highway improvements in the early part of the twentieth century came from state and local governments and from private organizations promoting particular highways. The first section of concrete highway in the country was a 1-mile section of Woodward Avenue in Detroit, Michigan, built by the Wayne County Road Commission. In 1913 a group of prominent automobile manufacturers, including Carl Graham Fisher of Prest-O-Lite, Roy D. Chapin of the Hudson Motor Car Company, and Henry B. Joy of the Packard Motor Car Company, established the Lincoln Highway Association. They proposed a hard-surfaced coast-to-coast highway named after Abraham Lincoln. In 1916 Congress changed the Office of Road Inquiry into the Bureau of Public Roads and gave it new responsibilities. The first federal spending on highways came with the Federal Aid Road Act of 1916, which provided $75 million to be spent over 5 years for the improvement of rural post roads. Administered by the Agriculture Department, funding took the form of grants to state highway departments on a 50-50 matching basis. The Federal Highway Act of 1921 was more ambitious. Congress appropriated $75 million for 1922 alone, with funds to go to the states on a 50-50 match-ing basis. Each state had to designate 7% of its highway mileage as "primary," with only those designated highways eligible for federal aid.[8]

Federal spending on highways, along with state and local spending, notably improved the condition of the nation's roads. Road building by the states was supported by gasoline taxes. Oregon, New Mexico, and Colorado imposed the first gasoline taxes in 1919, and the other states quickly followed suit. By 1931 the states enjoyed $526 million in revenues from gasoline taxes, with virtually all of the money earmarked for highway improvements. The quantity of "improved" (i.e., surfaced) roads, a mere 154,000 miles in 1904, stood at 447,000 miles in 1921 and 854,000 miles in 1930. By the end of World War II, 1.7 million miles of American roads were surfaced, and 1.6 million miles were not. There were plans in the works for a national system of highways as early as 1923. By then the federal Bureau of Public Roads, led by Thomas H. MacDonald, had developed a plan to link American cities with populations of ≥50,000 with a network of arterial highways.[9]

Improved roads certainly encouraged the widespread use of the automobile by millions of Americans through World War II. The improved reliability, ease of use, and comfort of automobiles, along with greater affordability over time, also fostered their use. Mass automobility came to the United States in the first half of the twentieth century because millions of individuals consciously decided to buy an automobile. They did so because they believed that an automobile would improve their lives, and for the most part it did. Aside from a few wealthy people who embraced the earliest cars, the first groups of Americans to enthusiastically adopt the automobile were farmers and people living in rural areas. The automobile (and the truck and tractor) had the greatest positive effect on the lives of farmers.

THE AUTOMOBILE AND RURAL AMERICA

Henry Ford marketed the Model T as "the farmer's car," and farmers made up a large and loyal group of Ford Motor Company customers. In 1908 the United States was still predominantly rural. One-third of the population lived on farms, and one-half lived in places with a population of <2500 people. Farmers initially bought cars to help with farm work and not for pleasure. They used Model Ts in particular to haul their commodities (e.g., milk and crops) to the nearest railroad line and modified them to plow their fields and to run other machines as well. A single car could replace two or three horses at less expense to the farmer.[7] In

1910 about 85,000 cars were in use on American farms, but the number climbed to 2.2 million in 1920 and 9.7 million in 1930. American farmers also operated 900,000 farm trucks and 920,000 tractors in 1930. The lightweight inexpensive Fordson tractor, the "Model T" of tractors, was the most popular model used. By 1950 American farmers operated 3.4 million tractors and 2.2 million farm trucks.[10]

Before the coming of the automobile to the farm, rural Americans were in most respects isolated from the mainstream of American culture. The automobile, combined with improved roads, made it possible for rural people to travel greater distances to visit relatives, attend church, see a doctor, or go into larger towns to shop. Itinerant preachers disappeared, as did many tiny village churches, replaced by expanding churches in larger towns and cities. With cars rural people attended church more often. The school bus brought the end of the one-room, one-teacher rural school. Larger regional schools, which could offer specialized courses and stronger academic programs, developed as a result. Some 86% of rural people were not served by a public library as late as 1926, but the automobile brought the branch library and the bookmobile. The automobile also improved the quality of medical services available to rural folks. Doctors were often the first people to buy cars, which made house calls much easier than with a horse and buggy. More importantly patients could drive some distance to the doctor's office or enjoy the benefits of urban hospitals. The automobile also brought the visiting nurse and the ambulance into the rural health care system. Among other things the number of amputations performed by rural doctors decreased with the coming of the automobiles. Finally, cars reduced the isolation and boredom of rural life. Rural Free Delivery improved contact with the outside world. Farmers and their families could enjoy shopping in larger towns, go to the movies, attend church and other social functions, and interact with people who were not farmers.[11]

MASS AUTOMOBILITY

In many respects, *mass automobility* did not come to dominate the American transportation system until the 1950s, when the decline in mass transit systems across the country made automobile ownership more of a necessity than a choice. In 1929 45% of American families did not own an automobile, and as late as 1950 the share of families without cars was still 40%. Poor and working class families in large cities did not own automobiles and did not need to own them, given reasonably reliable and inexpensive mass transit systems.

A survey done in the greater Pittsburgh area in 1934, for example, revealed that only 45% of chief wage earners owned cars, and only 22% of chief wage earners used their cars to get to work. One-half took mass transit, and 28% walked. The decline of urban mass transit systems in much of the United States starting in the 1920s and the demise of intercity rail passenger service starting in the 1950s made automobile ownership imperative. By 1981 only 13% of American households were without an automobile, and the household with multiple vehicles was common.[12]

THE AUTOMOBILE REPLACES THE STREETCAR

The appearance of the automobile and more importantly the bus in urban areas in the 1920s marked the start of the decline of most urban street railway systems. Ridership, which had reached about 13.6 billion in 1923, slipped nearly in half to 7.3 billion riders in 1942. The combined ridership of all streetcar systems was just under 10 billion passengers in 1945, when buses carried similar numbers. By 1960 bus patronage had decreased to 6.5 billion passengers, but streetcars were carrying only 463 million, with most of these in New York, Chicago, Boston, and a handful of other cities. Diesel buses replaced electric streetcar systems within cities and electric interurban lines, which went between cities. Electric streetcars ran on separate rights-of-way and normally ran faster than automobile and track traffic in most cities. However, diesel buses used the same traffic lanes as automobiles and trucks and so offered no advantage in terms of speed for urban travelers. In the 1950s and 1960s millions of city residents bought cars for the first time and stopped patronizing buses.[13]

THE AUTOMOBILE AND MASS TRANSIT

There is much evidence that the outcome (i.e., a sharp increase in automobile ownership in urban areas) was the result of a deliberate policy pursued by General Motors Corporation and a few allied companies to destroy mass transit systems. General Motors first entered the bus manufacturing business in 1925, when it bought the Yellow Coach Company and then established Greyhound as a long-distance bus transportation company. In 1935 General Motors established Omnibus, a subsidiary whose sole purpose was to buy up New York City's (surface) electric streetcar lines and convert them to bus operation. In 1936 General Motors, with partners Standard Oil and the Firestone Rubber Company, established National City Lines, a holding company that bought >100 electric transit lines during the next 20 years and converted all of them to buses. These included most of southern California's mass transit lines and the entire transit system of

St. Louis. Over time, as the quality of service declined on the bus lines, riders abandoned these mass transit systems and increasingly bought passenger cars.[13]

INTERCITY AND INTERSTATE TRANSPORTATION

The transportation systems providing intercity and interstate travel also changed dramatically after World War II. Railroad passenger traffic had peaked in 1920, increasingly replaced by buses. By 1948 buses carried more passengers between cities than did trains, but their combined numbers were already in decline. A growing system of high-speed interstate highways was already underway when Congress passed the Interstate Highway Act in 1956. The creation of the Interstate Highway System during the next quarter century only hastened the triumph of the automobile over alternative transportation systems. Motor vehicle registrations in the United States, some 49.2 million in 1950, reached 108.4 million in 1970 and came to dominate intercity travel.[3]

Plans for a nationwide system of express highways were well underway by World War II. A blueprint developed by Congress in 1944 envisioned the upgrading of 34,000 miles of main highways to limited-access express highway standards. Eastern states built a series of interconnecting high-speed toll roads to reduce congestion and to speed through traffic. The Pennsylvania Turnpike (1940) was the first, followed by the Maine Turnpike (1947), New Jersey Turnpike (1948), New York Thruway (1956), and the Massachusetts Turnpike (1957). With the completion of east-west toll roads through Ohio, Indiana, and Illinois in 1955 to 1958, cars and especially trucks could travel from New York to Chicago on these express toll roads. Once this system was completed, a truck traveling from Jersey City, New Jersey to Chicago could save 30 hours of elapsed time, 11 hours of travel time, and 30 gallons of gasoline using the toll roads instead of the state highways.[8]

The Interstate Highway Act of 1956
The passage of the Federal-Aid Highway Act of 1956, also known as the *Interstate Highway Act of 1956*, made a national system of express highways a reality. Federal gasoline taxes would be placed into a Highway Trust Fund, which could only be used for construction of interstate highways. The initial legislation that was proposed did not include expressways running through cities, but President Eisenhower agreed to add 5000 miles of urban freeways to garner support from members of Congress from urban districts. The federal government would pay 90% of the costs of these highways, and the states would pay the remaining 10%. The original plan called for 41,000 miles of express highways to be built at a cost of $27 billion.

The Interstate Highway System, still not entirely complete, has cost $70 billion for land acquisition and construction. This highway system further encouraged long-distance vacation travel. The numbers of recreational vehicles (travel trailers, campers, and motor homes) in use jumped sharply from 150,000 in 1956 to 728,000 in 1972. Automobile traffic in National Parks has reached such threatening numbers that the most popular parks have severely limited automobile access.[13]

IMPROVED TECHNOLOGY, FEATURES, AND COMFORT

Since World War II, the American automotive industry has produced a continuous stream of new features, which have made the automobile driving experience easier and more pleasant than ever. General Motors introduced tinted windshields on 1951 model Buicks, and tinted glass became a popular "improvement" in the 1950s. The reduced glare and improved driver vision during the day more than compensated for the loss of some vision at night. Power steering was first offered on 1951 Chrysler and Buick models. Cadillac followed suit in 1952, and 1 year later, power steering was available on most General Motors models. Comfort became more and more important for drivers, in part because trips grew longer in the postwar period. Air conditioning was first introduced on a number of makes in the 1953 model year. By 1967 nearly 40% of new cars had air conditioning. Today this feature is practically universal. Electric-powered features became all the rage in the 1950s. Packard had first introduced electric-powered windows in 1941, and these became standard equipment on luxury cars in the 1950s. Several makes first introduced six-way power seats and electric door locks on their 1956 models. In the early 1970s cruise control also became a popular option.[7]

FORM, FUNCTION, AND SAFETY CONSIDERATIONS

Many of the changes in automobile design and features that have appeared starting in the mid-1950s relate to safety. The automobile industry was already moving toward designing cars with "occupant safety" in mind when the publication of Ralph Nader's book *Unsafe at Any Speed: The Designed-In Dangers of the American Automobile* (1965) brought safety issues to the attention of the general public and Congress. The National Traffic and Motor Vehicle Safety Act of 1966 established the National Highway Traffic Safety

Administration (NHTSA), with the power to establish safety standards to apply to the 1968 model cars. Most of the initial set of standards reflected what the industry had already introduced on its own. Over time, a wide range of additional standards were applied to new automobiles.[3]

Safety improvements were designed to keep the driver and passengers inside the car in the event of a crash and to minimize injuries. Safety door latches to prevent doors from opening in a crash were standard equipment on most 1955 model American cars. In March 1963 the Studebaker Corporation installed front seat belts on all of its models, and the rest of the auto industry followed suit in the fall of 1963 with the 1964 models. The automakers then installed rear seat belts as standard equipment starting with the 1966 models. That same year General Motors, Chrysler, and American Motors installed collapsible steering columns on all of their models, and Ford introduced an energy-absorbing steering wheel.[7]

Improved tires and brakes also contributed to improved safety in the postwar period.

Packard first used tubeless tires as standard equipment in June 1954, and the other manufacturers followed suit by the end of the year. Studebaker introduced front-wheel disc brakes as an option on its 1963 models, and the rest of the industry followed Studebaker's lead within a few years. In the middle of the 1969 model year U.S. automakers installed bias-belted tires on roughly two-thirds of their cars, and the changeover to these improved tires was complete with the launch of the 1970 models. Within 3 years new cars were fitted with radial tires as standard equipment. Braking systems continued to evolve. The 1974 model Lincoln and Ford Thunderbird first offered antiskid brakes, but antilock brake systems (ABS) did not become a common option until the 1990s. The most important of the safety improvements was the requirement that automobiles be equipped with "passive restraint" systems to automatically protect passengers. These new rules, which finally took effect starting in 1987, brought the installation of air bags.[7]

ADAPTED DRIVING

With the first automobiles came the first instance of adapting the automobile so that people with disabilities could use cars more easily. Box 2-1 is an interview with Judge Quentin D. Corley, who adapted his Model T with great success (Figure 2-1).

BOX 2-1	Judge Quentin D. Corley: No One Is Helpless Unless He Allows Himself to Be

"A man with two good hands may be 'down and out,' but he doesn't have to be even though he has lost both hands. It's the way a man looks at life and his condition that makes for success or failure. Losing one's hands is a mighty big handicap, but even then a man is not helpless unless he allows himself to be; for such a misfortune handicaps its victim only in competition with manual laborers. The man who rises above the average does not do so by mere physical prowess but by mental development. A cripple can climb just as high as he will develop his brain power," said Judge Quentin D. Corley as we sat in his office looking out over the city of Dallas, where he has established himself as one of the leaders of his profession.

"To shrink from association with others is the first thing a cripple thinks of; but it is the most vital mistake he can make, because it tends to make him morose and puts him out of touch with human affairs. Without friends a cripple cannot live happily. I married after my accident, following a three-year courtship of the finest girl I knew. We have a son and a daughter and a happy home.

"When I lost my hands, I was helpless; but after several months I had an arm made and began to invent apparatus to help me become absolutely physically independent of the help of others. During the past twelve years I have invented a work hook, an automatic hand, an automatic self-locking elbow joint, and a machine for putting on my collar and tie. With these helps I am able to do everything I want to do and am just as independent as I would be if I had hands of the ordinary kind.

"I get up in the morning and light the gas fire, holding the match between the jaws of the hook.

"I shave every morning with a safety razor, held in my hook. I dress myself with the aid of my artificial arm, pulling on my shirt with the aid of my collar and tie machine, then put on my trousers and button them with my hook as quickly as one with hands can do.

"I comb my hair by holding the comb in the cuff of my arm; I can comb and dress in fifteen minutes.

"At the table I cut my meat with my fork and serve myself as anyone else with both hands does.

"In short, I endeavor to be a normal individual in every respect.

"When America entered the World War in 1917, I was busy attending to my duties as county Judge. I was soon called upon to aid the Surgeon General's Department in Washington in rehabilitation and 'cheer up' work among the wounded soldiers.

"My work with the Surgeon General's Department consisted of conferences in Washington, delivering of lectures on 'Overcoming Difficulties' to the wounded soldiers, and making a moving picture to show how I accomplish the many things I do in my everyday life.

"In March, 1919, I was called to New York by the Red Cross to deliver my lecture, 'Overcoming Difficulties,' before the International Conference, in Carnegie Hall. This conference was composed of delegates from the various allied nations engaged in the World War.

"In July, 1919, I was the guest of the Minister of War of Great Britain and of the British Red Cross, and spent two months in England and Scotland, lecturing and demonstrating before the wounded English soldiers. During this visit to England, I attended a garden party given by the late King George, and had the honor of being introduced to him and the pleasure of giving him a short demonstration of how I do things without hands.

"The British Red Cross, as a courtesy, sent me by auto over the entire northern battlefield of France. This was a wonderful trip, as we saw the battlefields just as they were when the war ended in 1918.

"On my return home, I went back to my duties as operator of an engraving plant which I had purchased before going to the Front; and for the next sixteen years was busy building up my business. I worked from ten to twelve hours everyday, during which time I trained twenty-five young men to be photoengravers. Although I could not do any of the actual work, I know the principles of the business so I could train my apprentices.

"When I started in the engraving business, I had two assistants; when I sold out last year, my assistants had increased to twenty-four.

"I do not pose as a rich man, but my financial condition is such that I can have all the necessities of life and many of the luxuries, if I never make any more money. However, fifty-two years of age is too young to retire, so I am working on some inventions which, if they are successful, will again put me 'in the harness.'

"I am now driving a v-8. You may wonder how I drive. When I am ready to leave home, I open the door with my hook, go to the garage, take the key to the car out of my pocket and put it in the lock. I steer my car by means of ring about five inches in diameter, fastened in the steering wheel, through which I place my arm. I feed the gas with my foot and the spark lever with my knee. I drive to the office, take the key from the car with my hook and put it into my pocket, go to my office, open the door, and begin my daily routine.

"I tear open my letters with my hook and read them handling all my books, papers, and letters myself.

"I hold my pen in my hook. When I took my law examination, I wore 140 pages of legal cap paper in three days and was not as tired as were the boys with hands.

"May I say in passing that my wife and I have taken several pleasure trips by auto. One summer I drove up Pikes Peak and all through the Rocky Mountain region. Since my accident I have driven more than 400,000 miles.

"I play any game that others play and after my accident decided to become an expert at croquet. Allow me to say without boasting that I have succeeded. I hold the handle of the mallet with my artificial hand and am able to defeat everyone with whom I have ever played. I made a device which enables me to roll tenpins and often enjoy this sport. I enjoy the beach and have as much fun diving and swimming as if I had both hands.

"In the afternoon, when I can get away from the office, I go home, get into my old clothes, and spend an hour in my garden. I spade, hoe, rake, and run a garden plow and lawn mower as well as any other person. I work in my garden for two reasons-because I need the exercise, and because I like to work among my flowers.

"After dinner my wife and I read the papers together if we are to have an evening at home; and after my wife has retired, I usually spend several hours in study.

"You ask me how I lost my hands? I am not proud to say that I lost them as a result of hopping on a moving train. I asked no recompense from the railroad company because I was to blame and did not deserve anything.

"I spend no time in vain regrets for what is past; the present and the future have enough to keep me busy. I am naturally proud of the fact that without hands, and without financial assistance from anyone, I have been able to accomplish what I have, and that without getting anything for which I did not give service.

"Should I like to have my hands back? Of, course I should, but I am not so foolish as to think about getting them again. Why should I worry over spilled milk? I am well and strong. I have a happy home, wife, children, friends, and the capacity to enjoy life. What more could anyone ask?

"One thing I want to make clear! No cripple ever succeeded by the 'booze route.' Any man who is willing to work and keep on working, to study and keep on studying, to live an upright life, and to meet every problem with a smile, will go 'over the top' just as surely as did the boys overseas, and will be just as deserving a credit as were they."

Quentin Corley
Los Angeles Times, April 14, 1918
And Interview with Author, March 19, 1936

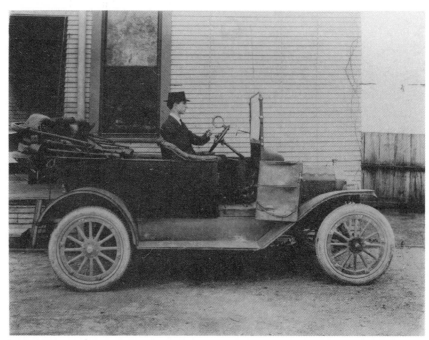

Figure 2-1 Judge Quentin D. Corley's adapted Model T. (Courtesy Brooke Penny.)

SECTION II

Pioneers in Driver Rehabilitation

Joseph M. Pellerito, Jr.

In the early era of driver rehabilitation much of what was considered to be the "standard of practice" was not evidence based but instead founded on the unique and creative problem-solving approaches that the early pioneers in the field had taken. Occupational therapists (OTs), driver educators, and "after-market" vendors who modified vehicles worked together to help ensure that anyone seeking driver rehabilitation services would be provided services that were professional and efficacious. However, little contact with automotive manufacturers took place, and concepts like ergonomics, human factors, and universal design were not widely developed or understood. Today driver rehabilitation specialists are not only members of their professional organizations (e.g., the National Mobility Equipment Dealer's Association, the Association for Driver Rehabilitation Specialists, and the American Occupational Therapy Association) but also they are actively involved in collaborating with other professionals who work for automobile manufacturers, governmental agencies (e.g., NHTSA), private businesses, and universities to improve the standard of care and maximize clients' driving independence, community mobility, and safety, as well as helping to ensure public safety.

OTs and driver educators comprised the first group to work with people with disabilities and the elderly population within the context of driver rehabilitation; both groups were eager to share their knowledge. OTs (i.e., registered and/or licensed OTs, as well as certified OT assistants) working as driver rehabilitation specialists have helped advance the field in many ways. One of the most important contributions came when OTs began insisting that clients should be seen by professional service providers as holistic beings and that an in-depth understanding of the complex and symbiotic body structures and functions is necessary to accurately assess and assist clients in achieving their driving and/or community mobility goals. OTs have also provided valuable information on what we refer to today as client factors (e.g., cognition, perception, sensory awareness, psychomotor status, cardiopulmonary status, and skin functioning) and how they provide a foundation on which meaningful occupations (e.g., activities of daily living, instrumental activities of daily living, education, play, leisure, and social participation) can occur.[14] Additionally, OT academics working with driver rehabilitation specialists in the field have joined researchers in other professions (e.g., psychology, neuropsychology, medicine, and engineering) in conducting research that is necessary to establish an evidence-based foundation for driver rehabilitation and community mobility service delivery. Driver educators also played an important role in helping mold the direction and future of driver rehabilitation as a legitimate profession, especially when the field was in its infancy. Driver educators helped to identify and articulate issues pertaining to optimizing driving safety and performance based on valuable field-tested methods. Some driver educators possessed a wealth of knowledge gained during years of dedicated service in an era that had only a handful of professionals working to meet clients' driver rehabilitation and community mobility needs. Finally, contemporary academics are working with specialists to advance the profession by conducting research that is beginning to define a "science of driving" and ensure that driver rehabilitation and community mobility services are evidence based, irrespective of a professional's background or years of experience.

SUMMARY

Today roughly 250 million cars, trucks, motor homes, and miscellaneous recreational vehicles ply America's streets and highways. Motor vehicles are the predominant form of transportation used by most people most of the time, in part because there are few practical, convenient alternatives. The popularity of motor vehicles has grown rapidly, starting in the first decade of the twentieth century. Part of this was the result of the growing affordability of gasoline-powered cars and trucks. Vast improvements in the nation's road and highway systems certainly facilitated "mass automobility." Over time automobiles became much easier to drive in terms of the strength and skills required of the driver. They also became more comfortable and safer. However, the fundamental root cause of the rapid spread of automobile ownership and use in the twentieth century was the fact that the automobile increased the freedom, choices, and mobility of its owner.

REFERENCES

1. Rae JB: *The American automobile: a brief history,* Chicago, 1965, The University of Chicago Press.
2. Flink JJ: *America adopts the automobile, 1895-1910,* Cambridge, MA, 1970, The MIT Press.
3. Flink JJ: *The automobile age,* Cambridge, MA, 1988, The MIT Press.
4. Mom G: *The electric vehicle: technology and expectations in the automobile age,* Baltimore, 2004, The Johns Hopkins University Press.
5. Rae JB: *American automobile manufacturers: the first forty years,* Philadelphia, 1959, The Chilton Company.
6. Eastman JW: *Styling vs. safety: the American automobile industry and the development of automotive safety, 1900-1966,* New York, 1984, University Press of America.
7. American Automobile Manufacturers Association: *Automobiles of America,* Sidney, OH, 1996, Cars and Parts Magazine.
8. Rae JB: *The road and the car in American life,* Cambridge, MA, 1971, The MIT Press.
9. Foster MS: *A nation on wheels: the automobile culture in America since 1945,* Belmont, CA, 2003, Wadsworth/Thomson.
10. Wik RM: *Henry Ford and grass-roots America,* Ann Arbor, MI, 1972, University of Michigan Press.
11. Berger MM: *The devil wagon in God's country: the automobile and social change in rural America, 1893-1929,* Hamden, CT, 1979, Archon Books.
12. Foster MS: *From streetcar to superhighway: American city planners and urban transportation, 1900-1940,* Philadelphia, 1981, Temple University Press.
13. St. Clair DJ: *The motorization of American cities,* Westport, CT, 1986, Praeger.
14. OT Practice Framework, 2002.

Chapter 3

THE ROLE OF THE AUTOMOBILE IN AMERICAN CULTURE

Joseph M. Pellerito, Jr. • *Catherine L. Lysack*

"It is probable that no invention. . .so quickly exerted influences that ramified through the national culture, transforming even habits of thought and language."

-The Presidential Committee Report on the impact of the automobile, 1934

KEY TERMS

- Efficient mobility
- Community mobility
- Cultural lag
- American Dream
- Car culture
- Marginalization

CHAPTER OBJECTIVES

After completing this chapter, the reader will be able to do the following:

- Explain how the automobile has affected American culture.
- Understand who has been marginalized by the American car culture.
- Understand why older drivers may not want to stop driving.

THE AUTOMOBILE IN AMERICAN LIFE

Our consumption of automobiles satisfies a real need for transportation, a need as basic as food, clothing, and shelter, but this need has changed as the social and spatial patterns of American culture have changed. This chapter builds on the historical perspective presented in Chapter 2 and examines the automobile as a historically situated form of transportation, one appropriate to a particular stage in capitalist development. We also suggest that the automobile was and continues to be simultaneously a cause and consequence of the rise of consumerism. This chapter discusses how the automobile came to be this indispensable method of transportation and a personal and meaningful symbol of what it means to participate fully in mainstream American life (Figure 3-1).

THE DISTANT PAST AND THEMES OF MOBILITY, MOVEMENT, AND PROGRESS

Throughout history civilizations have advanced in part by trading ideas, goods, and services. Transportation methods have thus been central to the success of cultures and generations for eons. Celebrating the creative ways humans have moved animate and inanimate objects with speed and efficiency has been a central theme throughout the millennia in cultural stories around the globe. Rich oral traditions and detailed written histories have emphasized accounts of efficient and even supernatural mobility as central themes within traditional stories meant to be instructive and edifying for members of the community. Examples include, but are certainly not limited to (1) the Exodus of the Jews from Egypt and their epic journey out of Egypt via (i.e., through) the Red Sea[1]; (2) Alexander the Great

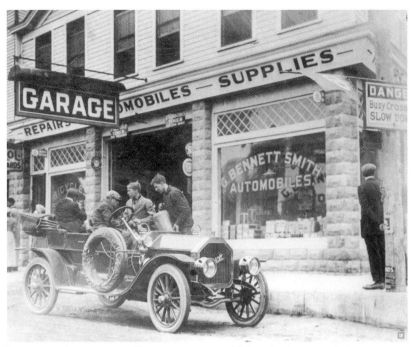

Figure 3-1 Automotive garages began to proliferate as motor vehicle sales increased. (Courtesy General Motors Media Archive, Detroit, Mich.)

and his army traversing the vast and often exigent topography of Europe and Asia to defeat innumerable tribes and kingdoms, profoundly changing human history[2]; (3) Christopher Columbus daring to travel beyond the edge of what was perceived by the masses to be a flat planet and discovering the New World, enabling him to establish trade routes connecting disparate and diverse societies; (4) the pioneers crossing the uncharted and sometimes hostile American frontier during the nineteenth century; (5) the Underground Railroad in North America that featured covert escape routes and support systems for enslaved African Americans and the abolitionists who opposed the cruelties associated with the slave trade during an era that saw a nation deeply divided and at war with itself[3]; (6) the wave of immigrants who left Europe in masses during the late nineteenth century and throughout the first half of the twentieth century, crossing the Atlantic Ocean with minimal personal and financial resources in hopes of finding a better life in North America; and finally (7) the creation and refinement of the assembly line that not only revolutionized how motor vehicles were built, but countless other products as well.

Moreover, the critical role *efficient mobility* has played throughout history and today is evident when examining how a person's life can depend on the speed and efficiency of public officials expeditiously arriving on the scene of an accident in order to intervene and ameliorate personal and public emergencies (e.g., an ambulance driver responding to motor vehicle crashes and fire-fighters to a forest or building fire). The critical role played by efficient mobility is also highlighted when one reflects on the many amazing structures and mobility systems that have been constructed throughout time, including the Great Pyramids, Stonehenge, the International Space Station, and the Autobahn, to name a few. These timeless symbols of humankind's ingenuity are also a testament to the efficient and purposeful movement of people and materials in extraordinary ways.

THE NOT-SO-DISTANT PAST AND THE EMERGENCE OF AN AMERICAN CAR CULTURE

Just as mobility has been instrumental in helping to ensure the survival of sentient and unconscious creatures throughout time, *community mobility,* in the form of driving a motor vehicle, has also been a critical aspect of the twentieth and contemporary twenty-first century living. Driving and community mobility have provided historians, sociologists, and other scholars a fertile topic that has been examined within a variety of contexts, and some have concluded that no invention in modern human history has had a more profound influence on how people work, play, and pursue and experience leisure-time activities than the automobile and the infrastructure that supports it. Despite the vast array of scholarship on the topic of the automobile and its many dimensions, there is disagreement on the origins of the automobile itself. For example many people still debate whether the automobile was invented in

Europe or the United States. It is generally accepted, however, that the drive, ingenuity, strength, and perseverance of the American inventors, designers, industrialists, and autoworkers ensured that the automobile would become a global phenomenon.[4]

The automobile has changed the lifestyle of the average American more than any other twentieth century innovation with the possible exception of television and perhaps computers and information technology. It has brought a flexible and individual form of transportation that makes everything from employment to leisure time pursuits easier and more enjoyable than it has ever been.

Moving from place to place with greater speed and efficiency has affected how and where people live, work, and spend their leisure time activities. In a gone-by era trolleys powered by electricity enabled urban centers to expand into suburbia; however, it was the automobile that got people and commodities from place to place much faster and according to individual schedules.[5] Coal- and wood-burning steam locomotives moved large numbers of people vast distances across rivers, over flat prairie lands, and even directly through mountains. The result was a network of railways crossing continents and connecting East and West and North and South, as well as rural with urban and suburban areas throughout North America and wherever there was land, people, and industrialization. However, railroads eventually gave way to the automobile because automobiles powered by the internal combustion engines eventually outpaced walking, running, bicycles, horse-drawn carriages, and steam- and electric-powered vehicles. Under the right circumstances, automobiles could meet and exceed speeds attained by some locomotive trains, and cars were certainly faster moving from a dead stop. The burgeoning infrastructure that supported the automobile empowered people to move from place to place with speed, efficiency, reliability, and a personal style that was previously unavailable to the general public. All of this was accomplished because the automobile enabled individuals to choose when and where to move based on their self-determined schedules versus depending on a predetermined and often unreliable train schedule or restricted by the limitations in speed and distance that were associated with the horse and carriage or even the earlier steam- or electric-powered vehicles.

The reasons why the automobile has assumed such a central place in the lives of Americans are complex, but it can be argued that at least two broad cultural beliefs helped to propel the ascendancy of the automobile to the heights it has attained today. These cultural beliefs go well beyond the practical advantages of horse-drawn carriages of the past and the numerous types of trolleys, buses, and trains that have been transporting people and things for more than a century. These are (1) the belief in the power of science and technology to bring progress and improvement for all in society; and (2) the individually held belief that through personal freedom and independence all individuals can achieve the *American Dream* (or some semblance of it). Both are powerful metaphors in the story of the automobile in American life.

Science and Technology

Vast infrastructure projects undertaken by the government provided major labor opportunities to assist America out of the Great Depression. The ensuing network of superhighways transformed the economy nationally and locally. Industry and manufacturing jobs brought wealth to average Americans during this period, but the shape of work life and commerce, not to mention family life, were radically reorganized to be accessible by automobile. The cultural view of the time was that "good old American know-how" could be applied to most any economic or social enterprise, and the result would be successful. There was an optimism that abounded, and a myriad of scientific discoveries and technologic innovations were made in arenas as diverse as medical treatments and kitchen appliances. At the foundation of this thinking was the belief that progress was possible through science. This sense of scientific optimism has fueled the automotive industry since its inception.

Freedom and Independence

The second broad cultural belief was that through personal freedom and independence all individuals could achieve the American Dream. The substance of that dream is found in the Declaration of Independence: "We hold these truths to be self-evident, that all men are created equal, that they are endowed by God, Creator, with certain inalienable Rights, that among these are Life, Liberty, and the pursuit of Happiness." The American Dream meant hope—an unshakable belief that happiness and security were truly possible for anyone who pursued it. Everyone knew, whether native born or immigrant, that they had a unique opportunity to make a better life for themselves, their families, and even whole communities (e.g., Little Italy in New York City, Chinatown in San Francisco, and other ethnic cleavages in the United States). The automobile assumed a critical place in the American Dream because it helped foster personal freedom and independence.

Over time automobiles have represented much more than convenient transportation; cars, and more recently trucks and recreational vehicles, are a status symbol. The type of car a person could afford and then the style chosen communicated status. In this way the automobile became a symbol of success (i.e., of having "made it" in American life), much like owning a house. If one worked hard enough, everything, including a beautiful house in the suburbs and a fine automobile with its own house we call a garage, would be the reward. A car in the driveway was a tangible statement to one's community that they belonged in the mainstream of American life, and the brand and model type, such as a luxury or sports car, often helped to place an exclamation point on that statement.

We will now briefly review the impact of the automobile on work and family life from the early twentieth century through the 1950s and up to the current day.

THE AUTOMOBILE IN THE EARLY TWENTIETH CENTURY

The early twentieth century ushered in a new era that was fueled by the public's imagination and desire for efficient and speedy land transportation. The aspirations of the inventors and industrialists who shaped the automotive culture changed the landscape of America and the world forever. The *cultural lag* (i.e., technologic advances often have unforeseen negative consequences, such as the need for increasingly sophisticated safety devices in cars and trucks to reduce injuries and fatalities) that came about reflected an industry that addressed issues pertaining to driver, passenger, and pedestrian safety, negative environmental consequences, and vehicle reliability as an afterthought and only when the public demanded greater accountability. Industrialists driven by a vision of widespread adoption of motor vehicles had to be willing and able to adapt to the changing needs of the growing worker and consumer bases. Building increasingly reliable, safe, and affordable motor vehicles ultimately helped capture the public's collective imagination, win their trust, and most importantly, persuade them that the benefits associated with motor vehicles outweighed the costs. One of the most influential figures in automotive history was Henry Ford. He offered the world more than a vision of ingenuity and a blueprint for a profitable automotive manufacturer. He influenced the methods and means of production that helped drive the industrial revolution and pave the way for workers on assembly lines in the United States and eventually around the world to afford the cars they were building with an investment of sweat, energy, and determination. Workers' pride was associated with sound workmanship and ownership. The impact of motor vehicles on public life also was pronounced in other ways.

The automobile soon influenced the speed and efficiency in which city services were carried out, leading to an improved quality of life, health, and well-being of the general population. Streets were cleaner and safer thanks to mechanized street cleaners and motorized police cars; fires were much less destructive because the horse-drawn or steam-powered fire wagons were replaced with speedy and reliable gasoline-powered rigs; and a person or animal with an injury or illness was better served thanks to ambulances and automobiles that transported sick and injured patients to hospitals and clinics or brought professionals to the patients in any number of diverse locations within a community or the outlying rural countryside. Irrespective of the situation, from transporting a pregnant woman in an ambulance to the hospital or carrying the deceased in a hearse to a cemetery, automobiles have played a key role in helping people as they experience what are often considered to be defining moments in any person's life (Figure 3-2).

HENRY FORD: AN INDUSTRIAL GIANT AND FORBEARER OF THE EMERGING CAR CULTURE

One name that is synonymous with serving as a catalyst in cultivating the seeds of a car culture when the auto industry was in its infancy is Henry Ford. Ford did not invent the automobile, design the internal combustion engine, or originate the creative and revolutionary methods of assembling automobiles on wheeled platforms that resulted in a quantum leap toward greater work efficiency and ultimately to the efficient and profitable mass production of automobiles. It was his contemporary and competitor Ransom E. Olds who first introduced mass-production techniques after he founded the Olds Motor Works in 1899 in Detroit, Michigan.[5] However, Henry Ford is responsible for something much more important than achieving any of these early and important automotive milestones; he built the most popular car in history and improved on the mass-production techniques that were initially pioneered by Olds. By moving parts along a conveyor belt, Ford was able to maximize efficiency that led to greater output. Ford explained in his autobiography in 1922, "The step forward in assembly came when we began taking the work to the men instead of the men to the work."[6] It was these production methods that perhaps first exemplified ergonomic and human factor principles being efficiently applied in the industrial work setting.

Most importantly Ford paid his Ford Motor Company employees who were working on the assembly line a wage that enabled them to purchase the products they were building. The 5-dollar per day wage was a bold and revolutionary step taken by Ford that affected worker retention, loyalty, and empowerment that continues to influence modern labor relations and consumer spending. Henry Ford, like Olds, was a visionary who understood that once automobiles were affordable for the average citizen, they would radically

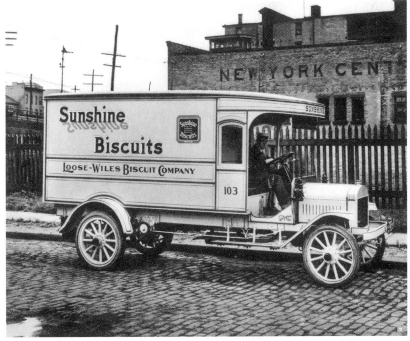

Figure 3-2 Motor vehicles enabled efficient and cost-effective transportation of goods, such as Sunshine Biscuits. (Courtesy General Motors Media Archive, Detroit, Mich.)

alter the ways in which people moved within and between communities.[5] Ford wrote that:

> I will build a motor car for the great multitude; it will be large enough for the family but small enough for the individual to care for. It will be constructed of the best materials, by the best men to be hired after the simplest designs that modern engineering can devise. But it will be so low in price that no man making a good salary will be unable to own one, and enjoy with his family the blessings of hours of pleasure in God's great open spaces.[6]

The Model T fulfilled Ford's goal and set the industry standard because most adults could drive it and maintain it with minimal skills and resources. The Model T provided its owner with a strong and durable chassis that was mounted higher than the vehicles that were being built by other manufacturers competing for the finite number of buyers at that time. The Model T's higher profile helped its owner to traverse the poorly maintained dirt roads, cow pastures, dry riverbeds, and any number of other pathways that were not initially designed with automobiles in mind. Because there were no dedicated automotive garages complete with certified automotive mechanics, owners of the Model T had to make any needed repairs themselves, and parts for the car could soon be found in "five-and-ten cent" stores throughout the country. It was not long before roads and bridges were expanding at an exponential rate to support the growing numbers of motorists who had given up their horse-drawn carriages, bicycles,

steamships, and trains as their preferred methods of community mobility (Figure 3-3).

Henry Ford and the other industrial giants may have influenced American culture and the economy of the early twentieth century more than anyone else working within the private sector. Ford was an individual with vision and imagination that not only transformed American culture and economy but also forever impacted how people around the world move from place to place. Perhaps his greatest achievements were paying his workers a wage that enabled them to purchase the products they were creating and offering those high-quality products at an accessible price to the general population, which moved them closer to realizing the American Dream. Although Henry Ford could not have imagined all of the ways his vision has impacted American culture, there is no question that he has left an indelible mark on global transportation for decades to come.

THE AMERICAN DREAM AFTER WORLD WAR II: FROM FACTORIES TO SUBURBS

The impact of the automobile was felt most acutely after World War II. The economic boom years after World War II provided a growing middle class eager to buy a car and buy into the American Dream. In addition, vast regions of the country were suddenly accessible to the average American through a system of new

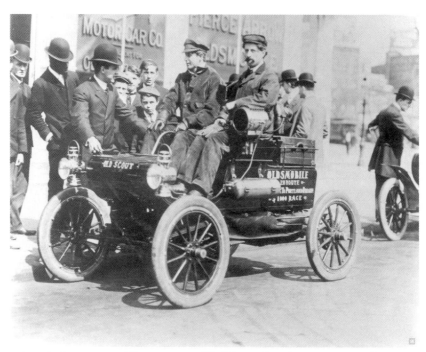

Figure 3-3 It was not long before automobiles were modified for racing. (Courtesy General Motors Media Archive, Detroit, Mich.)

interstate highways that extended personal travel over greater distances than ever before. Technologic developments of this time also made cars more comfortable and stylish. The automobile was therefore useful and efficient for commuting from home in the suburbs to work in the city. In time the automobile became the primary means by which families spent their leisure time. Although air travel has transformed personal travel over longer distances, the automobile nonetheless remains an overwhelmingly practical method of transportation and a symbol of personal success.

The motorcar was one of the major contributors if not *the* major contributor to suburbanization of America during the years 1920 to 1960. By sheer force of numbers, utility, and aesthetic appeal the automobile irrevocably transformed the geographic and socioeconomic landscape. In 1900 there were only 8000 cars in the entire country, owned naturally enough by the very rich. However, by 1925 a new Model T was rolling off the assembly line every 15 seconds, and by 1930 there were >26 million cars used by about one-half the U.S. population. Today it has been said there are more cars on the road in the United States than there are Americans under the age of 21: "There is a registered motor vehicle for every 1.3 persons in the USA, and the average American household has twice as many automobiles as it has children under the age of twenty"[7] (p 86). In 2003 it was reported in *Salon* magazine that there were 107 million U.S. households, each with an average of 1.9 cars, trucks, or sport utility vehicles

(SUVs) and 1.8 drivers. That equaled 204 million vehicles and 191 million drivers.[8] In large part the explosion of automobile ownership owes a debt of gratitude to Henry Ford's use of standardized parts and the widespread adoption of his revolutionary production methods such as the assembly line. This meant the purchase price of a car decreased even as wages increased throughout the country. Before World War I a car cost the average American worker the equivalent of 24 months' wages. By the late 1920s a car could be purchased for about 3 months' wages.[9] However, since then the cost of cars has increased significantly in conjunction with American's demands for bigger and more comfortable cars. The automobile industry estimates the average car today is purchased for about $25,000. This represents far more than 3 months' wages. Later in this chapter we will explore more of the reasons for the love affair with the automobile that must make the car worth buying (Figures 3-4 and 3-5).

SUBURBANIZATION: A TRANSFORMATION IN AMERICAN LIFE

The force of suburbanization has significantly reshaped American work and leisure. The 1950s and 1960s saw the birth of a new class of professional and managerial workers. Likewise the economy saw a transformation from industrial labor and blue-collar jobs to white-collar professional and management jobs. This new class of worker was distributed among the various strata

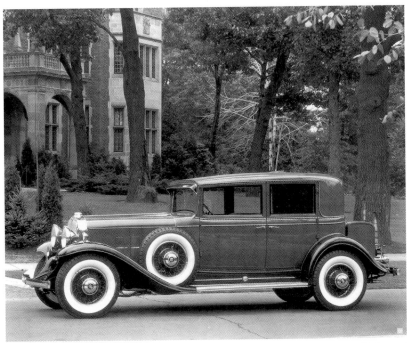

Figure 3-4 Automobiles often reflected a buyer's taste and social status. (Courtesy General Motors Media Archive, Detroit, Mich.)

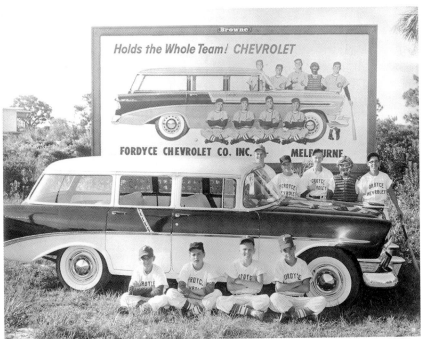

Figure 3-5 Automobiles soon were able to transport groups of people. (Courtesy General Motors Media Archive, Detroit, Mich.)

of the corporation to transmit instructions and information and to supervise directly the work process. The work process itself was broken down into numerous separate tasks and synchronized through the scientific management of individual and group worker behavior, which in many ways mimicked the technologic innovation of automated assembly line decades earlier. As the work process intensified, the length of the workday was shortened, and wage rates increased. Furthermore as manufacturing declined in central cities, the proportion of communications, finance, management, clerical, and professional services located there increased.

Moreover the socioeconomic relationship between suburbs and the central city changed. As downtown shopping districts were transformed into central government and corporate headquarters, small retail services that could not afford skyrocketing rents and were losing customers unwilling to face downtown traffic snarls relocated in the suburbs near their customers. Likewise large department stores set up branch stores in these satellite communities. Mail-order firms like Sears, Roebuck and Company and Montgomery Ward turned into suburban chains. Banks also established branches in suburban communities. Dentists, doctors, and a variety of other professional service providers opened offices near their clients' (and their own) homes. Popular forms of arts and entertainment and most professional sports teams eventually abandoned the heart of many American cities, leaving behind decaying shells of what were once attractive entertainment venues. In short, many formerly centralized institutions and services were relocated in the suburbs. See Chapter 22 for more information about the automobile and urban sprawl.

Automobiles also had a profound impact on the architecture and housing that continues to be built along the roads and highways that exist in every town, village, and city. The car culture created these roadways, as well as one-, two-, three-, and even four plus–car garages that are like small houses built to protect and preserve the beloved automobile. Wachs and Crawford,[7] in their book *The Car and City*, describe the unique relationship that has been cast between the automobile and American cities like Los Angeles, which embraced the automobile as a symbol of cultural liberation. Gas stations, motels, hotels, shopping malls, drive-in movie theaters, suburbia, and traffic jams would probably not exist, or not exist as we know them, if not for the automobile. It gave us the armored car and drive-by shootings and Hollywood movies featuring memorable (and not so memorable) car chase sequences. Cars have helped law enforcement and criminals alike, became props for film and television celebrities, and have influenced the global entertainment industry for generations. Cars have also provided people with hours of pleasure during Sunday afternoon drives and have helped to bring family and friends together to celebrate holidays and special occasions or provide comfort during times of hardship and tragedy. Auto racing has become the most popular sport in America, and automobiles continue to serve as a highly desired status symbol by much of the population.

More than one century ago and up to and including present day motorists, people began to identify with their automobiles in ways they never did with other modes of transportation; drive-in movie theaters gave way to drive-in banking, restaurants, pharmacies, and even wedding chapels.[5] Historically the personal mobility facilitated by the automobile has not only played a key role in improving overall personal and public health and well-being but also it has had a significant impact on our collective ability to laugh and love and express our personal individuality (Figure 3-6).

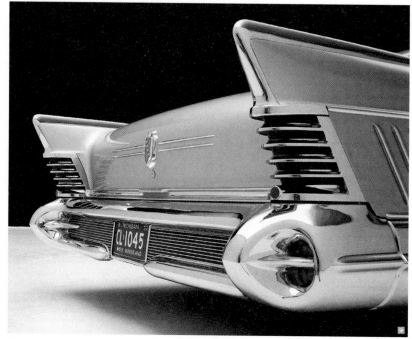

Figure 3-6 Automobile fins spoke volumes about a driver's style and panache. (Courtesy General Motors Media Archive, Detroit, Mich.)

THE PROLIFERATION OF ROADS AND HIGHWAYS IN AMERICA

In 1904 there were only 250 paved and gravel roads in the United States. During the first decade of the 1900s the pressure for more roads initially came from the 10 million registered bicyclists who were members of influential clubs, such as the League of American Wheelman, who persuaded Congress to establish the Bureau of Road Inquiry to investigate how the government could build a network of roads and highways.[5] People soon replaced their bicycles with automobiles, and local automobile clubs throughout the country that eventually merged to become the American Automobile Association (AAA), along with automobile manufacturers and oil companies, began to advocate for better and more numerous roads. In 1904 Congress approved the formation of the U.S. Office of Public Roads that provided financial assistance to the states for building new and improved roads. The Federal Highway Act was passed in 1909 and provided taxpayer dollars to begin building federal highways, organizing the country's roads into federal and state systems, and creating a system of numbering and marking the roads and highways—a system of paved roads that could accommodate millions of motorists by the 1920s.[5] As the affluent middle class grew, cars became much more important in terms of leisure and recreation rather than only for driving to work. The 1950s and 1960s, for example, brought the opening of the national park system, and camping became a financially accessible vacation option for the average suburban family. The national parks were also new and exciting. The automobile offered the opportunity to see what was exciting and new that only 20 years earlier was accessible only to the wealthy elite. Thus families purchased station wagons and bought camper trailers and went on family vacations crisscrossing the country. The car brought the family together, cementing family ties.

INTERSTATES: CATHEDRALS OF THE CAR CULTURE

That the rise of the automobile and suburbanization coincided with the building of freeways and interstates should be no surprise. There also is evidence that the car industry developed in the cities with the greatest number of paved miles, such as Cleveland and Detroit, but not Chicago, Philadelphia, or Washington, DC. Large-scale national projects, many of which began in the Depression era to stimulate the economy, funded by the government, eventually provided a massive system of interconnected roads and highways across the United States:

The interstates were the cathedrals of the car culture, and their social implications were staggering. Within a decade they would alter beyond recognize where and how Americans lived, worked, played, shopped and even loved.[10]

The interstate system took several decades to complete. Interstate designers followed the "form follows function" architecture typical of the 1950s (e.g., Albert Kahn who built the General Motors Building, the River Rouge factory, and others; Ludwig Mies van der Rohe whose spare clean lines inspired countless office towers; and modernist French architect Le Corbusier who designed buildings and furniture). There was sameness in the architecture of this period, but this sameness in design was the perfect metaphor for generations who welcomed consistency and quality control in their hotels, restaurants, and service stations.

The 1950s saw a massive growth of motels, drive-ins, and roadside diners to support interstate travel. McShane[11] describes how influential key automobile industrialists were in influencing transportation policy to their advantage. Laws were passed and changed to favor the car companies who argued their industry was fueling the American economy. Those early industrialists were hugely successful, and the landscape altered to accommodate the automobile. The shopping centers of the 1950s became malls in the 1960s. Car design and urban design moved in tandem. Cities and towns began to reshape themselves around the potential of the car to take people greater distances from home.[10] The "main streets" of America in the present continue in sharp decline as the shopping malls with ample free parking pull consumers into the suburbs.

THE AUTOMOBILE'S INFLUENCE ON WORK AND DAILY LIFE: HISTORICAL ROOTS

Sociologists Robert and Helen Lynd conducted a major study of American society during the 1920s. In 1929 they published their research in a book entitled *Middletown: A Study in Modern American Culture.* "Middletown" was the name used to disguise Muncie, Indiana, the actual place where they conducted their research. One of their findings was that the automobile had transformed the lives of people living in Middletown and by extension virtually everywhere else in the United States. The Lynds found that the car had become so important to Middletown residents that many families expressed a willingness to go without food and shelter, mortgage their homes, and deplete their bank savings rather than lose their cars. "We'd rather do without clothes than give up the car," a working-class mother of nine told the Lynds. "I'll go without food before I'll see us give up the car," another wife said emphatically. Other observers found that rural families were similarly attached to their cars. When a

U.S. Department of Agriculture inspector asked a farmwoman during the 1920s why her family had purchased an automobile before equipping their home with indoor plumbing, she replied, "Why, you can't go to town in a bathtub!"[12] For these urban and rural Americans alike, the car had become a basic social necessity.

Although the Lynds may not have fully appreciated it at the time, consumer goods, including the automobile, were slowly eroding class differences, actually leveling the socioeconomic playing field. Automobile ownership brought its own kind of democracy to American life. Automobility also was a strong contributor to women's liberation. Although the automobile did not lessen women's work, it nonetheless offered new possibilities for personal movement. It especially liberated women from the home. The automobile was a private vehicle, and that characteristic made it safer and more acceptable than public streetcars or trains. Even the most genteel women began traveling alone; some wealthier women took cross-country trips together unescorted by male relatives. This freedom, as many women described the experience of driving, was the positive side to the transformation of women's lives (Figure 3-7).

Historically, however, the primary use of the automobile was for husbands' transportation, primarily to work from home. Work was mostly downtown, and family life at home was in the suburbs. Decades ago the typical family consisted of two-parent households with a stay-at-home mom. Fathers were typically the sole breadwinner and really the only one to need a car. Of course this is much less the case today. However, in decades past grocery shopping did not always demand a car because groceries were often delivered directly to suburban homes. There were also many stores within walking distance of the family home. Children walked to school. Families walked to church. Thus mothers and children lived in their local neighborhoods and only used the car as part of family outings on weekends.

THE AUTOMOBILE AND ITS ROLE IN CHANGING PERSONAL AND PROFESSIONAL NETWORKS

Car culture has profoundly affected personal and professional networks. Reflection on the past 50 years confirms radical shifts in the ways we communicate with others and move through physical and social space. Most certainly our social and professional networks have expanded well beyond Cooley's[13] description of traditional primary and secondary groups that were synonymous with one's family, neighborhood, and self-contained communities that Ferdinand Toennies[14] referred to as *gemeinschaft*. The automobile industry helped fuel the rapid industrialization of the United States and much of Europe, which greatly influenced how and where people interacted. Pastoral *gemeinschaft* communities of place, belonging, and social reciprocity disintegrated, and societies emerged that reflected a *gesellschaft* existence.[14] Group members that previously interacted within smaller, tight-knit, and cohesive geographic communities now comprised citizens that no longer associated solely with a single primary community located in physical space but began interacting in and between multiple communities in which secondary or weak ties played an increasingly important role in defining social life.[15]

The automobile was originally designed to transport workers and goods, although it was soon after marketed as a means for the entire family to travel together. Recall the Lynd's research in Muncie, Indiana and the access to town that the automobile provided for relatively isolated rural families. Historically then the place of automobile in *gemeinschaft*-type communities was to provide efficient transportation of goods and people and sometimes to provide a means for family locomotion for leisure purposes. Today in stark contrast the use of the automobile is primarily a solitary activity. Look around the next time you are driving, and you will notice that people generally travel alone and are rarely in groups, especially when they are commuting between work and home. The automobile provides utility and functionality related to helping people fulfill their work and family obligations, fostering strong and weak ties, and meeting daily functional needs, but the car also serves as a dynamic (albeit expensive) form of self-expression of one's identity and even worldview.

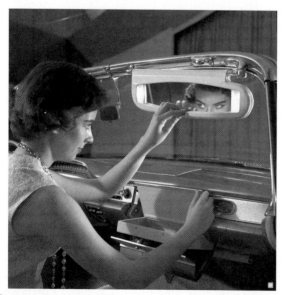

Figure 3-7 Automobiles soon featured amenities such as vanity mirrors and compartments designed to hold gloves and other items needed while on the road. (Courtesy General Motors Media Archive, Detroit, Mich.)

BORN TO BE WILD: CAR CULTURE AND THE AMERICAN TEEN

In the United States the automobile has become the quintessential icon of freedom and mobility. Not only do teenagers anxiously wait for the day they can obtain their driver's licenses so they can be mobile and free, but also the elderly dread the day they lose theirs and can no longer drive, no longer be independent, mobile, and free. It makes one wonder if before the automobile people young, old, and in between ever felt mobile and free. In this respect at least we can acknowledge the importance of the automobile in American life and its relationship to our identity throughout the life cycle (Figure 3-8).

In the 1950s the postwar boom produced a generation of teenagers with enough income to buy their own cars. These cars became so much more than just modes of transportation. They were reflections of a lifestyle. The ability to tune and soup-up muscle cars gave average Joes the opportunity to show off their power, their speed, and their style in a way that personified the car as character. American popular culture was never the same.

It must also be recognized that buying one's own first car and getting a license to drive may be two of the most significant moments in a young person's life after marriage and children. At the cusp of adulthood teenagers are exploring their identities and their futures. It is no wonder they are of great interest to the automobile industry. Research shows that brand loyalty occurs early in life. Therefore there is a great motivation on the part of the automotive industry to get a new driver for life. The success of that campaign rests

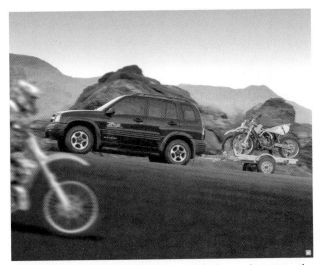

Figure 3-8 Automobiles have enabled people to travel farther distances and recreate in new and dynamic ways. (Courtesy General Motors Media Archive, Detroit, Mich.)

largely with advertising. Ford is one of the nation's largest advertisers. According to *Advertising Age*, an industry trade magazine, Ford's advertising budget has grown from about $13,500 in 1904 to an estimated $2.4 billion in 2001, the most recent figure available.[16]

At least in part because of advertising (Figure 3-9), the car has come to pervade American culture not only on the streets and in local drive-ins but also in entertainment. In movies the stars were often a combination of character and car. James Dean and his antiestablishment motorbike epitomized the *Rebel Without a Cause*. The blonde in her white T-Bird—Suzanne Somers' character in *American Graffiti*—was not even given a name, just credited "Blonde in T-Bird." Even the hit songs of the 1960s captured a generation and lifestyle focused on cars and girls. From the little Deuce Coupe to the '34 wagon, "Woody" to the little GTO, cars began to take center stage. Ever since, car culture has been a major niche lifestyle in America. In 2001 Universal Pictures' *The Fast and the Furious* opened number 1 at the box office, outperforming movies with bigger budgets, mega-stars, and expensive special events. The hot music, hip clothes, and flashy cars gave the film a uniquely broad appeal. Everyone could appreciate the high-performance machines and what they could do. The international music scene was similarly impacted. Do you remember the words to The Beatles song, "Drive My Car"?

Today teens are still a key market for advertisers, but marketing efforts and car buyers themselves are more diverse. Car campaigns are now selling minivans to "soccer moms" who shuttle kids between school, sports, lessons, and home; they sell reliable sedans to young professional women entering the workforce. They reach a broader market than just selling sports cars to aging male executives and half-ton trucks and muscle cars to young men. Advertisers, as well as automobile designers, have also become much more cognizant of the unique needs of various segments of the driving market, including older drivers and drivers with disabilities, enhancing their automobiles with more safety and convenience features, such as on-board navigation and security systems. Irrespective of car design, however, there is every sign that individual consumers continue to personalize and customize their cars to meet their individual needs.

One example of car customization is the bumper sticker and personalized license plates. Bumper stickers and other decals on motor vehicles proclaim any number of value statements, such as a driver's opinion about the pro-life versus pro-choice debate, his or her stand on a presidential election, or the pride associated with having a child on their school's honor roll, to name a few. A favorite vacation destination or sports team logos are other popular displays. Vehicle license plates

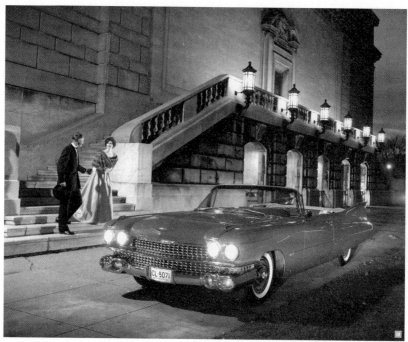

Figure 3-9   Advertisers reinforced the notion that there is nothing more American than owning an automobile. (Courtesy General Motors Media Archive, Detroit, Mich.)

are another example of personal expression. Vehicle plates originated during the Roman Empire, when anyone who owned a chariot was required to register his vehicle and affix an identification tag to it.[5] Today thousands of people subscribe to license plate catalogs, collect and trade license plates at conventions, and pay a premium for vanity plates that communicate creative personalized messages in a few letters or include images that reflect a driver's school or organizational affiliation.

THE AUTOMOBILE AND THE AMERICAN PUBLIC: IDENTITY SELLS

The type of motor vehicle a consumer chooses to drive is influenced by the brand image that is the result of a manufacturer's carefully orchestrated media campaign. For generations the vehicle type has provided consumers with a kind of symbol or badge designed to communicate a not-so-subtle message about one's perceived status, role, personal aesthetic (i.e., taste), or financial situation. Functionality and form also influenced who was able to drive the earliest automobiles. In 1911 Charles F. Kettering introduced the electric starter that was sold to the Cadillac Motor Company in 1912, facilitating women's ability to sit in the driver's seat because hand-cranking the engine was no longer required. However, it would take generations, a growing public concern, and legislation to begin effecting sufficient attitudinal change to achieve greater vehicle

accessibility and adapted driving solutions for people with disabilities.

> "The paramount ambition of the average man a few years ago was to own a home and have a bank account. The ambition of the same man today is to own and drive a car. . ." (Figures 3-10 and 3-11)
>
> -Moline, Illinois banker Wallace Ames, 1925

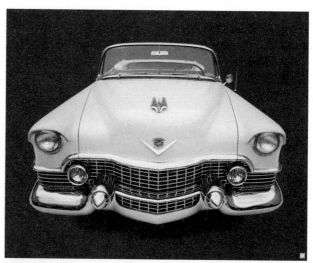

Figure 3-10   Form often upstaged function as designers mixed imagination and ingenuity to create what were considered by many to be works of art. (Courtesy General Motors Media Archive, Detroit, Mich.)

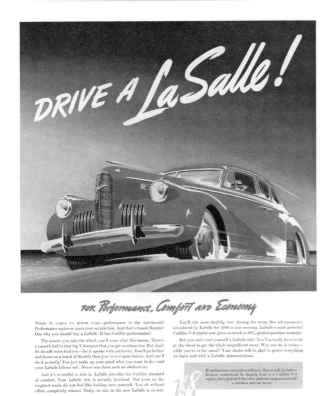

Figure 3-11 Automobile ownership has been marketed as a manifestation of the American Dream. (Courtesy General Motors Media Archive, Detroit, Mich.)

People have benefited from owning an automobile, and the automobile industry was instrumental in creating a large middle class within North America and other industrialized regions of the world. However, industry also contributed to myriad social problems that emerged as cities throughout North America matured. During the second half of the twentieth century in the United States access to affordable and reliable automobiles facilitated an efficient means for the mass exodus of people and industry away from tired urban centers, turning pastoral and rural settings into suburban America and further reinforcing dependence on the automobile and the proliferation of urban sprawl. The exodus from urban America has slowed somewhat, and today gentrification of varying degrees has taken place in the previously abandoned centers of many American cities. The reclamation of urban America by individuals, families, businesses, corporations, and institutions continues to largely depend on the existence of a viable infrastructure that enables efficient, reliable, and cost-effective transportation of people and the delivery of essential goods and services. Urban renewal has helped to expand and improve alternative transportation infrastructure (i.e., mass transit systems that offer citizens a variety of transportation options that are dependable, efficient, and economical)

in a few major metropolitan areas (e.g., Washington, DC, New York City, Boston, and San Francisco) but not in most urban or rural locations in the United States. For generations automobiles also have continued to be the way people prefer to move from place to place within and between their communities.[18,19] Individuals who possess the skills necessary to drive and the financial resources to own or lease a vehicle have helped to sustain the necessity in many parts of the world to possess a motor vehicle.

DRIVING: A RITE OR A RIGHT?

In contemporary industrialized societies in the United States and abroad driving is not considered an inalienable right but a privilege that is granted by the government and defined in legal terms.[20] However, driving is much more than a privilege, luxury, or *instrumental activity of daily living (IADL)* as some would suggest; it is an *activity of daily living (ADL)*[18] that is necessary for a full and productive social life in urban and rural areas around the world. Many people equate the possession of a driver's license with choice, freedom, and self-identity.[21] The European Conference of Ministers for Transport[22] studied the social costs of driving and reported that like most Americans, the adult European population largely held the belief that they possess a right to use a vehicle to meet their transportation needs.

America has always celebrated a kind of rugged individualism that is evident when one examines the compelling factors that influence people's preferred means (i.e., cars, trucks, vans, and SUVs) for community mobility. One contributing factor may be that the rite of passage associated with earning and keeping a driver's license is a universal symbol of autonomy and independence. Most Americans view driving as essential to their independence and quality of life.[18] Furthermore it is apparent that many Americans have developed a fascination with the automobile to the extent that is has become a celebrated image or dominant theme for television programs, movies, music, books and magazines, poetry, and even theatrical productions.

Unlike the European model that has facilitated efficient and cost-effective methods for moving people (i.e., the masses) within self-contained and vibrant urban areas, the American model has helped to foster the exponential growth of sprawling suburban communities that to some symbolize America's wealth and prosperity. To others suburbia represents unwarranted sprawl that necessarily dilutes municipal resources as city officials work to provide a range of public services to ever growing but much less densely populated suburban areas. The critical infrastructure required to support cities includes fire and police services, garbage collection, public transportation, school systems, and so on. Many cities in America today face a tremendous challenge in providing such services with a dwindling tax base. It is useful to note that U.S. highways, roads, and bridges that crisscross and dot the once pastoral American landscape provide transportation arteries for >140 million vehicles that move people and goods and facilitate the delivery of myriad services every day. Although the car culture around the world may differ in some important ways from the situation in the United States, nonetheless there is still a ubiquitous car culture and a complex infrastructure that supports it. There is also a global transportation infrastructure that has grown exponentially to facilitate the movement of people and goods around the planet. However, the negative consequences that are associated with the auto industry and the embrace of the personal automobile globally are significant, for example the potential effect vehicles have on global warming, diminished air quality, expanding health risks (e.g., asthma), and depleted natural resources. These factors and others have caused some people to promote the need for developing alternative and renewable energy sources, improved mass transit systems, and the next generation of clean vehicles. However, the vast majority of people in the United States continue to rely on traditional gas-burning vehicles without giving it a second thought.

The car culture in modern U.S. society demands that normative adult behavior include driving as the primary means for community mobility. Driving is an extraordinarily complex activity requiring complementary cognitive, sensoriperceptual, psychomotor, and functional abilities,[18,23] especially as vehicles continue to be engineered to move at higher rates of speed. Although driving can be an extraordinarily dangerous activity, it can also be a rewarding activity that adults and children, beginning in their mid-teen years, engage in. Individuals no longer capable of fulfilling societal expectations, including being able to independently and safely perform the tasks associated with driving, are sometimes seen as incompetent and are often stigmatized.[24] Driving cessation can lead to diminished spontaneity,[25] feelings of being a burden on family members,[26] and a perceived loss of social status.[27,28] Luborsky[29] used the cultural context as a backdrop against which he described popular cultural ideas of full adulthood and how they affect the social experiences, interpersonal interactions, and self-esteem of people with recently acquired disabilities. He asserted that every culture's model of adulthood includes the notion that the realization of competence and mastery occurs when language and the ability to achieve and maintain willful movement are successfully acquired. Duggan[30] expanded this idea and described how the loss of inde-pendent motor control threatens the experiences of full adulthood because social interaction and roles are negatively affected. Older adults and persons with disabilities are all too familiar with being marginalized and disenfranchised as a result of diminished personal and community mobility. Thus for individuals who are aging, contending with disabilities, or both, driving or the resumption of driving is a major goal toward maintaining community integration[31] and quality of life.

AMERICAN MODERNITY AND THE OPEN ROAD

During the twentieth century automobiles became part of our daily lives and an extension of ourselves—symbols of who we are as a people (or at least the image of people we wish to be). There are many indicators of the importance, meaning, and role of the automobile in our society; the fact that we have dedicated more land to cars (roads, parking, etc.) than to housing, for example, speaks loudly and forcefully about their place in modern American life. Other indicators include the number of magazines devoted to cars and car cultures (e.g., racing, low riding, and hot rodding) and the use of automobiles in movies (from *The Love Bug* to *Driving Miss Daisy, The Blues Brothers, Thelma and Louise,* and the ubiquitous *James Bond* movies), on television (*Starsky and Hutch, The Dukes of Hazzard;* and where would Batman and Robin be without their Batmobile?), in literature, and in the media in general. The automobile has deeply penetrated our psyche and our everyday language. Consider for example the phrases Sunday driver, backseat driver, joy ride, hitchhiking, and the information superhighway, to name a few.

The automobile has also been important to music, reminding us of the freedom, excitement, and promise of the open road. As early as 1899 Tin Pan Alley was turning out car-related hits such as *Fifteen Kisses on a Gallon of Gas* and *I'm Going to Park Myself in Your Arms.* The tradition of cars in songs continued throughout the twentieth century. In the 1960s in what was to become one of the most productive musical decades ever, we heard *Ramblin' Man* by the Allman Brothers Band, *Take Me Home* by Woody Guthrie, *Country Roads* by John Denver, and *America* by Simon and Garfunkel. However, no form of popular expression has celebrated the automobile with more passion and attention to nuance than rock and roll. From Chuck Berry to the Beach Boys and Bruce Springsteen to Steppenwolf, the glories and tragedies of the car culture are well documented. In *Ballad of Betsy* the Beach Boys described a car as "more loyal than any friend can be," and who can forget *Little Deuce Coupe* and *I Get Around*? Two of Bruce

Springsteen's hit songs about cars include *Born to Run* and *Cadillac Ranch*. Finally "car music" would not be complete without *Route 66*, composed by Bobby Troup and first recorded by the Nat King Cole Trio in 1946. This song has been recorded by every generation since, from the Andrew Sisters and Bing Crosby to Chuck Berry and the Rolling Stones.

The automobile has similarly influenced American literature and film. Perhaps John Steinbeck's classic *The Grapes of Wrath* is most well known. In the film version Henry Fonda stars as Tom Joad. In a most memorable scene Fonda is seen driving his family's run-down pickup truck away from their midwestern farm after being evicted by their landlord driving his new, luxury Duesenberg. The integration of narrative and material possession is seamless, the luxury car serving as an adjective describing social place and material wealth and power, and the old truck, the lack thereof. Thus cars in film, just as in music and literature before it, were used to reinforce the notion that dreams are possible. Perhaps going where you wanted and when you wanted was even an idea that evolved from our romantic notions of the cowboy and the West. In any event the car in all forms of popular culture underscores the idea of self-determination and self-reliance, fundamental values in the American cultural tradition.

THE CAR AND FAMILY LIFE

The world's population has stepped confidently into the new millennium. Expanding economies in China and India in particular are providing new markets for the consumption and production of automobiles. The challenge of automobility is sustainability (of the world's resources in the form of fossil fuels and raw materials) but also social. Does the organization of our world around the automobile really make economic sense, environmental sense, and social sense? See Chapter 22 for a more detailed discussion of the social costs of our reliance on the automobile. Although new technologies and advances in automobile engineering abound, not all is well with Henry Ford's dream. American life is radically different in 2005, and it appears that the limitations of automobility are becoming clearer. On one hand it appears life is virtually impossible without the car, although an increasingly vocal minority suggests it is precisely the car industry and political lobby surrounding the car industry that have put us in the situation we are now in.[32]

The past several decades have seen a sharp increase in the involvement in the paid labor force of women with young children. Much of the reliance on cars today reflects the way that two-worker and single-parent households juggle the complicated responsibilities of home and work. The car offers the convenience and flexibility essential to working parents, particularly mothers, who often carry the double burden of working at work and home. The car is absolutely essential in nearly every city and suburb and small town. In most urban areas and certainly in rural America there is simply no other efficient way of arriving to work and school on time. Unfortunately public transit service is not always available to connect suburbs and city, let alone suburb to suburb, the path of most commuters these days. Even if transit is available it takes two to three times longer to get to work than by car and is often inaccessible to people with mobility impairments. Related issues include the other ways cars are used. Research shows that driving today is increasingly linking work travel with children's activities and household errands. It is also the case that chauffeuring of children is a major focus of many local trips, and these trips vary daily and weekly, intensifying the need to have a car that offers this form of transportation flexibility.

In the past two decades teenagers have also come to need their own car because after-school employment has increased. In short, modern life is much more fragmented than in earlier decades. In fact, families today are almost too busy to eat traditional meals such as dinner together, let alone take vacations together. It was said that the 1970s were the "now generation," but it seems much truer today. North American society at least demands everything "right now" and "on demand." From e-mail and instant text messaging on cell phones to ubiquitous drive-through banking, pharmacies, and fast food restaurants, we have grown accustomed to and dependent on quick access to goods and services without having to leave the safety and comfort of our motor vehicles. In American society today taking a car trip to a national park is no longer exciting and new. Popular destinations for families with young children today are Disneyland or Disney World. College students vacation in Mexico, Florida, or the Gulf Coast. And neither group drives; they fly. Although the car has never been used more than it is today, the long-distance car vacation is essentially a vestige of the past.

MARGINALIZATION AND THE AUTOMOBILE: WHO IS LEFT BEHIND?

Ever since the advent of the automobile, there have been disenfranchised groups—mostly the poor and minorities—who could not afford an automobile and thus could not take part in the major economic and social transformations brought about by the automobile. One group who lost out was small family-run businesses. "Mom and Pop" businesses simply could not afford off-ramp locations adjacent to freeways, leaving mostly nationwide chains like Holiday Inn and McDonald's to flourish. Main Street America gave way to drive-through pickup windows on the off-ramps of interstates and freeways.

Others have lost out too, including entire towns that have suffered downturns in the automobile industry. One of the best-known examples is Flint, Michigan, made famous in Michael Moore's film *Roger and Me*. Flint was a sleepy village until the auto industry came to town and transformed it into an economic boomtown—only to take an economic nosedive after General Motors laid off 30,000 workers from its assembly plants in the early 1980s while the company was posting record profits. Today Flint is a ghost town with unemployment hovering around 40%, and the best option for many poor families is to see their sons and daughters join the military or leave town in search of employment elsewhere.

Others have analyzed the auto industry and its role in contributing to, not ameliorating, urban decay. Thomas Sugrue for example writes about Detroit as symbolic of rust-belt cities to show how deindustrialization and racial discrimination helped maintain and deepen the social and economic differences between blacks and whites living in and around Detroit.[9] Unsurprisingly Sugrue found that much of the postwar planning of the city—highways, land clearance for urban renewal projects, retail development, and the like—had a negative and disproportionate impact on poor blacks living in Detroit.[9]

Of course at the individual level many people never had a car and did not participate in the American Dream. The same is true today. The working poor must take the bus. The statistical profile bears this out. Jane Holtz Kay[32] reports in *Asphalt Nation* that in larger cities 60% of mass transit riders are women, and 48% are African American or Hispanic, more than twice their number in the population. Although many "haves" get good service, 38% of transit riders are "have-nots," surviving at just about the poverty level.

Today driving a motor vehicle is a critical aspect of modern living. Not only is the ability to drive an expression of autonomy and independence but also it contributes to the maintenance of our family and social ties, the daily operation of households, and the pursuit of a variety of recreational activities. Thus for aging individuals and people with disabilities, driving or the resumption of driving is a major goal toward achieving and maintaining optimal community integration.

CARLESSNESS BRINGS ISOLATION AND STIGMA

Persons who are carless are often viewed as aberrant and excluded from mainstream American life. Carlessness as a result of poverty is serious enough, but being unable to drive is likewise stigmatizing. If you do not drive there must be something wrong with you. Even choosing not to drive is viewed with some suspicion because of the variety of social disadvantages presumed attached. First, not being able to drive, not having access to a car, or both effectively removes you from bettering your economic position. Without a car it is difficult to get to a job. It also makes it far more difficult to live independently because automobile transportation is a necessity to enable all one's routine community activities—work, sports and leisure, a vast array of routine errands such as grocery shopping, church participation, doctors' appointments, and most social activities. There simply are no easy alternatives that offer the reliability, flexibility, and especially efficiency of intracommunity mobility and intercommunity travel. Individuals who cannot drive (for whatever reason) are at a huge disadvantage because our cities and towns are structured so there are no easy alternatives. Public transportation is often unavailable or inconvenient, and workplaces are too far from people's homes to make walking or other methods of transportation practical. See Chapter 22 for more information on urban planning and its effect on community mobility.

Older drivers and drivers with disabilities are at an even more pronounced disadvantage. Already marginalized by a society that devalues those who are "different" or "less able," disabled persons face the additional challenge of obtaining the requisite skills and technologies to enable them to drive. The impact of older drivers on the public consciousness is just beginning to be felt as the baby boomers age and confront a time when they may need to hang up the car keys. In 1983, 1 of every 15 licensed drivers in America was over the age of 70. By 1995 this had increased to 1 of every 11 drivers. By 2020, however, one of every five Americans will be over 65 years of age, and most of them will probably be licensed to drive.[34] What will these drivers need and demand as they confront limitations to their ability to continue to drive?

The reason older adults (and others) will not want to stop driving is because doing so has so many negative implications. First, not having ready access to an automobile means you cannot obtain basic necessities; cities and towns are so designed around the car that losing the ability to drive is a significant problem. Second, no car means greatly curtailed social activities. If your family and friends are not nearby, then social isolation is major risk when you are no longer able to drive. Thus when we take away the keys and inform our clients that they must cease driving, we are not only passing judgment on their physical and cognitive fitness but also we are dramatically reducing their social participation in society. In effect we are saying they lack the capacity to make decisions for themselves, and this is the ultimate affront to individual autonomy.

Once again our existing system of public transportation is simply not an adequate alternative for the frail elderly or people with disabilities. It is too slow and inconvenient and virtually inaccessible in many cities. The average speed of a local bus is about 7 miles an hour as opposed to 28 miles an hour for the car. The walk, wait, and walk times that are involved in a bus trip lower the speed to about 7 miles per hour. Buses also typically involve the possibility of difficult steps, exposure to bad weather, and delays from traffic congestion.[35] The time between losing a license because of frailty and being too frail to take a bus also is short; in fact many frail elderly people can probably drive long after they lose the ability and patience to take a bus. Private transportation services are prohibitively expensive for more than the most critical trips. Thus there are no generally recognized strategies for providing affordable alternatives to the private automobile. See Chapter 21 for more information on driving cessation and alternative mobility.

SUMMARY

Driving and the infrastructure that supports a worldwide car culture influence how we interact with others, view the world, imagine how others perceive us, and how that image influences the way we perceive ourselves.[36] The automobile and the generations of motor vehicles that have evolved from the early steam- and electric-powered horseless carriages have also profoundly influenced an American culture, which in turn has promoted a global car culture and impacted the ways people carry out their daily activities. In 1976 the United States was celebrating its two-hundredth anniversary, and General Motors Corporation (GM) marketed its Chevrolet brand of vehicles by using a patriotic advertising slogan that reinforced the notion that there is nothing more American than "hot dogs, apple pie, baseball, and Chevrolet" (i.e., cars and trucks manufactured by GM's Chevrolet auto brand). Automobiles continue to be the preferred method of personal or small group transportation by most Americans and people living in industrialized and developing countries around the world. Individuals who possess the necessary resources to own or lease a vehicle have more than an efficient means for intra-community and intercommunity mobility; cars and trucks are tangible symbols that remind us individually and collectively that with ownership comes the message that we are fully engaged in mainstream American life.

REFERENCES

1. Farstad A, editor: *Holy Bible: the new King James version: containing the old and new testaments,* Nashville, 1982, Thomas Nelson.
2. Smith SL: *Gold glass of the late Roman Empire: production, context, and function,* Ann Arbor, MI, 2000, University Microfilms, XLIII, p 432.
3. Brown K: personal communication, 2004.
4. Olson B, Cabadas J: *The American auto factory,* St. Paul, MN, 2002, MBI Publishing.
5. Sandler MW: *Driving around the USA: automobiles in American life,* New York, 2003, Oxford University Press.
6. Ford H, Crowther S: *My life and work (1922),* Whitefish, MT, 2003, Kessinger Publishing.
7. Wachs M, Crawford M, editors: *The car and the city: the automobile, the built environment, and daily urban life,* Ann Arbor, MI, 1992, University of Michigan Press.
8. Miller L: Cars, trucks now outnumber drivers, *Salon* August 29, 2003.
9. Berger ML: *The automobile in American history and culture: a reference guide,* Westport, CT, 2001, Greenwood Publishing.
10. Goddard SB: *Getting there: the epic struggle between road and rail in the American century,* New York, 1994, Basic Books.
11. McShane C: *Down the asphalt path: the automobile and the American city,* New York, 1994, Columbia University Press.
12. Lynd RS, Lynd HM: *Middletown: a study in modern American culture,* Orlando, FL, 1929, Harcourt Brace.
13. Cooley CH: *Human nature and the social order,* New York, 1902, Scribner's.
14. Tönnies F: *Geist der Neuzeit (1935),* ed 2, 1998.
15. Granovetter M: The strength of weak ties: a network theory revisited, *Sociological Theory* 1, 1983.
16. Dybis K: *Print, TV ad blitzes created classics: cars recognized for catchy slogans,* 2003, The Detroit News, Retrieved from *http://www.detnews.com/2003/specialreport/0306/09/f14-186972.htm.*
17. Reference deleted in pages.
18. Molnar LJ, Eby DW, Miller LL: Promoting independence and wellbeing: Successful approaches to enhancing elderly driving mobility, International Conference on Aging, Disability, and Independence, Washington, DC, 2003.
19. U.S. Department of Transportation: *Safe mobility for a maturing society: challenges and opportunities,* Washington, DC, 2003, Government Printing Office.
20. Wang CC, Kosinski CJ, Schwartzberg JG, et al: *Physician's guide to assessing and counseling older drivers,* Washington, DC, 2003, National Highway Traffic Safety.

21. Gillens L: Yielding to age: when the elderly can no longer drive, *J Gerontologic Nurs* 16(11):12-15, 1990.

22. European Conference of Ministers for Transport, 1994

23. Freund B, Szinovacz M: Effects of cognition on driving involvement among the oldest old: variations by gender and alternative transportation opportunities, *Gerontologist* 42:621-633, 2002.

24. Goffman E: *The presentation of self in everyday life,* Garden City, NY, 1963, Anchor.

25. Korner-Bitensky N, Sofer S, Kaizer F, et al: Assessing ability to drive following an acute neurological event: are we on the right road, *Revue Canadienne d'Ergothérapie* 61, 141-148, 1994.

26. Cook CA, Semmler CJ: Ethical dilemmas in driver reeducation, Am J Occup Ther 45:517-22, 1991.

27. Cynkin S, Robinson AM: Occupational therapy and activities health: toward health through activities, Boston, 1990, Little, Brown and Co.

28. Barnes MP, Hoyle EA: Driving assessment: a case of need, *Clin Rehabil* 9:115-120, 1995.

29. Luborsky M: Creative challenges and the construction of meaningful life narratives. In Adams-Price CE, editor: *Creativity and successful aging,* New York, 1998, Springer Publishing Company, pp 311-37.

30. Duggan CH: "God, if you're real, and you hear me, send me a sign": Dewey's story of living with a spinal cord injury, *J Religion Disabil Health* 4(1), 2000.

31. Ranney TA, Hunt LA: Researchers and occupational therapists can help each other to better understand what makes a good driver: two perspectives, *Work: A Journal of Prevention, Assessment Rehabilitation* 8:293-7, 1997.

32. Holtz KJ: *Asphalt nation: how the automobile took over America and how we can take it back,* New York, 1997, Crown Publishers.

33. Reference deleted in pages.

34. The Sheboygan Press: Editorial: Tighter licensing for senior drivers needed in state, July 23, 2003, Sheboygan, MI. Available at *www.wisinfo.com/sheboyganpress/print/print_11382735. shtml.* Accessed February 24, 2005.

35. Reno A: *Personal mobility in the United States, in a look ahead: year 2020,* Washington, DC, 1988, Transportation Research Board, National Research Council.

36. Vidich AJ, Lyman SM: Qualitative methods: their history in sociology and anthropology. In Denzin NK, Lincoln YS, editors: *Handbook of qualitative research,* Thousand Oaks, CA, 1994, Sage Schlegloff.

Chapter 4

THE DRIVER REHABILITATION TEAM

KEY TERMS

- Primary team members
- Key driver rehabilitation services
- Driver rehabilitation specialist (DRS)
- Community mobility
- Comprehensive driver rehabilitation evaluations
- Ancillary team members
- Certified driver rehabilitation specialist (CDRS)
- Occupational therapist specializing in driver rehabilitation
- Occupational therapy generalist
- Vehicle modifier
- Instrumental activities of daily living (IADL)
- Clinical reasoning
- Evidence-based practice
- Clinical screen
- Driver remediation plan
- Driver cessation plan
- Employment plan
- National Mobility Equipment Dealers Association (NMEDA)

CHAPTER OBJECTIVES

After completing this chapter, the reader will be able to do the following:

- Understand the difference between a driver rehabilitation specialist and a certified driver rehabilitation specialist.
- Recognize the primary and ancillary driver rehabilitation team members.
- Be familiar with the key driver rehabilitation and community mobility services.
- Realize that the driver rehabilitation specialist plays the central role in providing efficacious driver rehabilitation and community mobility services.
- Realize that the client is at the center of the driver rehabilitation team.
- Be familiar with the five service delivery models.
- Understand the National Mobility Equipment Dealers Association's role in the adaptive mobility industry.

SECTION I

Primary Team Members and Key Services

Joseph M. Pellerito, Jr. • Carol A. Blanc

DRIVER REHABILITATION SPECIALISTS

The services that are offered by a driver rehabilitation program are usually a good indicator of the professionals who comprise a particular program's team structure. Every driver rehabilitation program employs *primary team members* to provide *key driver rehabilitation services* irrespective of the program's service delivery model, team structure, or service offerings. Among the driver rehabilitation team members is the *driver rehabilitation specialist* (DRS); the DRS plays the central role in providing efficacious driver rehabilitation and more recently *community mobility* services to clients and their caregivers. DRSs conduct *comprehensive driver rehabilitation evaluations* with the aim of determining their clients' driver readiness. DRSs work with other health care professionals, including *ancillary team members*, to help ensure that clients achieve their driver rehabilitation goals, community mobility goals, or both. Table 4-1 lists key driver rehabilitation and community mobility serv-ices, as well as the professionals responsible for the services rendered. Any or all of these services are fea-tured within driver rehabilitation service delivery models in the United States.

DRSs often begin their careers by working as occupa-tional therapy generalists, driver educators, or in other health science fields before developing an expertise in

Table 4-1 Driver Rehabilitation and Community Mobility Key Services and the Professionals Who Provide Them

Services Provided by the Driver Rehabilitation Team Members	Professional(s) Responsible for Specific Service
Clinical screen	Occupational therapists and other health science professionals (e.g., pharmacists and physical therapists) specializing in driver rehabilitation services
Clinical evaluations	Occupational therapists and other health science professionals (e.g., pharmacists and physical therapists) specializing in driver rehabilitation services
On-road evaluations	Occupational therapists, driver educators, or other health science professionals (e.g., pharmacists and physical therapists) specializing in driver rehabilitation services
Off-street (e.g., driving range) training	Occupational therapists, driver educators, and other health science professionals specializing in driver rehabilitation services
On-road training	Occupational therapists, driver educators, and other health science professionals specializing in driver rehabilitation services
Recommendations for adapted driving aids	Occupational therapists, driver educators, and other health science professionals specializing in driver rehabilitation services
Recommendations for vehicle modifications	Occupational therapists, driver educators, and other health science professionals specializing in driver rehabilitation services
Client-vehicle fittings	Occupational therapists, driver educators, and other health science professionals specializing in driver rehabilitation services
Driving cessation planning	Occupational therapists, driver educators, and other health science professionals specializing in driver rehabilitation services
Counseling the driver who is no longer able to drive safely	Occupational therapists, driver educators, and other health science professionals specializing in driver rehabilitation services. Also physicians, neuropsychologists, psychologists, social workers, and others
Exploration of alternatives to driving for community mobility	Occupational therapists, driver educators, and other health science professionals specializing in driver rehabilitation services

driver rehabilitation and community mobility. Box 4-1 is a brief list of common professional credentials that have provided a foundation on which DRS careers have emerged.

Each of the groups presented in Box 4-1 comprises dedicated men and women who provide driver rehabilitation and community mobility services to people with disabilities and/or aging-related concerns. Occasionally individuals will have earned a combination of credentials and have professional experience that affords them multiple perspectives, such as occupational therapists who have become certified driver educators (or vice versa) and are working as DRSs or as *certified driver rehabilitation specialists* (CDRSs). It should also be pointed out that there is a distinction between the DRS

BOX 4-1	**Common Professional Credentials Held by Driver Rehabilitation Specialists**

- Registered and/or licensed occupational therapists (OTR or OTR/L)
- Occupational therapists who are also certified driver educators
- Professional credentials earned in other health science fields, such as pharmacy, physical therapy, and therapeutic recreation to name a few
- Certified driver educators

---

and CDRS credentials. Professionals who provide driver rehabilitation services may or may not have completed the requirements set forth by the Association for Driver Rehabilitation Specialists (ADED) to become a CDRS. Some DRSs practice in the United States and elsewhere around the world without having become certified because the process is currently voluntary. However, it is generally accepted that certification helps to improve the overall standards and quality of practice. Additionally a growing number of state vocational rehabilitation (VR) agencies now require that all of their clients' driver evaluations be performed by CDRSs; this may become a trend among other third-party payers as well. Recently the American Occupational Therapy Association's (AOTA) Representative Assembly (RA) voted to support the organization's development of its own certification programs in driver rehabilitation and community mobility, which will undoubtedly further expand and complicate the choices professionals and consumers must make with regard to professional training and seeking services, respectively. See Box 4-2 for more information on professional credentials in the field of driver rehabilitation and community mobility.

For clarity we have chosen to illustrate the differences and similarities throughout this chapter between the two largest groups of DRSs: occupational therapists and driver educators specializing in driver rehabilitation. We use the term *occupational therapist specializing in driver rehabilitation* to mean those professionals who have specialized in driver rehabilitation services and are working as DRSs, which should not be confused

---

BOX 4-2	**Professional Credentials**

The Association of Driver Rehabilitation Specialists (ADED), formerly the Association for Driver Educators of the Disabled, is an international and multidisciplinary association that provides education, training, and certification of DRSs. Specialists come from various disciplines, such as occupational therapy, driver education, physical therapy, kinesiotherapy, pharmacy, vocational rehabilitation, therapeutic recreation, rehabilitation engineering, and speech-language pathology, among others. Individuals wishing to become certified by ADED must have completed a specified period in the field on a full-time basis and pass a comprehensive certification examination. The requirements vary (e.g., hours of full-time practice) depending on the professional degree held by each prospective candidate. Individuals meeting the minimum requirements can sit for the certification examination at the organization's annual conference. Once certification is granted continuing education is required to remain in good standing within the organization.

Certification is not compulsory in the United States, and the American Occupational Therapy Association

(AOTA) is in the process of developing a process for occupational therapists interested in specializing in driver rehabilitation or community mobility. It is expected that there will be new standards of practice created along with a separate certification examination and guidelines that will outline expectations for continuing education. The provision of resources to assist practitioners, researchers, administrators, teachers, and students deliver efficacious driver rehabilitation services can already be found on AOTA's web site: www.aota.org.

The AOTA's representative assembly (RA) voted at their 2004 annual conference to support developing a specialty certification in driver rehabilitation or community mobility. At the time of this publication representatives from AOTA and ADED were exploring the need and feasibility for such a certification that would only be offered to occupational therapy professionals and how its implementation would help or hinder the advancement of the occupational therapy profession generally and driver rehabilitation specifically.

with occupational therapists who have not specialized in any single area of practice and are henceforth referred to as *occupational therapy generalists*. Also we refer to professionals who have specialized in driver rehabilitation services, irrespective of their specific professional credentials, as driver rehabilitation specialists, or DRSs, because as previously noted not all professionals working in the field of driver rehabilitation have been certified by ADED and thus do not hold the CDRS credential. See Box 4-3 for more information on the certification process offered by ADED that leads to earning a CDRS credential. Finally it is our assertion that DRSs have a professional and ethical responsibility to address community mobility issues in addition to the traditional services that have focused on driver evaluation and rehabilitation in the past. The importance of community mobility, within the context of this chapter and throughout this book, is centered on the notion that alternatives to driving that enable community mobility must be explored to help ensure optimal community participation and other desired outcomes. This is especially critical when a client must cease driving altogether and identify reliable and cost-effective alternative transportation.

CLIENTS AND THEIR CAREGIVERS

This chapter supports the view that the client is at the center of the driver rehabilitation team and that it is mutually beneficial for the client, DRS, and other team members when a client's full participation in the decision-making process is encouraged and expected. DRSs and other team members demonstrate that they value a client's perspective and input by actively listening to what is (or is not) being said and incorporating pertinent feedback and suggestions whenever possible. The client's caregiver(s) may take an active role in any aspect of the service delivery process and should be viewed as another important primary team member when applicable. The caregiver often "fills in the blanks" and provides valuable insight that the client may be lacking or unwilling to provide.

VEHICLE MODIFIERS

In addition to the DRS, client, and caregiver, the *vehicle modifier* (also known as the mobility equipment dealer or vendor) plays a primary role in the provision of driver rehabilitation and community mobility services. On the completion of a comprehensive driver rehabilitation evaluation, the vehicle modifier works closely with the DRS to review and perform the recommended modifications to a client's new or existing vehicle. The vehicle modifier often helps to refine the DRS's intervention plan by presenting a rationale for identifying alternative vehicle modifications to the DRS's and other primary team members' initial recommendations. However, vehicle modifiers do much more than their name implies; for example they often help the client and DRS identify the optimal vehicle type

---

BOX 4-3   Driver Rehabilitation Specialist Certification

Candidates may take the certification examination if they meet the education and/or experience requirements listed below:
A. An undergraduate degree or higher in a health-related* area of study with 1 year of full-time experience in degree area of study and an additional 1 year of full-time experience in the field of Driver Rehabilitation.†
B. Four-year undergraduate degree‡ or higher with a major or minor in Traffic Safety and/or a Driver and Traffic Safety Endorsement with 1 year of full-time experience in Traffic Safety and an additional 2 years of full-time experience in the field of Driver Rehabilitation.†
C. Two-year degree in a health-related* area of study with 1 year of experience in degree area of study and an

additional 3 years of full-time experience in the field of Driver Rehabilitation.†
D. Five years of full-time work experience in the field of Driver Rehabilitation.†
Full time means for ADED purposes 32 hours per week.
Examination content includes the following:
1. Program administration
2. The clinical evaluation
3. The in-vehicle assessment (i.e., preparing the vehicle for the on-road evaluation)
4. The on-road evaluation
5. Interpretation of the evaluation results
6. Planning and implementing recommendations

*Health-related degree means for ADED purposes: Occupational Therapy, Physical Therapy, Kinesiotherapy, Speech Therapy, Therapeutic Recreational Therapy, or other areas as approved by the Certification Committee.
†In the field of Driver Rehabilitation means for ADED purposes: Direct hands-on delivery of clinical (predriving evaluations) and/or behind-the-wheel evaluations and training with the client.
‡Undergraduate degree areas of study means for ADED purposes: Social Work, Vocational Rehabilitation, Health and Physical Education, Counseling, Psychology, or other areas as approved by the Certification Committee.
From The Association for Driver Rehabilitation Specialists: Association for Driver Rehabilitation Specialists exam fact sheet, Ruston, LA, http://www.aded.net/i4a/pages/ index.cfm?pageid=120#spot1.

and vehicle modifications that maximize the client's safety as a driver or passenger after accessing or exiting a vehicle with efficiency. Additionally vehicle modifiers and DRSs collaborate to identify ways to maximize a client's overall driving performance with or without adapted driving aids. Over the years vehicle modifiers have continued to develop customized adaptive driving equipment and vehicle modification procedures to meet the unique needs of clients who require more than off-the-shelf products (i.e., "turn-key" solutions). Reputable mobility equipment dealers are members of the National Mobility Equipment Dealers Association (NMEDA), which will be discussed later in this chapter. Box 4-4 provides a description of what constitutes a vehicle modification. Vehicle modifiers and the other primary driver rehabilitation team members continue to make major contributions to the rapidly evolving field of driver rehabilitation and community mobility.

THE CASE MANAGER

Driver rehabilitation services can be costly, especially if the client or caregiver must purchase or modify a vehicle and also participate in a comprehensive driver rehabilitation evaluation and training program. In some cases clients are fortunate to have the necessary insurance coverage or a relationship with an organization with a philanthropic mission that fully or partially pays for the costs associated with the procured driver rehabilitation and community mobility services and equipment. The professional who represents the funding entity is the last primary driver rehabilitation team member examined in this chapter. Generally these individuals have the title of case manager and often have a professional background in social work, nursing, or some other allied health profession. The case manager advocates for his or her clients and coordinates the client's overall care. The case manager also provides a communication link between the other driver rehabilitation team members and the third-party payer's professional who has the authority to authorize payment for services, vehicle modifications, and equipment (e.g., the insurance company's claims adjuster). For example, workers' compensation or auto insurance cases usually pay for driver rehabilitation and community mobility services and equipment that are necessary to enable the client to drive or ride as a passenger safely, which is considered reasonable and customary. We will now examine how community mobility, and particularly driving cessation planning and alternative transportation, have become critical components of the comprehensive driver rehabilitation evaluation.

DRIVING CESSATION AND ALTERNATIVE TRANSPORTATION

Collaboration between the DRS and the other ancillary driver rehabilitation team members (e.g., physiatrists, physical or occupational therapy seating specialists and generalists, neuropsychologists, social workers, nurses, therapeutic recreation specialists, educators, and others) provides the client with the best chance to learn or relearn foundational skills (i.e., client factors such as strength, endurance, vision, and cognition), obtain durable medical equipment (DME), and use technology required to safely drive a stock or modified van, car, or truck. However, if the primary driver rehabilitation team members determine that a client is no longer able to drive safely with or without restrictions, the DRS should be compelled to assist his or her client with identifying and using community mobility resources for dependable alternative transportation. Access to dependable alternative transportation is an essential *instrumental activities of daily living (IADL)* and is necessary to fully empower clients who no longer drive because of declining physical or mental health, socioeconomic status, aging-related concerns, or some other factor. When driving is no longer an option for safe, efficient, and dependable community mobility, the DRS should assist the client and his or her caregivers to develop strategies for accessing and using alternative transportation methods to help ensure full community participation, resumption of life roles, maintenance of personal and professional networks, and optimal health and well-being; these are some of the keys that promote quality living. Alternative transportation

| BOX 4-4 | What Constitutes a Vehicle Modification? |

Vehicle modifications are any mechanical or structural changes to a passenger car, van, truck, or other motor vehicle that permit an individual with a disability and/or aging-related concern to safely drive or ride as a passenger. Vehicle modifications also include wheelchair or scooter loaders, which are usually mounted on the roof, in the passenger area, in the trunk, or in other storage areas of a car, van, or truck. Automotive adaptive driving aids added to a stock motor vehicle enable an individual with mobility restrictions to control the vehicle's primary and secondary controls, such as accelerator, foot brake, turn signals, dimmer switch, steering wheel, and parking brake, to name a few.[1] See Chapter 11 for a complete listing of primary and secondary vehicle controls and Chapter 18 for an exploration of in-vehicle intelligent transport systems and driving.

options are often unfamiliar to clients and caregivers who have relied on driving a motor vehicle as their primary (and more often their sole) method of transportation.

Most driver rehabilitation programs in the United States are primarily set up to help clients safely drive a car, van, or truck with or without modifications. Only a few driver rehabilitation programs have adopted the notion that community mobility must be addressed by exploring alternative transportation options as an integral part of the comprehensive driver rehabilitation evaluation. This is especially true for the client who perceives failing a driver evaluation as a critique of his or her self-worth, which can lead to a decline in community participation. Clients who will no longer be driving need the services of a driver rehabilitation (and community mobility) team perhaps more than individuals who will be new or returning to driving. Clients deemed unsafe to drive require access to a dependable means of transportation if they are to successfully avoid the negative consequences often experienced after driving cessation.

To summarize, people with disabilities and aging-related concerns often require that their existing or prospective vehicles be modified before they can access them, stow their ambulation aids or secure their wheeled mobility devices, transfer into and out of their vehicles, and drive or ride as passengers with optimal safety and comfort. It is the DRS who plays the key role in performing the assessments that comprise the comprehensive driver rehabilitation evaluation. Evaluations should include recommendations for specific adapted driving aids, preferred vehicle type, structural modifications to the vehicle, and an on-road training regimen when applicable. If a client is deemed unsafe to drive, the DRS should develop a driving cessation plan to help preserve the client's quality of life by identifying safe and reliable alternative transportation to maintain community mobility and its associated benefits. It is true that in many instances the physiatrist may be seen as the team leader; however, the DRS possesses the necessary knowledge and skills that are required for completing the bulk of the professional tasks associated with a comprehensive driver rehabilitation evaluation and training program. See Chapters 6, 11, 12, 13, and 21 for more information on driver rehabilitation and community mobility services.

SECTION II

Service Delivery Models

Joseph M. Pellerito, Jr. • *Carol A. Blanc*

We will now turn to the key roles driver rehabilitation team members play within several distinct practice or service delivery models. It is important to note that the models presented here do not represent an exhaustive listing of the creative and credible driver rehabilitation models throughout North America and elsewhere around the world. Rather the models selected reflect the most common programmatic structures currently in existence in the United States.

Service delivery models will continue to change over time with the adoption of leading-edge technology and the emergence of driver rehabilitation evidence-based practice. (See Chapter 24 for more information on research and evidence-based practice in driver rehabilitation.) The driver rehabilitation team's collective aim remains the same today as it did at the profession's inception several decades ago: to continuously improve the standards of driver rehabilitation practice to effectively address clients' complex issues and challenges that preclude them from driving and/or accessing dependable alternative transportation. The kinds of services offered vary by program and typically include one or more of the key service areas presented in Table 4-1. Service delivery models provide the contexts or environments in which key driver rehabilitation and community mobility services are offered and delivered.

The service delivery models briefly presented in this chapter include the traditional medical model, the community-based model, the VR model, the university-based model, and the Veterans Affairs model.

In the United States, driving evaluations are often a part of a VR plan of care and are commonly conducted to determine driver readiness for clients who need to commute to and from a work setting, attend school as a means to secure a job after graduation, or are in the process of seeking employment. VR counselors can initiate a referral for driver rehabilitation and community mobility services and pay for the costs that are incurred, depending on whether VR funds are available at the time services are requested. (See Chapter 15 for more information on funding driver rehabilitation services and equipment.) VR counselors are generally aware of the services offered by a reputable driver rehabilitation and community mobility program and often enjoy an established relationship with the program's personnel. However, in some instances VR counselors may contact a driving program to inquire about the services offered and to become familiar with the steps their clients must take before undergoing a driver rehabilitation evaluation. Additionally if the client's disability is the result of a work-related injury, workers' compensation is another potential funding source that will pay for a driver evaluation as part of the client's life care plan. Another funding source is a branch of the state VR services called Independent Living Services (ILS). ILS provides services for clients who do not intend to return to work but want to participate more fully in the community with greater safety and independence. Each VR program's services and benefits vary from state to state, which requires health care professionals (and DRSs in particular) to stay abreast of the current VR practices in their respective states and counties. If a client does not qualify for any of these programs, the associated costs must be incurred by the client, which is commonly referred to as "private pay" or "self pay." However, not all clients are able to afford driver rehabilitation and community mobility services and may need assistance to identify people, organizations, and institutions that can help them identify alternative funding sources (e.g., philanthropic groups, religious organizations, and community groups).

THE TRADITIONAL MEDICAL MODEL

The medical model features programs that are housed within a hospital, rehabilitation center, and/or freestanding outpatient clinic. Depending on a particular state's requirements, these programs may or may not be required to maintain their licensure as a state-licensed driving school and are usually well suited to address the medical, psychosocial, and socioeconomic challenges that can impact driving and community mobility. These programs are usually well prepared because they subscribe to a client-centered and multidisciplinary team approach that usually includes one or more occupational therapists specializing in driver rehabilitation. DRSs who possess an occupational therapy background are educated and trained to view their clients holistically and are adept at bridging the gap between theory and practice; without that bridge, evidence-based practice would not exist. In other words, occupational therapists are uniquely positioned to use *clinical reasoning* that is founded on *evidence-based practice* and demonstrate competent skills that are often developed during years of experience in the field.

A combination of knowledge and skills is necessary for a DRS to perform a comprehensive driver rehabilitation evaluation and plan and execute an efficacious driver training program. DRSs use various tools to help their clients achieve their short- and long-term driver rehabilitation and community mobility goals. Technology can be used at any point during the evaluation—training—follow-up continuum of care. For example, DRSs may use driving simulators, virtual reality technology, or off-street areas set up as closed circuit courses; each of these tools affords clients opportunities to participate in training programs more fully because they can practice to remediate skills in a protected environment. Protocols that specify off-street in addition to on-road driver training in familiar and unfamiliar areas

under various environmental conditions can dramatically increase the effectiveness of the services rendered.

Occupational therapy generalists may perform a *clinical screen* and then refer their clients to an occupational therapist specializing in driver rehabilitation. However, the generalist should never make a definitive conclusion about a client's driver readiness that is based on a predriving screen alone. A DRS is the only professional prepared to perform a comprehensive driver rehabilitation evaluation that includes the clinical and on-road evaluations. Clients should be given the opportunity to demonstrate their ability (or lack of ability) to drive outside of the clinical environment while they are behind the wheel of a motor vehicle before they are told to cease driving. There are few exceptions to this rule (e.g., a client reporting that he or she experienced recent seizure activity). Recommending that a client cease driving or be given a restricted license is a serious proposition. Conversely if the team recommends continuance of driving, the public is depending on their collective knowledge and experience to ensure their safety. The DRS must be certain that the information gathered throughout the evaluation process is valid and complete. Only then can the driver rehabilitation team, and particularly the DRS, be confident in the documented recommendations.

Some facilities employ driver educators to perform some or the entire on-road portion of the comprehensive driver rehabilitation evaluation after the occupational therapist specializing in driver rehabilitation has completed a clinical evaluation. Team members must work closely together throughout each phase of the evaluation and training program to help ensure the client's goals are realized. Clinical evaluations generally consist of examining range of motion, coordination, strength, cognition and perception, visual acuity, and reaction time tests, such as brake reaction, to name a few. Other tests may be completed depending on the initial evaluation findings with the aim of assessing the client's knowledge about the rules of the road, topographic orientation, and his or her ability to read and interpret road signage. See Chapters 6, 12, 13, and 14 for more details about driver evaluation, training, and documentation.

The client should have already obtained a learner's permit or possess a valid driver's license to participate in the on-road portion of the evaluation. In some cases the Medical Review Program (MRP) at the Motor Vehicle Division (MVD) may issue a limited driver's permit to be used only while the client is being evaluated or trained by the DRS. Rules vary from state to state (e.g., California and Arizona can issue a temporary and limited permit), and it is the DRS's responsibility to stay abreast of current regulations, policies, and laws in his or her respective service area(s).

If the client has been referred for complementary services such as a wheeled mobility and seating evaluation, the DRS should communicate with the seating specialist to determine the type of mobility and seating system that was recommended (if any) and how it may impact the client's driving performance. Most importantly if a client is planning to drive while seated in a power wheelchair, the DRS must recognize that the type of wheelchair and seating components will impact the client's driving performance as much as the adapted driving equipment. Wheeled mobility and seating systems provide a client's foundation or base of support and must be integrated into the adapted vehicle in a complementary fashion, taking into consideration function and aesthetics. This is done to facilitate a successful van modification and promote optimal driving performance. The wheelchair vendor, seating specialist, occupational therapy generalist, vehicle modifier, DRS, and physician must communicate before generating the vehicle prescription or commencing with the vehicle modifications and training program.

If the medical model includes an occupational therapist and a driver educator who provide driver rehabilitation services, they should maintain an ongoing dialogue face to face, over the telephone, and on the Internet before, during, and after the on-road driving evaluation. If the driver educator is scheduled to perform the on-road evaluation, he or she should consult the occupational therapist to determine the preferred transfer method, preferred ambulation aid or wheeled mobility device, and adapted driving aids required for any aspect of the on-road evaluation, training program, or both. (See Chapter 11 for more information on preparing the vehicle before the on-road evaluation.) The driver educator and occupational therapist specializing in driver rehabilitation can initiate the behind-the-wheel evaluation of their client's on-road driving performance. In some cases the driver educator and occupational therapist will ride in the vehicle together during each session or at least during the first and last driving session. The driver educator is usually seated in the front passenger seat and the occupational therapist in the backseat. This configuration enables each professional to collaborate as the evaluation is occurring, which may help to increase validity and inter-rater reliability of the on-road evaluation. This strategy also helps each of the professionals to evaluate firsthand a client's performance and develop recommendations in a collaborative fashion.

The interpretation of the clinical evaluation and the on-road evaluation is typically presented to the client by the occupational therapist with the driver educator present to answer questions that may be raised by the client, his or her caregiver, or both. A report is generated by the occupational therapist; the driver educator may provide the on-road evaluation components by mutual agreement of the driver rehabilitation team in advance of the driving evaluation. Depending on the client's diagnosis or diagnoses, age-related concerns, previous driving history, social history, actual driving performance, and need for vehicle modifications and adapted driving aids, the recommendations are delineated by the primary evaluator (i.e., occupational therapist who receives feedback from the driver educator and client whenever possible) in the driver rehabilitation evaluation report.

A client may need additional on-road training to learn compensatory techniques, how to use unfamiliar adapted driving aids, and/or to improve his or her defensive driving techniques. Some clients may only need a driving evaluation for clearance to drive after completing their rehabilitation program designed to address specific needs that were associated with a particular diagnosis that was not expected to impact the client's long-term driving performance (e.g., total knee replacement). Conversely, some clients may not successfully pass the on-road driver evaluation and should be assisted with developing either a *driver remediation plan* or *driver cessation plan*, depending on the anticipated prognosis that is determined by the driver rehabilitation and community mobility team members. The remediation plans should include action steps that are meant to help a client improve his or her overall functional abilities related to the driving task. For example, a client can be referred for additional outpatient therapies or have a customized home program designed by the occupational therapy generalist and/or other allied health professionals. The driver rehabilitation primary team members can also seek out additional professional consultations, such as neuropsychology, neuro-ophthalmology, or an occupational therapy low-vision specialist. Alternative transportation resources can be explored, and a consultation with a physical or occupational therapist specializing in wheeled mobility and seating can be facilitated. A wheeled mobility and seating evaluation that addresses positioning for optimal comfort, safety, and independence in performing activities of daily living (ADL) is often a critical step to facilitate a successful driver evaluation outcome. This is especially important if the client intends to use his or her power wheelchair as the driver's seat "base" while driving a modified van. A new wheelchair prescription should be developed in collaboration with a physical or occupational therapy seating specialist and the DRS to help ensure the system is integrated properly into the adapted vehicle. If the client is working with a speech-language pathologist on improving cognitive skills, this is a great opportunity for the DRS to identify the specific executive function skills (e.g., recognition of roadway signage, route planning, problem solving, and interpretation of unfamiliar and unexpected situations) the client should focus on to achieve goals pertaining to driving or using alternative transportation services or both.

If remedial steps are not appropriate or prove to be ineffective and the client is no longer a candidate for driving, the DRS can do much more than simply provide a list of alternative transportation resources (e.g., city bus services, dial-a-ride, taxis, senior volunteer services, and mass transit) for the client and his caregivers to peruse. Actively helping clients and their caregivers to identify and use alternative transportation is an essential service that every DRS should be prepared to provide.

The occupational therapist and driver educator specializing in driver rehabilitation complete the vehicle prescription together, and depending on each specialist's knowledge level and experience, one person may take the lead in documenting the recommendations for adapted driving aids and structural modifications to the client's vehicle. Collaboration between the specialists, client, caregivers, and the vehicle modifier is the key to making certain that any concerns are addressed before the prescription is finalized and costly mistakes are made. In some programs occupational therapists specializing in driver rehabilitation may have completed additional education and training to become a driving educator. Under these circumstances professionals with dual perspectives perform the clinical and on-road evaluations, provide on-road driver training, complete the evaluation reports, develop the prescriptions for adapted driving controls and/or vehicle modifications, and assist the vehicle modifier with client-vehicle fittings. Programs that employ dual-credentialed specialists may also employ driver educators to assist with providing on-road training and developing equipment prescriptions.

Clients may be referred to a neuro-ophthalmologist for a consultation and vision therapy, an occupational therapist working as a low-vision specialist, a wheeled mobility and seating specialist, or for some other aspect of outpatient rehabilitation provided by therapy generalists, such as speech-language pathologists, neuropsychologists, physical therapists, or therapeutic recreation specialists (TRSs), to name a few. DRSs should remember that ancillary professional consultations and services can augment the driver rehabilitation evaluation and address pertinent issues that may arise that are relevant to driver rehabilitation and the client's overall health, safety, and well-being. Depending on the client's socioeconomic status and method of payment, communication is required between the payer (e.g., vocational rehabilitation counselor, case manager, or others) and the occupational therapist regarding the client's needs to gain preauthorization for driver rehabilitation and community mobility services.

On completion of a comprehensive driver evaluation the DRS develops a plan with specific action steps for the client and team to pursue. When a DRS determines that a client is not a good candidate for driving but could be safely transported as a passenger in an adapted vehicle, the DRS may be required to develop a set of recommendations that includes details for a modified passenger vehicle. Conversely if the DRS determines that driving is a realistic goal, the evaluation report will identify the steps that are required for the client to safely drive with or without driving restrictions, adapted driving aids, and vehicle modifications. The VR counselor and workers' compensation or auto insurance case manager will communicate with the DRS or the person responsible for scheduling the client's date for follow-up services and authorize an on-road driver's training program. On successful completion of an on-road training program that includes a thorough evaluation of a client's driving performance in traffic situations that begin with minimal challenges and increase gradually to more complex driving situations, a report is generated and prescriptions are written that describe the optimal vehicle type, structural modifications to the vehicle, and adapted driving aids that are required so that the client can achieve the goals outlined in the comprehensive driver rehabilitation evaluation report.

The VR counselor or case manager initiates the bidding process by requesting that bids be gathered for the proposed vehicle modifications and adapted driving aids. The decision to award a job to a particular vehicle modifier can be influenced by numerous factors, such as an existing relationship between the vendor and the payer, client, or other driver rehabilitation team members. Clients and/or caregivers' preferences are usually based on the fact that they have worked with the vendor at some time in the past. Many clients or caregivers can become overwhelmed during what is often viewed as a complex and sometimes taxing process and instead defer their opinion while looking to the physician, VR counselor, or DRS for guidance. Some states may award the vehicle modification job to the lowest bidder, whereas others may only award it to a state-authorized vehicle modifier. In any case it is usually the DRS who has the closest working relationships with the vehicle modifiers in the respective geographic service area. Therefore, the DRS is best positioned among the driver rehabilitation team members to accurately assess a vehicle modifier's level of competence and expertise.

Once the job is awarded to a vehicle modifier, the DRS is notified and informed about the chosen vendor. Once the vehicle modifications are completed, it is the responsibility of the vehicle modifier to contact the DRS, VR counselor, and case manager to schedule the client-vehicle fitting. The client, vehicle modifier, and DRS should be present at the client-vehicle fitting. The prescription is reviewed in detail while the client is inside of the vehicle to help ensure that the prescribed vehicle modifications and adapted driving aids are what was recommended by the DRS. If the vehicle is drivable at the time of the initial fitting, the DRS will often reassess the client's driving performance while on the road to determine whether any adjustments to the system are required. Vehicle modifiers make the necessary adjustments because they performed the installation and are familiar with how the equipment is integrated into a vehicle, which can significantly affect a client's driving performance or comfort and safety while traveling as a passenger. Because the DRS works closely with a client during the on-road training phase, he or she is in the best position to judge the overall client-vehicle fit and anticipate potential issues that can arise during this important juncture in the driver rehabilitation evaluation process.[2] Needless to say a strong collaborative relationship between the DRS, vehicle modifier, and the client is necessary throughout the vehicle modification process. Collaboration is the key to making certain that a proper client-vehicle fit is achieved. In more complex vehicle modifications there may be two or three separate fittings before the DRS and client approve the vehicle's configuration. The DRS should begin the training program in the client's vehicle to reinforce what has already been learned, to help ensure carryover, and to determine whether any other definitive adjustments need to be made by the vehicle modifier. The VR counselor, workers' compensation case manager, or auto insurance case manager may attend one of the fitting sessions to get further acquainted with the process and to see the modifications firsthand with the client present. A vehicle inspection is sometimes required by VR services, which should be completed by an engineer or occupational therapist specializing in driver rehabilitation. After the inspection has been completed the DRS secures the client's signature, which indicates his or her acceptance of the modified vehicle. It is the vehicle modifier's responsibility to educate the client about vehicle maintenance and equipment warranties. Emergency procedures are also reviewed, such as the mechanical operation of a lift in the event of an electrical failure. The vehicle modifier also must inform the client of the Federal Motor Vehicle Safety Standards (FMVSS) and any exemptions that apply to the completed modifications.

Many vehicle modifiers are active members of NMEDA and have become Quality Assurance Program (QAP) certified. NMEDA's QAP is a nationally recognized certification program for the adaptive mobility equipment industry. Some vehicle modifiers are QAP certified, which helps to ensure that vehicle modifications have been completed by a qualified vendor. The QAP was developed to promote safety, quality, and reliability within the industry. Some states will only engage a vendor with QAP certification to perform work for the VR programs.[2]

Additionally NMEDA members are required to follow their organization's guidelines for equipment installation and vehicle modifications. NMEDA is an organization committed to help ensure accountability and professionalism in the manufacturing and installation of safe and reliable transportation and driving equipment for people with disabilities and aging-related concerns. These guidelines are updated annually because of the rapid changes in vehicle infrastructures, adapted driving equipment, and other related technology. NMEDA members are also required to adhere to the safety standards published by the National Highway Traffic Safety Administration (NHTSA), which can be found on the World Wide Web (WWW).

On completion of the vehicle modification and the on-road training program, the DRS fills out a Medical Examination Report that lists the client's restrictions, such as driving only when using hand controls, driving during the daytime, and/or driving within a specified area. The form is completed by the client's physician and is forwarded to the Department of Transportation (DOT) MVD—Medical Advisory Board for review. In most cases the client is contacted for a special road test and has access to the appropriate adapted driving aids in the vehicle as necessary. If the client passes the road test with the DOT MVD road tester, he or she is issued a restricted driver's license.

THE COMMUNITY-BASED MODEL

Driver rehabilitation services provided within a community setting is the second practice model that we will now explore. Services within the community-based model are typically offered by driving schools that are state licensed and employ driver educators and/or driving instructors. Many of these programs in the private sector have added driver rehabilitation services to their core services; however, very few of these address alternatives to driving because community mobility and driving cessation are, in all likelihood, never formally addressed. Driving schools typically provide driving instruction to able-bodied young adults and occasionally older adults. Many driver educators and driving instructors have also become DRSs by becoming involved with ADED and earning a CDRS credential. In some instances commercial driving schools also hire occupational therapists specializing in driver rehabilitation to perform the clinical evaluation and provide other specialized driver evaluation and training services.

Many programs around the United States have added cars or vans to their fleet of stock vehicles that are equipped with adapted driving equipment and other vehicle modifications designed for people with disabilities. The community driving programs usually do not require a physician's referral to see a client for driver rehabilitation services. Referrals received by DRSs working in community-based programs can originate with VR counselors, family physicians, allied health therapists working as generalists or specialists, physiatrists, vehicle modifiers, ophthalmologists, and case managers, among others. Clients and caregivers also independently seek out driver rehabilitation services.

Traditionally driver educators specializing in driver rehabilitation services will travel to a client's home to conduct the predriving and on-road evaluations and the on-road training sessions. It should be noted that the clients seen by driver educators, and especially driving instructors, usually do not present the kinds of complex medical diagnoses that occupational therapists address on a routine basis. Minimally, driver educators should consult with an occupational therapist to help ensure that the clinical evaluation is adequately performed and interpreted, which can have a dramatic impact on determining a client's readiness to drive.

A vehicle prescription that highlights recommended adapted driving aids and vehicle modifications is provided on successful completion of the on-road evaluation. Training may commence before a client receives his or her modified vehicle or afterward, depending on a variety of factors. Some key questions the DRS should consider include the following:

• How complex are the modifications and adapted driving controls?
• Does the driver rehabilitation program own a vehicle type with the kinds of modifications and adapted driving aids that the client requires for optimal safety and competence while behind the wheel?
• Is the client medically stable?

The DRS will also work closely with the client and the vehicle modifier to help ensure a successful client-vehicle fit.

If the DRS notes any further problem areas, he or she should refer the client to the appropriate health care specialist for a consultation. For example if a client's low vision impacts his or her ability to drive safely, the DRS should initiate a referral to an ophthalmologist or an occupational therapist who specializes in assessing and treating low vision; clients who opt to drive a modified van from their power wheelchairs may require a referral to a wheeled mobility and seating specialist to explore ways to improve sitting balance while driving.

Community driving schools often contract with rehabilitation centers and community hospitals that employ occupational therapists who specialize in driver rehabilitation to provide driver rehabilitation services within their respective facilities. Driver educators and commercial driving school instructors should work closely with an occupational therapist when conducting a clinical evaluation to help select the best type of vehicle, vehicle modifications, and adapted driving equipment before the on-road evaluation begins. The occupational therapist or driver educator must be seated in the vehicle while the on-road driving evaluation is taking place. Each professional makes his or her own mental notes on the client's specific and overall performance. Additionally the occupational therapist also documents in writing the client's driving performance while riding in the backseat of the evaluation vehicle. Once the on-road driving evaluation is completed the DRSs discuss the results of the comprehensive evaluation and provide their recommendations to the client, caregivers, and other driver rehabilitation team members. The occupational therapist may take the lead in interpreting the data collected during the clinical evaluation and collaborate with the driver educator to interpret and report on the data collected and documented during the on-road portion of the evaluation. If additional on-road training is recommended the driver educator or occupational therapist will complete the training with the client and provide verbal and written feedback to the other team members. The driver rehabilitation team member with the most experience (and the most knowledge) usually generates the prescription that highlights the recommended vehicle modifications and adapted driving equipment. Of course the driver educator and occupational therapist work closely with the vehicle modifier throughout the entire process. Transition training can occur in the client's personal vehicle or in the vehicle owned by the community-based driver rehabilitation program.

The driver educator or occupational therapist can help to prepare the client for the MVD road test that is a requirement for securing a driver's license. A DRS from a community-based driving program often accompanies a client seeking licensure or relicensure through the MVD. The road test conducted by the MVD occurs in the client's or driving program's vehicle. When appropriate the driver educator or occupational therapist will provide the MVD with recommendations for specific driving restrictions the client must honor to maintain his or her driving privileges.

THE INDEPENDENT ENTREPRENEUR COMMUNITY-BASED MODEL

Another kind of community-based model is one that features a professional such as an occupational therapist who has opened a for-profit driving program. Private practices are state-licensed driving schools and require a physician's referral to work with clients and caregivers. In most instances this type of program features an occupational therapist who conducts the clinical and on-road evaluations, plans and implements driver training regimens, and generates prescriptions for vehicle modifications and adapted driving aids.

These programs follow the same format as the medical model except that many private practices employ DRSs who travel to a client's neighborhood to conduct the clinical and on-road evaluations and on-road training. Variations in staffing and service delivery reveal that occupational therapists may perform the clinical evaluation while a driver educator or certified occupational therapy assistant (COTA) performs the on-road evaluations with the occupational therapist sitting in the backseat at least during the first and last on-road evaluation and/or training sessions. In some programs driver educators complete the evaluations when the client's diagnosis or diagnoses are not considered complex. One example is when a client's diagnosis is not progressive and will remain constant over time. Still other private practice programs employ DRSs from other allied health fields, such as physical therapy, speech-language pathology, and pharmacy. Irrespective of the team's professional makeup in any given program, alternative transportation options must be formally addressed, especially when a client is no longer able to drive.

THE VOCATIONAL REHABILITATION MODEL

The VR model is a state-funded model that, like other service delivery models, employs DRSs credentialed in diverse professional fields of study. The DRS is usually an occupational therapist or a driver educator who may or may not have completed the voluntary certification process administered by ADED.

Clients work with VR counselors to develop an employment plan, which may or may not include driver rehabilitation services. If driving can assist a client in securing gainful employment, the VR counselor often refers the client to a DRS for a comprehensive driving evaluation.[1] On successful completion of a predriving and on-road evaluation, behind-the-wheel training commences. Once a prescription is submitted that includes details about the recommended vehicle type, adapted driving aids, and vehicle modifications, a bidding process (similar to the processes that occur in the other practice models) will determine which vendor will perform the necessary vehicle modifications and conduct the client-vehicle fitting session(s). VR programs generally require that there must be at least three bids received from qualified vendors. A growing number of states prefer that vehicle modifiers maintain a current membership in NMEDA and participate in NMEDA's QAP accreditation. This may help a vehicle modifier be recognized and become an approved vendor who can provide state-reimbursed services and equipment to clients or caregivers. The VR counselor will then notify the client and DRS when and to whom the bid was awarded.

The client may already own a vehicle that will be modified or may plan to purchase a new or used stock or modified vehicle. However, not all vehicles are compatible with the suggested modifications and adapted driving equipment. The vehicle modifier and DRS can provide information and counseling to assist the client in making an informed decision when selecting the vehicle's make and model. The prescription that was prepared by the DRS is used to guide the driver rehabilitation team involved in this process and to keep the various team members in agreement and focused on the needs of the client. When the vehicle modifications are at the stage when it is time for the initial fitting, the vehicle modifier will contact the client and the DRS to set up a date to conduct the initial client-vehicle fitting. The client must have his or her definitive wheeled mobility aid (e.g., scooter or wheelchair) at these fittings. Once again on completion of the vehicle modifications, a formal inspection by an engineer or occupational therapist is often required. The engineer or occupational therapist will approve the vehicle only if it passes the inspection. If there are any noncompliance issues with respect to the prescription specifications, the vehicle modifier will be required to make the necessary changes, no matter how complex, and schedule another inspection with the engineer or occupational therapist before the vehicle will be released and delivered to the client. Once the client-vehicle fitting is successfully completed the client is required to pay for any of the costs incurred that are not covered by VR before the sale is finalized and the client takes possession of the vehicle.[1] Box 4-5 lists vehicle modifications that are frequently reimbursed by state VR services.

EXAMPLES OF VR SERVICE DELIVERY MODELS

Connecticut has a unique driver rehabilitation program and on further inspection can provide insight into the functioning of one VR model. Once the client and counselor determine that driving will be essential to the completion of the client's employment plan, the client is referred to one or both of the following programs for a driver evaluation. Simple or low-tech modification needs will be referred to The Department of Motor Vehicles, Handicapped Driver Training Unit. The Handicapped Driver Training Unit conducts predriving and on-road assessments, on-road training and testing, licensing, and relicensing. The employees of the Department of Motor Vehicles, Handicapped Driver Training Unit are not

BOX 4-5	Vehicle Modifications Frequently Reimbursed by State Vocational Rehabilitation Services

Rooftop wheelchair carriers
Wheelchair lifts
Power door operators
Adaptive driving aids
Electronic control consoles
Low-effort steering and braking systems
Floor modifications to accommodate a wheelchair or scooter
Six- and eight-way power transfer seat bases
Raised roofs and raised door openings that enable a client to enter a vehicle from a wheelchair
Lowered floors for minivans and full-size vans
Modified floor covering (e.g., smooth surface) for those clients who enter a van from a wheelchair
Wheelchair tie-down systems

Data from Sidlovsky A: State of Connecticut vehicle modifications, *Hartford, CT, BSS Publication #03-02, pp 4-13.*

DRSs. The evaluation indicates whether the client meets the state's minimum standards for visual acuity required for driving and what equipment and vehicle modifications the client will need to drive safely. If the client does not meet these minimum standards, he or she cannot be licensed to operate a motor vehicle.[1]

Clients in Connecticut requiring access to vehicles that have undergone complex modifications are referred to the Easter Seals Mobility Center (i.e., subcontractor to VR services) for the clinical and on-road evaluations. The Easter Seals Mobility Center employs an occupational therapist and a driver educator. The Center's personnel also write vehicle prescriptions that highlight recommendations for the preferred vehicle type, vehicle modifications, adapted driving aids, and a driver-training program. The report that is generated also indicates whether the client has demonstrated competence with regard to operating a motor vehicle while on the road. The Easter Seals Mobility Center only reimburses comprehensive driver rehabilitation evaluations in cases in which a client is in need of high-tech driving equipment. Otherwise once clients obtain their modified vehicles, they are referred back to the Department of Motor Vehicles, Handicapped Driver Training Unit to complete the on-road testing and licensing process.

The Bureau of Rehabilitation Services appoints a consultant to oversee and expedite the vehicle modification process and facilitate timely communication with the consumer, VR counselor, and vehicle modifier when there are inquiries about the status of a particular vehicle's modifications.[1] This consultant communicates (along with the Department of Motor Vehicle's handicapped driver training consultant) with the occupational therapist specializing in driver rehabilitation or engineer to review, prescribe, approve, and evaluate the client's vehicle modifications.

In Kentucky a free-standing driving program employs a VR administrator, who is a DRS, and one driver educator. This Kentucky Driving Program contracts with the University of Kentucky Medical Center to subcontract three occupational therapists who provide full-time driver rehabilitation services. All of the employees have a formal driver education endorsement earned after successfully completing several college-level courses at Eastern Kentucky University.

The initial evaluations are performed by the occupational therapists, who together with the driver educator provide on-road evaluation and training. Once the client demonstrates proficiency using low-tech adapted driving aids, the occupational therapist completes all of the necessary documentation (including the equipment prescriptions) and participates in each of the client-vehicle fittings until the client takes possession of the vehicle and is taken off schedule. This program's DRSs travel to their clients' homes to conduct the evaluations and on-road training, which is thought to have improved outcomes in Kentucky. In addition other DRSs will be contracted to perform predriving or clinical evaluations and on-road training sessions because of location or client diagnosis and equipment needed.

In more complex cases that require using high-tech equipment and vehicles, the occupational therapist, driver educator, vehicle modifier, wheeled mobility and seating specialist, and other primary and ancillary team members must work closely together to help ensure timely and accurate communication so that the client's needs are sufficiently met. The other members of the driver rehabilitation team sometimes view the driver educator as the vehicle modification specialist. The occupational therapist and driver educator collaborate to document the client's status and develop the vehicle prescriptions that highlight recommended vehicle modifications, adapted driving aids, and specific training regimens, as well as conduct the client-vehicle fittings with the vehicle modifier present.

Vehicle prescriptions require bids that are provided by at least three vehicle modifiers who are QAP accredited. Once the work is awarded to a particular vehicle modifier, the client is notified and kept abreast of the progress made toward modifying the vehicle. The client-vehicle fitting is required, and in cases in which there are complex modifications, two or even three fittings may be required before the client can take possession of the vehicle. The client is responsible for purchasing his or her own vehicle as prescribed by the DRS. The VR program will pay for the modifications within the state guidelines. As a general rule the VR program requires the client to become a licensed driver with the recommended modifications before authorizing the vehicle modifications. The ultimate goal of the client's employment plan is to become gainfully employed, and driving to the job can be a viable component as decided by the client and the VR counselor.

The occupational therapist or driver educator helps prepare the client for the Kentucky Motor Vehicle licensure road test. In most cases the client takes the road test using the program's vehicle or his or her personal vehicle. Once successfully completing the road test the client's license will indicate any applicable adapted driving equipment or driving restrictions.

Another VR driving program is in California. This particular California Department of Rehabilitation Driving Program employs a VR counselor/administrator, a rehabilitation engineer, an occupational therapist, and two driver educators. The driver educators have completed a number of college-level courses that have earned them a certificate in traffic safety. This is a closed system because this program only sees clients who qualify for the services offered through the California Department of Rehabilitation. The clients must have a viable *employment plan* and be working toward finding a job, developing job skills, pursuing education as an avenue toward gainful employment, or obtaining job training in preparation for employment. Driving is viewed as a secondary goal that may or may not support employment directly (e.g., being hired as a truck driver) or indirectly (using a vehicle to commute to and from work).

The occupational therapist performs the clinical evaluations and recommends the adapted driving aids to be used by the client during the on-road evaluation. The driver educator sets up the vehicle and completes the behind-the-wheel evaluation with the occupational therapist riding in the backseat of the evaluation vehicle. Some additional functional assessment time and on-road training may be required during subsequent visits to compile the proper information for the following reports: (1) functional assessment, written by the occupational therapist and the driver educator; (2) on-road evaluation, written by the occupational therapist and driver educator; and (3) recommendations for vehicle modifications, written by the rehabilitation engineer. The client is referred for a wheeled mobility and seating or visual perceptual/low-vision evaluation as necessary before the vehicle prescription is finalized.

Behind-the-wheel training is offered to the clients served by the California Department of Rehabilitation as a service; however, because California is such a large state, access to services can become difficult for some clients. For example clients who live far away may be referred to a local driving school to complete their training. In cases in which high-tech vehicles are required, the evaluation and training may need to be extended (e.g., approximately 20 hours) to help the DRSs make a sound decision as to whether the client should drive. The final on-road training occurs in the client's adapted vehicle on-site or at a local driving school.

The client-vehicle fitting is completed by the driver educators (i.e., occupational therapist and driver educator) or with the rehabilitation engineer. Of course the vehicle modifier and the client are always present at the fittings. The occupational therapist attends the client-vehicle fittings only if an adjustment or change is required, for example, the client's needs have changed because of diminished functioning that is related to a progressive disease. After the fittings have been completed the state vehicle inspector examines the vehicle, signs off, and approves an invoice to pay for the completed modifications. Currently the California VR system does not require vehicle modifiers to participate in the QAP; however, they are expected to implement that requirement in the near term. If the client is unable to complete the driver rehabilitation program successfully, the vehicle is recalled and reassigned to another client who may need the vehicle further modified to meet his or her unique needs.

THE UNIVERSITY MODEL

The University Model is often state- and/or federally funded and located either on a university campus or within a university-affiliated teaching hospital setting. This model usually employs occupational therapists who specialize in driver rehabilitation. Some programs also employ a driver educator. A doctor's referral is required for a client to enroll in the program, and the evaluation and training format is much the same as the Medical Model in terms of the services provided. The predriving or clinical evaluation and the on-road evaluation occur usually in an adapted car or van that is owned and maintained by the university. Vehicle prescriptions that include detailed recommendations for vehicle modification, adapted driving aids, behind-the-wheel training regimens, and vehicle fittings are featured services within this program model. University-based programs are generally provided on a fee-for-service basis and may be supported in part by grant funding.

Universities place importance on research, education, and service; therefore, driver rehabilitation programs can potentially assist faculty members and DRSs in these endeavors. For example programs offer access to prospective clients for dynamic teaching opportunities and potential research and grant activities. Programs may also offer some kind of pro bono services to clients living in the respective communities that are underserved and would otherwise be unable to receive driver rehabilitation services.

A good example of the numerous university-based programs found in the United States is located on a campus in Louisiana. This program employs an occupational therapist and a driver educator who specialize in providing driver rehabilitation services. The clinical evaluation is performed by the occupational therapist, who recommends the preferred vehicle type and modifications and applicable adapted driving aids that are required to optimize the client's performance during the on-road evaluation. The driver educator and the occupational therapist ride in the vehicle together to evaluate the client's driving skills; the driver educator usually rides in the front passenger seat, and the occupational therapist rides in the backseat. The driver educator or occupational therapist generates the vehicle prescription, with input provided by the professional playing the secondary or supportive role. Vehicle fittings are conducted with the occupational therapist, driver educator, vehicle modifier, and the client present. Sometimes the rehabilitation engineer also participates in the vehicle fittings. Most of the comprehensive driver rehabilitation evaluations locally are performed at the university setting; however, for some of the challenging high-tech van evaluations or for clients who live far from the university, driving program personnel will conduct the evaluation in or near the client's home. Because of time constraints the driving program does minimal on-road training. In most cases clients are referred to qualified driving instructors who are employed by reputable commercial driving schools and have experience working with people with disabilities and/or aging-related concerns. Behind-the-wheel training with high-tech vans is only referred to highly experienced DRSs who travel to see the clients at their locations of choice. In addition to providing driver evaluations, this program has been active in securing grant funding that has enabled continuing education workshops for DRSs locally and nationally.

THE ACUTE CARE HOSPITAL MODEL

Another example of a university model is an acute rehabilitation hospital located in the northeastern part of the United States. This program is not required by state law to have a driving school license. The administrator of the program is an occupational therapist specializing in driver rehabilitation; other team members include a driver educator specializing in driver rehabilitation and an occupational therapist who is certified as both a driving instructor and as a DRS. In this program the employees have cross-trained and collaborate on most cases. Each team member performs the clinical and on-road evaluations, documents the results, and generates modification/equipment prescriptions as needed. The driver educator performs basic assessments and routinely consults with the occupational therapist for advice on a range of issues, such as standardized testing procedures, understanding the implications that certain diagnoses can have on driving, strategies to optimize client-vehicle fittings, functional assessments, and intervention approaches to help clients plan for, and contend with, driving cessation. A rehabilitation engineer or occupational therapist conducts the vehicle inspections. This program subscribes to the notion that all clients should be evaluated while on the road with very few exceptions (e.g., recent seizure activity, vision restrictions, or both). In addition to clinical and on-road evaluations, team members also provide all behind-the-wheel training services and accompany clients when they are seeking licensure or relicensure. In some cases clients require additional therapy before they can successfully return to or begin driving. In such cases, primary driver rehabilitation team members can initiate a referral to a therapy specialist or generalist for remediation of skills and techniques that support safe driving (e.g., improving client factors such as upper extremity strength, endurance, and range of motion). Clients return to complete the driving program once the ancillary therapy services have been provided. This center is also active in research, education, and service-oriented programs, which is common within university models.

THE VETERANS AFFAIRS MODEL

The Veterans Affairs (VA) model features federally funded driver rehabilitation programs for American veterans who are either service connected or nonservice connected. The service-connected veteran is generally viewed as a higher priority than non–service-connected veterans. For a veteran to be considered service connected, his or her disability (e.g., health condition, traumatic injury, disease) must have occurred or be traceable to the time period when he or she was enlisted in the military. Driver rehabilitation programs are offered in 40 of 225 veterans' hospitals in the United States and Puerto Rico.

Therapists capable of performing comprehensive driver evaluations and on-road training within the VA system must have a minimum of a baccalaureate degree in adapted physical education, occupational therapy, kinesiotherapy, physical therapy, or a related health science field of study and specialize in driver rehabilitation. The VA DRSs attend a special 2-week course offered by the Long Beach Veterans Hospital in Long Beach, California, to hone their skills in the areas of clinical and on-road driver evaluations, client education, and on-road training. This course employs a problem-based and hands-on approach to learning and helps to prepare the participants to provide efficacious driver rehabilitation services.

Each driving program throughout the country has one primary therapist and one alternate DRS per program per facility. About one-half of the occupational therapists who provide driver rehabilitation services at veterans' hospitals are CDRSs. They are encouraged to obtain the experience required to be eligible to sit for the CDRS examination through ADED; however, not unlike other programs around the country, certification remains an optional requirement for DRSs employed by the VA.

In the past the VA administration would only approve a prescription for adapted driving aids if the recommended equipment could be found on a VA-approved adaptive driving equipment list. The rationale was based on the VA's independent testing of various kinds of adaptive driving equipment. Now prescriptions are submitted through the Prosthetics Department in the VA Central office where the requests are reviewed and either approved or denied. If the recommended adapted driving equipment is in compliance with the Society of Automotive Engineers (SAE) and NHTSA standards, the VA will usually approve the DRS's recommendations. However, the DRS must clearly document the veteran's needs and demonstrate that the recommendations are reasonable and medically necessary to meet his or her driving needs and optimize his or her safety and performance while behind the wheel of a motor vehicle. The DRS presents his or her recommendations to the VA's Acquisition and Material Management Service for completing the equipment procurement process.

For the veteran to obtain a driver rehabilitation evaluation, on-road training, adapted driving aids, and vehicle modifications, no employment plan is required. However, after the veteran's legal eligibility has been determined he or she then is referred to the physical medicine and rehabilitation department for a physical and/or psychological examination to determine whether the veteran is able to undergo special driver training. If the client is service connected, then he or she can apply for a vehicle grant for $11,000 (one-time grant). This grant is reevaluated every 2 or 3 years and adjusted accordingly because of inflation. Vehicle modifications will be provided to enable the client to drive independently or ride as a passenger in a vehicle with optimal comfort and safety. A veteran can have two vehicles modified in a 4-year period. The VA also covers maintenance of the vehicle's automatic transmission, power steering, power brakes, and vehicle modifications only if the veteran is service connected and received the grant to help pay for a vehicle. Generally the VA driving programs are a closed system (i.e., serving veterans only); however, there are two programs open to the general public on a fee-for-service basis in Richmond, Virginia, and Dallas, Texas.

CONCLUSION

Professionals who comprise the driver rehabilitation team provide a solid foundation upon which driver rehabilitation programs can operate. Each member of the driver rehabilitation team performs a vital role during clinical and on-road evaluations, the vehicle modification process, the client-vehicle fitting, and on-road driver training. The primary team members include the client, DRS, vehicle modifier, and funding source agent. Ancillary services also support the primary team by providing complementary evaluation and interventions that enable driving and/or community mobility goals to be achieved. The particular service delivery model that any given program subscribes to is often a good indicator of the kinds of services they offer. Irrespective of the program and service delivery model, however, there is a common goal that is shared by every DRS: to continuously improve the standards of driver rehabilitation practice to effectively address the complex issues and challenges that preclude clients from driving and/or accessing dependable alternative transportation. See Box 4-6 for information on locating a driver rehabilitation service provider.

SECTION III

The Role of the Vehicle Modifier: A Closer Look

Linda McQuistion • *Dana L. Roeling*

Mobility equipment dealers are people who own or operate facilities known as vehicle modification shops or mobility equipment dealerships. Their technicians work with individuals with disabilities and/or aging-related concerns who need vehicle modifications or adaptive equipment to drive independently or to be transported as a passenger. As such they fill an extremely pivotal role in the driver rehabilitation team. Not only do they serve the primary role of vehicle modifier and adaptive equipment installer, but also they assist the DRS in the vehicle selection and fitting phases of the driver rehabilitation and vehicle modification process.

| **BOX 4-6** | **Locating a Driver Rehabilitation Service Provider** |

Clients or caregivers wishing to locate a comprehensive driver rehabilitation program often begin their search by speaking with their family physician. The physician is usually aware of the local or regional driver rehabilitation programs and can write a prescription requesting a formal driving evaluation for his or her client as necessary. The referral is often as succinct as a phrase (or even a word or two) that simply requests that a "driver evaluation" be completed; he or she usually does not specify the need for a clinical versus an on-road evaluation that is followed by on-road training using appropriate adaptive driving equipment or exploration of alternatives to driving to enable community mobility.

Another way clients and caregivers seek out driver rehabilitation services is by either directly calling or stopping by a facility where a driver rehabilitation program is offered or a mobility equipment dealer's (i.e., vehicle modifier) shop is located. In the latter case the mobility equipment dealer should encourage the client to seek out a driver rehabilitation specialist (DRS) who can provide a comprehensive driver evaluation. If the client or caregiver is unclear about what kinds of services should be offered, the dealer should refer them to Table 4-1, which presents

a succinct listing of driver rehabilitation and community mobility key services and the professionals who provide them. Clients undergoing rehabilitation as inpatients or outpatients to address an injury or illness may also be referred by the occupational therapist working in the capacity as a generalist or by any one of the other driver rehabilitation team members (e.g., physiatrist, physical therapist, speech-language pathologist, nurse, social worker, neuropsychologist, or therapeutic recreation specialist) for a comprehensive driver evaluation. Many community-based organizations (e.g., religious organizations, centers for independent living, and assisted-living centers) also search for driver rehabilitation programs suitable to address their clients' driving needs, community mobility needs, or both.[1] In any case prospective clients and caregivers can be referred to the ADED's or AOTA's Web sites for a state-by-state listing of driver rehabilitation service providers. Finally it is crucial that professionals also assist prospective clients to explore funding options to help ensure they get the services they need to achieve their driver rehabilitation and community mobility goals related to being a driver, passenger, or both.

NATIONAL MOBILITY EQUIPMENT DEALERS ASSOCIATION

Founded in 1988 the *National Mobility Equipment Dealers Association* (NMEDA) is an essential part of the adaptive mobility industry. NMEDA is primarily composed of Dealer Members; however, the association also has manufacturers as a secondary membership—Associate Members. A third component of the membership is known as the Professional Members. These individuals are more diverse. They include DRSs, rehabilitation engineers, vehicle modification inspectors, state and federal government employees with a role in the industry, and others.

Many of the advances in this industry can be attributed to the association. NMEDA has developed a comprehensive set of guidelines to "direct the mobility equipment industry toward consistency, quality and compliance,"[3] as it states in its Preamble. It goes on to say that the "guidelines are established to ensure that adaptive vehicle equipment is installed and vehicle modifications are completed according to the highest level of industry standards and business practices."[3] The guidelines are considered to be a living and useful document and are therefore updated annually. This is done by a committee of highly qualified individuals, including mobility equipment dealers, adaptive equipment manufacturers, engineers, and representatives

from the original equipment manufacturers (OEMs [e.g., Ford, General Motors, and DaimlerChrysler]). The document is extensive; the 2004 edition contained 32 chapters plus terminology, illustrations, and reference sections. Each chapter provides guidance on the proper installation or modification related to one topical area, such as power door openers, extended doors, reduced effort steering, and electrically powered seat bases.

QUALITY ASSURANCE

NMEDA created a QAP for its dealers. Under this program a dealer's shop can be accredited in any or all of three categories, depending on the types of work being done at that shop. The types of accreditation are Mobility Equipment Installer, Structural Vehicle Modifier, and High-Tech Driving System Installer. To receive the accreditation the shop must meet certain standards regarding, among other things, accessibility, documentation, liability insurance, and employee training. They must track and label every vehicle that is modified under the QAP and agree to submit to periodic independent inspections of their facility and vehicles they have modified. It is no wonder that many state VR agencies now require NMEDA's QAP as a condition of funding a vehicle modification for one of their consumers. The VA has now added the QAP to its list of requirements as well.

DYNAMIC TESTING

NMEDA has also undertaken a vigorous dynamic testing program that includes crash testing of full-size Ford vans and pull testing of seat bases. The ultimate purpose of this testing is to supply members of NMEDA with manuals that contain guidelines to be followed for installing such items as lowered floors, aft-of-axel fuel systems, and raised roofs and doors that are compliant with Federal/Canadian Motor Vehicle Safety Standards (FMVSS/CMVSS) promulgated by NHTSA/Transport Canada.

SERVICE SCHOOLS

Service schools have been set up by NMEDA in conjunction with the various manufacturers of adaptive mobility equipment. Technicians must learn proper installation methods. At the same time dealers cannot afford to send their technicians all over North America for periodic training. Nor can they afford to be without them for the extensive amount of time that it would require; technicians would have to be sent to many different places to be trained to install all of the different types of adaptive equipment or to earn factory certifications from the different manufacturers. Therefore NMEDA developed service schools where multiple manufacturers come together at one location with the aim of enabling technicians to earn several certificates at one time and in one place.

THE PRIMARY ROLE: VEHICLE MODIFIER AND MOBILITY EQUIPMENT INSTALLER

The primary role of the mobility equipment dealer within the context of the driver rehabilitation team is that of vehicle modifier and mobility equipment installer. Using NMEDA's QAP accreditation standards provides a convenient framework for categorizing the types of adaptive mobility work performed at the dealers' shops. This also helps to facilitate the selection process for consumers and third-party payers. The categories of work responsibilities, which correspond to the types of QAP accreditation, are listed in Table 4-2. The specific modifications and equipment installation methods that reflect the accreditation process also are presented.

Based on the level of training of the technicians, the dealer may be qualified in one or more of the categories listed in Table 4-2. It is also expected that dealers require their technicians to keep their manufacturers' certificates current and that standards of practice are adhered to, such as structural vehicle modifiers employing only certified welders to perform the structural vehicle modifications.

Whenever vehicles are being altered mobility equipment dealers must be knowledgeable of any applicable standards or guidelines that may be impacted by such modifications. Dealers must have an understanding of the FMVSS/CMVSS. They must also have a working knowledge of what vehicle structures can be altered and what cannot be altered (also known as the make inoperative prohibition).

To help ensure drivers remain safe on the road U.S. safety standards prohibit vehicle modifiers from disengaging federally required safety equipment installed by automobile manufacturers. This prohibition inadvertently limits the mobility of people with disabilities and/or aging-related concerns. Part 49, Section 30122, of the U.S. Code of Federal Regulations contains a make inoperative prohibition to prevent vehicle modifiers from altering federally required safety equipment as defined in the FMVSS. NHTSA, which is part of the U.S. DOT, sets and enforces these standards. NHTSA set up a system to address modification requests on a case-by-case basis; however, this had been a cumbersome solution. To streamline the process and enable NHTSA to provide guidance to modifiers on the types of modifications that can be made without unduly decreasing the level of safety, the agency published its "Exemption from the Make Inoperative Prohibition" in the Federal Register on February 20, 2001.[4] The new rules allow certain modifications to be made for persons with disabilities and others without the delays of detailed written requests and case-by-case analysis. To take advantage of the exemption mobility equipment dealers must register with NHTSA. Table 4-3 lists examples of FMVSS for which NHTSA does and does not grant an exemption.

NMEDA has assisted its membership in understanding what can and cannot be modified by holding workshops at its annual conference, including articles in its newsletter the *Circuit Breaker*, and by publishing its own set of comprehensive guidelines. This, coupled with the dynamic testing program and how-to manuals, enables dealers to remain NHTSA/Transport Canada compliant. All NMEDA dealer members agree to follow the NMEDA guidelines. Failure to comply can result in possible action through the mediation committee. QAP-accredited shops must follow the guidelines as a condition of their accreditation. Failure to do so could result in serious consequences as levied by the QAP compliance committee.

The ultimate goal during the installation phase is to provide the consumer with safe, reliable transportation.

Table 4-2 National Mobility Equipment Dealers Association Categories and Modifications Included in the Accreditation Process

Type of Accreditation	Modifications or Installation Included in Process
Mobility equipment installer	Trunk lifts for wheelchairs and scooters Portable ramps Power and manual wheelchair tie-downs Simple nondriver devices Manual hand control Steering devices Left foot accelerator Pedal extensions Rooftop carriers Low- and zero-effort steering systems with backup Low- and zero-effort braking systems with backup Driver and passenger power and manual transfer seats Wheelchair lifts Secondary driving aids (nonelectrical) Driver training brakes Power seat bases
Structural vehicle modifier	All structural modifications including the following: • Lowered floors • Power pans • Raised roofs • Raised doors • Support cages
High-tech driving systems installer	All high-tech primary driving systems including the following: • Electronic and pneumatic gas/brake • Horizontal, joystick, hydraulic, and electronic steering systems • Touch pads/secondary controls (requiring electrical)

Table 4-3 National Highway Traffic Safety Administration Exemptions and Nonexemptions

Federal Motor Vehicle Safety Standards	Example
Exempt	124 Accelerator Control Systems 209 Seat Belt Assemblies 301 Fuel System Integrity 302 Flammability of Interior Materials
Not exempt	135 Passenger Car Brake Systems S5.3-1: Only if removal of OEM foot pedal is required. 202 Head Restraints: Entire standard for wheelchair-seated drivers or right front passenger or S4.3 (b) (1) and S4.3 (b) (2) minimum height specifications only if seat back/head restraint must be modified for the driver with a disability. 204 Steering Control Rearward Displacement: Entire standard when modification requires structural change to or removal of OEM steering shaft. 208 Occupant Crash Protection: S4.1.5.1 (a) (1), S4.1.5.1 (a) (3), S4.2.6.2, S5, S7.1, S7.2, and S7.4—installing air bag on/off switch or removal of the air bag or knee bolster for the seating position modified, only when type 2 or 2A seat belt meeting FMVSS 209 and 210 is installed.

Thus the final step in the modification/installation phase is to deliver the finished product to the consumer. It is beneficial for the occupational therapist specializing in driver rehabilitation to be present at delivery. The delivery process involves the following:

- Warranties: The dealer will make sure that all dealer and manufacturer warranty information is appropriately transferred to the consumer.
- Owner's manuals: The dealer provides copies of owner's manuals and reviews this information with the consumer, paying special attention to required maintenance. The dealer also provides other appropriate technical information (e.g., wiring diagrams).
- Check-out: The dealer reviews all systems with the consumer, once again paying special attention to emergency features (e.g., warning buzzers and egress).
- NHTSA requirements: If applicable the dealer explains to the consumer the concept of the exemption to the make inoperative prohibition and informs the consumer that his or her vehicle may no longer be in compliance with all FMVSS.

The dealer must then affix a permanent label to the consumer's vehicle that states: "This vehicle has been modified in accordance with 49 C.F.R. 595.6 and may no longer comply with all Federal Motor Vehicle Safety Standards in effect at the time of its original manufacture." The dealer is also required by NHTSA to provide a list of FMVSS affected to the consumer. He or she also provides a load-carrying capacity reduction disclosure, a statement based on the vehicle's gross vehicle weight rating (GVWR), in compliance with 49 C.F.R. 595, indicating any reduction in load-carrying capacity of the vehicle of >220 pounds after the modifications are complete. The dealer must inform the consumer whether the weight of his or her wheelchair is included in the available load capacity.

ANCILLARY ROLE: FITTING

As part of the driver rehabilitation team the dealer/technician works closely with the DRS and consumer during the client-vehicle fitting. This is to ensure that all equipment is positioned to optimize the functional recommendations of the DRS, consumer choice, and technical feasibility. The dealer or technician works with the team to fine-tune such items as the exact location for a remote-axis steering system or a switch site for a secondary control. The more high tech the item, the greater the number of fittings with which the dealer/technician will assist.

ANCILLARY ROLE: VEHICLE SELECTION

Not every vehicle modification or equipment installation is compatible with every stock vehicle. The dealer can assist in answering such questions as the following:

- Will this particular scooter hoist fit in my trunk?
- Can I drive a van while seated in a power wheelchair?
- Has the modified van that I will be receiving been crash tested?
- Will this high-tech driving system fit in a minivan with a lowered floor?

It is important that the consumer be advised to wait on making a vehicle purchase until after his or her adaptive driving equipment and vehicle modification needs have been fully identified and documented by the DRS, if one is required for third-party payment. The consumer certainly does not want to make an expensive mistake, like purchasing a vehicle that cannot be modified to meet his or her needs. The dealer can be a valuable resource in helping the consumer and DRS identify and even locate the right vehicle.

ANCILLARY ROLE: EQUIPMENT TRIALS

Once the DRS has determined that certain pieces of adaptive mobility equipment are needed by the consumer, he or she may want the consumer to be able to experience a trial using this technology to be certain that the consumer is able to benefit from the device before purchasing it. If the DRS does not have the exact piece(s) of equipment as part of his or her evaluation vehicle, he or she should take the consumer to a dealer's shop for an equipment trial. One example may be the use of a trunk-mounted scooter hoist for which the consumer will be required to remove the scooter seat in order to load the mobility device into his or her trunk. The DRS may have already determined that the hoist plus the scooter in question will fit nicely into the trunk of the consumer's existing vehicle. However, the DRS may want to be able to observe the consumer's ability to use the device before generating an equipment prescription.

SUMMARY

The mobility equipment dealer's primary role is that of vehicle modifier and mobility equipment installer.

This is a complicated and multifaceted role that requires the mobility equipment dealer and the dealer technicians to be appropriately educated and trained in an ongoing fashion to maintain a high level of knowledge and competence related to technical issues, government regulations, and modification procedures and techniques. NMEDA plays a pivotal role in assisting dealers and dealer employees in remaining current in their technical knowledge and skills, which is necessary to maintain NHTSA/Transport Canada compliance.

REFERENCES

1. Sidlovsky A: *State of Connecticut vehicle modifications,* Hartford, CT, BSS Publication #03-02, pp 4-13.
2. Roeling D, NMEDA: Why you need to know who we are! *Assoc Driver Rehabil Specialists NewsBreak Newsl* Summer:10, 2002.
3. NMEDA: Preamble.
4. NHTSA: *Exemption from the make inoperative prohibition,* Federal Register, February 20, 2001.[4]

Part II

MEASURING DRIVING POTENTIAL BEFORE HITTING THE ROAD

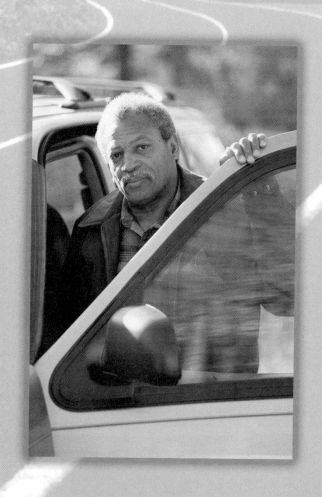

Chapter 5

THE ADAPTED DRIVING DECISION GUIDE

Joseph M. Pellerito, Jr. • *Cynthia J. Burt*

KEY TERMS

- Comprehensive driver rehabilitation evaluation
- Clinical evaluation
- On-road evaluation
- Client-centered approach
- Decision-making process
- Technology abandonment
- Comprehensive driver rehabilitation services
- Specialists
- Generalists
- Driver readiness
- Compensatory techniques
- Driving controls
- Secondary driving controls
- Risk factors
- Performance tools

CHAPTER OBJECTIVES

After completing this chapter, the reader will be able to do the following:

- Understand who can benefit from the Adapted Driving Decision Guide.
- Be aware of the primary driver rehabilitation services and the professionals responsible for providing them.
- Know the primary assessments that comprise a comprehensive driver rehabilitation evaluation.
- Appreciate how consumer involvement in the decision-making process can reduce the

occurrence of technology abandonment within the context of assistive technology and driver rehabilitation.

- Recognize the role the clinical evaluation plays in helping to determine a client's readiness to drive.
- Understand how vision, sensorimotor factors, cognitive factors, and the caregiver's role can impact driver readiness.
- Understand how a client's mobility aid and its efficient management can impact the vehicle selection and modification processes.
- Recognize how a client's transfer status can influence the vehicle selection and modification processes.
- Recognize the benefits and limitations of adapted driving from sedans, coupes, sport utility vehicles, trucks, minivans, and full-sized vans.
- Recognize how functional impairments can influence driving performance and the selection of proper adaptive driving aids.
- Recognize the role that the on-road evaluation plays in helping to identify potential adaptive driving aids, appropriate vehicle types, and vehicle modifications that can enhance a client's driving performance.
- Understand the importance of addressing alternatives to driving for community mobility when recommending that a client cease driving.
- Understand the risk factors that contribute to driving cessation, including diminished cognitive, psychomotor, and sensoriperceptual skills.

OVERVIEW

The *Adapted Driving Decision Guide* (henceforth referred to as "the guide") was produced in cooperation with health care and industry professionals, consumers, and their caregivers. The guide should not replace a *comprehensive driver rehabilitation evaluation* conducted by a driver rehabilitation specialist (DRS). Rather the guide is intended to provide DRSs, clients, caregivers, and others with information about (1) practical ways to assess an individual's driver readiness; (2) the steps involved in selecting an appropriate vehicle type that can meet a client's unique set of needs and wants; (3) structural vehicle modifications and adaptive driving aids that can enhance vehicle accessibility and a driver's on-road driving performance; and (4) the potential impact that driving cessation and access to alternative community mobility can have on improving a client's quality of life and other desired outcomes.

NAVIGATING THE GUIDE

If driver evaluation, rehabilitation, and alternative community mobility services are unfamiliar to prospective clients, professional health care providers, or both, the guide can provide a helpful tool for exploring these and other interesting topics pertaining to the rapidly changing profession of driver rehabilitation. It is recommended that the reader explore the guide in a linear fashion. That is, start from the beginning, and progress through each subsequent topic area. However, individuals who are either familiar with the field of driver rehabilitation or are wanting to find an answer to a specific question or set of questions may want to navigate through the guide in a nonlinear fashion; that is, start by selecting topics of interest, and peruse applicable content irrespective of its location within the guide. This approach can be helpful when the entire scope of the guide is not applicable to a particular reader's specific interests, needs, or both. The guide is organized in a logical fashion, with key topic areas presented in Table 5-1.

DRIVER REHABILITATION SERVICES AND A CLIENT-CENTERED APPROACH

Clients who do not drive because of functional impairments resulting from accidental injury, illness, aging-related changes, or some other cause have similar needs to maintain their community mobility (including driving a motor vehicle) as those of the general population. The DRS assesses a client's predriving status by performing a *clinical evaluation*. Once the clinical evaluation has been completed, an *on-road evaluation* is conducted by the DRS to assess the client's actual driving performance with the purpose of recommending an appropriate vehicle type, structural vehicle modifications, adaptive driving equipment, and a regimen for off-road (e.g., driving simulator) or on-road (also known as behind the wheel) driver training. DRSs can

also assist their clients with planning for, or contending with, driving cessation and exploring alternative transportation options when required.

By exploring the guide with their clients, DRSs are subscribing to a *client-centered approach*, which reinforces the belief that clients should participate fully in the decision-making process. Accessing relevant information enables clients to make informed choices and possess greater insight into how those choices may impact their health and well-being generally and driving performance or alternative community mobility outcomes specifically. The notion of clients taking a more active role in the *decision-making process*, especially within the traditional medical model, has been examined by numerous researchers; many scholars have asserted that although the idea of client involvement is a familiar concept, many professionals in the field of rehabilitation continue to function within the old medical model and support a role of passivity for the client versus the role of decision maker for the rehabilitation professional.[1-4] Moreover, findings from a number of studies have supported the importance of client involvement, but that client involvement has not become a practice fully implemented into the rehabilitation process. A client-centered approach can decrease the rate of discontinuance of assistive technology devices and increase user satisfaction because the client is involved in the selection, acquisition, training, implementation, and ongoing use of assistive technology devices.[1]

Irrespective of whether the client is a new driver or is preparing to return to driving, DRSs can use the guide to help clients make some important predriving decisions that often mark the beginning of addressing their personal needs as they are formulating their driving or alternative community mobility objectives. Of course neither clients nor DRSs should rely solely on the guide when making important decisions about driving, alternative community mobility, or both. Each client must undergo a comprehensive driver rehabilitation evaluation to fully explore the factors that can help determine whether safe and efficient driving, access to alternative transportation, or both are realistic goals. Comprehensive driver rehabilitation evaluations include the clinical and on-road evaluations.

As a DRS and client navigate the guide, content pertinent to driver assessment, rehabilitation, and training is presented that highlights key considerations and potential solutions for a variety of driving needs. Once readers have finished reading the guide's introduction (Overview), they are afforded the opportunity to respond to a series of questions in the following three sections (Driver Readiness, Vehicle Selection, and Driving Controls). Questions are presented with the aim of facilitating discussion between a client and

Table 5-1 Index of Topics

Index of Topics	Description of Topic Areas
Overview	This section provides the reader with an introduction to the *Adapted Driving Decision Guide*. Information is presented on the client-centered approach, primary and ancillary driver rehabilitation team members, tips on selecting the best driver rehabilitation program, and other content that could be considered foundational
Driver readiness	This section enables the reader to identify how visual, sensorimotor, cognitive, and psychosocial factors can impact driver readiness
Vehicle selection	This section helps the reader to understand how specific mobility aids can impact the transfer techniques used by clients when entering and exiting a vehicle and the vehicle selection process; readers will also recognize the benefits and limitations of driving different types of vehicles (e.g., sedans, coupes, SUVs, trucks, minivans, full-sized vans)
Driving controls	This section also presents questions about primary and secondary adaptive driving controls and describes how they function; the reader will examine how functional impairments can impact driving performance and how adaptive driving controls can help a client compensate for specific impairments while driving a motor vehicle; a series of client profiles that features prospective adaptive driving aids also is presented
Driving cessation	This section facilitates the reader's understanding of some of the risk factors that can contribute to driving cessation; risk factors include but are certainly not limited to decreased sensoriperceptual and psychomotor skills; the reader will also be able to explore strategies and resources for identifying alternative transportation options
Performance tools	This section presents the reader with a list of performance tools that are designed to enhance a DRS's knowledge level and professional competence; the tools included on the CD-ROM that was provided with this book include case studies, evaluation tools, and research articles, as well as a glossary of terms, materials that help define driver rehabilitation and alternative community mobility, and other information that can increase a DRS's knowledge base

DRS, Driver rehabilitation specialist; *SUV,* sport utility vehicle.

DRS about a range of driver rehabilitation and alternative community mobility topics of interest. The client's responses (and more importantly the discussion between the client and DRS that follows) will enable the DRS to more fully examine the client's driver readiness, prospective vehicle features that could potentially improve the overall client-vehicle fit, transfer techniques for getting into and out of the vehicle, storage options for personal mobility aids, and potential structural vehicle modifications and adaptive driving controls. DRSs are encouraged to document their clients' feedback to give their clients a voice, develop and refine goals and objectives, and improve the overall evaluation process.

The guide can also help clients become knowledgeable about the processes associated with driver evaluation and rehabilitation. Informed decision making

starts with educated clients who can articulate their needs and wants to DRSs and other members of the driver rehabilitation team. Maintaining clear lines of communication between clients and DRSs will not only lead to clients becoming more knowledgeable about driver rehabilitation and alternative community mobility but also will help to facilitate a culture within the field of driver rehabilitation and community mobility in which DRSs and other health care professionals value a client's full participation in the decision-making process. Reimer-Reiss and Wacker[1] reinforced this point by asserting that the best service delivery models acknowledge that clients and professionals are a part of the same team. Initially clients should be educated about their choices, financing options, training, and resources for long-term vehicle and equipment maintenance. Clients then should articulate their personal needs, goals, values, and preferences so that solutions can be formulated through an open exchange of information with the DRS and the other driver rehabilitation team members. Clients should work with their DRSs to identify preferred vehicles, structural modifications to the vehicle, adaptive driving aids, and a training regimen that will best fit their specific needs. Finally Reimer-Reiss and Wacker[1] concluded that clients must be involved in the entire evaluation process and that the identified technology must meet an important functional need or set of needs.

DRIVER REHABILITATION AND ENHANCED QUALITY OF LIFE

Assistive technology devices, including modified vehicles with adaptive driving aids, can assist people with disabilities, aging-related concerns, or both to participate in their respective communities more fully, which often results in an improved quality of life. Driver rehabilitation is also credited with helping clients achieve higher levels of functional ability and independence.[5] Assistive technology, including adaptive driving technology, is recognized as a means for individuals with disabilities to access mainstream society[6] and as a mode to potentially level the playing field[7] between clients receiving driver rehabilitation services and their peers. According to the National Center for Health Statistics,[8] >17 million Americans used an assistive technology device in 1994 to compensate for an impairment. Some researchers have attributed the increase in the initial adoption of assistive technology to the passage of federal laws that increased the funding for assistive technology devices and services during the 1980s and 1990s.

TECHNOLOGY DISCONTINUANCE

These laws have increased access to assistive technology for some people in need; however, many of those same recipients are dissatisfied and become disillusioned with devices, services such as training to use a device, or both soon after they are provided. Dissatisfaction typically results in discontinuance (sometimes referred to as abandonment) of assistive technology devices according to Reimer-Reiss and Wacker.[1] A national survey conducted about a decade ago on *technology abandonment* found that 29.3% of all devices obtained by clients were eventually abandoned.[5] In a more recent study Scherer[9] reported that despite the assistance and enhanced independence offered by many assistive devices and the growth in assistive technology options in general, the rate of assistive technology nonuse, abandonment, and discontinuance remains high; that is, on average, nearly

one-third of all devices provided to consumers are not used soon after they are provided. The rate of technology abandonment as reported at the 1999 California State University, Northridge (CSUN) conference was as high as 80%, and others such as Philip and Zhao[5] suggested technology abandonment is at a rate of ≥29%.

Rogers[10] found that professional support is one of the variables most highly correlated to appropriate and continued use of technology. Research on assistive technology has reinforced this finding and contends that individuals with disabilities and elderly people without support are typically less successful than those who are supported. The following excerpt from Reimer-Reiss and Wacker[1] further reinforces the need to involve clients in the decision-making process to reduce the likelihood of them rejecting adaptive driving solutions recommended by the DRS and driver rehabilitation team:

> Consistent with the literature on assistive technology, consumer involvement was related to assistive technology continuance/discontinuance. The literature demonstrated that consumers who do not believe that they are involved in the selection of their assistive technology devices are more likely to discontinue using them than individuals who feel involved.... The significant inverse relationship between consumer involvement and discontinuance of assistive technology provides further justification for professionals to involve individuals with disabilities in all aspects of decision making. Consumer involvement is not a new concept in the field of rehabilitation and has been discussed extensively in the literature. Several authors noted that a consumer-driven model provides the consumer with a sense of ownership and responsibility which often leads to continued use of assistive technology.

KEY DRIVER REHABILITATION SERVICES

There are numerous service delivery models presented in Chapters 1, 4, and 26, and these models reflect current standards of practice in the United States and abroad. However, irrespective of the service delivery model that is being examined, driver rehabilitation programs that claim to offer *comprehensive driver rehabilitation services* must either provide the key services listed in Box 5-1 to be considered a one-stop shop or collaborate with other providers in their service areas to provide a full continuum of services. For example it is important that DRSs who solely provide clinical evaluations (Table 5-2) should collaborate with an established driver rehabilitation program that can augment the clinical evaluation with other important driver rehabilitation services, such as on-road evaluations and training. It is also important to note that alternative community mobility services, such as developing and implementing a driving cessation plan, strategizing how to access and use alternative transportation, or both should be addressed during a comprehensive driver rehabilitation evaluation whenever necessary. DRSs also should address issues pertaining to driving cessation and alternative community mobility (irrespective of their professional training and experience) when applicable to ensure that they are comprehensive in their delivery of driver rehabilitation and community mobility services.

DRIVER REHABILITATION TEAM MEMBERS AND KEY SERVICES

In Chapter 4 the reader learned that the services offered by a driver rehabilitation program are usually a good indicator of the professionals who comprise a particular program's driver rehabilitation team. Every driver rehabilitation program employs primary team members to provide key driver rehabilitation services, irrespective of the program's service delivery model, team structure, and services. Among these dedicated professionals is the DRS; the DRS plays the central role in providing efficacious driver rehabilitation and more recently alternative community mobility services to clients and their caregivers. DRSs work with other health care professionals, including ancillary driver rehabilitation team members, to help ensure that clients achieve their driver rehabilitation goals, alternative community mobility goals, or both. See Box 5-2 for a list of driver rehabilitation primary and ancillary team members and Table 4-1 for key driver rehabilitation and alternative community mobility services and the professionals responsible for providing these services.

EVALUATING A DRIVER REHABILITATION PROGRAM

Clients may require the assistance of their caregivers, health care workers, or both to recognize the key factors that should be considered when evaluating prospective driver rehabilitation programs. In addition to helping their clients identify reputable driver rehabilitation programs and DRSs, professionals can counsel them on how to advocate for themselves with regard to accessing services, equipment, and funding. To be an effective advocate, a client or caregiver must be able to ask the right questions when attempting to discern whether a particular program would meet the client's specific needs. See Box 5-3 for a list of key questions that a client or caregiver should ask when evaluating a driver rehabilitation program. The Association for Driver Rehabilitation Specialists (ADED), the organization that certifies DRSs, and the American Occupational Therapy Association (AOTA) can suggest a qualified program or specialist in a client's geographic area, especially if the client lives in or near a medium- to large-sized city.

DRIVER READINESS

The sections on Driver Readiness, Vehicle Selection, and Driving Controls of the guide present questions meant to stimulate discussion between the client and DRS. Individuals can also benefit from perusing these sections independently to contemplate the questions presented, the answers provided, and the implications

---

BOX 5-1 | Key Driver Rehabilitation Services

Driver evaluation and rehabilitation services may include the following:
- Predriving screenings during an occupational therapy generalist's activities of daily living or instrumental activities of daily living assessment
- Clinical evaluations that entail assessing a client's physical, sensory, and cognitive abilities (see Table 5-2 for a succinct list of common clinical assessments that are combined to create the clinical evaluation)
- In-vehicle assessments to help determine the best vehicle type, adaptive driving aids, and structural modifications to the vehicle before taking a client on the road. See Chapter 11 for more information on preparing for the on-road evaluation.
- Off-road assessments and training can be conducted on a driving range or in an isolated parking lot, which enables the client to learn and practice driving skills in a protected physical environment

- The on-road driving evaluation examines the client's ability to access a vehicle, stow and secure an ambulation aid as necessary, and drive a vehicle with or without structural modifications, adaptive driving equipment, or both
- A driving simulator can be used as a tool to assess driver readiness or as a means for driver remediation and training in a protected virtual environment
- Assistance with the vehicle selection process
- Recommendations for structural vehicle modifications
- Recommendations for adaptive driving aids
- On- or off-road driver training while using a specific vehicle with or without structural vehicle modifications, adaptive driving controls, or both
- Developing and implementing driving cessation plans and providing counseling that includes exploring alternative community mobility options and coping strategies
- Exploring funding options for driver rehabilitation and community mobility services and equipment

Table 5-2   **The Clinical Assessments Used by DRSs While Conducting the First Part of a Comprehensive Driver Rehabilitation Evaluation**

The Clinical Evaluation Components	Client Factors	Assessment Tools
Initial interview with client, caregivers, and family	• Client's medical and social history • Caregiver and family input	• Interview guide that is program specific
Physical assessments	• ROM • Strength • Fine motor coordination • Muscle tone	• Goniometric ROM measurements (procedure available in Norkin, 2003; norms available in Pedretti, 2001) • MMT (procedure available in Hislop & Montgomery, 2002) • Hand-held dynamometry (norms available in Mathiowetz, et al, 1985; positioning available in Pedretti, 2001) • Hand-held pinch gauge (positioning available in Pedretti, 2001; Adult Norms available from Mathiowetz et al, 1985) • Nine Hole Peg test (tool available from Sammons Preston P.O. Box 5071 Bolingbrook, IL 60440 (1-800-547-4333; Adult Norms available from Oxford et al, 2003) • Examination and observation
	• Proprioception and Kinesthesia	• Examination and observation
	• Endurance	• Observation
	• Balance (static and dynamic) • Sitting balance • Standing balance • Ambulation status • Primary ambulation aid used • Wheeled mobility and seating	• Berg Balance Scale (Available at www.chcr.brown.edu/Balance.html). • Tinetti Assessment Tool (including balance test and gait test) (information available at www.injuryresearch.bc.ca/Publications/Repository/Tinetti%20Balance%20Scale.pdf). See also Tinetti, 1986 • Dynamic Gait Index (see http://r-sports.hp.infoseek.co.jp/siryou/blance/dgi.doc) • Interview and observation • Consultation with the primary OT and PT generalists and seating specialists as needed
	• Tactile sensation • Light and deep pressure • Stereognosis	• Sensation kit
	• Brake reaction time	• Brake reaction test (see www.neuropsychonline.com/loni/jcrarchives/vol06/v6i5(engum).pdf page 6 of 18)
Visual assessments	• Visual acuity • Peripheral vision • Depth perception • Color perception • Road sign recognition • Binocular glare testing • Contrast sensitivity	• Optec Vision Tester (see Optic Vision Tester: Reference and Instruction Manual, 1993) • Snellen Chart (available at www.mdsupport.org/snellen.html) • TVPS-R (Test of visual perceptual skills) (available at http://www.slosson.com/productCat7054.ctlg) • Hooper Visual Organization Test available (at http://buros.unl.edu/buros/jsp/reviews.jsp?item=06001167)

Table 5-2 The Clinical Assessments Used by DRSs While Conducting the First Part of a Comprehensive Driver Rehabilitation Evaluation—cont'd

The Clinical Evaluation Components	Client Factors	Assessment Tools
	• Stereopsis • Contrast sensitivity • Peripheral vision • Tracking • Convergence • Saccades • Pursuits	• UFOV test available to purchase (at http://www.psychcorp.com.au/otprod.htm#Adol) • Beery-Buktenica Developmental Test of Visual-Motor Integration (VMI) (available at http://www.pearsonassessments.com/tests/vmi.html) • Benton Visual Retention Test (available at http://buros.unl.edu/buros/jsp/reviews.jsp?item=06000306) • Dynavision (available from Performance Enterprises, 76 Major Button's Drive, Markham, Ontario, Canada L3P 3G7 Phone 905-472-9074 Fax 905-294-6327 www.dynavision2000.com blackjones@home.com)
Cognitive and visual perceptual assessments	• Form constancy • Visual memory • Visual closure • Visual discrimination	• Motor-Free Visual Perceptual Test (MVPT-3) (available at www.proedinc.com/store/index.php?mode=product_detail&id=10081) • Trail Making Test (available at www.medicine.uiowa.edu/igec/tools/assets/trail_making_test.pdf) • CLOX 1 CLOX 2 (instructions available at http://geriatrics.uthscsa.edu/educational/med_students/clox_admin.html) • Rivermead Behavioral Memory Test (available at http://www.nss-nrs.com/cgi-bin/WebObjects/NSS.woa/wa/Products/detail?id=1000073) • Cognitive Linguistic Quick Test (CLQT) (available at http://www.psychcorp.com.au/clqt.html)

DRS, Driver rehabilitation specialist; *ROM*, range of motion; *MMT*, manual muscle testing; *PT*, physical therapist.

of the two. This process of course can and should occur when clients are available and according to their own schedules. The concepts contained within the guide may be more readily acquired because the reader can approach the learning process when he or she is perhaps most ready to learn, irrespective of the time of day. Finally a high degree of privacy is afforded to the learner, which can also more effectively engage clients and caregivers as compared with other educational methods that are sometimes used, such as group lectures, the dissemination of printed materials, and even informal dialogue between the client and DRS.

HAS MAXIMUM RECOVERY POTENTIAL BEEN REACHED?

Physicians and other health care professionals consider a client's diagnosis, past and current health status, and response to treatment after an injury or illness (among other factors) when formulating a prognosis and trajectory for recovery. For example timing is important in

determining when to initiate a comprehensive driver rehabilitation evaluation because it can be prudent (in some cases) to wait until the client has reached his or her maximum recovery potential before investing limited human and financial resources on a comprehensive driver rehabilitation evaluation, purchasing or leasing a vehicle, and/or performing vehicle modifications that may not be required at some point in the near future because the client's status is steadily improving. It is the DRS's responsibility to help coordinate the evaluation and training processes, and that includes working with the other driver rehabilitation team members to determine when driver rehabilitation services can best be rendered.

DOES THE CLIENT POSSESS OR PLAN TO OBTAIN A VALID DRIVER'S LICENSE?

Most states require clients who are diagnosed with one or more health conditions that negatively affect their ability to drive to report them on their driver's license

---

| **BOX 5-2** | **Driver Rehabilitation Primary and Ancillary Team Members** |

PRIMARY TEAM MEMBERS
- The client
- The client's chief caregivers
- The primary driver rehabilitation specialist (DRS) assigned to the client's case, such as an occupational therapist, driver educator, or other health care professional who has specialized in driver rehabilitation (e.g., pharmacists, physical therapists, and rehabilitation engineers)
- Vehicle modifier (also known as the mobility equipment dealer)
- Physicians such as the client's physiatrist or general practitioner
- Case managers

ANCILLARY TEAM MEMBERS
- The client's friends and extended family members
- Occupational therapy generalists
- Occupational therapy assistants
- Neuropsychologists/psychologists
- Other allied health professionals working as *generalists* in their respective areas of practice (e.g., speech-language pathologists, audiologists, physical therapists, therapeutic recreation specialists, social workers, nurses, physicians, orthotists, and prosthetists)
- Other allied health professionals working as *specialists* in their respective areas of practice (e.g., occupational or physical therapy wheeled mobility and seating specialists, occupational therapy low vision specialists, surgeons, ophthalmologists, and geriatricians)
- Occupational therapists or other allied health professionals specializing in driver rehabilitation who are not assigned to a particular client's case but are consulted for input by the primary DRS
- Personnel working in state departments responsible for licensing and relicensing driver applicants

---

| **BOX 5-3** | **Key Questions to Ask Before Selecting a Driver Rehabilitation Program** |

Health care providers can help their clients make informed decisions about which prospective programs and driver rehabilitation specialists (DRSs) could potentially meet their individual driving needs, alternative community mobility needs, or both. Making the right selection depends on whether clients and their caregivers are aware of some of the important questions to ask, including the following:
- Does the program provide a full spectrum of driver rehabilitation and alternative community mobility services? Are descriptions of the services offered and other key information, such as hours of operation and days the program is open for business, readily available in print and on the program's web site?
- Is the program easily accessible in terms of its physical location; that is, where is the program's storefront located in relationship to the client's residence? Will the DRS visit the client near or at his or her home to provide professional services?
- Are the program's personnel, including the DRS and the person responsible for scheduling the appointments, readily available to answer any questions the client or caregiver deems important?
- Does the DRS promptly return telephone inquiries and thoroughly answer any questions the client has pertaining to the requested services?
- Does the DRS's professional background lend itself to ensuring that he or she views clients holistically and that he or she is competent with conducting evidence-based evaluations and training?
- How extensive is the DRS's experience in driver rehabilitation? Has he or she had experience in conducting clinical evaluations and on-road evaluations and training?
- Has the DRS voluntarily completed the requirements to become a certified driver rehabilitation specialist (CDRS) through the Association of Driver Rehabilitation Specialists (ADED) or attained an equivalent credential offered by the American Occupational Therapy Association (AOTA)?
- Does the DRS adequately address driving cessation and explore alternative community mobility versus simply providing a list of potential resources or not address them at all?
- Does the DRS maintain his or her memberships in the professional organizations that promote evidence-based practice and a client-centered approach, such as ADED and AOTA?

applications they submit to their respective state licensing authorities. Moreover states usually indicate on the licenses of people who use modified vehicles that they are competent to do so. DRSs can help their clients determine whether they meet their respective state's licensing criteria by helping them understand the legal, ethical, and practical implications of public policy such as laws and state agency notification requirements. See Appendix A for more information on state licensing requirements and reporting laws. See also Chapters 7, 21, and 23 for more information on driver readiness, driving cessation, and driver rehabilitation legal and professional ethics. ADED, the organization that certifies driver rehabilitation specialists (CDRSs), and the AOTA provide information on their respective web sites on how to locate a qualified driver rehabilitation program by state and geographic area.

IS THE CLIENT'S VISION STABLE?

Many diagnoses, such as stroke, acquired brain injury, cerebral palsy (CP), brain tumors, diabetes mellitus (DM), macular degeneration, and multiple sclerosis (MS), among others, can affect an individual's visual acuity, cognition, and visual perception,[11] which can in turn impair an individual's ability to drive safely. For example Fisk et al.[12] found that survivors of stroke had impaired contrast sensitivity, peripheral vision, and useful field of view, which can decrease driving performance. Brain injuries often include a whiplash injury component that can result in oculomotor complications.[13,14] Some researchers have reported that visual acuity, oculomotor abnormalities, and refractive errors have been observed in patients with CP.[15,16] Research has also shown that DM can affect vision in dramatic ways, including macular degeneration[11,17] and diabetic retinopathy, which can also negatively affect driving performance.[18] Of course vision can also be affected by the aging process.[19-21] Clients demonstrating difficulty with personal mobility when using a wheelchair or ambulation aid because of decreased visual acuity, visual perception, and/or cognition are not likely to be able to operate a motor vehicle safely. See Chapters 6, 12, and 21 and Appendix A for more information on vision and driving.

IS THE CLIENT'S HEARING INTACT?

Hearing plays an important role in overall driving performance. If there are functional limitations because of impaired hearing, compensatory strategies must be used. See Chapters 6, 12, and 13 for more information on how hearing impairments impact driving and compensatory strategies DRSs frequently use to address this problem.

CAN THE CLIENT MAINTAIN BALANCE?

To drive a car while sitting on an original equipment manufacturer's (OEM) seat, a driver must be able to stow his or her ambulation aid while maintaining his or her balance so that the ambulation device, such as a manual wheelchair, does not interfere with being able to open the vehicle's door. Possessing the ability to maintain one's sitting or standing balance while stowing a mobility aid is another important factor that can impact the type of vehicle that is recommended and the client's safety. For a client who will not be using a modified van and will not be driving while seated in a manual wheelchair, adequate sitting balance is required to be able to safely disassemble, load, and secure the wheelchair into a vehicle. This is often the case if there is no one else to assist with this task or if a rooftop electromechanical wheelchair storage system is not a viable solution.

Clients who use motorized scooters for near-distance community mobility and are not planning on using adapted vans will most likely benefit from an electromechanical hoist that is designed to enable them or their caregivers to lift and load their wheeled mobility aids into a full-sized car's trunk, a pickup truck's payload area, or a sport utility vehicle (SUV). The client or caregiver is then required to secure the scooter by securing it to a docking device before transferring into the vehicle. The docking device is designed to secure the scooter while the vehicle and its occupants are en route. Once this task has been accomplished, the client must be able to ambulate a short distance to the driver's side door and transfer into the vehicle. Functionally intact standing balance may mean the difference between driving from an OEM driver's seat in a stock vehicle versus having to use a wheeled mobility device with a more expensive and confining seating and positioning system in an adapted vehicle, such as a structurally modified minivan or full-sized van with a wheelchair lift or ramp.

Medical conditions that are the result of illness, injury, the aging process, or any combination of these and other factors can impair clients' sensorimotor status and preclude them from driving, using alternative transportation, or both. The following "yes or no" questions address some of the important factors to consider before making a determination about *driver readiness*. In many instances the answers to these questions are more complex and therefore require more than a concrete "yes" or "no" response. Often they require thoughtful dialogue between the DRS and client because the answer is sometimes "maybe" or even "I don't know." These questions are also important to consider before initiating a predriving clinical evaluation or on-road driving evaluation. Possible answers to these questions also should be contemplated before the DRS and client make decisions about a preferred vehicle type, structural vehicle modifications, and adaptive driving equipment.

HAS THE CLIENT MAXIMIZED ACTIVE RANGE OF MOTION, STRENGTH, AND SENSATION IN THE HEAD AND NECK, UPPER EXTREMITIES, AND TRUNK?

Being able to move one's head and arms, maintain a functional sitting posture, and sense one's position in space (proprioception), and having awareness of movement (kinesthesia) are important factors that can make a difference when determining whether a client has some of the foundational skills that are necessary to drive with or without vehicle modifications. However, there are no standardized anthropometric data that provide the quantitative thresholds required to perform the myriad tasks associated with driving preparation (e.g., accessing the vehicle, securing the seat belt, and adjusting the mirrors and seat) and actual driving performance tasks with efficiency and safety for people with disabilities, aging-related concerns, or both.

DRSs must combine objective assessments that have been shown to provide meaningful and valid data with clinical reasoning that is grounded in evidence-based practice when making judgments about clients' driver readiness. Ultimately it is experience and professional networking that provides the critical link between theory and practice. Finally DRSs must view each client holistically. For example not every client uses one or both upper extremities to drive, which underscores the need to assess lower and upper extremity function and the other client factors (e.g., cognition, visual perception, and visual acuity) that provide the foundation on which activities, habits, and occupations such as driving or using alternative transportation can be successfully performed.

HAS THE CLIENT MAXIMIZED BASIC ACTIVITIES OF DAILY LIVING, ABILITY TO PERFORM TRANSFERS, AND MOBILITY STATUS?

If the client's prognosis is expected to decline because his or her condition is deteriorating (e.g., amyotrophic lateral sclerosis), rather than remaining static (e.g., upper extremity amputation) or improving in the short term (e.g., right total knee arthroplasty), the DRS should recognize that the client's needs will inevitably change in time, making equipment recommendations and driver training strategies potentially obsolete and ineffective. Therefore the client's functional capacity

status should be reevaluated at regular and predetermined intervals that are agreed on by the DRS, client, and other driver rehabilitation team members. Recommendations can then be updated accordingly to reflect the client's current status and anticipated needs for the short and long term.

IS THE CLIENT TOPOGRAPHICALLY ORIENTED IN FAMILIAR COMMUNITY ENVIRONMENTS?

A driver generally should be independent navigating a motor vehicle throughout familiar community settings. Drivers must possess adequate memory, problem solving, complex attention, orientation, and visual acuity and perception (among other factors) to be topographically oriented.[22] Otherwise problems may arise, such as getting lost and becoming increasingly confused or frustrated or venturing into areas that have high crime rates or that lack critical services such as hospitals, gas stations, and police and fire services. DRSs may need to assist their clients with input from their caregivers when appropriate to weigh the benefits versus risks associated with driving if they require supervision because they lack topographic orientation when attempting to navigate through familiar areas. If clients only become confused in unfamiliar areas, DRSs must assess whether their clients can use *compensatory techniques* (maps) or technology (e.g., OnStar [General Motors, Detroit, MI], dashboard compasses, global positioning satellite navigational systems, and cellular phones) to reach their desired destinations safely and within reasonable amounts of time.

DOES THE CLIENT HAVE AN APPOINTED LEGAL GUARDIAN? DO THE CLIENT'S CAREGIVERS SUPPORT DRIVING?

Many states will not permit individuals to acquire or keep driver's licenses if they have legal guardians. Clients who require 24-hour supervision are usually advised not to drive (or to drive minimally) or not to drive without another adult, such as their legal guardian, who can assist with navigation, especially through unfamiliar areas, during inclement weather, and in other instances in which increased stress can negatively impact driving performance. In states that do allow adult clients with guardians to drive, however, guardians should be aware of the applicable laws within the states where they reside and be aware of their own liability if their loved one is involved in a traffic accident.

DRSs should consider whether a client's caregivers are in support of the client's desire to drive a motor vehicle with or without modifications.[23] For example a disagreement between a client and his or her family member over the family member's perception of the client's lack of readiness to drive can become emotionally charged and counterproductive for everyone involved. In some instances caregivers may not want to be the bearer of bad news and will encourage their loved ones to undergo a comprehensive driver rehabilitation evaluation because they suspect the client will not successfully pass the evaluation. The DRS should ask for the client's approval to speak with his or her family member or members about their concerns and opinions about the client's readiness to drive before initiating the clinical and on-road evaluations. The DRS should also consider the fact that a comprehensive driver rehabilitation evaluation takes place in a relatively short time period, but the client's family has observed the client's behavior for a much longer period and usually possesses insight that can help the DRS make a more informed assessment of the client's readiness to get behind the wheel of a motor vehicle. Regardless of the family member's opinion, however, DRSs must come to their own conclusions based on thorough clinical evaluations and on-road evaluations.

It is also important to keep in mind that family members in some instances have ulterior motives for wanting their loved ones to fail a driving evaluation. For example driving cessation may result in the family members realizing some tangible gain, such as possession of the client's vehicle, which explains their opposition to assisting the client to drive. Moreover a family member may harbor biases about his or her loved one's ability to drive simply because he or she is elderly. The caregiver may believe that everyone older than a certain age should stop driving, irrespective of their ability to drive safely, and no argument that is bolstered with facts based on the client's successful driving performance and research will influence the caregiver to alter his or her position. This may sound peculiar to most people but underscores the fact that many caregivers who are also family members may not be able to be objective when it comes to making their own assessments of their loved one's ability or inability to drive. Finally a caregiver may not want to assume the responsibility or expend the necessary time commitment to help his or her loved one enjoy the benefits associated with alternative community mobility, such as full community participation (e.g., shopping, attending church, and visiting relatives and friends), if driving cessation is determined to be necessary to help ensure the safety and well-being of the client and other road users. In the event that a client does not successfully complete a driver rehabilitation evaluation, it is critical that the DRS address the issue of alternative community mobility if the client is going to be able to enjoy sustained community participation, age in place, and engage in meaningful and life-affirming activities. For more information on driving cessation,

see the section on Driving Cessation of this guide and Chapter 22 and Appendices G and H.

VEHICLE SELECTION

DOES THE CLIENT NEED ASSISTANCE ENTERING OR EXITING A VEHICLE FROM THE DRIVER'S SIDE?

In some cases a client may be able to transfer onto the OEM driver's seat from outside the vehicle but will require additional assistance stowing his or her mobility device. For example a client who has sustained a spinal cord injury (SCI) and is diagnosed with tetraplegia (quadriplegia) will require assistance with stowing a manual ultralightweight wheelchair and perhaps some aspect of transferring into and out of the vehicle using a sit-pivot or sliding board style transfer technique. The associated costs of modifying a vehicle that would enable greater access while the client remains in his or her wheeled mobility device could be justified and should be strongly considered. This is especially true when considering the fact that the client requires assistance with entering and exiting the vehicle, stowing his or her manual wheelchair, and performing the transfer task safely and efficiently.

The client should also consider that the person who is assisting him or her could also be the driver. In this scenario, the client would be the passenger and could save the money that would have been spent on structural modifications to the vehicle and adaptive driving controls. Of course driving may be the client's ultimate goal, and he or she may possess the financial resources or have access to other funding sources that would help procure a modified vehicle designed to facilitate easier and safer vehicle accessibility and driving for independent community mobility. The DRS may consider referring the client to receive ancillary therapy services to improve the client's balance, strength, and endurance that are required to perform the predriving and postdriving tasks, such as transferring into and out of the vehicle and loading and unloading a wheeled mobility device or ambulation aid safely and efficiently. See Chapter 15 for more information on funding driver rehabilitation and community mobility services and equipment.

DOES THE CLIENT NEED ASSISTANCE WITH COMMUNITY MOBILITY THAT DOES NOT INVOLVE DRIVING?

Clients who require supervision, physical assistance, or both for alternative community mobility (e.g., ambulating to the bus stop) because of low endurance or being at risk for falling should compare the costs of modifying a motor vehicle for adapted driving versus the potential cost savings that could be realized if the client's caregiver providing the necessary assistance could be identified as the driver instead of fulfilling the role of the helper and perhaps passenger. Referring the client to receive ancillary therapy services from occupational and physical therapy generalists with the aim of evaluating the client's rehabilitation potential and implementing intervention plans that are designed to help the client perform community mobility tasks with improved endurance and safety may also be warranted. Therapy generalists are well-prepared to evaluate the client's rehabilitation potential and implement interventions that are designed to improve the client factors, such as strength, endurance, and cognition, that support the performance of driving and community mobility tasks with adequate endurance, safety, and efficiency.

DOES THE CLIENT USE A MOBILITY AID WHEN TRAVELING THROUGHOUT THE COMMUNITY?

If the client uses more than one mobility aid, consider the primary mobility aid to be the one that is most often used when he or she is away from home and traveling short distances in the community. Outside activities typically require more effort and stamina than indoor activities. Therefore most people consider their primary mobility aids to be the ones that help them conserve the greatest amount of energy and extend their endurance while moving about in the community. The following is a list of mobility aids and a brief explanation of each.

Power Wheelchairs

There are numerous reasons why people use power wheelchairs. For example individuals who cannot ambulate with or without using an ambulation aid for community distances or who cannot propel a manual wheelchair with their upper extremities, feet, or both often benefit from power wheelchairs. Power wheelchairs require less energy expenditure than other types of mobility aids (e.g., manual wheelchairs, walkers, and canes) and extend the endurance of those who use them because of the reduced physical effort required for personal mobility. Clients with musculoskeletal complications, such as arthritis, and those who are at risk for repetitive stress injuries or have neuromuscular deficits[24] also can benefit greatly from using a power wheelchair for personal community mobility. However, it is important that clients do not become deconditioned as a result of no longer ambulating short community distances. Therefore a therapeutic exercise regimen should be developed for the client by an occupational or physical therapy generalist to compensate for the decreased physical activity.

Power chairs can be classified many different ways. Conventional power wheelchairs can resemble a manual wheelchair frame that has been modified to include motors that drive the rear wheels by belts or gears.[24] However, contemporary power chairs have a power base and feature a separate seating system, such as a tilt-in-space, recliner, or tilt-and-recline system. Power wheelchairs with such bases feature front-, mid-, or rear-wheel drive with numerous wheel diameter options.[24] Mid-wheel drive chairs by and large have a smaller turning radius that can improve overall maneuverability, especially in confined areas. Power base wheelchairs also enable rehabilitation engineering technologists (RETs) and durable medical equipment (DME) dealers to work with occupational and physical therapy seating and wheeled mobility specialists to modify the seating system as a client's stature changes in time (e.g., a growing child or an adult who gains weight because of a reduced activity level or as a result of a particular drug therapy regimen's side effects). These power wheelchairs are dependable indoors and outdoors for community mobility over short distances. Clients who use power wheelchairs for community mobility must obey the same laws that apply to pedestrians, such as not driving in the street, making sure to cross a street at a crosswalk when available, and obeying street lights.

To simplify the presentation of the general types of power wheelchairs, four categories from the least complex to the most advanced are presented here:

1. Manual wheelchairs with add-on units (Medicare miscellaneous reimbursement code K0108 because Medicare does not recognize this type of wheelchair as a reimbursable item): These chairs feature a power pack that is added on to the existing manual wheelchair. These wheelchairs and some of the so-called hybrid wheelchairs can be disassembled and folded to stow away in a vehicle when not in use.
2. Low-end power wheelchairs, including scooters (Medicare reimbursement code K0010): These chairs are not programmable, have a potentiometer that can adjust the preset speed setting up to a 3% variation, and typically include a joystick control of the wheelchair's speed and direction. Some standard power wheelchairs have folding frames for easier storage when not in use; however, this usually requires the assistance of a caregiver who can lift the wheelchair's components and stow them in the vehicle, which is not a simple task.[25]
3. High-end power wheelchairs (Medicare reimbursement code K0012): These chairs are oper-

ated with a joystick driving control or alternative driving control device, such as a sip-and-puff control, chin control, or proportional head control. High-end power wheelchairs have programmable electronics for fine-tuning performance adjustments, such as forward, reverse, acceleration, and deceleration. These chairs may also be equipped with tilt-in-space, recline, or a combination of tilt-and-recline features that enable the client to perform pressure relief and achieve a reclined position in the event of the onset of orthostatic hypotension. This class of power wheelchairs does not have a folding frame and requires clients to use modified full-sized vans or minivans for vehicle accessibility.

4. Ultrahigh-end power wheelchairs (Medicare reimbursement codes K0012 and K00014 depending on weight limitations of the power base and available electronic options): These chairs offer functionality beyond mobility, such as seat elevation or the ability to lift the user to a standing or near-standing position. Ultrapower chairs are not collapsible and often require a specialized tiedown system for securing them in the vehicle. It is important that the wheelchair manufacturer confirms that the power wheelchair is compatible with the selected tiedown securement system, irrespective of whether the client will be a driver or passenger. The client may also not be able to drive from some ultrahigh-end power wheelchairs because they may not be compatible with existing vehicle types and tiedown systems. Certain systems may not facilitate adequate line of sight, which depends on proper positioning of the client.

Manual Wheelchairs

Manual wheelchairs are available with rigid frames for greater maneuverability in tight spaces and a stiffer ride or with folding frames that add weight but may be easier to load and stow for some people when the wheelchair is not in use. Folding manual wheelchairs have only a few removable parts that usually include a seat cushion, footrests, and armrests. Most clients who use folding wheelchairs and drive elect to stow their wheelchairs by lifting them into the backseat of a two-door car while seated on the OEM driver's seat. Rigid-frame manual chairs enable clients to remove and stow the wheels, fold down the wheelchair's backrest compactly, and place the individual pieces of the wheelchair into the vehicle. The frame of a rigid wheelchair is often small enough for a client to pull it over his or her lap between the steering wheel and his or her chest and place it on the passenger's seat or backseat.

There are five basic types of manual wheelchairs:

1. Lightweight manual wheelchairs (Medicare reimbursement K0004 and weighs between 26 and 36 lb): Multipurpose chairs that are constructed with lighter-weight materials, such as aluminum, for reduced effort and easier transportation
2. Ultralightweight manual wheelchairs (Medicare reimbursement K0005 and weighs <26 lb): Made of strong but lightweight materials, such as titanium, and are designed for active clients who may or may not participate in adapted sports and recreation, such as competitive racing or wheelchair basketball[26]
3. Economy manual wheelchairs (standard Medicare reimbursement K0001, weighs >36 lb, and supports clients weighing ≤250 lb): The no-frills version of a standard folding manual wheelchair is heavier and bulkier than the lightweight or ultralightweight models and features simple sling upholstery and steel and chrome parts.
4. Heavy-duty specialty manual wheelchairs (Medicare reimbursement K0001, weighs >36 pounds, accommodates seat widths >22 inches, and supports up to 350 lb): Offer features that address clients' special needs, such as bariatric clients who require wheelchairs that can support >250 lb; obese clients may also need manually tilting and/or reclining wheelchair backs for pressure relief with the aim of reducing the risk of developing a pressure ulcer, managing orthostatic hypotension, or both; these clients may require a specialty manual wheelchair that would enable them to stand while supported with appropriate seating and positioning devices, which can help to improve circulation, skin integrity, renal function, and bone density, as well as reduce muscle spasms.
5. Specialty manual wheelchairs (Medicare reimbursement code K0009): Include manual tilt and manual recline wheelchairs and other wheelchairs that are activity or environment specific, such as for use on a sandy beach[24]

Walking Aids

Walking aids provide a single-point, dual-point, or multipoint base of support for clients who have difficulty ambulating on level or uneven surfaces. Walking aids can improve balance and enhance forward and lateral stability and safety while ambulating. Some types of ambulation aids are made of durable and lightweight materials, such as aluminum or titanium, for easier handling and can be folded for easier storage.

Canes

A standard (single-point) cane comprises a single shaft of wood or aluminum tubing with a handle that helps to steady the user's gait. Quad canes (four-point) provide increased stability because they feature four rubber-tipped prongs located at the end of the cane's shaft. Quad canes come in two sizes, depending on the client's needs, including canes with a small or large base of support. Just as the name implies, large-base quad canes provide clients with a slightly larger base of support than the small-base version but can make a big difference in assisting a client to maintain his or her balance while ambulating on level and uneven surfaces, such as tiled or carpeted floors, ramps, grassy hills with a mild slope, and stairs with or without handrails.

Crutches

Crutches provide two additional points of support for the client. Axillary crutches are the most commonly recognized type of crutches. Loft-strand (forearm) crutches have handgrips and rigid cuffs that wrap around the user's forearms to reduce arm strain and provide added stability.

Walkers

Walkers provide a multipoint (four points) base of support. Standard walkers are lifted and moved forward with each subsequent step. Rolling walkers are simply modified standard walkers with two wheels attached on the bottom of the front legs so they can be rolled forward with each step, therefore eliminating the need for a client to lift the walker as he or she is ambulating. Hemiwalkers are similar to standard walkers but are designed specifically for one-handed use by adding a handle between the standard handle grips.

Three- or four-wheeled walkers also offer greater maneuverability and special features, such as built-in seats for resting and tote baskets for carrying one's belongings. However, three- and four-wheeled walkers may require increased strength and balance to fold, lift, and safely stow in a vehicle.

Scooters

Individuals who can walk short distances but have limited endurance often benefit from motorized scooters. However, the seat on a scooter does not provide a great deal of rear or lateral support; therefore scooter users must be able to maintain their sitting balance and safely ascend from a sitting to a standing position (and vice versa). Scooters are available in three- or four-wheel configurations, vary in overall size and weight, and can be disassembled for transport. Scooters can also offer special features, such as powered height-adjustable seats, large baskets for carrying items such as groceries, and accessories such as lights, horns, and brightly colored flags that enhance the client's visibility and safety when traveling about in his or her community.

CAN THE CLIENT STOW THE MOBILITY AID?

The driver must be able to maintain his or her sitting or standing balance to stow a mobility aid safely. For example if the client is a wheelchair user, he or she must have adequate dynamic sitting balance to disassemble a wheelchair and stow the chair's components while seated on the OEM driver's seat. If the client uses a scooter, he or she may need to use a device that can lift the scooter and help position it into a docking device while he or she is standing. Then the client must walk a short distance to open the driver's side door, access the vehicle, and close the door. Therefore the client's balance status (and in this case dynamic standing balance) may mean the difference between driving from the driver's seat of an unmodified vehicle versus requiring a structurally modified vehicle (i.e., a full-sized van or minivan) that can accommodate a client who must access the vehicle while seated on a scooter or wheelchair.

CAN THE CLIENT TRANSFER TO THE DRIVER'S SEAT FROM INSIDE THE VEHICLE?

When a client is unable to transfer into the driver's seat from outside the vehicle or stow a wheelchair or ambulation aid, he or she will need a structurally modified van with a ramp or lift. Once the client is inside the vehicle and the wheelchair is secured, the client should transfer onto a six- or eight-way power seat base, which is a motorized base on which the OEM seat is secured. Power seat bases are on a track that enables the OEM seat to slide and rotate into a variety of positions that are closer to the client and his or her wheeled mobility device. Power seat bases come in parallel or scissor style configurations. The scissor style power seat base allows for greater adjustability that often results in easier and safer transfers when using a sliding board or sit-pivot technique from inside a minivan or full-sized van.

WILL THE CLIENT BE DRIVING FROM A WHEELCHAIR?

Clients should decide whether they will be driving from a wheelchair or transferring to a power seat base. They should consider the strength, endurance, and energy that are required for each potential transfer and the associated risks, such as soft tissue injuries (e.g., tendonitis, bursitis, and shearing effects) and the risk of falling. They should also consider the number of times they will transfer from a wheelchair onto and off of the vehicle's seat in a single day. For example a client who intends to complete three errands within 1 hour, including going to the bank, grocery store, and pharmacy, will be required to perform up to eight transfers in less than 60 minutes! Clients who drive modified vans eliminate all but two transfers (i.e., getting into and out of their wheeled mobility devices), irrespective of the number of errands completed.

Driving from a power wheelchair usually requires the vehicle's floor to be lowered or its roof to be raised, as well as the installation of some type of seating system that can elevate the driver with the purpose of allowing him or her to have the proper line of sight through the windshield and access to the *driving controls*. An automatic electromechanical wheelchair tiedown system is required to secure the wheelchair and its occupant. Hybrid power wheelchairs, which can be operated in power or manual modes, may be too lightweight to permit safe driving. If the client uses this type of wheelchair, the DRS should follow the options available for manual wheelchair users with regard to vehicle accessibility, tiedown systems, and if necessary stowing the wheelchair. See Chapters 9 and 18 for more information on seating, occupant restraints, and tiedown systems.

HAS THE CLIENT MAXIMIZED TRANSFER STATUS?

In some cases a client may be able to transfer onto the driver's seat from outside of the vehicle but may require assistance with stowing the wheelchair or ambulation aid or with some aspect of the transfer task, such as managing his or her involved lower extremities. If a client requires assistance when entering or exiting the vehicle, he or she should consider the cost of modifying a vehicle with the aim of making driving a viable goal versus the caregiver fulfilling the role of the driver while the client rides as a passenger. This approach is appropriate when a client is not a viable candidate for driving and he or she should be focusing on driving

cessation and alternative community mobility. Transfer status also affects whether a person can drive from a wheelchair or the OEM seat. Driving from a wheelchair requires a structurally modified vehicle. If the client has not maximized his or her transfer status, purchasing a modified vehicle may not be advisable because it may not be needed in the near term. Conversely if the client's condition is deteriorating, it will be difficult for the DRS to recommend vehicle modifications that will be appropriate as the client's status changes in time.

Box 5-4 lists some general points to keep in mind when the client is transferring into and out of a vehicle. Box 5-5 lists some basic instructions for transferring onto a vehicle's seat while inside of a vehicle from a power wheelchair using a sit-pivot transfer technique.

The DRS should make sure that the client considers the energy expenditure required and the potential wear and tear on his or her body during the transfer task. Also the DRS should help the client to realize that a driver transfers into and out of the driver's seat a minimum of four times for every one errand. If the client completes three errands, he or she would perform as many as eight transfers! A wheelchair user may want to drive from his or her wheelchair if the potential energy expenditure is a concern; added physical and mental stress can increase the likelihood of the client becoming injured, experiencing an exacerbation of an existing health condition, or both.

IF THE CLIENT OWNS A VEHICLE, CAN HE OR SHE DRIVE IT?

Before recommending an optimal vehicle class, the DRS must first determine whether the client owns a vehicle and whether he or she could potentially drive it

---

BOX 5-4	**Vehicle Transfer Techniques**

- The client should never use the vehicle's door for support because it could swing open or closed as he or she shifts his or her weight while getting into or out of the vehicle. The client should support himself or herself by holding onto the vehicle's frame or allowing a healthy adult caregiver to provide whatever level of assistance is required to help ensure safety during the transfer.
- It is always easier for a client to transfer to the front seat of a vehicle because the adjustability of the seat allows for more legroom than the back seats.
- The client should always position the seat as far back as possible before he or she transfers to create more room to maneuver when getting into or out of the vehicle.

- When entering the vehicle from standing, the client should have his or her back to the vehicle, sit down, and then swing his or her legs into the vehicle; then simply reverse this procedure when exiting the vehicle to maintain good postural alignment and minimize the risk of falling.
- If the client's existing vehicle has upholstered seats, the driver rehabilitation specialist can suggest that the client consider wearing clothing that reduces friction, such as silk or polyester, which can help make the transfer easier. Leather seats provide the best surface for reducing friction during the transfer task.

BOX 5-5 | **Transfer Techniques Inside the Vehicle from a Power Wheelchair to a Vehicle's Seat**

1. Once the client has driven his or her wheelchair onto the vehicle's ramp or lift and has accessed the van, ask him or her to remove the wheelchair footrest and armrest on the side from which he or she will be transferring; alternatively he or she can swing the footrest and armrest out of the way versus removing them altogether.
2. Have the client position the wheelchair as close to the driver's seat as possible. It should be pointed out that some vans might have an original equipment manufacturer swivel seat or a power-assisted six- or eight-way adjustable seat that can be positioned to minimize the distance between the wheelchair and the driver's seat.
3. The driver rehabilitation specialist must be certain the client's wheelchair is properly positioned and secured by the wheelchair tiedown device.
4. The client should turn the wheelchair's power off, and a transfer belt should be secured around the client's waist.
5. The client should then be cued, as needed, to scoot as far forward in the wheelchair as possible while being provided contact guard assistance to reduce the risk of him or her falling.
6. The client should place one hand on the vehicle's seat and the other hand on the edge of the wheelchair cushion for support.
7. The driver rehabilitation specialist should make sure the client's feet are positioned flat on the floor and that his or her knees are flexed at a 90-degree angle; this is necessary for the client's lower extremities to provide a base of support throughout the transfer. The driver rehabilitation specialist should use joint protection and proper body mechanics, such as flexing his or her knees and maintaining an erect upper body posture, before, during, and after the transfer task. A driver rehabilitation specialist can practice in the vehicle without the client during a "dry run" to get acclimated to the vehicle's interior (e.g., available head room, trip hazards).
8. The client should use both arms to push up from a seated position while swiveling over and onto the car seat; alternatively the client can use a sliding board to provide a bridge between the wheelchair's and vehicle's seating surfaces.
9. The driver rehabilitation specialist should make sure the client is securely on the driver's seat, has fastened his or her seat belt including a chest strap if needed for additional support, has adjusted the mirrors for optimal visibility, and is positioned to properly operate the vehicle. The client should be able to access all of the primary and secondary driving controls without straining or losing his or her balance.

---

with or without vehicle modifications including adapted driving aids. Several considerations must be addressed before the DRS and client can decide on the best type of vehicle, including the following:

• Can the client transfer into and out of the existing vehicle from either outside or inside of the vehicle?
• Will an adaptation to the vehicle's seat allow him or her to safely and independently transfer into and out of the vehicle?
• Is the client using the most appropriate mobility aid for personal mobility?
• Can the client transfer and stow his or her mobility aid within a reasonable amount of time without compromising safety and/or using up available energy reserves?
• Will a hoist lift or other adaptation allow the client to stow the mobility aid independently in the vehicle?
• Are there musculoskeletal/soft tissue issues that should be considered?
• Is it likely that the client will be exposed to inclement weather?
• Where does the client park the vehicle? Is the vehicle parked in an attached garage or some other protected parking area, such as a parking garage? Will the client use valet parking services on a regular basis?

• If the client currently owns a vehicle, is it compatible with the recommended adaptive driving equipment? A vehicle generally should minimally have automatic transmission, power steering, and power brakes to be compatible with even the most basic adaptive driving aids. Clients who are able to transfer easily and stow their own mobility aids but have vehicles with manual transmissions may need to purchase a different vehicle.
• Is the client's vehicle in good working condition? Are the vehicle's systems operational, such as electrical, exhaust, brakes, and *secondary driving controls*?
• Is the vehicle reliable?
• What is the vehicle's repair history? Has the vehicle ever "broken down" or failed to start? If yes, why did it break down? What was done to remedy the situation?
• Does the vehicle pose a threat in any way to the client's or the client's prospective passengers' safety, health, and well-being?
• Will the client be able to call for assistance from his or her vehicle? For example, does the client own a cell phone? Subscribe to a roadside assistance program?

The client must also consider the condition of his or her vehicle because most reputable vehicle modifiers will refuse to adapt a vehicle if it is not in reasonably good condition.

CAN THE CLIENT DRIVE A CAR OR SUV OR IS AN ADAPTED VAN REQUIRED?

If the client is not able to transfer independently into and out of a car or SUV and stow his or her mobility aid, the DRS and client should consider selecting an adapted van (minivan or full-sized van). Individuals who are at risk for musculoskeletal or soft tissue injuries associated with performing transfers and stowing their mobility aids may also want to consider an adapted van. Clients who live in areas that experience inclement weather, especially snow and freezing rain, should consider driving an adapted van because stowing their mobility aids in cars would expose them needlessly to the elements and place them at a higher risk for a weather-related injury or illness. Finally clients who have decreased energy, strength, and endurance, such as a client diagnosed with rheumatoid arthritis, could also benefit from an adapted van because it would help to conserve limited energy reserves and provide joint protection by eliminating the need for excess transfers. Clients should assess how comfortable they are in cars and SUVs versus full-sized vans or minivans. If a client is used to driving a full-sized car, becoming acclimated to the look and feel of a van can complicate the evaluation process. In the final analysis, however, clients will usually adapt to the subtle (and not so subtle) nuances of driving a van versus a car or SUV if it means that they can drive.

DOES THE CLIENT HAVE ACCESS TO THE FINANCIAL RESOURCES TO PURCHASE AND/OR MODIFY AN ADAPTED VAN?

The client's preference should be a consideration when selecting a vehicle; however, the DRS and client must be realistic about the client's functional status and his or her ability or inability to secure the funding that is necessary to pay for a vehicle, vehicle modifications, or both. Therefore although a van may be considered to be the optimal vehicle type for the client, the following questions should be considered:

- What is the client's functional status?
- What are the client's personal financial resources?
- Does the client have access to funding through workers' compensation, auto insurance, or self-pay resources?
- Does the client have access to a governmental agency for funding of equipment and services, such as state vocational rehabilitation programs, the Veterans Administration, or the victims of crime compensation funds?
- Does the client have access to donations from charitable organizations, such as churches, synagogues, Optimist Clubs, private foundations, and others?

SHOULD THE CLIENT DRIVE A FULL-SIZED VAN OR MINIVAN?

A client's seated height can help determine whether a minivan or full-sized van is needed. Seated height is the distance from the floor to the top of the client's head when he or she is sitting in a wheelchair. Seated height will determine a driver's line of sight, overall visibility, and the available clearance and headroom within a vehicle. If the client's seated height generally is >54 inches, he or she will most likely need a full-sized van. If the client's seated height is <53 inches, a minivan may work. If the client's seated height is 54 inches exactly, either vehicle type may be suitable. The DRS should keep in mind that these numbers are approximate and could (and often do) vary in terms of client-vehicle fit from individual to individual.

PLATFORM LIFTS

Platform lifts fold out from a frame that has been mounted to the van. The frame raises and lowers the platform, and when it is not in use, the lift typically rests in an upright position on the inside of the van's side doors.

UNDER-THE-VEHICLE LIFTS

Under-the-vehicle lifts are attached beneath the body of the van and housed in a protective enclosure to prevent damage from road debris. When an under-the-vehicle lift is activated, it extends outward, raises to the level of the van's floor, and retracts underneath the van when it is not in use. These lifts require that the vehicle be stored in a garage when not in use in areas that use salt on the roads because of snow and ice during cold weather.

TRANSFER SEAT BASES

Transfer seat bases come in two styles: parallel or scissor style. The scissor style transfer seat base can be used for clients performing sliding board transfers. It also is a preferred seat style when clients require the driver's seat to have a finer adjustment for positioning the seat closer to their wheeled mobility devices when transferring. The OEM seat should always be used in conjunction with a power seat base. A major study by the Transportation Development Centre of Canada[27] (1998) reported the following:

> All three of the transfer seat bases tested withstood a static load equivalent to 20 times the combined weight of the entire seat assembly, applied horizontally (in both the forward and rearward direction) through the combined center of gravity

location. The seat assembly comprised a representative OEM seat weighing 15.5 kg (34 lb) and the six-way transfer seat base. None of the three six-way transfer seat bases tested was able to sustain the simultaneous application of the 20 times combined seat assembly weight and the 26,688 N (6,000 lb) seat belt assembly load comprising 13,344 N (3,000 lb) applied to both the pelvic and torso body blocks. In conclusion, there is a significant probability that current state-of-the-art six-way transfer seat bases, when installed in conjunction with OEM seats, which retain the original inboard seat belt buckle assembly, will experience structural failure when subjected to loads commensurate with a 48 km/h (30 mph) frontal crash impact.

ROTARY LIFTS

Rotary lifts are mounted on a single vertical post on the inside of the van's side or rear doors. The lift platforms rotate in and out of the doors and travel vertically between the ground and the van floor, resting on the vehicle's floor when not in use.

HOIST LIFTS

Hoist style lifts do not have platforms and feature an "arm" that swings in and out of the van's side doors. The hoist's arm is connected to a docking device that is attached to a wheelchair frame that allows a client to raise and lower an unoccupied wheelchair or scooter into and out of the vehicle.

TIEDOWN SYSTEMS

For the wheelchair user who prefers to remain in his or her wheelchair while driving or riding as a passenger, tiedown devices are necessary to keep the chair securely in place while the vehicle is in motion. Some tiedown systems are manually operated and use belts to fasten and secure a wheelchair's frame to a floor-mounted track. Drivers who use manual tiedown systems should have good static and dynamic sitting balance, upper extremity strength, endurance, and manual dexterity. There are also power lockdown devices that allow the wheelchair user to drive directly over an automatic latching mechanism that secures the lower part of the chair's frame in place. If the wheelchair is a folding manual wheelchair, the power lockdown device may disable the folding mechanism. Users of manual wheelchairs should consider the additional weight that the lockdown mechanism adds to the wheelchair. DRSs working with power wheelchair users should contact the wheelchair manufacturer and work with a vehicle modifier to determine whether the wheelchair is compatible with the power lockdown device being considered as an option. For example some wheelchairs have a bottom clearance that is too low to accept these devices.

DRIVING CONTROLS

STEERING DEVICES

The effort that is required for anyone to turn a steering wheel can be a potential barrier to driving. Physical abilities vary, and limited range of motion, strength, endurance, and hand function may make it difficult to grasp or turn a standard steering wheel, especially for an extended period. The following adaptations and modifications can provide assistance with steering:

- Spinner knob: Drivers with full hand function who can grip the knob firmly with either the left or right hand to control the steering wheel can use this device. The knob may be placed in any number of positions depending on the DRS's recommendation. For example the traditional 2 o'clock position may cause stress and fatigue by requiring the driver to maintain his or her shoulder in a flexed position that is close to 90 degrees. Placing the spinner knob at the 6 o'clock position, for example, may help to remedy this problem because the driver's shoulder would be in a position that is close to neutral while driving in a straightforward direction. The traditional 2 o'clock position for mounting a steering device such as a spinner knob is no longer preferred because of the increased risk of injury associated with an airbag inflating upon impact and potentially causing an individual to strike himself or herself in the head and neck.
- Single pin/post: Drivers with functional cylindrical handgrip and good upper extremity strength and endurance of the arm that will be used to steer the vehicle may benefit from this device. This device also keeps the client's wrist and forearm in a neutral position while steering.
- Tri-pin: Drivers with little or no finger function can use this device. It is a three-post device that holds the driver's wrist and fingers in position while he or she controls the steering wheel. This device enables the client to slide his or her hand into and out of position without having to contend with a strap or any other securement method.
- Quad fork, palm spinner, V-grip: These devices are designed for a driver with limited hand function, such as reduced grip strength.
  - Palm grip: This device can benefit drivers with adequate grip strength by helping to keep the forearm in a pronated position.
  - Amputee ring: This device is designed for drivers with prosthetic limbs and enables a hook-style terminal device to interface with the steering wheel. This device is shown in the picture of Mr. Quentin Corley, who helped devise one of the

first adaptive driving aids in the United States (see Figure 2-1).

A common modification to compensate for a driver's limited arm strength is to reduce the effort required to turn the steering wheel. The standard power steering system of a vehicle can be modified to make turning the wheel even easier. However, the driver must still have good range of motion to use this type of advanced power steering.

Reduced effort steering can be described as a 40% reduction in effort (approximately) that is required for a driver to turn the steering wheel as compared with standard power steering. As power steering effort is reduced, the natural recovery effect when completing a turn is also reduced, but some of this effect will still be apparent.

Minimal effort steering (also known as zero effort steering) can be described as a 70% reduction in effort (approximately) that is required to turn the steering wheel as compared with standard power steering. Minimal effort steering virtually eliminates the recovery effect of standard steering and therefore requires greater vigilance when "recovering" from a turn. For safety, alternate drivers must be warned about and ideally trained to compensate for the lost recovery effect.

A back-up or emergency electric pump should be used in conjunction with modified effort steering systems for those instances when the engine is unable to provide power to the power steering system, such as when an engine stalls.

ACCELERATION AND BRAKING

Mechanical hand controls are manually operated devices that attach to a vehicle's steering column or instrument panel and feature a handle that is directly connected to the brake and indirectly connected to the accelerator. The primary difference between different mechanical hand control styles is the way in which the control handle is moved to operate the accelerator. A list and brief descriptions of the most common hand controls used in the United States are presented here:

- Push/right angle style: The client must push the handle upward toward the instrument panel to brake and pull downward at a right angle to accelerate. Clients with limited finger dexterity can operate this type of mechanical hand control.
- Push/pull style: The client must push forward on the handle to brake and pull it backward to accelerate. Clients with limited finger dexterity can operate this type of mechanical hand control. A three-post hand interface also can be installed to allow the user to maintain contact with the handle at all times while driving.

- Push/rock style: The client must push the handle forward to brake and rock it back to accelerate. Clients with no finger dexterity can operate this type of hand control.
- Push/rotate style: The client must push the handle forward to brake and twist it to accelerate. Clients with full or limited finger function can operate this control.

Power-assisted hand controls are used to compensate for limited strength, range of motion, or both by reducing the effort required for accelerating and braking. There are two types of assisted hand controls available: mechanical assisted and power assisted.[25] These controls can usually be installed in a convenient location within reach of the client. The handles of these devices can be modified to allow a client with limited or no finger function to maintain contact with the control handle at all times while driving the vehicle. There are various systems available in electronic, pneumatic, or vacuum-powered models.

SECONDARY DRIVING CONTROLS

An extension handle can be attached to the vehicle's gear shift lever to bring the lever closer to the driver on the right side of the steering wheel. This provides the client with improved leverage and easier access to the gearshift. The handle can also be extended to the left side of the steering wheel to allow shifting operations to be performed with the left hand. Minimal to no finger dexterity is required to use these devices if they are configured properly.

The turn signal stalk can be modified with a mechanical extension that attaches to the steering column and allows the turn signals to be operated from the left side of the steering wheel. A similar device can also be used to bring the turn signal lever closer to the steering wheel on the right side of the steering column. This device requires that the client have adequate finger dexterity.

Rigid key holders can be used to provide a larger surface area to grip while inserting the key into the ignition. These devices also provide the client with increased leverage while turning the key and ignition. Some finger dexterity is required to insert the key into the ignition, whereas little or no finger dexterity is required to turn the key holder.

Electronic auxiliary controls can be operated with electronic switches that are located in convenient locations that are readily accessible within the vehicle's interior. Controls are configured individually or in combination so that clients can control the following: HVAC (heater/air conditioning), ignition, gearshift, horn, turn signals, wipers, radio, emergency brake, and others. The switches required to operate each auxiliary control are typically mounted on a single internally lighted control panel located within reach of the driver. The switches are designed to operate without the need for finger dexterity; they are generally light touch switches that can be further modified with small raised rubber bumpers if necessary. Some controls use a scanner-type selection interface, allowing multiple devices to be operated with a limited number of switches or even a single switch. Voice activation enables the client to activate secondary driving controls by speaking. Commands are typically single words that activate the operation of desired controls, such as turning the vehicle's lights or windshield wipers on and off. Voice recognition systems must be programmed to recognize the client's unique vocal patterns as requests for the activation or deactivation of various secondary driving controls.

Special mirrors can be added to sideview mirrors or to replace the rearview mirror to assist with blind-spot management. Spotting mirrors are commercially available convex mirrors that are placed on sideview mirrors that expand the periphery and allow the driver to locate blind spots with greater ease. Lane-changer mirrors are commercially available and supplement or replace the rearview mirror and allow the driver to locate the blind spots with greater ease. Lane-changer mirrors can help the driver decide whether it is safe to change lanes. SmartView Mirrors (Cheshire, Connecticut) are supplemental sideview mirrors and come in pairs (i.e., one right and one left mirror). There is a delineated area on each mirror that assists the driver in deciding whether it is safe to change lanes and to check blind spots. Panoramic mirrors provide a wide-angle view of the traffic environment and can be applied to the vehicle's sideview mirrors.

Supplemental restraints are the final type of secondary driving control. Chest straps provide additional postural support for clients with decreased sitting balance. Wheelchair restraints include a variety of tiedown devices that automatically or manually secure a wheeled mobility device.

ADAPTIVE DRIVING AIDS

The following questions can help the DRS and client begin to assess which adaptive driving aids could potentially address the client's specific functional deficits related to the driving task. These questions are certainly not exhaustive and are not meant to replace the comprehensive driver rehabilitation evaluation. These questions are meant to help the DRS to begin assessing the client's functional status as it relates to some of the basic driving tasks and to facilitate discussion about adaptive driving aids.

Once the reader has reached this point in the guide, it is assumed the client's cognition, visual perception, and visual acuity are intact. If this is not the case, however, then the reader is advised to refer to Chapters 6, 7, and 22 for more information on the comprehensive driver rehabilitation evaluation, driver readiness, and driving cessation. The guide focuses on potential solutions that address pathokinesiology (i.e., impaired movement) and other related factors that can diminish or preclude driving performance. It is recommended that the DRS record the client's responses and use the documented feedback to identify prospective adaptive driving aids. Finally the following questions feature supporting content that is meant to help clarify the meaning of the questions presented and to provide functional tasks that are designed to help clients answer the questions posed to them. All of the following activities are performed while the client is in a seated position unless otherwise noted.

Does the Client Have Functional Use of the Right Foot? Of the Left Foot?

Can the client perform the following tasks with ease? Ask the client the following questions:

- Can you point your foot and toes downward (plantar flexion) as if you are using an accelerator pedal of a motor vehicle?
- Can you point your toes and foot upward (dorsiflexion) as if you are easing off of the accelerator pedal?
- Can you move your foot from side to side as if you are alternately using the accelerator pedal and brake pedal?

Does the Client Have Normal Feeling in the Feet?

Can the client perform the following tasks with ease? Ask the client the following questions:

- Can you accurately sense water temperature with your feet when you step into a shower, take a bath, or swim in a pool or lake?
- Are you aware if a small object, such as a pebble or twig, is in your shoe?
- Are you aware of the position of your feet without looking at them?
- Have you ever had a pressure ulcer or ulcers on your feet?
- Can you sense deep pressure with your feet, such as differentiating the amount of pressure you exert when depressing the brake pedal?

Performing these tasks with ease and reporting a medical history that does not include pressure ulcers may indicate that the client can drive with the manufacturer's standard accelerator and brake pedals. Some people who cannot easily perform these tasks or report a history of skin breakdown, decreased sensation, or both may still be able to drive with the manufacturer's standard equipment; however, in any case, clients should always seek a professional driver rehabilitation evaluation that is conducted by a DRS working in a reputable driver rehabilitation and community mobility program. The client's sitting balance, upper extremity movement, and head and neck movement now are examined.

Does the Client Have Functional Use of the Right Arm and Hand? Of the Left Arm and Hand?

Can the client perform the following tasks with ease? Ask the client the following questions and to perform the following tasks:

- Can you raise your right arm to shoulder height as if you were reaching out in front of you to place your hand on someone's left shoulder?
- Can you raise your left arm to shoulder height as if you were reaching out in front of you to place your hand on someone's right shoulder?
- Can you raise your right arm to shoulder height as if you were reaching out in front of you to place your hand on someone's left shoulder (if he or she was facing you) and move it 180 degrees along a horizontal plane?
- Can you raise your left arm to shoulder height as if you were reaching out in front of you to place your hand on someone's left shoulder (if he or she was facing you) and move it 180 degrees along a horizontal plane?
- With your shoulder in a neutral position and your elbow flexed 90 degrees can you sustain functional cylindrical grasp of a soda pop can and maintain it just above your waist with your right hand?
- With your shoulder in a neutral position and your elbow flexed 90 degrees can you sustain functional cylindrical grasp of a soda pop can and maintain it just above your waist with your left hand?

Does the Client Have Normal Feeling in the Arms and Hands?

Can the client perform the following tasks with ease? Ask the client the following questions and to perform the following tasks:

- Can you accurately sense water temperature with your hands when you reach into a shower, a bath, a pool, or a lake?
- Are you aware if you sustain a paper cut or bruise your arms and hands?
- Are you aware of the position of your arms and hands without looking at them?
- Can you discern what is in your hands (e.g., coin, pencil, key, paper clip) with your vision occluded?
- Have you ever had a pressure ulcer or ulcers on your arms, hands, or both? If your answer is yes, was it because you lacked sensation, circulation, or both? Are you at risk for developing pressure ulcers? If your answer is yes, why?

Does the Client Have Functional Movement of the Neck?

Can your client perform the following tasks with ease? Ask your client to perform the following tasks:

- Can you look over your right shoulder as if to see who is approaching you from behind on the right?
- Can you look over your left shoulder as if to see who is approaching you from behind on the left?

Does the Client Have Good Unsupported Sitting Balance?

Can the client perform the following tasks with ease? While providing the client with contact guard assistance and using a transfer belt, ask the client if he or she can perform the following tasks:

- Can you flex (bend) your trunk forward and retrieve a small object (such as a slipper or tennis ball) from off of the floor?
- Can you laterally flex your trunk to your left side and retrieve a small object from off of the floor?
- Can you laterally flex your trunk to your right side and retrieve a small object from off of the floor?

CLIENT PROFILES

1. If the client is able to use all extremities except his or her left arm to drive, here are some suggestions for adaptive equipment that may be considered:
   - Steering devices such as a spinner knob
   - Left crossover turn signal
   - Emergency brake extension
2. If the client is able to use all extremities except his or her right arm to drive, here are some suggestions for adaptive equipment that may be considered:
   - Crossover left hand gearshift
   - Steering devices
   - Key assist for ignition
   - Electronic adaptations
3. If the client is able to use his or her left foot and left arm to drive, here are some suggestions for adaptive equipment that may be considered:
   - Crossover left hand gearshift
   - Left crossover turn signals
   - Steering device
   - Key assist for ignition
   - Electronic adaptations
   - Left foot accelerator
4. If the client is able to use his or her right foot and right arm to drive, here are some suggestions for adaptive equipment that may be considered:
   - Right crossover turn signals
   - Steering devices
   - Electronic adaptations

5. If the client is able to only use both upper extremities to drive, here are some suggestions for adaptive equipment that may be considered:
   - Steering devices
   - Hand controls
   - Parking brake extension
6. If the client is able to use only one upper extremity to drive, here are some suggestions for adaptive equipment that may be considered:
   - High-tech driving solutions
   - Joystick driving controls
7. If the client is able to use only one lower extremity to drive, here are some suggestions for adaptive equipment that may be considered:
   - High-tech driving solutions
   - Remote steering wheel
   - Secondary controls in headrest
   - Voice activated scanning system for secondary driving controls

DRIVING CESSATION

The rite of passage associated with earning and keeping a driver's license after demonstrating driving competence is a universal symbol of autonomy and independence. Driving and the infrastructure that supports the worldwide car culture influence how we interact with others, view the world, and imagine how others perceive us, and how that image influences the way we perceive ourselves.[28] When age-related physical or mental limitations or both impair safe driving, driving cessation becomes necessary to ensure the safety of drivers with disabilities, aging-related concerns, or both and the public at large; a growing body of literature shows that without proper planning and intervention (e.g., counseling the client who is no longer fit to drive, exploring alternatives to driving for community mobility) there are many negative consequences associated with driving cessation.

ELDERLY DRIVERS

The proportion and number of elderly drivers have increased dramatically during the past two decades,[29] and it is widely anticipated that this trend will continue.[30] There are 35 million Americans aged ≥65 years, which is approximately 13% of the total U.S. population; the number of elderly drivers is expected to double and reach 70 million by the year 2030.[31] Drivers aged ≥55 years comprised 28% of the driving population in 2000, and that number is expected to increase to 39% by the year 2050.[32,33] More than 80% of trips undertaken by people aged >65 years in the United States are in passenger vehicles that are usually their own.[34]

Elderly Americans resemble the broader population when it comes to their dependence on privately owned automobiles.[31] It is no wonder then that elderly people continue to drive even after experiencing the cumulative effects of aging and chronic disease or the instantaneous disabling effects that are often associated with traumatic injuries, chronic disabilities, and impairments associated with the aging process.[35] However, there is significant variation in the functional abilities of elderly drivers. Although it has been estimated that approximately one-third of the population aged >65 years have limitations that render them unable to perform a significant number of activities of daily living, it is still the case that more than two-thirds of these persons continue to drive.[36]

Motor Vehicle Accidents and Elderly Drivers

There is also mounting evidence that older drivers account for a disproportionate number of traffic accidents and mortality.[37] The oldest drivers, that is, individuals who are ≥75 years of age, experience traffic accidents at a rate second only to the youngest drivers between 15 and 24 years of age.[38] More than 7000 elderly drivers die in automobile accidents on highways and roads in the United States annually, and the number of elderly drivers ≥70 years of age killed in vehicular accidents nationwide has increased 39% during a 10-year period.[39] Florida had the most auto fatalities in 1999, followed by Texas, California, Pennsylvania, and Michigan.[39] Motor vehicle accidents are the leading cause of accidental deaths for people aged 65 to 74 years and the second leading cause for older people in general (after falls).[40] By age group, drivers aged ≥80 years have the highest fatality rate, drivers aged 65 to 79 years have the third highest, and drivers aged 16 to 24 years have the second highest.[41] Physiologic changes, concomitant medical conditions, and medications associated with aging can impair driving ability.[35] Thus as the number of elderly drivers increases, their competence to drive has become a growing concern for their families, caregivers, and physicians; medical doctors possess an added responsibility because they have the legal authority and responsibility to report individuals they deem unsafe to drive. Safe driving is similarly the concern of the general public, the automobile manufacturing industry, researchers, the insurance industry, and health care providers including occupational therapists working as DRSs.

Risk Factors That Contribute to Driving Cessation

Multiple chronic and acute medical conditions secondary to injury, illness, or the aging process often result in declining cognition, psychomotor skills, and vision and hearing (i.e., sensoriperceptual) functioning that are *risk factors* decreasing an individual's ability to drive safely.[42-46] Driving cessation is influenced by the presence of numerous physical and cognitive health challenges associated with aging because people are seen as holistic beings; that is, there are complementary systems, structures, and functions[47] that are required to be functioning properly to perform complex tasks such as driving.[35] The implications of compromised body systems on driving cessation and elderly persons are reviewed in brief below.

Cognition

Studies have documented how cognitive deficits affect driving outcomes among elderly persons. Freund and Szinovacz[30] reported that people diagnosed with cognitive impairments and Alzheimer's disease significantly reduce the miles they drive, although it is unclear as to when and at what level of cognitive impairment individuals start to self-restrict or cease driving. Odenheimer[48] writes that with the aging of our nation's population and the strong association of aging with dementing disorders, there is reason to be concerned. Keplinger[49] reported that dementia of the Alzheimer's type is the most common cause of cognitive impairment; its prevalence is estimated to be as high as 11.6% in persons ≥65 years and 47.8% in persons >85 years. Cerebrovascular disease is another important factor. Legh-Smith et al[50] report that as many as 58% of patients do not resume driving after a stroke because of the severity of their residual cognitive disability. Studies have also focused on specific gender when examining cognitive impairment and alteration of driving habits. Foley et al[51] found that driving cessation was positively correlated with cognitive impairment and estimated that nearly 4% of male drivers ≥75 years of age (i.e., 175,000) have dementia in the United States.

Psychomotor Skills

Aging leads to decreased strength, coordination, reaction time, extremity range of motion, and trunk mobility, all of which are key components of driving ability.[35] Musculoskeletal conditions such as rheumatoid arthritis and osteoarthritis, neurologic conditions such as stroke and Parkinson's disease, and other medical conditions such as diabetes mellitus can adversely affect driving performance.[49,52] Functional disability leads to elderly persons modifying their driving patterns, such as limiting or refraining from highway driving or driving to fewer destinations that are viewed to be more essential than other surrendered destinations[53]; for example the grocery store and church may be seen as essential, whereas the monthly visit with the in-laws may no longer be seen as viable or desirable.

Sensoriperceptual Skills

Most of the sensory input for driving comes from vision, and many ophthalmologic conditions that are common among elderly persons produce visual impairment, including cataracts, glaucoma, and diabetic retinopathy. Although most states have standard vision screening as a part of the overall driving assessment process to obtain a driver's license for the first time, there are no standards related to subsequent reevaluations of driving fitness. Furthermore as Shipp and Penchansky[53] report, even in the states in which screening takes place, there is significant variation in the frequency and level of vision testing. Thus there is much controversy over and discussion about the question of driving continuation.[54] On the one hand there is evidence that poor performance on simple paper and pencil perceptual tests is predictive of poor driving performance.[55] For example in an historical cohort study[56] of 84 individuals with stroke, it was demonstrated that the Motor Free Visual Perception Test (MFVPT) was clearly predictive of on-road driving performance. Using the MFVPT in combination with the Trail Making B test resulted in the most efficient screening model, such that those scoring poorly on both tests were 22 times more likely to fail the on-road evaluation. That being said, it is also the case that older drivers may become aware of their decreased cognitive and physiologic status and adjust their driving behavior accordingly. Kosnik et al[57] reported that older drivers are often aware of their decreased functional capacity and voluntarily cease driving or adjust their driving patterns by driving less frequently, for shorter distances, during daylight hours, more slowly, and during non–rush hours. As an individual's abilities decline gradually over time (e.g., dementia) or suddenly (e.g., cerebrovascular accident), access to dependable and economic alternative transportation becomes a central factor in determining his or her quality of life.

PASSENGER INFORMATION: DRIVING CESSATION AND ALTERNATIVE TRANSPORTATION

The absence of alternative transportation including an available family member or friend in possession of a driver's license and a vehicle who is willing to assist, the lack of comprehensive systems of public and mass transportation in many cities and most rural areas, and the absence of a copilot makes driving cessation more complicated and devastating than it may be otherwise. Why some individuals continue to drive with cognitive, kinesthetic, visual perceptual, and/or functional deficits may be explained in part by the fact that people rely on the automobile for their primary means of transportation, and this is also true for older adults[58] and people with disabilities. When clients have access to other drivers they are more likely to accept driving cessation; however, more often than not there are no other drivers in their households who are available and willing to provide reliable alternative transportation.[59]

Table 5-3   **Performance Tools on CD-ROM**

Performance Tool	Format	Source
Chapter 5 (*The Adapted Driving Decision Guide*), which features digital images of structurally modified vehicles and adaptive driving aids	PDF document featuring digital images.	Pellerito JM (ed.): *Driver rehabilitation and community mobility: principles and practice*, St. Louis, 2005, Elsevier
Driver Rehabilitation and Community Mobility Assessment Forms	PDF documents	Center for Biomedical Engineering and Rehabilitation Science at Louisiana Tech University
Driving Cessation Decision Guide	PDF document	Eby DW, Molnar LJ, Shope JT: *Driving decisions workbook*, Report No. UMTRI-2000-14. Ann Arbor, MI, 2000, University of Michigan Transportation Research Institute
Promising Approaches to Enhancing Elderly Mobility	PDF document	Molnar LJ, Eby DW, Miller LL: *Promising approaches to enhancing elderly mobility*, Report No. UMTRI-2003-14. Ann Arbor, MI, 2003, University of Michigan Transportation Research Institute
Driving and Dementia: A Review of the Literature	PDF document	Brown LB: *Journal of Geriatric Psychiatry and Neurology* 17:232-240, 2004
Physician's Guide to Assessing and Counseling Older Drivers: American Medical Association	PDF document	Wang CC, Kosinski CJ, Schwartzberg JG, et al: *Physician's guide to assessing and counseling older drivers*, Washington, DC, 2003, National Highway Traffic Safety Administration
Safe Mobility for a Maturing Society: Challenges and Opportunities	PDF document	US Department of Transportation (November 2003). *Safe Mobility for a Maturing Society: Challenges and Opportunities.* Washington, DC.
Driver rehabilitation and community mobility web sites	PDF document	WWW
Auto manufacturers' mobility assistance programs	PDF document	WWW
Organizations that focus on driver rehabilitation and community mobility	PDF document	WWW

PDF, Portable document file.

However, driving cessation can also lead to a heavy dependence on informal support systems, resulting in caregivers missing work or giving up working altogether to care for and provide transportation services for their elderly loved ones.[30] Consequences such as these may account for some of the hesitancy to stop driving among some impaired elderly drivers.[30] In some instances elderly men who do not have driving spouses receive help from their wives who fill the role of copilot.[60] Fulfilling the role of a copilot may include assisting with topographic orientation and navigation through unfamiliar areas or by watching the traffic environment and offering verbal guidance to elderly driving partners that can serve an early warning when there is impending danger. Foley et al[51] confirmed that 10% of elderly men with incident dementia reported to have continued driving with the help of a copilot. Copiloting has received some scrutiny during the past several years[51,61,62]; however, copiloting as a driving compensation strategy has not been studied in a systematic fashion.[30]

Drivers are not the only ones who can benefit from the use of adaptive driving equipment and structural vehicle modifications. Passengers can also use the same types of devices that help drivers enter and exit a vehicle and make the ride safer and more comfortable.

PERFORMANCE TOOLS

The CD-ROM included with this book features a number of *performance tools* that are meant to enhance a DRS's knowledge base and effectiveness when providing driver rehabilitation and community mobility services. The performance tools can also benefit clients and caregivers wishing to access additional information about driver rehabilitation and community mobility. Electronic copies of numerous documents are available in portable document format (PDF) and can be downloaded and saved as an electronic document, printed, and saved as a hard copy or opened and read as a PDF document. Table 5-3 shows the tools available on the CD-ROM.

REFERENCES

1. Reimer-Reiss ML, Wacker RR: Factors associated with assistive technology discontinuance among individuals with disabilities, *J Rehabil* 66(3), July-Sept, 2000. Available at: *www.findarticles.com*. Accessed January 4, 2005.
2. Gradel K: Customer service: what is its place in assistive technology and employment services? *J Vocat Rehabil* 1:41-54, 1991.
3. Reed BJ, Fried JH, Rhoades BJ: Empowerment and assistive technology: the local resource team model, *J Rehabil* 61:30-35, 1995.
4. Williams RR: Assistive technology in the eye of the beholder, *J Vocat Rehabil* 1:9-12, 1991.
5. Phillips B, Zhao H: Predictors of assistive technology abandonment, *Assist Technol* 5:36-45, 1993.
6. Uslan MM: Barriers to acquiring assistive technology: cost and lack of information, *J Visual Impairment Blindness* 86:402-407, 1992.
7. Scherer MJ: *Living in the state of stuck*, Cambridge, MA, 1993, Brookline.
8. National Center for Health Statistics, 1997, November 13. Trends and differential use of assistive technology devices: United States. Available at: *www.cdc.gov/nchswww/*. Accessed January 4, 2005.
9. Scherer MJ: The importance of assistive technology outcomes, 2002. Available at: www.e-bility.com. Accessed October 12, 2004.
10. Rogers EM: *Diffusion of innovations*, ed 4, New York, 1995, The Free Press.
11. Owsley C, McGwin G Jr: Vision impairment and driving, Survey Ophthalmol 43:535-550, 1999.
12. Fisk GD, Owsley C, Mennemeier M: Vision, attention, and self-reported driving behaviors in community-dwelling stroke survivors, *Arch Phys Med Rehabil* 83:469-477, 2002.
13. Burke JP, Oreton HP: Whiplash and its effect on the visual system, *Graefes Arch Clin Exp Ophthalmol* 230:335-339, 1992.
14. Ciuffreda KJ, Suchoff IB, Marrone MA, et al: Oculomotor rehabilitation in traumatic brain-injured patients, *J Behav Optom* 7:31-38, 1996.
15. Hertz BG, Rosenberg J: Effect of mental retardation and motor disability on testing with visual acuity cards, *Dev Med Child Neurol* 34:115-122, 1992.
16. Schenk-Rootlieb AJF, van Nieuwenhuizen O, van der Graaf Y, et al: The prevalence of cerebral visual disturbance in children with cerebral palsy, *Dev Med Child Neurol* 34:473-480, 1992.
17. Klein R, Klein BEK: Blood pressure control and diabetic retinopathy, *Br J Ophthalmol* 86:365-367, 2002.
18. Szlyk JP, Mahler CL, Seiple W, et al: Relationship of retinal, structural, and clinical vision parameters to driving performance of diabetic retinopathy patients, *J Rehabil Res Dev* 41(3A):347-358, 2004.
19. Klein R, Klein BE, Moss SE, et al: The Wisconsin Epidemiologic Study of Diabetic Retinopathy. III. Prevalence and risk of diabetic retinopathy when age at diagnosis is 30 years or older, *Arch Ophthalmol* 102:527-532, 1984.
20. Klein R, Klein BE, Linton KL: Prevalence of age-related maculopathy. The Beaver Dam Eye Study, *Ophthalmology* 99:933-943, 1992.
21. Klein R, Rowland ML, Harris MI: Racial/ ethnic differences in age-related maculopathy. Third National Health and Nutrition Examination Survey, *Ophthalmology* 102:371-381, 1995. [Published erratum appears in *Ophthalmology* 102:1126, 1995].
22. Parasuraman R, Nestor P: Attention and driving, *Clin Geriatr Med* 9:377-386, 1993.
23. Drachman DA: Who may drive? Who may not? Who shall decide? *Ann Neurol* 24:787-788, 1988.
24. Trombley CA, Radomski MV, editors: *Occupational therapy for physical dysfunction*, ed 5, Philadelphia, 2003, Lippincott Williams & Wilkins.

25. Cook A, Hussey S: *Assistive technologies: principles and practice*, St. Louis, 2002, Mosby.

26. Angelo J: *Assistive technology for rehabilitation therapists*, Philadelphia, 1997, FA Davis.

27. Transportation Development Centre of Canada: TP 13246E, *Evaluation of six-way transfer seat bases*, 1998, TES Ltd. Available at: *www.tc.gc.ca/tdc/projects/access/c/9299.html*. Accessed January 4, 2005.

28. Blumer H, Lyman SM, Vidich AJ: *Selected works of Herbert Blumer: a public philosophy for mass society*, Champaign-Urbana, IL, 2000, University of Illinois Press.

29. Lundberg C, Hakamies-Blomqvist L, Almkvist O, et al: Impairments of some cognitive functions are common in crash-involved older drivers, *Accid Anal Prevent* 30:371-377, 1998.

30. Freund B, Szinovacz M: Effects of cognition on driving involvement among the oldest old: variations by gender and alternative transportation opportunities, *Gerontologist* 42:621-633, 2002.

31. U.S. Department of Transportation: *Safe mobility for a maturing society: challenges and opportunities*, Washington, DC, 2003, U.S. Department of Transportation.

32. Cushman LA: Cognitive capacity and concurrent driving performance in older drivers, *IATSS Res* 20:38-45, 1996.

33. Marottoli RA, Ostfeld AM, Merrill SS, et al: Driving cessation and changes in mileage driven among elderly individuals, *J Gerontol Social Sci* 48:S255-S260, 1993.

34. National Research Council: *Transportation in an ageing society*, Washington, DC, 1988, Transportation Research Board.

35. Molnar LJ, Eby DW, Miller LL: *Promising approaches for enhancing elderly mobility*, Ann Arbor, MI, 2003, University of Michigan Transportation Research Institute.

36. Rosenbloom S: Transportation needs of the elderly population, *Clin Geriatr Med* 9:297-310, 1993.

37. Friedland RP, Koss E, Kumar A, et al: Motor vehicle crashes in dementia of the Alzheimer type, *Ann Neurol* 24:782-786, 1988.

38. Williams AF, Carsten O: Driver age and crash involvement, *Am J Public Health* 79:326-327, 1989.

39. Aging News Alert: *Fatalities rise among older drivers*. Silver Spring, Maryland, Oct. 20, 2000, CD Publications, p 11

40. U.S. Department of Health and Human Services (1991).

41. U.S. Department of Commerce (1995).

42. Graca J: Driving and aging, *Clin Geriatr Med* 2:583, 1986.

43. Lucas-Blaustein MJ, Filipp L, Dungan C, et al: Driving in patients with dementia, *J Am Geriatr Soc* 36:1087-1091, 1988.

44. Ray WA, Thapa PB, Shorr RI: Medications and the older driver, *Clin Geriatr Med* 9:413-438, 1993.

45. Sivak M: Vision, perception and attention of older drivers. The safety and mobility of older drivers: what we know and promising research issues, *UMTRI Res Rev* 26:7-10, 1995.

46. McKenna P: Fitness to drive: a neuropsychological perspective, *J Mental Health* 7:9-18, 1998.

47. World Health Organization: *ICF International Classification of Functioning, Disability and Health*, Geneva, 2001, World Health Organization.

48. Odenheimer GL: Dementia and the older driver, *Clin Geriatr Med* 9:349-364, 1993.

49. Keplinger 1998

50. Legh-Smith J, Wade DT, Hewer RL: Driving after a stroke, *J Royal Soc Med* 79:200-203, 1986.

51. Foley DJ, Masaki KH, Ross GW, et al: Driving cessation in older men with incident dementia, *J Am Geriatr Soc* 48:928-930, 2000.

52. Underwood M: The older driver, *Arch Intern Med* 35 (1):33-41, 1992.

53. Kline DW, Kline TJ, Fozard JL, et al: Vision, aging, and driving: the problems of older drivers, *J Gerontol* 47:27-34, 1992.

54. Shipp MD, Penchansky R: Vision testing and the elderly driver: is there a problem meriting policy change? *J Am Optom Assoc* 66:343-351, 1995.

55. Wilkinson M: A discussion with Mark Wilkinson, M.D. Topic: rehabilitation & driving, December 19, 1998. Available at: *http://www.mdsupport.org/clinic/wilkinsonsession.html*. Accessed January 4, 2005.

56. Gallo JJ, Rebok GW, Lesikar SE: Driving habits of adults aged 60 years and older, *J Am Geriatr Soc* 47:335-341, 1999.

57. Korner-Bitensky N, Sofer S, Gélinas I, et al: Evaluating driving potential in persons with stroke: a survey of occupational therapy practices, *Am J Occup Ther* 52:916-919, 1998.

58. Kosnik WD, Sekuler R, Kline DW: Self-reported visual problems of older drivers, *Hum Factors* 32:597, 1990

59. Jette AM, Branch LG: A ten-year follow-up of driving patterns among the community-dwelling elderly, *Hum Factors* 34:25-31, 1992.

60. Kington R, Reuben D, Rogowski J, et al: Sociodemographic and health factors in driving patterns after 50 years of age, *Am J Public Health* 84:1327-1329, 1994.

61. Burkhardt JC, Berger AM, Creedon MA, et al: *Mobility and independence. Changes and challenges for older drivers*, Washington, DC, 1998, Final report to U.S. Department of Health and Human Services and the National Highway Traffic Safety Administration.

62. Bedard M, Mollowy DW, Luel JA: Factors associated with motor vehicle crashes in cognitively impaired older adults, *Alzheimer Dis Assoc Disord* 122:135-139, 1998.

63. Shua-Haim JR, Gross JS: A simulated driving evaluation for patients with Alzheimer's disease, *Am J Alzheimer Dis* 11:2-7, 1996.

Chapter 6

THE CLINICAL EVALUATION

KEY TERMS

- Clinical evaluation
- Comprehensive driver rehabilitation evaluation
- On-road evaluation
- Instrumental activities of daily living
- Team approach
- Proprioception
- Kinesthetic awareness
- Visual function
- Visual acuity
- Field of view
- Peripheral vision
- Central field of view
- Contrast sensitivity
- Scanning
- Tracking
- Sight
- Vision
- Orientation and mobility specialist
- Bioptics
- Executive function

CHAPTER OBJECTIVES

After completing this chapter, the reader will be able to do the following:

- Understand the benefits and limitations of the clinical evaluation.
- Know the range of assessment tests to administer during the clinical evaluation.
- Recognize that a comprehensive driver rehabilitation evaluation is comprised of both the clinical evaluation and the on-road evaluation of driving performance.
- Understand the role of the driver rehabilitation specialist in assessing drivers with visual impairments.
- Understand what role orientation and mobility specialists can play in the clinical evaluation and how it complements the contributions of the driver rehabilitation team members.
- Understand the role of the driver rehabilitation specialist in assessing drivers with hearing impairments.
- Know how to work with a psychiatrist to identify and assess people at risk for driving impairments due to psychosocial factors.

SECTION I

The Clinical Evaluation

Carol J. Wheatley • Joseph M. Pellerito, Jr.
Susan Redepenning

The *clinical evaluation* entails assessing clients' discrete fundamental performance areas that are considered to be critical to the task of operating a motor vehicle. The word "clinical" refers to the frequent practice of administering driver rehabilitation tests or assessments in an occupational therapy clinic and has been used to differentiate this portion of the *comprehensive driver rehabilitation evaluation* from the on-road (i.e., behind-the-wheel) evaluation.

The clinical evaluation can serve a variety of purposes, including helping the driver rehabilitation specialist (DRS) to do the following:

- Establish the client's ability to meet basic criteria (e.g., visual acuity) set by the driver licensing agency for securing or maintaining a driver's license
- Develop a client profile that highlights existing strengths and weaknesses related to predriving activities (e.g., transferring into the vehicle and stowing a mobility aid) and basic driving skills
- Identify the need for initiating referrals to other specialists (e.g., neuropsychologists, wheeled mobility and seating specialists, low-vision specialists)
- Prepare to conduct an individualized on-road evaluation
- Determine the client's potential to learn new skills and benefit from adaptive driving equipment options
- Develop compensatory strategies for driving or alternatives to driving that enable community mobility
- Develop a customized driver training plan that is tailored to meet the unique needs of the client

The predictive value of the clinical evaluation has not been well established in the professional literature. (See Chapters 7 and 24 for more information about driver rehabilitation and community mobility evidence-based practice.) However, researchers and practitioners are collaborating to develop evaluation protocols that are both reliable and valid. There is not a consensus among DRSs as to which clinical tests can most effectively predict driver readiness; however, there are numerous assessments that are used by DRSs. See Table 5-2 for a comprehensive list of frequently used tests by DRSs while conducting clinical evaluations.

Data collected during the clinical evaluation are almost never sufficient to provide a definitive recommendation that a client is safe or unsafe to drive, with a few exceptions to be discussed later in this chapter. Rather the clinical evaluation is most beneficial in helping the DRS to analyze and understand the client's on-road driving performance. Therefore, a comprehensive driver rehabilitation evaluation must include both the clinical evaluation and the *on-road evaluation*. This section will focus on the following topics: (1) the importance of health care providers, such as occupational therapy (OT) generalists, recognizing the importance of screening clients in order to determine when it is appropriate to initiate referrals to qualified DRSs; (2) the value of the driver rehabilitation *team approach*; and (3) the component tests comprising the clinical evaluation that provides the foundation upon which the on-road evaluation of a client's driving performance can be conducted.

DRIVING AND COMMUNITY MOBILITY

Community mobility includes traveling about the community under one's own power (e.g., walking, biking, roller skating), using a wheeled mobility device (e.g., motorized scooter) or ambulation aid (e.g., walker, crutches, cane), operating a motor vehicle, and accessing alternative transportation such as riding as a passenger in a motor vehicle with a family member or friend who is driving, taking the bus, and using a form of mass transit, to name a few. Community mobility should be considered an activity of daily living (ADL) for most people in the United States and elsewhere around the world.[1] However, because of its complexity, most consider community mobility generally, and driving specifically, to be an *instrumental activity of daily living* (IADL). Before a DRS can evaluate a client's ability to drive a motor vehicle, he or she must first assess the prerequisite skills that enable a person to get behind the wheel of a motor vehicle and drive safely. After all, driving is without question one of the most complicated, dangerous, and meaningful activities that human beings engage in on a regular basis! (See Box 6-1.)

THE TEAM APPROACH

Driver rehabilitation and community mobility is a growing service area and has expanded beyond the traditional boundaries that were once demarcated by the field of physical medicine and rehabilitation. Professionals with diverse education, training, and credentials are becoming DRSs and expertly perform evaluations to determine whether a client can safely drive or whether intervention is warranted. Teamwork between the primary and ancillary driver rehabilitation team members is critical to ensure that a comprehensive driver rehabilitation evaluation of the client's capacity to perform the driving task is completed. In order to

BOX 6-1	Stages of the Driver Rehabilitation Process

1. Initial client screening and referral to a driver rehabilitation specialist
2. The clinical evaluation
3. The on-road evaluation of driving performance
4. On-road training
5. Long-term follow-up

accomplish this, DRSs assess the client's skills as they relate to driving at a variety of points along the rehabilitation continuum and, when the client is ready, validate the results through the on-road evaluation. Hopewell asserted that "Rehabilitation professionals should always work together as a team and should be aware of effective interventions for their profession, as well as the limitations of working in this area"[2] (p. 55). See Chapter 4 for more information on the driver rehabilitation team.

Clients, caregivers, DRSs, and the other driver rehabilitation team members work collaboratively to gain insight into the following:

- Clients' skill level prior to the onset of their disability that was secondary to an illness, injury, or the aging process
- The value that clients place on driving, alternatives to driving that enable community mobility, or both in the context of maintaining their preferred lifestyles
- Current deficits that negatively impact driving performance
- The feasibility of driving as a goal for community mobility
- The feasibility of clients to efficiently use alternative transportation

It is important for driver rehabilitation professionals, clients, and caregivers to understand the complexity of skills required to safely operate a motor vehicle. The professional driver rehabilitation team members can help clients recognize their strengths and limitations and carefully formulate a plan designed to help them begin or return to driving if possible. It is important for each of the team members to understand the importance of the on-road evaluation that is conducted by the DRS. To help facilitate the client's understanding, DRSs often recruit family members to participate in the evaluation process because the key to a successful or failed course of therapeutic intervention is family and caregiver participation.[3]

Rehabilitation professionals play an important role in helping to ensure that driving is included in the early development of the general rehabilitation intervention plan. Many rehabilitation facilities have added driving and community mobility to the initial evaluation checklist that is used by OT generalists and other rehabilitation team members. This usually marks the beginning of the data collection process to establish clients' predriving baseline status. Baseline information is used by DRSs to be better prepared to conduct formal clinical driver evaluations. It is often helpful if the DRS has some notion about a client's interests, history, and baseline skills before initiating the formal evaluation process.

How can rehabilitation and other health care professionals, such as physicians and OT generalists, accurately determine the role that driving, alternative community mobility, or both plays in the lives of their clients within the context of clients' IADL? Generalists can interview their clients with the aim of answering the following questions because answers to these and other basic questions about a client's past and current driving history can help health care professionals determine when to initiate a referral to a DRS.

- Does the client possess a valid driver's license? If not, did they ever possess a valid license? When and why was it forfeited?
- Does the client currently own a vehicle? If yes, what are the vehicle's make and model and what year was it manufactured? If no, has the client ever owned a motor vehicle?
- Is driving a motor vehicle necessary for the client to participate in work, self-care, and/or leisure activities in his or her community?
- Where did (or does) the client typically go when driving a motor vehicle?
- How would the client handle driving in inclement versus clement weather?
- Does the client need to consider storing a mobility aid or ambulation aid in the vehicle, such as a scooter or walker, respectively?

Answers to these questions can help the DRS gain insight into the role and function that driving has played, and could potentially play, for the client. Although during the early stages of rehabilitation it is characteristically premature for generalists to request that a DRS conduct a comprehensive driver rehabilitation evaluation, the long-term goal of driving will be indirectly addressed when OT generalists assist their clients with achieving more basic treatment objectives that are foundational to, and necessary for, safe and efficient driving and community mobility. This is important for the clients' peace of mind and can serve to motivate them to complete the smaller steps (e.g., improved strength, endurance, visual perception, cognition) that are required to attain their IADL goals, including driving. OT generalists should help their clients to connect the dots and realize the importance that client factors play in enabling the skills that are prerequisites to driving a motor vehicle.

Throughout the rehabilitation process, professionals can then continue to link clients' treatment goals to the long-term goal of driving. For example the physician will consider the impact of medications; the OT relates the client's level of independence with his or her personal care, cooking, housekeeping, visual perceptual, and executive skills; the physical therapist (PT) works on balance and gait training and identifies appropriate mobility aids; and the speech-language pathologist addresses language and cognition such as executive functioning. This process will support the client's desire to drive or use alternative transportation methods and will help health care professionals determine when a referral to the DRS should be initiated.

THE SCREENING PROCESS

As described in the previous section, the rehabilitation team can perform an on-going assessment of the client's skills related to driving. In some settings, such as an outpatient OT clinic, however, a client may be referred specifically for an assessment to determine his or her readiness to participate in a comprehensive driver rehabilitation evaluation. Two options are listed below for rehabilitation specialists and caregivers that can be used in the predriving screening process.

GROSS IMPAIRMENTS SCREENING (GRIMPS)

A Gross Impairments Screening (GRIMPS) battery has been developed as a tool for driver licensing agency staff to provide early detection of driving impairments in the well elderly population.[4] The battery consists of tests in two domains:

- Physical measures: Rapid pace walk, foot tap, head-neck rotation, and arm reach
- Perceptual-cognitive measures: Motor-Free Visual Perception Test (visual closure subtest; MVPT), Trail Making Test Part B, cued/delayed recall, scan test, dynamic trails, computer-based test, and Useful Field of Vision (UFOV) test–subtest 2 (processing speed and divided attention)[4]

ASSESSMENT OF DRIVING-RELATED SKILLS

The Assessment of Driving-Related Skills (ADReS) is designed for use by physicians. It is comprised of brief assessments designed to target essential functions that are required for safe driving including the following: vision, cognition, and motor skills. Any impairment in these functions may increase the client's risk for crash[4]; however, the ADReS does not claim to predict crash risk. The ADReS uses the Snellen chart to test visual acuity, confrontation testing to evaluate visual field of view, Trail Making Test Part B, Clock Drawing Test (CDT), rapid pace walk, manual range of motion (ROM) testing, and manual muscle strength testing. The test is fully described and a score sheet is provided in the *Physicians Guide to Assessing and Counseling Older Drivers.*[5]

Some OT clinics coordinate efforts with their local driver rehabilitation service providers to develop a screening instrument for their settings. The battery of tests covers the essential skill areas of physical abilities, attention, visual perception, and cognition but uses different testing instruments to avoid a practice effect with evaluations conducted by the DRS.

For the active driver and caregivers there are many resources, driving self-screens, and impairment indicators. One example is the Association for Driver Rehabilitation Specialists (ADED), which has published warning signs listed by disability on its web site. The Safe Mobility for Life project also has the "How Is Your Driving Health?" brochure (Figure 6-1), Self-Awareness Checklist, and Tips to Help You Drive Safely Longer, to name a few. These invaluable resources (Box 6-2) are available at no cost to OT generalists, DRSs, clients, caregivers, and others.

THE CLINICAL EVALUATION

Clinical evaluations are conducted by DRSs such as occupational therapists specializing in driver rehabilitation and community mobility services. The clinical evaluation is comprised of a series of tests that are by and large accepted by the professional community within the United States. As previously mentioned, the clinical evaluation is the first of two components that make up the comprehensive driver rehabilitation evaluation and must be completed before on-road evaluations can be initiated. DRSs use the clinical evaluation to analyze clients' strengths and limitations in a variety of skill areas. The on-road evaluations of actual driving performance require clients to integrate these skills in a smooth, coordinated manner with quick speed of response. It is also critical that the rehabilitation specialist and DRS are aware of the state statutes regarding driving, reporting procedures, and the level of expertise that is required of the DRSs practicing in their respective states.

BOX 6-2	Driver and Caregiver Resources

Association for Driver Rehabilitation Specialists' web site: Fact sheets, with warning signs listed by client's disability
    www.aded.net
    Safe Mobility for Older Drivers
    http://www.nhtsa.dot.gov/people/injury/olddrive/safe/01a.htm
    The Safe Mobility for Life project
    How Is Your Driving Health? A Self-Awareness Checklist and Tips to Help You Drive Safely Longer
    http://www.nhtsa.dot.gov/people/injury/olddrive/modeldriver/1_app_c.htm

How Is Your Driving Health?

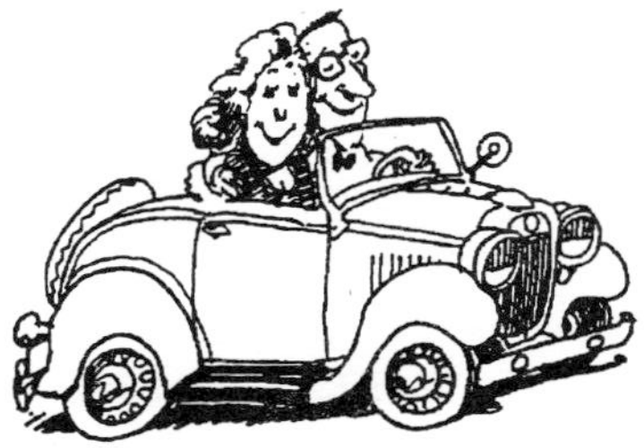

A Self-Awareness Checklist

&

Tips to Help You Drive Safely Longer

A product promoting *Safe Mobility for Life* from the Maryland Research Consortium on older drivers, and the National Highway Traffic Safety Administration.

SELF AWARENESS: THE KEY TO SAFE DRIVING

While we all want to keep driving for as long we can, none of us wants to be a threat to ourselves or to others because we are no longer able to drive safely. A leading cause of accidental death among older persons is automobile crashes.

— ☀ —

It's important to remember that most seniors *are* capable, and have a lifetime of valuable driving experience. Decisions about a person's ability to drive should never be based on age alone.

— ☀ —

Fortunately, most seniors take appropriate steps when they detect a problem with their driving. But it's not always obvious when a general health problem, vision problem, or a side effect of medications will lead to a driving impairment.

— ☀ —

Self awareness is the key. People who can accurately assess their fitness to drive can adjust their driving habits, and stay safe on the road. They will retain the personal mobility that comes with driving, while limiting the risks to themselves and to others.

— ☀ —

This brochure can increase your awareness about different problems that lead to unsafe driving. It also gives you tips to help keep you behind the wheel. For more information, contact:

To find a driver rehabilitation specialist in your area:
- Association of Driver Educators for the Disabled (608) 884-8833
- Maryland Board of Occupational Therapy Practice (410) 764-4728

To find a mature driver education class in your area:
- AARP/55-Alive Toll Free: 1-888-AARP-NOW (1-888-227-7669)
- AAA Safe Driving for Mature Drivers (Call your local AAA club for availability of classes)

For information about benefits & services for older persons provided by the Agency on Aging in your area:
- Senior Information & Assistance Programs Toll Free: 1-800-AGE-DIAL (1-800-243-3425) TTY-410-767-1083

DON'T IGNORE THE WARNING SIGNS

HAS THIS HAPPENED TO YOU?

◊ A friend or family member has expressed concern about your driving.

◊ You sometimes get lost while driving on routes that were once familiar.

◊ You have been pulled over by a police officer and warned of poor driving behavior, regardless of whether or not you received a ticket.

◊ You have had several moving violations, near misses, or actual crashes in the past three years.

◊ Your doctor or other health care giver has advised you to restrict or stop driving.

— ☀ —

✓ Listen to what people tell you who know you best and care the most about you.

✓ Discuss driving with your doctor—he or she can evaluate the interactions and side effects of all the medications you may be taking.

✓ Refresh your knowledge of safe driving practices and learn about new traffic control & roadway design features through a mature driver class.

✓ Begin planning for alternative ways of meeting your mobility needs. Now is the time to learn about mobility options in your community -- try them out...see what works best for you.

Figure 6-1 How Is Your Driving Health? brochure. (From the Maryland Research Consortium on older drivers and the National Highway Traffic Safety Administration.)

Continued

VISION

Good driving health begins with good vision. With declining vision, your responses to signals, signs, and changing traffic conditions become slower, increasing your crash risk.

Warning Signs

- You have problems reading highway or street signs, or recognizing someone you know across the street.
- You have trouble seeing lane lines & other pavement markings; curbs & medians; and other vehicles & pedestrians, especially at dawn or dusk, and at night.
- You are experiencing more discomfort from the glare of oncoming headlights at night.

Tips

✓ Make sure your corrective lenses have a current prescription, and always wear them. If you lose or break your glasses, don't rely on an old pair; replace them right away with your new prescription.

✓ Do **not** wear sunglasses or tinted lenses at night. This reduces the amount of light that reaches your eyes, and makes driving much more hazardous.

✓ Keep your windshield and headlights clean, and make sure your headlight aim is checked when your vehicle is inspected.

✓ Sit high enough in your seat so that you can see the road within 10 feet in front of your car. This will make a big difference in reducing the amount of glare you experience from opposing headlights at night. Use a cushion if your car seats don't have vertical adjustment.

✓ People age 61 and older should see an optometrist or ophthalmologist every year to check for cataracts, glaucoma, macular degeneration, diabetic retinopathy, and other conditions for which we are at greater risk as we grow older.

PHYSICAL FITNESS

Diminished strength, flexibility, and coordination can have a major impact on your ability to control your vehicle in a safe manner.

Warning Signs

- You have trouble looking over your shoulder to change lanes, or looking left & right to check traffic at intersections.
- You have trouble moving your foot from the gas to the brake pedal, or turning the steering wheel.
- You have fallen down in the past 3 years.
- You walk less than 1 block per day.
- You can't raise your arms above your shoulders.
- You have difficulty climbing stairs.

Tips

✓ With your doctor's approval, do some stretching exercises, and start a walking program. Walk around the block, or in a shopping mall. Also, check your local health clubs, YMCAs, senior centers, community colleges, and hospitals for fitness programs geared to the needs of seniors.

✓ Get examined by a podiatrist if you have pain or swelling in your feet. If you have pain or stiffness in your arms, legs, or neck, your doctor may prescribe medication and/or physical therapy.

✓ An occupational therapist or a *certified driving rehabilitation specialist* may be able to prescribe special equipment for your car to make it easier to steer and to use your pedals.

✓ Eliminate your driver's side blind spot by re-aiming your mirror. First, lean your head against the window, *then* adjust your mirror outward so that when you look at the inside edge you can barely see the side of your car. If you use a wide-angle mirror, get *lots* of practice judging distances to other cars before using it in traffic.

ATTENTION AND REACTION TIME

Driving often requires quick reactions to safety threats. As we grow older, it becomes more difficult to divide attention and to make rapid responses.

Warning Signs

- You feel overwhelmed by all of the signs, signals, markings, pedestrians, and other vehicles that you must pay attention to at intersections.
- Gaps in traffic are harder to judge, making it more difficult to turn left at intersections, or to merge with traffic when turning right.
- You take medications that make you drowsy.
- You often get lost or become disoriented.
- You aren't confident that you can handle the demands of high speeds or heavy traffic volumes.
- You are slower in recognizing cars coming out of driveways or side streets, or realizing that another car has slowed or stopped ahead of you.

Tips

✓ Plan your route. Drive where you are familiar with the road conditions and traffic patterns.

✓ Drive during the day, and avoid rush hours.

✓ A passenger can serve as a "second pair of eyes." But don't get distracted in conversation!

✓ When approaching intersections, remember to stay alert for cars and pedestrians entering from the side unexpectedly.

✓ Leave enough distance between you and the car ahead to react to a sudden stop, but understand that *too large* a gap will invite others to cut in front of you in heavy traffic. A gap of 3 seconds or more is most desirable, conditions permitting. Look for a tree, sign, etc. When the car ahead of you passes this point count "1001, 1002, 1003." If you can count to 1003 by the time you get to the same point, this equals a 3-second gap.

Figure 6-1 cont'd

TEST SELECTION

Driving is a complex task requiring efficient and accurate use of physical, sensory, and cognitive skills; therefore, the assessment of driving skills is an equally complex process[3] (p 17). The battery of tests that comprise the clinical evaluation can be expanded and abbreviated based on the issues that are specific to the client. For example a client with an incomplete spinal cord injury (SCI) would require a detailed investigation of his or her physical capacities and deficits and the long-term potential for further recovery. By contrast a physical assessment may not be needed for an individual with a diagnosis of attention deficit disorder (ADD) who has no history of sensorimotor limitations. Using these same examples, a brief screening of cognitive skills (versus a full cognitive evaluation) may be all that is needed for the individual with SCI; by contrast a far more thorough assessment of visual perception, cognition, and academic skills would be warranted for the client with learning disabilities.

McKenna[6] offered the following suggestions for preferred characteristics of tests if they are to be included in the battery of clinical assessments. The assessment tools should require basic skills and could be easily passed by the majority of the population and should not depend on intelligence level. Each of the tests should have a direct functional correlate to the driving task and most importantly should be validated by the on-road evaluation.

ADED[7] published the *Best Practices for the Delivery of Driver Rehabilitation Services* and lists the following components as parts of the clinical evaluation:
- Interview and medical history
- Physical assessment
- Visual assessment
- Cognitive assessment

Interview and Medical History

The interview can begin with the DRS providing a brief overview of the stages of the comprehensive driver rehabilitation evaluation and training (i.e., clinical evaluation, on-road evaluation, and on-road training) or by addressing driving cessation by identifying alternative community mobility. The current status of the client's driver's license must be addressed by the DRS and discussed with the client, as this may determine possible limits to the behind-the-wheel assessment. The DRS must be familiar with the licensing requirements for his or her state; for example an on-road evaluation may not be conducted if the individual's driving privilege has been revoked or refused by the licensing agency. Also, a state may require the readministration of the law test if the client's license has been expired beyond a specified length of time. This would indicate the need to include an assessment of the client's ability to demonstrate his or her knowledge of the rules of the road by passing a paper and pencil test that is often presented in a multiple-choice format.

The state's licensing and medical reporting regulations should be discussed with the individual. See Appendix A for a listing of licensing laws and reporting requirements by state. Many clients who have been referred for a driver rehabilitation evaluation may be unaware of the specific laws pertaining to driving with a disability, aging-related concern, or both. A release of information form may be completed by the DRS for the licensing agency, the physician, and other relevant parties. The possible outcomes of the driver evaluation should be clearly defined, as well as the policy of the driver rehabilitation program regarding reporting drivers who may present a danger to themselves, to the public, or both.

The DRS performs a thorough assessment of the client's driving habits. Several questionnaires are available to serve this purpose and often include items such as typical distances traveled by motor vehicle, times of the day when the client is most often behind the wheel, the kinds of traffic environments he or she is accustomed to driving in, and crash history.[3,8] Questions can be included to address the client's ability to analyze his or her own strengths and weaknesses and tendency to self-limit his or her driving, such as avoiding high-volume traffic or not driving at night. If a cross-check of the client's insight and awareness of deficits is needed, the questionnaire can also be given to a family member to complete.

Physical Assessment

An assessment of the client's physical skills enables the DRS to anticipate possible problems in vehicle control and to guide the decision-making process for adapted driving equipment, vehicle modifications, and driver training strategies. See Chapter 11 for a description of the ways that the information acquired during the clinical evaluation can be used to determine the preferred vehicle type and equipment fit.

Height and Limb Length

For clients of short stature or who have limbs that are shorter than the normal range, the DRS should consider the implications for vehicle modifications. A seating system may be needed to position the individual for enhanced line of sight to help ensure correct viewing of the traffic environment. Modifications may be needed to resize or reposition the steering wheel or to add an on/off switch to the driver's front airbag. A vehicle with power-adjustable brake and accelerator pedals, after-market extensions, or the use of hand controls may be viable options. A client of above average height may need to make careful choices as to the type of vehicle (e.g., van, sport utility vehicle [SUV], or truck) for ease of entering and exiting and for proper positioning and line of sight once inside of the vehicle. Measurements of the length of the client's limbs and trunk may be useful. Digital photographs of the client seated in the mocked-up vehicle are valuable for design purpose, to establish a visual baseline measurement, for formulating recommendations, and to illustrate the client's needs for third-party reimbursement.

Range of Motion and Strength

The client's ability to turn his or her head from side to side is important for visual scanning and searching techniques, especially while in traffic, stopped or yielding at an intersection, or both. Neck ROM tends to decrease as people age.[9] The DRS should ask the client to look to the right and left and measure and document any limitations. If the limitation in the client's neck range is not likely to improve, the DRS should consider the possibility of an enhanced mirror system in the vehicle. Barry et al[10] found that the use of a cervical brace had a negative impact on driving performance, with an increase in the driver's blind spots. Moreover drivers were observed to compensate by decreased speeds and slower acceleration when executing lane changes, which can increase the likelihood of a traffic accident.

The DRS should measure any limitations in the client's upper extremity joint ROM. Limitations in ROM may indicate the need to increase the client's seat height in the vehicle or to modify the size or position of the steering wheel. Limited reach may also affect the client's ability to access secondary controls, such as lights, turn signals, windshield wipers, and heating and air-conditioning controls.

A manual muscle test (MMT) may be warranted for a thorough assessment of the client's arm strength. Because operation of the vehicle controls involves a coordination of movements, the action of steering or of hand control use can be imitated and the degree of strength noted. Reduced effort steering or electronic gas and brake may be needed. A dynamometer, muscle testing, or both can be used to assess grip strength. Various steering devices may be considered for individuals with grasp weakness.

Joint ROM and strength of the lower extremities (especially the right leg) should also be assessed. Limitations in hip, knee, and ankle motion may affect the client's ability to enter and exit the vehicle and may influence recommendations for the type of vehicle to be selected. Limitations in lower extremity ROM may affect proper positioning that is necessary for the client to safely reach the controls and to sit at a proper viewing height. The client's ability to move his or her foot

from the gas pedal to the brake pedal can be further assessed during brake reaction testing.

There will likely be joint ROM restrictions after a total hip replacement, which may make it difficult for the client to get into and out of the vehicle safely. The client may also be at risk for falling when walking to and from the vehicle and when entering or exiting the vehicle. If the surgery was performed on the right hip, there may be interference with accelerator to brake reaction time. The client may also need an assistive device for walking, such as a walker or cane. He or she would need to be able to stow the ambulation aid safely in the vehicle and learn how to get into and out of the car in a way that does not require flexing the hip greater than 90 degrees or externally rotating the hip. The client may need to look at alternative ways to drive if his or her right lower extremity ROM, coordination, or strength is not sufficient for safe driving with the involved extremity or foot. A left foot gas pedal may be a consideration for adapted driving.

Limitations in right ankle motion, such as a status post-ankle fracture or the use of a right ankle-foot orthosis, would hinder the client's ability to apply the correct amount of pressure on the accelerator and brake pedals. A client may intend to compensate by lifting his or her leg from the hip; however, this maneuver is fatiguing and could compromise foot pedal control in time. A better alternative would be to use the uninvolved left leg with a left foot gas pedal. If both legs are limited, hand controls may be a consideration.

Sensation

Proprioception and *kinesthetic awareness*, or the knowledge of the position of the extremity and its movement, respectively, are critical to driving. Clients with decreased position sense and kinesthetic awareness may have difficulty with accurate foot placement on the pedals and movement even if their feet are positioned properly. Other important sensory input would be the ability to sense light and deep pressure, which would allow the client to judge the amount of force he or she is exerting on the accelerator and brake pedals.

Sensation of the upper and lower extremities should be considered. For example a client diagnosed with right hemiplegia after a cerebrovascular accident (CVA) might have good recovery of arm motion but might have decreased sensation in the involved extremities. Consequently steering may be more accurate using the left arm only with a steering (i.e., spinner) knob.

Another consideration would be whether the client's health condition is progressive or static. For example consider a person with diabetes mellitus (DM) who underwent a right leg amputation because of circulatory problems. Although he or she may demonstrate satisfactory sensation in the left lower extremity, brake reaction speed, and driving skill with a left foot accelerator, the DRS, after consultation with the physician, may recommend hand controls in anticipation of further sensory loss in the left leg.

Coordination

Coordination of arm and leg motion is critical to control a motor vehicle. Because the vehicle becomes an extension of the driver, the vehicle amplifies difficulty in coordination. For example a client with Parkinson's disease (PD) may only be exerting slight tremulous motion on the steering wheel; however, the vehicle may be moving from side to side in the lane. An individual with cerebral palsy (CP) may exert excess force on the brake, resulting in a harder stop than is desired.

Muscle Tone

An assessment of muscle tone will help the DRS to appreciate the degree of the individual's motor control for handling the vehicle. An example would be an individual diagnosed with a traumatic brain injury (TBI) that resulted in a mild left hemiparesis who wishes to steer the vehicle using both hands. However, as the client drives and muscle tone increases, the left hand begins pulling the steering wheel to the left, causing the vehicle to cross the centerline. In this example the client may be able to better control his or her steering using a right spinner knob. The DRS can then assess the client's ability to use his or her left hand for operation of the turn signals.

Intermittent spasm activity can be a problem for individuals with SCI. Sudden severe spasms affecting the client's legs, trunk stability, or arm motion can seriously impact vehicle control. Typically an individual with SCI learns to avoid the motions that can trigger a spasm, but sometimes hitting a speed bump while driving or riding as a passenger in a vehicle, for example, can initiate spasm activity. A referral to the physician for medication management may be indicated.

Clients with CP may experience the effect of reflexes impacting on their voluntary movement. For example head turning to the right or left may elicit arm extension to that side, resulting in a tendency to steer in that direction. There may be associated reactions from one extremity to another. A client using hand controls may notice that steering to the left results in a similar motion in the left arm, thereby increasing acceleration via the hand controls during the turn. One extreme example is the client who was unable to apply the brake without eliciting a startle reaction that caused him to release his grasp on the steering wheel. Typically an extended in-vehicle evaluation period is needed to determine whether the individual can develop the ability to inhibit these reflexive motions to maintain control over the vehicle. Another consideration would be the client's ability to access the secondary controls of the vehicle, such as the turn signals, lights, and the heating and air-conditioning system. An alternate access method may need to be considered.

Apraxia, or deficits in motor planning, can be a factor in clients with TBI, stroke, or dementia. Individuals with autism spectrum disorders also can have deficits in motor coordination.[11] These deficits can have serious implications for the client's ability to control the motor vehicle, depending on the severity of the apraxia noted.

Endurance

The DRS can observe the client's endurance for activity during the span of the clinical evaluation and interview the client about his or her awareness of his or her stamina and the changes in his or her movement capacity when fatigued. Motor and cognitive fatigue can be a particular problem for individuals with multiple sclerosis (MS). It may be advisable to schedule the assessment for several sessions, with at least one appointment in the afternoon hours, so that the client's limitations can be noted and compensation strategies considered. This factor can be further assessed during the on-road evaluation. For example an individual may be able to drive satisfactorily with standard controls during the morning hours but may experience a decrease in vehicle handling abilities later in the day, indicating the need to assess the use of adapted driving equipment on an as-needed basis. Clients' sensitivity to their own endurance limitations is key because they will need to self-limit their driving to shorter trips, specified times of the day, or have a back-up plan for support.

Reaction Speed

The time required to identify and respond to a stimulus can be critical to safe driving in the dynamic, complex traffic environment. A decrease in response time has been documented in clients with acquired brain injury,[12,13] stroke,[14] and MS[15,16] and in the elderly population.[17,18]

Some state licensing agencies have set criteria for brake reaction speed. In Maryland, for example, the Motor Vehicle Administration (MVA) requires a minimum reaction speed of 0.5 second (0.5/sec), tested on the American Automobile Association (AAA) Brake Reaction Timer. The AAA instruction manual indicates that a reaction time of 0.39 second falls at the fiftieth percentile for men and women, with ages ranging from 21 to 80 years.[19] Unfortunately the AAA no longer offers this equipment; therefore alternative reaction speed testing equipment must be used.

Porto Clinic

The Porto Clinic provides an assessment of simple and complex reaction time and near- versus far-point vision and depth perception. The client is instructed to apply pressure to the accelerator in response to a green light on the control panel. When the light changes to yellow, the client should reduce pressure on the accelerator and apply the brake in response to the red light. The instrument then measures the speed of the client's response, which is judged against the norms provided. It is worthwhile to note that brake reaction testing does not assess the client's ability to control the amount of pressure placed on the accelerator or brake pedals. These skills would be further assessed in the vehicle.

Vericom

The Vericom braking reaction timer (Vericom Computers, Inc., Rogers, MN) is an in-vehicle assessment tool. The Vericom draws power from the vehicle's battery via the accessory power outlet. It has a suction-mounted control panel just above the center dashboard, which is used by the DRS. A small display is mounted within the view of the driver but without blocking visibility of either the road environment or the vehicle's dashboard gauges.

This test is conducted in a large, vacant parking lot or a designated driving range. Driving practice is provided to allow the driver to become familiar with the handling of the vehicle and to demonstrate sufficient vehicle control skills. The driver is instructed to accelerate beyond a minimum of 25 mph. At a random interval the DRS activates a red light, indicating a need for a hard brake. The Vericom will measure reaction time, stop time, brake speed, reaction distance, stop distance, and peak G (i.e., the maximum G force pulled). Vericom suggests that the average reaction time is normally considered to be 0.75 second.[20]

It has been noted that reaction time in the vehicle is generally slower than the rate measured during the clinical evaluation. Response time is also likely to be slowed when the driver is surprised or the driving situation is stressful, or both.[21]

Several visual perceptual/cognitive tests also provide a means to rate visual processing speed, notably the MVPT-3 and the Trail Making Test. These provide a useful comparison with the client's performance on the brake reaction speed tests and may indicate a client's potential to improve. For example an individual who has an average response time on the MVPT-3 but fails the brake reaction test may have a specific impairment of lower extremity functioning and may respond well to treatment. By comparison a client who scores low on both measures is demonstrating a more global deficit in processing and response rate, and remediation may not be as successful.

Balance

A client's balance affects his or her ability to travel to and from the vehicle and to safely enter or exit the vehicle.

The client's sitting balance can be a factor when making turns, particularly for individuals with SCIs and other diagnoses that impact sitting balance. Decreased sitting balance may be compensated for by seating systems, additional seat belts, or both. A preliminary assessment of balance can be done during the clinical evaluation by interviewing the client and by pushing slightly on his or her shoulder from the right or left and then observing his or her ability to maintain an erect sitting posture or his or her need to compensate by arm or leg motion. Of course the DRS is advised to provide clients with close supervision and use a transfer belt during these assessment procedures to minimize the risk of a client falling.

Considerations Regarding Wheelchairs

The client's skill in wheelchair to and from vehicle transfers would be more specifically assessed in the vehicle, but an initial discussion of techniques, adaptive equipment, and endurance could be held during the clinical evaluation. The DRS should note that the act of transferring to the driver's side of the vehicle presents different challenges than transferring to the passenger's side. Many clients who have been passengers since the onset of their injuries may not have as much experience in transferring on the driver's side of the vehicle.

It is also important to note the make and model of the wheelchair or scooter and to discuss plans for storage of the equipment in the vehicle. Another significant issue is the individuals' indication of their need and intention to acquire a new wheelchair or scooter because this may be a critical factor in current and future vehicle modification recommendations. An OT or PT wheeled mobility and seating specialist consult may be needed to fully address this issue. See Chapters 9 and 17 for more information about wheeled mobility and driving.

Visual Skills

Several screening tools are available, and if the DRS notes problems in a client's visual skills, a referral to a vision specialist is warranted.

Optec

The Optec is a vision screening tool.[22] The slide package designed for driving includes an assessment of near-point vision (to assess acuity for the dashboard controls of a vehicle or to adequately view the clinical evaluation tests), distance vision, peripheral vision, color discrimination, depth perception, and sign recognition. The Optec also has tumbling E slides, which can be useful to assess far-point acuity for clients with aphasia. A recommended addition, because of its importance to driving, is the contrast package.[23] This measures an individual's contrast sensitivity, which would indicate his or her vision during poor lighting conditions (e.g., at night, at dusk, on a cloudy day, on a rainy day).

Titmus Vision Screener

The Titmus Vision Screener, like the Optec, provides assessment of near and distance acuity, traffic color recognition, depth perception, and peripheral vision. For clients with language impairment, visual acuity slides using number stimuli or tumbling Es are available. Slides also are provided for traffic sign recognition set at 20/40 or 20/70 visual acuity. The ability to recognize common traffic signs can be one pertinent indicator of driver readiness for clients with dementia.[24] Note that the Porto Clinic also provides a means to assess acuity and depth perception as previously stated.

Cognitive Skills

A complex array of cognitive skills is considered relevant to the function of driving, notably attention, scanning, visual perception, judgment, memory, and executive skills.[2,25] See Chapters 1, 7, 12, and 21 for more information.

Visual Perception Tests

The MVPT was designed and standardized for adults for the normal population and the brain-injured population.[26] It has norms for people aged 18 to 80 years and is a motor-free test of visual perceptual abilities, including spatial relationships, visual discrimination, figure-ground, visual closure, and visual memory.[27] This test provides a profile of basic visual perceptual skills needed to drive, as well as an indication of a client's speed in processing visual information, and has been correlated to driving performance.[28]

MVPT-3[29] is the version of the test that is available at the time of this writing. The test has been expanded to 65 items. Several subsections have been added (e.g., spatial orientation and figure-ground, as well as more difficult items requiring visual closure and visual short-term memory). The test norms now extend to ages ≥94 years. A means to record and judge response speed has also been included,[30] which is critical for responding to the rapid processing of traffic interaction.[12] This version of the test was recently introduced and is markedly more difficult. Test norms also do not exist as of yet to correlate test performance with the determination of driving risk.

The Test of Visual Perceptual Skills—Revised (TVPS-R) is similar in format to the MVPT but provides a consistent number of test items for each of its seven subtests: visual discrimination, visual memory, visual-spatial relationships, visual form constancy, visual sequential memory, visual figure-ground, and visual closure. The test offers an upper level (UL) version that provides norms for young people aged 12 to 18 years.

The test has recently been revised to add less difficult items and to refine the norms.[31]

The Hooper Visual Organization Test provides 30 drawings of common objects that have been cut apart and rearranged. The client is asked to name the object and so must mentally rotate the parts into a recognizable whole. The test was normed on subjects ranging in ages from 13 to 80 years.[32]

In the UFOV test, the concept of "useful field of view" refers to the brain's ability to comprehend visual information with the head and eyes in a stationary position.[33] The UFOV test is administered on a computer using a touch screen. The test involves a series of slides and objects the client must remember amid background visual distractions. It tests visual memory, visual attention, and divided attention with structured and unstructured components. The test differs substantially from standard eye examinations that measure visual acuity or visual function and the ability to see an object at a given distance.[34] The UFOV has been shown to be a strong predictor of crash risk in older drivers.[35]

Inclusion of a visual-motor test in the clinical evaluation is advisable because driving is not a motor-free task. The test also should be used for the population for which it has been designed. For example a test that assesses the developmental level of a skill, such as visual-motor coordination, is valuable for use with individuals with developmental disabilities such as CP, mental retardation (MR), and spina bifida (SB). By contrast a test such as the Benton Test of Visual Retention has been designed for individuals with acquired deficits such as TBI and CVA. This test does not provide developmental norms; however, it does provide an indication of memory for visual stimuli and a measure of visual inattention. In contrast, unilateral neglect would not be a likely deficit noted with a client with CP for example.

The Beery-Buktenica Developmental Test of Visual-Motor Integration (VMI) consists of 27 geometric forms of increasing complexity. The client is required to copy each form without erasing. The results are analyzed by specific criteria, and norms are provided for young people aged 3 to 18 years.[36]

The Benton Visual Retention Test provides three sets of 10 geometric designs and allows for four methods of administration. It assesses the client's ability to copy the designs and demonstrate recall in one of three different conditions. The versatility of the test allows for repeated administration while minimizing the practice effect. The test is also sensitive to inattention, demonstrated by an increased number of errors for designs on the right or left of the page. The norms can be adjusted for age and education level; norms are provided for those aged 8 to 89 years.[37]

The Dynavision has a series of lights arranged in a large circle on a metal board. The board is adjustable so that a client can be tested at different heights or from a seated position. The large size helps to ensure that a significant portion of the client's visual field is stimulated. The lights are illuminated in a random pattern, and the client is required to touch each light to turn it off or to cause another light to activate.[38] There are several modes of increasing complexity that require various response patterns by the client. There has been some evidence that visual-motor training using this tool can result in improvement of a client's on-road driving performance.[39]

Cognition and Memory

The Trail Making Test has been highly correlated with driving performance.[2] The Trail Making Test was initially designed as part of the U.S. Army Individual Test Battery[40] and is now in the public domain. The administration instructions are provided in detail in *A Compendium of Neuropsychological Tests: Administration, Norms and Commentary*[41]; they are reproduced in Box 6-3.

Norms are available for persons aged 18 to 89 years, and it has been noted that scores decrease for individuals with advanced age or lower education levels.[42] A government study[4] suggested that a timed score of 100 seconds on the Trails B subtest would indicate a need for further testing of driving performance because it correlated with increased crash risk.

CLOX is a clock drawing test that is designed to differentiate executive function and visual-spatial praxis.[43] In CLOX 1 the client is requested to draw a clock, and in CLOX 2 the client copies a clock drawn by the evaluator. Standardized instructions are provided: "Draw me a clock that says 1:45. Set the hands and numbers on the face so that a child could read them"[43] (p. 589). For CLOX 2 the evaluator draws a clock in a circle printed on the scoring sheet, following a specific sequence. The client is then asked to copy the evaluator's drawing. The two drawings are then scored, and the client's performance for the two testing conditions is compared. The test is particularly valuable for clients with dementia and Alzheimer's disease.

The Rivermead Behavioral Memory Test is a test of everyday memory skills, including the ability to remember names, faces, pictures, appointments, a brief story, a short route within the room, and the location of a personal object hidden in the room. Normal performance would result in one or two errors on the 12-test items.[44]

In the Cognitive Linguistic Quick Test (CLQT) five domains of cognitive function can be comparatively assessed with this instrument: attention, visual-spatial skills, language, memory, and executive function. The test is criterion referenced for two age ranges, 18 to 60 and 70 to 89 years, and is designed for clients who are experiencing cognitive deficits as a result of CVAs, acquired brain injuries (ABIs), and dementia.[45]

Tests of driving knowledge are informal tests that demonstrate the client's knowledge of the rules of driving. They test the client's ability to recognize road signs, familiarity with vehicle laws, and practical applications of the rules of the road. A familiar example would be the law test provided by many driver-licensing agencies to qualify an individual for a learner's permit. Similar tests are also available from driver education courses. For experienced drivers, tests of defensive driving techniques are available. Although these tests provide an indication of the client's knowledge of information pertinent to driving, they do not assess or predict the client's functional driving skills or ability to integrate knowledge and performance skills when on the road.

A Driver Performance Test (DPT) consists of 40 brief videotaped driving scenes, each taken from the perspective of the driver in the vehicle. Each video is followed by a multiple-choice question. The test items are given point scores for the best to the least acceptable answer. The scores can be compared with those of experienced drivers of automobiles and light trucks and can be analyzed for strengths and weaknesses in the skills of Search, Identify, Predict, Decide, and Execute, which are the critical skills for safe operation of a motor vehicle.[46]

INTERPRETATION OF TEST RESULTS

As previously stated the primary value of the clinical evaluation is to prepare the DRS for the on-road testing and to provide a possible explanation of the client's on-road performance. It has also been stressed throughout this chapter that a decision to "pass" or "fail" the client should not be based on the clinical evaluation alone. However, there are a few exceptions to this rule. A recommendation against driving that is based on clinical evaluation results is appropriate in the following situations:

• The client does not meet the standards set by the driver-licensing agency. If the client does not meet the vision criteria, brake reaction speed, if applicable, or various medical qualifications (e.g., a seizure disorder that is controlled by medication for a specified time period), a referral to a specialist (e.g., vision care or neurologist) or for further therapy may be considered.

• The client scores in the severely deficient ranges on all or most of the tests included in the clinical evaluation.

BOX 6-3 | Instructions for the Trail Making Test Parts A and B

ADMINISTRATION—PART A

Sample A. When ready to begin the test, place the Part A test sheet in front of the subject. Give the subject a pencil, and say: *"On this page* (point) *are some numbers. Begin at number 1* (point to "1") *and draw a line from one to two,* (point to "2"), *two to three* (point to "3"), *three to four* (point to "4"), *and so on, in order, until you reach the end* (pointing to the circle marked "END"). *Draw the lines as fast as you can. Do not lift the pencil from the paper. Ready! Begin!"*

If the subject makes a mistake on Sample A, point it out, and explain it. The following explanations of mistakes are acceptable:

1. "You started with the wrong circle. This is where you start (point to "1")."
2. "You skipped this circle (point to the one omitted). You should go from number one (point) to two (point), two to three (point) and so on, until you reach the circle marked 'END' (point)."
3. "Please keep the pencil on the paper, and continue right onto the next circle."

After the mistake has been explained, the examiner marks out the wrong part and says: *"Go on from here"* (point to the last circle completed correctly in the sequence).

If the subject still cannot complete Sample A, take the subject's hand and guide the pencil (eraser end down) through the trail. Then say: *"Now you try it. Put your pencil, point down. Remember, begin at number one* (point) *and draw a line from one to two* (point to "2"), *two to three* (point to "3"), *three to four* (point to "4"), *and so on, in order until you reach the circle marked 'END'* (point). *Do not skip around but go from one number to the next in the proper order. If you make a mistake, mark it out. Remember, work as fast as you can. Ready! Begin!"*

If the subject succeeds this time, go on to Part A of the test. If not, repeat the procedure until the subject does succeed, or it becomes evident that he or she cannot do it.

If the subject completes the sample item correctly and in a manner that he or she knows what to do, say: *"Good! Let's try the next one."* Turn the page, and give Part A of the test.

Test. Say, *"On this page are numbers from 1 to 25. Do this the same way. Begin at number one* (point) *and draw a line from one to two* (point to "2"), *two to three* (point to "3"), *three to four* (point to "4"), *and so on, in order until you reach the end* (point). *Remember, work as fast as you can. Ready! Begin!"*

Start timing. If the subject makes an error, call it to his or her attention immediately, and have the subject proceed from the point where the mistake occurred. Do not stop timing.

If the examinee completes Part A without error, remove the test sheet. Record the time in seconds. Errors count only in the increased time of performance. Then say: *"That's fine. Now we'll try another one."* Proceed immediately to Part B, sample.

ADMINISTRATION—PART B

Sample B. Place the test sheet for Part B, sample side up, flat on the table in front of the examinee, in the same position as the sheet for Part A was placed. Point with the right hand to the sample and say: *"On this page are some numbers and letters. Begin at number one* (point) *and draw a line from one to A* (point to "A"), *A to two* (point to "2"), *two to B* (point to "B"), *B to three* (point to "3"), *three to C* (point to "C"), *and so on, in order until you reach the end* (point to circle marked "END"). *Remember, first you have a number* (point to "1"), *then a letter* (point to "A"), *then a number* (point to "2"), *then a letter* (point to "B"), *and so on. Draw the lines as fast as you can. Ready! Begin!"*

If the subject makes a mistake on Sample B, point it out, and explain it. The following explanations of mistakes are acceptable:

1. "You started with the wrong circle. This is where you start (point to "1")."
2. "You skipped this circle (point to the one omitted). You should go from one (point) to A (point), A to two (point), two to B (point), B to three (point), and so on, until you reach the circle marked 'END' (point)." If it is clear that the subject intended to touch the circle but missed it, do not count it as an omission, but caution him or her to touch the circle.
3. "You only went as far as this circle (point). You should have gone to the circle marked 'END' (point)."
4. "Please keep the pencil on the paper, and go right onto the next circle."

After the mistake has been explained, the examiner marks out the wrong part and says: *"Go on from here"* (point to the last circle completed correctly in the sequence).

If the subject still cannot complete Sample B, take the subject's hand and guide the pencil (eraser end down) through the circles. Then say: *"Now you try it. Remember you begin at number one* (point) *and draw a line from one to A* (point to "A"), *A to two* (point to "2"), *two to B* (point to "B"), *B to three* (point to "3"), *and so on until you reach the circle marked 'END'* (point). *Ready! Begin!"*

Test. If the subject completes the sample item correctly, say: *"Good. Let's try the next one."* Turn the page over and proceed immediately to Part B, and say: *"On this page are some numbers and letters. Begin at number one* (point) *and draw a line from one to A* (point to "A"), *A to two* (point to "2"), *two to B* (point to "B"), *B to three* (point to "3"), *three to C* (point to "C"), *and so on, in order until you reach the end* (point to circle marked "END"). *Remember, first you have a number* (point to "1"), *then a letter* (point to "B"), *and so on. Do not skip around, but go from one circle to the next in the proper order. Draw the lines as fast as you can. Ready! Begin!"*

Start timing. If the subject makes an error immediately, call it to his or her attention and have the subject proceed from the point where the mistake occurred. Do not stop timing.

If the subject completes Part B without error, remove the test sheet. Record the time in seconds. Errors count only in the increased time of performance.

From Spreen O, Strauss E: A compendium of neuropsychological tests, ed 2, New York, 1998, Oxford University Press.

This situation may occur with clients who have severe deficits from such diagnoses as TBI or stroke or from progressive diseases such as dementia, PD, MS, and amyotrophic lateral sclerosis (ALS), to name a few. In the cases of such conditions as head trauma or stroke, consideration may be given to a recommendation for further therapy if the onset is relatively recent or if therapeutic efforts have been minimal in the client's past. The potential for improvement may be limited in those with progressive disorders. It is also advisable to discuss the recommendations with the physician to gather additional understanding of the client's prognosis.

The DRS may choose to perform the on-road evaluation to provide additional concrete feedback to the client who is disputing the recommendations of the clinical evaluation. It would be advisable that the on-road evaluation be carried out in an off-street, protected environment before moving to evaluate the client's on-road driving performance. A driving simulator may also provide the client with an opportunity to practice driving in a protected virtual environment. See Chapters 10, 12, 13, and 21 for more information on off-street evaluation and remediation, driving simulators, and driving cessation.

COORDINATION WITH THE ON-ROAD EVALUATION

In some settings the DRS may perform the clinical evaluation and the on-road evaluation. In other models of driver rehabilitation service provision, different individuals handle the two phases of the comprehensive evaluation. If there are two DRSs involved in the evaluation, an open line of communication between the two practitioners is essential. The information learned from the clinical tests needs to be conveyed to the on-road evaluator so that he or she can be prepared to observe the client performing certain aspects of the driving task that are expected to be challenging and to be ready for possible problems that may arise. The point has been made throughout this text that the clinical evaluation is not necessarily predictive of on-road performance; therefore the practitioner who sees only the clinical evaluation needs to be mindful of a possible discrepancy between clinical and on-road performance. Conversely the practitioner who only observes a client's on-road driving performance needs to appreciate the value of standardized testing of abstract measures, such as subtle visual perceptual and cognitive functions. There needs to be mutual respect between each of the respective DRSs and an acknowledgment that every client must receive both components of the comprehensive driver rehabilitation evaluation. It is only by joining efforts that a meaningful analysis can be completed, producing the best possible recommendations for the client being served.

SECTION II

The Clinical Evaluation of Vision

Patrick T. Baker

The DRS sees clients of driving age for many reasons. Any illness or injury that affects the body's ability to function physically or cognitively may have an affect on the ability to drive or access alternative transportation. Many individuals seek rehabilitation specifically for low vision driving. Some require bioptic lenses as driving aids. However, it is more common that the DRS encounters vision-related driving issues through routine screening and testing of clients who are referred to the DRS for a variety of reasons (e.g., clients who are contending with impairments caused by illness, injury, or aging-related concerns). Clients seeking assistance because of a particular primary diagnosis may also have underlying symptoms of macular degeneration, cataracts, glaucoma, visual field loss, and other eye conditions that may or may not be related to the primary condition and may or may not have even been diagnosed and treated in the past. Because vision plays an enormous role in enabling clients to safely operate a motor vehicle, it is the responsibility of the DRS to carefully evaluate the client's functional visual ability as a key assessment component that is a part of the comprehensive driver rehabilitation evaluation. For example the DRS needs to be able to distinguish whether a person's driving difficulty comes not from an issue related to turning the wheel physically but from not being able to perceive the lane markers. An evaluation of visual acuity, contrast, and visual fields will assist the DRS in isolating the cause of the difficulty. It is also important to note that the DRS is unqualified for and should not attempt to diagnose the etiology of visual impairments.

The vision screening process enables the DRS to identify and describe observed symptoms that should cue him or her to generate recommendations and referrals to a qualified ophthalmologist, optometrist, or other medical professionals for in-depth evaluation, intervention, and follow-up evaluation. Although symptoms of vision loss may be observed and reported by many health care professionals, formal diagnosis and medical treatment must be left to those professionals who are fully qualified to do so.

THE ROLE OF VISION IN THE OPERATION OF A MOTOR VEHICLE

Visual function is an essential component of driving. Up to 95% of all information comprehended by the driver while operating a motor vehicle is obtained through the visual sense.[47] Visual function includes acuity, visual field of view (central and peripheral), contrast sensitivity and glare recovery, scanning and tracking, and visual perceptual skills. The successful driver must be able to integrate all of these components to comprehend fully the ever-changing environment through which he or she is moving.

PARAMETERS FOR LICENSURE BY THE BUREAU OF MOTOR VEHICLES

Visual acuity and peripheral visual field are the primary factors used by state governments to determine whether a person has the visual skills necessary to operate a motor vehicle with competence. The law governing the operation of a motor vehicle in the United States is prescribed by each state and varies somewhat between states. Some degree of acuity between 20/20 and 20/200 generally is required. Some states also require a minimal peripheral field of view in one or both eyes of between 70 degrees (monocular) and 140 degrees with biocular vision. Acuity of 20/40 or poorer may require corrective lenses, whereas acuity poorer than 20/100 may require specialized aids and training.[48] Some states have a minimum peripheral field of view requirement, and some do not. Many states have conditional or restricted licensing for a variety of issues, including visual impairments. The most common is the need for corrective lenses while driving, but some states restrict drivers to driving during daylight hours only, and several states allow bioptic driving.

A policy statement by the American Academy of Ophthalmology suggests that visual acuity may not be the most reliable indicator of driving ability.[49] There is ongoing research exploring the best methods of assessing a client's visual ability to drive, and tests such as the UFOV may provide a more thorough assessment of visual function relative to the operation of a motor vehicle. Table 6-1 gives a state-by-state review as prepared by the National Transportation Safety Board.[50] Currently detailed information regarding state driving vision requirements should be obtained from the Bureau of Motor Vehicles or Department of Public Safety for the particular state in question.

VISUAL SKILLS

Visual acuity is the ability of the visual system to recognize detail at various distances. Sufficient acuity is needed to read text, recognize faces, and identify objects near and far. Some degree of visual acuity is required to read signs and dashboard instruments and recognize objects such as other vehicles and pedestrians while driving. Various professionals administer the most common tests of visual acuity using eye charts. The most frequently used charts are the Snellen Eye Chart, Colenbrander 1-m Chart, Early Treatment of Diabetic Retinopathy Study (ETDRS), Bailey-Lovie, and LEA charts.

The client is asked to read a series of letters of known height at a prescribed distance, with the smallest legible letters read indicating the degree of near or far acuity. Snellen described the standard eye as being able to read letters subtending 5 degrees of arc and developed his chart to test acuity. Used as the standard for years, the Snellen chart has several flaws, such as lack of geometric progression, a variable number of letters per line, and lack of proportional spacing to letter size. Current charts, such as the ETDRS, use a geometric progression of the symbols used on the chart called a logarithmic minimum angle of resolution (logMAR). Each line contains the same number of symbols, with each line value equaling 0.1 log unit, or 25%, smaller than the preceding line (when starting at the top of the chart). This standardization allows for consistency in evaluation of acuity levels. Charts are designed for assessing near and far distance acuity. The terms 20/20, 20/40, and so on are the notations derived from the Snellen chart and are the most commonly recognized visual acuity values. Most of the other eye charts provide a Snellen equivalent, which is a conversion of the metric measurement of acuity into the more familiar Snellen terminology.

Field of view is the portion of the viewing area that can be perceived by the client without turning his or her head, irrespective of acuity. The field of view has natural limitations defined by the eyebrows and cheekbone structure and the shape and size of the nose. Other natural limitations depend on the shape and structure of the eye itself, particularly as it relates to visual images entering the eye from the periphery and subsequently where the image falls on the outer edge of the retina. Because of these natural limitations, the normal field of view is approximately 90 degrees temporally or toward the ear, 60 degrees nasally or toward the nose, 70 degrees below the horizontal plane, and 45 degrees

Text continued on p 124.

Table 6-1 Guidelines for Motor Vehicle Administrators: License Renewal Requirements

State/Province	2001 Licensing Renewal Requirements and Distinctions for Older Drivers*
Alabama	4-year renewal cycle (in person). No tests for renewal. Minimum acuity 20/60 in one eye with/without corrective lenses. May *not* use bioptic telescopic lens to meet acuity standard. *No special requirements for older drivers.*
Alaska	5-year renewal cycle (mail in every other cycle). No renewal by mail for drivers aged 69+ and for drivers whose previous renewal was by mail. Vision test required at in-person renewal. Minimum 20/40 in one eye for unrestricted license. 20/40 to 20/100 needs report from eye specialist; license request determined by discretion. May use bioptic telescopic lens in certain conditions.
Arizona	12-year renewal cycle. At age 65, reduction of interval to 5 years. New photograph and vision test at renewal; no renewal by mail after age 70 (available to active duty veterans and dependents only). Minimum acuity 20/40 in one eye required; acuity of 20/60 restricted to daytime only. May *not* use bioptic telescopic lens to meet acuity standard.
Arkansas	4-year renewal cycle. Vision test required at renewal, with minimum 20/40 required for unrestricted license. Acuity of 20/60 restricted to daytime only. Bioptic telescopes permitted in certain circumstances. *No special requirements for older drivers.*
California	5-year renewal cycle (may be mail in for no more than two sequential cycles) with vision test and written knowledge test required. No renewal by mail at age 70. Minimum visual acuity is 20/200 (best corrected) in at least one eye as verified by an optometrist or ophthalmologist. Bioptic lenses are permitted for driving but may not be used to meet 20/200 acuity standard.
Colorado	10-year renewal cycle (mail in every other cycle). At age 61, reduction in renewal to 5 years. No renewal by mail at age 66. Vision test required at renewal. Written test required only if point accumulations result in suspension (12 points in 12 mo, or 18 points in 24 mo, for nonminor and noncommercial drivers). Minimum acuity must be 20/70 in the better eye if worse eye is 20/200 or better, 20/40 if worse eye is worse than 20/200. Bioptic telescopes are permitted to meet acuity standard.
Connecticut	4-year renewal cycle (in person). Vision test required in person. 20/40 required in better eye for unrestricted license; 20/50 to 20/70 restricted license; in some circumstances, a license may be issued when acuity is 20/200. No license may be issued to drivers using telescopic aids. Reduction of interval to 2 years may be requested by drivers aged 65+.
Delaware	5-year renewal cycle (in person). No tests required for renewal. Minimum acuity 20/40 for unrestricted license, restricted license at 20/50; beyond 20/50 driving privileges denied. Bioptic telescopes treated on case-by-case basis. *No special requirements for older drivers.*
District of Columbia	4-year renewal cycle (in person). Unrestricted license for 20/40 acuity; 20/70 in better eye requires 140E visual field for restricted license. At age 70, vision test required and physician signature attesting to physical and mental capability to drive; a medical report plus reaction test may also be required. At age 75 written knowledge and road tests may be required.
Florida	6-year renewal cycle for clean driving record; 4-year renewal cycle for unclean record. In-person renewal required every third cycle. Vision test at in-person renewal. Must have 20/70 in either eye with or without corrective lenses. Monocular people need 20/40 in fellow eye. Bioptic telescopes are *not* recognized to meet acuity standard. *No special requirements for older drivers.*

Table 6-1 **Guidelines for Motor Vehicle Administrators: License Renewal Requirements—cont'd**

State/Province	2001 Licensing Renewal Requirements and Distinctions for Older Drivers*
Georgia	4-year renewal cycle (in person). Vision test required for renewal (within previous 6-month period). Acuity 20/60 in either eye with or without corrective lenses. Bioptic telescopes permitted for best acuity as low as 20/200, with restrictions. *No special requirements for older drivers.*
Hawaii	6-year renewal cycle for drivers ages 18 to 71 (in person). Vision test required, with 20/40 standard for better eye. Bioptic telescopes permitted for driving but not for passing vision test. Reduction of interval to 2 years for drivers aged 72+.
Idaho	4-year renewal cycle (mail in every other renewal). Vision test required: 20/40 in better eye for no restrictions; 20/50-20/60 requires annual testing; 20/70 denied license. Use of bioptic telescopes is acceptable, but acuity must reach 20/40. Driving test may be required if examiner thinks it is needed. No renewal by mail after age 69.
Illinois	4-year renewal cycle for ages 21 to 80 (mail in every other cycle for drivers with clean records and no medical report review requirements). Vision test at in-person renewal: 20/40 in better eye for no restrictions, 20/70 in better eye results in daylight-only restriction. May have 20/100 in better eye and 20/40 through bioptic telescope. Written test every 8 years unless clean driving record. From ages 81 to 86 reduction of interval to 2 years. At age 87 reduction of interval to 1 year. No renewal by mail, vision test required, and on-road driving test required at age 75+.
Indiana	4-year renewal cycle (in person). Vision screening at renewal, including acuity and peripheral vision. 20/40 in better eye for no restriction; restricted license for 20/50. Bioptic telescope lenses permitted for best acuity as low as 20/200, with some restrictions, if 20/40 achieved with telescope. At age 75 renewal cycles are reduced to 3 years. (Mandatory drive test for people age 75+ eliminated 1/19/00). Drive test required for people with 14 points or 3 convictions in 12-month period.
Iowa	Renewal cycle of 2 years or 4 years at driver's option. Vision screening at renewal: 20/40 in better eye with or without corrective lenses; 20/50 in better eye results in restricted license for daylight only; 20/70 in better eye results in restricted license for daylight only up to 35 mph. Bioptic telescopes are not permitted to meet acuity requirement. At age 70 renewal cycle is 2 years.
Kansas	6-year renewal cycle for ages 16-64 (in person). Vision and knowledge test at renewal. Minimum acuity: 20/40 better eye; 20/60 better eye with doctor report; worse than 20/60 must demonstrate ability to operate vehicle safely and have safe record for 3 years. At age 65 renewal every 4 years.
Kentucky	4-year renewal cycle (in person). No tests required for renewal. Minimum visual acuity 20/200 or better with corrective lenses in better eye; 20/60 or better using a bioptic telescopic device. *No special requirements for older drivers.*
Louisiana	4-year renewal cycle (mail in every other cycle). Vision test at renewal. Minimum acuity 20/40 in better eye for unrestricted; 20/50-20/70 with restrictions; 20/70-20/100 possible restricted license; less than 20/100 in better eye, referred to Medical Advisory Board (MAB). No renewal by mail to drivers age 70+ or those with a conviction of moving violation in 2-year period before renewal.

Continued

Table 6-1   Guidelines for Motor Vehicle Administrators: License Renewal Requirements—cont'd

State/Province	2001 Licensing Renewal Requirements and Distinctions for Older Drivers*
Maine	6-year renewal cycle. At age 65 renew every 4 years. Vision screening test at renewal for age 40, 52, and 65; every 4 years after age 65. Minimum acuity 20/40 better eye without restrictions; 20/70 better eye with restrictions.
Maryland	5-year renewal cycle. Vision tests required for renewal (binocular, acuity, peripheral). Minimum acuity of at least 20/40 plus continuous field of vision at least 140E in each eye for unrestricted license; at least 20/70 in one or both eyes for restricted but requires continuous field of view of at least 110E with at least 35E lateral to the midline of each side; 20/70-20/100 requires special permission from MAB. Medical report required for new drivers age 70+. (Maryland law specifies that age alone is not grounds for reexamination of older drivers).
Massachusetts	5-year renewal cycle (in person). Vision screening at renewal: 20/40 better eye for unrestricted; 20/70 better eye for restricted; 20/40 through telescope, 20/100 through carrier. *No special requirements for older drivers.* (Massachusetts law prohibits discrimination by reason of age for licensing issues.)
Michigan	4-year renewal cycle (mail in every other cycle if free of convictions). Vision and knowledge test at renewal; renewal denied for visual acuity of 20/100 or less in one eye and less than 20/50 in the other eye. Minimum acuity 20/40 better eye for unrestricted; 20/70 better eye with daylight only restriction; 20/60 if progressive abnormalities or diseases of the eye. *No special requirements for older drivers.*
Minnesota	4-year renewal cycle. Vision test at renewal: 20/40 in better eye for no restrictions; 20/70 in better eye for speed limit restrictions; 20/100 better eye referred to driver evaluation unit. *No special requirements for older drivers.* (Minnesota law specifies that age alone is not justification for reexamination.)
Mississippi	4-year renewal cycle (in person). Vision test at renewal: 20/200 best corrected without telescope; 20/70 with telescope. *No special requirements for older drivers.*
Missouri	6-year renewal cycle (in person). At age 70, reduction in renewal cycle to 3 years. Vision test and traffic sign recognition test required at renewal. Minimum acuity: 20/40 in better eye for unrestricted; up to 20/160 for restricted.
Montana	8-year renewal cycle for ages 21-67. Vision test at renewal: 20/40 in better eye for no restrictions; 20/70 in better eye with restrictions on daylight and speed; 20/100 in better eye possible restricted license if need is shown. For ages 68-74, renewal cycle reduced to 1-6 years. At age 75 renewal cycle reduced to 4 years.
Nebraska	5-year renewal cycle. Vision test at renewal: Knowledge test if violations on record. Acuity 20/40 required in better eye, but 17 restrictions are used, depending on vision in each eye. *No special requirements for older drivers.*
Nevada	4-year renewal cycle (mail in every other cycle if qualified). Minimum acuity 20/40 in better eye. Bioptic telescopes permitted to meet acuity standard: 20/40 through telescope, 20/120 through carrier, 130E visual field. Vision test and medical report required to renew by mail at age 70.

Table 6-1 Guidelines for Motor Vehicle Administrators: License Renewal Requirements—cont'd

State/Province	2001 Licensing Renewal Requirements and Distinctions for Older Drivers*
New Hampshire	4-year renewal cycle (in person). Vision test at renewal: 20/40 better eye for unrestricted; 20/70 in better eye with restrictions. At age 75 road test required at renewal.
New Jersey	4-year renewal cycle (10-year in-person digitized photo licenses will be implemented in 2003). Periodic vision retest: 20/50 better eye; 20/70 in better eye with restrictions. Bioptic telescope permitted to meet acuity standard. *No special requirements for older drivers.*
New Mexico	4- or 8-year renewal cycle. Drivers may not apply for 8-year license if they will reach the age of 75 during the last 4 years of the 8-year period. Vision test required for renewal; knowledge and driving test may be required Minimum acuity: 20/40 better eye; 20/80 better eye with restrictions.
New York	5-year renewal cycle. No tests for renewal. Minimum best corrected acuity 20/40 in one eye; 20/40-20/70 best-corrected one eye requires minimum 140E horizontal visual field; 20/80-20/100 best corrected in one eye requires minimum 140E horizontal visual field plus 20/40 through bioptic telescopic lens. *No special requirements for older drivers.*
North Carolina	5-year renewal cycle (in person). Vision and traffic sign recognition tests required for renewal. Acuity 20/40 in better eye required for unrestricted; 20/70 better eye with restrictions. Bioptic telescopes are *not* permitted for meeting acuity standard but are permitted for driving. *No special requirements for older drivers, except that people age 60+ are not required to parallel park in the road test.*
North Dakota	4-year renewal cycle. Vision test required for renewal: 20/40 better eye for unrestricted; 20/70 in better eye with restrictions. Bioptic telescopes permitted to meet acuity standard: 20/130 in carrier, 20/40 in telescope, full peripheral field. *No special requirements for older drivers.*
Ohio	4-year renewal cycle. Vision test required for renewal: 20/40 better eye for unrestricted; 20/70 better eye with restrictions; bioptic telescopes permitted to meet acuity standards. *No special requirements for older drivers.*
Oklahoma	4-year renewal cycle (in person). No tests for renewal. Minimum acuity: 20/40 better eye for unrestricted; 20/100 better eye with restrictions. Bioptic telescopes *not* permitted to meet acuity standard but may be used for driving. *No special requirements for older drivers.*
Oregon	8-year renewal cycle (mail in every other cycle). Vision screening test once every 8 years at age 50+. Minimum acuity: 20/40 better eye for unrestricted; 20/70 better eye with restrictions. Bioptic telescopes *not* permitted to meet acuity standard but may be used for driving.
Pennsylvania	4-year renewal cycle. Drivers age 65+ may renew every 2 years. Random physical examinations for all drivers age 45+; most selected are age 65+. Minimum acuity: 20/40 better eye for unrestricted; up to 20/100 combined vision with restrictions. Bioptic telescopes *not* permitted to meet acuity standards but may be used for driving.
Rhode Island	5-year renewal cycle. Vision test required for renewal: 20/40 better eye. At age 70 renewal cycle reduced to 2 years.

Continued

Table 6-1   Guidelines for Motor Vehicle Administrators: License Renewal Requirements—cont'd

State/Province	2001 Licensing Renewal Requirements and Distinctions for Older Drivers*
South Carolina	5-year renewal cycle (in person). Renewal by mail if no violations in past 2 years and if license is not suspended, revoked, or canceled. Vision test and knowledge test required if >5 points on record. Minimum acuity: 20/40 better eye for unrestricted; 20/70 in better eye if worse eye is 20/200 or better; 20/40 if worse eye is worse than 20/200. Bioptic telescopes *not* permitted to meet acuity standard but may be used for driving. *No special requirements for older drivers.*
South Dakota	5-year renewal cycle. Vision test required for renewal: 20/40 better eye for unrestricted; 20/60 better eye with restrictions. *No special requirements for older drivers.*
Tennessee	5-year renewal cycle (mail in every other cycle). Minimum acuity: 20/30 better eye; 20/70 better eye with restrictions; 20/200 better eye requires bioptic telescopes with 20/60 through the telescope. Bioptic telescopes are permitted to meet standard. No tests required for renewal. *No special requirements for older drivers.*
Texas	6-year renewal cycle (effective 01/01/02; staggered 4-6 years until 2002). Vision test required for renewal: 20/40 better eye; 20/70 better eye with restrictions. Bioptic telescopes are permitted to meet acuity standard, and driver must pass a road test. *No special requirements for older drivers.*
Utah	5-year renewal cycle (mail in every other cycle if no suspensions, no revocations, no convictions for reckless driving, and no more than 4 reportable violations). Vision test required for drivers age 65+ every renewal. Minimum acuity: 20/40 for unrestricted; 20/100 in better eye with restrictions. Bioptic telescopes are *not* permitted to meet acuity standard.
Vermont	2- or 4-year renewal cycle. Minimum acuity: 20/40 in better eye; bioptic telescopes are permitted to meet visual acuity standard, and driver must pass road test. No tests for renewal. *No special requirements for older drivers.*
Virginia	5-year renewal cycle (mail in every other cycle unless suspended or revoked, 2+ violations, seizures/blackouts, DMV medical review indicator on license, failed vision test). Vision test required for renewal. Minimum acuity: 20/40 better eye for unrestricted; 20/200 with restrictions; bioptic telescopes are permitted with 20/200 through carrier, 20/70 through telescope. Knowledge and road test required if 2+ violations in 5 years. *No special requirements for older drivers.*
Washington	5-year renewal cycle (in person). Vision test required for renewal. Minimum acuity 20/40 better eye; 20/70 better eye with restrictions. Bioptic telescopes are permitted to meet acuity standards. Other tests may be required if License Service Representative deems it necessary. *No special requirements for older drivers.*
West Virginia	5-year renewal cycle. Minimum acuity: 20/60 better eye; if worse than 20/60, optometrist or ophthalmologist must declare ability to be safe. Bioptic telescopes are *not* permitted to meet acuity standard but may be used for driving. No tests required for renewal. *No special requirements for older drivers.*
Wisconsin	8-year renewal cycle (in person). Minimum acuity: 20/40 better eye; 20/100 better eye with restrictions. Bioptic telescopes are *not* permitted to meet acuity standards but may be used for driving. Vision test required for renewal. *No special requirements for older drivers.*

Table 6-1   Guidelines for Motor Vehicle Administrators: License Renewal Requirements—cont'd

State/Province	2001 Licensing Renewal Requirements and Distinctions for Older Drivers*
Wyoming	4-year renewal cycle (mail in every other cycle). Vision test required for renewal (for mail in and in person). Minimum acuity; 20/40 better eye; 20/100 better eye with restrictions. Bioptic telescopes are permitted to meet acuity standard. *No special requirements for older drivers.*
Alberta	No mandatory retesting; medical review and vision test at ages 75, 80, and every 2 years thereafter.
British Columbia	No mandatory retesting; medical review at age 80 and every 2 years thereafter.
Manitoba	Annual license renewal. No mandatory retesting; no periodic medical review. Minimum acuity of 6/12 (20/40) −2 in the better eye with or without correction. May drive with restrictions with acuity of 6/12 (20/40) −3, to 6/18 (20/60) −2 in the better eye. Telescopic lenses not eligible for any class of license. Minimum horizontal field requirement of 120° with both eyes tested together or tested separately and results superimposed. Visual fields to be measured at or 10° above or below fixation. Standards exist for hemianopsia and quadratic field defects, color perception, and diplopia. Drivers with depth perception and diabetic retinopathy impairments must meet visual acuity and field standards. On recommendation from a physician, mature drivers can be requested to complete medical, vision, or oral test.
New Brunswick	4-year renewal for passenger vehicle license (may be renewed by mail). No tests required for renewal. Minimum visual acuity (corrected) must be at least 20/40 in at least one eye. *No special requirements for older drivers.*
Newfoundland and Labrador	5-year renewal cycle (may be by mail if current photo is on file). No tests required for renewal. Drivers age 75 must present a medical exam form from their physician to renew their licenses. Drivers age 80 must provide a medical report every 2 years.
Northwest Territories	No mandatory retesting; medical review at ages 75, 80, and every 2 years thereafter.
Nova Scotia	No mandatory retesting; no periodic medical review; drivers 65+ involved in a collision must take a written and on-road test.
Nunavut	5-year renewal cycle (in person). No tests required for renewal unless medical concerns have been identified. *No special requirements for older drivers.*
Ontario	5-year renewal cycle (in person). At age 80, renewal every 2 years. Mail-in renewal is an option for drivers with no testing requirements who have had photo taken within past 2 years. Mandatory written knowledge test, vision test, and participation in a 90-minute group education session on safe driving at age 80 and every 2 years thereafter; includes driver record review. Senior drivers may be required to pass a road test before being relicensed if they have an excessive number of demerit points showing on their record. Some drivers may be required to pass a road test before being relicensed if, in the opinion of the instructor, they may represent a safety risk. Collision-involved drivers aged 70+ who are convicted of a collision-related offense must take mandatory vision, knowledge, and road tests. Vision requirements include 20/40 acuity in better eye, with or without corrective lenses, and 120° peripheral vision. No periodic medical review requirement under Section 203 of Highway Traffic Act; physicians required to report any patient aged 16+ with a medical condition that may make driving dangerous. Medical report may be required on a cyclical basis if there is evidence of a medical condition that may eventually interfere with safe operation of motor vehicle.

Continued

Table 6-1 **Guidelines for Motor Vehicle Administrators: License Renewal Requirements—cont'd**

State/Province	2001 Licensing Renewal Requirements and Distinctions for Older Drivers*
Prince Edward Island	3-year renewal cycle (may be renewed by mail, but regular renewal is in person). No tests required for renewal. Minimum acuity for original license 20/40 in better eye. *No special requirements for older drivers.* On recommendation from the police, physician, or family member, mature drivers can be requested to complete medical, vision, or oral test.
Quebec	2-year renewal cycle (may be renewed by mail, but driver must come to a service center every 4 years to have a picture taken). At ages 75, 80, and every 2 years thereafter, drivers must present a medical examination and optometric report (with acceptable exam results) when renewing. No tests required for renewal, but a declaration of illness or impairment that has not been previously reported must be reported upon renewal. Visual requirements for licensing include 20/40 vision with or without glasses in at least one eye, and minimum field of vision of 120 degrees.
Saskatchewan	Annual renewals required for all drivers (may be renewed by mail). No tests required for renewal unless driver's license indicates that an annual vision, road, or medical exam is required. When a license is issued or renewed, any medical condition that may affect a driver's ability to drive must be reported to SGI. If the license indicated that an annual medical exam report is required, then a medical report must be presented at the time of renewal. Minimum visual requirements for passenger vehicle driver license: 20/50 with both eyes examined together (aided or unaided); field of vision must measure a minimum of 120 degrees (both eyes measured together). *No special requirements for older drivers.* On recommendation from the police, physician, or family member, mature drivers can be requested to complete medical, vision, or oral test.
Yukon	No mandatory retesting; medical review and vision test at age 70, every 2 years to age 80, annually thereafter.

*Information about each jurisdiction was obtained from one or more of the following sources: DMV licensing official, DMV website, DMV Driver's Manual, research report, Insurance Institute for Highway Safety.
Staplin L, Lococo KH, Gish KW, et al: *Model driver screening and evaluation program final technical report: DOT HS 809 581. Guidelines for motor vehicle administrators,* Washington, DC, 2003, National Highway Traffic Safety Administration. Available at: *http://www.nhtsa.dot.gov/people/injury/olderdrive/modeldriver/.* Accessed January 5, 2004.

above the horizontal plane, as shown in Figure 6-2. Part of the total field of view is binocular, accounting for approximately 120 degrees in the middle of the field of view because the visual fields of both eyes overlap. Because the visual fields overlap, each of the eyes views an object from a slightly different angle, providing stereoscopic or binocular vision, a key component of depth perception.

Peripheral vision is that portion of the field of view along the outer limits of the entire field and is the second aspect of vision that is most frequently tested by state licensing bureaus. Although commonly referring to the field of view in a horizontal plane at an angle of approximately 90 degrees temporally from each eye, the peripheral field also includes the vertical plane above and below the visual center. Peripheral vision is important to recognize movements approaching from the far left or right, such as a vehicle at an intersection or a vehicle passing from behind in another lane. It is

also important in the detection of street signs and traffic lights above the center of vision and in responding to the instruments on the dashboard, such as a flashing warning light that is located below the center of view. Peripheral vision is not used to identify objects so much as it is used as a cue to shift central vision from one object to one coming into the field of view to identify it and initiate a process of assessing potential reactions to the visual stimulus.

Another important aspect of the field of view is that portion of the visual field seen by the macula, the *central field of view.* This portion of the retina, with a radius of approximately 30 degrees, is used for detail and color and is responsible for visual acuity. The retina is a specialized layer of photoreceptor cells on the posterior portion of the eye (Figure 6-3) that converts light into nerve impulses that are sent to the occipital lobes of the brain for processing and interpretation. The retinas, made up of two types of receptors called

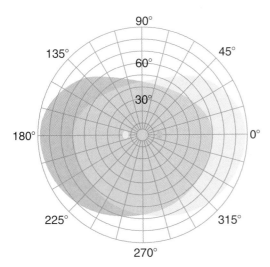

Figure 6-2 Normal visual fields for the two eyes, superimposed on each other. (From Nolte J: *The human brain: an introduction to its functional anatomy,* ed 5, St. Louis, 2002, Mosby.)

rods, detect light and dark shades and movements, whereas the cones detect color and detail. Rods are found more predominantly around the outer portion of the retina and are useful for night vision and detecting objects along the periphery of the field of view. The cones are found in the central macula area of the retina,

culminating at the fovea. Reading, as well as recognition of object detail, including the color and texture of objects, depends on the function of the cones in the macula. Diseases such as macular degeneration damage areas of the macula, leaving crucial areas of the most important part of the central field of view distorted, hazy, or blank. These damaged areas are called scotomas. Imagine trying to read this sentence or the instrumentation on the dashboard when the very word or number you look at is missing because of macular damage. A more detailed discussion of photoreceptor cells follows in the section on visual anatomy.

Contrast sensitivity, scanning, and glare recovery are other aspects of visual function that are vital to driving skill that are not evaluated by state licensing bureaus. *Contrast sensitivity* describes the ability of the eye to detect various shades of gray or color shades. The ability to differentiate subtle shadings or detect details in poor lighting conditions greatly impacts acuity. Contrast is the measure of visual perception between light and dark, whether that is black and white, various shades of gray, or various shades of color. The black print on the white page you are reading is a distinct contrast, but most of our visual images are composed of less sharply defined tones and shades. The beauty we find in many things, such as a rose petal, comes from the delicate and subtle shades of coloring inherent in

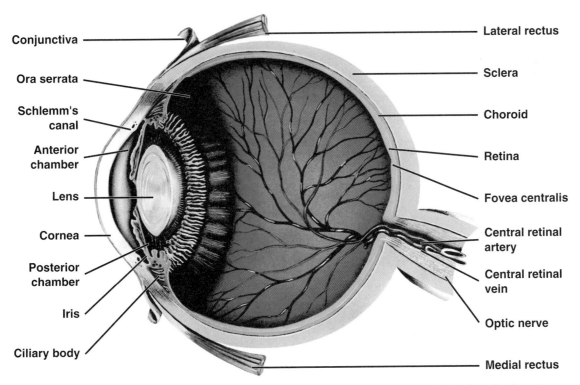

Figure 6-3 The major anatomic structures of the eye. (From Palay DA, Krachmer JH: *Ophthalmology for the primary care physician,* St. Louis, 1997, Mosby.)

their features. Contrast sensitivity within the context of the visual aspects of driving skill is important for object recognition, reading of road signage, location of the curb and dividing lanes, and recognition of lights, such as brake and traffic lights. People demonstrating difficulties with contrast, such as those with cataracts, have increased difficulty with these and other driving tasks. This can be compounded when driving in less than optimum lighting conditions. Even though the client may have adequate acuity in the clinical or community setting where the clinical evaluation has taken place, the DRS must ask how acuity is affected by glare, rain, fog, overcast skies, or driving at dusk or at night. Early morning and at dusk are the two most difficult times of the day to perceive objects because there is often insufficient light for the cones of the eyes to see color and detail but too much light to benefit from the rods that are designed for night vision.

Scanning is the ability of the eyes to search within the field of view to locate an object. For this to be successful, the person must be able to move the eyes (and the head) in a coordinated, purposeful pattern horizontally, vertically, and diagonally to locate objects. The client must then be able to hold his or her gaze on the selected object and focus the lens to maximize acuity for recognition of that object. *Tracking* is scanning plus motion; the person must find and fixate on an object and if it is a moving object, such as a vehicle or pedestrian, follow its movement. Another example is the necessity of a driver to follow a line, such as the dividing line on a highway.

Glare is a common distraction for all drivers. Sunlight reflecting from another vehicle, from wet or icy pavement, and from headlights or even the sun itself can momentarily affect anyone's ability to see. When the driver has cataracts or perhaps some type of retinal disease, recovering visual function after encountering a glare situation can last for many seconds or even minutes. Visual acuity can be greatly reduced in these circumstances and can lead to loss of control of the vehicle and worse.

VISUAL PERCEPTUAL SKILLS AND HOW THEY RELATE TO DRIVING

Visual perceptual skills are the result of the ability of the brain to correctly interpret what the eyes see (assuming the visual function is normal) and correctly develop a visual understanding of what this interpretation means. That is, the person has to first see what is in the visual field and send the correct information to the occipital lobes. Then the brain has to organize, interpret, and understand the visual images it has received. Finally the brain must correctly integrate this visual image with

other skills (e.g., bilateral upper and lower extremity gross motor movements, fine motor grasp and release, cervical rotation in conjunction with proprioception, stereognosis, and vestibular skills) to use vision to coordinate the movements necessary to make a left turn at an intersection. This of course is happening at the same time the driver should be monitoring his or her rate of speed, the actions of other vehicles and pedestrians, and avoiding any potholes and obstructions in the path of travel. These skills are vital to the operation of a motor vehicle and are compounded by the fact that, in addition to a myriad of visual details to observe, integrate, and act on, the speed required to process these actions is constantly influenced by the relative speed of the moving vehicle and the speed of other moving objects. Visual perception is also affected by the quality of the person's visual acuity, visual field, contrast sensitivity, ability to recover from glare, and ability to scan and track efficiently through the environment.

Figure-ground refers to the ability to discern an object relative to its background. For example the driver should be able to detect the shape of the hood of the automobile relative to the roadway or perceive a deer crossing the road ahead and gauge its distance from the vehicle. Figure-ground is an important aspect of depth perception and, like acuity, is affected by contrast sensitivity.

Visual closure is the ability to see a portion of an object or to see it briefly and to be able to recognize it correctly by mentally completing the image (e.g., being able to recognize that the tousled red hair "floating" from right to left "on top" of the parked vehicle ahead is actually the top of the head of a child who has just chased a ball into the street between two vehicles). Another example would be the correct recognition of objects in the image seen from a quick glance into the rearview mirror without requiring a prolonged look into the mirror to memorize the view.

Visual memory is the ability to recall what was seen, such as the view from that quick glance in the mirror or the ability to remember that the McDonald's sign was after the Wendy's and Burger King signs ahead, without having to look again to recall the order.

Spatial relations involve correctly interpreting the distances between objects visually and the ability to judge the relative distances of moving objects to each other in a three-dimensional perspective. Binocular vision is a key component in successfully interpreting spatial relationships. Binocular vision occurs because of the relative positions of the two eyes and the object being perceived. Because of the distance between the forward-facing eyes and the object, each eye sees it from a slightly different perspective. The brain synthesizes the separate visual images into one and is able to interpret the subtle differences between each image to determine distance to the object. For the brain to interpret this information successfully, the acuity of each eye needs to be similar. A person who has acuity in one eye greater than two Snellen equivalents of the other eye is said to have biocular (bi = two; ocular = eye) vision. For example a client may have 20/30 vision in one eye and 20/60 in the other, a difference of three Snellen equivalents. The brain has difficulty blending the disparate visual information of each eye; therefore the client may have difficulty with near distance acuity because one eye is blurry. The brain may choose to ignore the information from the weak eye; therefore the client effectively uses only one eye in certain circumstances. Refractive correction of the weak eye may equalize the acuity of each eye. Other clients may have a condition in which, for a variety of reasons, only one eye functions. This is called monocular vision. When a person develops biocular or monocular vision as an adult, depth perception may be an issue. People born with one functioning eye or having been monocular for some time often acclimate to this condition and have adequate depth perception. Many states have regulations governing the licensing of a person with monocular vision that should be reviewed by the DRS evaluating such a client.

Visual discrimination is the ability to detect a specific object or shape among others. Locating a speed limit sign, pedestrian, or another vehicle among all the other surrounding visual images is an example of visual discrimination.

Most vision testing, whether done by a medical professional, a state licensing bureau, or a DRS, is done in a clinical setting with optimum lighting conditions. Rarely is lighting optimum for any period while driving. The DRS is the only service provider trained to evaluate visual driving skills in a real life setting; therefore he or she has a unique opportunity and responsibility to make a thorough assessment of the visual skills of clients.

VISUAL FUNCTION

The terms *sight* and *vision* are two words that appear to be interchangeable; however, they refer to two distinct parts of visual function. *Sight* refers to the information gathered by the photoreceptor cells of the retina and the resulting nerve impulses transmitted by the optic neural pathway. *Vision* refers to how the brain converts these neural impulses into what we perceive and how the brain interprets this information. The eyes capture a series of light wavelengths in a pattern and convert them into electrical impulses; the brain perceives these impulses as an automobile traveling in the same lane 20 feet ahead for example.

THE ANATOMY OF THE EYE

To understand the information provided in the medical chart of an eye examination or to discuss the results with a physician, the DRS must have a working knowledge of the visual system. The DRS should be able to synthesize this information and relate it to what he or she observes functionally with clients. The following discussion is not meant to be a detailed anatomy and physiology lesson of the visual pathway; there are many superb texts on this subject for the person who is interested in the complexity of this system. Rather it is meant as a general overview of anatomy, with an emphasis on those anatomic and physiologic aspects that may affect the driving skill. Figure 6-3 identifies the location of the eye structures discussed in this section.

Exterior Structures

The eyelids cover the exterior portion of the eyes, protecting them from injury and dryness, and serve to limit light entry into the eye. Blinking of the eyelids provides lubrication for the exterior of the eye. When the eyelids are closed, the entire eye should be covered. With the eyes opened, the upper lids should be even with the superior margin of the cornea; if the upper portion of the cornea is covered, this is described as ptosis. Ptosis may affect the client's ability to locate and react to overhead visual cues, such as stoplights, or may affect lateral peripheral vision. Irregularities of the external eye, including discharges from the eye, should be noted for their potential to affect the field of view or acuity.

Extrinsic Muscles of the Eye and Cranial Nerves

The globe of each eye is located in the front of the skull, situated in a protective bony orbit. Each orbit is composed of parts of seven skull bones, creating a rounded, cone-shaped cavity with the apex of the cone at the posterior of the cavity. At the apex an opening (foramen) exists to allow blood vessels and nerves to enter and exit the orbit. Connective tissues (fascia), fat deposits, and the extraocular muscles (EOMs) line the eye orbit; the fat deposits cushion the globes of the eyes, whereas the fascia and the EOMs support, move, and stabilize the eye. The six EOMs are the superior rectus, inferior rectus, lateral rectus, medial rectus, and superior and inferior oblique (Figure 6-4). Eye movement is a complex skill, involving the coordinated contraction and relaxation of the EOMs of each eye, the plane of each muscle (as determined by the origin and insertions), and the effects of each on the rotation of the globe within the orbit. Specific cranial nerves innervate each muscle of the eye. There are 12 pairs of named and numbered cranial nerves leading from the brain and brainstem to particular areas of the body, mostly in the head and neck regions, the heart, lungs, and digestive tract. We are concerned primarily with four cranial nerves: the optic (II), the oculomotor (III), the trochlear (IV), and the abducens (VI). The optic nerve serves as the visual pathway from the retina to the optic chiasm, whereas the other three are important for extraocular eye movements. In addition to these four, the trigeminal (V) nerve provides sensory innervations for the eye and other nearby tissues, and the facial (VII) nerve initiates reflexive tearing of the eye and is involved in blinking of the eyelids. The spinal accessory nerve (XI), although not directly related to vision, is important for postural control of the head and neck and head rotation, important features in the ability to focus gaze on an object.[51-53]

Some familiarity with the musculature, innervation, and movement of the eyes is important to the DRS because the visual skill of driving requires the ability to scan the environment, track moving objects, and focus one's gaze on specific items in the field of view. The inability to look in a certain direction may limit the driver's ability to avoid dangerous objects or situations within the path of travel. Table 6-2 consolidates the most relevant information regarding the muscles of the eye and eye movement.

Structures of the Eye

The sclera, commonly known as the white of the eye, is composed of collagen and does not contain blood vessels. The sclera forms the exterior eyeball, protecting interior contents. Rheumatoid arthritis, lupus, sarcoidosis, and other autoimmune diseases may damage tissues composed of collagen; congenital glaucoma and external environmental pressure changes can damage the sclera.

Like the sclera, the cornea is composed of collagen; however, because of the lattice arrangement of the fibers, the cornea is clear rather than opaque white. The five layers of the cornea provide roughly two-thirds of the total refractive power of the eye. The central 4 mm of the cornea, directly over the pupil, are crucial for central vision. Uneven curvature of this area leads to a condition known as astigmatism, which, along with other corneal changes, may require corrective lenses or surgical procedures, such as radical keratotomy.

Anterior Cavity

The interior of the eye is divided into the anterior and posterior cavities. The anterior cavity is composed of the anterior and posterior chambers. The anterior chamber refers to the space and structures lying between the interior cornea and the anterior portion of the iris. In the anterior and posterior chambers, aqueous humor is the clear fluid produced by the ciliary process, contributing to corneal metabolism, and

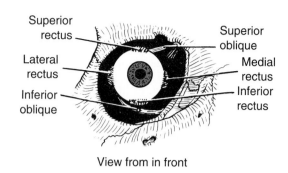

View from in front

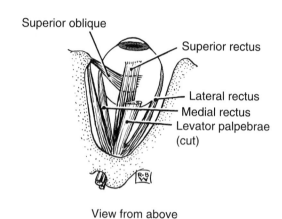

View from above

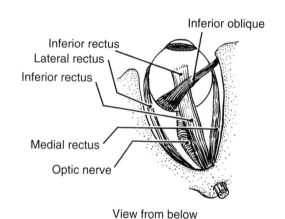

View from below

Figure 6-4 Anterior, superior, and inferior views of the extraocular muscles of the right eye. (From von Noorden GK: *Atlas of strabismus*, ed 4, St. Louis, 1983, Mosby.)

is part of the pathway on which light travels to the retina. Aqueous humor provides intraocular pressure (IOP) contributing to the shape and safety of the eye. Made continually in the posterior chamber, aqueous humor flows to the anterior chamber and exits through the angle, a complex area at the juncture of the iris and cornea containing the trabecular network and the canal of Schlemm (see Figure 6-3). Any change in the angle affecting the flow of aqueous

Table 6-2 Muscles of the Eye and Eye Movement

Extraocular Muscle	Innervation	Muscle Action
Superior rectus (SR)	Superior division of the oculomotor (CN III)	Elevation, intorsion, and adduction
Inferior rectus (IR)	A branch of the inferior division of CN III	Depression, extorsion, and adduction
Medical rectus (MR)	A branch of the inferior division of CN III	Adduction
Lateral rectus (LR)	The abducens (CN VI)	Abduction
Superior oblique (SO)	The trochlear (CN IV)	Intorsion, depression, and abduction
Inferior oblique (IO)	CN III	Extorsion, elevation, and abduction

Looking to the RIGHT		Looking to the LEFT	
S. Oblique	I. Oblique	I. Oblique	S. Rectus
L. Rectus	M. Rectus	M. Rectus	L. Rectus
I. Rectus	S. Oblique	S. Oblique	I. Rectus

humor can lead to conditions known as closed-angle or open-angle glaucoma. Normal IOP ranges from 10 to 21 mm Hg. Glaucoma, a condition that can cause damage to the retina and optic nerve, may be caused by prolonged excessive IOP.

The colored, muscular center of the visible part of the eye is the iris. The pupil is the open space in the center of the iris, through which light enters the eye, leading to the retina. The autonomic nervous system controls the contraction of the dilator and sphincter muscles of the iris, which regulates the amount of light entering the pupil. The dilator muscle increases the pupil size, allowing in more light, and is controlled by the sympathetic system. The parasympathetic system regulates the sphincter muscle, which restricts light by narrowing the pupil. The color of the iris is genetically determined and restricts light additionally through light absorption. Fair-skinned people with blue or gray eyes often have a decreased tolerance for bright light because brown pigment provides greater absorption than blue. Albinism, defined by a significant lack of pigmentation throughout the body, seriously affects the person's ability to tolerate light. Inflammation of the iris is called iritis and may interfere with vision.

The space between the posterior side of the iris and the anterior side of the lens is called the posterior chamber. Surrounding the lens is the ciliary body that produces aqueous humor. This flows from the posterior chamber to the anterior chamber and is eliminated through the Isle of Schlemm. The ciliary muscle is attached to the lens through the ciliary body by fibers called zonules. The ciliary muscle alters the lens shape to change the focal distance for near and distance viewing called accommodations. The ciliary body comprises two parts, the pars plicata and the pars plana. The pars plicata is made up of ciliary processes that constitute the attachment site for the zonules and produce the aqueous humor. The posterior portion of the ciliary body is called the pars plana and attaches to the ora serrata, which is the anterior boundary of the retina.[53]

Functioning to focus light onto the retina, the lens is a biconvex transparent structure situated directly behind the iris. The lens is composed of the anterior capsule, an epithelial cell layer, and the lens cortex and nucleus. The lens is held in place by the zonule fibers attached to the ciliary muscle. This muscle regulates the shape of the lens. In childhood the lens is pliable, allowing a wide focal range. The lens continues to grow throughout life, becoming more compact with age. When people reach their mid-40s, the lens often loses flexibility; therefore it can no longer focus light sufficiently at near distances, a condition called presbyopia. Reading glasses are a common treatment option for this condition. By age 55 years, the lens may lose its ability to accommodate; bifocal lenses can correct for near and far acuity deficits. Cataracts are a clouding or opacity of the lens, resulting in reduction or distortion of light transmitted through the lens. Trauma, changes in metabolism, chemical or radiologic contamination, and normal aging may cause cataracts. Surgical correction of cataracts is effected by removal of the interior lens material and insertion of an intraocular lens (IOL) into the anterior capsule.[51,53]

Posterior Cavity

The posterior cavity is the part of the eye posterior to the lens, including the vitreous humor, posterior sclera, choroid, and the retina. Vitreous humor is a clear, gelatinous fluid that fills the globe of the eye between the lens and retina, composed of 99% water with a small amount of collagen. The primary function of the vitreous humor is to provide volume to the eye, maintain the shape of the globe, and transmit clearly light refracted by structures toward the front of the eye. Unlike the aqueous humor, the vitreous humor is not continually renewed; once mature the production of vitreous humor is finished. The vitreous humor may shrink slightly with aging, pulling away from the interior of the sclera or retina. The resulting space fills with fluid. When this detachment occurs at the retina, an individual may see light flashes or floaters. Other types of floaters occur naturally as bits of protein or pigment floating freely in the vitreous humor and may be seen as shadowy forms when viewing a highly illuminated background. A sudden onset of many floaters or a loss of a noticeable area of the visual field could be a sign of a retinal detachment, which would require immediate medical attention.[51]

The retina lines the posterior two-thirds of the posterior cavity with a complex nine-layer tissue. Only 0.5 mm thick, it operates like the film of the eye camera, converting light stimulation into neural transmissions to the brain. The sclera forms the outer globe of the eye. The choroid is a network of blood vessels between the retina and the sclera, nourishing the neural cells of the retina and the retinal pigment epithelium (RPE). The choroid extends from the ora serrata (anterior margin of the retina) to the margin of the optic nerve. Branches of the ophthalmic artery, long and short posterior arteries, and the ciliary artery provide arterial blood supply. Understanding the arterial blood supply to the ocular system is important for appreciating the effects a stroke or CVA in one artery may have on the tissues supplied by it or one of its branches. In surgical procedures important landmarks are seen in the veins in each quadrant of the choroid that form a single, larger vein. Bruch's membrane (a so-called "basement" membrane) is located on the anterior portion of the choriocapillaris (capillaries in the choroid). This allows nutrients to pass from the capillaries to the photoreceptor layer of the retina. Examination of the eyes of elderly people may disclose drusen, yellowish deposits of waste products from the RPE. Inflammation of the retinal capillaries and RPE is called chorioretinitis and may be caused by toxoplasmosis, syphilis, sarcoidosis, histoplasmosis, and tuberculosis. The RPE is the outer of the two underlying layers of the retina. When examining and viewing the retina one can see through the transparent neural layers of the retina to the pigmented RPE. This pigment absorbs excess light and is genetically determined. Blonde-haired and redheaded people usually display minimal pigmentation, whereas brunettes normally have a brownish-orange-pink coloration. Asians and Indians are usually found to have a bluish-black coloring in the RPE. People with albinism not only lack pigment in the iris but also have no pigment in the RPE. The RPE provides nourishment for the neural retinal tissues and functions in waste removal in that area. A common location for retinal detachments is in the space between the RPE and inner neural cell layers.[51,52]

The neural part of the retina that converts the light stimulation into nerve transmissions is composed of three layers. From outside to inside, these layers are arranged as follows. The photoreceptor cell layer containing the rods and cones lies next to the RPE. The 130 million rods of the retina are located at the retinal periphery and thus are useful for peripheral vision and night vision or in reduced light conditions. Most important about the rods is their production of rhodopsin, a pigment that absorbs specific wavelengths of light. The nerve impulses are formed by chemical reactions caused by the absorption of light by the rhodopsin. Rhodopsin is regenerated in the dark; in healthy persons complete regeneration (dark adaptation) takes approximately 30 minutes. Once the rods have regenerated the rhodopsin, they can function again at optimum level. The inability to adapt fully or a significant delay in adaptation may be a sign of congenital stationary night blindness. Night blindness may also be caused by a lack of vitamin A, necessary for rhodopsin to carry out its task effectively. Retinitis pigmentosa (RP) is a congenital disease that damages the rods in time, leading to increasing loss of peripheral vision, night blindness, and tunnel vision, in which the individual is left with predominantly a central field of view (a tunnel) provided by only the cones in the macula of the retina. Decreased ability to adapt to light and dark results in difficulty adapting to certain conditions, such as glare on entering a darker building on a bright sunny day or when driving into and out of a tunnel or into and out of shadows, because the light/dark adaptation is too slow.

The photoreceptor cells responsible for color and detail visual ability are called cones. Testing acuity is really testing cone cell function. Located primarily in the macula, the six million cones function best in full but not excessive light conditions. The cones appear to manifest in three varieties, each able to absorb specific wavelengths of light (red, green, and blue) with its own specialized pigment to detect colors. Similar to the rhodopsin in the rods, erythrolabe (red), chlorolabe (green), and cyanolabe (blue) are activated by the specific wavelengths of light associated with their color. Specific wavelengths of light determine the stimulation of each type of cone. The occipital lobes process this information, resulting in the ability to perceive an almost infinite range of colors in the visible spectrum. Serious color vision deficiency affects approximately 8% of the population. In the more common type all three pigments are produced, but one does not function sufficiently. This may lead to a washed-out color, or one of the pigments may be used ineffectively. The most common instance of this type of color blindness is an inability to identify red and green correctly, called red/green color blindness, which is a sex-linked recessive trait. In other types of color blindness one or more pigments may be missing altogether. In a condition called rod monochromatism, the person is born without functioning cones, leading to poor acuity, no color vision, nystagmus, and photophobia. Color vision dysfunction of one eye indicates retinal or optic nerve disease, whereas dysfunction of both eyes indicates a congenital defect. There is also the factor of hysterical color blindness caused by emotional trauma, which is well attested and documented. Optic neuritis is another disease that significantly influences the transmission of color vision along the optic nerve.[51,52] Faulty color vision may cause the driver to fail to recognize the indication of traffic or brake lights. Traffic signs such as stop, yield, and directional and speed limit signs are color- and shape-coded for easy recognition. Although there is no research to support increased driving risk from color vision deficiency, limited color vision decreases the options available for the timely detection and observation of important traffic sign information.

The macula and fovea are located in the central retina. Surrounding the fovea, the macula accounts for only 1.5 mm of the retinal surface. Other than the fovea itself, the macula has the greatest concentration of cones and together with the fovea forms that portion of the retina responsible for the greatest clarity, detail, and color vision. Age-related macular degeneration (ARMD or AMD) is a condition frequently occurring in older adults. AMD results from a gradual breakdown of the RPE, causing central vision loss. Symptoms include blurring of details, distortions of straight lines or edges, and tiny patches of complete vision loss. Although these patches, called scotomas, of destroyed macula are a small percentage of the total retinal area, they cause significant loss of detail vision because of their location on the macula. Peripheral vision remains intact, and portions of the macula may be unaffected. Depending on the location of the scotomas(s), clients may be able to use their remaining vision to compensate for the lost areas of vision using a technique called eccentric viewing. Less commonly called exudative or wet macular degeneration is caused by blood oozing from an abnormal growth of blood vessels into the macula. Although people with macular degeneration may be able to observe objects and the roadway in the distance, vision becomes problematic for near distance tasks, such as attempting to stop at a sufficiently close distance to the vehicle in front at a traffic light, when negotiating a lane change, parking, or reading dashboard instruments.

The second of the neural transmitting layers is the bipolar cell layer, serving to connect the photoreceptor cell layer to the ganglion cell layer. Other cells in this layer provide integration of neural transmission and structural/nutritional support.

The innermost of the three retinal cell layers features the ganglion cells. The axons from these cells combine to form the optic nerve, thus providing the necessary link from the retina to the occipital lobes of the brain. The ganglion cells will be discussed further with the optic disc.

The optic disc is the gathering point for the millions of axons of the ganglion cells and the beginning of the optic nerve. Visual information is ultimately received and analyzed by the occipital lobes. To send the information, the photoreceptor layer of the retina converts the light stimulation into neurotransmitters, which in turn stimulate other layers of retinal nerves. The ganglion cells of the innermost cell layer have axons that form a nerve fiber layer (NFL). These axons are the individual fibers of the optic nerve. Each axon bundles with others in the vicinity, following a specific universal path to the optic disc or optic nerve head to the point where the ganglion cell axons converge to form the optic nerve. Because there are no photoreceptor cells in the optic disc, this results in a minute physiologic blind spot. During an ophthalmic eye examination, the 1.5-mm disc may be seen as a lighter, pink area with an even lighter center called the optic cup, a depression in the center of the disc, the observation of which is important in diagnosing the health of the eye. In a healthy eye the cup is normally approximately one-third the size of the disc, or a ratio of 0.3 C/D, although this can vary between individuals. Changes in this ratio over time or between eyes may signal damage to the nerve fibers forming the optic disc. IOP from glaucoma or other damage may cause the nerve fibers to die; the cup appears larger because of decreased mass of the nerves in the optic disc.[51,52]

Blood Supply to the Visual System

The ophthalmic branch of the internal carotid artery supplies arterial blood to the eye and surrounding structures. The central retinal artery (CRA), a branch of the ophthalmic artery, supplies the inner two-thirds of the retina. The CRA and the central retinal vein (CRV), which removes blood from the eye to return to the heart, enter the eye at the optic disc and branch into four smaller vessels, the superior and inferior nasal and temporal branches, each branch servicing a quadrant of the retinal ganglion and bipolar cells. A serious ocular emergency is created if a vessel of the CRA or CRV becomes occluded (blocked) because blockage of the artery means loss of oxygen and nutrients, whereas occlusion of the vein causes the vessel to become distended, leading to hemorrhage.

The internal carotid artery, the middle and posterior cerebral arteries, the cerebellar artery, and the vertebrobasilar artery system supply blood to various parts of the brain containing the visual pathway. Trauma or occlusion in one of these vessels or branches may result in damage to the visual pathway or negatively impact the synthesizing of visual neural impulses into useful information. Table 6-3 summarizes the major arteries and symptoms of damage to them.

Injury to the blood supply to the brain is the most frequent cause of a CVA or stroke. A stroke emanating from the arterial supply serving the visual system can cause a visual field loss called a homonymous (corresponding) hemianopia (hemi = half, anopia = no vision). CVA or stroke is a relatively common diagnosis seen by the DRS. The client suffering from the effects of a CVA referred for a driving evaluation may have loss of motor function on the left or right side that may affect either or both and the upper and lower extremities. The client may experience postural deficits and motor planning and cognitive changes. The DRS must evaluate all of these symptoms. In addition to the more obvious symptoms, the post-CVA client may have visual deficits that are not readily observable and may have not been diagnosed. The client may be unaware of visual changes or loss of visual field. As a result of the stroke, the client loses part or all of the visual field from the nasal side of one eye and the temporal side of the other eye. A stroke affecting the right side of the body (i.e., right hemiplegia) accounts for approximately 36% of right hemianopias, and 25% of left-side strokes (i.e., left hemiplegia) result in left hemianopia. The damage does not affect eye function; rather it damages the neural pathway to the occipital lobe or the lobe itself. It should be recalled that the nerve fibers from the ganglion cells of the retina cross or desiccate at the optic chiasm. As the optic tract leaves the chiasm, each tract contains fibers from the right and the left. Therefore damage to the visual pathway posterior to the optic chiasm affects the visual field of both eyes. Depending on the severity and location of the insult, the field loss may be only a portion of a quadrant of the visual field, or the trauma may result in total field loss of one-half of the field of view in both eyes. A condition known as homonymous hemianopsia also may occur, which means with neglect. This occurs more frequently with a stroke affecting the left side of the body. Besides having the loss of physical and sensory function of the left arm, leg, or both, postural deficits, cognitive changes, and possible speech (aphasia) and swallowing problems (dysphagia), the client may frequently lose awareness of the left side of the body. With neglect means that the client no longer attends to that side of the body and may not even be aware that his or her left arm for example is his or her own. The client with left neglect tends to lean to the right with his or her head and eyes turned toward the right. Visually the eyes move from midline to the right but do not cross midline to the left.[51,53]

AFFERENT PATHWAYS TO PRIMARY VISUAL AREA IN OCCIPITAL LOBE

As light enters through the pupil, it is focused on the retina by the lens (Figure 6-5). The retina is a complex layer of cells on the rear inner surface of the eye capable of turning light energy into nerve impulses, which are then sent to the occipital lobes of the brain. The occipital lobes visualize the object in question by interpreting the neural impulses received from the retina. The impulses travel along the ganglion cell axons to the optic nerve head, the beginning of the optic nerve. The optic nerves of each eye leave the orbital socket of the skull and lead posteriorly to the optic chiasm, located in the middle of the underneath side of the brain, slightly anterior to the center.

Table 6-3   Blood Supply to the Visual System

Major Artery Supplying Brain	Potential Symptoms
Middle cerebral artery (MCA)	Contralateral hemiplegia (weakness or paralysis of opposite side), involving face, tongue, arm, and leg. Contralateral homonymous hemianopsia, aphasia (if the dominant hemisphere is affected), sensory deficits, and perceptual deficits including anosognosia, unilateral neglect (usually the left side), impaired vertical perception, visual spatial deficits, and perseveration (if the nondominant hemisphere is affected).
Internal carotid artery (ICA)	Contralateral hemiplegia, hemianesthesia, and homonymous hemianopsia. Involvement of the dominant side includes aphasia, agraphia, dysgraphia, acalculia, right-left confusion, and finger agnosia. Nondominant involvement effects include visual-perceptual dysfunction, unilateral neglect, anosognosia, constructional apraxia, attention deficits, and loss of topographic memory.
Anterior cerebral artery (ACA)	Contralateral weakness or paralysis of the lower extremity, which is greater than the upper extremity, lower extremity spasticity, and severe weakness of the face and tongue. Apraxia, mental changes, confusion, disorientation, abulia, whispering, limited verbal output, perseveration, and amnesia. Primitive reflexes, bowel and bladder incontinence.
Posterior cerebral artery (PCA)	Effects are varied and may include a broad area of the brain; however, more common effects are involuntary movement disorders (hemiballism, postural tremor, hemichorea, hemiataxia, and intention tremor). Memory loss, alexia, astereognosis, dysesthesia, akinesthesia, contralateral homonymous hemianopsia or quadrantopsia, anomia, topographic disorientation, and visual agnosia.
Cerebellar artery	Ipsilateral (same side) ataxia, contralateral loss of pain and temperature sensitivity, ipsilateral facial analgesia, dysphagia and dysarthria, nystagmus, and contralateral hemiparesis.
Vertebrobasilar artery system	Affects brainstem functions with bilateral sensory and motor involvement, loss of proprioception, hemiplegia, quadriplegia, and involvement of cranial nerves III-XII.

It is at the optic chiasm where the nerve fibers from the nasal side of one retina cross over to join the temporal fibers from the other eye. The crossing, or decussation, of these fibers is important to blend the information from each eye into one scene. The retinal nerves exiting the retina on the side of the eye closer to the body midline (therefore closer to the nose) are called the nasal fibers. Because of the curvature of the eye and the inversion of the image caused by the focalization of the image by the lens onto the retina, these fibers perceive the temporal or outer side of the field of view. The temporal fibers, which are the fibers farther away from the body midline, receive input from the nasal or middle of the field of view. The field of view from the temporal side of each eye overlaps slightly in the middle, resulting in the ability to perceive distance and depth perception. If the crossing of the optic nerve fibers did not occur, then the brain would perceive two separate images from slightly differing angles.

The nerves leaving the optic chiasm are called the optic tracts and extend to the lateral geniculate body of both hemispheres of the brain, which begins to synthesize the separate images into one and helps to integrate information from other senses, such as the vestibular (balance) system, so that the brain can begin to interpret the environment more fully. Leaving the lateral geniculate body, the optic tracts, now called optic radiations, travel to the visual (occipital) cortex. Damage anywhere along this pathway can cause significant loss of vision in the area of the visual field that is affected.

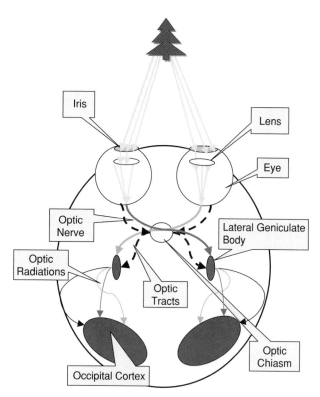

Figure 6-5 Afferent pathways to the primary visual area in the occipital lobe. (Courtesy Patrick T. Baker.)

For purposes of examination and diagnosis, the field of view of each eye is divided into quadrants. Injury anywhere along the visual pathway, from the retina to the occipital lobes, can cause decreased or complete loss of vision in the quadrant(s) affected by the injury or illness.[52,53]

VISUAL DYSFUNCTION AND THE EFFECT ON THE DRIVING SKILL

The DRS should be aware of some of the more common medical conditions and their effect on visual function. Table 6-4 includes some of the more common conditions the DRS may encounter.

THE CLINICAL EVALUATION OF VISION

The task of the DRS in the evaluation, treatment, and recommendation process of the client referred for driving rehabilitation is a multifaceted and complex undertaking. First and foremost the DRS must remember that the safety of the client, potential passengers riding with the client, other motorists and pedestrians, and the DRS himself or herself is paramount. The operation of a motor vehicle even in optimum conditions by fully capable and highly qualified individuals is a risky endeavor. The DRS must have sufficient knowledge of physical, cognitive, psychological, and visual function and know how illness and injury affect function to accurately assess a client's ability to operate a motor vehicle safely. Most driver evaluations take place in a two-step process: the clinical evaluation and the on-road evaluation.

Table 6-4 Medical Conditions and Their Effect on Visual Function

Effect on Visual Function	Condition
Vision conditions affecting acuity	Amblyopia, astigmatism, myopia, hyperopia, presbyopia, cataracts, glaucoma, iritis, macular degeneration, optic neuritis, nystagmus, diabetic retinopathy, retinopathy of prematurity (RP), retinitis pigmentosa, retinal tears and detachment and conditions affecting the blood supply to the eye and retina, including the central retinal artery and veins
Vision conditions affecting field of view	Cerebrovascular accident, ptosis, strabismus, nystagmus, RP, cataracts, glaucoma, retinal detachment or tears, optic neuritis, and diabetic retinopathy
Vision conditions affecting contrast sensitivity and glare	Cataracts, glaucoma, optic neuritis, iritis, and albinism
Vision conditions affecting scanning ability	Traumatic brain injury, stroke, tumors or other diseases that affect the cranial nerves serving the extraocular muscles and muscles of the neck that permit postural control and head movements

SCREENING VERSUS EVALUATION AND DIAGNOSIS

The clinical evaluation is composed of an evaluation of ROM, strength, cognition, and visual function performed in generally optimum conditions. This testing usually is done via the use of screening tools that quickly give the examiner an overall clinical picture of function but are not designed to be an exhaustive physical and psychological evaluation. For example the DRS may determine that the client has decreased upper extremity ROM and strength by assessing ROM and strength but cannot determine by these methods the cause of the deficit. Similarly a vision screen may suggest symptoms of loss of peripheral vision but will not distinguish whether this is the result of cataracts, glaucoma, ptosis, RP, or other conditions that can affect peripheral vision. Cognitive screens may indicate decreased memory skills or limited focus of attention, but the DRS is not, nor need be, sufficiently trained to diagnose whether this is the result of dementia or simply a case of a nervous client who is anxious about failing the driving evaluation. The function of the clinical screening process is to provide the DRS with clues and insights as to potential issues affecting the client's functional performance on the road. It is the responsibility of the DRS to report symptoms of deficits in function to the referring physician or to make appropriate referrals so that the client may receive a complete examination and diagnosis of the cause of the dysfunction.

Typically the driving evaluation should begin with a chart review and medical history of the client if the medical record is available. If unavailable the DRS must take an oral medical and functional history from the client. A review of the medical record should include the presenting diagnosis, secondary diagnoses, surgical history, recent visual examinations, cognitive assessment, and the prescribed and over-the-counter medications being taken. The DRS should be sufficiently conversant with medical terminology and anatomy to interpret the information recorded in the chart and to recognize medications that may interfere with cognitive and visual function. The DRS should not be hesitant to refer to a medical or pharmacologic dictionary or call the client's physician to discuss questions about the client's medical, pharmacologic, or ocular history.

On those occasions when the client's medical chart is unavailable, the DRS needs to ask thoughtful, appropriate questions regarding the client's overall health and function. Frequently clients may be reluctant to offer information regarding personal health challenges because of a fear that disclosing such facts may negatively affect the evaluation and recommendations. They may have forgotten some aspect of the health history or even be unaware of other issues. In some cases, and with the client's permission, interviewing a close family member or friend may provide additional information and insight regarding the client's past and current health and functional capabilities. In addition to a review of medical history, a discussion of functional performance will provide useful information. For example if the client reports difficulty reading and finding things in the home or is bumping into objects, there may be some undiagnosed visual conditions affecting acuity, visual perceptual skills, or peripheral vision that may also affect driving. Asking appropriate indirect questions regarding ADL skills can elicit important useful information, whereas a direct question about visual or cognitive function may be met with an evasive "Good!" as the reply.

COMMONLY USED TOOLS FOR EVALUATING VISION

There are numerous methods used clinically to evaluate the client's visual function. Tools used in the assessment process can vary from the use of the evaluator's finger or pen that the client tracks visually while the evaluator observes eye movements to expensive computer programs and equipment. Expenditures for sophisticated equipment need to be weighed against the potential value of the information gained, again with the understanding that the role of the DRS is to identify symptoms and evaluate the effect on driving performance, not to diagnose conditions. Another factor when choosing assessment methods is time. Sophisticated equipment and procedures take additional time, which in turn affects the cost involved for the client being evaluated. For example driving assessments conducted in a hospital-based setting may bill for services in 15-minute increments. A complex, lengthy assessment process may be interesting and enlightening for the clinician but is so long as to be cost prohibitive to the potential client who needs the evaluation. An intense evaluation process may provide a wealth of clinical information but may be far more information than is necessary to determine functional ability to operate a motor vehicle. It should also be remembered that although significant, the vision assessment is only a part of the total driving evaluation; there are other important screens of physical and cognitive abilities that need to be assessed. Time is a major factor in the evaluation, not only for cost effectiveness but also because of the fatigue factor of the client.

The following are some examples of relatively easy, quick, and effective assessment instruments that are frequently used and have demonstrated reliability in research projects conducted on the assessment of functional visual performance and driving. Several of the following assessment tools have been used by the American Medical Association's Assessing and Counseling Older Drivers Program and the National Highway Traffic Safety Administration's (NHTSA's) Model Driver Screening and Evaluation Program and have demonstrated correlations between driving performance and outcomes of these tests.

Useful field of view is a phrase that describes a functional assessment of visual skill and a computer program designed to assess it. Field of view, as described earlier in this chapter, refers to the area, in degrees, of the environment a person can visually detect without moving his or her head and is not dependent on acuity. Useful field of view represents that portion of the field of view that the client is capable of effectively using in a variety of conditions. For example as a person is driving, he or she is able to shift his or her visual focus of attention to all points within his or her field of view and is aware of all relevant visual information. In these conditions the driver's useful field of view and actual field of view are similar. During high stress conditions, such as driving on a rainy, foggy night or on an unfamiliar road, the driver's anxiety level may increase, and his or her focus of attention becomes riveted on the road directly in front of the vehicle. He or she may become visually unaware of movements or objects in the periphery of his or her normal field of view; therefore in effect the driver's useful visual field is reduced to some fraction of that described in optimum conditions. Other common examples of situations that can reduce the effective useful field of view while driving are the use of cellular phones, adjusting the radio channel, changing tapes or compact discs, eating, and talking. Certain medical conditions also affect portions of the field of view, reducing the size of the useful portion.

A computer program of the same name requires the client to locate randomly flashing symbols on a computer screen, which appear at an increasing rate, thereby increasing the visual demands and stress level of the person being evaluated. Eventually the frequency of the appearance of the symbols on the screen becomes so rapid that the client cannot keep up. The results of this test have been evaluated in a number of research studies and have been found to have some validity in the appraisal of visual driving performance. Older drivers with ≥40% impairment in their useful field of view, which stems from decreases in visual sensory function, visual processing speed, and/or visual attentional skills, appear to be at an increased crash risk.[54]

The MVPT is a widely used assessment tool adaptable for many purposes. It is called motor free because the client does not need to move physically to take the test. The test has several versions but generally consists of a series of pages containing specially designed images. This tool is designed to test the visual perceptual skills, figure-ground, visual memory, closure, visual discrimination, and spatial relations. The evaluator provides instruction for each section of the test, and the client chooses the correct answer. In addition to visual skills the clinician can also observe secondary issues, such as ability to understand and recall the instructions, focus of attention, and the effects of stress of the client's behavior. The National Transportation Safety Board program used a subsection of the MVPT, Visual Closure (VC), which provided statistically significant results.

Freund Clock is another quick assessment tool that has demonstrated validity with regard to assessment of driving dysfunction. This tool gives the examiner indications regarding long- and short-term memory, visual perception, visual spatial skills, selective attention, and *executive function.* The client is given a sheet of paper and a pencil and asked to draw a clock face, include all the numbers, and set the time to 7:10. The DRS scores the completed task looking for eight specific points, grading "yes" or "no" to each point.

1. All 12 hours are placed in correct numeric order with the "12" at the top.
2. Only the 12 numbers are present, no duplicates, omissions, or extraneous marks.
3. The numbers are drawn inside the clock face.
4. The numbers are equally, or nearly equally, spaced from each other.
5. The numbers are equally, or nearly equally, spaced around the clock.
6. One clock hand points to the number 2.
7. The other clock hand points to the number 7.
8. There are only two clock hands.

If the client misses any component of the test, this may signal the need for intervention.[55] Trail Making Test Part B is the second part of the Trail Making Test Parts A and B. It is another paper and pencil test that takes only a few minutes to administer and has been shown to evaluate working memory, visual processing, visual spatial skills, selective and divided attention, and psychomotor coordination. Research has shown that poor performance on the Trail Making Test Part B correlates with decreased driving skills. The test consists of a preprinted sheet with the numbers 1 through 12 and the letters A through L placed randomly about the page. The client is asked to connect the numbers and letters with a pencil line, with the instruction "starting with 1 draw a line to A, then to 2, then to B, and so on, alternating back and forth between numbers and letters until finishing with the number 12." The test is timed. Should the client make an error, the administrator corrects the client immediately, and the time for correction is counted in the total score. In the prepilot study conducted in Maryland for the NHTSA "Model Driver Screening and Evaluation Program" project, the present *Notebook* authors found that subjects who took ≥5 minutes to complete the Trail Making Test Part B protocol were 1.41 times more likely to be involved in a crash compared with subjects who completed this test in <5 minutes. The mean time to complete the Trail Making Test Part B protocol was 161.14 seconds for the crash-free drivers and 180.57 seconds for the crash-involved drivers. Subjects ranged in age from 68 to 89 years (mean age, 75.7 years); 131 of the 363 subjects were involved in at least one crash in the previous 6-year period (1991 through 1997).[54]

The DRS should be sensitive to the client's feelings regarding an evaluation of his or her abilities. A client who is active, is independent, works, or is responsible for his or her family may resent submitting to the Mini-Mental Status Examination, Freund Clock, MVPT, or other tests that do not readily appear relevant to driving. The client who does not wear corrective lenses, has no difficulty reading, and does not report any visual deficits may not be appropriate for a full vision assessment. Some clients coming for a driving evaluation may not be receptive to anything other than getting in the vehicle and driving because their perception is that this is what they are there to do. In all situations the DRS should observe the client's behavior while he or she is filling out paperwork, walking, during the clinical assessment, and in the vehicle to detect any subtle indications of visual, cognitive, or physical problems that may be present.

OCULAR HISTORY AND EYE EXAMINATION

In addition to the physical portions of the driving evaluation, the visual examination is vitally important. Successful operation of a motor vehicle cannot be accomplished if the driver cannot scan the environment sufficiently, track objects, or does not have the acuity or peripheral visual skills to identify objects in or near the path of travel that may be relevant. Even if the client does not appear to require a formal assessment of ocular function, the DRS should observe and note behaviors that may indicate the presence of a subtle deficit. If a recent eye examination is available from a physician, the DRS should review it and ask for additional information from the client. For example occasionally clients report having received a new lens prescription, but "they just do not seem to work right." The client may have other insight as to functional visual performance that is not found in a clinical evaluation. After reviewing the chart and obtaining the client's own assessment of his or her visual function, the DRS can begin the clinical screening process. We will review some basic concepts and simple procedures that can be easily used to determine a baseline of useful information.

Seated in front of the client, with ample lighting, the DRS can begin with an exterior observation of the face and eyes, looking for any obvious discharges from either eye and noting the shape and position of the eyelids. Any discoloration or irritation of the sclera or clouding of the cornea should be noted, as well as the apparent focus of attention or irregular movements (nystagmus) of the eyes. While seated in this position, a method can be used to evaluate extraocular movements. Using a pen, small light, or even his or her own finger, the evaluator asks the client to follow the object with his or her eyes while not moving the head. With the use of horizontal, vertical, and diagonal moments, the clinician observes the client's eye movements while he or she tracks the object. The client's ability to track the object in all planes should be noted, and the DRS should observe the ability of the eyes to cross midline and the fluidity of the movement (saccades). While holding the object approximately 14 to 16 inches away from the client directly in front of the nose and then moving slowly toward the nose, the client should be able to maintain focal attention on the moving object through convergence. Both eyes should turn slightly inward, so that they appear crossed, until the object reaches just a few inches away, when one eye loses focus and reverts to its normal, centered position. With instruction to continue to attend to the object, it is retracted slowly, until both eyes are again focused on the object, known as divergence.

Peripheral vision can be assessed similarly. Slowly move an object or fingers from behind the client into his or her field of view with instructions to the client to indicate when the moving object is first seen. This should be done from the sides at eye level, below eye level, and above eye level to assess the entire perimeter of the peripheral field. Significant deficits may suggest a referral for a formal evaluation of peripheral vision by a qualified physician.

Acuity is easily tested using a number of charts and devices such as the Snellen Eye Chart, Colenbrander 1-m Chart, ETDRS, Bailey-Lovie, and LEA charts. Distance between the client and the chart and lighting are critical factors when testing acuity. The individual chart should have instructions regarding optimum distance for use, and the light should be appropriate without reflection or glare on the chart or the client. The client is asked to cover first one eye, then the other and read the letters or symbols on the chart, with the smallest letters that are legible corresponding to the level of acuity. Charts such as the Colenbrander permit the use of both eyes while reading sentences. The sentences decrease in size line by line. Acuity should be tested for near and far, with the understanding that for the purposes of driving, far acuity is more important. Asking the client to locate objects at various distances in the environment is another test of functional acuity. This can be done indoors, outdoors, and in the automobile. Two advantages of this type of testing are that the DRS can observe visual function at far greater distances than is possible clinically and can observe functional acuity in a variety of lighting conditions.

Another method to test acuity and other aspects of visual function uses a compact, relatively inexpensive piece of equipment. The Optec 2000 is one brand used for vision assessment and looks similar to those devices used by state testing offices to assess vision. These are usually portable, self-contained units with internal lighting and a series of plates imprinted with tests for acuity, color, fusion, phorias, depth perception, peripheral vision, and contrast. The client looks into a viewfinder and reads or describes the information on the plate. The evaluator can switch plates with a dial. Although there are limits to the sensitivity of this device, it is an efficient method of screening for a number of conditions quickly and provides sufficient information to indicate potential issues and to suggest the need for a referral for more professional evaluation.

Fusion is the ability of the brain to blend the information seen by each eye into one scene. The inability to do so may result in double vision (i.e., observing two of the same object side by side). This can be tested with the Optec 2000, checking for phorias when testing convergence and divergence, and by simply asking the client whether he or she ever has double vision.

Phorias are the tendency of one eye to drift away from the focal point in certain circumstances (i.e., the inability to fixate the gaze of both eyes onto a specific object). Significant phorias, called tropias, limit the ability to fuse the separate images into one, resulting in double vision.

Depth perception is the ability to determine the relative distances between objects at various points in the environment. The ability to perceive relative distances is possible because of binocular vision. The visual fields of both eyes overlap approximately 120 degrees in the central area of the visual field. Because of the location of the eyes (and the retina) in the skull and the visual axis of the eye, each retina perceives an object from a slightly different angle, and the brain is able to triangulate the object location and the image in each eye to determine its distance. Other factors used to judge distance include relative size. An object of known size appears smaller at a greater distance. When one object is situated in front of another, it is superimposed; therefore one object has to be closer than the other one. Linear objects, such as railroad tracks, appear to converge as the distance increases. Moving objects, such as vehicles, appear to move more quickly at near distance

than at far. Good acuity and contrast sensitivity allow the viewer to more accurately gauge the shape and size of an object, thereby permitting one to distinguish more accurately a close object from one farther away. There are tools available that allow the examiner to measure the client's degree of depth perception. The client is asked to observe two points on a sliding scale, usually measured in millimeters, with one point stationary, while the client moves the other point into a position of side-by-side alignment. The person with normal depth perception will be able to recognize and make precise adjustments to align the two points. The Optec 2000 uses plates imprinted with pictures that are designed to make some of the designs appear to float above or appear closer to the viewer than others, a three-dimensional effect.

Contrast sensitivity is the ability to perceive various shades of black and white, as well as color. Tests such as Pelli-Robson Contrast Sensitivity Chart and the LEA Vision Screening Card are designed to assess the ability of the eyes to detect variances in spatial frequencies of gray.

Glare refers to the comparison of a light source with its background. Glare is produced if the light source, such as automobile headlights or the sun reflecting from a snowy groundcover, is more than three times as bright as the background. Discomfort glare causes pain and fatigue, whereas disability glare interferes with vision by blinding or dazzling the client and results in reduced visual performance. Many eye conditions such as cataracts, macular degeneration, RP, aphakia, retinal cone dystrophies, optic neuropathy, and albinism affect the person's ability to tolerate not only glare but also normal lighting conditions. Glare recovery is the time required for the person affected by glare to recover visual function after the glare is removed. Typically the recovery time for a healthy adult is 50 to 60 seconds, although with age this may become slightly increased. This effect can be noted when entering a building from outdoors on a bright, sunny day. The eyes need time to adjust, and as they do acuity returns to normal. People who are acutely affected by glare or bright conditions may require several minutes to recover. During the recovery time they may have little or no functional vision. This can be catastrophic if it occurs during the operation of a motor vehicle. Glare recovery can be tested by asking the client to determine his or her best-corrected acuity using an eye chart while wearing corrective lenses and occluding the better eye. The client is then asked to read the next line above. The evaluator then shines a penlight into the nonoccluded eye for 10 seconds, followed by instruction to read the line above his or her acuity level as soon as he or she can perceive it. Timing begins when the penlight is removed. A significant delay in recovery should suggest a referral to a vision specialist for further evaluation. People significantly impaired because of intolerance of light may become photophobic and avoid highly illuminated situations whenever possible. There are a number of companies that manufacture filters and lenses designed to reduce the impact of excessive light and glare entering the eye. The composition and color of the lens reduce or block various wavelengths of light as it passes through the lens. People reporting significant concerns or problems with glare or photophobia should consult an eye specialist to determine the cause and seek professional assistance in choosing the correct protective lens, such as amber or yellow-orange filters.

Color vision is typically tested using the Ishihara color plates or other similar instruments that can be obtained on a series of printed cards, or with mechanical devices such as the ones noted earlier. The client is asked to look at the card or plate. A person with normal color vision will be able to see colored numbers, letters, or symbols within the design on the card. People with deficits will be unable to perceive one or more of the imbedded designs. The Ishihara plates detect red/green deficits only. Another test, the American Optical H-R-R, detects red/green and blue/yellow deficits. The Farnsworth Panel D-15 and Farnsworth-Munsell 100 hue tests use colored caps, which the client arranges in correct order to assess color vision. Functional color vision may be assessed by asking the client to identify various colors in the environment, such as different road signs and vehicles, while driving. People with red/green color vision deficits may have trouble recognizing the color of traffic lights; however, they are typically consistently sequenced throughout geographic regions, such as red at the top, then yellow, with green on the bottom. The DRS should be concerned not so much as to whether the client can determine red from green but whether this deficit limits the ability to determine which light is activated.

Field losses refer to the absence of vision in some part of the visual field. Typically these are designated as either central visual field or peripheral visual field losses, depending on the location. Field loss can occur from structural changes, such as ptosis of an eyelid obstructing the field of view, but more commonly refers to damage to the retina or optic pathway. Retinal damage may affect the field of view but only in the damaged eye. Optic pathway damage can result from TBI, tumors, infection, and disease, or as the result of a stroke. The location and nature of the injury determine the effect it has on the visual field; however, this damage occurs to the visual field of both eyes. This is a serious condition that takes months of physical rehabilitation to overcome. Clients are usually left with some permanent residual loss of functional motor, cognitive, and visual skills. In addition to PT and OT interventions, the use of optical devices, such as Fresnel prisms, yoked prisms, the Visual Field Awareness System, the Inwave Field-Expanding Hemispheric Lens, and mirror systems, can expand the field of view for the client.[56] Many clients can be taught scanning and tracking techniques that improve the ability to locate objects in the environment. Although there are some interventions that can improve functional vision, the actual field loss is usually permanent. Even without neglect a driver with field loss has to constantly scan the environment with his or her remaining vision. A client with a left visual field loss cannot monitor traffic to the left while tracking the path of travel during a right turn at a four-way intersection and may be at risk from traffic approaching from the opposite side of the intersection and the left. Field loss can be assessed using confrontation visual field testing. Another test used by eye professionals is the Humphrey's Visual Field Test.

The other field loss is known as central vision loss and most often results from AMD. The central 30 degrees of the field of view, the primary domain of the cones cells, is used for detail, color, and daylight vision. AMD causes tiny portions of the macula to be destroyed, resulting in a scotoma, or loss of a portion of the visual field. Loss of central vision affects acuity and contrast sensitivity. The client perceives scotomas as distortions or as a dark spot(s) in the visual field. These may be a central, paracentral (adjacent to the fixation point), or pericentral (surrounding the fixation point) scotoma.

Scotomas are not just caused by AMD; they can occur as the result of glaucoma and RP (ring scotomas). Depending on the location and density of the scotoma(s), visual function can be drastically impaired. Reading, writing, watching television, and identification of medications can become difficult or impossible. Driving is affected when the client cannot observe road signs, read the dashboard instruments, perceive oncoming vehicles or pedestrians, or judge distances as objects come close. Because AMD is a progressive condition, people with AMD frequently are trained to assess their vision daily with the use of an Amsler Grid. The Amsler Grid is similar to graph paper. The client looks at the grid and marks where the lines are distorted or absent. A comparison of grids over time can indicate changes in the retinal scotomas.

Visual motor skills refer to the ability of the client to use the EOMs to efficiently move his or her eyes to observe objects in the visual field and to fixate the eyes on specific objects successfully. Scanning allows the person to move the eyes in a pattern over the field of view to locate fixed objects, such as looking for a particular business sign along the road. Tracking requires the ability to move the eyes to follow a moving object, such as another vehicle, pedestrian, or animal, or to follow a path of travel, such as the curve of the road.

Saccadic eye movements are short rapid eye movements used to continually refixate the gaze while reading a line of print or to track a moving object. Saccadic movement is also used to retain fixation on an object while the head is turning. The examiner can watch the client's eyes while he or she reads printed material or while the client follows the examiner's moving finger or pen. Smooth pursuits define efficient saccadic eye movement, whereas irregular saccades appear as jerky movement. With irregular saccadic movements, the client may lose fixation on an object and have difficulty regaining fixation. Nystagmus is defined as a rhythmic oscillation of the eyes and can be vertical, lateral, or rotational. There are many types of nystagmus that can be caused by ocular or vestibular conditions or as the result of brainstem lesions. Certain types of nystagmus can be induced by looking laterally to the edge of the periphery and holding the gaze or by rapidly spinning the person, stopping quickly, and asking him or her to fixate on an object. Nystagmus limits acuity by affecting the person's ability to fixate on an object and can be compounded when trying to attend to other moving vehicles while driving. The DRS can observe eye movements, such as pursuits, saccades, scanning, and tracking, when asking the client to follow an object or light source with his or her eyes without turning the head. In the vehicle a small mirror strategically placed on the dashboard will permit the DRS to watch driver eye movements while continuing to observe road conditions.

SUMMARY

Vision is the critical factor used by a driver to gather information about the environment and objects moving in and out of the driver's vicinity. The DRS has to be proficient in understanding the visual system and assessing symptoms of injury and disease that have an effect on driving performance. Corrective lenses, surgery, adaptive viewing techniques, and vehicle adaptations are some of the interventions that can improve functional visual deficits. Several states allow the use of bioptic lenses while driving. These are small telescopic lenses set into the regular frame or lens of the client above the central field of view. The client is trained to use these lenses to briefly observe details of an object in the distance. They are not meant to substitute for regular prescription lenses, nor are they to be used for more than a brief glance of the object in question. Because these are magnification lenses, the field of view is reduced, and actual distance to the object appears decreased. An in-depth review of bioptic lenses and their use in the operation of a motor vehicle is provided in the following section.

The Clinical Evaluation of Bioptic Drivers

Charles P. Huss

The acquisition of restrictive driving privileges has become a reality for thousands of individuals with low vision nationwide. Many states also allow certain individuals with low vision to use bioptic telescopic lens systems as an accommodative device for driving. As more states develop and implement formalized programs of low vision driver services, *orientation and mobility* (O & M) *specialists* are being sought to play a contributing role in the screening and training process of individuals with low vision who want to drive. However, most people are not aware of the O & M profession or what such professionals do. Once included as a member of a multidisciplinary team involved in low vision driving, the role and services of the O & M specialist provide a critical link between those who fall under the responsibility of the low vision clinician and the DRS.

This section will provide readers with an overview of the O & M profession, including, but not limited to, what such professionals do, the type of coursework included in their professional preparation programs that makes them suitable for working with individuals with varying degrees of vision loss on travel-related tasks, and the type of complementary services that some O & M specialists can provide as a part of the screening process of prospective drivers with low vision who use bioptic lenses. Some of this author's past professional experiences as an O & M specialist involved the screening process of young novice bioptic drivers, as a part of the West Virginia Low Vision Driving Study (1985 through 1996), and this also will be commented on in this chapter.

ORIENTATION AND MOBILITY AS A PROFESSION

College- and university-level professional preparation programs for people wanting to become O & M specialists originated in the 1960s. The first two programs to graduate O & M specialists were graduate-level programs located at Boston College, Chestnut Hill, Massachusetts, and Western Michigan University, Kalamazoo, Michigan.[57]

From an O & M professional's perspective, orientation is defined as the ability to use one's remaining senses in establishing one's position and relationship to all other significant objects in one's environment.

Establishing one's relationship to objects in the environment includes all remaining visual function that is pertinent to the discussion at hand. Mobility is defined as the ability to navigate from one's fixed position to a desired position in another part of the environment.[58]

Since this profession's inception, the primary or intended role of the O & M specialist has been to provide instruction in a sequential nature to individuals with varying degrees of vision loss on specific techniques, strategies, and modifications necessary to ensure safe and efficient mobility in familiar and unfamiliar indoor and outdoor environments.[59] Some of the more traditional skills taught by O & M specialists include precane skills, cane skills, street-crossing skills, environmental awareness skills (including related concept and sensory development), map reading skills, and distance low vision aid skills.[60]

Many of the first graduates to enter the field obtained jobs at agencies or hospital rehabilitation centers that served blinded war veterans and other adults with significant vision loss. By and large the other adults' cases of sight loss were the result of congenital anomalies, hereditary factors, accidents, or systemic disease(s). Some O & M specialists opt to become dually certified in other related fields to enhance their future employability. They earn the credentials associated with titles such as rehabilitation teacher of the adult blind, teacher of children with visual impairments, or low vision rehabilitation therapist. The latter two professions also require college or university undergraduate- or graduate-level training and are certified and regulated by professionals' respective state departments of education. All new and most former graduates of the professional programs are now certified through the Academy for Certification of Vision Rehabilitation and Education Professionals (ACVREP), except for classroom teachers of children with visual impairment. There were approximately 3000 certified professionals in the ACVREP database as of the first quarter of 2004.[60]

In addition to blinded war veterans and the adult blind and visually impaired, O & M specialists provide valuable services to children and adolescents who are blind or visually impaired, multihandicapped blind and visually impaired, deaf-blind and low vision, and the aging blind and low vision. Professionals can find employment in public and private institutions, such as residential school systems, residential and outpatient rehabilitation facilities, and hospital or private practice clinics. Itinerant, homebound, or extension services in students' homes, work, or school settings are other types of ancillary and optional services provided by O & M professionals.

A major misconception about the O & M profession is that, as rehabilitation specialists, they only work with blind persons or those who have no functional vision whatsoever. This notion is incorrect and in fact could not be further from the truth. Approximately 80% to 90% of the individuals served by O & M specialists possess some degree of residual vision. Some students can learn to use and benefit from a long cane or become guide dog users, whereas others benefit from the use of special optical devices known as low vision aids when standard corrective lenses alone are insufficient to meet their needs.

COURSEWORK INVOLVED IN BECOMING AN O & M SPECIALIST

There are approximately 20 college-level or university-level professional preparation programs located worldwide that prepare people to become O & M specialists. A list of the graduate- and undergraduate-level O & M professional preparation programs is available for review at the Association for Education and Rehabilitation of the Blind and Visually Impaired (AERBVI) web site (www.aerbvi.org). Most programs are for 1 to 2 years. Typical coursework is listed in Box 6-4. The coursework places O & M specialists in a favorable position to better understand and objectively critique the functional performance of assigned students on travel-related tasks and community mobility.

BOX 6-4 | **Typical Coursework for Orientation and Mobility Specialist Programs**

- Ocular anatomy, physiology, and pathology
- Use of low vision and low vision aids (including functional assessment and training)
- Orientation and mobility techniques (travel training under blindfold and simulation of visual impairment)
- Dynamics of blindness and visual impairment (including exposure to coping skills, preconceived attitudes, and stereotypes)
- Fundamentals of orientation and mobility (including environmental awareness training and classes that review key concepts)
- Education of children with visual impairments (adaptations, special needs)
- Gerontology
- Statistics and research methods
- Practicum experiences
- Internships
- Independent research

BIOPTICS AND RESTRICTED DRIVING PRIVILEGES

Within the past 30 years, many states have amended their vision standards for driving and have permitted some people with mild to moderate levels of central vision loss to be considered for restricted driving privileges. As of 1999, 47 states had issued restricted driving privileges to select individuals with low vision. A wide variance in accepted visual acuity for such restrictive driving privileges exists nationwide and ranges from 20/50 visual acuity in some states to as low as and including 20/200 visual acuity in others.[61]

As of 2003, 34 of the states that grant restricted low vision driving privileges also permitted the use of special optical accommodative devices known as bioptic telescopic lens systems, or more commonly known as *bioptics*, for visual assistance while driving.[62] In some states the use of bioptics is an option up to the discretion of the low vision specialist who conducts the vision examination of the student in question. In other states it is a requirement by law that such devices be situated in place and used by select individuals with low vision who are granted a driver's license and the privileges that go with it.

The concept of bioptics and several of the original patented prototypes are the results of years of pioneering low vision prostheses research conducted by William Feinbloom, O.D., dating back to the 1930s.[63] Bioptics are prescribed by optometrists or ophthalmologists who specialize in low vision practice. These special lens arrangements are a combination, two-lens optical device (Figure 6-6) consisting of a pair of standard ophthalmic or carrier lenses and a miniature telescopic lens unit mounted permanently at a 10-degree angle to the carrier lens.

The photograph in Figure 6-6 reveals a frontal view of a Designs for Vision (DVI), Inc. (Ronkonkoma, NY) 2.2× Galilean BIO II binocular mock-up bioptic telescopic lens system in a standard black yeoman frame (note the physical location of the telescopic units,

which are above the normal viewing area through the carrier or support lenses). People using bioptics (Figure 6-7) look through the lower carrier lenses for general nonmagnified viewing purposes (e.g., for gross object awareness or orientation to the driving environment) and briefly through the telescopic lens unit (i.e., ≤0.5 second per fixation) for spotting distant detail, color, or movement of critical objects or forms in or near one's path of travel while driving.[64]

Figure 6-7, *A* presents a lateral view of a person looking through the carrier lens of a DVI 2.2× Galilean BIO II mock-up bioptic telescopic lens system. It is important to note that a student's view through the carrier lens is directly below and within close proximity to the telescopic housing. This is an advantage of using frames with adjustable nose pads, which optimize the viewing area and minimize the fixation time from the carrier to the telescopic lens and back again. Figure 6-7, *B* presents a lateral view of a person looking through the telescopic portion of a DVI 2.2× Galilean BIO II mock-up bioptic telescopic lens system. It is also important to note that the average time spent looking through a telescope should be ≤0.5 second per fixation to prevent a lack of full-field awareness, resulting in the possibility

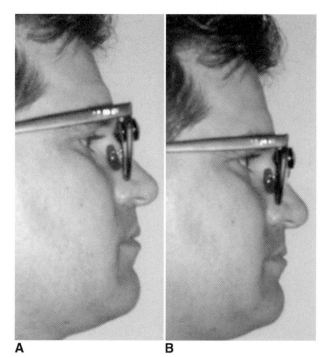

A   **B**

Figure 6-7   A, A lateral view of a person looking through the carrier lens of a DVI 2.2× Galilean BIO II mock-up bioptic telescopic lens system. **B,** A lateral view of a person looking through the telescopic portion of a DVI 2.2× Galilean BIO II mock-up bioptic telescopic lens system.

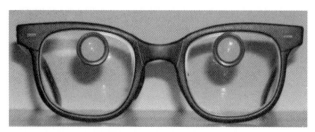

Figure 6-6   Bioptic glasses.

of weaving in or out of a traffic lane or losing control of the vehicle. More illustrative and in-depth descriptive information on bioptics and bioptic driving can be found at the BiOptic Driving Network's web site (www.biopticdriving.org).

The proliferation of restrictive driving privileges for some individuals with low vision and the use of bioptics as an accommodative device have been in part the result of two major factors:

- Long- and short-term research efforts undertaken during the past 40 years[65-75]
- Federal statutes such as Section 504 of the Federal Rehabilitation Act of 1973, the Americans with Disabilities Act, and the NHTSA Office of Civil Rights, which has been delegated the responsibility to protect in part the rights of persons with low vision who want to drive[76]

WEST VIRGINIA LOW VISION DRIVING STUDY

In 1983, shortly after being employed at the West Virginia Rehabilitation Center (WVRC), this author was invited to be part of a multidisciplinary research group that was positioned to explore and formulate methods for screening, training, and assessing the driving potential of a select group of people with visual impairments. Other principal team members included an optometrist specializing in low vision practice, a DRS, a psychologist, an OT generalist, and an audiologist.[77] All of the staff who were involved in this research endeavor were employees or under contractual work agreements with the West Virginia Division of Rehabilitation Services (WVDRS). The WVRC, which operates under the auspices of the WVDRS state agency, is one of nine state-operated comprehensive rehabilitation centers in the United States and is located in Institute, West Virginia.[78]

The impetus for initiating this pilot study was the realization that no programs were available at that time in West Virginia that were designed to enable people below the legal vision limits to be screened, trained, and licensed to drive using appropriate low vision aids. The project staff conducted an in-depth review of related literature, explored current standards of practice in the field, examined the legal aspects of this issue in West Virginia, and identified a sufficient number of individuals who could potentially qualify for participation in the West Virginia study. Once these tasks were completed, it was determined that the proposed pilot study was feasible and should continue with its primary aim of making a contribution to the knowledge and practice of enabling visually challenged individuals to drive using low vision aids.

VISION REQUIREMENTS FOR INCLUSION IN THE STUDY

Students with visual challenges who participated in the center's initial 3-year pilot study (1985 through 1988) or identical low vision driver services that followed for the next 7 years (1989 through 1996) met and maintained the following visual requirements:

- Distance visual acuity between 20/50 and 20/200 inclusive, with best standard spectacle or contact lens correction in the better eye
- Visual field of 120 degrees horizontally and 80 degrees vertically or greater in the same eye as used for the visual acuity determination
- Distance visual acuity of 20/40 or better using distance optical low vision aids prescribed by either a licensed optometrist or ophthalmologist
- No ocular diagnosis or prognosis that was likely to result in significant deterioration of vision below the protocol levels of visual acuity and visual fields as stated below

All of the candidates who volunteered to continue in this pilot study or the full continuum of services were also required to submit to other evaluations administered by the multidisciplinary team of professionals.[77]

ROLES AND RESPONSIBILITIES

In addition to serving as project coordinator, this author's assigned O & M role and responsibilities during the ongoing screening process were to assist in determining the level of predriver readiness and gathering background information about the prospective project participants enrolled in this study. To collect background information, we conducted a comprehensive interview, conducted and assessed students' functional performance on two routes, and assessed the students' functional performance while another student was positioned as a passenger.

The first step was to conduct a comprehensive interview with each project participant. In some cases the referring field counselor may have already completed this task, and an interview transcript was available in the participant's case file. Case files included information related to the following:

- Vision condition history
- Family history
- Residence history
- History of past travel experiences, including driving history (if any)
- Education history
- Past participation in sports or other recreational activities
- Reasons or rationale for wanting to drive

The information was relevant and often provided insight into the project participant's long-term adjustment to vision loss, functional vision limitations, functional abilities learned from observing others, environmental awareness of his or her surroundings, capability of learning the complexities of the driving task, use of his or her remaining intact vision for related dynamic tasks, the need for intensive and individualized training if voids exist, and his or her need to drive. Understanding the participant's need to drive is extremely important, especially if a third-party funding source, such as vocational rehabilitation, is paying the bill for optical aids and training.

The second step was to conduct and assess students' functional performance on two outdoor routes, including the following:

• The first route featured a staircase-shaped multiblock two-directional route of travel and its reverse route that transitioned from a quiet residential setting into a small town with two-way traffic and stop sign–controlled intersections.
• The second route started as a staircase-shaped multiblock two-directional route of travel and transitioned from a small-sized business setting to a medium-sized business setting and then back to the student's original starting point via an alternate L-shaped route of travel that presented stop sign– and traffic light–controlled intersections and two-way and one-way traffic patterns.

Students were requested to execute these routes in the same manner as if they were not being observed or as if they were traveling independently in their home surroundings. One to two sets of simple verbal directions were given at a time as students executed the respective routes. The students were given no additional assistance in executing these routes other than to have verbal instructions or directions repeated as necessary. While the participants negotiated these routes, this instructor observed the students' driving performance in terms of noted strengths and areas needing improvement relative to pedestrian safety and community mobility.

The final step was to assess the students' functional performance, which was completed while another student was positioned as a passenger in a vehicle driven by this author. Such passenger-in-car evaluations entailed observation and evaluation of students' visual search patterns and narrative driving abilities while traveling on a variety of roadways through different environmental settings. For example this author would instruct a student to look out in front of the vehicle as far as he or she could see and verbalize information about the type of intersection he or she was approaching (e.g., cross-shaped or T-shaped to the left or right), respective types of traffic control devices (e.g., road markings, signs, or signals), and other road users (i.e., stationary or moving) that he or she was able to detect in, along, or approaching our path of travel. This instructor also attempted to determine a student's preexisting knowledge and his or her understanding and rationale for using such basic skills as the following:

• Defensive driving skills, such as eye lead time, head and eye scanning, ample following distance, leaving oneself an out, and use of a vehicle's horn, lights, and turn signals
• Critical object or condition awareness skills, such as roadway characteristics, traffic control devices, and other road users that influence a driver's speed, lane position, or both
• Yielding procedures at approaching intersections to avoid collisions

RESULTS OF O & M SCREENING PROCESS

There were 107 individuals identified by low vision rehabilitation specialists as meeting the study's visual protocol and 69 individuals returned voluntarily to participate and complete the series of evaluations conducted by the multidisciplinary research team.[79] Because some candidates never imagined that someday they would be given the opportunity to demonstrate their functional competence behind the wheel of an automobile, evaluation results revealed that most of the student participants had problems relating to the dynamics of travel or the driving task, and these are presented below.

The first problem was poor vision skills. For example some students consistently directed their line of sight downward instead of ahead and laterally (i.e., back and forth along a horizontal plane) toward their intended path of travel. Subsequently such students were not able to correctly state the distances they had traveled in terms of linear blocks, the shapes of the routes traveled, the types of traffic control encountered at intersections, or any significant number of major landmarks for orientation purposes when requested by this author at the completion of the routes traveled initially on foot. Some of the students also demonstrated conceptual deficits in understanding terms such as a linear block of land, a street marker, or route shape.

The second problem was a lack of knowledge and understanding of basic motor vehicle yielding procedures, pavement markings, common roads signs, and wording typically used to differentiate traffic control at respective intersections. For example this author would ask the student the following question: "Was the first intersection that you crossed an example of a two-way or four-way stop sign–controlled intersection?" Some students responded with a blank stare or shrugged their shoulders to indicate a lack of knowledge and understanding.

The third problem was a lack of decision-making skills or demonstrated poor independent decision-making skills when crossing multiple-lane roadways. For example some students waited until a break in traffic to cross a street or crossed midsequence without 180 degrees of head rotation and eye scanning before stepping down from the curb during the respective street crossings.

The fourth problem was a demonstration of a lack of hazard perception skills. For example some students did not demonstrate the ability to detect (or did not respond) to the errors made by other motor vehicle operators, such as turning the wrong way on a one-way street, turning from the wrong lane of one street onto another street, and changing lanes incorrectly or at illegal times or locations.

Lastly there were demonstrated problems with identification of distance detail, color, or movement of objects or forms. For example some students were unable to consistently identify the names of streets on street marker signs located at different corners of the intersection from where they were standing; whether a distantly located traffic light was green, amber, or red; or the nonverbal communication of a driver who had stopped and was yielding or waving them on to cross first in front of the other driver at an intersection. This author gathered the latter observations without the student participants using any type of distant low vision aid.

Of the 69 student participants 56 individuals demonstrated acceptable performance scores and were invited to return to the center at a later date to initiate formalized programs of low vision driver training.[77] The formalized programs that address low vision driver training are addressed in Chapter 12.

BASIC LOW VISION ORIENTATION AND MOBILITY TRAINING

The 13 individuals who were not found to be ready for driving by this author and other project staff were invited to return to the center at a later date to participate in an individualized program of basic survival low vision orientation and mobility training on foot and as a passenger in a car. The passenger-in-car mobility training would seek to enhance and improve their skill development and conceptual understanding of the following tasks:

- Receive, retain, and follow route instructions: Mental mapping skills, basic conceptual development of orientation skills (including block distance, position, street marker, street continuity, basic math, body turns, route shape, laterality, directionality, parallel versus perpendicular, numbering systems, and reverse versus alternate routes), and basic map reading and map usage skills

- Travel a designated path or route: Eye lead, scanning ability, static versus dynamic orientation, sampling one's environment, object avoidance, awareness of textural and gradient change, and visual recall

- Detect, identify, and react in time to critical objects or conditions located outdoors within various environmental settings: Functional acuity abilities[80] (including awareness acuity, identification acuity, sure acuity, or preferred viewing distance), functional field abilities[80] (including static visual field, dynamic visual field, and preferred visual field), conceptual development (including time and distance, sun clues, facing, compass directions, and route shape), and critical object or condition awareness (including roadway characteristics, traffic control devices, and other road users)

- Detect, analyze, and cross intersections (i.e., controlled and noncontrolled): Scanning ability before and during crossing; conceptual development (including shape; size; signage; pavement markings; position and direction of signs, traffic lights, and traffic; and parallel and perpendicular); method of crossing; object, speed, and depth perception; walking speed; collision trap awareness; color identification and discrimination; yielding procedures; object avoidance; sound detection, differentiation, and localization; confidence and safety; turn right or left on red laws

- Distance low vision aids (e.g., handheld and/or spectacle mounted): Related definitions (bioptic, Plano lens, scotoma—area of complete or relative loss of vision, and vertex distance), purpose (rapid nonmanual interchange; detection of distant detail, color, or activity; and increased margin of safety), types (Galilean, expanded field prism [EFP], behind-the-lens, visual-enhancing systems [VES], bilevel telemicroscopic apparatus [BITA], M-Lens system, and Beecher Mirage), comparison features (actual magnification, restricted field of view, adjustability of focus, portability, appearance, weight, chromatic aberration, image quality, and cost), basis use (short-term spotting skills, scanning skills, and extended viewing), and areas of concern (forward and backward head tilt, difference in image size and distance, vertical displacement, fixation time, field[s] of view, Jack-in-the-box effect, halo effect caused by angle of sunlight, ring or rectangular scotoma, apparent movement of objects or forms opposite the direction of head and neck, movements when viewing through telescopic lens unit, and reference point maintenance through carrier and telescopic lens units)

The individuals who returned, voluntarily participated, and completed this remedial program of basic travel training satisfactorily (i.e., 3 to 4 weeks for most students) were then reevaluated for admission into the formalized low vision driver education training at the center. Those students who did not complete the basic travel training satisfactorily or elected not to return for adaptive driver education and training were advised of their right to be reconsidered for such services at a future date, once such prerequisites were achieved.

ALTERNATIVE TO DRIVER EDUCATION

The Finding Wheels program is an alternative to driver education and training for students with visual disabilities who are not ready to drive or elect not to drive but want to address their transportation issues. The Finding Wheels curriculum was designed for nondrivers with visual impairments for gaining control of their transportation needs.[81] It was created as a tool for teachers of students with visual disabilities, O & M specialists, other rehabilitation professionals, and parents who assist adolescents and young adults during the transition process from home to an active and independent lifestyle, including their pursuit of gainful employment. The printed advertisement for this book indicates that it will help address concerns faced by individuals seeking employment, such as how one chooses or arranges transportation, hires or fires a driver, exchanges services for rides, prepares a transportation budget, and how one determines the best way of approaching a co-worker and asking for a ride. It can be used as a stand-alone program, offered collectively, or as a complementary component to existing O & M curricula.

SUMMARY

This section provided readers with an overview of O & M, the academic coursework needed to teach in the mobility area, and how O & M specialists can become actively involved in the provision of low vision driver services. When included the O & M specialist plays a key role that complements the contributions of the other team members by helping the team determine which individuals meet a state's visual requirements for restrictive driving and are likely to be successful in a low vision driver education and training

program. O & M specialists can also offer alternative community mobility education and training programs to students who do not see themselves or are not seen by others (i.e., the driver rehabilitation team) as viable candidates for driving at that point in their lives.

Until additional training becomes part of the academic preparation for rehabilitation professionals like O & M specialists, professionals interested in working with individuals with low vision who want to drive can obtain the specialized evaluation and training by attending one of the related preconference workshops offered occasionally in advance of the annual conference of the international organization known as the Association for Driver Rehabilitation Specialists that retained the acronym ADED and was formerly called the Association of Driver Educators for the Disabled. For more information on ADED, see Chapters 1,2, and 4, Appendices C and E, and ADED's web site (www.driver-ed.org).

The role and responsibilities of the O & M specialist in the training of bioptic drivers will be one of those areas discussed in Chapter 12, the on-road evaluation and training section of this book.

SECTION IV
The Clinical Evaluation of Hearing
Marilyn Di Stefano

Our sense of hearing helps us maintain an awareness of our environment, contributes to our state of arousal and alertness, and enables us to communicate via speech. Although adequate visual skills are acknowledged as the primary prerequisite sensory function related to safe driving abilities,[82] our hearing also plays an important, although perhaps more subtle, role in impacting overall driving performance. If our hearing or speech perception abilities are altered or absent, strategies must be used to help compensate for these functional limitations.

HEARING: A BRIEF REVIEW

The ability to hear depends on the integrity of our auditory system. This comprises the sensory organs responsible for detecting sound (i.e., the ears that comprise the outer, middle, and inner segments), the nervous pathways leading from the ear to the brain, and the brain itself. The ear converts the energy from sound waves into nervous impulses, which are then processed in the brain, resulting in the perception of sound and recognition of auditory patterns.[83]

Closely related to the hearing apparatus are the organs responsible for maintaining orientation, balance, gaze stabilization, and modulating autonomic responses (i.e., the semicircular canals and related neural system). Impairments that lead to dysfunction of the balance/orientation system also can sometimes be associated with hearing loss. Recent research has noted that disorders associated with dizziness and balance can impact driving abilities[84]; however, these issues are beyond the scope of this chapter.

CAUSES OF HEARING LOSS

Hearing impairments associated with the sensory component of the system are generally of two main types: conductive hearing loss related to the outer or middle ear, and sensorineural hearing loss, which is usually linked to problems with the neural cells of the inner ear. Mixed hearing loss can result from disorders of the conductive and neural mechanism of the ear.

Impairments relating to the nervous system beyond the ear are of two types, depending on the characteristics of the underlying disorder. If they are related to structural lesions of the nervous system (e.g., damage caused by a CVA or traumatic injury), they are called retrocochlear disorders. If the disorder is associated with lesions of the nervous system (e.g., deficits associated with the diffuse changes accompanying the aging process or a developmental disability), it is termed a central auditory processing disorder. These types of conditions usually have an impact on communication, including speech perception.[85] Central auditory processing disorder will not be discussed further in this chapter, which instead will focus predominantly on issues related to hearing loss.

Permanent hearing impairments may result from a number of health conditions. Although age-related hearing loss is the main contributor to hearing loss in adults,[85] there are many other causes that can be added to the following nonexhaustive list:

- Intake of certain medications or exposure to particular chemicals
- Congenital conditions (e.g., craniofacial malformations such as an absent ear canal)
- Injuries at birth, complications associated with prematurity, or both
- Head and neck injuries
- Middle ear disease
- Ménière's disease
- Bone disorders (e.g., otosclerosis)
- Exposure to loud noise (e.g., occupationally related noise resulting in induced hearing loss)
- Genetic abnormalities
- Viruses (e.g., mumps and measles)
- Tumors

- Temporary interruptions to the blood supply either at the ear or within the brain (e.g., stroke)
- Other causes with unknown etiologies[83,86,87]

TREATMENT OF HEARING LOSS

Treatments available to assist individuals with a hearing loss include surgery, removal of obstructions such as earwax, medication such as antibiotics or drugs that control fluid buildup in the ear, and the prescription of hearing aids and devices. When there is a problem in the external or middle ear, a conductive hearing impairment occurs. In most people with sensorineural hearing loss (i.e., because of significant damage to the cochlea, the hair cells, or the nerve) the damage is permanent and cannot be corrected with surgery or drug therapy.

The ability to treat certain types of hearing loss makes establishing an accurate diagnosis an important first step when considering whether hearing loss will impact driving or community mobility. Regular medical evaluations of hearing status are recommended for people with an existing hearing impairment or for those with chronic, deteriorating, or neurologic conditions in which hearing function may be affected. Regular medical evaluations that include a hearing assessment also may be important for older clients or people with disabilities who may be contending with multiple health issues.

COCHLEAR IMPLANTS

Clients referred for a comprehensive driver rehabilitation evaluation may present with cochlear implants. Cochlear implants may be offered to some individuals with profound sensorineural deafness who cannot benefit from even the most advanced and powerful hearing aids. The implants consist of a small battery-operated speech processor and a microphone worn outside the ear that converts sound waves into electrical signals. The signals are transmitted to electrodes that are surgically implanted in the cochlea, and the electrodes stimulate the nerve in the ear so that sounds can reach the brain. Because the procedure does not restore normal hearing and is not reversible, extensive preoperative screening is required. After surgery the client requires a long period of rehabilitation support, and hearing aids can no longer be used in the ear with a cochlear implant. Clients who have had cochlear implant surgery can hear some sounds and often report that the implants help them to speak and speech read better.[88] Understanding which sounds can be heard by individuals with a cochlear implant may be important in terms of vehicle modifications and communication requirements for evaluation and retraining interventions.

FREQUENCY OF HEARING LOSS

It has been difficult to establish the prevalence of hearing loss that reflects the general population primarily because differences in research methodologies make aggregating the results problematic. For example studies vary in relation to what age groups are investigated and the selection criteria used to operationally define what constitutes an individual with hearing loss (e.g., use of hearing aids and decreased hearing under specified threshold levels). Some studies also have used information about hearing function from survey or self-reporting methods rather than data from established and valid hearing tests or other clinical assessments. It also has been difficult to determine how many people with hearing loss have remained unaccounted for because they have not sought assistance from a medical professional. In the United States between 40% and 50% of Americans aged ≥75 years are estimated to experience such sensory impairment.[89] In Australia it has been conservatively estimated that hearing loss affects 20% of the total population.[87] It is generally accepted that hearing loss prevalence rates increase as the population ages.[90] DRSs are likely to encounter individuals with decreased hearing who are requesting a comprehensive driver rehabilitation evaluation; therefore it is important to understand how best to address their particular needs.

GENERAL EFFECTS OF HEARING LOSS

The type and extent of hearing dysfunction will ultimately impact an individual's ability to perform the functional tasks associated with driving or alternative community mobility. Others may not detect mild hearing loss if an individual uses appropriate compensatory skills, especially if the hearing loss only affects one ear.

Individuals with hearing impairment commonly face difficulties with the following issues[83,87,89,91]:
- Distinguishing speech from background noise
- Distinguishing one consonant from another
- Hearing their own speech and monitoring speech volume
- Hypersensitivity to loud sounds
- Hearing various sounds made by appliances and machinery (e.g., alarms and timers)
- Psychological and social functioning impacted by the consequences of hearing impediments

Clients also may experience depression, social isolation, and cognitive changes.[92,93]

COPING WITH HEARING LOSS

According to Davis[90] and Fozard,[91] individuals differ substantially in relation to how well they cope with the sequelae of hearing impairments depending on the following interrelated factors:
- The nature of the condition
- Whether one or both ears are affected
- The age of onset
- Whether the loss was sudden or gradual
- The communication demands experienced by the individual

There also may be associated difficulties related to symptoms of hearing loss; one of the most common is tinnitus. Tinnitus has been described as any sound heard in one or both ears or the head that does not originate from the environment. Many people temporarily experience tinnitus at some point in their lives, for example as an initial and temporary response to being exposed to a loud noise. Approximately 17% to 30% of the population in Australia experience permanent (i.e., constant) tinnitus.[87] Tinnitus affects people in different ways depending on its frequency, the nature of the sounds (i.e., ringing, whooshing, or clicking), and the degree of personal adaptation to the condition.[94,95] There is little research that supports efficacious medical treatment for tinnitus. However, some success has been achieved through interventions such as the following:
- Coping skills training, relaxation therapy
- Optimizing hearing and suppressing tinnitus by using a hearing aid
- Using a tinnitus masker, which is a device worn like a hearing aid that produces pleasant sounds that mask the buzzing, ringing, humming, or whistling noise associated with tinnitus[88]

IMPACT OF HEARING LOSS ON COMMUNICATION

Individuals with anything more than a mild hearing loss usually experience communication difficulties. The nature of the sensory hearing impairment and the degree and effect of speech perception disorders can be variable.[96] Table 6-5 depicts, in general terms, the effects on communication experienced by individuals with different degrees or categories of hearing loss. It is often difficult to place individuals neatly within these categories because hearing loss patterns vary depending on the thresholds and frequencies affected. Health care professionals and people with hearing impairments use these groupings as a point of reference that can help others understand a client's general level of disability.

IMPACT OF HEARING LOSS ON DRIVING

Loss of hearing abilities may influence a driver in a number of ways. Considering the environment within

Table 6-5   Hearing Loss and Its Impact on Communication

General Category of Hearing Loss	Impact on Communication
Minimal	May have difficulty hearing speech in noisy environments
Mild	Has some difficulty with speech even in quiet environments
Moderate	Needs to be in close proximity to others to hear conversational speech and may require frequent repetition
Moderately severe	Able to hear only loud conversational speech
Severe	Cannot hear conversational speech
Profound	Hearing cannot be used as the primary form of communication and may only hear very loud sounds

Data from Stach B: *Clinical audiology: an introduction*, San Diego, 1998, Singular Publishing Group Inc.; VicDeaf HEAR Service: *Understanding hearing loss*, 2002. Available at: http://www.vicdeaf.com.au/informationResources. Accessed January 5, 2005.

the vehicle, the driver may experience difficulties with the following:

- Hearing sounds associated with "feedback systems" from primary or secondary controls (e.g., engine noises and indicator clicks)
- Conversing satisfactorily with DRSs, driving instructors/assessors, or passengers
- Recognizing any malfunctions with the vehicle that are usually evident through auditory feedback (e.g., climate control/heating fans)

Reduced abilities to hear sounds relating to changing environmental factors originating from outside the vehicle may have a significant impact on a driver. This could influence the speed and appropriateness of responses and therefore may have a greater impact on driving safety.[97] For example a driver with a hearing impairment may have reduced abilities to do the following:

- Hear emergency alarms, horns, or other sounds coming from nearby vehicles
- Hear traffic management signals, such as warning bells associated with railway crossings
- Localize where sounds are coming from; for example it may be difficult to identify the location of an emergency vehicle within the surrounding traffic in the absence of visual cues
- Maintain awareness of other less visible road users such as motorcyclists

There also may be other less obvious negative effects of hearing loss related to the reduction in auditory sensory stimuli. For example on long and monotonous drives, drivers with hearing impairments may experience difficulty with remaining alert and vigilant because some of the strategies used to help maintain arousal, such as listening to the radio, rely on hearing. It has also been reported that individuals with hearing impairments require more concentration when attempting to hear, particularly in noisy backgrounds.[87] This may place an additional load on the mental workload of such drivers and suggests that for example they may fatigue more readily compared with non–hearing-impaired drivers when conversing with passengers while traveling.

From a predriver assessment perspective, clients may present with additional health issues that can interact with or compound the consequences of hearing loss. For this reason it is important to consider each client's particular needs and requirements with reference to the interaction between presenting problems. For example the existence of a moderate hearing loss may not by itself pose a major functional barrier to driving. However, in combination with a visual decrement and a memory problem (such as forgetting to wear hearing aids, glasses, or both), overall functional abilities may be far less compared with the loss associated with any of the impairments on their own.

HEARING IMPAIRMENT AND INCREASED CRASH RISK

There is a paucity of research investigating hearing loss and its impact on driving performance. One Australian study did report an increased risk of crash associated with moderate hearing loss or loss of hearing in one ear.[98] Anecdotal evidence suggests that most of the individuals with a significant hearing loss who drive are aware of their impairment and modify their driving behavior accordingly, compensating for their hearing loss by restricting when and where they drive and by increasing the frequency of visually checking the traffic environment around them. The drivers' ability to respond to critical events in the driving environment still needs to be evaluated, particularly for clients with high driving exposure, those towing trailers or caravans, and those driving vehicles such as trucks or vans, the design of which impedes the use of internal mirrors to assist in monitoring the surrounding traffic. Of particular concern to licensing authorities are those individuals who seek licensure to drive commercial vehicles; in such instances jurisdictions may restrict licensing privileges depending on the degree of loss or may recommend the installation of additional mirrors to optimize visual compensatory strategies.[99] See Chapters 5, 11, and 12 for more information on vehicle modifications, including adapted driving controls.

OFF-ROAD ASSESSMENT FOR HEARING LOSS

As previously discussed elsewhere in this text, the off-road assessment is performed for a number of reasons, including the following:
- To ensure the driver has the basic capacities required to demonstrate driving skills, and to check that all relevant medical and licensing criteria or guidelines are met
- To identify any impairment factors amenable to intervention to optimize function (e.g., use of hearing aids to ensure optimal auditory abilities)
- To identify any functional limitations that may improve with either remediation or compensation strategies
- To collect information that is applicable to clinical reasoning regarding interpreting the client's on-road performance
- To determine the timing of the on-road evaluation in relation to training or other interventions required as part of the driver rehabilitation process
- To understand personal and lifestyle factors relevant to independent community mobility

BOX 6-5	Hearing Function Issues That Need to Be Evaluated by the DRS During the Clinical Evaluation

- Optimal hearing status and need to review treatment or use of hearing aids
- Interaction between hearing problems and any other presenting issues (e.g., visual deficits)
- Driver training needs
- On-road evaluation requirements
- Licensing issues (e.g., conditional requirements)

- To seek information regarding funding sources should driver rehabilitation and/or vehicle modifications be required

With specific reference to hearing function, the clinical evaluation will seek to identify issues listed in Box 6-5.

Hearing loss may or may not be evident by simply observing the client. The client should be asked to report any preexisting health condition that has caused either short- or long-term hearing loss. Documentation contained within the medical or allied health referral information also should be thoroughly reviewed because it may make reference to the use of hearing aids or other hearing augmentation devices. The DRS must then identify how the nature and degree of hearing loss may impact on the driving tasks, assessment procedures, and any intervention processes that may be warranted.

When there is no such specific documentation, the DRS should still assess the individual for the existence of any hearing impairment. This can be done in various ways, including by identifying any risk factors that may be related to the existence of a hearing loss (e.g., occupational history issues, previous head injury, and medical conditions that may impact on hearing abilities) and by carefully observing the client and monitoring the communication process throughout the clinical evaluation.

MEDICAL HISTORY AND RISK FACTORS

Consideration should be given to medical conditions that can result in hearing loss. If any such conditions are relevant, further detailed questioning may be required. For example if the driver has sustained trauma to the head or a closed head injury, it is worthwhile checking whether he or she experienced any temporary or permanent auditory or visual losses associated with these events. Because coping with a hearing loss relies on adequate alternative sensory function, cognitive abilities, and maintenance of arousal/attentional capacity, particular attention needs to be directed toward other aspects of the medical history that may indicate potential decrements in these areas, such as other medical diagnoses, medications, and alcohol or drug use. Drugs (illicit and prescribed) and alcohol have the potential to impair driving in a number of ways, including causing drowsiness, blurred vision, or dizziness.[100]

THE CLINICAL INTERVIEW

Standard clinical evaluation protocols may include specific questions asked verbally and presented concurrently in writing that will elicit relevant hearing-related information from the client, such as the following[101]:
- Do you have a history of being hard of hearing?
- Do you use a hearing aid or any other hearing amplification devices?
- Do you ever experience difficulties with hearing conversational speech or environmental sounds or noise while driving?

Such interview questions may not be helpful if clients have other cognitive or behavioral issues that can decrease insight. In such cases seeking the opinion of collateral sources (e.g., family members, caregivers, spouses, and significant others) and information about previous accidents or incidents could be helpful.[97] A client's answers in response to questioning about daily activities can also serve as a means to identify potential indicators of hearing difficulties. Clients may report difficulties with hearing in noisy environments, needing increased volume on the television and radio as compared with others in the same room, increased occurrences of headaches and feelings of fatigue and malaise after engaging in social interaction within a noisy environment, or an imbalance in hearing abilities (i.e., one ear hears better than the other). They also may refer to a family history of hearing loss, ringing or other noises within the ears or head that do not originate in the environment, wax buildup or discharge from the ear or ears, a previous injury to the ear or ears, prolonged exposure to loud noise in a work or recreational context (recently or in the past), or episodes of vertigo or feeling dizzy and sensations of falling or overbalancing.[86,102] In such instances it may be worthwhile referring the client to his or her primary medical practitioner for further investigation of these signs and symptoms before the on-road evaluation or training.

OBSERVATION OF THE DRIVER AND MONITORING OF THE COMMUNICATION PROCESS

Clinical evaluation procedures usually involve an interview and various screening tests undertaken in an envi-

---

BOX 6-6	Clinical Evaluation Indicators of Possible Hearing Loss

- Difficulty hearing and responding to speech, even in a quiet environment
- Frequent requests to repeat instructions
- Needing to see the speakers' face to follow instructions
- Speaking loudly (people who are hard of hearing may have difficulties determining how loudly they speak)
- Background noise interfering significantly with hearing speech
- Unusual head posture or leaning toward the speaker
- Gestures indicating difficulty with hearing, such as cupping a hand behind the ear to direct sound into the ear canal

---

ronment that is preferably quiet and free from distractions. Irrespective of whether the clinical evaluation is conducted in a traditional clinical setting versus somewhere in the community, careful observation of the client's abilities to respond to questions and instructions is a key to identifying difficulties with hearing and other key factors that enable safe driving. Observations indicative of a hearing loss that may emerge during the clinical evaluation are listed in Box 6-6.

Individuals with certain behavioral or cognitive problems (e.g., affective disorders or health conditions that lead to decreased memory) may also present in similar ways; therefore these factors need to be ruled out as a possible explanation of such behavior.

Sometimes uncomplicated types of hearing screening tests are used within the contexts of health care or driver assessments (e.g., "speech" or "whisper" tests). Such tests are extremely difficult to implement in a standardized way, and their value over and above what can be gained from attending to a client's responses during the interview and evaluation process is questionable.[103] Depending on the degree of functional impairment, it may be worthwhile referring the client for further investigation of the presenting issues. The goal of such an intervention is to help ensure that the client's health status is optimal for proceeding to the next stage of the driver evaluation process, which after the clinical evaluation is usually the on-road evaluation. See Chapters 11, 12, and 13 for more information about on-road evaluation and training.

OPTIMIZING THE DRIVER'S HEARING

If the client reports or demonstrates a significant hearing impairment, it is worthwhile exploring and determining the following:

- The time since the client has been seen by his or her primary medical doctor
- The last time he or she had his or her hearing status evaluated by a medical specialist or relevant allied health professional
- Whether he or she wears a hearing aid in one or both ears, or if he or she uses other types of hearing devices
- If the client has had any problems with using his or her hearing device(s)
- Whether he or she has had surgery to address a hearing problem
- The length of time that the hearing problems have had an impact on his or her daily communication needs
- The nature of any specific driving-related hearing difficulties
- If he or she is in contact with local groups or agencies that provide resources for people who are hard of hearing (e.g., counselors or self-help groups that assist individuals to explore strategies to cope with their disability and compensate for the challenges associated with hearing loss)
- Whether he or she has undertaken any formal training designed to help people cope with hearing loss, adapting to its negative effects, or both

Learning to adapt to living with a hearing loss can take some time, especially for a client with a newly acquired injury or illness that has led to a major loss of hearing. If the client has only recently acquired a hearing aid and he or she reports difficulties with it, it is worthwhile addressing basic issues to help ensure the client has achieved an optimal level of hearing. For example the DRS should determine the following: Is the client's hearing aid inserted in the correct ear? Does it fit properly? Is the volume setting correct? Does the battery need to be replaced?

It is not unusual to encounter individuals with a hearing loss who are not aware of the range of devices available to assist them in managing hearing impairment. There is a range of communication devices (apart from hearing aids) that can amplify sound, which are suitable for use when the client with a hearing impairment converses with either one or two individuals or a group of people. There also are task-specific devices used when undertaking particular aspects of a job; for example a modified stethoscope with an amplifier can be used by a health professional with a hearing impairment. Moreover there are devices that can be used to amplify the sound of a voice over significant background noise while in a car; this aid could be useful for drivers with significant hearing loss who require on-road driver evaluation, training, or both.[88] Such devices may be worthwhile with the aim of optimizing the client's hearing before undertaking further driver rehabilitation.

PREPARING FOR THE ON-ROAD EVALUATION

Clients who have not addressed significant hearing loss issues should be referred to a physician, allied health professional, or a specific community-based agency that provides advice and resources to clients who are hard of hearing. This may be appropriate to ensure that they undertake any on-road evaluation or training program with their hearing status optimized. For some DRSs working within rehabilitation settings, this process may be as simple as requesting that the physiatrist initiate a referral to the in-house speech and language pathologist or audiologist. In other situations it may be appropriate to directly refer the client to the nearest resource center for a review of available equipment and strategies designed to address hearing loss. In all cases in which hearing loss is suspected, and especially in the absence of medical documentation, it is important to refer the client to the treating medical practitioner so that a thorough medical review of the person's current hearing status is completed.

INTERACTIONS BETWEEN HEARING LOSS AND OTHER HEALTH ISSUES

As previously stated a key purpose of the clinical evaluation is to help ensure that the DRS has the opportunity to check for any impairments or other factors that may interact with the hearing loss to further limit driving function. For example the client may have had his or her hearing status reviewed recently; however, the client may not have had his or her vision checked for many years despite a history of significant visual impairment. In such instances it would be important to make sure that the client has his or her visual status reviewed and optimized before the on-road evaluation. This is because many compensatory strategies used with hearing loss rely on vision.

In some situations it may not be appropriate for individuals with a significant hearing loss and other health factors to proceed to the next stage of the comprehensive driver evaluation process. Although each individual needs to be considered on a case-by-case basis, some contraindications to driving may include the presence of a major hearing loss in conjunction with the following conditions:

- Major visual function decrements (e.g., related to acuity, visual fields, eye movements or coordination, and visual perception)
- Severe restriction in neck and/or upper spine ROM limiting head movement
- An acquired brain injury or other condition that results in limited insight into the functional implications of the existing impairments

- Significant difficulties with tasks requiring intact cognitive/perceptual functioning (e.g., attentional capacity, memory, spatial awareness, judgment, and problem solving)
- Behavioral disturbances that may influence the implementation of compensatory strategies
- Advanced chronic neurologic conditions (e.g., dementia, PD, MS, Alzheimer's disease, and ALS)
- Untreated epilepsy, dizziness, or fainting
- Seizure disorders
- Major side effects related to medication (e.g., fatigue and reduced coordination)
- Unmanaged alcohol consumption, drug abuse, or both
- Conditions associated with difficulty maintaining arousal or attentional capacity

This list is not exhaustive, and the DRS would be advised to liaise closely with the primary physician, other health care personnel, and family members when clients have complicated or advanced major health issues before making a determination that the client is or is not an appropriate candidate for an on-road evaluation.

COMMUNICATION REQUIREMENTS

Before commencing driver rehabilitation services, the DRS and the client with a hearing impairment must identify the best communication method to be used during the predriving evaluation, on-road evaluation, and training interventions. The driving assessor may require further information or training related to devices used for sound and speech amplification, as well as speech communication alternatives or supplements such as sign language, written communication, and the use of symbols, diagrams, or pictures. Such an exploration is especially important to enable the on-road evaluation and training to occur in an optimal environment where communication between the driver and the assessor is unambiguous and consistent. These communication issues are discussed more fully in the chapters pertaining to the on-road evaluation, including Chapters 12 and 13.

SECTION V

The Clinical Evaluation of Psychosocial Factors

Annette Lavezza • *Susan L. Martin*

Mental illness can be profound and devastating, greatly affecting an individual by impairing motivation, concentration, and performance. It can impact one's life

roles and change a person's ability to perform routine ADL and IADL, such as using a computer at work, completing a homework assignment, organizing a shopping list, and driving, to name a few. This section will explore symptoms commonly associated with mental illnesses, as well as the impact mental illness may have on cognitive function as it relates to driving and a client's performance during the clinical evaluation. We will also explore issues that pertain to the on-road evaluation and training of people who are contending with mental illness.

Driving is an IADL that integrates multiple sensory systems and requires prompt effective responses from an individual. In the general population 95% of all crashes are caused by human error.[104] These errors include executive dysfunction, impaired cognition, inattention, distractibility, perceptual deficits, and misinterpretation of the actions of others.[104] *Executive function* is the ability to coordinate multiple brain areas to achieve a goal.[105] Executive function includes solving novel problems, changing actions based on previous behavior, developing strategies, and sequencing a series of complex tasks.[105] These skills are crucial to the driving task and have been shown to be deficient for people with mental illness.

Having a mental illness does not mean a person is unsafe to drive. It is important to examine functional status and behavior rather than view the person as a singular diagnostic group or label.[104] The American Psychiatric Association (APA) concurs that the diagnosis of a mental illness alone does not indicate impaired driving.[106] Nonetheless 13% of clients who have a mental illness are considered unsafe to drive,[107] and 49% of people with mental illness are given medications that affect the skills of driving.[108] Therefore each person must be examined individually to make a determination about fitness to drive.

Over time the role of the psychiatrist in the realm of driving for people with mental illness has evolved. It has been noted that psychiatrists have been reluctant to become involved in driving issues because of limited knowledge of regulations and laws.[107] Specifically Wise and Watson[107] completed a survey of psychiatrists' knowledge of driving and mental illness, identifying the following additional reasons for limited discussion of driving fitness between the psychiatrist and individuals with mental illness, as it relates to driving fitness[107,109]:

- Driving is required for the person's employment
- The person may be reluctant to continue medications or attend therapy appointments
- The situation may damage the client-practitioner relationship
- Some psychiatrists view the discussion as inappropriate

In 1993 the APA published a position statement titled *The Role of the Psychiatrist in Assessing Driving Ability*.[106] Although the APA agrees that determining fitness to drive is not the sole responsibility of psychiatrists, they should have a role in counseling patients regarding this subject to maintain driver safety.[106] Psychiatrists should discuss the symptoms of the mental illness that may affect driving, discuss the side effects of medications including their interaction with alcohol, and choose medications with side effects that have a lesser impact on the skills required for driving when clinically appropriate.

It is necessary for the DRS to work together with the psychiatrist to identify people with risk factors for driving impairment and then perform the assessments required to determine a client's fitness to drive. The DRS must also work closely with the psychiatrist to be educated about the person's pharmaceutical regimen, length of treatment on particular medications, and potential side effects. There are a variety of medications for mental illness that may impact driving skills and therefore should be monitored closely by the client and professional driver rehabilitation team members.

There are several classes of medications that are used to treat depression. Monoamine oxidase inhibitors (MAOIs) may cause significant side effects, including daytime drowsiness and blurred vision in some people.[110] Conversely medications called selective serotonin reuptake inhibitors (SSRIs) generally cause fewer side effects, and the person only requires counseling about the most common side effects.[110] Side effects may include nausea, nervousness, insomnia, diarrhea, rash, and decreased sex drive. The most concerning class of antidepressants are the tricyclic antidepressants, which have been shown to contribute to a doubling of the risk of crash,[110,111] with the risk continuing to increase as the dosage increases.[111] These drugs impair function in the areas of attention, memory, motor coordination, and on-road driving tests.[111-119]

Benzodiazepines are used to treat anxiety but are also used for treatment of headaches, muscle spasms, arthritis, high blood pressure, and menopausal or menstrual problems. These medications generally may impair function or cause symptoms in multiple areas,[111,120-140] including vision, slurred speech, attention, hyperactivity, processing, confusion, memory, headaches, coordination, dizziness, vertigo, and tremors.

These functional impairments can have a great impact on driver safety. The identified impairments affect function in a dose-related manner[111]; therefore communication with the prescribing physician/psychiatrist is necessary. Specifically it is important to note the time of day the medication is taken. Long-acting benzodiazepines taken at night have been shown to have marked psychomotor impairments the next day versus short-acting benzodiazepines for which there is no identified impact after 5 to 9 hours.[110] Young adults who were tested on an open-road test after an injection of long-acting diazepam and the morning after receiving flurazepam demonstrated impairment consistent with having a blood alcohol content of 0.1%, which is equivalent to a sixfold increased crash risk.[111] The AMA recommends no driving during the initial dosing phase with these medications, and driving should only resume after education and counseling about the side effects.[110]

Finally medications for schizophrenia or antipsychotics vary and should be reviewed with the prescribing physician. Antipsychotics that are considered typical are often sedating and cause other side effects, including tremor and muscle tone changes. Atypical antipsychotics tend to have fewer side effects and are less sedating. See Chapter 8 for more information on medications and driving.

DEPRESSION

Depression is the overwhelming feeling of sadness that is persistent and altered from baseline personality. It impacts the individual's social, occupational, and educational roles. Depression is more than just sadness or grief; it is a chemical imbalance in the brain.

According to the *Diagnostic and Statistical Manual*, fourth edition (DSM-IV),[141] people with depression must have a period of at least 2 weeks with depressed mood, loss of interest or pleasure in activities, and four of the following symptoms:
• Change in appetite or weight
• Change in sleep
• Change in psychomotor activity
• Decreased energy
• Feelings of worthlessness or guilt
• Difficulty thinking, concentrating, or making decisions
• Thoughts of death or suicidal ideation

There is no single cause of depression. Research shows that there are a variety of different factors that may lead to depression, including heredity, medication side effects, medical conditions, environmental factors, life events, loss, trauma, or other medical conditions.[141] No matter the cause, research has established that depression is a biological disorder of brain chemistry. Depression may occur at any age but is most likely to develop during early adulthood. Women are more than twice as likely as men to experience depression, with a risk of 10% to 25% for women and 5% to 12% for men.[141]

There are a variety of treatments, including different therapies and medications. Regardless of the method, when depression is fully treated and in remission, symptoms such as memory and cognitive problems greatly improve and often are resolved altogether.[141,142] If left untreated, depression may last ≥6 months.[141] Once a diagnosis is made and treatment begins, there is a direct relationship between the overall treatment duration and improvement in cognitive function.[143]

People with depression may have a variety of symptoms,[141] including anhedonia, anxiety, complaints of pain, changes in sleep patterns, distractibility, decreased memory, decreased speech, decreased eating, delusions, difficulty with executive functioning, excessive worrying, indecisiveness, irritability, lack of emotion, poor concentration, ruminating thoughts, sadness, slow movements, tearfulness, and thoughts of death or suicide. Of these symptoms the cognitive impairments experienced by people with depression are the most detrimental to safe driving. There have been a variety of studies published examining the cognitive changes experienced by people with depression. A study completed by Austin et al[144] examined cognition and depression and found that cognitive impairments in depression affect a person's ability to function at work and that impairments in depression are similar to those seen in schizophrenia and neurologic disorders. Although the studies examined different parts of cognitive functioning, they all agreed that people with depression have a high risk of experiencing changes in thinking and overall cognitive functioning (Box 6-7).

Although impairments in cognitive functioning can significantly impair safe driving, changes in motor activity experienced by people with depression can also further increase the impact this diagnosis has on safe driving skills. People with depression have also been found to have psychomotor slowing. This may include longer movement duration, longer pauses, and lower velocities.[154,155] Changes also include requiring increased time to brake, decreased ability to respond to hazards, and difficulty turning the steering wheel. Psychomotor slowing also has been found to impair simple reaction time.[153] Decreased movement time coupled with slowed decision making is significantly impaired in individuals with depression.[156,157] The risk of psychomotor impairments increases with the severity of depression and age of the client. Changes in motor movements also may be a side effect of certain medications prescribed to treat depression.

Research has identified a variety of factors that impact the degree of cognitive impairment, including automatic versus effortful tasks, sustained effort, age, length of depression, severity of the illness, motivation, and sometimes even the time of day.

Research completed by a variety of groups found that although there are observable impairments in automatic (recognition) and effortful tasks (such as verbal recall), as a group, people with depression do worse on effort-demanding cognitive tasks versus automatic tasks.[147-151,158,159] Therefore a person with depression may be successful with routine activities like housekeeping but have trouble managing driving during situations that force an individual to problem solve and promptly respond to changing, unpredictable vehicles and other potentially dangerous stimuli in the traffic environment. See Chapter 19 for more information on traffic safety.

A study completed by Cohen[147] examined the change in motor and cognitive function in people with depression. Cohen[147] completed a study that found people with depression demonstrated the greatest level of cognitive impairments and motor deficits when engaged in activities that required sustained effort. Therefore people with depression may be more likely to demonstrate symptoms of cognitive impairments when engaged in the sustained activity of driving, especially when confronted with a stressful driving environment. Driving requires sustained cognitive and motor skills.

Studies show that there is a direct relationship between age and cognitive impairments for individuals with depression.[160,161] Rabins et al[162] found that elderly people with depression have similar cognitive symptoms as those with dementing illness. Several studies support this finding by linking cognitive deficits in depression to frontal lobe abnormalities, the same region affected by some forms of dementia.[160,163,164] It is important to note that the occurrence of cognitive impairments together with major depression is not a predictor of progressive dementing illness.[162] Cognitive impairments are reversible after successful treatment of depression.* However, people

---

BOX 6-7	**Possible Changes in Cognitive Functioning Because of Depression**

- Attention[145]
- Executive dysfunction[145,146]
- Visuospatial learning[145]
- Pattern recognition[145]
- Spatial recognition[145]
- Spatial working memory[145]
- Memory, including long term and recall[143,145,147-151]
- Paired associated learning[145]
- Consolidation[147]
- Initiation[147]
- Maintenance of behavior[147]
- Impaired ability to switch focus of attention, set-shifting such as needed for Trail Making Test Part B[152,153]
- Impaired inhibition or behavioral response[152]

---

*References 142,143,147,160,162,165.

aged >60 years with depression have been found to demonstrate a slower recovery from cognitive impairments related to depression.[142]

Older adults with depression demonstrate the following patterns of impairments[142,154,160,166]: psychomotor slowing, required increased time to complete complex task, decreased attention, decreased visuospatial skills, decreased memory processing, delayed recall memory, decreased executive functioning, delayed language and verbal fluency, delayed planning, delayed sequencing, decreased abstract thinking, and slowed attention shifting.

Younger people between the ages of 20 and 40 years with depression are more likely to demonstrate cognitive impairments with updating, shifting, and inhibition processes.[167] Younger people with moderate depression also demonstrated less impairment with working memory when compared with people in older age groups.[169,170]

The severity of depression experienced by the individual may also impact the level of cognitive impairment. Cohen[147] and Harvey et al[167] found as the severity of the depression increased, so did the impairment of motor and cognitive performance. The level of motivation may similarly impact the level of cognitive dysfunction. Miller and Lewis[171] and Henriques et al[172] found that people with depression are more likely to demonstrate lower motivation, and this in turn has been found to impair cognitive performance.

For some individuals with depression, even time of day may impact cognitive performance. Moffoot et al[173] examined changes in mood and neuropsychological function based on time of day. They observed people with diurnal variation, in whom depression was worse earlier in the day. These subjects demonstrated greater impairments with cognitive testing when evaluated in the morning. They demonstrated deficits with comprehension, attention, concentration, working memory, episodic memory, and reaction time.

THE CLINICAL EVALUATION

For people with depression the clinical interview becomes an important part of the clinical evaluation. The DRS should use this time to build rapport with the client and increase understanding of how the mental illness impacts his or her life. During the clinical evaluation interview, the DRS should also ask about whether the client has ever been diagnosed with depression and other mental illnesses. Many times people will come into the office because of another medical condition and neglect to mention the diagnosis of a mental illness. This may occur because they may not be thinking about the potential impact mental illness can have on safe driving. There also are individuals who are reluctant to volunteer information about depression and

---

BOX 6-8	**Medical History Questions Regarding Mental Health**

GENERAL QUESTIONS
- Have you ever been treated or diagnosed with a mental illness?
- Have you ever experienced prolonged periods of sadness?
- How long have you been treated for depression?
- What symptoms are you experiencing?
- Have you been formally diagnosed or treated for depression?
- Do you receive medication? Do you participate in therapy?

QUESTIONS TO ASK IF THE CLIENT IS TAKING AN ANTIDEPRESSANT
- How long have you been taking this medication?
- Why are you taking it?
- How much, how often, and what time of day do you take the medication?
- Do you experience any side effects?
- What kind of doctor prescribed this medicine?

---

other mental illnesses because of stigma. Therefore when asking about medical history, make sure to ask about history of depressive symptoms and treatment of depression (Box 6-8).

Next, be sure to review medications used to treat depression. Again, it is helpful to be up to date and familiar with common antidepressants. Clients may deny history or symptoms of depression but report taking a medication commonly used to treat depression. Consider a client who denied symptoms of depression and anxiety but is taking an antidepressant for his or her headaches. On further questioning it may be determined that he or she has been taking this mediation for several years; it was prescribed by a psychiatrist and is helpful for balancing mood. All clues may indicate the person has been diagnosed with a mental illness. If a DRS has a client who reports taking an antidepressant, the DRS should ask the client the questions listed in Box 6-8.

Cognitive impairments secondary to depression may be severe enough to affect a person's ability to function at work. During the clinical interview the DRS should ask clients whether they are currently working. If they are not working because of cognitive impairments they are experiencing, it may not be the best time to test on-road driving skills.[144] However, the DRS should be careful not to jump to conclusions. The DRS again should ask clients about circumstances surrounding return to work issues and ask them about how they spend their days. For example clients may report that they are not currently working but spend the day running and organize their homes and families. Even though they are not working, they continue to participate in their communities and manage high-level life roles.

During cognitive and visual perceptual testing, the DRS should watch for decreased concentration, decreased attention, and task set shifting difficulties. Cognitive impairments from depression may become apparent during the Trail Making A and/or B test, visual perceptual testing, processing speed, problem solving, and memory testing. The DRS should also check for delayed motor responses with reaction time testing and diadochokinesia. The DRS must keep in mind that deficits may not always be found when tested individually but are more easily recognized when the client is asked to coordinate functions.[105]

The DRS should also think about the commonly observable symptoms of depression, such as tearfulness, irritability, and slowed movements. The DRS should watch for and pay attention to these symptoms. Someone who easily cries when frustrated may not be ready to drive. People who are easily irritated or angered also may not yet have the patience needed for safe driving, especially during stressful situations.

The DRS must remember to be careful not to jump to conclusions about driver readiness with an older client who is demonstrating cognitive impairments. Depression in older adults presents similarly to dementia. If the client reports a history of depression, the DRS should be sure to contact the referring physician and report the cognitive impairments observed and assessed. Successful treatment of depressive symptoms can help to reverse cognitive impairment even in older adults. In this situation the client may greatly benefit from medical attention for treatment of depression before proceeding to the on-road portion of the comprehensive driver rehabilitation evaluation.

With the client's permission, the DRS should be sure to use secondary sources such as doctors, family members, and friends to gain insight and information about the client. Spouses and family members are particularly helpful sources of information for elderly clients with depression. Invite family members into the facility during the clinical evaluation and speak with them separately while the client is completing testing. Secondary sources are helpful in providing information about how the client functions at home and can provide observations of any changes in function and behavior.

If the client with depression is demonstrating cognitive impairments that are evident in the clinical evaluation, it may be beneficial to recommend that the client receive treatment for symptoms and provide him or her with a predriving reassessment before pursuing the on-road evaluation.

OTs play a vital role in providing holistic treatment to their clients. Therefore if a DRS has a client who seems to be impacted by symptoms of depression or any other mental illness, it is important to notify the client's referring doctor and encourage the client to get help. Successful treatment will not only improve his or her driving performance but also will help to improve the overall value and role performance in the client's life.

ANXIETY

Anxiety is a normal health emotion. It is the feeling a person may get before a big test or before a presentation to an unknown audience. Anxiety can help to motivate a person to perform better and work harder. However, for people with anxiety disorders, this normal, healthy emotion becomes so extreme that it often paralyzes and negatively impacts their functional performance. People with anxiety disorder experience anxiety that is disproportionate to what could potentially happen as a result of an event or a situation. A person with anxiety generally fears the worst and feels all situations will become a catastrophe.[141] Many people still believe that anxiety disorders are a character flaw or something that can just be fixed, but anxiety disorder is much more than a character flaw. It is a serious mood disorder that affects a person's ability to function in everyday activities.

Although there are several different forms of anxiety disorders, they have a common base of symptoms. Anxiety disorder is when someone experiences excessive worry for at least 6 months and may be related to a number of events or activities.[141] According to the DSM-IV,[141] people with anxiety disorder must have three of the following symptoms: restlessness, easily fatigued, poor concentration, increased irritability, muscle tension, and sleep disturbances.

Other complaints or symptoms reported by people with anxiety disorder may include shortness of breath, dizziness, unsteadiness, increased heart rate, trembling or shaking, sweating, choking, nausea, diarrhea, numbness or tingling sensations, chest pain or discomfort, or fear of dying.

Research has found that anxiety disorders may be caused by a variety of different factors, including motor vehicle accidents, family history, genetics, increased stress, inadequate coping, or traumatic life experiences. According to Norris[174] and Dougal et al[175] motor vehicle accidents are one of the most common causes for anxiety disorders. Interestingly, according to Bryant and Harvey,[176] females are more likely to display increased anxiety or develop posttraumatic stress disorder as a result of a vehicle crash. Passengers who have been in a vehicle crash also are more likely than drivers to demonstrate symptoms of anxiety and acute stress disorder. Bryant and Harvey[176] explain this by the decreased feeling of control experienced by the passenger.

People with anxiety disorders experience a variety of changes in cognitive performance. Because the anxiety is often related to a psychologically traumatic event, it is no surprise that the client may experience disability in several areas of function.[141,175] Clients may demonstrate any one of the following changes with cognitive performance[176]: impairments in awareness, avoidance of thoughts, irritability, decreased concentration, motor restlessness, or exaggerated startle response.

PREDRIVING ASSESSMENT

As with people with depression, the clinical interview is an excellent time to build rapport with the client with anxiety. The DRS should be sure to ask the client about anxiety or other mental illnesses. The DRS must remember that people may not volunteer this information because of the stigma often associated with mental illness.

Many clients who present to the driving program report symptoms of anxiety related to a vehicle crash. Therefore the DRS should make sure to ask clients about recent driving habits and any traffic tickets and crashes. If the client reports a recent crash, especially one that resulted in injury, the DRS should make sure to ask him or her about the details surrounding the event. The DRS must remember that research shows that women and passengers are more likely to experience anxiety as a result of vehicle crashes. Also consider

the previous list of signs and symptoms in this chapter. Box 6-9 contains a list of questions to ask.

The DRS next should be sure to take a through inventory of all medications the client is currently taking, including prescribed and over-the-counter drugs. The DRS should be familiar with common medications used to treat anxiety. The DRS should keep in mind that drugs have multiple uses. Therefore the DRS must be careful not to jump to conclusions. If the DRS has a client who reports taking medication for anxiety or is taking a medication commonly used for anxiety, the DRS should ask him or her the questions listed in Box 6-9.

Often the client will come into the office without being formally assessed or treated for the anxiety disorder, and it is not until the DRS begins the clinical evaluation process that signs and symptoms of anxiety begin to appear. Furthermore, for many clients symptoms of anxiety will not appear until the anxiety-causing stimulus is present. For example a client who reports increased anxiety because of being injured in a crash with a tractor-trailer may not display symptoms of anxiety until the car that he or she is driving is in close proximity to a tractor-trailer.

There are a variety of ways cognitive impairments from anxiety may impact performance during the clinical evaluation. Performance anxiety may lower test scores, particularly on cognitively challenging tests, such as visual perceptual testing and cognitive testing. Clients also may demonstrate a slower processing speed because of worries about being right. Decreased confidence may also result in slowed response time during testing. Clients with anxiety also are sometimes so focused on getting the answer right that they forget the directions and subsequently forget what they are supposed to be doing.

DRSs should also be able to recognize symptoms of anxiety, including poor concentration, fear, shortness of breath, diaphoresis (i.e., sweating), and negative self-talk, to name a few (see a more comprehensive list previously presented in this chapter). The DRS must make sure he or she talks to clients about their performance and make an effort to specify how the observed anxiety impacted performance outcomes during the clinical evaluation, on-road testing, or both. Of course DRSs must document their observations and the client's performance to establish a baseline or to document reassessment data that are compared with previously established performance outcomes. The DRS also should be supportive of the client and during testing minimize pass/fail responses. If the client is demonstrating symptoms of anxiety or cognitive impairment that are interfering and preventing the completion of testing, it may be beneficial to recommend the client receive treatment of the existing symptoms before pursuing a clinical reassessment or on-road evaluation.

BOX 6-9	**Questions to Ask a Client Who Reports a Recent Crash**

GENERAL QUESTIONS
- When did the crash occur?
- Who was driving?
- How did the crash happen?
- What injuries did you sustain from the crash?
- Are you experiencing anxiety or increased stress when placed in situations similar to the crash?
- Have you been formally diagnosed, or are you receiving treatment for depression?
- What symptoms of anxiety do you experience?
- What tends to cause anxiety symptoms?
- What helps to decrease anxiety?

QUESTIONS TO ASK IF THE CLIENT IS TAKING ANXIETY MEDICATION
- How long have you been taking this medication?
- Why are you taking it?
- How much, how often, and what time of day do you take the medication?
- Do you experience any side effects?
- What kind of doctor prescribed this medicine?

SCHIZOPHRENIA

Schizophrenia is a chronic mental illness that is usually first diagnosed in a person's late teens to mid-30s.[141] Although symptoms may be controlled, people diagnosed with schizophrenia often experience exacerbations. Seventy to 80% of people with schizophrenia who do not receive treatment will experience intensified symptoms and relapse within 1 year.[177] With treatment the chance of relapse decreases by 30% but still remains at 40% to 50% of the overall relapse rate.[177] The disorder is devastating to families and clients because 60% to 70% of people with schizophrenia never marry, have children, or find meaningful employment; they have limited social contacts during a period in their lives when others in their age group are experiencing many of these milestone activities and more.[141]

To be diagnosed with schizophrenia, the symptoms must be present for a significant portion of 1 month.[141] The symptoms of schizophrenia generally are categorized as either positive or negative. The positive symptoms are generally the psychotic symptoms, such as hallucinations and delusions. These symptoms usually respond to antipsychotic medication therapy. A person with schizophrenia experiences perceptual changes through auditory or visual hallucinations that include seeing or hearing things that other people do not experience.[141] The second positive symptom is the presence of delusions, which are fixed, false beliefs.[141] At least one-half of the people with schizophrenia who experience delusions act on their belief that their delusions are real; unfortunately this action (or reaction) may include the use of a motor vehicle.[104] Any additional positive symptoms are related to impairments in communication and language. There are people with schizophrenia who also demonstrate disorganized speech,[141] such that their conversation is often difficult to follow because of the loose connections and free associations. The final positive symptom relates to behavior disorders in which the person with schizophrenia has disorganized behavior or becomes catatonic.[141]

People with schizophrenia also display negative symptoms, which are more pervasive and tend to remain after the positive symptoms are controlled. First the person with schizophrenia often displays a flattened affect,[141] meaning the person displays a limited, if any, range of facial expressions. Second the person may display decreased fluidity of speech and a decreased vocabulary, resulting in terse responses that reflect a poverty of thought.[141] People with schizophrenia also often have decreased motivation and thus spend much of the day in bed.[141] Likewise they have difficulty gaining pleasure from meaningful activities.[141] Finally these people experience impaired attention.

Driving a vehicle may be problematic for people with schizophrenia because of the cognitive impairments associated with the disorder. First deficits of executive dysfunction have been noted with people who have schizophrenia, particularly those deficits related to impaired working memory. Working memory is the ability to hold information for brief periods so it can be further processed to create a meaningful response.[178] This type of memory is required for learning, reasoning, planning, and comprehension.[178] Therefore people with schizophrenia may have difficulty managing complex problem-solving tasks that occur when driving. Second people with schizophrenia experience impairments with visual perceptual skills,[178] although Tek et al[178] identified that the visual perceptual deficits relate more to object visual perception rather than spatial visual perception.

THE CLINICAL EVALUATION

During the clinical evaluation it is important to evaluate attention, visual perception, problem solving, and reasoning. There may be a greater focus on divided attention such as the Trail Making Test or UFOV. Clients also should be screened for impulsivity and threat recognition. General observations made by the DRS during the clinical evaluation will be as valuable as the actual test results. The DRS will need to document the client's level of alertness and the content of his or her conversations with the client before, during, and after the evaluation. General organizational abilities also can be assessed by paying attention to things such as whether the client arrived on time with the proper paperwork for the appointment. It is important to screen the client for delusions and hallucinations, especially when he or she is planning to use a motor vehicle. Box 6-10 has a list of questions to ask the client's caregiver, physician, or both.

BOX 6-10	Assessment Questions Regarding Schizophrenia

Questions to ask a client's caregiver, physician, or both may include the following:
- Is the client chronically delusional?
- Has the client ever acted on the delusions?
- What is the degree of the client's compliance with taking his or her medications?
- What are the current medication side effects?
- How long has the client been taking the particular medication regimen?

SUMMARY

A diagnosis of a mental illness should be considered when evaluating the entire person and should not immediately lead the DRS to conclude a person is unsafe to drive. The DRS should modify the clinical evaluation to determine the impact of cognitive and motor deficits on driving performance. The medications for these conditions also should be closely reviewed. It is the responsibility of the DRS to be alert for symptoms of mental illness and work collaboratively with the client, his or her psychiatrist, and the rest of the driver rehabilitation team to develop an effective evaluation and treatment approach.

REFERENCES

1. Davis ES: Defining OT roles in driving, *OT Practice* 8:15-18, 2003.
2. Hopewell CA: Driving assessment issues for practicing clinicians, *J Head Trauma Rehabil* 17:48-61, 2002.
3. Stav WB: *Driving rehabilitation: a guide for assessment and intervention*, San Antonio, 2004, The Psychological Corporation.
4. National Highway Traffic Safety Administration: Model driver screening and evaluation program: final technical report. Volume 1: *Project summary and model program recommendations (DOT HS 809 582)*, Washington, DC, 2003, U.S. Department of Transportation.
5. Wang CC, Kosinski CJ, Schwartzberg JG, et al: *Physician's guide to assessing and counseling older drivers*, Washington, DC, 2003, National Highway Traffic Safety Administration.
6. McKenna P: Fitness to drive: a neuropsychological perspective, *J Mental Health* 7:9-18, 1998.
7. Association for Driver Rehabilitation Specialists: *Best practices for the delivery of driver rehabilitation services*, Ruston, LA, 2004, Association for Driver Rehabilitation Specialists.
8. Owsley C, Stalvey B, Wells J, et al: Older drivers and cataract: driving habits and crash risk, *J Gerontol Med Sci* 54A:M203-M211, 1999.
9. Isler RB, Parsonson BS, Hansson GJ: Age related effects of restricted head movements on the useful field of view of drivers, *Accid Anal Prevent* 29: 793-801, 1997.
10. Barry CJ, Smith D, Lennarson P, et al: The effect of wearing a restrictive neck brace on driver performance, *Neurosurg* 53:98-102, 2003.
11. Capo LC: Autism, employment, and the role of occupational therapy, *Work* 16:201-207, 2001.
12. Brower WH, Withaar FK, Tant MLM, et al: Attention and driving in traumatic brain injury: a question of coping with time-pressure, *J Head Trauma Rehabil* 17:1-15, 2002.
13. Groeger JA: *Understanding driving: applying cognitive psychology to a complex everyday task*, East Sussex, UK, 2000, Psychology Press.
14. Klavora P, Gaskovski P, Martin K, Forsyth, et al: The effects of dynavision rehabilitation on the behind the wheel driving ability and selected psychomotor abilities of persons after stroke, *Am J Occup Ther* 49:534-542, 1995.
15. Shawaryn MA, Schultheis MT, Garay E, et al: Assessing functional status: exploring the relationship between the multiple sclerosis functional composite and driving, *Arch Phys Med Rehabil* 83:1123-1129, 2002.
16. Schultheis MT, Garay E, DeLuca J: The influence of cognitive impairment on driving performance in multiple sclerosis, *Neurology* 56:1089-1094, 2001.
17. Marottoli RA, Drickamer MA: Psychomotor mobility and the elderly driver, *Clin Geriatr Med* 9:403-411, 1993.
18. Korteling JE: Perception-response speed and driving capabilities of brain-damaged and older drivers, *Hum Factors* 32:95-108, 1990.
19. American Automobile Association: *Automatic brake reaction timer: instructions for use*, Heathrow, FL, undated, American Automobile Association.
20. Vericom: *Vericom Manual VC3000, Version 3.2.5*, 2004.
21. Sanders MS, McCormick EJ: Human factors and the automobile. In Sanders MS, McCormick EJ, editors: *Human factors in engineering and design*, New York, 2003, McGraw-Hill, Inc.
22. Stereo Optical Co., Inc: *Vision tester slide packages and instructions*, 2004, Stereo Optical Co., Inc.
23. Stereo Optical Co., Inc: *Functional Acuity Contrast Test F.A.C.T. Appendix*, 2000, Stereo Optical Co., Inc.
24. Carr DB, LaBarge E, Dunnigan K, et al: Differentiating drivers with dementia of the Alzheimer type from healthy older persons with a traffic sign naming test, *J Gerontol Med Sci* 53A:M135-M139, 1998.
25. Radford KA, Lincoln NB: Concurrent validity of the stroke drivers screening assessment, *Arch Phys Med Rehabil* 85:324-328, 2004.
26. Bouska MJ, Kwatny E: *Manual for the application of the motor-free visual perception test to the adult population*, ed 6, Philadelphia, PA, 1982, Temple University Rehabilitation Research and Training Center.
27. Colarusso RP, Hammill DD: *Motor-free visual perception test manual*, ed 1, Novato, CA, 1972, Academic Therapy Publications.
28. Korner-Bitensky N, Mazur BL, Sofer S, et al: Visual testing for readiness to drive after stroke: a multicenter study, *Am J Phys Med Rehabil* 79:253-259, 2000.
29. Colarusso RP, Hammill DD: *Motor-free visual perception test manual*, ed 3, Novato, CA, 2003, Academic Therapy Publications.
30. Martin NA: *Use of the response time index with the motor free visual perception test*, ed 3, Novato, CA, 2003, Academic Therapy Publications.
31. Gardner MF: *Test of visual perceptual skills manual*, rev ed, Hydesville, CA, 1996, Psychological and Educational Publications.
32. Hooper HE: *The Hooper visual organization test manual*, Los Angeles, 1979, Western Psychological Services.
33. Mestre DR: *Dynamic evaluation of the useful field of view in driving*, Marseilles, France, 2004, Cognitive Neurosciences Centre.

34. National Institute on Aging: *New test predicts crash risk of older drivers*, 1998, Science Blog.

35. Owsley C, Ball K, McGwin G Jr, et al: Visual processing impairment and risk of motor vehicle crash among older adults, *JAMA* 279:1083-1088, 1998.

36. Beery KE: *The Beery-Buktenica developmental test of visual-motor integration manual*, rev ed, Parsippany, NJ, 1997, Modern Curriculum Press.

37. Sivan AB: *Benton visual retention test manual*, ed 5, San Antonio, 1992, The Psychological Corporation.

38. Klavora P, Warren L, Leung M: *Dynavision handbook and treatment manual for rehabilitation of visual and motor deficits*, Lenexa, KS, 1996a, visABILITIES Rehab Services.

39. Klavora P, Gaskovski P, Forsyth R: Test-retest reliability of three Dynavision tasks, *Perceptual Motor Skills* 80:607-610, 1995.

40. Army Individual Test Battery: *Manual of directions and scoring*, Washington, DC, 1944, War Department, Adjutant General's Office. Cited in Lezak MD: *Neuropsychological assessment*, New York, 1995, Oxford University Press, pp. 381-384.

41. Spreen O, Strauss E: *A compendium of neuropsychological tests: administration, norms and commentary*, New York, 1998, Oxford Press.

42. Tombaugh TT: Trail Making Test A and B: normative data stratified by age and education, *Arch Clin Neuropsychol* 19:203-214, 2004.

43. Royall DR, Cordes JA, Polk M: CLOX: an executive clock drawing task, *J Neurosurg Psychiatr* 64:588-594, 1998.

44. Wilson B, Cockburn J, Baddeley A: *The Rivermead behavioral memory test manual*, Reading, UK, 1985, The Thames Valley Test Company.

45. Helm-Estabrooks N: *Cognitive linguistic quick test: examiner's manual*, San Antonio, 2001, The Psychological Corporation.

46. Safe Performance Associates: *Driver performance test manual*, Clearwater, FL, undated, Safe Performance Associates.

47. Shiner D, Schieber F: Visual requirements for safety and mobility of older drivers, *Hum Factors* 33:507-519, 1991.

48. Fletcher DC: *Low vision rehabilitation: caring for the whole person*, San Francisco, 1999, American Academy of Ophthalmology.

49. American Academy of Ophthalmology: *Policy statement: vision requirements for driving*, Approved by the Board of Trustees, October 2001. Available at: *http://www.aao.org/aao/member/policy/driving.cfm*. Accessed January 14, 2004.

50. Staplin L, Lococo KH, Gish KW, et al: *Model driver screening and evaluation program final technical report: DOT HS 809 581. Guidelines for motor vehicle administrators*, Washington, DC, 2003, National Highway Traffic Safety Administration. Available at: *http://www.nhtsa.dot.gov/people/injury/olderdrive/mod eldriver/*. Accessed January 5, 2004.

51. Lens A, Langley T, Nemeth SC, et al: *Ocular anatomy and physiology*, Thorofare, NJ, 1999, SLACK Inc.

52. Nolte J: *The human brain*, ed 3, St. Louis, 1993, Mosby.

53. Tortora GJ, Grabowski SR: *Principles of anatomy and physiology*, ed 7, New York, 1993, HarperCollins College.

54. Staplin L, Lococo KH, Gish KW, et al: DOT HS 808 853. *Safe mobility for older people notebook. I.C. Develop tools needed to implement model programs*. Washington, DC: National Highway Traffic Safety Administration Model Driver Screening and Evaluation Program, April 1999. Available at: *http://www.nhsta.dot.gov/people/injury/olddrive/safe/0 1c02.htm*. Accessed November 3, 2004.

55. Freund B, Gravenstein S, Ferris R: *Use of the clock drawing test as a screen for driving competency in older adults*. Presented at the Annual Meeting of the American Geriatrics Society, Washington, DC, May 9, 2002.

56. Brilliant RL: *Essentials of low vision practice*, Woburn, MA, 1999, Butterworth-Heinemann.

57. Weiner W, Siffermann E: The development of the profession of orientation and mobility. In Blasch B, Wiener W, Welsh R, editors: *Foundations of orientation and mobility*, ed 2, New York, 1997, AFB Press, pp. 553-579.

58. Lydon WT, McGraw ML: *Concept development for visually handicapped children: a resource guide for teachers and other professionals working in educational settings*, rev ed, New York, 1973, AFB Press.

59. Children Accessing Travel Situations, Project CATS: Definitions section, Indiana Deafblind Services Project, 2002. Available at: *http://cats.indstate.edu/ ttdefinitions.html*. Last accessed November 14, 2004.

60. Mikrut SL: Personal communication, *ACVREP information* to members of the American Academy of Ophthalmology Vision Rehabilitation List Serve. Available at: *visionrehab@lists.aao.org*. Accessed February 6, 2004.

61. Peli E, Peli D: State vision requirements. In *Driving with confidence: a practical guide to driving with low vision*, River Edge, NJ, 2002, World Scientific, pp. 122-181.

62. Shuldiner RJ: *Vision and driving: state rules, regulations and policies, 2003*. Available at: *www.lowvisioncare.com/visionlaws.htm*. Accessed October 23, 2004.

63. Collins C: Profile of Dr. William Feinbloom, *J Rehabil Optom* 1:3-5, 1983.

64. Feinbloom W: Driving with bioptic telescopic spectacles, *Am J Optom Physiol Opt* 54:35-42, 1977.

65. Burg A: Some preliminary findings concerning the relation between vision and driving performance, *J Am Optom Assoc* 38:372-377, 1967.

66. Chapman BG: Techniques and variables related to driving—Part I, *J Rehabil Optom* Summer:18-20, 1984.

67. Chapman BG: Techniques and variables related to diving—Part II, *J Rehabil Optom* Fall:12-14, 1984.

68. Corn AL, Lippmann O, et al: Licensed drivers with bioptic telescopic spectacles: user profiles and perceptions, *Review* 21:221-230, 1990.

69. Huss CP: Model approach: low vision driver's training and assessment, *J Vision Rehabil* 2:31-44, 1988.

70. Jose RT, Butler JB: Driver's training for partially sighted persons: an interdisciplinary approach, *New Outlook Blind* 69:305-311, 1975.

71. Newman JD: A rational approach to license drivers using bioptic telescopes, *J Am Optom Assoc* 47:510-513, 1976.

72. Park W, Unatin J, et al: A driving program for the visually impaired, *J Am Optom Assoc* 64:54-59, 1993.

73. Szlyk JP, Seiple W, et al: Measuring the effectiveness of bioptic telescopes for persons with central vision loss, *J Rehabil Res Develop* 37:1-13, 2000.

74. Taylor DG: Telescopic spectacles for driving: user data satisfaction, preferences and effects in vocational, educational and personal tasks: a study in Illinois, *J Vision Rehabil* 4:29-59, 1990.

75. Vogel GL: Training the bioptic telescope wearer for driving, *J Am Optom Assoc* 62:288-293, 1991.

76. National Highway Traffic Safety Administration, Office of Civil Rights: Complaint Processing, U.S. Department of Transportation Report No. DOT HS 809 350, 2001.

77. Huss CP: *Driving with bioptic telescopic lens systems.* Paper Presentation at the Eye and The Auto International Forum, Daimler Chrysler Technology Center, Auburn Hills, MI, 2001.

78. West Virginia Division of Rehabilitation Services Driving in the 21st century: specialized driver's training for the most severely disabled, *WVDRS Workable News* 2:1-5, 2003.

79. Huss CP: Training the low vision driver. In Stuen C, Arditi A, Horowitz A, et al, editors: *Vision '99: vision rehabilitation: assessment, intervention and outcomes,* New York, 2000, Swets & Zeitlinger Publishers, pp. 264-267.

80. Geruschat DK, Smith AJ: Low vision and mobility. In Blasch BB, Wiener W, et al, editors: *Foundations of orientation and mobility,* ed 2, New York, 1997, AFB Press, pp. 63-103.

81. Corn AL, Rosenblum LP: *Finding wheels: a curriculum for non-drivers with visual impairments for gaining control of transportation needs,* Austin, TX, 2000, ProEd Publishers.

82. Shinar D, Schieber F: Visual requirements for safety and mobility of older drivers, *Hum Factors* 33:507-519, 1991.

83. Davis P: *Listen up! Overcoming hearing loss,* Woollahra, Australia, 1996, Gore and Osment Publications.

84. Cohen HS, Wells J, Timball KT, et al: Driving disability and dizziness, *J Safety Res* 34:361-369, 2003.

85. Stach B: *Clinical audiology: an introduction,* San Diego, 1998, Singular Publishing Group Inc.

86. Ballantyne J: Deafness: types and clinical characteristics. In Ballantyne J, Martin MC, Martin A, editors: *Deafness,* ed 5, London, 1993, Whurr Publishers Ltd., pp. 62-65.

87. VicDeaf HEAR Service: *Understanding hearing loss, 2002.* Available at: *http:// www.vicdeaf.com.au/ informationResources.* Accessed June 16, 2004.

88. Doyle J: Sound and hearing. In Doyle J, Bench J, Day N, et al, editors: *Practical audiology for speech-language therapists,* London, 1998, Whurr Publishers, pp. 11-31.

89. National Institute on Deafness and Other Communication Disorders: *Statistics about hearing disorders, ear infections and deafness, 2004.* Accessed June 16, 2004.

90. Davis A: The prevalence of deafness. In Ballantyne J, Martin MC, Martin A, editors: *Deafness,* ed 5, London, 1993, Whurr Publishers Ltd., pp. 1-11.

91. Fozard JL, Gordon-Salant S: Changes in vision and hearing with aging. In Birren JE, Warner Schaie K, Abeles RP, et al, editors: *Handbook of the psychology of aging,* ed 5, San Diego, 2001, Academic Press.

92. Abyad A: In office screening for age-related hearing and vision loss, *Geriatrics* 52:45-57, 1997.

93. Gething L: Ageing with long-standing hearing impairment and deafness, *Int J Rehabil Res* 23:209-215, 2000.

94. Freeland A: *Deafness: the facts,* Oxford, 1989, Oxford University Press.

95. Hallam R: *Living with tinnitus: dealing with the ringing in your ears,* Northamptonshire, UK, 1989, Thorsons Publishers Limited.

96. Fisk AD, Rogers WAE: *Handbook of human factors and the older adult,* San Diego, 1997, Academic Press.

97. Dolinar TM, McQuillenn AD, Ranseen JD: Health, safety and the older driver, *Patient Care* 15:22-34, 2001.

98. Ivers RQ, Mitchell P, Cumming RG: Sensory impairment and driving: the blue mountains eye study, *Am J Public Health* 89:85-87, 1999.

99. Austroads: *Assessing fitness to drive: for commercial and private vehicle drivers: medical standards for licensing and clinical management guidelines,* ed 3, Sydney, 2003, Austroads Incorporated.

100. Roller L, Gowan J: Drugs and driving, *Curr Ther* February:65-71, 2001.

101. School of Occupational Therapy, LaTrobe University: *Driver education and rehabilitation course manual for occupational therapists,* Melbourne, 2003, School of Occupational Therapy, La Trobe University.

102. Shimon DA: *Coping with hearing loss and hearing aids,* San Diego, 1992, Singular Publishing Group, Inc.

103. Ballantyne J: The functional examination of hearing. In Ballantyne J, Martin MC, Martin A, editors: *Deafness,* ed 5, London, 1993, Whurr Publishers Ltd., pp. 65-89.

104. Harris M: Psychiatric conditions with relevance to fitness to drive, *Adv Psychiatr Treat* 6:261-269, 2000.

105. Elliott R: Executive functions and their disorders, *Br Med Bull* 65:49-59, 2003.

106. American Psychiatric Association: *The role of the psychiatrist in assessing driving ability: position statement.* Document reference number 930004, Arlington, VA, 1993, American Psychiatric Association.

107. Wise MEJ, Watson JP: Postal survey of psychiatrists' knowledge and attitudes towards driving and mental illness, *Psychiatr Bull* 25:345-349, 2001.

108. Elwood P: Driving, mental illness and role of the psychiatrist, *Irish J Psychol Med* 15:49-51, 1998.

109. Brown P: Mental illness and motor insurance, *Psychiatr Bull* 17:620-621, 1993.

110. American Medical Association: *Physician's guide to assessing and counseling older drivers,* Chicago, 2004, AMA.

111. Ray WA, Thapa PB, Shorr RI: Medications and the older driver, *Clin Geriatr Med* 9:413-438, 1993.

112. Deputal D, Pomara N: Effect of antidepressants on human performance: a review, *J Clin Psychopharmacol* 10:105-111, 1990.

113. Hindmarch I: A pharmacological profile of fluoxetine and other antidepressants on aspects of skilled performance and car handling ability, *Br J Psychiatry* 153:99-104, 1988.

114. Moskowitz H, Burns MM: Cognitive performance in geriatric subjects after acute treatment with antidepressants, *Neuropsychobiology* 15:38-43, 1986.

115. Mattila MJ, Saarialho-Kere U, Mattila M: Acute effects of sertraline, amitriptyline and placebo on the psychomotor performance of healthy subjects over 50 years of age, *J Clin Psychiatry* 49:52-58, 1988.

116. Mattila MJ, Liliquist R, Seppala T: Effects of amitriptyline and mianserin on psychomotor skills and memory in the man, *Br J Clin Pharmacol* 5:53S-55S, 1978.

117. Scott DB, Tiplady B: Effects of amitriptyline and zimelidine in combination with ethanol, *Psychopharmacology* 76:209-211, 1982.

118. Seppala T, Linnoila M: Effects of zimeldine and other antidepressants on skilled performance: a comprehensive review, *Acta Psychiatr Scand* 68:135-140, 1983.

119. Swift CJ, Haythorne JM, Clarke P, et al: Cardiovascular, sedative and anticholinergic effects of amitriptyline and zimelidine in young and elderly volunteers, *Acta Psychiatr Scand* 63:425-432, 1981.

120. Betts TA, Birtle J: Effect of two hypnotic drugs on actual driving performance next morning, *BMJ* 285:852, 1982. In Ray WA, Thapa PB, Shorr RI: Medications and the older driver, *Clin Geriatr Med* 9:413-438, 1993.

121. Bliwise D, Seidel W, Karacan I, et al: Daytime sleepiness as a criterion in hypnotic medication trials: comparison of triazolam and flurazepam, *Sleep* 6:156-163, 1983.

122. Campbell AJ, Somerton DT: Benzodiazepine drug effect on body way in elderly subjects, *J Clin Experiment Gerontol* 4:341-347, 1982.

123. Carskadon MA, Seidel WF, Greenblatt DJ, et al: Daytime carryover of triazolam and flurazepam in elderly insomniacs, *Sleep* 5:361-371, 1982.

124. Castleden CM, George CF, Marcer D, et al: Increased sensitivity to nitrazepam in old age, *BMJ* 1:10-12, 1977.

125. Cook PJ, Huggett A, Graham-Pole, et al: Hypnotic accumulation and hangover in elderly inpatients: a controlled double-blind study of temazepam and nitrazepam, *BMJ* 286:100-102, 1983.

126. Greenblatt DJ, Harmatz JS, Shapiro L, et al: Sensitivity to triazolam in the elderly, *N Engl J Med* 324:1691-1698, 1991.

127. Laurell H, Tornros J: The carry-over effects of triazolam compared with nitrazepam and placebo in acute emergency driving situations and in monotonous simulated driving, *Acta Pharmacol Toxicol* 58:182-186, 1986.

128. Linnoila M, Erwin CW, Logue PE, et al: Psychomotor effects of diazepam in anxious patients and healthy volunteers, *J Clin Psychopharmacol* 3:88-96, 1983.

129. Moskowitz H: Attention tasks as skills performance measures of drug effects, *Br J Clin Pharmacol* 18:51S-61S, 1984.

130. Moskowitz H, Limmoila M, Roehrs T: Psychomotor performance in chronic insomniacs during 14-day use of fluzaepam and midazolam, *J Clin Psychopharmacol* 10:44S-55S, 1990.

131. Moskowitz H, Smiley A: Effects of chronically administered busiporne and diazepam on driving-related skills performance, *J Clin Psychiatry* 43:45-55, 1982.

132. O'Hanlon JF, Blaauw GJ, Riemersma JBJ: Diazepam impairs lateral position control in highway driving, *Science* 217:79-81, 1982.

133. O'Hanlon JF, Volkerts ER: Hypnotics and actual driving performance, *Acta Psychiatr Scand* 74:95-104, 1986.

134. Palva ES, Linnoila M, Saario I, et al: Acute and subacute effects of diazepam on psychomotor skills: interaction with alcohol, *Acta Pharmacol Toxicol* 45:257-264, 1979.

135. Robin DW, Hasan SS, Lichtenstein MJ, et al: Pharmacodynamics and drug reaction: dose-related effects of triazolam on postural sway, *Clin Pharmacol Ther* 49:581-588, 1991.

136. Rothenberg SJ, Selkoe D: Specific oculomotor deficits after diazepam. I. Saccadic eye movements, *Psychopharmacology* 74:232-236, 1981.

137. Rothenberg SJ, Selkoe D: Specific oculomotor deficits after diazepam. I. Smooth pursuit eye movements, *Psychopharmacology* 74:237-240, 1981.

138. Schmidt U, Brendemuhl D, Ruther E: Aspects of driving after hypnotic therapy with particular reference to temazepam, *Acta Psychiatr Scand* 74:112-118, 1986.

139. Stapleton JM, Guthrie S, Linnoila M: Effects of alcohol and other psychotropic drugs on eye movement: relevance to traffic safety, *J Study Alcohol* 47:426-432, 1986.

140. van Laar MW, Volkerts ER, Willigenburg APP: Therapeutic effects and effects on actual driving performance of chronically administered buspirone and diazepam in anxious patients, *J Clin Psychopharmacol* 12:86-95, 1992.

141. American Psychiatric Association: *DSM IV: diagnostic and statistical manual of mental disorders*, ed 4, Washington, DC, 1994, AMA.

142. Tarbuck AF, Paykel ES: Effects of major depression on the cognitive function of younger and older subjects, *Psychol Med* 3:33-40, 1995.

143. Sternberg DE, Jarvik ME: Memory functions in depression: improvements with antidepressant medication, *Arch Gen Psychiatry* 33:219-224, 1976.

144. Austin MP, Mitchel P, Goodwin GM: Cognitive deficits in depression: possible implications of functional neuropathology, *Br J Psychiatry* 178:200-206, 2001.

145. Porter RJ, Gallagher P, Thompson JM, et al: Neurocognitive impairment in drug free patients with major depressive disorder, *Br J Psychiatry* 182:214-220, 2003.

146. Schatzberg AF, Posener JA, DeBattists C, et al: Neuropsychological deficits in psychotic versus nonpsychotic major depression and no mental illness, *Am J Psychiatry* 157:1095-1100, 2000.

147. Cohen RM, Weingartner H, Smallberg SA, et al: Effort and cognition in depression, *Arch General Psychiatry* 39:593-597, 1982.

148. Frith CD, Steven M, Johnstone EC, et al: Effects of ECT and depression on various aspects of memory, *Br J Psychiatry* 142:610-617, 1983.

149. Wolfe J, Granholm E, Butters N, et al: Verbal memory deficits associated with major affective disorders: a comparison of unipolar and bipolar patients, *J Affect Disord* 13:83-92, 1987.

150. Golinkoff M, Sweene J: Cognitive impairments in depression, *J Affect Disord* 17:105-112, 1989.

151. Brown RG, Scott LC, Bench CJ, et al: Cognitive function in depression: its relationship to the presence and severity of intellectual decline, *Psychol Med* 24:829-847, 1994.

152. Murphy FC, Sahakian BJ, Rubinstein JS, et al: Emotional bias and inhibitory control processes in mania and depression, *Psychol Med* 29:1307-1321, 1999.

153. Austin MP, Mitchell P, Wilhelm K, et al: Melancholic depression: a pattern of frontal cognitive impairment, *Psychol Med* 29:73-85, 1999.

154. Beats BC, Sahakiah BJ, Levy R: Cognitive performance in tests sensitive to frontal lobe dysfunction in the elderly depression, *Psychol Med* 26:591-603, 1996.

155. Sabbe B, Hulstijn W, Van Hoof J, et al: Retardation in depression: assessment by means of simple motor tasks, *J Affect Disord* 55:39-44, 1999.

156. Byrne DG: Choice reaction times in depressive states, *Br J Soc Clin Psychol* 15:149-156, 1976.

157. Cornell DG, Saurez R, Berent S: Psychomotor retardation in melancholic and non-melancholic depression: cognitive and motor components, *J Abnorm Psychol* 932:150-157, 1984.

158. Weingartner H, Cohen RM, Murphy DL, et al: Cognitive processes in depression, *Arch Gen Psychiatry* 38:42-47, 1981.

159. Roy-Byrne PP, Weingartner H, Bierer LM, et al: Effortful and automatic cognitive processes in depression, *Arch Gen Psychiatry* 43:265-267, 1986.

160. Kramer-Ginsberg E, Greenwald BS, Krishnan KRR, et al: Neuropsychological functioning and MRI signal hyperintensities in geriatric depression, *Am J Psychiatry* 15:438-444, 1999.

161. Goodwin GM: Neuropsychological and neuroimaging evidence for the involvement of the frontal lobes in depression, *J Psychopharmacol* 11:115-122, 1997.

162. Rabins PV, Merchange A, Nestadt G: Criteria for diagnosing reversible dementia caused by depression: validation by 2-year follow-up, *Br J Psychiatry* 144:488-492, 1984.

163. Hickie I, Scott E, Mitchell P, et al: Subcortical hyperintensities on magnetic resonance imaging: clinical correlates and prognostic significance in patients with severe depression, *Biol Psychiatry* 37:151-160, 1995.

164. Cummings JL: The neuroanatomy of depression, *J Clin Psychiatry* 54:14-20, 1993.

165. Fromm D, Schopflocher D: Neuropsychological test performance in depressed patients before and after drug therapy, *Biol Psychiatry* 19:55-72, 1984.

166. Lockwood KA, Alexopoulos GS, Kakuma T, et al: Subtypes of cognitive impairment in depressed older adult, *Am J Geriatr Psychiatry* 8:201-208, 2000.

167. Harvey PO, Le Bastard G, Pochon JB, et al: Executive functions and updating of the contents of working memory in unipolar depression, *J Psychiatry Res* 38:567-576, 2004.

168. Reference deleted in pages.

169. Channon S: Executive dysfunction in depression: Wisconsin card sorting test, *J Neurol Neurosurg Psychiatry* 66:162-171, 1996.

170. Channon S, Green PS: Executive function in depression: the role of performance strategies in adding depressed and non-depressed participants, *J Neurol Neurosurg Psychiatry* 66:162-171, 1999.

171. Miller E, Lewis P: Recognition memory in elderly patients with depression and dementia: a signal detection analysis, *J Abnorm Psychol* 86:84-86, 1977.

172. Henriques JB, Glowacki JM, Davidson RJ: Reward fails to alter response bias in depression, *J Abnorm Psychol* 103:460-466, 1994.

173. Moffoot APR, O'Carroll RE, Bennie J, et al: Diurnal variation of mood and neuropsychological function in major depression with melancholia, *J Affect Disord* 32:257-269, 1994.

174. Norris FH: Epidemiology of trauma: frequency and impact of different potential traumatic events on different demographic groups, *J Consult Clin Psychol* 60:409-418, 1992.

175. Dougall AL, Ursano RJ, Posluszny DM, et al: Predictors of posttraumatic stress among victims of motor vehicle accidents, *Psychosomat Med* 63:402-411, 2001.

176. Bryant RA, Harvey AG: Gender differences in the relationship between acute stress disorder and posttraumatic stress disorder following motor vehicle accident, *Aust N Z J Psychiatry* 37:226-229, 2003.

177. Berkow R, et al, eds. *The Merck manual of medical information home edition*, Whitehouse Station, NJ, 1997, Merck Research Laboratories.

178. Tek C, Gold J, Blaxton T, et al: Visual perceptual and working memory impairments in schizophrenia, *Arch Gen Psychiatry* 59:146-153, 2002.

Chapter 7

DETERMINING FITNESS TO DRIVE: NEUROPSYCHOLOGICAL AND PSYCHOLOGICAL CONSIDERATIONS

Renee Coleman Bryer • Lisa J. Rapport • Robin A. Hanks

KEY TERMS

- Acquired brain disorder
- Driving fitness
- Attention
- Processing speed
- Language functioning
- Memory functioning
- Visuospatial and visuomotor functioning
- Executive functioning

CHAPTER OBJECTIVES

After completing this chapter, the reader will be able to do the following:

- Name and describe the six conceptual domains of cognitive functioning.
- Identify factors that are useful for predicting accidents.
- Explain why evaluation of driving skills alone is not enough to assess driving ability, and explain what other evaluations should be made.
- Explain why research on driving assessment in older adults is an important area of research.
- Explain how to approach the possibility of driving cessation.

NEUROPSYCHOLOGY OF DRIVING RISK

Neuropsychology is the study of the relationship between brain functioning and behavior. Neuropsychologists make use of a number of information sources, including behavioral observation, an individual's self-report, medical records, and results from performance tests to better understand the interplay between an individual's cognitive/emotional status and his or her daily functioning. Driving is a complex behavior that can be affected by an individual's emotional and/or cognitive status in many different ways. Cognitive functioning generally can be categorized into six broad conceptual domains: attention, processing speed, language functioning, memory functioning, visuospatial and visuomotor functioning, and executive functioning. Emotional/personality functioning is another domain of neuropsychological functioning that plays an important role in driving fitness. Although these domains are not entirely independent, statistical analyses examining commonly used neuropsychological tests have demonstrated that these areas of cognitive functioning are fairly distinct entities. *Acquired brain disorder* is a term that we will use in this chapter to refer to any medical event or pathologic process that causes damage to the brain resulting in neuropsychological impairment (e.g., traumatic brain injury [TBI], stroke, or dementia). Depending on the type and severity of the disturbance, impairment may be evident in one or all of the cognitive domains. Ability to drive safely, or *driving fitness*, is one of the aspects of everyday functioning that may be substantially affected by neuropsychological impairment.

The first conceptual domain, *attention*, is hierarchical and captures many different aspects of cognition, including the ability to focus for short or long periods on a single stimulus (i.e., simple or sustained attention) and the ability to attend to multiple pieces of information simultaneously (i.e., complex or divided attention). The highest component of the attentional hierarchy, working memory, is thought to involve complex attentional processes that involve executive functioning; therefore it will be discussed in that section of this chapter. Impairment in visuospatial attention, such as unilateral visual neglect or the tendency to be inattentive to stimuli in one of the lateral visual fields, often results from damage to the right parietal lobe of the brain. This phenomenon, which is relatively common after a right hemisphere stroke, also is described in the section on visuospatial functioning. Impaired attention may adversely affect driving in several ways: an individual may miss important, unforeseen obstacles or events on the road entirely; be easily distracted while driving; or be unable to process several events simultaneously. Any of these behavioral manifestations of attentional impairment could pose serious problems for an individual's ability to drive safely. Attentional abilities have long been recognized as predictive of driving fitness.[1]

Processing speed refers to the latency in verbal or motor responses to a stimulus. Although impairments in processing speed often accompany attentional deficits, a deficit in either of these domains individually may be problematic in the context of driving resumption. For example a person with a processing speed deficit may be able to attend to an unexpected stimulus on the road adequately (i.e., recognize the hazard) but may not be able to process the stimulus in sufficient time to produce an appropriate response and react to it (i.e., avoid the hazard). Deficits in processing speed are a common consequence of acquired brain disorders, and slowing of processing speed is a common consequence of normal aging.

Language functioning involves an individual's ability to communicate by comprehending verbal information (in an auditory or written modality) and responding to such information through the use of verbal or nonverbal expression. Although the relationship between driving and language disruption is not immediately apparent, alexia (the inability to read) or aphasia (the inability to understand or express language) may hinder driving fitness. For example an individual with alexia may be unable to interpret road signs, particularly those that cannot be immediately identified by shape, and an individual with aphasia may be unable to ask for or respond to directions or assistance. Although language functioning is not commonly cited as pivotal in decisions regarding driving fitness, some studies have indicated that left hemisphere damage, including sequelae such as aphasia,[2,3] is sufficient to substantially compromise fitness to drive.

Memory functioning can have a considerable impact on driving ability. Memory can be conceptualized as occurring in three stages: encoding (the ability to acquire new information), consolidation (the transformation of new information to permanent storage), and retrieval (the ability to recall learned material). The most obvious manifestation of problems in this domain entails being unable to learn new driving routes and/or to recall these routes without extensive rehearsal. Research suggests that among individuals with Alzheimer's disease (AD), which is characterized by memory impairment, as dementia advances from a severity level of "very mild" to "mild," driving impairment becomes a significant traffic safety problem.[4] Although memory problems are most commonly associated with dementia, deficits in memory also are common after TBI or stroke, and in disorders such as multiple sclerosis. Decreased memory functioning also is characteristic of normal aging but is not considered to be problematic unless there is a diagnosis of dementia.

Visuospatial functioning and visuomotor functioning are instrumental to driving.[5] Visuospatial disorders can be grouped into four basic categories[6]: defective localization of points in space, difficulties judging direction and distance of or length of stimuli (often related to impaired depth perception), impaired topographic orientation (knowledge of geographic location), and unilateral visual neglect. Deficits in visuospatial functioning can affect an individual's ability to assess the location of visual stimuli while driving (i.e., curbs, pedestrians, street lights, and other vehicles) and increase the likelihood that an individual may become disoriented or lost. Visuomotor disturbances refer to any deficit in making movement directed by visual stimuli. Visual scanning is the most notable aspect of visuomotor functioning related to driving. In a cognitively intact individual, visual scanning occurs in an organized fashion, and the systematic approach to examining the visual environment plays an important role in how the environment is perceived or how the brain processes the information. Many persons with acquired brain disorders have abnormal eye movements that result in a disorganized or inaccurate translation of the visual world. Risk for crashes while driving even a wheelchair increases substantially when these impairments arise.[7,8]

Executive functioning represents the highest level of cognitive functioning and is especially susceptible to impairment after brain damage. There is growing recognition that this domain of cognition has a tremendous impact on functional outcomes such as driving. Executive functioning includes a broad spectrum of abilities, including anticipatory behavior, problem solving, self-monitoring, and self-assessment, all of which are critical aspects of risk and fitness to drive.[9] The term can also encompass other high-level aspects of cognitive functioning that sometimes overlap with the domain of attention, including multitasking, mental flexibility, inhibitory ability, and attentional vigilance functions. Other aspects of executive functioning include abstract thinking, insight, and preserved personality functioning. Often neuropsychological test batteries for driving assessment have been brief, largely neglecting important domains such as executive functioning.[10-13] Although the ability to drive a motor vehicle relies heavily on perception, motor skills, and information processing speed, numerous investigators have emphasized the special importance of executive functions in making determinations about an individual's driving ability.[14-16]

THE ROLE OF EXECUTIVE FUNCTIONING IN DRIVING

Various studies indicate that risk for accidents is moderated by higher-order cognitive abilities[17-20] and that performance on tasks of executive functioning is predictive of on-road driving ability. Coleman et al[21] reported that performance on tasks of executive functioning, combined with years postinjury and disability at discharge from a rehabilitation hospital, predicted postdischarge traffic accidents and violations after TBI. Similarly Daigneault et al[17] reported that older drivers with a history of accidents performed more poorly than control subjects on tasks of executive functioning. The standard versions of the *Trails B*[22] and the *Stroop*[23] tests, both commonly used neuropsychological tasks evaluating executive function, have shown strong correlations with driving ability.[18,20] Other commonly used tests of executive functioning that have shown strong predictive utility include the *Matrix Reasoning* and *Letter-Number Sequencing* subtests of the Wechsler Adult Intelligence Scale (WAIS)–III,[24] the *Colored Trails Test*,[25] the *Tower of London*,[26] and the *Wisconsin Card Sorting Test*.[27]

Executive functions also play a major role in the functional capacity of other cognitive and motor functions. Perceptual and motor skills may be intact but functionally hindered by the complexity of the stimulus challenge. The *Useful Field of Vision* (UFOV)[28] test illustrates this point by combining assessment of simple peripheral vision with assessment of functional visual capacity during conditions of increased cognitive load.

Selective and divided attention tasks are included to mimic real world conditions in which stimulus fields may be complex and cluttered. Research using the UFOV test generally has demonstrated that the functional range of peripheral vision is inversely related to cognitive load.[29] The UFOV test has shown strong predictive validity for crashes and driving evaluations[30-34] and 86% accuracy predicting the outcome of driving evaluations[35] among older adults. The test is gaining popularity in the driving evaluation process; however, generalizability of UFOV validity research to persons with acquired brain disorders, such as stroke and TBI, has been limited.

Two studies indicated that the UFOV test might be useful in assessing driving readiness in TBI survivors.[36,37] TBI survivors performed more poorly on the UFOV test than did college students, and the authors interpreted this finding as possibly indicative of a higher risk for crashes[37]; however, no actual assessment of driving safety was conducted. In fact only 9% of the TBI survivors scored above the UFOV test cutoff associated with increased risk of crash among healthy older adults. Considering that TBI survivors fail driving evaluations at rates of 30% to 60%, it may not have good predictive validity in this population. Fisk et al[37] and Calvanio et al[36] found that the UFOV test correlated strongly with several standard visual attention tests, including *Trails A and B*, but neither study directly examined the relationship of performance on the UFOV test and actual driving ability. Although these findings provide some support for generalizing crash-risk research on the UFOV test to persons with TBI, a high correlation between the UFOV test and *Trails B* highlights the importance of simultaneously examining the unique predictive powers of measures used to assess fitness to drive.

SELF-AWARENESS OF DEFICIT, EXECUTIVE FUNCTIONING, AND COMPENSATORY STRATEGIES

A number of theorists have proposed that executive function is a complex phenomenon made up of a variety of cognitive processes or modules. Research findings support the notion that executive functions may be made up of a number of overlapping elements that dissociate during certain cognitive and behavioral tasks.[38] Any number of these executive processes or modules may be differentially impaired in any patient with brain damage, and each damaged process/module may manifest its own unique behavioral and cognitive sequelae.[38] Self-reflection or self-awareness is one such module of executive functioning. Persons with neurologic disorders frequently evidence poor self-awareness of their impairments as indicated by a discrepancy between self-ratings and observer ratings of their functioning.[39-42] Tests of executive functioning show strong correlations with observer ratings of dysexecutive problems in everyday life,[38,43] and these tasks are better predictors of lack of insight than are tests of premorbid intellectual functions, intelligence quotient (IQ), memory, or language.[38]

Issues of self-awareness have been identified as important in predicting accidents, further emphasizing the importance of assessing various aspects of executive functioning in the standard driving evaluation. In three studies Rapport et al[44-46] examined risk for in-patient fall among right hemisphere stroke, elderly, and TBI samples. Each study found that tests of executive functioning better predicted risk for accidents than did measures of physical impairment or motor ability. In essence, self-regulatory aspects of executive control may moderate fall risk associated with impairment in other cognitive domains, such as visuospatial functioning.

In the context of resumption of driving, the relationship between cognitive impairment and driver safety can be conceptualized as a curvilinear distribution with mildly impaired and profoundly impaired individuals least likely to be at risk. Risk of accident for the former group is low because of their minimal level of impairment, whereas risk of accident for the latter group is low because their profound level of impairment makes it unlikely that they will attempt to drive. In the spectrum that lies between these groups, self-awareness acts as the critical moderating variable. Individuals with intact self-awareness of deficit, regardless of the extent of their neurocognitive and physical limitations, are less likely to act in ways that place themselves and others in jeopardy. In contrast underappreciation of even mild deficits can increase risk substantially. A study investigating the relationship between neuropsychological test results and on-road driving performance among patients with neurologic disorders (i.e., cerebrovascular accident, TBI, and multiple sclerosis) indicated that awareness of cognitive impairment, in addition to performance on measures of visuoconstructive ability, reaction time, and visual attention, was able to discriminate between groups with varying levels of driving ability.[20]

Self-awareness plays an important role in the ability to adopt compensatory behaviors. An individual who is unaware of his or her limitations has no reason to change his or her behavior; recognition of a "problem" is the first step toward adaptation or the use of strategies to compensate. For example Hanks et al[47] showed that objective (i.e., behaviorally anchored) measures of ability were strongly related to performance on tasks of executive function and that higher-level cognitive abil-

ities influence the ability to compensate for unresolved impairment in these domains.

Several studies of driving resumption in individuals with neurologic disorders underscore the importance of compensatory potential. van Zomeren et al[48] found no relationship between neurologic status and driving skill, and they discuss their results in terms of patients' compensatory potential. Similarly Cotrell and Wild[49] concluded that awareness of deficit might be critical to restricting driving behavior among patients with AD because the ability to adapt driving behavior to cognitive limitations might prolong their status as drivers. The potential for compensatory behavior to moderate on-road accident risk is supported by other investigators as well.[9,50-52]

COGNITIVE PERFORMANCES AS A PREDICTOR OF FITNESS TO DRIVE

Overall relicensing rates for disabled drivers in a rehabilitation setting are as high as 72%, with 90% of persons with noncognitive disabilities (e.g., spinal cord injury, congenital disability, and muscular dystrophy) resuming driving and 50% of persons with cognitive impairments (e.g., stroke, cerebral palsy, and closed head injury) achieving this goal.[16,53,54] Literature on disability and driving generally indicates that disabilities per se are not related to increased rates of crashes or violations. In fact most disabled drivers are highly motivated to be good drivers,[16] and according to Schultheis et al[55] persons with TBI who complete a comprehensive driving evaluation reintegrate into the driving community without increased risk for accident.

Historically there has been an assumption that psychomotor abilities, including visual scanning, attention, and reaction time, comprise the basis of a construct characterized as driving skill.[15] The implicit assumption based on this construct is that degree of driving skill is directly related to driver performance. Unfortunately, although driving skill has been shown least predictive of actual driving behavior or accident risk,[56] most state licensing examinations have been based on this notion. A large body of literature suggests that knowledge of driving regulations and basic psychomotor abilities, such as coordination and reaction time, are among the least predictive factors of accident risk. For instance young drivers, who typically possess optimum physical abilities, are those with the highest risk for accident and traffic violation.[57,58] Conley and Smiley[59] performed a comprehensive study of driving records of 22,253 drivers during a 4-year period and failed to find any consistent relationship between "knowledge" examinations and the frequency or type of accidents and moving violations. Based on their review Hopewell and van Zomeren[15] asserted that neither knowledge of driving nor skill level is an adequate predictor of driving behavior. Therefore driving skills may be more accurately viewed as *necessary* rather than *sufficient* for safe driving.[18]

Because evaluating driving skills alone is not an adequate assessment of driving ability, neuropsychological testing serves to augment the standard driving evaluation. Cognitive impairments identified as playing a significant role in poor driving include reduced awareness, inadequate scanning, disinhibition, impulsivity, reduced information processing, concrete thinking, poor judgment, impaired problem solving, impaired executive function, distractibility, and attentional deficits.[1] Memory deficits, reduced endurance, impaired sequencing, and visual and spatial impairment are also commonly identified.[1,5,60] In a review of driver's training programs,[54] deficits in judgment and reasoning and/or the inability to follow direction often prevented patients from successfully obtaining relicensure.

There are several well-recognized driving assessments in which standard neuropsychological testing is incorporated. The *Cognitive Behavioral Driver's Inventory* (CBDI)[1] includes computerized and standardized psychometric tasks. Standardized psychometric tests in this battery include *Picture Completion* and *Digit Symbol* from the *WAIS–Revised*[61] and *Trails A and B*.[22] Predictive accuracy of on-road evaluation based on the cognitive and perceptual test performance of the CDBI was as high as 89% in a neurologically disordered sample; however, for patients in the borderline range there was not a significant relationship between the test performance and the on-road evaluation. The two subgroups with weak relationships between performance on the CBDI and the on-road evaluation were young TBI patients, who drive worse than the CBDI predicted, and elderly patients, who drive better than the CBDI predicted. Nonetheless the creators of the CBDI recommend that the on-road test be part of the evaluation of fitness to drive in young TBI patients and elderly patients.

The *Coorabel Program*[62] is another popular driving inventory that has shown considerable success in the prediction of on-road driving performance. The Coorabel neuropsychological battery includes *Visual Form Discrimination*,[6] *Judgment of Line Orientation*,[6] *Trails A and B*,[22] *Benton Visual Retention Test*,[63] *Picture Completion, Block Design*, and *Digit Symbol*.[61] The Coorabel Program yielded a slightly better rate of prediction compared with the CBDI.[62] Only 3 of 129 cases passed the neuropsychological assessment and subsequently failed the road test; however, the authors conceded that a multidisciplinary assessment of driver

competence, inclusive of on-road testing, is necessary and that medical guidelines alone are insufficient to predict driver fitness.

In another study[64] a standard neuropsychological battery was administered to a diverse clinical population of drivers and nondrivers. The authors used discriminant function analysis to compare the neuropsychological performance of the two groups. Driving status was well predicted by neuropsychological tests of general function (*Information, Digit Symbol, Token Test*, and *Rey Complex Figure Test*). Motor skills (*Finger Tapping* and *Rey Complex Figure Copy Time*) and visual recognition skills (*Rey Complex Figure False Negative and Recognition*) were also valuable predictors. The authors concluded that it is possible to predict driving status in a real-life clinical sample from neuropsychological assessment.

A variety of outcome criteria may be used in evaluating the utility of neuropsychological testing in driving assessment, including performance on a driving simulator or in an on-road evaluation, driving records, or family member reports. Each of these criteria has advantages and disadvantages, but none is a perfect measure of fitness to drive. Often the final decision regarding driving competency is based on a comprehensive driving evaluation that includes a simulator and an on-road and/or parking lot evaluation. In these types of studies neuropsychological tests have shown predictive value in the assessment of fitness to drive.[5,10,65,66] One study using family member reports of driving ability as the criterion found that a short neuropsychological battery that included the *Token Test, Rey Complex Figure, Finger Tapping*, and several subtests of the *WAIS* was able to identify individuals who were deemed competent to drive and those who were not.[64] In sum, although some studies have yielded mixed findings,* many studies conducted during the past two decades using a variety of outcome criteria (on-road evaluations, driving records, and family member reports) lend credence to the ecological validity of neuropsychological testing in the assessment of fitness to drive. Nonetheless the overwhelming consensus is that neuropsychological evaluations should supplement on-road tests rather than serve as the sole criterion of fitness to drive.†

Although the combined findings of previous research support the validity of neuropsychological assessment in evaluating fitness to drive, methodological problems limit the clinical application of most of the individual studies. Selection bias in archival studies of convenience samples, small sample sizes, or investigations that are limited to a single neuropsychological

---

*References 12,13,16,48,67,68.
†References 11,16,62,67,69,70.

predictor are frequently encountered.[3,9,52,71-77] Although multivariate methods are essential to facilitate prediction of driving outcome, the majority of studies using these methods violated important assumptions of the statistical models, primarily because of inadequate ratio of cases to variables, which leads to overfitting and spuriously high prediction models.*

There has been no consensus among clinicians about the selection of tests or normative databases used to determine who should pass a comprehensive driving evaluation,[80] and it is apparent that a standard test battery designed to be sensitive to general cognitive dysfunction is not well suited for identifying specific functional capacities, such as driving.† Furthermore clinical settings and empirical research investigating fitness to drive have largely neglected to compare the relative predictive values of the neuropsychological measures administered.

In addition to these methodological weaknesses, generalizability from studies conducted in Europe and other countries outside of the United States is also questionable. Return to driving and driving habits may be affected by various cultural and environmental factors, such as the availability and use of public transportation. Compared with European countries, the United States has a higher proportion of eligible persons who drive, as well as a higher proportion of women who drive.[81-83] For example in two studies conducted in the United Kingdom, only one-third of survivors drove before their stroke,[82,83] and men represented >90% of poststroke drivers.[82]

The frequent use of mixed populations is also highly problematic, given well-established differences in the physical and cognitive sequelae of the various acquired neurologic disorders. In many studies the neurologic sample is a diverse clinical group (i.e., including stroke, TBI, cerebral palsy, seizure disorders, and multiple sclerosis). This approach dilutes subtle test patterns and significant findings that may be unique to a particular clinical population. For example stroke survivors generally are older than other populations of persons with neurologic disorders. Problems with visuoperceptual abilities and slowed reaction time increase with age[34,84] and are commonly observed after stroke.[31] Older drivers[84-88] and stroke survivors[3,29] are known to use compensatory strategies that may moderate risk observed in younger counterparts with similar functional impairments.[89,90] Considering that individuals within particular diagnostic categories possess a unique neuropsychological, demographic, and medical profile, it is important to examine the relationship between neuropsychological performance and driving ability within

each of the following clinical subgroups individually: TBI survivors, stroke survivors, individuals with dementia, and healthy, older drivers.

TBI SURVIVORS

Visuospatial deficits and psychomotor retardation, as well as longer posttraumatic amnesia and lower IQ scores, have been identified as reasons that TBI survivors are unable to resume driving.[91] Several of the early driving studies evaluating risk for accident after TBI suggested that TBI survivors posed an increased risk even after a considerable recovery period and compared with their age- and driving experience–matched counterparts. Hopewell and Price[91] found that approximately 25% of brain-injured drivers who were able to return to driving were considered potentially "high-risk" drivers. Stokx and Gaillard[92] reported that patients 2 years after severe concussion responded more slowly than did healthy adults on reaction time tasks and on driving tasks. van Zomeren et al[48] found that TBI survivors performed worse than a healthy control group matched for age and driving experience with regard to lateral position control on a highway track in an instrumented vehicle and during rides in the subjects' own vehicles with professional observers. Notably they found no relationship between neurologic status, as measured by length of posttraumatic amnesia and Glasgow Coma Scale (Box 7-1), and driving skill.

BOX 7-1	Glasgow Coma Scale

EYES OPEN
4 Spontaneously
3 On request
2 To pain stimuli (supraorbital or digital)
1 No opening

BEST VERBAL RESPONSE
5 Oriented to time, place, person
4 Engages in conversation, confused in content
3 Words spoken but conversation not sustained
2 Groans evoked by pain
1 No response

BEST MOTOR RESPONSE
5 Obeys a command ("Hold out three fingers.")
4 Localizes a painful stimulus
3 Flexes either arm
2 Extends arm to painful stimulus
1 No response

From Phipps WJ, Monahan FD, Sands JK, et al: Medical-surgical nursing: health and illness perspectives, ed 7, St. Louis, 2003, Mosby.

---

*References 5,35,52,66,71,73-75,78,79
†References 3,9,13,52,71-77.

Many TBI survivors who resume driving do have residual deficits that may impair the knowledge and skill necessary to drive safely.[5,8,10,16,54] However, it is important to note that low estimated fitness percentages concern patients with severe TBI.[93] Brain-injured individuals who restrict their driving activity may mitigate their increased risk for accident.[94] Katz et al[68] examined the driving safety of TBI and stroke survivors who passed a comprehensive driving evaluation and who were followed for up to 5 years and found no difference between patient and control groups in type of driving, incidence of speeding tickets, near accidents, accidents, or the cost of vehicle damage when accidents occurred.

In the few studies that evaluate the utility of neuropsychological testing in evaluation of fitness to drive among samples comprising exclusively TBI survivors, results have been mixed. van Zomeren et al[48] found that although TBI survivors evidenced significant impairment on the neuropsychological battery and drove worse than a healthy control group that was matched on age and driving experience, the only relationships found between neuropsychological test performance and actual driving ability involved visuomotor impairment as measured by the *Benton Visual Retention Test* and *Trails A* and slower performance on the *Minnesota Rate of Manipulation Test* and lateral position control. Although TBI survivors performed worse than control subjects on measures of attention (as measured by the *Bourdon, Stroop, Digit Symbol,* and *Choice Reaction Time*), there was no relationship between their performances on these measures and actual on-road driving ability. In another study evaluating the predictive ability of four neuropsychological tests (*Perceptual Speed* test, *WAIS Symbol-Digit Substitution* subtest, *Tracking-Reaction* dual task, and a *Time Estimation* task) to performance on an open-road driving test, only the tests of perceptual speed and time estimation were significantly correlated with driving performance.[11] When combined with coma duration and driving experience, performance on these two tasks explained a significant proportion of performance on the open-road evaluation. Nonetheless these authors concluded that neuropsychological tests were insufficient to completely replace an open-road driving evaluation; however, these authors' conclusions regarding "neuropsychological" testing seem rather broad considering that their test battery was extremely limited. Brooke et al[95] found a significant relationship between the sum of rated scores of the *Tactual Performance Test*[96] and *Trail Making Test*[22] and the global pass/fail ratings of the open-road evaluation, but it was not linearly related to the driving performance score on which those final ratings were based.

In contrast to these negative findings regarding the relationship between neuropsychological performance

and on-road driving ability, Gouvier et al[12] found that all of the neuropsychological measures they administered to a sample of brain-injured (and spinal cord–injured) patients were significant predictors of driving ability and that some were highly predictive. Their neuropsychological battery included several subtests from the *WAIS–Revised,*[61] the *Motor Free Visual Perception Test,*[97] the *Baylor Adult Visual Perceptual Assessment,*[98] *Trail Making Tests,*[22] and the *Symbol-Digit Modalities Test.*[99] They found that the oral version of the *Symbol-Digit Modalities* test accounted for 70% of variability in performance observed on a full-sized vehicle driving score. Although the authors did not advocate replacing an on-road evaluation with a neuropsychological battery alone, they strongly supported the use of neuropsychological testing to screen for on-road evaluation. Similarly in our research[21] there were significant differences between drivers and nondrivers on measures including the *Colored Trails Test* and two subtests of the *WAIS-III* (*Letter-Number Sequencing* and *Matrix Reasoning*) in an urban sample of TBI survivors.

STROKE SURVIVORS

Research investigating individuals with a history of stroke indicates that, similar to TBI survivors, these individuals may have residual deficits that compromise their driving ability. However, those stroke survivors who resume driving may compensate for residual impairments by strategically limiting their exposure (e.g., avoiding night driving, heavy traffic, and long trips).[3,37] These findings are supported by general research on older drivers.[84-88] Additionally survivors with history of at-fault accidents tend to limit their driving more than do survivors without histories of such events.[85] Thus self-monitoring, including cessation of driving among 50% to 70% of stroke survivors, is one successful mechanism to manage risk. Driver retraining and education regarding risk reduction also have been shown to be effective among persons with neurologic disorder[10,31,55,68] and high-risk older drivers.[84,100] Therefore, although cessation is an effective manner to limit risk, the personal cost of that decision may be unnecessarily high for the sizable number of (traumatic and nontraumatic) brain injury survivors who could resume driving safely.

A body of research supports the value of neuropsychological assessment in predicting fitness to drive after stroke.* In one study, tests involving complex reasoning skills showed a significant relationship with the overall grading of driving performance.[104] Another study of 84 stroke survivors[19] reported that individuals who passed

---

*References 19,52,74,75,79,101-103.

the on-road evaluation had better scores on the majority of perceptual tests than did those who failed. Those patients who performed poorly on the combination of tests determined most predictive, including the *Motor-Free Visuoperceptual Test* (MVPT)[97] and *Trails B*,[22] were 22 times more likely to fail the on-road evaluation than were patients who performed well on the neuropsychological measures. Studies of mixed samples that included stroke survivors confirm the value of neuropsychological tests in enhancing classification accuracy for on-road evaluations.*

Examination of *stroke-specific* factors associated with driving fitness has been limited and has yielded mixed findings. For example some studies indicate that survivors of right hemisphere strokes have greater risk for automobile accident than do survivors of left hemisphere strokes[10,19,102,107] and may be more difficult to retrain to drive.[108] These findings make intuitive sense because visual and attentional deficits are more commonly observed with right hemisphere insult, as is denial of illness.[109] For example previous studies found that survivors of right hemisphere stroke who show unilateral neglect or rightward-orienting bias are more prone to accidents in wheelchair driving than are their left hemisphere counterparts on in vivo obstacle courses[7,8,110] and in computer-simulation wheelchair-driving paradigms.[111,112] However, several studies have found no association between side of brain lesion and the decision to drive or pass rates on driving evaluations.† Some studies have indicated that left hemisphere damage,[29] including sequelae such as aphasia,[2,3] is sufficient to compromise fitness to drive substantially. Unfortunately the relative risks associated with classic symptoms of left and right hemisphere insults are difficult to determine because many studies excluded persons with aphasia. Archival and convenience samples drawn from driver evaluation centers[19,30,78,101,102] also typically suffer from referral and selection bias. Persons whose deficits are obviously relevant to driving, more frequent in right versus left hemisphere damage, are referred for evaluation more often than are persons with deficits such as aphasia and impaired comprehension.

INDIVIDUALS WITH DEMENTIA

Most studies evaluating driving and dementia have examined individuals with AD. Presumably individuals with vascular dementia are included in studies of stroke and driving, adding another methodological problem to this body of literature. Retrospective surveys have suggested that many individuals with AD continue to

drive[115,116] and have a higher risk of crashes.[117,118] Several studies have taken the severity of AD into account when making recommendations regarding whether an individual can demonstrate a reasonable level of driving competence. The University of Washington developed a Clinical Dementia Rating scale (CDR)[119,120] that taps a wide range of cognitive abilities based on a 90-minute interview with the patient and a collateral source. A study of the risk of driving and AD based on a systematic review of the literature using the National Library of Medicine's MEDLINE database indicated that driving is mildly impaired in those drivers with probable AD at a severity level equivalent to a CDR score reflecting "very mild dementia" and is no greater than that tolerated in other segments of the driving population (e.g., drivers age 16 to 21 years and those driving under the influence of alcohol at a blood alcohol concentration of <0.08%); however, driving ability becomes a significant traffic safety problem based on crashes and other driving performance indices when AD has progressed to a CDR score reflecting "mild dementia."[4]

Considerable evidence suggests that deficits in selective attention are particularly important to impaired driving performance among persons with AD.[121,122] One study examining the relationship between cognitive test scores and driving performance in individuals with very mild and mild AD indicated that error rate and reaction time on a visual search task were the best predictors of driving performance.[123] Moreover visual search performance provided incremental predictive ability beyond level of dementia severity and performance on several traditional psychometric tests. In addition to providing support for the use of neuropsychological testing in helping to identify "at-risk" drivers, this study underscores the importance of assessing visual attention in the driving evaluation because it was correlated with on-road driving performance.

There is not consensus in the literature regarding the specific neuropsychological deficits that place a patient with dementia "at risk" on the road, but there is mounting evidence that neuropsychological test performances are related to driving outcomes that are considered important. For example a meta-analysis of 27 studies that examined the relationship between neuropsychological functioning and driving ability for adults with dementia found a significant relationship between performance in many cognitive domains, including attention, visuospatial functioning, attention, memory, executive functioning, and language, and on-road or nonroad driving measures.[124] Cognitive decline as indicated by neuropsychological testing was related to decline in driving ability.

A study using single-photon emission computed tomography (SPECT) to examine driving ability in

---

*References 5,10,20,35,65,66,70,105,106.
†References 30,31,51,78,101,113,114.

individuals with AD found that impaired driving ability was associated with reduction in cortical perfusion. Specifically, reduction of perfusion was noted in the right hemisphere, particularly in the temporo-occipital area.[125] With increased severity of driving impairment, frontal cortical perfusion was also reduced. Based on these findings the authors advocated the use of measures of visuoperceptual and executive functions in identifying those at greatest risk for driving impairment rather than rely on measures tapping left hemisphere–based verbal tasks.

A number of studies have indicated that neuropsychological evaluation and even neuroimaging may be useful in driving assessment of patients with AD; however, some mixed findings have been reported. Bieliauskas et al[89] found that certain global cognitive measures predicted some driving errors for patients with AD; however, neuropsychological tests demonstrated relatively weak overall power in predicting driving errors. These authors speculated that driving requires relatively overlearned skills (e.g., procedural memory) that are somewhat independent of many specific neuropsychological measures. However, the battery of neuropsychological measures administered was limited and did not include measures of higher-order executive functioning or self-awareness. Trobe et al[69] examined the relationship between neuropsychological test scores and driving record in a large sample of individuals with AD. These authors reported that neuropsychological test scores did not predict crashes or violations; however, their neuropsychological battery also was brief and did not include any measures of executive functioning or self-awareness.

Although neuropsychological tests to date have been found to be insufficient predictors of fitness to drive in persons with AD, results have been useful in screening candidates for the on-road evaluation. Other driving experts suggest that cognitive evaluation be used in conjunction with standardized driving performance evaluation.[78,95]

HEALTHY, OLDER DRIVERS

There are an increasing number of licensed drivers aged ≥70 years. Some reports suggest that between 1987 and 1997 the number of older drivers increased 45%.[126] There has been a corresponding increase in the number of older drivers involved in fatal crashes, making driving assessment in older adults a particularly important area of research. Similar to studies evaluating the predictive ability of neuropsychological testing in diverse clinical populations, the findings in geriatric populations tend to be mixed. However, the notion that driving may require relatively overlearned skills[89] may have bearing on older persons' fitness to drive despite

known decrements in reaction time and complex attention that accompany aging. Older persons generally show poorer driving-related skills, including increased eye movements and slower driving speeds in a driving simulator, although they do not show significantly higher on-road accident rates than younger groups, which suggests that they are able to behaviorally compensate for their visuocognitive and motor deficits.[127] Given the considerable driving experience amassed by most older drivers, Brouwer et al[128] reported that driving programs should be aimed at providing older drivers with information regarding their psychological abilities and driving skills to give them the opportunity to adopt compensatory strategies. However, Daigneault et al[17] compared older drivers who had a history of accidents with those who did not and found that despite their records the higher-risk drivers reported using compensatory strategies and adopting less-risky driving behavior. These authors emphasized the importance of measuring executive functions, apart from willingness to adopt compensatory strategies, in the driving assessment of older persons.

Visual deficits are common in elderly patients and are a predictor of vehicle crashes in older adults.[33] Therefore visual attention must be carefully evaluated during driving assessment. The UFOV test has been found to be a reliable and valid indicator of visual information-processing deficits in the elderly population.[28] In another study of elderly patients[129] significant correlations were obtained between in-traffic and a test of global cognitive functioning. Measures of problem solving, response inhibition, general anxiety, and variability in attention have been found to be significant predictors of relative decline in successful obstacle avoidance among healthy older adults.[130] A review on assessment of fitness to drive in older drivers with cognitive impairment[131] reported that cognitively impaired persons as a group performed significantly worse than did healthy control subjects on neuropsychological and driving measures. However, only low to moderate correlations could be established between neuropsychological test results and on-road driving performance, making it difficult to discriminate between cognitively impaired patients who were fit or unfit to drive. Nonetheless the authors advocated the use of the *Trail Making Test*, visual attention tests, and tests of visuoperceptual abilities as a means to screen for an on-road evaluation (i.e., older drivers who performed well would receive their license without further examination). Although chronological age and cognitive status, particularly executive functions, are correlated with crashes, they may be relatively poor at discriminating between those who are fit or unfit to drive.[17,33] See Chapters 6, 12, and 21 for more information on vision and driving.

PSYCHOLOGICAL CHARACTERISTICS AND TBI

A review of the literature suggests that personality and behavioral disturbances also have been implicated in driving safety.[132] Personality changes, such as emotional lability, reduced insight, and increased irritability, in conjunction with decreased impulse control, a high rate of driving exposure, and a widespread lack of driving fitness testing may compound the issue of safety to drive after TBI.[133] The relationship between substance use and risk for motor vehicle accidents is also widely appreciated. Similarly aggression (i.e., "road rage") is widely recognized as a hazard associated with increased risk for accident and mortality.[134-136] Hopewell et al[15] reviewed the literature and concluded that beyond the primary functional abilities required for safe driving, psychological factors, including pattern and severity of substance abuse and nature and extent of psychiatric and executive disturbance, accounted for a great deal of driving skill and driving risk. Matthews et al[137] found that the aggression dimension of a driver stress inventory predicted frequent and error-prone overtaking on a driving simulator. Several authors have suggested that measures of aggression and substance use should be included in standard driving assessment batteries.[15,138] Thus far, however, although they are recognized as important, measures of this nature have not been thoroughly examined in the context of a standard driving assessment or in the prediction of long-term driving safety among persons with neurologic disorder.

DRIVING RESUMPTION POSTREHABILITATION

THE CAREGIVER HOLDS THE KEYS

Family support has been identified as among the most critical factors in achieving rehabilitation success, including return to driving.[20] Brain injury survivors who resume driving often report that their decision to do so was dependent on advice they received from family members, physicians, or other health care professionals.[133] Unfortunately survivors and family members rarely have sufficient knowledge to form opinions on an empirical basis. Furthermore patients and caregivers place differential emphasis on cognitive and physical abilities in their judgment of the patient's level of functioning.[47]

Our research indicated that although neuropsychological functioning was the strongest predictor of actual driving safety among 60 brain injury survivors, caregiver perceptions of the survivors' driving ability was the strongest predictor of their driving status and number of miles driven postinjury.[21] In other words the caregivers of brain injury survivors "hold the keys to the car." Unfortunately the relation between caregiver perceptions and survivor neuropsychological functioning was modest at best. Thus caregivers and significant others may be making this important determination based on inadequate or inaccurate information. A meta-analysis indicated that the relationship between neuropsychological functioning and driving ability for adults with dementia indicated a significant relationship between cognitive measures and driving, but caregiver reports of driving ability and cognitive variables were correlated significantly only on measures of mental status and visuospatial skills.[124] The relation between survivor perceptions of restrictions and actual medical contraindications to driving is also weak[139]; thus many individuals who could resume driving safely may not do so because they misinterpret information about their medical fitness to drive. In literature on stroke, research indicates the presence of a similar phenomenon to TBI: professional advice on driving is frequently absent or inaccurate.[133,139,140] Most survivors report that they received no driving advice from health professionals after their stroke.[133,140]

OTHER POTENTIAL OBSTACLES

In addition to caregivers' perceptions, a number of other factors may preclude brain injury survivors' return to driving, including physical disability, cognitive impairment, psychological issues, and limited resources (e.g., limited or no access to a motor vehicle). Anxiety is one such psychological factor that has recently been identified as influencing the decision to resume or cease driving.[141] Schultheis et al[55] explored some of these issues among 47 TBI survivors who had successfully completed a comprehensive driving evaluation; however, the influences of these factors on resumption of driving have not been investigated among the broad population of individuals completing rehabilitation who do and do not resume driving.

Clearly some barriers to driving are legitimate factors that should limit or terminate driving privileges; however, many individuals with acquired brain disorder resume driving despite increased risk associated with impairments for which they cannot compensate safely. It is unclear whether these individuals inaccurately believe that they are fit to drive[9] or drive despite knowledge that they are at high risk.[51] The accuracy of perceptions regarding barriers to driving has a direct bearing on the validity of decisions regarding driving behavior. In sum many persons with neurologic disorder who are competent to drive do not do so. Others may have impairments that could be addressed with adaptive equipment or remediated through retraining. It is essential to identify barriers to driving and their influence on community integration, as well as factors that do and do not affect fitness to drive so that interventions to improve access and safety can be enhanced to maximize independence and community integration of persons with acquired disabilities.

DRIVING AND COMMUNITY INTEGRATION

The ability to drive a motor vehicle may be regarded as an activity of daily living (ADL) because it directly affects level of independence and membership in a community. The ramifications of having driving privileges restricted or removed are immense. Driving privileges affect the ADL of the driver (e.g., accessibility to work, shopping, banking, and childcare responsibilities) and may have a significant impact on the families and significant others of those people. Of all of the potential life consequences of sustaining a brain injury, the possibility of facing driving restriction is of greater concern to patients than are any other functional limitations.[18] Rehabilitation professionals must balance concern for maximizing community reintegration of patients with the increasingly higher legal and ethical standards to which they are held with respect to protection of public interest.[18]

Several studies indicate that independence in driving is important to aspects of community integration. Research on persons with disabilities indicates that independent driving has a substantial influence on outcomes such as social participation, occupation, and social mobility, as well as feelings of connectedness and freedom from social limitations.[142-145] For example among persons with spinal cord injury, driving has independent effects on return to work and maintaining a job[142,143] and restrictions on social activities.[143] Similarly among persons with TBI, independence in driving has a substantial relation to job stability; persons who drive independently are four times more likely to find stable employment than those who do not.[144] Cessation of driving hinders access to social participation and decreases out-of-home activity (i.e., social mobility), which are essential aspects of community integration and have been linked directly to increased rates of physical and psychological morbidity, mortality, and depression.[3,82,146-148] It is noteworthy that Legh-Smith[82] found that cessation of driving adversely affects social activities and risk for depression among stroke survivors, even among persons having easy access to alternative transportation. Cessation of driving also has been linked to connectedness and social role via feelings of loneliness,[149] anger and frustration associated with new limitations on vocational and recreational activities,[150] adverse changes in personal roles,[150] and feelings of diminished autonomy and mobility.[149]

PARADIGM SHIFT IN THE FIELD OF DRIVING ASSESSMENT

REDEFINING DRIVING ASSESSMENT

Rather than viewing the driving assessment as a means of predicting safety, driving assessment has shifted to a focus on risk assessment. Brouwer and Withaar[54] emphasize that assessment of fitness to drive must examine the degree to which impaired cognitive functions affect ADL and level of insight. According to Hopewell[18] the task of rehabilitation professionals is less about determining whether someone can drive and more about emphasizing the identification of those drivers at "high risk" for accidents and developing treatment or management strategies that will maximize their independence while minimizing their risk. Similarly Galski et al[80] urge clinicians, lawmakers, and researchers to consider viewing the goal of driving evaluations as "determining who manifests an unacceptably high risk of making errors in human performance that cause accidents, near accidents, and/or property damage" rather viewing them as a tool of predicting who is a "safe driver."

To advance the field of driving assessment with the ultimate goal of maximizing our accuracy in assessment of driving risk, clinicians and scientists alike will eventually use measures in a neuropsychological battery that have been validated specifically for the purpose of assessing driving risk. Based on the current state of the literature, this battery would include tasks of visuospatial functioning, processing speed, visual attention, and multiple executive tasks including those that tap self-awareness of deficit and ability to adopt compensatory strategies. Additionally collection of a variety of biographical, medical, and psychological data would be routine (i.e., driving history, current driving exposure, substance use, current medications, and a brief personality screen). Similarly the on-road driving evaluation would be standardized.

Standardization of the driving assessment would have multiple advantages. From a clinical perspective it would lend itself to more thorough, accurate driving assessment; from the standpoint of research the validity of commonly administered tests could be easily examined across a wide sample of individuals. Standardization would also provide the foundation to begin investigating the various, unique aspects of different diagnostic groups and "customization" of the driving evaluation accordingly. The notion that a neuropsychological battery that adequately evaluates risk in one group of rehabilitation patients (e.g., stroke) may not be appropriate for another group (e.g., TBI) must be promoted and practiced. Until there is recognition that individuals in different diagnostic categories have special characteristics that influence their driving, research in driving assessment will be hampered considerably, and individuals interested in resuming driving may be wrongly denied.

RETRAINING AND NEW TECHNOLOGIES

In a single case study examining the "anatomy of a crash" in an individual with AD using an Iowa Driving Simulator, Reinach et al[151] urge for greater emphasis on driver training because "it has the potential to improve driver performance by reinforcing safe driving behaviors, alerting drivers to their own deficiencies, and improving response time by means of cognitive intervention" (p 26). For example Ball et al[33] show that reduction of the UFOV test can be expanded with training that may have implications for driving remediation. Reinach et al[151] also discuss the possibilities of intelligent transportation systems (ITSs) that may be able to provide information to drivers to increase their awareness (e.g., side object detection system that warns a driver when there is an object obstructing the path as the driver attempts to change lanes). Modifications to current highways and medians may be another means by which prevalence and severity of accidents may be reduced while allowing individuals with mild cognitive deficits to maintain their independence on the road. Taylor and Tripodes[152] also emphasize the importance of developing alternative transportation options for individuals with disabilities, particularly those with dementia, and underscore the impact of lack of public transportation on caregivers and patients. In their survey targeting California households in which an elderly driver recently had his or her license revoked because of dementia, they found that caregivers frequently reported missing work or stopping work entirely to act as chauffeurs. See Chapters 17 and 19 for more information on ITSs and traffic safety.

COUNSELING THE CESSATION OF DRIVING

Counseling the cessation of driving is a difficult and often uncomfortable task. Most adults plan for retirement from work and many other activities; however, few adults consider a time at which they may retire from driving. After an acquired brain disorder this issue arises suddenly, providing little time to prepare for the pragmatic or emotional sequelae of the change in status from independent driver to passenger.

EMPOWERMENT AND COLLABORATIVE TONE

Clearly the best result of the counseling process occurs when the adult who should cease driving owns the decision. Individuals who consider the decision to stop driving on their own are more likely to adhere to the conclusion and feel better about it.[153] Viewing the patient as a collaborator in the decision-making process and respecting the emotional meaning of the loss are important aspects of the process. Although admittedly aspirational, this is the best scenario.

Resistance to a prohibition on driving would be an expected response from most adults. Furthermore accepting the need for change relies heavily on believing that one's driving skills are no longer adequate to drive safely. Like many personality traits, the "driving self" is an enduring self-view that becomes increasingly entrenched and resistant to change over time and with experience.[154] Moreover even most healthy adults overrate their driving abilities and have difficulty evaluating their skills objectively.[154-156] The accuracy of an individual's self-assessment of his or her driving abilities may be hindered by impairments such as poor self-monitoring and unawareness of deficit, as well as by the positive self-bias observed in most adults. Thus traditional theoretical and clinical models of behavior change may be helpful in some regards; however, most psychotherapies that would be relevant to voluntary cessation of driving require some insight and accurate self-assessment. Nonetheless we believe that the first and best approach to counseling the cessation of driving is one that emphasizes a collaborative tone and encourages empowerment of the survivor to make this difficult decision on his or her own behalf. To that end education of the driver with an acquired brain disorder is essential.

EDUCATION

Education about the cognitive, sensory, and various physical abilities affected by the injury may help the survivor understand the reasons for concern about safety and sets the stage for the rationale of this difficult decision. Neuropsychological testing results can be valuable in determining the amount and nature of information to convey, given the survivor's level of cognitive ability. Explanations should explicitly link the survivor's specific deficits to requisite skills for safe driving, using evidence from available neuropsychological, medical, and driver evaluations. Address the responsibilities of driving, as well as how the survivor's brain injury affects the skills and abilities necessary to drive safely. Accidents, incidents, or near accidents that may have occurred since the injury also may be useful in making the reality of personal risk concrete. However, even repeated presentations of evidence that the driver is now unsafe may be met with great resistance. Evaluation of readiness for change is an ongoing process.

PLANNING FOR THE FUTURE AND PROBLEM SOLVING

Many patients will become more receptive to the change if the counseling process includes some modeling of problem solving to address meeting needs that were previously met via independent driving. Reassure the patient that transportation can be made available when it is needed, and demonstrate in concrete examples how this can be achieved. For example early in the counseling process have the patient select an important activity or event for which he or she previously relied on independent driving, and model the active problem solving required to accomplish the goal using alternative transportation.

Research with older drivers indicates that establishing specific plans for alternative transportation increases the likelihood that driving cessation will be voluntary[157] and decreases the driver's feelings of dependency.[158] Compensating for cessation of independent driving typically will involve the use of several alternatives rather than a single primary source. Alternative transportation options may include riding with friends or relatives, using public transportation, using available community resources that offer ride services, taxis or other private transport services, and walking. Relocating to an area with adequate public transportation or to an assisted living center that provides transportation also can be considered. Relocating to live in closer proximity to friends and relatives who can provide rides may ease the burden on the social network. Preferably relocation would be within the patient's current community.

During the counseling process the survivor should be provided with a list of helping resources that offer transportation services or links to transportation services. Social work services can be a particularly valuable asset to the team in identifying and maximizing available transportation options. Local and regional transportation authorities and local chapters of the American Association of Retired Persons (AARP) typically have a wealth of information about transportation options. The American Automobile Association (AAA) Foundation for Traffic Safety[159] advises having family or friends accompany persons new to public transportation on their initial journeys to increase the likelihood of having a positive experience that seems workable to the person and to decrease the likelihood of becoming overwhelmed or negative about the experience.

If possible, incorporate the survivor's available support network in the planning process. Family, friends, and community members can learn from their involvement this process in terms of helping the survivor in future problem solving and identifying specific contexts in which they can provide assistance in the form of rides, maintaining social visits, and so on. Involvement of persons in the support network also provides an opportunity to educate those individuals about the survivor's needs and the potential consequences of the survivor lacking support to compensate for the loss of independent driving.

THE MULTIDIMENSIONAL EFFECTS OF DRIVING CESSATION

Cessation of driving has consequences on a variety of life domains, and counseling should address each of these in a direct and proactive manner. Psychological sequelae are common, and it is important to be sensitive to issues including the survivor's grief regarding the loss and effects on self-identity and self-esteem.[153,160] Availability of alternative transportation does not eliminate the adverse psychological effects of driving cessation.[161] Because of the high risk of depression and decreased life satisfaction after the cessation of independent driving, it seems prudent to proactively address these issues and monitor the survivor over time.

The counseling process should take into account patient-specific factors that may underlie resistance and concern about driving cessation. According to Burkhardt et al[158] considerable evidence supports the notion that men are generally much more resistant to relinquishing their licenses than women are. Men are less likely to cease driving voluntarily[162] and are more likely to be ego invested in driving privileges. Some of the disproportionately adverse response observed in men may be culturally bound to gender identity (e.g., the symbol of driving as masculine); however, other aspects of the response, such as a more marked impact on the role of family provider for men than women, also may play an important role. Other common psychological responses include distress regarding loss of independence, feeling humbled and reluctant to ask for help, and concerns about isolation. Uncovering and openly processing the personal meaning of this loss to the survivor are essential.

A change in driving status may adversely affect the survivor's social functioning considerably. The counseling process should assess the extent to which cessation of driving will affect the patient's access to and involvement in his or her social network and community. Social contacts typically made via the patient traveling to friends and family should be monitored to minimize lessening of amount and quality. Problem solving to maintain continued access to the social community is essential. Strategies for enlisting and maintaining support and common concerns about burdening the social network can be reviewed. For example having family and friends visit and making regular schedules of visits can help to maintain social contacts. Feelings of burdening family and friends for rides may be lessened by offering the driver reimbursement for expenses incurred. Helping the patient organize errands and tasks to consolidate outings that require rides may help to reduce the number of times he or she needs to ask for help. The survivor should be encouraged to discuss these issues and concerns with members of his or her social network.

The economic consequences of driving cessation are a common pragmatic concern. In the United States access to usable public transportation varies widely, and private transportation such as taxis and private van services may be expensive alternatives. However, given the large expense of automobile ownership and maintenance it may be that carefully planned use of alternative transportation is a more economical option than is independent driving. See Chapter 21 and Appendices G and H for more information on driving cessation.

Presenting a Unified Front

When possible a team model of counseling the cessation of driving may be most effective. If the intervention includes cooperation by the entire rehabilitation team (e.g., physician, neuropsychologist, psychologist, social worker, occupational and physical therapy generalists, and driver rehabilitation specialists), as well as family members or other persons in the supportive network, patients may be more convinced of the reality and necessity to stop driving. A unified opinion and multiple presentations of the information may help to move the survivor toward accepting the change in status. This approach also shares the burden of blame that may be assigned by the survivor. Alternatively a staged response could be adopted, in which one person initiates the recommendation and other members of the rehabilitation team and the social network enter the process as needed. Some families prefer to have the patient's physician or another health care provider with authority initiate the process to minimize resentment of caregivers. At some point, however, their involvement in the process may be necessary. Regardless it is essential that the survivor hear a consistent message about the necessity to cease driving.

When All Else Fails

If the ideal outcome does not occur and the survivor refuses to relinquish his or her driving privileges volun-

tarily, a responsible health care professional must consider the option of forced cessation. Intrusive actions, such as confiscating car keys and selling or disabling the patient's automobile, may be necessary but should be considered a last resort.

Reporting of unsafe drivers to government licensing agencies is a complex issue. Survey research indicates that the public believes that physicians should be responsible for the reporting process; however, most physicians are unfamiliar with laws and regulations regarding such reports.[83,139,140] Ethical and legal responsibilities of physicians and other health care workers to protect the public interest must be balanced against ethical and legal obligations to maintain patient confidentiality. Although driver's licenses are issued by individual states, the privileges extended by those licenses extend across states; thus some federal regulations also may apply.

Laws and regulations regarding reporting vary widely across states and can be difficult to interpret with certainty.[163,164] In some states failure to report high-risk patients to the state licensing agency is considered malpractice,[164] and health care professionals may be liable if such patients are involved in crashes.[165] Nearly all states have laws that restrict driving privileges of persons with history of seizures or loss of consciousness from other medical etiologies, whereas some states have additional requirements regarding reporting of persons with various other cognitive disorders. For example California established legislation requiring physicians to report persons with diagnoses of AD and related conditions.[165] Conversely in some states (e.g., New York) a breach of confidentiality by a health care worker associated with notification of a government licensing agency is illegal. Lastly some state policies encourage reporting of unfit drivers and provide protection from liability for doing so but do not require such reporting by law.

Given the extreme variation in responsibilities and regulations on reporting unfit drivers, it is essential that all persons involved in the counseling process are intimately familiar with expectations applicable to their location. Sources of information regarding legal requirements and restrictions on reporting unfit drivers include applicable state Departments of Motor Vehicles (DMVs) and State Attorneys General offices.[160] The Internet web sites maintained by each state's DMV post information applicable to eligibility and reporting criteria. Internet web sites hosted by sources other than the state government may provide legal regulations for individual states, but it is important to ensure that the information posted is current. It also is important to note that regulations posted by government driver's licensing agencies may not fully account for legal requirements set forth regarding confidentiality by health care providers or institutional policies. Kakaiya et al[160] refer to these combined responsibilities as "medical standards for driver's licensure" and recommend obtaining detailed information regarding legal requirements and "permissible voluntary actions" that may apply to health care workers with knowledge of a patient who is not fit to drive. Kakaiya et al[160] also include the following Internet resources, which as of this date were still available to the public: (1) http://www.carbuyingtips.com/driver-licenses.htm, a site that provides links to DMV web sites for most U.S. states; and (2) http://www.povertylaw.org/links/statlink.htm, a site that provides links to access specific state statutes. We strongly recommend consultation with an attorney who is familiar with state laws governing health care and driving before taking action to report. Many institutions retain counsel expressly for these purposes.

An attractive option for health care workers is to enlist a family member (or other person authorized for access to the survivor's health care information) to complete a formal report to the government agency. These persons generally do not have legal obligations regarding the survivor's confidentiality and can make reports of unfit drivers to the DMV without legal consequences. However, the emotional consequences of such an action to the family system may be high. See Chapters 21 and 23 as well as Appendix A for more information on driving cessation, ethical considerations, and state driver licensing requirements and reporting laws, respectively.

SUMMARY

Driving is a complex activity that is affected by a variety of cognitive, emotional, social, environmental, and legal factors. Each of these aspects deserves full consideration when an individual expresses an interest in resuming or beginning driving. The combination of these factors becomes especially important when an individual experiences an acquired brain disorder. In these instances neuropsychological evaluation is useful in identifying the cognitive and emotional factors that may impact an individual's driving fitness, as well as providing a framework for family education and counseling.

A greater appreciation of the objective driving evaluation is of particular importance given current research findings that indicate that family members and health professionals often make decisions regarding an individual's ability to drive without sufficient information. Presently assumptions and subjective perceptions may misguide the decision-making process. Although neuropsychological evaluation is still in its early stages

of development in the context of driving assessment, there is enough empirical support to legitimize its use among health professionals as a screen for an on-road driving evaluation and as an educational tool for the individual, family members, and the multidisciplinary team.

The shift in driver's assessment from prediction of fitness to drive to risk assessment highlights an increasing awareness that ability to drive is better understood as being on a continuum than as falling into a discrete category. As such, research investigating driving assessment is evolving to define fundamental neuropsychological and social aspects of driving behavior, as well as general personality factors that affect an individual's ability to perform this activity. Eventually subtleties in an individual's driving assessment profile will be delineated to systematically inform decisions concerning assessment of driving risk, including an individual's propensity to adopt compensatory strategies. Computer technology, neuroimaging, and driving simulators will play a larger role in the comprehensive driver rehabilitation evaluation process, and increased standardization of driving assessment protocols will allow for comparison between research findings and the development of focused test batteries for specific clinical populations.

Review of the neuropsychological and psychological factors in driving is impressive. For a field that is in its infancy, findings in this area are encouraging in their applicability. However, much of the present research lacks the level of scientific rigor it deserves considering the impact of decisions concerning driving. From the perspective of the individual and the public, few decisions carry more weight than those concerning fitness to drive. With the advent of evidence-based medicine and increased accountability of clinical services to third-party payers, the demand for empirically sound research and accurate decision making concerning assessment of driving risk is high. Ultimately the individual, the public, and the neurosciences at large will benefit greatly from the revolutionary advances that are occurring in this field.

REFERENCES

1. Engum E, Cron L, Hulse C, et al: Cognitive behavioral driver's inventory, *Cogn Rehabil* September/October:34-50, 1988.
2. Golper LA, Rau MT, Marshall RC: Aphasic adults and their decisions on driving: an evaluation, *Arch Phys Med Rehabil* 61:34-40, 1980.
3. Mackenzie C, Paton G: Resumption of driving with aphasia following stroke, *Aphasiology* 17:107-122, 2003.
4. Dubinsky RM, Stein AC, Lyons K: Practice parameter: risk of driving and Alzheimer's disease (an evidence-based review), *Neurology* 54:2205-2211, 2000.

5. Galski T, Bruno R, Ehle H: Driving after cerebral damage: a model with implications for evaluation, *Am J Occup Ther* 46:324-332, 1992.

6. Benton AL, Hamsher KS, Varney NR, et al: *Contributions to neuropsychological assessment*, New York, 1983, Oxford University Press.

7. Webster JS, Rapport LJ, Godlewski MC, et al: Effect of attentional bias to right space on wheelchair mobility, *J Clin Exp Neuropsychol* 16:129-137, 1994.

8. Webster JS, Rhoades LA, Morrill B, et al: Rightward orienting bias, wheelchair maneuvering, and fall risk, *Arch Phys Med Rehabil* 76:924-928, 1995.

9. Heikkilä VM, Korpelainen J, Turkka J, et al: Clinical evaluation of the driving ability in stroke patients, *Acta Neurol Scand* 99:349-355, 1999.

10. Sivak M, Olson P, Kewman D, et al: Driving and perceptual/cognitive skills: behavioral consequences of brain damage, *Arch Phys Med Rehabil* 62:476-483, 1981.

11. Korteling JE, Kaptein NA: Neuropsychological driving fitness tests for brain-damaged subjects, *Arch Phys Med Rehabil* 77:138-145, 1996.

12. Gouvier WD, Maxfield MW, Schwietzer JR, et al: Psychometric prediction of driving performance among the disabled, *Arch Phys Med Rehabil* 70:745-750, 1989.

13. Rothke S: The relationship between neuropsychological test scores and performance on driving evaluation, *Int J Clin Neuropsychol* 11:134-136, 1989.

14. McKenna P: Fitness to drive: a neuropsychological perspective, *J Ment Health* 7:9-18, 1998.

15. Hopewell CA, van Zomeren AH: Neuropsychological aspects of motor vehicle operation. In Tupper DE, Cicerone KD, editors: *The neuropsychology of everyday life: assessment and basic competencies*, Boston, 1990, Kluwer.

16. van Zomeren A, Brouwer W, Minderhoud J: Acquired brain damage and driving: a review, *Arch Phys Med Rehabil* 68:697-705, 1987.

17. Daigneault G, Joly P, Frigon JY: Executive functions in the evaluation of accident risk of older drivers, *J Clin Exp Neuropsychol* 24:221-238, 2002.

18. Hopewell CA: Driving assessment issues for practicing clinicians, *J Head Trauma Rehabil* 17:48-61, 2002.

19. Mazer BL, Korner-Bitensky NA, Sofer S: Predicting ability to drive after stroke, *Arch Phys Med Rehabil* 79:743-750, 1998.

20. Schanke A, Sundet K: Comprehensive driving assessment: neuropsychological testing and on-road evaluation of brain injured patients, *Scand J Psychol* 41:113-121, 2000.

21. Coleman RD, Rapport LJ, Ergh TC, et al: Predictors of driving outcome after traumatic brain injury, *Arch Phys Med Rehabil* 83:1415-1422, 2002.

22. Reitan RM, Davison LA: *Clinical neuropsychology: current status and applications*, New York, 1974, Halstead Press.

23. Trenerry MR, Crosson B, Deboe J, et al: *Stroop Neuropsychological Screening Test*, 1989, Psychological Assessment Resources.

24. Wechsler D: *Wechsler Adult Intelligence Scale*, ed 3, San Antonio, TX, 1997, Psychological Assessment Corp.

25. D'Elia L, Satz P, Uchiyama C, et al: *Color Trails Test*, Odessa, FL, 1996, Psychological Assessment Resources.

26. Culbertson WC, Zillmer EA: *Tower of London, Drexel University*, Odessa, FL, 2001, Psychological Assessment Resources.

27. Heaton RK: *Wisconsin Card Sorting Test Manual*, Odessa, FL, 1981, Psychological Assessment Resources.

28. Ball K, Owsley C: The useful field of view test: a new technique for evaluating age-related declines in visual function, *J Am Optom Assoc* 63:71-79, 1992.

29. Fisk GD, Owsley C, Mennemeier M: Vision, attention, and self-reported driving behaviors in community-dwelling stroke survivors, *Arch Phys Med Rehabil* 83:469-477, 2002.

30. Cushman LA, Cogliandro FC: On-road driving post-stroke: cognitive and other factors, *Arch Clin Neuropsychol* 14:799, 1999.

31. Mazer BL, Sofer S, Korner-Bitensky N, et al: Effectiveness of a visual attention retraining program on the driving performance of clients with stroke, *Arch Phys Med Rehabil* 84:541-550, 2003.

32. Owsley C, Ball K, McGwin G Jr, et al: Visual processing impairment and risk of motor vehicle crash among older adults, *JAMA* 279:1083-1088, 1998.

33. Ball K, Owsley C, Sloane ME, et al: Visual attention problems as a predictor of vehicle crashes in older drivers, *Invest Ophthalmol Vis Sci* 34:3110-123, 1993.

34. Goode K, Ball K, Sloane M, et al: Useful field of view and other neurocognitive indicators of crash risk in older adults, *J Clin Psychol Med Settings* 5:425-440, 1998.

35. Myers RS, Ball KK, Kalina TD, et al: Relation of useful field of view and other screening tests to on-road driving performance, *Percept Mot Skills* 91:279-290, 2000.

36. Calvanio R, Williams R, Burke DT, et al: Acquired brain injury, visual attention, and the Useful Field of View Test: a pilot study, *Arch Phys Med Rehabil* 85:474-478, 2004.

37. Fisk GD, Novack T, Mennemeier M, et al: Useful field of view after traumatic brain injury, *J Head Trauma Rehabil* 17:16-25, 2002.

38. Burgess P, Alderman N, Evans J, et al: The ecological validity of tests of executive function, *J Int Neuropsychol Soc* 4:547-558, 1998.

39. Prigatano G, Ogano M, Amakusa B: A cross-cultural study on impaired self-awareness in Japanese patients with brain dysfunction, *Neuropsychiatry Neuropsychol Behav Neurol* 10:135-143, 1997.

40. Prigatano GP, Bruna O, Mataro M, Munoz JM, Fernandez S, Junque C. Initial disturbances of consciousness and resultant impaired awareness in Spanish patients with traumatic brain injury, *J Head Trauma Rehabil* 13:29-38, 1998.

41. Prigatano G, Altman I: Impaired awareness of behavioral limitations after traumatic brain injury, *Arch Phys Med Rehabil* 71:1058-1064, 1990.

42. Prigatano G, Altman I, O'Brien K: Behavioral limitations that brain injured patients tend to underestimate, *Clin Neuropsychol* 4:163-176, 1990.

43. Prigatano GP, Leathem JM: Awareness of behavioral limitations after traumatic brain injury: a cross-cultural study of New Zealand Maoris and Non-Maoris, *Clin Neuropsychol* 7:123-135, 1993.

44. Rapport LJ, Webster JS, Flemming KL, et al: Predictors of falls among right-hemisphere stroke patients in the rehabilitation setting, *Arch Phys Med Rehabil* 74:621-626, 1993.

45. Rapport LJ, Hanks RA, Millis SR, et al: Executive functioning and predictors of falls in the rehabilitation setting, *Arch Phys Med Rehabil* 79:629-633, 1998.

46. Rapport LJ, Lichtenberg PA, Vangel S: *Cognition and fall risk among geriatric rehabilitation patients,* Paper presented at the meeting of the American Psychological Association, 1998, San Francisco, CA.

47. Hanks RA, Rapport LJ, Millis SR, et al: Measures of executive functioning as predictors of functional ability and social integration in a rehabilitation sample, *Arch Phys Med Rehabil* 79:629-633, 1999.

48. van Zomeren AH, Brouwer WH, Rothengatter JA, et al: Fitness to drive a car after recovery from severe head injury, *Arch Phys Med Rehabil* 69:90-96, 1988.

49. Cotrell V, Wild K: Longitudinal study of self-imposed driving restrictions and deficit awareness in patients with Alzheimer disease, *Alzheimer Dis Assoc Disord* 13:151-156, 1999.

50. Brouwer WH, Ponds RW: Driving competence in older persons, *Disabil Rehabil* 16:149-161, 1994.

51. Lings S, Jensen PB: Driving after stroke: a controlled laboratory investigation, *Int Disabil Stud* 13:74-82, 1991.

52. Lundqvist A, Gerdle B, Ronnberg J: Neuropsychological aspects of driving after a stroke—in the simulator and on the road, *Appl Cog Psychol* 14:135-150, 2000.

53. Shore D, Gurgold G, Robbins S: Handicapped driving: an overview of assessment and training, *Arch Phys Med Rehabil* 61:481, 1980.

54. Brouwer WH, Withaar F: Fitness to drive after traumatic brain injury, *Neuropsychol Rehabil* 7:177-193, 1997.

55. Schultheis MT, Matheis RJ, Nead R, et al: Driving behaviors following brain injury: self-report and motor vehicle records, *J Head Trauma Rehabil* 17:38-47, 2002.

56. Wallace JE, Crancer A: Licensing exams and their relation to subsequent driving record, *Behav Res Highway Safety* 2:53-65, 1971.

57. Johnson HM: Detection and treatment of accident prone drivers, *Psycholog Bull* 43:489-532, 1946.

58. McFarland RA, Moore RC, Warren AB: *Human variables in motor vehicle accidents: a review of the literature,* Cambridge, MA, 1954, Harvard School of Public Health.

59. Conley JA, Smiley R: Driver licensing tests as a predictor of subsequent violations, *Hum Factors* 18:565-574, 1976.

60. Owsley C, Ball K, Sloane M, et al: Visual/cognitive correlates of vehicle accidents in older drivers, *Psychol Aging* 6:403-415, 1991.

61. Wechsler D: *Wechsler Adult Intelligence Scale-Revised,* San Antonio, TX, 1981, Psychological Assessment Corp.

62. Fox GK, Bashford GM, Caust SL: Identifying safe versus unsafe drivers following brain impairment: The Coorabel Programme, *Disabil Rehabil* 14:140-145, 1992.

63. Benton AL: *Revised Visual Retention Test,* ed 4, New York, 1974, The Psychological Corporation.

64. Meyers J, Volbrecht M, Kaster-Bundgaard J: Driving is more than pedal pushing, *Appl Neuropsychol* 6:154-164, 1999.

65. Galski T, Ehle HT, Williams JB: Off-road driving evaluations for persons with cerebral injury: a factor analytic study of pre-driver and simulator testing, *Am J Occup Ther* 51:352-359, 1997.

66. Galski T, Bruno R, Ehle H: Prediction of behind-the-wheel driving performance in patients with cerebral brain damage: a discriminant function analysis, *Am J Occup Ther* 47:391-396, 1993.

67. Boake C, MacLeod M, High WM, et al: Increased risk of motor vehicle crashes among drivers with traumatic brain injury, *J Int Neuropsychol Soc* 4:75, 1998 (abstract).

68. Katz RT, Golden RS, Butter J, et al: Driving safety after brain damage: follow-up of twenty-two patients with matched controls, *Arch Phys Med Rehabil* 71:133-137, 1990.

69. Trobe JD, Waller PF, Cook-Flannagan CA, et al: Crashes and violations among drivers with Alzheimer disease, *Arch Neurol* 53:411-416, 1996.

70. Lundqvist A, Ronnberg J: Driving problems and adaptive driving behaviour after brain injury: a qualitative assessment, *Neuropsychol Rehabil* 11:171-185, 2001.

71. Klavora P, Gaskovski P, Martin K, et al: The effects of Dynavision rehabilitation on behind-the-wheel driving ability and selected psychomotor abilities of persons after stroke, *Am J Occup Ther* 49:534-542, 1995.

72. Marshall SC, Grinnell D, Heisel B, et al: Attentional deficits in stroke patients: a visual dual task experiment, *Arch Phys Med Rehabil* 78:7-12, 1997.

73. Nouri F, Tinson D: A comparison between a driving simulator and a road test in the assessment of the stroke driver, *Int J Rehabil Res* 10:349-350, 1987.

74. Nouri F, Tinson D, Lincoln N: Cognitive ability and driving after stroke, *Int Disabil Stud* 9:110-115, 1987.

75. Nouri F, Lincoln N: Predicting driving performance after stroke, *BMJ* 307:482-483, 1993.

76. Quigley FL, DeLisa JA: Assessing the driving potential of cerebral vascular accident patients, *Am J Occup Ther* 37:474-478, 1983.

77. Szlyk JP, Brigell M, Seiple W: Effects of age and hemianopic visual-field loss on driving, *Optom Vis Sci* 70:1031-1037, 1993.

78. Jones R, Giddens H, Croft D: Assessment and training of brain-damaged drivers, *Am J Occup Ther* 37:754-760, 1983.

79. Klavora P, Heslegrave RJ, Young M: Driving skills in elderly persons with stroke: comparison of two new assessment options, *Arch Phys Med Rehabil* 81:701-705, 2000.

80. Galski T, Ehle HT, McDonald MA, et al: Evaluating fitness to drive after cerebral injury: basic issues and recommendations for medical and legal communities, *J Head Trauma Rehabil* 15:895-908, 2000.

81. Fisk GD, Owsley C, Pulley LV: Driving after stroke: driving exposure, advice, and evaluations, *Arch Phys Med Rehabil* 78:1338-1345, 1997.

82. Legh-Smith J, Wade DT, Hewer RL: Driving after a stroke, *J R Soc Med* 79:200-203, 1986.

83. Nouri F: Fitness to drive and the general practitioner, *Int Disabil Stud* 10:101-103, 1988.

84. Owsley C, Stalvey BT, Phillips JM: The efficacy of an educational intervention in promoting self-regulation among high-risk older drivers, *Accid Anal Prev* 35:393-400, 2003.

85. Ball K, Owsley C, Stalvey B, et al: Driving avoidance and functional impairment in older drivers, *Accid Anal Prev* 30:313-322, 1998.

86. Lyman JM, McGwin G, Sims RV: Factors related to driving difficulty and habits in older drivers, *Accid Anal Prev* 33:413-421, 2001.

87. Marottoli RA, Ostfeld AM, Merrill SS, et al: Driving cessation and changes in mileage driven among elderly individuals, *J Gerontol* 48:S255-S260, 1993.

88. Owsley C, Stalvey B, Wells J, et al: Older drivers and cataract: driving habits and crash risk, *J Gerontol A Biol Sci Med Sci* 54:M203-M211, 1999.

89. Bieliauskas LA, Roper BR, Trobe J, et al: Cognitive measures, driving safety, and Alzheimer disease, *Clin Neuropsychol* 12:206-212, 1998.

90. Heikkilä VM: Relationship of laboratory and on-road tests for driving-school students and experienced drivers, *Percept Mot Skills* 90:227-235, 2000.

91. Hopewell CA, Price RJ: Driving after head injury, *J Clin Exper Neuropsychol* 7:148, 1985.

92. Stokx L, Gaillard A: Task and driving performance of patients with severe concussion of the brain, *J Clin Exper Neuropsychol* 8:421-436, 1986.

93. Brouwer WH, Withaar F, Tant M, van Zomeren A: Attention and driving in traumatic brain injury: a question of coping with time-pressure, *J Head Trauma Rehabil* 17:1-5, 2002.

94. Priddy D, Johnson P, Lam C: Driving after severe head injury, *Brain Inj* 4:267-272, 1990.

95. Brooke MM, Questad KA, Patterson DR, et al: Driving evaluation after traumatic brain injury, *Am J Phys Med Rehabil* 71:177-182, 1992.

96. Reitan RM, Wolfson D: *The Halstead-Reitan Neuropsychological Test Battery*, Tucson, AZ, 1985, Neuropsychology Press.

97. Colarusso R, Hammill D: *Motor Free Visual Perception Test*, Novato, CA, 1972, Academic Therapy Publications.

98. Dykes V, et al: *Baylor Adult Visual Perceptual Assessment*, Dallas, TX, 1980, Baylor University Medical Center, Department of Occupational Therapy.

99. Smith A: The symbol-digit modalities test: a neuropsychological test for economic screening of learning and other cerebral disorders. In Hellmuth J, editor: *Learning disorders*, Seattle, WA, 1968, *Special Child Publications*, pp 83-91.

100. Klavora P, Heslegrave RJ: Senior drivers: an overview of problems and intervention strategies, *J Aging Phys Activity* 10:322-335, 2002.

101. Akinwuntan AE, Feys H, DeWeerdt W, et al: Determinants of driving after stroke, *Arch Phys Med Rehabil* 83:334-341, 2002.

102. Korner-Bitensky NA, Mazer BL, Sofer S, et al: Visual testing for readiness to drive after stroke: a multi-center study, *Am J Phys Med Rehabil* 79:253-259, 2000.

103. Lundberg C, Caneman G, Samuelsson SM, et al: The assessment of fitness to drive after a stroke: the Nordic Stroke Driver Screening Assessment, *Scand J Psychol* 44:23-30, 2003.

104. Nouri FM, Lincoln NB: Validation of a cognitive assessment: predicting driving performance after stroke, *Clin Rehabil* 6:275-281, 1992.

105. Engum ES, Lambert EW, Scott K: Criterion-related validity of the cognitive behavioral driver's inventory, *Cogn Rehabil* 8:20-26, 1990.

106. Schultheis MT, Hillary F, Chute DL: The Neurocognitive Driving Test: applying technology to the assessment of driving ability following brain injury, *Rehabil Psychol* 48:275-280, 2003.

107. Mayor A, Junque C, Vendrell P, et al: Driving again after stroke: influence of clinical variables and reaction-time performance, *J Clin Exp Neuropsychol* 9:275, 1987.

108. Bardach J: Psychological factors in the handicapped driver, *Arch Phys Med Rehabil* 52:328-332, 1971.

109. Heilman KM, Valenstein E: *Clinical neuropsychology*, ed 4, Oxford, 2003, Oxford University Press.

110. Webster JS, Rapport LJ: Wheelchair accidents associated with hemispatial neglect, *J Clin Exp Neuropsychol* 15:50, 1993.

111. Webster JS, McFarland PT, Rapport LJ, et al: Computer-assisted training for improving wheelchair mobility in unilateral neglect patients, *Arch Phys Med Rehabil* 82:769-775, 2001.

112. Rhoades L, Webster JS, Morrill B, et al: Hemispatial neglect in simulated wheelchair obstacle course performance, *Clin Neuropsychol* 8:347-348, 1994.

113. Chaudhuri GA: Predictors for driving ability in stroke patients, *Arch Phys Med Rehabil* 68:664-665, 1987.

114. Sundet K, Goffeng L, Hofft E: To drive or not to drive: neuropsychological assessment for driver's license among stroke patients, *Scand J Psychol* 36:47-58, 1995.

115. Gilley DW, Wilson RS, Bennett DA, et al: Cessation of driving and unsafe motor vehicle operation by dementia patients, *Arch Intern Med* 151:941-946, 1991.

116. Logsdon RG, Teri L, Larson E: Driving and Alzheimer's disease, *J Gen Intern Med* 7:583-588, 1992.

117. Friedland RP, Koss E, Kumar A, et al: Motor vehicle crashes in dementia of the Alzheimer type, *Ann Neurol* 24:782-786, 1988.

118. Lucas-Blaustein MJ, Filipp L, Dungan C, et al: Driving in patients with dementia, *J Am Geriatr Soc* 36:1087-1091, 1988.

119. Hughes CP, Berg L, Danziger W, et al: A new clinical scale for the staging of dementia, *Br J Psychiatry* 140:566-572, 1982.

120. Morris JC: The clinical dementia rating (CDR): current version and scoring rules, *Neurology* 43:2412-2414, 1993.

121. Duchek JM, Hunt L, Ball K, et al: The role of selective attention in driving and dementia of the Alzheimer's type, *Alzheimer Dis Assoc Disord* 11:48-56, 1997.

122. Parasuraman R, Nestor P: Attention and driving skills in aging and Alzheimer's disease, *Hum Factors* 33:539-557, 1991.

123. Duchek JM, Hunt L, Ball K, et al: Attention and driving performance in Alzheimer's disease, *J Gerontol* 53:130-141, 1998.

124. Reger MA, Welsh RK, Watson GS, et al: The relationship between neuropsychological functioning and driving ability in dementia: a meta-analysis, *Neuropsychology* 18:85-93, 2004.

125. Ott B, Heindel W, Whelihan W, et al: A single-photon emission computed tomography imaging study of driving impairment in patients with Alzheimer's disease, *Dement Geriatr Cogn Disord* 11:153-160, 2000.

126. U.S. Department of Transportation (USDOT), National Highway Traffic Safety Administration

(NHTSA): *Traffic Safety Facts 1998: Older Population, DOT HS 808 955.* Available at *http://www.nhtsa.dot.gov/people/ncsa/pdf/Older98.pdf* p. 1, as of June 22, 2000.

127. Szlyk JP, Seiple W, Viana M: Relative effects of age and compromised vision on driving performance, *Hum Factors* 37:430-436, 1995.

128. Brouwer W, Rothengatter T, van Wolffelaar P: Compensatory potential in elderly drivers. In Rothengatter T, de Bruin R, editors: *Road user behaviour: theory and research,* Assen, The Netherlands, 1988, Van Gorcum.

129. Odenheimer GL, Beaudet M, Jette AM, et al: Performance-based driving evaluation of the elderly driver: safety, reliability, and validity, *J Gerontol* 49:M153-M159, 1994.

130. Persad CC, Giordani B, Chen HC, et al: Neuropsychological predictors of complex obstacle avoidance in healthy older adults, *J Gerontol* 50:272-277, 1995.

131. Withaar F, Brouwer W, van Zomeren A: Fitness to drive in older drivers with cognitive impairment, *J Int Neuropsychol* 6:480-490, 2000.

132. Galski T, Ehle HT, Williams JB: Estimates of driving abilities and skills in different conditions, *Am J Occup Ther* 52:268-275, 1998.

133. Fisk G, Schneider J, Novack T: Driving following traumatic brain injury: prevalence, exposure, advice and evaluations, *Brain Inj* 12:683-695, 1998.

134. Gulian E, Matthews G, Glendon AI, et al: Dimensions of driver stress, *Ergonomics* 32:585-602, 1989.

135. Martinez R: The Statement of the Honorable Recardo Marinez, M.D., Administrator, National Highway Traffic Safety Administration before the Subcommittee on Surface Transportation, Committee on Transportation and Infrastructure, U.S. House of Representatives, July 17, 1997.

136. Snyder D: Statement of David S. Snyder, Assistant General Counsel, American Insurance Association, representing advocates for highway and auto safety before the House Committee on Transportation and Infrastructure, Surface Transportation Subcommittee, July 17, 1997.

137. Matthews G, Dorn L, Hoyes TW, et al: Driver stress and performance on a driving simulator, *Hum Factors* 40:136-149, 1998.

138. Jackson H, Hopewell C, Glass C, et al: The Katz Adjustment Scale: modification of use with survivors of traumatic brain injury and spinal injury, *Brain Inj* 6:109-127, 1992.

139. Kelly R, Warke T, Steele I: Medical restrictions to driving: the awareness of patients and doctors, *Postgrad Med J* 75:537-539, 1999.

140. Goodyear K, Roseveare C: Driving restrictions after stroke: doctors' awareness of DVLA guidelines and advice given to patients, *Clin Med* 3:86-87, 2003.

141. Taylor J, Deane F, Podd J: Driving-related fear: a review, *Clin Psychol Rev* 22:631-645, 2002.

142. Anderson CJ, Vogel LC: Employment outcomes of adults who sustained spinal cord injuries as children or adolescents, *Arch Phys Med Rehabil* 83:791-801, 2002.

143. Kiyono Y, Hashizume C, Matsui N, et al: Car-driving abilities of people with tetraplegia, *Arch Phys Med Rehabil* 82:1389-1392, 2001.

144. Kreutzer JS, Marwitz JH, Walker W, et al: Moderating factors in return to work and job stability after traumatic brain injury, *J Head Trauma Rehabil* 18:128-138, 2003.

145. Siosteen A, Lundqvist C, Blomstrand C, et al: The quality of life of three functional spinal cord injury subgroups in a Swedish community, *Paraplegia* 28:476-488, 1990.

146. Glass TA, de Leon CM, Marottoli RA, et al: Population based study of social and productive activities as predictors of survival among elderly Americans, *BMJ* 319:478-483, 1999.

147. Marottoli RA, de Leon CFM, Glass TA, et al: Consequences of driving cessation: decreased out-of-home activity levels, *J Gerontol B Psychol Sci Social Sci* 55:S334-S340, 2000.

148. Marottoli RA, Mendes de Leon CFM, Glass TA, et al: Driving cessation and increased depressive symptoms: prospective evidence from the New Haven EPESE. Established Populations for Epidemiologic Studies of the Elderly, *J Am Geriatr Soc* 45:202-206, 1997.

149. Johnson JE: Urban older adults and the forfeiture of a driver's license, *J Gerontol Nurs* 25:12-18, 1999.

150. Hallett JD, Zasler ND, Maurer P, et al: Role change after traumatic brain injury in adults, *Am J Occup Ther* 48:241-246, 1994.

151. Reinach SJ, Rizzo M, McGehee DV: Driving with Alzheimer disease: the anatomy of a crash, *Alzheimer Dis Assoc Disord* 11(Suppl 1):21-27, 1997.

152. Taylor BD, Tripodes S: The effects of driving cessation on the elderly with dementia and their caregivers, *Accid Anal Prev* 33:519-528, 2001.

153. Bahro M, Silber E, Box P, et al: Giving up driving in Alzheimers disease: an integrative therapeutic approach, *Int J Geriatr Psychiatr* 10:871-874, 1995.

154. Groeger JA, Grande GE: Self-preserving assessments of skill? *Br J Psychol* 87:61-79, 1996.

155. Glendon AI, Dorn L, Davies DR, et al: Age and gender differences in perceived accident likelihood and driver competences, *Risk Anal* 16:755-762, 1996.

156. Marottoli RA, Richardson ED: Confidence in, and self-rating of, driving ability among older drivers, *Accid Anal Prev* 30:331-336, 1998.

157. Central Plains Area Agency on Aging: *A positive approach to retirement from driving: Senior Transportation Project,* Guidebook 3 in a series of 5, Wichita, KS, 1995, Central Plains Area Agency on Aging.

158. Burkhardt J, Berger AM, McGavock AT: Chapter 22: The mobility consequences of the reduction or cessation of driving by older women. In Womens Travel Issues: *Proceedings from the second national conference,* October 1996, U.S. Department of Transportation, Federal Highway Administration. Office of Highway Information Management, HPM 40. Publication No. FHWA-PL-97-024, pp 439-454.

159. AAA Foundation for Traffic Safety 2000: *Retiring from driving.* Available at: *www.aaafoundation.org.* Accessed December 6, 2004.

160. Kakaiya R, Tisovec R, Fulkerson P: Evaluation of fitness to drive, *Postgrad Med* 107:229-236, 2000.

161. Fonda SJ, Wallace RB, Herzog AR: Changes in driving patterns and worsening depressive symptoms among older adults, *J Gerontol B Psychol Sci Soc Sci* 56:S343-S351, 2001.

162. Jette AM, Branch L: A ten-year follow-up of driving patterns among the community dwelling elderly, *Hum Factors* 34:25-31, 1992.

163. McLachlan RS: Medical conditions and driving: legal requirements and approach of neurologists, *Med Law* 16:269-275, 1997.

164. Shua-Haim JR, Gross JS: The co-pilot driver syndrome, *J Am Geriatr Soc* 44:815-817, 1996.

165. Reuben D, George P: Driving and dementia: California's approach to a medical policy dilemma, *West J Med* 164:111-121, 1996.

Chapter 8

MEDICATIONS, DISABILITIES, AND DRIVING

Renee Tyree

KEY TERMS

- Pharmacology
- Drug
- Therapeutic use
- Functional classification
- Pharmacokinetics
- Administration site
- Side effects
- Pharmacodynamics
- Therapeutics
- Adverse reactions
- Food and Drug Administration (FDA)
- Addiction
- Tolerance
- Physical dependence

CHAPTER OBJECTIVES

After completing this chapter, the reader will be able to do the following:

- Explain why the driver rehabilitation specialist should be familiar with the categories of drugs, whether prescribed, over the counter, or illegal.
- Know what information is important to ascertain when taking a client's medical and drug history.
- Understand the different classifications of drugs.
- Understand why it is important to be aware of what effect medications may have on one's ability to be a safe and functional driver.

The use of medications, prescribed by a physician or purchased over the counter (OTC), has become prevalent in American society and in developed countries throughout the world. Driver rehabilitation specialists (DRSs) must recognize that their clients' driving performance can be, and often is, impacted by the medication or medications they are taking for any number of medical conditions known or unknown to the client and professional treatment team members. Drug therapy is instrumental in helping countless people enjoy longer and better lives, provided they have access to prescribed and OTC medications. For people with disabilities and elderly persons, medications such as antiseizure regimens can help to foster competence and safety when driving a motor vehicle. Conversely medications and illegal substances can also dramatically impair driving performance and community mobility. This chapter will explore various facets of medications and disabilities and how they impact driving.

Most people are likely to feel unwell at some point in their lives, and each medical condition's unique etiology and the resulting symptoms often act as the impetus for people to consume some kind of OTC remedy, with or without the advice of a doctor or pharmacist. People with disabilities and elderly persons receiving driver rehabilitation services are likely to be taking two or more classes of medications concurrently, which can increase the likelihood of unwanted medication effects. DRSs may gain valuable insight into a client's driving performance, or lack thereof, with an understanding of the medications he or she may be taking. Because the DRS interacts with people who take one or more medications it is important to be aware of the desired, as well as the undesired, effects of these preparations. However, because there are thousands of medications and hundreds of facts about each of them, it is a nearly impossible task (as well as unnecessary) for the DRS to memorize every fact associated with prescribed, OTC, and illegal drugs. The DRS should instead learn to identify general categories of drugs and predict the overall impact each drug will have on driving performance by focusing on a few facts and understanding key pharmacologic principles. The content in this chapter presents the basic principles of pharmacology and pertinent information about those medications most often used by people with disabilities and elderly persons.

PHARMACOLOGY

Pharmacology is the study of the preparation, properties, uses, and actions of drugs. The DRS should be familiar with how medications work in the body, how drugs are named, and how drugs are classified.

HOW MEDICATIONS WORK IN THE BODY

A *drug* can be defined as any substance that is natural or synthetic that when taken into the body results in a change in medical, behavioral, or perceptual states for either medically therapeutic or nonmedical purposes. People are often not aware that they are ingesting a drug when they drink alcohol or consume a cup of coffee or when they apply popular OTC products, such as topical ointments to reduce pain or eye drops to reduce redness. The formulation of a drug depends on the following key factors:
- The physiologic barriers the drug is capable of permeating
- The setting in which the drug will be used
- The urgency of the medical situation that requires administering a drug or drugs
- The disposition of the drug within the body after administration
- The stability of the drug

DRUG NAMES

Most drugs are known by several names (Table 8-1): chemical, generic, trade, and official, each of which serves a specific function. However, the use of multiple drug names often contributes to confusion among the general public and at times the medical community as well. A drug's names (i.e., chemical, generic, and official) are established at different phases of drug development and serve different but equally important functions. A drug's chemical name describes its atomic and molecular structure. Once several clinical trials have been completed successfully and the Food and Drug Administration (FDA) has deemed a drug efficacious, it is given a generic name, also known as a nonproprietary name. Before FDA approval is granted, the manufacturer must create and register a trade name (or brand name). Trade names are copyrighted, and their use is restricted to the drug manufacturer. Once the patent has expired, any manufacturer may produce the drug and market it using the drug's generic name.

DRUG CLASSIFICATIONS

Drugs are classified in various ways to assist physicians, pharmacists, other allied health professionals (e.g., DRSs), and more recently clients and caregivers in understanding the prescription and proper use of pharmaceuticals (Table 8-2). Drugs can be classified by their *therapeutic use*, such as antibiotics or antidepressants. Prescription drugs may be further divided into subgroups that focus on a particular drug's mechanism of action. Drugs can also be classified by their *functional classification*.

PHARMACOKINETICS

Pharmacokinetics is the study of a particular drug's concentration in various parts of the body as it passes

Table 8-1   An Example of Different Names for the Same Drug

Type of Name	Name
Chemical	γ-Amino butyric acid (GABA) chlorophyll derivative
Generic	Baclofen
Trade	Lioresal

Table 8-2 An Example of Different Classifications for One Drug

Classification	Name
Therapeutic use	Antidepressants
Subgroup	Tricyclic antidepressants (Elavil) Serotonin reuptake inhibitors (Prozac)
Functional classification	Psychotherapeutics

through the body during the absorption, distribution, metabolism, and excretion phases.

ABSORPTION

Before a drug can begin working, it must be transformed from its pharmaceutical dosage form to a biologically available substance that can reach its site of action. The rate at which a drug is absorbed depends on several factors, including site of administration, circulation route throughout the tissues into which the drug was administered, and the solubility of the drug.

Absorption begins at the site of administration. Depending on the chemical composition of a drug, it may be better absorbed at one *administration site* versus another. Medications generally enter the body by one of the following ways:

- Oral: Oral agents must be able to withstand the acidic environment of the stomach and must permeate the gastrointestinal lining before entering the bloodstream.
- Rectal: Usually administered as a suppository. This route is used when there are swallowing problems, vomiting, or unresponsiveness; however, absorption by this route is often unreliable and less effective than other sites.
- Parenteral: Involving skin puncture. Intravenous (IV) administration has a rapid onset of action because the agent is injected directly into the bloodstream. Intramuscular (IM) rate of absorption will depend on the drug formulation. Subcutaneous injection beneath the skin is absorbed into the bloodstream at a rate also controlled by the formulation of the drug in question.
- Topical: Useful for the local delivery of agents. Used for most dermatologic and ophthalmologic agents, as well as some dental and sports medicine preparations.

- Inhalation: Generally is rapidly absorbed and is used for drugs that can be delivered and absorbed as an inhalant, including drugs that can be smoked (e.g., cigarettes, marijuana, and crack cocaine).
- Transdermal: Through the skin. A few drugs can be formulated such that a "patch" containing the drug is applied to the skin. The drug can then "seep" out of the patch and be absorbed through the skin into the capillary bed.

DISTRIBUTION

Distribution is the process by which a drug is transported by the circulating fluid to various sites within the body. This is the factor that accounts for most of an agent's unintended effects, also known as *side effects*. For example a medication that is intended for action in the brain often travels through the body, resulting in unintended effects on other body structures (e.g., liver) along the way. These side effects may be benign or can result in a negative effect on the client's health and functional capacity that may or may not be evident to the client or others.

METABOLISM

Drugs, chemicals, and toxins are all foreign to the human body. The body attempts to rid itself of foreign chemicals, regardless of whether they are therapeutic or harmful. Drug metabolism is the conversion of a drug's chemical structure into a molecule that is more readily excreted from the body. Although drug metabolism often creates a new compound with less biological activity, drugs can also be metabolized into more active compounds. Most drugs must be metabolized before they are excreted from the body, and the metabolism process is highly individualized and influenced by many factors, including the client's general nutritional status, inherited genetic factors, age, gender, and level of physical activity.

EXCRETION

Excretion describes how a drug leaves the body. Some drugs are excreted from the body after they have been metabolized, whereas others are excreted unchanged. Most drugs, toxins, and metabolites are excreted in the urine, and others are excreted in feces or through the air. The primary organ for drug elimination is the kidney.

PHARMACODYNAMICS

Pharmacodynamics is the study of the biochemical and physiologic effects of drugs and their mechanism of action. A drug's actions may be structurally specific or nonspecific. Most drugs bind to extracellular receptors where they initiate a series of biochemical reactions that alter the cells' physiology. This is a specific action, whereas a nonspecific drug action does not combine with cell receptors to produce a biological response within a cell's interior.

THERAPEUTICS

Therapeutics is the study of how drugs are used to prevent and manage disease. Whether a drug is useful for therapy is crucially dependent on its ability to produce the desired effect without undesirable effects or, minimally, with tolerable side effects that are outweighed by the drug's benefits. A desired effect is the intended or expected clinical response to a drug. This is the response that is evaluated when a drug is given to a client, and a dosage adjustment, along with the continuation of a particular drug therapy, is based on this effect. Conversely *adverse reactions* are any unintended responses to a drug that occur when a client is receiving therapeutic doses of that drug for prophylaxis, diagnosis, or therapy purposes. An adverse reaction associated with excessive amounts of a drug is considered a drug overdose. Idiosyncratic responses are excessive or abnormal responses to a drug that are genetically determined and may be difficult to distinguish from an adverse reaction. An allergic reaction is an adverse response as a result of a previous exposure to the same drug or one that is chemically similar to it. The first exposure triggers the generation of antibodies to the drug. On the second exposure the immune system reacts to the drug in question as if it was a foreign invader and may produce a hypersensitivity reaction. A drug interaction (Table 8-3) occurs when one drug is given concurrently with another and alters the pharmacokinetics or pharmacodynamics of the other drug. Some known drug interactions are beneficial, such as those that increase the effectiveness of one when taken together, whereas other interactions may lead to undesired toxicities. Drug interactions may occur by one of the following mechanisms:

- Altering absorption: The presence of one compound may alter the environment necessary for another drug to pass into the body.
- Altering how a drug is metabolized: Some drugs may stimulate enzymes that break them down, thereby increasing the overall rate of drug metabolism. This occurs while other drugs compete for the metabolizing enzymes, thereby slowing the rate of metabolism of both drugs.
- Competing for protein binding sites: Drugs that bind to proteins may compete with other drugs for that protein site, which can lead to an increased concentration of either drug.

Table 8-3   Drug Interactions and Potential Outcomes

Type of Interaction	Mathematical Model
Addition: The response elicited by the two drugs is equal to the combined responses of the individual drugs.	$1 + 1 = 2$
Synergism: The response elicited by the two drugs is greater than the combined responses of the individual drugs.	$1 + 1 = 3$
Potentiation: A drug that has no effect enhances the effect of the other drug.	$0 + 1 = 3$
Antagonism: One drug inhibits or reduces the effect of another drug, and the antagonist usually has no inherent activity.	$1 + 1 = 0$

Possessing knowledge about the way drugs are absorbed, distributed, and excreted by the body is important to the understanding of expected drug effects and to the ability to identify possible adverse reactions and unexpected effects. This is a complex science that can generally predict a drug's effects and potential side effects because of rigorous clinical trials before a manufacturer is granted permission by the *Food and Drug Administration (FDA)* to bring a drug to the market in the United States. However, benefits and unwanted side effects vary for each person examined because there are genetic differences in drug disposition and metabolism pathways, as well as in how a client handles a drug. Drugs are more likely to cause difficulty in certain groups because of the way their members' body chemistry interacts with particular substances; however, most healthy adults have had some unexpected outcomes from taking medications that were prescribed or purchased OTC.

Every drug has a usual dosage range; however, many factors, such as weight, ethnicity, gender, pregnancy status, and liver and kidney function, can alter the effective dose in these situations. Children, older adults, people with disabilities, and people with chronic health conditions also can respond differently to medications. Primary explanations for these inconsistencies include differences in body stature and physiology that impact the absorption rate and elimination of medications. People with chronic health conditions are often at a higher risk if there is a decrease in liver or kidney function because they are unable to eliminate the medications they are metabolizing. Any condition that alters the typical functioning of the body may change the course of drug therapy and result in an unwanted response to a medication.

OLDER ADULTS

There are many changes in the ability of the body to absorb, metabolize, and excrete medications as the body ages. This can be caused in part by the overall and generalized slowing of the aging person's metabolism. The older adult is more likely to be taking multiple medications and have a higher incidence of chronic health conditions that can also reduce the ability to absorb, distribute, and eliminate medications. People with disabilities often also must contend with chronic health conditions; however, persons with certain disabilities are more likely to have chronic health conditions that require a variety of medications. For example immobility can lead to decreased physical activity and general slowing of blood flow through the body, resulting in oral medications remaining in the stomach for longer periods than

usual. These factors can lead to changes in the absorption, distribution, and metabolism of a drug and result in either a decreased or increased response to the drug in question. Some developmental disabilities are associated with altered function of the kidneys and liver, which are vital organs responsible for the metabolism of medications. Finally some disabilities involve problems with metabolizing proteins and carbohydrates that can also impact an individual's response to a medication.

THERAPEUTIC DRUG CLASSIFICATIONS

DRSs commonly see clients who are taking medications to treat or manage symptoms associated with a single condition or multiple diagnoses. Medications can be divided into drug classifications, and each drug can be associated with the characteristics of a particular classification. Each drug that falls within a particular classification has a specific mechanism of action for its intended therapeutic effect; each medication in a given therapeutic class will have a similar mechanism of action and side effect profile. Based on these characteristics, the DRS may be able predict the actions, side effects, and potential interactions of a drug or drugs. Categories such as antibiotic, cardiovascular, and hormonal drugs are examples of therapeutic classes. The following section comprises a discussion of different categories of drugs.

CARDIOVASCULAR DRUGS

The therapeutic goal of this class of drugs is to manage cardiovascular disorders, including hypertension (Table 8-4), heart failure (Table 8-5), angina (Table 8-6), and arrhythmia (Table 8-7).[1-4]

DRUGS THAT AFFECT THE CENTRAL NERVOUS SYSTEM

Thousands of neuronal signals fire through our brains each moment of every day and control breathing, movements, thoughts, and even emotions. Because numerous pathways in the brain use the same neurotransmitters, treating a damaged pathway also can unintentionally affect synapses of normal neurons. This is why central nervous system (CNS) drugs are notorious for causing a variety of unwanted side effects. Dispensing medication that acts on the CNS is most often associated with managing depression, anxiety, seizures, acquired brain injury, stroke, and Parkinson's disease, to name a few.

Table 8-4 **Hypertension Drugs**

Drug	Mechanism	Undesirable Effects	Drug Interactions
Furosemide (Lasix) Hydrochlorothiazide	Diuretic	Dehydration, decreases sodium and potassium, hyperglycemia	Enhance effects of antihypertensive drugs
Clonidine (Catapres) Methyldopa (Aldomet)	Agonist	Drowsiness, dry mouth, headache	TCA, alcohol, increase CNS depression
Prazosin (Minipress) Terazosin (Hytrin)	α-Blocker	Hypotension, dry mouth, edema, congestion	Enhance actions of other antihypertensives
Atenolol (Tenormin) Metoprolol (Lopressor)	β-Blocker	CNS depression, sedation	Enhance the effects of digoxin
Captopril (Capoten) Lisinopril (Prinivil) Enalaparil (Vasotec)	ACE inhibitor, adrenergic	Hypotension, dizziness, headache, dry unproductive cough	Increased hypotension with diuretics

TCA, Tricyclic antidepressant; *CNS*, central nervous system; *ACE*, angiotensin-converting enzyme.

Table 8-5 **Heart Failure Drug**

Drug	Mechanism	Undesirable Effects	Drug Interactions
Digoxin (Lanoxin)	Inhibits sodium pump	Bradycardia, arrhythmias, nausea, diarrhea	Diuretics, corticosteroids

Table 8-6 **Angina Drugs**

Drug	Mechanism	Undesirable Effects	Drug Interactions
Nitroglycerin (nitrates)	Dilates myocardial arteries	Hypotension, bradycardia	Alcohol, other antihypertensive agents
Diltiazem (Cardizem) Verapamil (Isoptin)	Calcium entry blocker	Headache, dizziness, edema, decreased cardiac output	β-Blockers, digoxin

ANTICONVULSANTS

There are many different types of seizures that are divided into two main types: partial and generalized. Drugs used to manage seizures are chosen by their abil-ity to control certain types of seizures. A suitable single agent's dose is increased until the desired effect is achieved or until toxicity prevents further increase. A second drug may be added if maximal doses of the initial drug fail to promote the desired outcome. Abrupt

Table 8-7 Arrhythmia Drugs

Drug	Mechanism	Undesirable Effects	Drug Interactions
Quinidine Procainamide (Pronestyl) Disopyramide (Norpace)	Slows conduction	Nausea, vomiting, diarrhea	Phenobarbital, digoxin, phenytoin
Lidocaine (Xylocaine) Mexiletine (Mexitil)	Decreases automaticity of A-V node?????	Drowsiness, paresthesias	β-Blockers, Tagamet

discontinuation of an anticonvulsant may actually induce seizures and therefore is contraindicated. Adverse side effects among the anticonvulsants are CNS suppression and dermatologic, hematologic, and hepatic changes. Box 8-1 lists a few of the anticonvulsant drugs available.[1-4]

ANTIDEPRESSANTS

Antidepressants alter the flow of certain chemicals that are thought to be deficient in the brain cells of people with depression. Tricyclic antidepressants (Table 8-8) are commonly used, as are serotonin-specific drugs, such as fluoxetine. Because of its side effect and drug interaction profile, the class of antidepressants known as monoamine oxidase inhibitors is less commonly used.

BOX 8-1	Anticonvulsant Drugs

Phenytoin (Dilantin)
Carbamazepine (Tegretol)
Phenobarbital
Benzodiazepines
Valproic acid (Depakote)
Gabapentin (Neurontin)
Topiramate (Topamax)

SEROTONIN REUPTAKE INHIBITORS

Medications in this class include fluoxetine (Prozac), paroxetine (Paxil), and sertraline (Zoloft) and work by blocking the reuptake of the neurotransmitter serotonin. This class of medications was considered to have fewer side effects than tricyclic antidepressants and is still considered the least sedating; however, recent evidence points to a possible link with increased suicide, violence, and mania.[5]

ANTIPSYCHOTIC DRUGS

Antipsychotic medications are used to manage the behaviors and symptoms of psychotic illnesses such as schizophrenia. There are a number of antipsychotic medications available. These medications typically affect the neurotransmitter dopamine and include chlorpromazine (Thorazine) and thioridazine (Mellaril). Because these drugs block the dopamine receptors, they suppress all dopamine receptor-mediated actions in the brain. Specific neurologic side effects include tardive dyskinesia, akathisia, and parkinsonism.

ANTIANXIETY DRUGS

Benzodiazepines (diazepam [Valium], flurazepam [Dalmane, Roche], and lorazepam [Serax]) and

Table 8-8 Tricyclic Antidepressants

Drug	Mechanism	Undesirable Effects	Drug Interactions
Amitriptyline (Elavil) Nortriptyline (Pamelor) Imipramine (Tofranil)	Not clear, but most increase levels of monoamine neurotransmitter	Highly sedating, hypotension, weight gain	Monoamine reuptake inhibitor, additive effect with other central nervous system depressants

barbiturates (phenobarbital and barbital) are the most common antianxiety medications used in Western medicine. Both drugs enhance the actions of the neurotransmitter γ-aminobutyric acid. Physicians typically prescribe benzodiazepines more frequently because they have fewer side effects. Both agents are also effective muscle relaxants, sleep agents, and anticonvulsants; drowsiness, sedation, "clouding" of consciousness, ataxia, dysarthria, and behavioral disinhibition are sometimes unwanted side effects associated with these drugs. Finally buspirone is different from other anxiolytics because it has few if any typical antianxiety side effects, such as sedation and physical impairment. However, this drug may impair mental or physical ability required for the performance of potentially hazardous tasks, such as driving or operating heavy machinery. Drug interaction effects for each of these drugs would be additive effects with anything that also causes sedation.

CNS Stimulants

In children, attention deficit disorder (ADD) is characterized by a short attention span, restlessness, distractibility, impulsivity, and emotional lability. Amphetamine-like drugs reduce these symptoms in most children. Referring to this class of drugs as stimulants is a misnomer because although these drugs were first noted for their ability to stimulate the CNS, the effects of these drugs are complex (Table 8-9). It is theorized that the beneficial effects of amphetamines in hyperkinetic children are caused by inhibition of "fast-rate" behavior and that the amphetamine-induced acceleration of "slow-rate" behavior in children with ADD may account for improved learning, memory skills, and overall scholastic performance.

Drugs that Treat Parkinson's Disease

Parkinson's disease essentially is caused by a decrease in the dopamine neurotransmission secondary to the degradation of the dopaminergic neurons. Treatment consists of either increasing dopamine neurotransmission or blocking cholinergic neurotransmission (Table 8-10).

Drugs that Treat Alzheimer's Disease

Changes in the brain that characterize Alzheimer's disease begin long before people develop clinical symptoms, such as memory loss. Patients with Alzheimer's disease show behavioral consequences (e.g., decline in memory and learning) that are partially related to cholinergic deficits. Treatments have focused on maintaining the acetylcholine levels in the brain. Medications used are considered cholinesterase inhibitors. It is not fully understood how cholinesterase inhibitors work to manage Alzheimer's disease, but current research has shown that this class of inhibitors prevents the breakdown of acetylcholine. Acetylcholine is an important chemical in the brain that is widely believed to be instrumental in memory and other cognitive processes. However, as Alzheimer's disease progresses, the brain produces less and less acetylcholine, and cholinesterase inhibitors may eventually lose their effectiveness altogether. Galantamine (Reminyl), Rivastigmine (Exelon), Donepezil (Aricept), and Tacrine (Cognex) are cholinesterase inhibitors.[1-4] Nausea, vomiting, and diarrhea are common side effects associated with these medications, and drug interactions are usually minimal.

Table 8-9 CNS Stimulants

Drug	Mechanism	Undesirable Effects	Interactions
Amphetamine (Dexedrine)	CNS stimulant	Overstimulation, restlessness, insomnia, anorexia	Monoamine oxidase inhibitors, tricyclic antidepressants, barbiturates
Methylphenidate (Ritalin) Pemoline (Cylert)	Mild CNS stimulant	Overstimulation, restlessness, insomnia, anorexia	Monoamine oxidase inhibitors, tricyclic antidepressants, barbiturates

CNS, Central nervous system.

Table 8-10 Drugs That Treat Parkinson's Disease

Drug	Mechanism	Undesirable Effects	Drug Interactions
Levodopa/carbidopa	Increased dopamine	Nausea, vomiting	Antipsychotic drugs, antidepressants
Amantadine (Symmetrel)	Releases dopamine	At high doses hallucinations, confusion	Enhance CNS side effects
Pergolide (Eldepryl)	Inhibits degradation of dopamine	Nausea, hallucinations, hypotension, dizziness, confusion	Fatal reactions with MAO inhibitors
Trihexyphenidyl (Artane)	Cholinergic antagonist	Urinary retention, CNS disturbances	Decreases levodopa because of decreased GI motility

CNS, Central nervous system; *MAO,* monoamine oxidase; *GI,* gastrointestinal.

DRUGS THAT TREAT MULTIPLE SCLEROSIS

Although no cure has been found for multiple sclerosis (MS), there are medications available to slow the progression and ease the symptoms of the disease. These medications are considered disease-modifying agents and are all taken by injection (Table 8-11).

ANTITHROMBUS DRUGS

A thrombus is a clot that forms in a blood vessel or heart chamber. Thrombus formation depends on blood flow, blood coagulation, and the vessel wall. Platelet adhesion to a vessel wall initiates the formation of an arterial thrombus, whereas venous thrombi develop in areas of slow blood flow. Anticoagulants inhibit blood coagulation; antithrombotic agents prevent platelet aggregation; and thrombolytic agents degrade clots that have already formed. Blood coagulation occurs as a cascade. Several clotting factors require vitamin K for activation; therefore inhibition of vitamin K is a pharmacologic strategy for preventing clots (Table 8-12).

Table 8-11 Multiple Sclerosis Drug Therapy

Drug	Mechanism	Undesirable Effects	Drug Interactions
Interferon 1a (Avonex) Interferon 1b (Betaseron) Interferon β-1a (Rebif)	Biologic response modifier	Flulike symptoms, depression, anxiety	
Glatiramer (Copaxone)	Biologic response modifier	Runny nose, tremor, weakness, weight gain	
Mitoxantrone (Novantrone)	Antineoplastic	Urine may change color, nausea, hair loss, menstrual disorders	Many

Table 8-12 Antithrombus Drugs

Drug	Mechanism	Undesirable Effects	Drug Interactions
Heparin Warfarin (Coumadin)	Anticoagulant blocking vitamin K–dependent clotting factors	Bleeding, hemorrhage	Aspirin, ibuprofen, high doses of vitamin C or K, Tagamet, and many others
Aspirin Ibuprofen Dipyridamole Ticlopidine Clopidogrel (Plavix)	Antithrombotic	Gastrointestinal bleeding, ulceration, headache	Coumadin, β-blockers, prazosin, captopril

MUSCLE RELAXANTS

There are three types of muscles in the body:

- Skeletal muscles that are controlled by the voluntary part of the brain and provide postural support and help to make movement possible
- Smooth muscles that line the digestive tract and enable the eyes to move and other involuntary activities of the body for example
- Cardiac muscles

Skeletal muscle relaxants are used to relax certain muscles in the body with some direct effect on the CNS. Centrally acting muscle relaxants act in the CNS to produce their muscle relaxant effect. The actions on the CNS are also responsible for some of this class of medication's side effects, such as drowsiness, decreased appetite, dizziness, ataxia, headache, dry mouth, double vision, diminished concentration, and decreased coordination. Box 8-2 lists the medications commonly used.[1-4]

BOX 8-2	Commonly Used Muscle Relaxants

Carisoprodol (Soma)
Cyclobenzaprine (Flexeril)
Methocarbamol (Robaxin)
Lioresal (Baclofen)
Tizanidine (Zanaflex)
Dantrolene (Dantrium)
Diazepam (Valium)

DRUGS THAT TREAT GASTROINTESTINAL DISORDERS

Gastrointestinal problems that can be corrected with medication include diarrhea, constipation, acid reflux, and the formation of peptic ulcers. Gastroesophageal reflux disease (GERD) and peptic ulcer disease are often treated using the same medications. Drug therapy usually consists of neutralizing stomach contents or reducing gastric acid secretions. Histamine receptor blockers are used to reduce histamine-induced acid release by competing for histamine receptors. Antacids also reduce acidity but require higher and more frequent doses as compared with histamine blockers. Medications in this category include Tagamet, Zantac, and Axid and generally have few side effects. Tagamet is associated with more side effects than the others. Tagamet increases the blood levels of many other medications, such as theophylline, Dilantin, and anticoagulants.

ANALGESICS

Analgesics are a broad therapeutic category with several subcategories described by their mechanism of action. The therapeutic goal generally is to reduce a patient's level of pain and discomfort. Analgesics have the following subcategories:

- Opioid analgesics (narcotic; e.g., morphine, codeine, oxycodone, and meperidine): Opium, derived from poppies, relieves pain and induces euphoria by binding to opiate receptors in the brain. Narcotic analgesics can be effective in relieving pain and are often used when nonnarcotic options have failed. All drugs within this category produce respiratory depression, constipation, hypotension, and CNS depression, and the effects will be compounded with the addition of anything that decreases the CNS's ability to function.

- Nonnarcotic analgesics (e.g., acetaminophen): This class has little or no antiinflammatory activity, and it is thought that their mechanism of action is achieved by inhibiting prostaglandin synthesis. Prostaglandins modulate components of the inflammation process, body temperature, pain transmission, and platelet aggregation. Acetaminophen has few side effects and drug interactions except at high doses. Liver toxicity can also occur when combined with alcohol.

- Nonsteroidal antiinflammatory drugs (NSAIDs; e.g., aspirin, ibuprofen, and naproxen): These medications reduce inflammation, pain, and fever by inhibiting the sensation of pain. Their mechanism of action is also related to an effect on prostaglandins. All medications in this class can cause gastrointestinal bleeding, an upset stomach, and/or interact with anticoagulant and antidiabetic agents.

ANTIINFECTIVES

Bacteria are a constant factor in the world. The body's natural defenses ordinarily protect against invasion by bacteria and viruses; an infection occurs when this relationship and the balance are disturbed. Symptoms of an infection may be localized, such as with a cut, or generalized, such as when a client has a fever. The primary goal of antimicrobial therapy is to destroy destructive organisms without harming other healthy tissues. Many drugs offer selective toxicity, which can be effective against certain bacterium and cause few side effects. The identity and the drug sensitivity must be determined when choosing the most effective antiinfective agent. Box 8-3 lists the many broad classes of antiinfective and antibiotic drugs.[1-4]

Antibiotic, antibacterial, and antifungal drugs are among the most commonly used medications by people with disabilities and elderly persons. They are also some of the most complex to manage because of their adverse drug effects and interactions.

DRUGS THAT TREAT RESPIRATORY CONDITIONS

Bronchoconstriction, inflammation, and loss of lung elasticity are the three most common processes that result in bronchial obstruction, and drug therapy is usually prescribed to reverse or prevent these

| BOX 8-3 | Classes of Antiinfectives and Antibiotics |

Penicillin: Penicillin G, amoxicillin, and ampicillin
Cephalosporins: Cefaclor and cefoxitin
Aminoglycosides: Gentamicin and tobramycin
Tetracyclines: Tetracycline and doxycycline
Sulfonamides: Sulfisoxazole and trimethoprim-sulfamethoxazole
Urinary antiseptics: Nitrofurantoin
Antifungals: Nystatin and miconazole

processes. Bronchoconstriction results from the effects of inflammatory agents released within the bronchial walls. Chronic inflammation is caused by prolonged exposure to airway irritants, such as cigarette smoke. The result is airways that are constricted, with increased secretions of mucus. In patients with reactive airway disease (i.e., asthma) the trachea and bronchi are sensitive to stimuli, which results in wheezing, coughing, and chest tightness. Treatment methods include using inhaled agents that relax the bronchial cell walls, oral agents that dilate the bronchioles, inhaled agents that inhibit the release of the inflammatory mediator, or oral corticosteroids to abate the inflammation present (Table 8-13).

DRUGS THAT TREAT ENDOCRINE DISORDERS

Endocrine disorders usually result in either an oversupply or undersupply of hormones. Several glands that are found throughout the body produce hormones. These substances are released into the blood and act on target organs or structures at sites other than those in which they are produced. Drugs used to compensate for hormonal disorders are generally designed to replace insufficient hormone production and typically have minimal deleterious side effects. Some of the endocrine organs and the hormones they produce include the following:

- Pituitary gland: Produces hormones that control growth, metabolism, fluid balance, and certain types of reproductive functions.
- Thyroid gland: Produces thyroxin that controls metabolism, growth, and maturation. Calcitonin is also produced by the thyroid gland and facilitates new bone growth.
- Adrenal glands: Secrete hormones that control the autonomic fight or flight mechanism, epinephrine and norepinephrine, cortisol, aldosterone, and androgens.

Table 8-13 Respiratory Medications

Drug	Mechanism	Undesirable Effect	Drug Interactions
Albuterol (Ventolin) Metaproterenol (Alupent), inhaled	Bronchodilator	Tachycardia, central nervous system stimulation	Tricyclic antidepressants
Theophylline (Theo-Dur), oral	Dilate bronchiole	Nausea, vomiting, headache, tachycardia	Many: antibiotics, contraceptives, Tagamet
Dexamethasone (Decadron) Triamcinolone (Azmacort), inhaled	Decreases inflammation	Increased risk of mouth fungal infection	

- Pancreas: A large and important gland located behind the stomach close to the duodenum that helps to digest food and produce insulin, the main chemical for breaking down and balancing the sugar level in the bloodstream.

DIETARY SUPPLEMENTS

Vitamins, herbal supplements, and alternative medicines are becoming more prominent today as evidenced by people who are self-medicating with OTC supplements in greater numbers than ever before. Vitamins, dietary supplements, and herbs are much like prescription medications and can have unwanted side effects and drug interactions. Natural does not necessarily mean that a particular dietary supplement is safe. Many vitamins, supplements, and herbal home remedies can have a strong pharmacologic effect on the body, especially in individuals who already have a compromised immune system, other health challenges, or both. Herbs and dietary supplements also may have chemical components in variable concentrations based on plant genetics, plant parts, and growing and processing conditions. The FDA regulates dietary supplements under a different set of regulations than those covering conventional medications that are either purchased OTC or prescribed by a physician. Manufacturers of dietary supplements generally are not required to register with the FDA or obtain FDA approval before producing and selling their products. Therefore documented adverse effects and drug interaction information are minimal at best. Because of the potential for supplement–drug interactions, it is important that DRSs are as aware of a client's dietary supplement usage as they are of their client's prescription drug use.

MEDICATION HISTORY

A drug history is a critical component of a client's medical history. The information obtained can assist the DRS to determine whether medications may influence the client's performance during the clinical evaluation, on-road evaluation, or both. It is advised that clients present to the DRS a current list of medications that includes the name(s) and dosage(s), as well as when and how often a medication is taken. This list should be exhaustive and include herbals, vitamins, home remedies, and OTC medications.

The DRS should inquire about each drug (i.e., prescription, OTC, and herbal) taken. Box 8-4 lists what pertinent information the DRS should ascertain.

SPECIAL CONSIDERATIONS

Although every drug has a usual dosage range, certain factors, such as client's age, weight, culture, gender, and

BOX 8-4	Information the DRS Needs to Obtain About Each Drug

Name of medication
Indication/reason for taking
Administration route
Frequency of administration
Duration of therapy: Are there any recent changes, and how long on the current combination of medications and why?
Adverse reactions or side effects the client may be experiencing
The physician who prescribed the medication(s)

ethnicity, may contribute to impacting kidney or liver function, resulting in the need for a dosage adjustment.

AGE

Age produces certain changes in body composition and organ function and presents unique dosing requirements. Again, elderly clients also are more likely to have multiple illnesses and to take multiple drugs; therefore the DRS should be cognizant that there is an increased risk of drug interactions for these clients.

COMPLIANCE

Medication treatments are not effective if the drugs are not taken. The DRS should determine whether the client has any other problems that may affect his or her compliance with the medication treatment plan. It also should be noted that a person out of work or without health insurance might fail to fill prescriptions because he or she lacks the financial resources. In these cases the DRS should work with the client and other professional team members (e.g., social worker) to identify alternative funding sources as necessary.

Proper medication usage is another critical factor for achieving the full benefits of the prescribed medication and improved driving performance and safety. Response time, visual acuity and perception, and possession of the necessary skills to interact with other drivers can all be affected negatively or positively by medications. To achieve the desired effect and decrease the potential for unwanted side effects, all prescribed medications need to be taken correctly and consistently. DRSs should ask their clients the following questions about medication usage: How and when do you take your medication(s)? Do you alter or change the dosage(s) from the prescribed dosage(s)? Do you alter the type of medication(s) or dosage(s) depending on what your plans for the day happen to be? Have you taken your medication(s) today?

SUBSTANCE ABUSE

Substance abuse can be defined as being physically dependent, psychologically dependent, or both on any substance, such as alcohol, prescription medications, or drugs taken without being prescribed by a physician. People with disabilities experience a substantially higher substance abuse risk than people without disabilities. Moreover the prevalence of alcoholism is higher among elderly people treated in health care settings than among the general elderly population in the United States. There are also disability-specific risk factors (e.g., prescribed medications, chronic medical problems, social isolation, and behavioral problems).

ADDICTION

Addiction occurs when a person's behavior is negatively affected or controlled by the urge to obtain and use legal or illegal substances because of the gratification experienced on a physical, emotional, and/or psychological level. Addictions to prescribed medications can result when a client is attempting to minimize his or her pain and discomfort that is often associated with a medical condition by taking prescription pain medications such as codeine, Dilantin, OxyContin, and others.

TOLERANCE

Tolerance occurs when a person becomes less responsive to a medication's intended action or effect, which results in decreased or absent benefits as compared with the benefits derived from the medication when the client first took it. Tolerance may develop much more rapidly in some individuals than others and requires close monitoring by the client's physician who prescribed the medication(s).

DEPENDENCE

Physical dependence means that the person will have withdrawal symptoms if the medication is suddenly discontinued. Psychological dependence means the user believes that he or she cannot function without a drug and therefore craves it even if withdrawal symptoms are not experienced on cessation. Certainly alcohol and illicit drugs can affect the ability to drive. The question of alcohol and drug use history is another component of the client's broader medication history. Some states may require documentation from a substance abuse professional for medical clearance to obtain a driver's license.

Questions that may be asked include the following:
- How often do you drink alcohol?
- How many drinks do you have in a typical week?
- Has anyone told you to cut down on your drinking or not to drink?
- Have you recovered from a substance abuse treatment program?
- Do you take any medications that are not prescribed for you, even occasionally?
- Do you use any illicit drugs?

HOW MEDICATIONS CAN IMPAIR DRIVING

Most people today recognize that consuming alcohol impairs safe driving; however, fewer people are aware that taking medications, irrespective of whether they are prescribed or OTC (e.g., codeine, Valium, antihistamines, cough syrups, and pain relievers), can also impair an individual's ability to safely operate a motor vehicle. Combining OTC and prescription medications also can further complicate and undermine driving performance. Box 8-5 presents some of the medication types that can impair a person's ability to drive.

The aging process, as well as disabling conditions, can change a person's metabolism and affect muscle tone and organ function, requiring a longer period for the body to rid itself of medications. Drugs can accumulate, and a small amount may have a large effect. The same drug that did not impair a person when younger can suddenly do so as he or she ages. The same medications also impair people differently and impair our bodies in a variety of ways. Box 8-6 lists the different effects medications can have on an individual.

The effects of drugs on driving abilities can also continue many hours after a drug is taken. Being impaired by a drug, intentionally or not, increases the potential for a crash. Medications are a complex piece of the comprehensive driver evaluation process. The DRS must use the medication and medical history of his or her clients along with the observations made clinically and during an on-road evaluation to establish whether there is a possible link between medications and poor or inconsistent driving performance. DRSs usually are not pharmacologists; however, each specialist must be aware of the role and effects medications have in their clients'

lives and what effect medications may have on the clients' ability to become safe and functional drivers.

MEDICATION RESOURCES

Because this is not a pharmacy textbook or a complete drug reference manual and because medications are constantly changing, consulting drug reference materials that are updated on a regular basis is necessary when evaluating a client's medication history. There is certainly a lot of information available on the Internet and in reference books. The difficulty lies in evaluating the information for usefulness and relevance. Not all side effects associated with a given drug will inevitably be experienced; furthermore, a particular medication may cause a side effect not commonly attributed to it. In addition to other reference sources, the client's physician, a pharmacist, or local drug information center can be beneficial resources for the DRS, client, and caregiver.

REFERENCES

1. Loeb S, Blanchard R, editors: *2002 drug handbook*, Blue Bell, PA, 2001, Blanchard & Loeb.
2. Berkow R: *Merck manual of medical information*, Whitehouse Station, NJ, 1997, Merck & Co., Inc.
3. Ellsworth AJ, Witt DM, Dugdale DC, et al: *Mosby's medical drug reference*, St. Louis, 2000, Mosby.
4. Griffith HW: Complete guide to prescription and nonprescription drugs, New York, 2002, Berkley Publishing.
5. Breggin PR: Suicidality, violence and mania caused by selective serotonin reuptake inhibitors (SSRIs): a review and analysis, *Int J Risk Safety Med* 16:31-49, 2003/2004.

BOX 8-6   Potential Effects of Medication

Slower reaction time
Difficulty visually tracking objects
Alteration of depth perception
Diminished coordination while steering the vehicle and accessing the braking system
Hyperactivity
Lack of attention
Reduction of peripheral vision
Confusion
Drowsiness
Lack of awareness of surroundings
Decreased accuracy of movements
Decreased ability to perceive hazards and identify risks

BOX 8-5   Medications That Can Impair Driving

Alcohol-containing medicines
Allergy medicines
Amphetamines
Antianxiety medications
Antibiotics
Antidepressants
Antinausea medicines
Antiseizure medicines
Barbiturates
Blood pressure medicines
Blood sugar medicines
Caffeine-containing medicines
Cough syrups
Decongestants
Motion sickness medicines
Narcotic pain medications
Sedatives
Stimulants
Tranquilizers
Ulcer medication

Chapter 9

THE IMPACT OF POSITIONING AND MOBILITY DEVICES ON DRIVING AND COMMUNITY MOBILITY

Beth E. Anderson • Chris Maurer

KEY TERMS

- Wheeled mobility and seating evaluation
- Mobility device
- Wheeled mobility and seating specialists
- Loading device
- Seating components
- Proximal stability
- Balance
- Wheelchair lift

CHAPTER OBJECTIVES

After completing this chapter, the reader will be able to do the following:

- Understand the role of the wheeled mobility and seating specialist within the context of driver rehabilitation and community mobility.
- Understand the impact that wheeled mobility and seating evaluations can have on driving and community mobility.
- Explain the equipment considerations concerning wheeled mobility and seating options and vehicle modifications.

INTRODUCTION

Driving is a treasured occupation for many persons, providing independence and a sense of empowerment.

Optimal seating and positioning are required to make driving or riding as a passenger in a motor vehicle a safe reality for people of all ages with and without disabilities. Many people have had the experience of sitting in a vehicle that "fits like a glove": visibility is perfect; the controls are within easy reach; and everything feels right. Although some persons with disabilities, aging-related challenges, or both have no special needs beyond the adjustability available in the original manufacturer's equipment (OEM), others require careful evaluation to configure the seating space for optimal performance and safety. Health conditions that are frequently associated with manual or power wheelchair use are spinal cord injury, acquired brain injury, multiple sclerosis, amyotrophic lateral sclerosis, muscular dystrophy, Parkinson's disease, cerebral palsy, spina bifida, osteoarthritis, rheumatoid arthritis, heart and lung disease, and spinal deformities.[1] Motor skill deficits likely to require a specialized seating and positioning evaluation (henceforth referred to as a *"wheeled mobility and seating evaluation"*) for driving and community mobility include limited or fixed range of motion of the upper or lower limbs, impaired balance or posture, decreased endurance, and abnormal tone.

PRACTITIONER ROLES IN SEATING AND POSITIONING

In-vehicle seating and positioning evaluations for safe driving and traveling are performed by a driver rehabilitation specialist (DRS). A thorough evaluation of the client's mobility impairment and need for a *mobility device*, current and potential, is also required. After the evaluation, interventions may include modifications to

199

the client's wheelchair to accommodate optimal driver positioning, the recommendation of a device for loading and stowing the client's wheelchair or motorized scooter, and suggestions for modifying the client's vehicle to optimize accessibility, independence, and safety.

However, the process to determine safe mobility begins with the determination of the optimal seating and positioning with regard to the client's personal mobility device, such as a manual or power wheelchair, motorized scooter, or ambulation aid. A *wheeled mobility and seating specialist* typically performs this evaluation. The role of the seating specialist is to choose and modify the primary mobility device to allow the client the greatest level of independence and safety in all activities of daily living (ADL) and instrumental activities of daily living (IADL). This includes personal mobility within indoor living spaces and the community at large. Because independence and safety in daily living activities are critical, these basic functions must be preserved when seating and positioning recommendations for driving are offered. Therefore collaboration between the driver rehabilitation and seating specialists is imperative.

Collaboration allows each specialist to offer insights that aid in a client's return to successful driving or alternative community mobility. During the seating and positioning evaluation for mobility the DRS can provide guidance concerning the ease with which a particular device can be transported. This advice can help avoid situations in which a mobility device is not used because it cannot be transported or is not compatible with other necessary technology, such as a wheelchair tiedown system. The DRS also can identify changes in the size and configuration of a replacement wheelchair that can adversely affect the client's driving performance. For instance height changes in a wheelchair or seat cushion could result in costly additional vehicle modifications because the client's line of sight could be dramatically altered. During the comprehensive driver rehabilitation evaluation conducted by the DRS, the seating specialist can give advice regarding components that will give the client added stability and support within the dynamic environment of the vehicle. A seating specialist can also assist in designing specialized seating systems for a variety of vehicles to help meet the client's needs. For example a client with short stature or significant fixed postural deformities of the trunk or pelvis may need specialized seating to provide adequate visibility, stability, and comfort while in the vehicle.

The use of a mobility device raises the following questions for the DRS:
- How can the device be transported?
- Does the device break down into component parts?

- How difficult is it to disassemble, and how much does each part weigh?
- Will the device provide the stability the client needs to operate a motor vehicle while seated in it, or must he or she perform a transfer to and from the driver's seat?

All of these questions must be answered as part of a mobility and seating evaluation for driving.

COMPONENTS OF A DRIVER REHABILITATION EVALUATION

The driver rehabilitation evaluation requires a thorough evaluation of seated mobility needs, as may be performed by a wheeled mobility and seating specialist. Therefore information is presented here about both types of mobility evaluations to help the reader determine how best to accommodate a mobility device within the broader context of a comprehensive driver rehabilitation evaluation.

The nature of the client's disability has long-term implications for seated or wheeled mobility and driving. The prognosis must be considered for understanding and predicting the possible direction of the disease process and its impact on the client being assessed. Key questions include the following:
- Is it likely that the condition will deteriorate, remain stable, or improve over time?
- What is the projected timeframe for anticipated changes, if any?
- What, if any, secondary complications are present that could affect either the client's need for a mobility device or ability to use one?

In life-care planning a modified vehicle is usually projected to last 7 to 10 years. If a client's condition is progressive, a wheeled mobility device may be needed in the future, and the DRS should carefully consider the client's potential and long-term needs. Conversely if the client with a progressive condition currently uses a specific mobility device, that piece of durable medical equipment (DME) may become obsolete during the 7- to 10-year period and require the client to obtain a new device. However, if a client's condition is progressing slowly, it may not be necessary for the DRS to address potential changes in the client's mobility during the lifetime of the vehicle. In this case client and caregiver education about potential accommodations that may be needed later and the assurance that a reevaluation can be scheduled if the client's medical status changes are sufficient. When a rapid progression of symptoms is anticipated, it may be more appropriate and cost-effective to select a vehicle that can be further modified in response to the changing needs of the client. This approach is sometimes preferred even if the vehicle modifications are more extensive than the client initially requires because it can be more costly to retrofit a vehicle at a later date.

Seating and driving evaluations include assessing the client's range of motion and strength, as well as coordination of upper and lower extremities. Examples of lower limb deformities are decreased hip flexion, excessive hip abduction or adduction, decreased knee flexion and extension, and ankle plantar flexion with inversion or eversion contractures. Common limitations of upper limb range of motion that affect seating include decreased elbow and wrist extension and shoulder external rotation. In addition to influencing the client's ability to operate the primary and secondary driving controls or mobility device, limited range of motion, strength, and coordination skills also affect the client's ability to load and unload the mobility device in a vehicle. In some cases a *loading device* or lift can be used to compensate for a lack of strength, but this may not be useful if the client does not have the coordination to operate switches or attach the loading device to the mobility aid.

Additional issues that negatively affect safe driving include impaired balance, hypertonicity, or both. Frequently observed pelvic and trunk deformities include a posterior pelvic tilt with thoracic kyphosis, a pelvic obliquity with an associated scoliosis, and pelvic and trunk rotation.[1] A neutral pelvis, trunk, and lower extremity alignment is the ideal goal for functional positioning and stable posture.[2] To promote a stable posture, identification and correction of flexible (versus fixed) orthopedic deformities may be necessary.[1] If that is not possible, fixed deformities must be stabilized to decrease the potential for further deformity and to provide stability.[1] In the presence of a flexible skeletal deformity *seating components* are typically placed to correct the deformity. Conversely seating components for fixed deformities approximate the deformity to prevent it from worsening. Common seating components that aid trunk and pelvic positioning include lap belts, chest straps, and lateral thoracic support and pelvic guides.[1] Lower extremity positioning components include lateral thigh supports, abductor pommels, pivot pads, angle adjustable footplates, and toe and ankle straps. Upper limb positioning options include arm troughs, lap trays, and wrist or forearm straps.

Abnormal muscle tone is common with neurologic impairments such as acquired brain injury, spinal cord injury, cerebral palsy, muscular dystrophy, and multiple sclerosis. Muscle tone is graded by the amount of resistance to velocity-dependent passive muscle elongation.[3] Increased or decreased tone or hypertonicity or hypotonicity, respectively, of the limbs or trunk can affect a client's ability to function. Often clients with decreased tone, such as occurs with muscle dystrophy, cannot maintain their body positioning voluntarily against gravity. In this case maximizing the contours of the seating system and using gravity through tilt or recline of the wheelchair can provide additional external support. The use of a shock-absorbing wheelchair base can also help stabilize the client. Increased tone, such as occurs with acquired brain injury, spinal cord injury, cerebral palsy, and multiple sclerosis, can limit a client's voluntary motion at a joint and pose a challenge for proper and safe positioning. Uncontrolled hypertonicity, or rigidity, which involves constant resistance to stretching by a muscle, with heightened deep tendon reflexes[3] can continuously alter a client's position in a seating system, potentially leading to postural deformities, skin breakdown, and decreased function and comfort. When dealing with hypertonicity the DRS may suggest increasing the seat angle so that the angle formed by the hip and knee is >90 degrees. Ankle dorsiflexion may also be recommended. Power wheelchair bases with shock absorption features can also assist in creating a smoother ride for the client with hypertonicity.

Ambulation is an additional evaluation component. Many clients prefer to ambulate even if they have impaired gait or limited endurance. Some will resist the use of any mobility device because of the image they imagine it projects. However, safe ambulation within the community presents specific challenges, such as increased walking distances, the need for continuous balance while walking, and the presence of limiting factors such as pain or fatigue. It is important for the driving and seating specialist to make the client aware of these potential limitations. For example a client with multiple sclerosis may resist using a mobility device. However, if the client becomes too fatigued from the summer heat, for example, his or her ability to ambulate may be affected, as well as the ability to drive safely, because of decreased lower extremity function. The ability to ambulate will also influence where and how a device can be stowed in the vehicle. If the client cannot ambulate, the device must be within reach of the driver's seat or door so that he or she can be independent with stowing and retrieving the device. Another issue occurs when the client is independent at home with a manual wheelchair or without any device. However, in the community, weather patterns, distances typically traveled, and terrain must also be taken into consideration. In this setting the client may lack the endurance to ambulate for more than a few minutes at a time and may have difficulty with different terrain. The seating specialist must address these issues so that the client chooses a mobility device that will permit the achievement of all preferred goals, such as working or shopping.

Transfer skills also must be assessed for safety and efficiency. If a transfer takes too much time or requires the expenditure of limited energy reserves, the transfer process will have a negative impact on the client's day-to-day functioning. To emphasize this point the DRS may ask the client to imagine that he or she had just gotten into the car before realizing that something important had been left in the house, like a wallet or a briefcase with an important project, something so vital that he or she cannot leave without it. Now the client must transfer out of the car, go back into the house to retrieve the necessary item, exit the home, and then transfer back into the car to leave. How difficult would that be? How much time would it add? How much energy would it consume? Another scenario that can be explored is the need to run errands. Is it worthwhile to stop and pick up a few items if an extra 25 minutes are added just to get in and out of the car? How will weather affect entering and exiting the vehicle? Extremes of heat or cold can make transfers more difficult. In the final analysis the client must decide how reasonable and realistic it is to get in and out of the car several times a day. If the time and difficulty of each transfer is too great, it may cause the client to limit how often he or she ventures out, thus negatively impacting his or her community participation, interaction, and independence.[4]

The possibility exists for a client to be able to transfer to a power transfer seat in a modified van but not to a standard car seat because of the relative position of the wheelchair seat to the vehicle seat. A transfer performed within a van allows the client to be protected from the weather and also provides greater privacy. However, seating components may make it more or less difficult to transfer from a particular mobility device. The seating specialist should consider the ease with which the seating and positioning components are removed and replaced when the client will be performing independent transfers.

Specific questions should be asked of the person who uses a wheelchair or ambulation aid. Is it used on a full-time or part-time basis? Is more than one mobility device used? If more than one mobility device is used, it may be necessary for the client to choose which device is most practical in the community because it is frequently not possible or practical to accommodate more than one style of mobility device in the same vehicle. Clients with tetraplegic (quadriplegic) injuries, such as C5-7, are often faced with this decision. The client may be able to propel a manual wheelchair indoors but may require assistance to push up a ramp or steep incline, or traverse rough terrain. Often the seating specialist will recommend both a power and a manual wheelchair; however, in many instances the client's vehicle will not have the versatility to transport both wheelchairs interchangeably[5] or at the same time. Scooter users must be cautioned that they should never ride as passengers or drive from their scooters because

of problems with stability. The scooter user also must be able to perform an independent transfer if it is to be the primary mobility device.

EQUIPMENT CONSIDERATIONS

Once the primary mobility device has been identified the DRS must address the following factors:
• Weight of the device
• Combined weight of the client and the device if the client will enter the vehicle while in the device
• Dimensions of the device, such as length, width, and height. The seated height of the user is also necessary if the client will enter the vehicle or will be driving while in the device. Seat height is especially important in identifying the driver's line of sight and potential positioning challenges while behind the wheel of a motor vehicle.

Optimizing function is the overall goal of any seating and mobility system for an individual. Two requirements that are especially important to driving include *proximal stability* and *balance*. A therapeutic principle commonly used in driver evaluations is to provide proximal muscular stability to promote controlled distal mobility.[6] Further optimization of function occurs through the equipment recommendations of the DRS in consultation with the vehicle user. In the remainder of the chapter driving issues related to manual and power wheelchairs, loading devices, and vehicle selection are identified and explored.

MOBILITY DEVICES

Mobility devices mainly comprise the wheelchair base and the seating system (Figure 9-1). The wheelchair base is typically the frame of the wheelchair and includes the drive wheels, casters, and any motors. The primary seating components include the seat pan and cushion, backrest, and back cushion. A headrest, armrests, legrests, and footplates are part of the postural support system, as are any other positioning devices, such as a seatbelt, adductor wedge, and lateral supports. There are now numerous commercial solutions to achieve a fully customized contoured seating system designed to meet a client's unique needs. The variety of seating systems, wheelchair bases, and postural support options currently available allows greater numbers of clients with mobility impairments to experience increased independence, improved quality of life, and greater community participation in daily activities.

Manual Wheelchair Considerations

Most people who use manual wheelchairs have sufficient upper extremity strength to propel the wheelchair

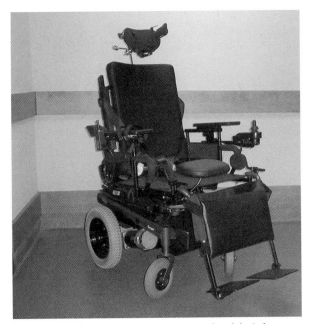

Figure 9-1 Rear wheel drive power wheelchair base with power tilt seating system.

for functional mobility. Alternate power can come from both legs or one leg, as is sometimes seen in clients with central cord injury, or from one arm combined with one leg, as seen in clients with hemiplegia. Manual tilt, recline, or tilt and recline wheelchairs are typically used for people who are completely dependent for mobility and pressure relief. In addition to these issues the type of manual wheelchair and seating system

selected should address the client's postural goals; home, work, and community needs; and the need for dependable community mobility or transportation. These needs can include the ability to load the wheelchair into and out of a vehicle, the use of alternative transportation, or the ability to tie down the wheelchair for van transport. Independent driving from a manual wheelchair is feasible, but at this time manufacturers of automatic tiedown systems do not recommend the practice. If possible, using the OEM is preferred for safety versus driving from the wheelchair.

Wheelchair Frames

Folding Frames. There are two types of manual wheelchair frames: folding (Figure 9-2, *A*) and rigid (Figure 9-2, *B*). The overall width of most manual wheelchairs is affected by the seat width of the chair needed to accommodate the client's physique. The overall width of the chair, rim to rim, is a necessary consideration when determining whether the chair will fit onto a lift platform or a minivan ramp (Figure 9-3). Folding-frame chairs have a cross-brace that allows the frame of the wheelchair to fold up into a relatively narrow shape.

The width and the height of manually folding wheelchairs are important factors for loading and storage. There are several options for transportation of manual wheelchairs. Depending on the height of the car roof, a driver may or may not be able to lift the folded wheelchair frame across his or her body to self-load it because of the height of the chair's back posts. However, most folding wheelchairs will fit into the trunk of most cars currently being driven in the United States (Figure 9-4).

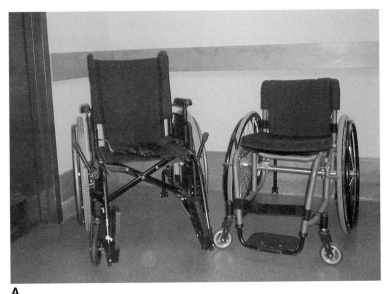

A

Figure 9-2 **A,** Manual folding wheelchair *(left)* and manual rigid wheelchair *(right).*

Continued

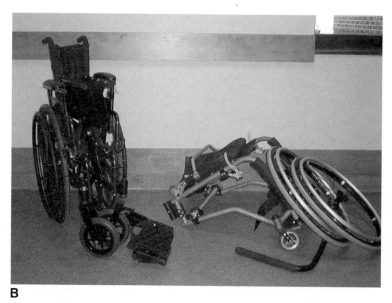

B

Figure 9-2 cont'd **B,** Folding-frame wheelchair *(left)* and rigid frame wheelchair *(right)* disassembled for transport.

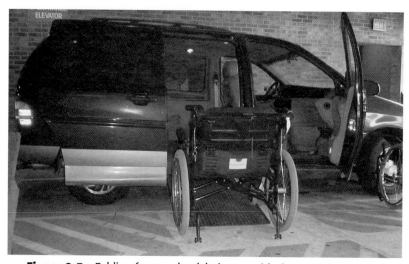

Figure 9-3 Folding-frame wheelchair, too wide for a minivan ramp.

One drawback, though, is that the wheelchair may be too long to fit into a trunk when laid on its side, depending on the height of the back posts.

Another commonly used option for wheelchair transportation is to place the wheelchair behind the driver's seat. In this case the key factor for success is the overall width of the folded chair (Figure 9-5). Folding wheelchairs that can accommodate bariatric clients do not fold as narrowly as standard chairs and weigh more because they are designed to accommodate the clients' increased weight. The weight of the chair will impact a client's ability to self-load or the caregiver's ability to lift the chair and place it into the trunk. In all cases removing separate parts, such as armrests, legrests, wheels, and antitip bars, can decrease the overall weight of the wheelchair. Disadvantages to this solution include the difficulty of keeping track of all the parts when the wheelchair is disassembled and the increased time needed to remove and replace all of the parts during the transfer period.

Rigid Frames. Rigid frame wheelchairs have a fixed frame. The back posts typically fold down, and quick-release wheels are removed to allow for easier loading and storage. The dimension of the frame with the back folded down is a consideration for dependent and independent loading (see Figure 9-2, *B*). The height of the frame frequently is too great to allow it to fit into most car trunks. Therefore, the chair is usually placed inside the car, which will limit the number of passengers the vehicle can accommodate. Depending on the size of

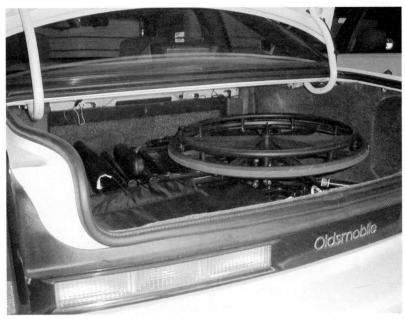

Figure 9-4 Folding wheelchair loaded into the trunk of a car.

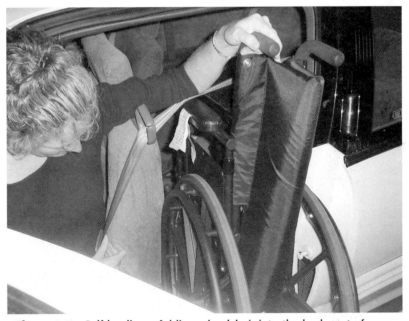

Figure 9-5 Self-loading a folding wheelchair into the back seat of a car.

the driver and the width of the wheelchair frame, the frame also may not fit between the driver and the steering wheel when self-loading (Figure 9-6).

Frame Material. Most contemporary wheelchairs are made of either aluminum or titanium. Titanium is a lighter metal than aluminum. Titanium frames are frequently preferred by self-loaders and caregivers because of the decreased weight of the frame compared with aluminum frames. Consideration of the back post style

and the type and height of the back support for rigid and folding wheelchairs is necessary when addressing transportation. The back height of a manual wheelchair may need to be higher for a client driving from his or her wheelchair to provide more postural support during dynamic situations, such as accelerating and braking. Additional positioning devices, such as lateral trunk supports and chest straps, may be necessary to provide stability under the same circumstances. In

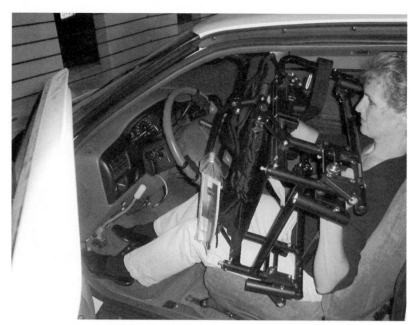

Figure 9-6 Self-loading a rigid wheelchair into a car.

some instances a different type of back device that provides more stable posterior support may be necessary for the safety of a driver.

Rigid frame wheelchairs have two options of back posts: fixed or folding. The back posts can be fixed to the frame of the wheelchair, as is standard in folding wheelchairs. This eliminates the weight of hardware that is required for the back posts to fold, but it also creates a taller frame, which may limit the ease with which it can be loaded into the vehicle. Because of limited space in cars people who choose fixed back posts frequently drive vehicles such as sport utility vehicles (SUVs), trucks, or vans. Folding back posts on rigid frame wheelchairs make the chair shorter and therefore increase ease of loading. However, the greater number of moving parts on the frame creates the potential for additional maintenance needs. The client loading the wheelchair into a vehicle also must be able to operate the release mechanism, which may be problematic for clients with limited upper limb range of motion, coordination, or both.

Wheelchair Options

Wheelchair Backs. For folding and rigid wheelchairs, the standard upholstery back is the lightest option and will fold with the frame of the chair, which decreases the number of steps required to load the wheelchair. However, the standard upholstery back more often than not offers the least trunk support, especially laterally, which may impact the stability of a driver or passenger who remains in the wheelchair while en route.

Removable solid backs are frequently used to provide appropriate support and balance for clients with limited trunk control, pain, endurance, or a combination of these or other factors. These backs interface with the back posts of the wheelchair with either fixed or quick-release hardware. Many of the solid back supports provide adjustability of the seat angle, which can assist with stable, gravity-assisted positioning, especially because most folding-frame back posts are fixed to the wheelchair frame. The maximum height of most folding- and rigid frame back posts is 20 inches. A solid back can be mounted to the back posts to allow for higher back support and therefore more stability. The disadvantage of a solid back support is that it must be removed to fold a folding-frame wheelchair. This is also true for most rigid frame chairs with folding back posts. A removable back adds an extra step in loading and unloading a wheelchair into a vehicle and requires sufficient manual dexterity to manage the release mechanisms.

Push Handles. Push handles allow someone else to push a person in a manual wheelchair; some wheelchair users also use them to provide additional sitting balance support during reaching tasks. Push handles can be integrated into the back post or bolted onto the rigidizer bar that is present on rigid frame wheelchairs (Figure 9-7, *A*).

When people become independent with propulsion they may no longer need or want assistance pushing their wheelchair. Most push handles integrated onto the back posts have to be cut off for removal. On rigid wheelchairs, push handles that bolt onto the rigidizer bar extend more posteriorly than those integrated onto the back post, creating a taller frame when folded down (Figure 9-7, *B*). However, many people like the idea that they can be unbolted if no longer needed.

Either type of push handle will increase the amount of space necessary for loading a wheelchair into a vehicle (Figure 9-7, *C*). There is an option of quick-release push handles but that requires an extra step during wheelchair loading and is another item to keep track of during the transfer process and while on the road.

Armrests. Armrests are used for upper extremity support and may be fixed, removable, flip back, or swing away. The armrest selected may depend on whether the client can independently remove the armrest for transferring or for loading the wheelchair. This requires not only an evaluation of the client's upper limb strength and fine motor skills but also a review of the situations in which the armrest will need to be removed. For example clients who drive must remove the wheelchair armrest before transferring to the driver's seat in a van. There may not be enough room to

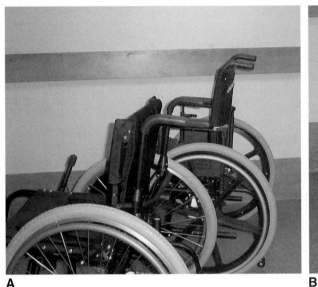

A

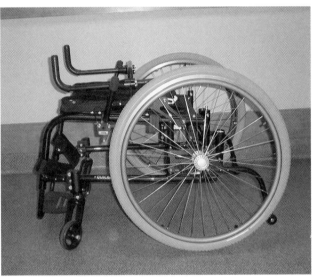

B

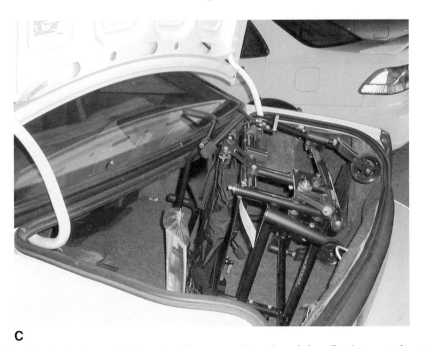

C

Figure 9-7 *A,* Push handles bolted onto rigidizer bar *(foreground),* and push handles integrated onto back posts. **B,** Rigid wheelchair backrest folding down with push handles bolted on rigidizer bar. **C,** Push handle interfering with rigid wheelchair being loaded into the trunk of a car.

perform a stand or squat pivot (i.e., modified stand pivot) transfer unless the armrest is removed, even though a fixed armrest is not problematic for the client under other circumstances. Whereas a swing-away and removable armrest is a popular option for daily tasks, during lateral movement it may impinge on the driver's seat, preventing it from being removed. Figure 9-8 provides an example of a swing-away and removable armrest.

The length of the armrest is a consideration mainly for clients who will be driving from their wheelchairs. The armrest may interfere with driver controls if the armrest or components on the armrest extend too far; for example, the armrest may come in contact with the vehicle's dashboard, affecting optimal positioning.

Front End Style

Swing-Away Legrests. Swing-away legrests (Figure 9-9) are available on almost all folding-frame wheelchairs but are uncommon on rigid frame wheelchairs. The advantage to these legrests is that they can swing out of the way to allow foot contact with the ground for stand or squat pivot transfers into a vehicle. Swing-away legrests are also removable, which decreases the weight of the frame when lifting it during loading and shortens the length of the frame. As with all removable parts, increased loading time will be needed, as well as the ability to remove and replace the part.

Rigid Front Hanger. All rigid wheelchairs and a few folding-frame wheelchairs offer a rigid front hanger so that the legrest is a part of the frame and cannot be removed. The footrests can be one solid piece, have one flip-up solid piece, or have two separate flip-up footplates. These types of configurations eliminate the hardware to swing away the legrests, which decreases the weight of the wheelchair slightly. The overall length of the wheelchair frame cannot be shortened to increase the ease of loading a wheelchair with fixed front hangers.

Legrest/Hanger Angle and Taper. The angle of the legrest or hanger is a choice when configuring manual wheelchairs. Most common options are 60, 70, 80, 85, and 90 degrees. A greater angle at the knee creates a shorter frame length, which impacts loading the wheel-

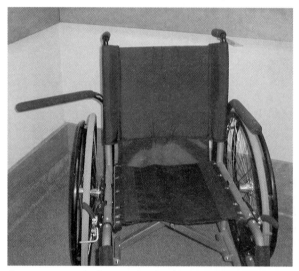

Figure 9-8 Tubular armrest in the swing-away position.

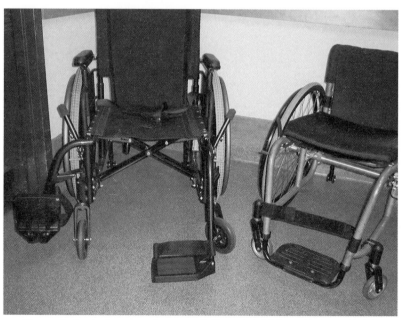

Figure 9-9 Swing-away legrests *(left)* and rigid front hanger *(right)*.

chair. It will also allow a wheelchair driver to get closer to the steering wheel before the legrests or front hanger interferes with driving components. Figure 9-10 illustrates this.

When the overall footrest width is smaller than the seat width, the legrest component or front hanger is considered to be tapered. A tapered legrest component or front hanger is primarily advantageous to wheelchair drivers (Figure 9-11). Tapered legrests may allow the driver to get close enough to the steer-ing wheel in a van without extra modification to the driver's space.

Wheel Considerations

Wheel Types. There are numerous wheel options available for manual wheelchairs. Weight of the wheel, maintenance requirements, and shock absorption capabilities are factors to consider when choosing the wheel type. The feature of wheels that impacts loading into a vehicle is weight. The most common wheel types are

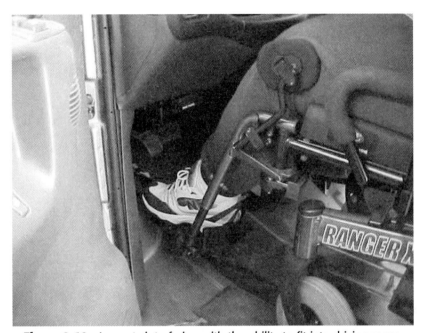

Figure 9-10   Legrests interfering with the ability to fit into driving space.

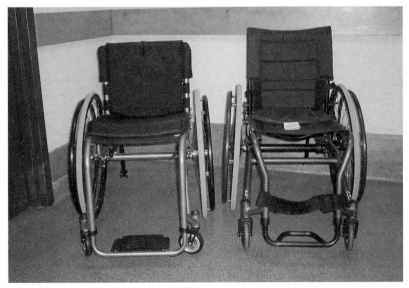

Figure 9-11   Nontapered *(left)* versus tapered *(right)* front hanger.

spoke and mag or molded wheels. Spoke and other high-performance wheels are lighter than mag or molded wheels, which not only make the chair easier to propel but also decrease the overall weight of the chair.

Axle Options. Wheels can either be bolted onto the frame of the chair or attached with a quick-release mechanism. Quick-release axles are always used on rigid wheelchairs to allow for loading; they are an option on most folding-frame wheelchairs. The capability to remove the wheels decreases the overall width and weight of the wheelchair. The client loading the wheelchair must have the ability to remove quick-release axles. Figure 9-12 illustrates quad release axles, which may be used to compensate for poor fine motor control, limited strength, or incoordination.

Wheel Locks. Wheel locks are used to stabilize the manual wheelchair during transfers or transportation. Wheel lock options include high mount push/pull locks or scissor locks (Figure 9-13, *A*). Push/pull locks require the least manual dexterity and sitting balance to operate. When the wheels are removed for loading into a vehicle, the push/pull locks extend laterally from the frame of the chair, increasing the width of the frame as well as the potential for getting caught either on the client loading the wheelchair or on parts of the vehicle. Push/pull locks are shown in Figure 9-13, *B*.

Scissor locks fold under the frame of the wheelchair when not in use and therefore do not add to the frame width when the wheels are removed. However, people with decreased hand function or impaired sitting balance have more difficulty managing scissor locks. Scissor locks also tend to be less effective than push/pull locks in sta-

bilizing tires, especially polyurethane tires, which can impact the stability of the wheelchair during transfers.

Wheel Camber. Wheel camber is the angle of the wheel as seen in a frontal plane and is increased when the point of wheel contact with the floor is greater than the point of the wheel near the top. A greater degree of wheel camber increases the stability of the wheelchair and improves the turning response. However, increasing the camber of the wheels may affect the ability of a wheelchair to fit onto a lift platform or minivan ramp because of the increased overall width of the chair (Figure 9-14).

Power-Activated Power Assist Wheels
Power assist wheels (Figure 9-15) can be used in place of standard wheels on manual wheelchairs to increase the ease of propulsion and decrease upper extremity stress. These wheels may assist a client with impaired upper extremity strength to independently propel the wheelchair up a ramp or onto a lift for loading. However, these wheels can be heavy, weighing up to 26 pounds per wheel. Therefore these wheels are harder to remove and greatly increase the weight of the wheelchair. Furthermore power assist wheels may not be compatible with some tiedown systems, such as a standard cam lock.

Casters
Casters are the small front wheels on manual wheelchairs. They come in a variety of sizes depending on the user's needs. Suspension casters are an option to absorb shock from the ground, in order to create a smoother

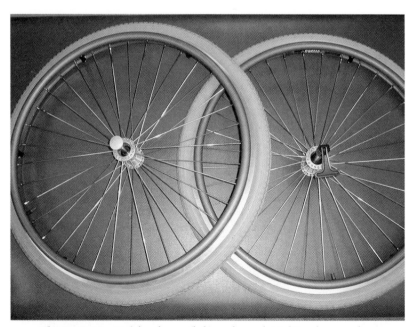

Figure 9-12 Quick-release *(left)* and quad *(right)* release axles.

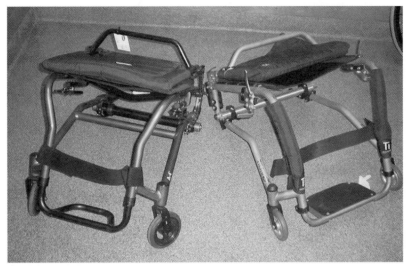

A

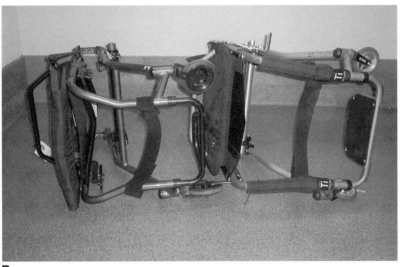

B

Figure 9-13 **A,** Push/pull wheel locks *(left),* and scissor wheel locks *(right).* **B,** View of wheel locks with the wheelchairs on their side to imitate loading into a vehicle. Push/pull wheel locks extend laterally, creating potential to interfere with objects in the car when loading the wheelchair.

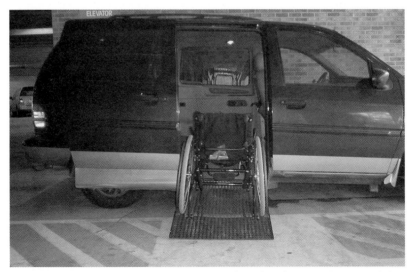

Figure 9-14   A wheelchair with 6 degrees of camber that does not fit on a minivan ramp.

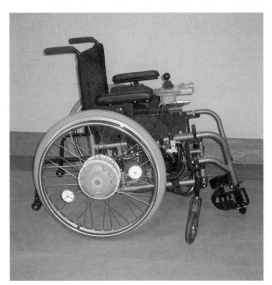

Figure 9-15 Example of power assist wheelchair.

ride for the community wheelchair user. The primary disadvantage of driving a vehicle from a wheelchair with suspension casters is that the frame of the wheelchair moves with the suspension device, creating a potentially unstable situation, especially when braking.

Quick-release casters are an option to allow for storage of a rigid frame wheelchair in a car trunk because the depth of the frame after the rear wheels are removed becomes smaller. Without the casters attached to the frame of the chair, loading a chair across the driver's seat also becomes less cumbersome.

Tiedown Options for Manual Wheelchairs

Occupied Wheelchair. A wheelchair must always be secured for transport whether it is occupied or not. Two common tiedown options available for manual wheelchairs being transported in a van are the strap (manual) and automatic tiedowns. Strap tie downs can only be used with a wheelchair passenger because a wheelchair driver cannot access the straps while seated in a wheelchair. The straps must be attached to the wheelchair frame and not to any removable parts, such as legrests and armrests. Automatic tie downs must be used with clients who will be driving from their wheelchairs and are an option for passengers, depending on the position of the wheelchair within the vehicle. Unfortunately there are few rigid frame wheelchairs that can accept an automatic tie down; however, automatic tiedowns can be used with most folding-frame wheelchairs. Discussion with the manual wheelchair user about the potential for driving in the future is therefore necessary when a wheelchair prescription is being finalized. It is recommended that if an automatic tie down is used for a manual wheelchair, there should

also be a manual tie down back-up system. This will still allow the wheelchair user to drive even if using a different wheelchair that does not have the required bracket for the automatic tiedown system. Finally, the automatic tiedown bracket adds weight to the frame of the wheelchair and will prevent folding because it is bolted across the wheelchair frame.[1]

Unoccupied Wheelchair. A cam lock is also available to secure an unoccupied wheelchair in a van. Loading devices, which can be used to lift an unoccupied wheelchair into a vehicle, provide some measure of stability because the wheelchair is attached to the device; however, most loading devices would not secure the chair in a stationary position in the event of a vehicular accident. See Chapter 17 for more information on tiedown systems.

Power Wheelchair Considerations

People who do not possess the strength or endurance to propel a manual wheelchair functionally often use power wheelchairs for personal mobility. Power wheelchairs are commonly driven with a joystick controlled by one hand; however, there are numerous alternative devices that allow a client to maneuver a power wheelchair if sufficient hand or arm function is not available. Power wheelchairs can have standard frames in which the seating system is part of the frame of the power chair. Power bases that can accommodate separate seating systems are also now widely available. The overall width, weight, and turning radius of the power wheelchair are considerations that can impact driving and alternative community mobility, such as riding as a passenger in a van.

Width

The overall width of a power wheelchair will impact accessing van-lift platforms or van ramps. Wheelchairs with power bases and separate seating systems are frequently narrower than the same seat width of a manual wheelchair frame.

Weight

The weight of an unoccupied power wheelchair may approach the weight limit of external lift devices. Weights of power wheelchairs can exceed 300 pounds unoccupied! Knowing the overall weight of the power wheelchair combined with the client's weight is important when addressing ramps or lifting devices that the client may require to be able to maneuver his or her wheelchair iinto the vehicle.

Turning Radius

The turning radius and length of a power wheelchair affect its ability to maneuver inside a vehicle. There are three configurations of power wheelchair drives: front-, mid/center-, and rear-wheel drive (Figure 9-16).

Front- and mid-wheel drive wheelchairs offer the smallest turning radii. Rear-wheel drive power wheelchairs and scooters tend to have the widest turning radii. The space necessary to turn a device is an important consideration because vans have limited areas in which to maneuver.

Armrests

Most clients who require power wheelchairs for mobility also require armrests for additional upper extremity and trunk support. When a client presents with limited or no functional upper extremity movement, additional components, such as arm troughs and contoured or flat hand pads, may be required. Flat components allow for easier lateral movement to access and manipulate the wheelchair's driving controls. The length of the armrest also becomes a consideration for drivers because it may interfere with driving controls, such as limiting access to the steering wheel, hand-controls, or both. Armrests can have an adjustable height option or be fixed at a standard height. A wheelchair user may need an adjustable height armrest when driving a vehicle to provide added resistance and upper extremity support. This is especially true with driving systems that feature advanced technology.

Joysticks, used to control the wheelchair, are usually placed at the end of an armrest. The placement of the joystick may interfere with positioning of the vehicle's adaptive driving equipment. Swing-away joystick mounts (Figure 9-17) are available to allow the joystick to be swung to the side of the armrest to decrease such potential interference. When driving, extra care must be taken to ensure that the joystick is locked in the swing-away position so that it does not release unexpectedly. If the joystick is mounted on the left side of the wheelchair, there may be insufficient room between the door and the armrest to allow the joystick to be swung away.

Legrest/Hanger Angle and Taper
The legrest/hanger angle and taper considerations are the same for people who drive from power wheelchairs as for those who drive from manual wheelchairs.

Tiedown Options for Power Wheelchairs
Two tiedown options are available to secure power wheelchairs being transported in vans: strap and automatic. Strap tie downs can only be used for a wheelchair passenger, as is the case with manual wheelchairs. Also, as with manual wheelchairs, the straps must be attached to the frame and not to removable parts, such as legrests and armrests, or any other part of the seating system. Ease of use of strap tie downs is differently affected by two power wheelchair options. Plastic shrouds or base covers are currently popular features of many power wheelchairs, making it difficult to access the power base frame for the straps. Conversely there are some power wheelchairs that have tiedown brackets welded to the frame for increased ease of use. There are instances in which particular wheelchair components must be ordered for power wheelchair drivers to help ensure optimal safety and success. For example steel rather than plastic tower seat attachments may be needed for the seating system. If the wheelchair is configured for occupied transport, the unoccupied wheelchair back

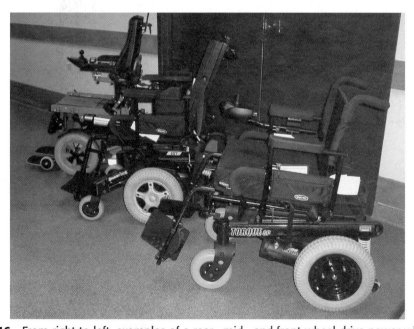

Figure 9-16 From right to left, examples of a rear-, mid-, and front-wheel drive power wheelchairs.

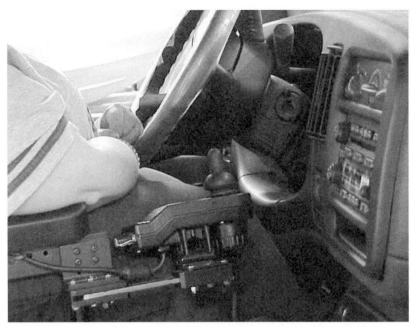

Figure 9-17 The position of a joystick in relation to the dashboard of a vehicle.

also must be able to be secured in an upright position (Figure 9-18).

Automatic tie downs must be used for wheelchair drivers and are an option for passengers, depending on the position of the wheelchair in the vehicle. Wheelchairs should be forward facing during transportation. As with manual wheelchairs suspension systems of power wheelchairs may dampen the shock felt by the user and improve one's ability to negotiate uneven terrain but may compromise the stability of the wheelchair and client when in a moving vehicle.

Additional modification to the lockdown system may be necessary to stabilize the wheelchair sufficiently for driving. It may not be possible to dampen the suspension enough to provide adequate stability for a user of a sensitive driving system involving sophisticated technology. Unfortunately some power wheelchair bases are not compatible with the commercially available automatic lockdown systems, therefore eliminating the ability of clients to drive safely from these wheelchairs.[1]

A driver should not drive from a scooter or remain seated on a scooter when riding in a vehicle as a

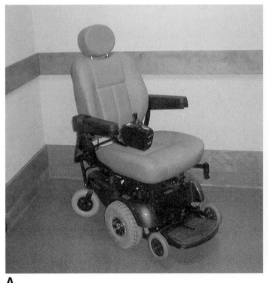
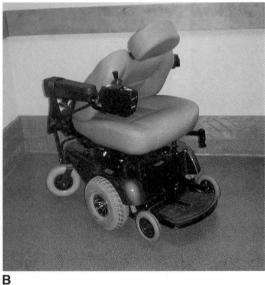

A   B

Figure 9-18 **A,** Example of a van seat back in the upright and folded-down positions. **B,** For occupied transport the wheelchair back must be fixed in an upright position.

passenger (Figure 9-19). Automatic tiedowns for scooters are designed to be used with scooters that are unoccupied. The Scooter Station by Creative Controls Inc. (Troy, MI) acts much like a vise grip with large pads that press in from each side. This device can also accommodate some power chairs that are incompatible with other automatic tiedown systems. As with other tiedowns the Scooter Station is only appropriate for stabilization of an unoccupied scooter or wheelchair. Scooters can be disassembled to allow a lifting device to load the base into the interior of a vehicle or trunk. Scooter seats are more problematic. Captain's seats are frequently used with scooters and can be awkward and difficult to properly lift in and out of a vehicle. Scooter

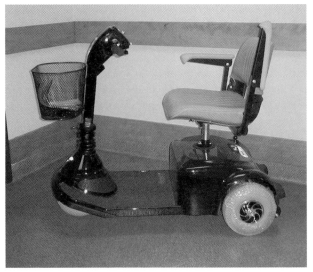

Figure 9-19 Power scooter.

seat removal is required for loading into the trunk of a car. Additional bar-style devices are commercially available to secure a deck-type scooter to the vehicle for added stability and safety.

Power Seating Systems for Power Wheelchair Users

Power seating systems allow gravity-assisted positioning, pressure relief of the ischial tuberosities and other bony prominences, and improved functional ability. The most common types of power seating systems are power tilt, power recline, combined power tilt/recline, and power seat elevators.

Power Tilt. In a power tilt-in-space seating system the entire seating system may tilt backward while maintaining the optimal back-to-seat angle (Figure 9-20). However, for optimal safety while a client is driving or riding as a passenger in a vehicle all seating systems should be in the upright position.

Adding a power tilt to some power bases increases the seat-to-floor height, which may affect the client's line of sight and interfere with steering wheel clearance. This change also will increase the client's overall seated height in the upright position, which may interfere with van door clearance. This occurs because power chairs have switches preventing tilt or recline beyond a certain point or angle (e.g., 45 degrees). Unless the limit switches can be modified this situation may prevent the client from independently accessing the van.

Power Recline. Power recline seating systems allow the seat-to-back angle to increase through use of an actuator. As a result the client's seated posture can vary from upright to nearly supine (Figure 9-21). A power recline seating system provides independence in pressure

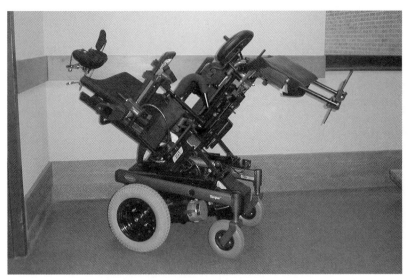

Figure 9-20 Power tilt seating system.

relief and positioning for daily needs. However, as with the power tilt systems, the addition of a power recline may increase seat-to-floor height and the client's overall seated height versus a power wheelchair without a power recline or tilt system.

As already discussed with power tilt seating systems the safest way to be transported in a power recline wheelchair is with the seating system in the upright position. The placements of secondary seating components, such as lateral trunk supports and the headrest, are usually fixed on a seating system. The position of these postural supports relative to the user will change as the wheelchair is reclined. Care must be taken to ensure that the changes in position of these supports are not detrimental to either the user or driver safety. Lap trays should be removed for safety during transport.

Most power recline systems have elevating legrests that raise when the wheelchair back is reclined to maintain stable positioning of the client and prevent circulatory pooling in his or her lower extremities. Elevating legrests at their lowest position protrude farther forward than standard legrests, which increases the overall length of the wheelchair. Increasing the length of the chair may interfere with maneuvering inside a vehicle and positioning within the driver's space. The length of the wheelchair becomes even greater if the legrests elevate when the back is reclined. For the client riding as a passenger, legrests can interfere with front seat passengers or with gas and brake pedals or the motor cover if the client is the driver.

Deactivating the tilt/recline mechanism when the wheelchair power is off will prevent accidental activation while the vehicle is in motion. However, interference with the driving controls must be avoided when placing the switch to activate the tilt/recline mechanism on the wheelchair.

Power Seat Elevator. Power seat elevators improve a wheelchair user's ability to reach high objects and to level the transfer surfaces for improved safety and independence when transferring. Most power seat elevators use a single post design to raise and lower the seat. As with the previous power seating systems addition of a seat elevator can increase the seat-to-floor height distance of the system. The user may have to drive a vehicle from the lowest wheelchair position for stability, which may impact vehicle modifications. As with the other power supports seat elevation must be avoided or disabled while the client is driving or riding as a passenger.

Seating Components

Additional external seating components, such as chest straps and lateral thoracic supports, are often necessary to provide appropriate client stability during daily activities. At times these components are only needed during dynamic situations, such as driving. These seating components can be used on manual and power wheelchairs.

Chest and Lap Straps. Chest straps provide lateral and anteroposterior postural support to clients with impaired trunk stability and sitting balance. The client must be able to secure and remove the chest strap in order to perform independent transfers. The use of Velcro (Velcro USA Inc., Manchester, NH) and thumb loops can assist the client with impaired hand function to don and doff the chest strap. A torso support strap, such as the Grandmar (International Medical Equipment Corporation, Chico, CA), is frequently used for drivers to provide added trunk stability. This strap can be used on the vehicle seat or on the wheelchair seat. It has a figure-eight design with one loop circling the client's trunk and the other portion attached to the wheelchair or vehicle seat. Adjustable lateral straps provide lateral stability. This support is available in custom lengths and with various closure styles that accommodate a variety of body types and different degrees of hand function (Figure 9-22).

Lap belts help maintain stable pelvic positioning for clients with limited trunk, pelvic, or lower limb control. They also aid pelvic stability during periods of clonus or spasticity-related hyperextension of the lower limbs. The position of the lap belt under the anterior superior iliac spines (ASISs) of the pelvis is especially important while driving a motor vehicle to minimize the potential for sliding forward during braking.

Lateral Thoracic Supports. Thoracic supports are used either to provide lateral stability for a client with decreased trunk stability or to correct or accommodate a spinal scoliosis. Thoracic supports may also provide

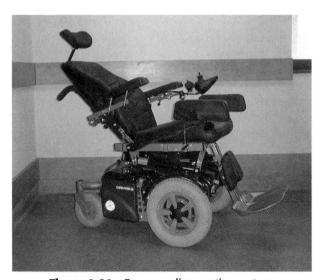

Figure 9-21   Power recline seating system.

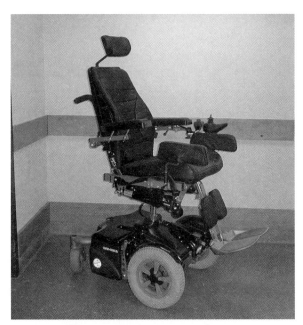

Figure 9-22 Power seat elevator.

lateral stability for the client who experiences excessive lateral trunk spasticity when performing voluntary movements of the upper or lower limbs. If trunk supports are required only during driving, the client must be able to don and doff the supports independently.

Headrests. A headrest may be necessary to provide head and neck support, especially when the client is in a tilted or reclined position. Headrests do not typically provide anterior support; therefore additional components may be necessary if the client has weak posterior neck musculature. Headrests may also be required for clients wanting to access public transportation and school buses.

Wheelchair Cushions. Wheelchair cushions aid postural support and redirect pressure from bony prominences, such as the ischial tuberosities and coccyx to the hamstrings, to decrease the risk of skin breakdown. The user's ability to perform upper extremity tasks and transfers from a particular cushion should be assessed. Driving a vehicle typically is a bimanual task, and adequate trunk and pelvic stability is critical for independent and stable upper extremity function. Solid seat inserts may increase stability while seated, but a solid seat weighs more than an upholstered seat. This will affect the overall weight of a manual wheelchair and the force required to propel it. The weight of a cushion also can impact the ability of a wheelchair user to stow and retrieve the cushion.

Cushions are available in many different heights. Occasionally a wheelchair driver uses more than one cushion or changes the cushion because of skin compromise. Again, the driver must use caution in this circumstance because differences in cushion height may alter his or her position in relation to the driving controls, fit beneath the steering wheel, head clearance, and visibility.

LOADING DEVICES

A loading device is used to lift a wheelchair or motorized scooter onto or into a vehicle. Interior and exterior loading devices have different advantages and disadvantages. For the purpose of this chapter the term loading device will be used to describe only those products used to lift and transport unoccupied wheelchairs or scooters. The term *wheelchair lift* will be used to describe interior mounted lifts that raise the client and his or her mobility device together into a van. When looking at manufacturers' literature these two terms are often used interchangeably. A few automotive terms need to be defined because they must be understood before a DRS can attempt to recommend these devices.

There are several terms associated with loading devices. The following is a short list:
- *Original Equipment Manufacturer (OEM).* Equipment installed by the company that first manufactured the product.[7] This term is used to describe the standard or stock factory-installed equipment available for a vehicle. Over the years adaptive equipment, such as power door openers, have become standard OEM options because they make tasks easier for all consumers. See Chapter 16 for more information on motor vehicles and universal design.
- *Gross Vehicle Weight Rating (GVWR).* The GVWR is the rating of a vehicle's carrying capacity.[7] This includes the weight of the vehicle, fuel, fluids, and full payload. If the gross vehicle weight is higher than the GVWR it is considered overloaded. This can result in damage to the vehicle and can adversely affect vehicle handling, leading to potentially dangerous situations.
- *Interior Payload Weight.* The amount of weight a vehicle can carry, including the weight of all occupants, options, cargo, and other equipment,[7] such as a wheelchair and loading device. This is an important consideration, especially when lifts are needed. For example although an exterior lift may free up interior space, the total amount of payload available for passengers and cargo is decreased. An interior mounted lift will reduce available payload and cargo room and may require the sacrifice of some seating space to accommodate the mobility device.
- *Tongue Weight.* The weight that can be supported by a trailer hitch.[7] Too much tongue weight causes overloading of the rear axle, which results in lifting of the front suspension and reduced steering response. A vehicle's tongue weight is usually 10% to 15% of its

loaded trailer weight, which is determined by the class of hitch it can support.

- *Hitch Class.* Trailer hitches are classified by the capacity of trailer weight that can be towed and by the amount of tongue weight that can be supported. The hitches for noncommercial vehicles fall into four classes[8]:

    Class 1: 2000 lb loaded trailer weight with 200 lb tongue weight

    Class 2: Up to 3500 lb loaded trailer weight with 300/350 lb tongue weight

    Class 3: Up to 5000 lb loaded trailer weight with 500 lb tongue weight

    Class 4: Up to 10,000 lb loaded trailer weight with 1000 to 1200 lb tongue weight. Class 4 may also include any hitches with capacities >5000 lb.

A class 1 hitch can be mounted on almost any vehicle. Class 2 hitches are usually found on midsize or larger cars. Class 3 hitches are found on minivans and midsize SUVs and larger vehicles. Class 4 hitches may be found on some full-sized cars, pickup trucks, vans, and larger vehicles. The vehicle owner's manual will list the type of hitch it can accept. The age and condition of the vehicle must also be taken into account. A high-mileage vehicle may have worn suspension, decreasing the amount of weight it can support despite the weight identified in the owner's manual.

A loading device is not the same as a trailer of course. A trailer has its own axle and wheels to partially support the load, whereas there is no similar support for an exterior loading device, which extends outward from the vehicle. This cantilevered load places a torque load on the rear of the vehicle, which it was not designed to handle. Even an interior mounted loading device loads the suspension more than the average vehicle user would on a consistent basis. These factors may result in premature wear issues that are not covered by the OEM warranty. Some vehicle models have optional load-leveling features, which can help to compensate for the added load on the suspension.

Issues affecting rear-loading devices relate to rear vision, vehicle dimensions, and weather. The driver's vision to the rear will be partially blocked by the external loading device and the mobility device. It may also make access to the trunk or rear storage more difficult. The vehicle will be longer, which may make it difficult to fit into a parking space or garage. Additionally the entire car may sit lower because of compression of the suspension, or the loading device may have a lower ground clearance than the chassis of the vehicle. This can result in scraping on speed bumps or bottoming out on hills and steep driveways. Weather presents other issues. An exterior lift, even with a cover, cannot fully protect a mobility device from road debris, rain,

salt, snow, ice, and mud. There will be only minimal protection of the device from road spray kicked up by the tires. The electronic components on a scooter or power wheelchair can be damaged by exposure to these elements. Finally the loading device should be equipped with a system to keep the wheelchair or scooter secure in the dynamic driving environment.

Even with the identified disadvantages these devices offer significant assistance to the disabled driver or passenger. Ideally a loading device is selected only after analysis of the client's limitations and skills, selection of the most appropriate mobility device, and recommendations for the most accommodating vehicle to purchase. In practice, however, the client plans to keep an existing vehicle and currently uses a mobility device that may or may not be compatible with his or her driving needs. Therefore the loading device may need to be selected to accommodate these issues rather than the needs of the wheelchair driver or passenger.

The loading device may assist the client who can transfer to a vehicle independently but is unable to independently load his or her mobility device into that vehicle. It can also be used when the client is a dependent passenger and the driver is unable to load the mobility device in the vehicle independently because of size or weight. This may occur, for example, when elderly spouses are faced with limited mobility. The DRS must determine whether the user can operate the loading device, which may include partially dismantling the mobility device and even partially dismantling the loading device. The Space Saver lift by Bruno (Oconomowoc, WI) is an example of a lift that can be dismantled.

There are several loading devices that are designed to work with a broad variety of vehicles and mobility devices. Size and weight limitations of the various loading devices will affect the dimensions of the mobility device being loaded and the size of the vehicle in which it will be used. If the client does not know the weight of his or her mobility device and a wheelchair scale is not available, the manufacturer should be able to give a weight estimate. If a client is unable to bring the mobility device to the driving evaluation, specific measurements should be obtained, in advance if possible, so that compatible loading devices can be recommended. These include length, width, and height of the device. If the client cannot bring his or her vehicle, the trunk or door opening also should be determined.

The weight limitations of the loading device or the size limitations of the vehicle opening may necessitate the mobility device have folding or removable components. The primary disadvantages of removable parts are increased time, the need for greater dexterity and/or strength, potential loss, and part degradation from excessive use.

Loading Devices for Sedans

Sedans come in a variety of shapes and sizes. Although there is a relatively large variety of loading device options for sedans, most are compatible primarily with either folding manual wheelchairs or scooters. These devices can place chairs on the roof, in the trunk, or suspended from the rear bumper. Because of the weight of most power wheelchairs, only the largest sedans can be considered and then only for rear bumper–mounted lifts.

Car Top Loading Devices

Car top loaders are compatible only with folding manual wheelchairs. The driver must be able to transfer independently and remove his or her wheelchair cushion. There are currently two main car top devices on the market: the Tip Top Mobility Wheelchair lift (Minot, ND) and the Braun Chair Topper (Winamac, IN). The Tip Top Mobility Wheelchair lift requires the user to fold the wheelchair, whereas the Braun Chair Topper folds the seat as it lifts the wheelchair. Both require the user to unfold the chair independently. The manufacturers provide charts with the maximum folded dimensions of the wheelchair. Camber in the wheels adds to the folded width, as do tire and push rim style. Removable legrests reduce the length of the chair, if that is a problem, but add to the loading and reassembly time. Clients needing a solid seat back must be able to independently remove and replace the back. Like the removable legrests, this adds time and complicates the overall transfer process. As the lifting capacity may be as low as 45 pounds, the weight of the wheelchair at the time of lifting must be known. Fortunately many wheelchairs currently on the market can be lifted by these two examples of wheelchair lifts.

The folded width of the wheelchair can be a limiting factor. Older wheelchair models fold to a thinner dimension than newer ones. This can present a problem for the client who must replace an older style of folding chair and already uses a car top loader. It will be critical to work with the seating specialist to find a wheelchair that fits in the existing car top loader.

Rear Bumper Loading Devices

There is a greater variety of rear bumper loading compared with car top loading devices. They are diverse in design and operation. The simplest models are manual and use a crank or spring mechanism to raise a folding manual wheelchair to the height of the rear bumper after it is rolled into a holder. The more complex models have platforms with tie downs to secure the mobility device and power lifting mechanisms. The independent driver must be able to ambulate from the driver's door to the rear bumper of the car, and he or she must have adequate strength and balance to maneuver the device onto and off the loader. These factors may not be immediately obvious to the user and can result in disappointment. As an example an evaluation was completed recently for a client who intended to transport her upright power chair on the rear of her full-sized sedan. Her vocational counselor had endorsed this plan because it would not require significant expense and the client could use her existing vehicle. She did not have the funds to purchase a modified van. Neither the client nor the counselor had considered her limited mobility. She did not have the balance to stand and load the wheelchair on the device, and she was unable to walk around to the driver's door of the car. When questioned about her ability to ambulate, she stated that the last time she had walked was 2 years ago when she fell because of impaired balance and broke her shoulder. Her driving control needs were minimal, involving just a set of mechanical hand controls and a steering knob. Unfortunately because of her inability to ambulate, she could not pursue her plan to load the chair onto the back of the car and therefore did not become an independent driver.

Despite model differences most of the rear bumper–mounted lifts share the same advantages and disadvantages. The major advantage is that the loading device does not take up any passenger or cargo space in the vehicle. If the client has a large enough sedan, SUV, or minivan to accommodate the combined weight of the mobility and loading devices, he or she will not need to change vehicles. Although the idea of a device on the back of a sedan seems to provide a simple solution, several factors must be considered. These devices can dramatically alter the handling characteristics of a vehicle. The combined weight of the devices compresses the rear suspension and takes weight off the front of the vehicle, reducing front wheel traction. If the vehicle has front wheel drive, it can become unpredictable on wet or slippery pavement, rough road surfaces, or with cross winds. Furthermore the driver may have more difficulty executing an evasive maneuver because there is less road contact with the drive wheels. If the driver's disability makes it more difficult to handle difficult steering maneuvers or if the client's reaction time is slower than normal, this could create hazardous driving conditions.

Tongue weight and the trailer hitch rating of the client's vehicle must be determined before a rear-mounted device can be recommended. Manual wheelchairs are relatively light, with most <50 pounds and several <25 pounds. Even with the weight of the loading device this should not adversely affect the handling of the vehicle. Scooters and power wheelchairs, including captain's seats and batteries, can weigh between 110 and 350 pounds, with some wheelchairs even heavier. A heavy mobility device can cause safety problems. In the worst case the combined weight of a power wheelchair and loading device could cause the sedan to exceed the GVWR, adversely affecting the handling of the vehicle. At the very least passenger and cargo capacity must be limited to avoid exceeding the limit. Therefore there is a dilemma for the rear bumper loading device user. Although mounting the device on the rear is appealing to allow more interior space for passengers and cargo, the weight of the devices may make it unsafe to operate the vehicle with passengers or cargo. Therefore it is critical that the vehicle and device be well matched and that the client is aware of any hazards and limitations before finalizing this decision.

In-Trunk Loading Devices

This category of loading device can be used with folding manual wheelchairs and some scooters. A deep trunk is needed, and some models of the loading devices have to be partially disassembled when stowed. The scooter seat must be removed and loaded into the trunk by the user because the loading device only lifts the scooter base. The seat weighs approximately 35 pounds. All models use power from the car battery to raise and lower the mobility device. Some loaders require the user to manually swing the device into the car once it has been raised; a few have power swing features. As with the rear bumper loader the user must ambulate to the driver's side door. The main advantage of in-trunk loading devices is that the device is protected within the trunk.

Loading Devices for Pickup Trucks

Some clients prefer a pickup truck to a car or van. The truck may be needed for their job, their driving environment, or simply their lifestyle. Today's trucks are more versatile and varied than ever. Powered seat lifts, such as the Glide 'n Go by Access Unlimited (Binghamton, NY) and the Bruno EZ-Rizer (Pasadena, TX), assist the client's transfer to a higher truck seat. The client must transfer to the seat lift at ground level. The loading device then raises the client to the level of the driver's seat, where the driver transfers onto the truck seat. A chair loader will then pick up the chair from the driver's door area of the vehicle and stow it. The client's ability to balance on the driver's seat or seat lift while attaching the mobility device to the loader must be assessed.

The easiest truck body style to use for a client with a folding manual wheelchair is an extended cab with rear-hinged doors. The Bruno Cab-Sider (Pasadena, TX) loads the folded chair behind the driver's seat. Rigid frame manual wheelchairs, scooters, and some power wheelchairs can be loaded into the bed of a pickup truck using the Bruno Out-Sider. The driver transfers into the driver's seat and attaches the arm of the lift to the wheelchair. Different styles of attachments are available for use with clients who have impaired fine motor coordination. The height clearance requirements for the lift arm may make it impossible to use the truck inside a parking deck or a family garage, which can be a major disadvantage. The Out-Sider works with trucks with standard or extended cabs. If a quad cab style is used, the lift arm will not extend far enough to reach the driver's door area. In this case the client would have to take a few steps from the wheelchair to the driver's seat after attaching the wheelchair to the docking device. Various styles of docking hardware are available to accommodate different degrees of hand function.

The issue of protecting the loading device and wheelchair from the elements also arises with a pickup truck. Rain or snow can damage power wheelchair and scooter electronic systems. Additionally the seat upholstery may get wet, making it uncomfortable for the client to sit in the wheelchair when he or she exits the truck. Wet upholstery is a significant risk because it can also contribute to skin breakdown. It is possible to purchase a powered lift cap, the Bruno POW'R Topper (Pasadena, TX), to use in conjunction with the Out-Sider. The top opens and closes like a clamshell, adding to the overall height and width of the mechanism. This can be a problem particularly on a full-sized truck. The cap does not form a weather-tight seal with the sides of the truck bed; therefore water can still enter the bed of the vehicle. Because of the opening mechanism the driver must park in uncovered parking and be exposed to the elements when transferring and loading the wheelchair. As with every loading device there are limits on the size and weight of the mobility device. The height of the seat and back determines whether the lift arm will be able to lift the wheels high enough to clear the side of the bed. The back height is an issue when adding a cap to the bed.

Other Options

In many cases the final vehicle recommendation is primarily influenced by a client's need to accommodate a mobility device rather than by the actual adaptive driving equipment used to operate the vehicle. Vehicles with large rear and side door openings can more easily accommodate a loading device. Depending on the location of the lift and the size of the mobility device, some of the passenger seating positions may be eliminated. The car top loaders may be used with minivans and SUVs, but they do add to the height of the vehicle; therefore garage door clearance and clearance for parking decks and drive-through structures must be considered. Chain extension kits can be added to lengthen the lift's chain when used with a vehicle taller than 58 inches.

Loaders for larger vehicles can be classified by their mounting location: rear hatch, driver's side sliding door, and passenger side sliding door.

Rear hatch loaders accommodate manual and power wheelchairs and scooters. The main limiting factor is the height of the available door opening at the rear of the vehicle. In some instances a fold-down seat back or folding tiller can be used to decrease the overall height of the mobility device. The independent driver must be able to ambulate from the rear of the vehicle to the driver's door, bend and attach the terminal device to the mobility device, operate the lift mechanism, and have the strength and balance to guide the mobility device into the vehicle. The independent driver must also be able to open and close the rear door. A few vehicles have a powered rear hatch as an option, but most rear doors are manual. After-market, or non-OEM, power hatch mechanisms exist but are not compatible with all vehicles. Because the rear doors are larger they are often more difficult to open and close. Hatches that open upward may be too high for a client with limited shoulder flexion, decreased hand function, or limited muscle strength for closing or reaching. Hatches may have a gas piston to help open them, but this can be dangerous for a client with impaired balance. The DRS needs to assess these skills before a loading device is considered. If a new vehicle is being chosen, the ease with which the rear hatch can be opened and the size of the opening are important criteria.

Some loading devices have manual swing mechanisms, whereas others are fully powered. The operator will still have to guide and steady the mobility device as it enters the vehicle with most lifts. The Vantage Mobility Elite (Phoenix, AZ) differs because it has a telescoping platform that raises the device and pulls it into the vehicle.

Devices for side doors are used primarily with minivans. Side-loading devices are typically paired with a power sliding door, with the center row of seats in the minivan removed. The device will sit behind the driver's seat and in front of the rear bench. For clients with children this can be a problem because access to the rear bench is compromised. The driver's side door is narrower than the passenger side door; therefore fewer devices can be loaded on that side. Scooters and folding manual wheelchairs are most commonly loaded through the driver's side door. The driver must still take several steps to the driver's seat after loading the mobility device. Devices can be loaded in the wider passenger side door, but this would require an independent driver to walk around the car to get to the driver's seat. This location is more commonly used when a caregiver is loading a mobility device. As always securing the mobility device inside the vehicle is a critical issue because a 200-pound wheelchair is a hazard to all vehicle occupants in the event of a crash if it is not properly secured.

Structurally Modified Vans

Clients who cannot transfer independently from their mobility device or who cannot load it independently with one of the devices already mentioned will need to use a structurally modified van. Some makes and models of full-sized vans and minivans can be modified to have greater interior heights and taller door openings. This is needed so that the client can enter the vehicle seated in the mobility device. Minivans are usually modified with lowered floors. Full-sized vans can have lowered floors and/or raised roofs with or without raised doors. Full-sized vans with 3/4-ton capacity are used because they have an adequate GVWR to accommodate the added weight of the modifications, equipment, and wheelchair. This helps the vehicle retain the OEM handling characteristics. Once again, large power wheelchairs with power seating systems can weigh >300 pounds. Most adaptive driving equipment can be used in either the modified minivan or the full-sized van; the dimensions of the client while in the mobility device are usually the determining factor for minivan or full-sized van selection.

These dimensions must be carefully measured. The client's seated height, from the floor to the top of the head, is the first measurement. The interior height of the van should be at least 2 inches greater than the client's seated height. A client whose seated height is ≤54 inches can use a 10-inch lowered floor minivan or a full-sized van with either a raised roof with raised doors or a 6-inch lowered floor. A client whose seated height is ≥55 inches will usually need a full-sized van with a lowered floor and a raised roof with raised doors. A client who sits 55 inches tall may fit in a 12-inch lowered floor minivan, but visibility out the windshield must be carefully evaluated before this can be confirmed. As more makes and models of vans are modified these guidelines may change.

If the client is going to drive from the wheelchair, the depth of the floor is critical. The client's knees must clear the base of the steering wheel, and his or her eye level should fall between the top and bottom of the rearview mirror. Whereas the need for knee clearance is intuitively obvious to drivers, the issue of line of sight may not be immediately apparent. However, if the driver is sitting too low, the steering wheel or dashboard will interfere with visibility; if the seat is too high, the tint band and roof line may prevent the driver from seeing overhead traffic signals or signs.

Lowered floors for full-sized vans can vary in depth from 1 to 10 inches below factory floor height. Floors deeper than 6 inches require vehicle frame modifications. The body of the van is frequently raised with any floor >4 inches deep. If the driver is going to transfer out of the wheelchair to the driver's seat, head clearance for the transfer is critical. More or less room may be needed depending on the client's transfer style. This must be assessed before recommendations can be made. Minivan floor depths are standard but can be built up slightly if needed. However, the most important issues to consider when choosing a vehicle for a wheelchair driver or passenger include adequate head clearance in the doorway, in the passenger area, and in the driver's area; adequate visibility through the windshield and side windows; and adequate knee/footrest clearance under the steering wheel and dashboard areas.

Wheelchair lifts are used to access the interior of full-sized vans. The length and width of the wheelchair are used to determine the platform size. At this time 29 inches is the most common functional platform width. Side door lifts have a maximum platform width of 32 inches. Wider lifts can be obtained to mount in the rear door opening of a van. When this location is used the floor of the van cannot be lowered. A van floor can only be lowered from the firewall in the front to an area just forward of the rear wheel wells. If a rear entry lift is used, a flat floor should be combined with a transfer seat or possibly a power driver floor pan. In most cases a client large enough to require an oversized lift will not have space to maneuver into the driver's area. Transfer seat bases also have weight limits. The combined weight of the client and his or her mobility device must be known to help ensure that it does not exceed lift capacity. Most lifts have a capacity between 600 pounds and 800 pounds.

Lowered floor minivans have folding ramps for access. The usable width is currently <30 inches. Many lowered floor minivans are equipped with a power kneel feature that lowers the rear end of the van to decrease the angle of the ramp. This is not critical for most power wheelchair users but may be necessary to allow a manual wheelchair user to push up the ramp independently. Chairs with camber in the wheels may not fit on the minivan ramp. The GVWR and the available interior turning space of a minivan are less than for a full-sized van.[9]

SUMMARY

The success of being transported or driving a vehicle for people for whom a wheelchair is the primary means of mobility depends on many factors, including types of mobility and vehicle access devices, dimensions of the seated user, wheelchair and loading/lifting device, and structural elements of the vehicle. The size of the wheelchair in its folded position, the weight of the wheelchair, and the number of removable components and types of release mechanisms will impact a user's ability to self-load a manual wheelchair. The height of a power chair, the weight of the chair, and the overall width will impact the ability to fit onto a lift or ramp and maneuver through the door opening into the interior of a modified minivan or full-sized van. The length of the wheelchair, the location of the joystick, the seat height, the degree of tilt or recline, the presence of custom arm troughs, and the compatibility with automatic tiedown systems can impact the client's ability to drive a van from a wheelchair. The types of loading devices available for a specific vehicle may dictate the type of mobility device recommended. The ability of a client to manipulate the loading device also will have an impact on the type of vehicle and mobility device recommended.

The myriad of issues to consider when recommending a mobility or transportation device can be complicated. To help ensure the client successfully achieves his or her driving and community mobility goals, communication between the seating specialist, the DRS, and the mobility equipment dealer is paramount.

REFERENCES

1. Cook AM, Hussey SM: *Assistive technologies: principles and practice*, ed 2, St. Louis, 2002, Mosby.
2. Bergen AF, Presperin J, Tallman T: *Positioning for function: wheelchairs and other assistive technologies*, Valhalla, NY, 1990, Valhalla Rehabilitation Publications.
3. Miller BF, O'Toole MT: *Miller-Keane encyclopedia and dictionary of medicine, nursing, and allied health*, ed 6, Philadelphia, 1997, Saunders.
4. Strano CM: Physical disabilities and their implications for driving, *Work: A Journal of Prevention Assessment Rehabilitation* 8:261-266, 1997.
5. Anderson BE: Driving assessment in spinal cord injury patients. In Kirshblum S, Campagnolo DI, DeLisa JA, editors: *Spinal cord medicine*, Philadelphia, 2002, Lippincott Williams & Wilkins.
6. Sullivan PE, Markos PD, Minor MA: *Techniques. An integrated approach to therapeutic exercise: theory and clinical application*, Reston, VA, 1982, Reston Publishing.
7. *SRO dictionary of automotive terms.* Available at: http://www.srodictionary.com/index.htm. Accessed January 1, 2005.
8. *Hitch information.* Available at: http://www.uhaul.com/hitches/selectahitch.pdf. Accessed January 1, 2005.
9. Holicky R: Big vans, minivans: pros and cons, *New Mobility* 6:50-53, 1995.

Chapter *10*

DRIVING SIMULATORS

Erica B. Stern • Elin Schold Davis

KEY TERMS

- Driving simulation
- Computerized graphic imagery (CGI)
- Mapped simulation
- Route-based simulation
- Field of view (FOV)
- Simulator sickness

CHAPTER OBJECTIVES

After completing this chapter, the reader will be able to do the following:

- Understand the role of driving simulation in driver rehabilitation and broader occupational therapy evaluation and intervention.
- Understand the benefits and limitations of driver simulation.
- Identify factors that contribute to simulator sickness and how to minimize those effects.

Driving simulation is a process in which technology creates an impression that one is driving a vehicle.[1] Simulation systems vary in size, realism, and cost, but each provides a safe, controlled, repeatable simulated driving experience in which errors can be made without cost to life, health, or property. Because of these qualities, driving simulation can be used in several aspects of occupational therapy, especially for therapists working as driver rehabilitation specialists (DRSs). It can be part of driver evaluation, allowing the DRS to see how clients may respond to roadway events that range from the commonplace to the dangerous before an on-road evaluation is initiated. Driving simulation may help DRSs

and clients decide the optimal timing for on-road evaluation. Simulation can help teach or improve driving skills by allowing clients to practice compensatory driving strategies in a less expensive and risk-free environment. Because driving is an activity that is challenging, age appropriate, and purposeful, driving simulation also can afford involvement in a richly meaningful clinical activity through which clients can work on more general goals, such as strengthening muscles or improving attention and reaction time, as well as better self-awareness of their driving or more general abilities. This chapter will introduce the reader to driving simulation as a modality and discuss its potential as one part of driver evaluation, intervention, and general occupational therapy evaluation and intervention.

BACKGROUND

In today's world of evolving technology one could be excused for assuming that driving simulation is a new idea. In actuality driving simulation began approximately 90 years ago.[1] Many early driving simulations "used a conveyor belt on which were mounted scale model vehicles on a painted image of a roadway."[1] A driver displayed his or her driving skill by controlling speed, maintaining lane position, and avoiding objects that appeared on the conveyor belt.

By the 1950s driving simulators were using moving photography to create a more visually realistic driver's view of the roadway and surrounding environment.[1] In those driving simulations the driver viewed a film of a roadway on a monitor or screen. As the film of the roadway played, the driver drove the route from a mock-up vehicle or a complete or a disarticulated cab of a real car. The driver's errors were recorded for a final report, but steering and pedal actions had no effect on the images being shown representing the drive.

As technology improved, simulation developers strove to make photographically based simulations more interactive. Early efforts allowed the filmed drive to speed, slow, or stop in response to the driver's use of accelerator and brake pedals.[1] Later some photographically based simulations used videodisk technology to permit driver route selection at each intersection.[1] Currently a widely used photographically based driving simulation offers digital videodisk (DVD)- and video-based systems. In both cases the drive is of a fixed video route that does not change in response to a driver's actions. Instead the system uses a separate feedback display (Figure 10-1) to inform the driver of errors during the drive and provides a record of the error. Because of this feedback the simulation is considered semiinteractive.

In the current decade there has been dramatic growth in computerized driving simulations. These simulations trade the visual realism of photographically based systems for the less visually realistic but more dynamically interactive options offered by *computerized graphic imagery* (CGI) (Figure 10-2).

CGI driving simulations are interactive, altering in response to a driver's input (i.e., dynamically changing the computer-generated visual environment based on a driver's steering, acceleration, and braking responses). Several manufacturers offer interactive driving simulations, with systems varying in their visual realism from flat cartoons to more detailed and textured images. These driving simulations also vary in the fidelity they offer between driver action and CGI changes. In interactive driving simulations the environment is flexible, and actions taken by a driver produce a change in the displayed driving scene. Although the visual and auditory realism is important in driving simulation, it is believed that the accuracy of the virtual environment has greater impact on a driving simulation's verisimilitude.

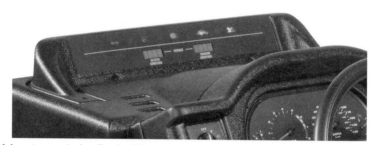

Figure 10-1 Doron Precision System's feedback display activated. (Courtesy Doron Precision Systems, Inc., Binghamton, New York.)

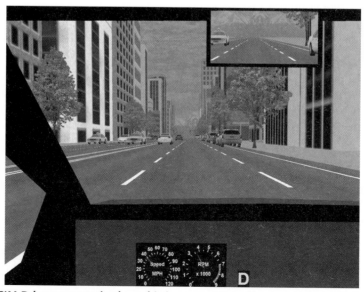

Figure 10-2 Current STISIM Drive computerized graphic imagery (CGI). (Courtesy Systems Technology, Hawthorne, Calif.)

SIMULATOR USE IN EVALUATION AND INTERVENTION

Interactive driving simulation offers unique and varied opportunities for occupational therapy and driver rehabilitation evaluation and intervention at various points across the rehabilitation timeline.

SIMULATOR USE AS A STEP IN DRIVING EVALUATION

Imagine that at your next driver's license renewal the worker behind the counter informs you that you will no longer be allowed to drive because your application failed to pass review. You left a number off of your address (demonstrating inattention), had several erasures (demonstrating poor real-time decision making), and failed to indicate your return address on the envelope (demonstrating inappropriate risk taking). Would you be persuaded by the worker's assertion that research had shown these measures to be good predictors of on-road behaviors, or would you remain unconvinced that these were reliable ways to measure your driving abilities? It seems likely that you would argue against their decision. Although research indicates that combinations of clinical tests are able to predict failure of on-road evaluation and elevated crash risk[2,3] (see Chapters 6 and 7), clients typically struggle to understand this relationship and may feel unreasonably judged if these tests are used to determine their appropriateness for an on-road evaluation. As a result DRSs often choose to take almost all clients onto the road for evaluation. Unfortunately this policy can increase the risks to the driver, the DRS, and the community.

Driving simulation does not replace traditional clinical evaluation nor does it replace an on-road driving evaluation. However, it does offer a no-risk experience that can provide additional objective and subjective data and an experience that may help a driver to understand the decisions made about his or her driving privileges. For example clinics may use driving simulation when deciding whether an on-road evaluation is appropriate at the current time. Clients who perform poorly on driving simulation may be more likely to understand why they are not ready for an on-road evaluation and less likely to feel that the decision to defer that evaluation is unfair.

Driving simulation systems differ in their strengths, weaknesses, and limitations, and each should be carefully and cautiously considered before it is included as part of a clinical driving evaluation. Until research demonstrates that a driving simulation is a reliable and valid prediction of on-road performance, performance in a driving simulator should be considered as only one part of a comprehensive driver rehabilitation evaluation. At present we know of no research that can support using even the most sophisticated driving simulation systems as the sole assessment tool for making decisions about driving, even if delivered by an occupational therapist working as a DRS.

SIMULATOR USE TO IMPROVE OCCUPATIONAL PERFORMANCE SKILLS

Like many other engaging and motivating clinical activities, driving simulation offers an occupational task that can be adapted to improve a wide variety of occupational performance skills. For example:

1. A simulated drive with numerous curves and turns may be used to challenge and improve sitting balance, upper extremity endurance, or sitting tolerance.
2. A simulated route can be devised to provide experiences to challenge and improve attention, divided attention, or stress control.
3. Vehicle color, signage, and physical settings (e.g., urban versus rural) can be manipulated so that driving simulation provides a range of challenges that clients can practice addressing in a safe and controlled environment.
4. Types and numbers of curves and turns can be set to work on upper extremity range of motion, strength, and endurance.
5. A route can be filled with significant challenges originating from the left side to reinforce real-time scanning for persons with hemianopsia and hemineglect.
6. A driving simulator could offer a safe opportunity for repeated, age-appropriate practice of treatment strategies for adolescents with attention deficits associated with attention deficit disorder (ADD), attention deficit hyperactivity disorder (ADHD), or Asperger's syndrome.

In summary, driving simulation can provide a dynamic assessment and training tool that can be altered and used to improve specific physical, cognitive, and perceptual performance skills within the broader context of driving and community mobility.

USING DRIVING SIMULATION TO PRACTICE DRIVING SKILLS AND BEHAVIORS

Driving simulation offers a less expensive, less constrained way to practice driving skills when on-road practice is too dangerous, too costly, or simply unavailable. For example a driving simulator may be adapted with trial equipment for hands-only driving by someone with paraplegia or offer opportunities to experiment with different styles of equipment before spending the time and money to modify a real vehicle. Driving simulation also gives a person who may be anxious about any number of driving issues a low stress experience that can help to reinforce that driving is a viable and worthwhile goal for that individual.

USING DRIVING SIMULATION TO IMPROVE SELF-AWARENESS

Interactive driving simulation can provide a challenging context in which clients perform in real time and make quick judgments and decisions, sometimes with serious (albeit simulated) consequences that can be quite sobering. Drivers experience the effects of their actions, providing a clear link between cause and effect and affording the opportunity to improve a client's insight and self-awareness of driving errors. Once errors are recognized clients may be able to generalize, producing better insight into their functional strengths and deficits. A client's understanding of his or her current strengths and limitations generally improves his or her willingness to accept therapeutic decisions (such as deferring an on-road evaluation), use compensatory strategies (such as selecting intersections with protected left turns), and adhere to driving limitations (such as avoiding driving at night). This improved understanding of one's deficits related to driving also helps position the client as an informed member at the center of the driver rehabilitation team.

Some simulators allow replay of a driving segment. Although the DRS can give feedback while a client is driving, the replay option allows a client to play out choices without distraction or interruption and then review his or her driving performance while guided by a DRS's feedback. This review can help a client recognize errors and facilitates the collaborative process between the client and DRS as they interpret the client's performance together. The DRS is the critical link to improving self-awareness because it is the DRS's feedback that encourages a client to realize that functional deficits affect driving and nondriving performance. It is also worthwhile to point out that there is no evidence supporting the assertion that accessing a driving simulator improves insight among clients with impaired self-awareness.

FAMILIARIZATION DRIVES

Each use of interactive driving simulation, whether for assessment or treatment purposes, should begin with a familiarization drive. The familiarization drive meets three objectives: (1) to reduce simulation sickness; (2) to improve driving simulation comfort and performance; and (3) to demystify driving simulation to encourage a willingness to accept simulation experiences as valid representations of driving behaviors and abilities. In short the familiarization drive allows a client to adjust to the simulated experience.

The familiarization drive should provide 5 to 15 minutes of drive time. Several shorter drives are better than one longer one,[4] and best results are achieved when the client is introduced to the familiarization gradually. Box 10-1 summarizes the steps that should be taken in the familiarization protocol.

BOX 10-1   Steps in a Familiarization Protocol

1. Seat the driver in the simulator, and ask him or her to adjust the seat to his or her comfort (upright and distance from steering wheel).
2. To minimize simulator sickness, turn on fan and encourage the driver to sit as far as possible, while still comfortable, from the simulation screen(s).
3. Orient the driver to the basic components (e.g., steering wheel, gas, brake, rearview and sideview mirrors, and speedometer).
4. Without alarming the driver, explain early symptoms of simulation sickness (dizziness or nausea), and ask the driver to inform you immediately if he or she experiences these or other similar symptoms. Emphasize that it is not good to try to "tough through" these symptoms. It is better to take a brief break or discontinue. Complete a Simulator Sickness Questionnaire (optional).
5. Lead the driver through a series of driving experiences to allow him or her to get used to the icons used in the simulation and the speed and types of reactions that the driving simulation offers. We generally recommend that one progress as follows, although familiarization drives will differ across simulations:
   a. Accelerate to 25 miles per hour (mph) for several minutes, and then hit the brake. (This demonstrates typical minimum driving speed and its stopping distance.)
   b. Drive straight roads, with gentle curves and hills.
   c. Ask the client to identify objects as he or she drives. This orients to icons of posted speeds, road signs, trees, driveways versus roadways, and pedestrian crossings and allows the driver to focus on how these icons appear at full distance.
   d. Introduce intersection turns or sharper curves only toward the end of the familiarization drive.
   e. Encourage the driver to view the driving simulation in real terms from the start. As a result drivers are not encouraged to "play with the simulation" or to intentionally participate in dangerous driving activities such as speeding, driving off road, or intentional crashes. The familiarization drive should be relatively simple, without challenges, to shield clients from likely crash situations until the client is comfortable and familiar with the simulator.

The DRS plays a key role in a successful familiarization experience because he or she sets the tone. The DRS's instructions and corrections of driving errors must be calm and directive. A motivational interviewing model can successfully guide the client receiving driver rehabilitation services toward more accurate self-assessment of his or her driving. An overly strident corrective approach is likely to increase a client's defensiveness and create an adversarial atmosphere.

It is common for drivers to complain that a simulation does not feel the same as their motor vehicle. We begin the familiarization with the statement that a driving simulation is *not* the same as driving a real vehicle but that it can provide an opportunity to assess and improve driving skills. We also note that real vehicles differ from one another in their feel and response; therefore it is unlikely that a simulated drive will feel exactly as they remember their own car, van, truck, or SUV.

CASE STUDY #1: LOUISE KOROL

Diagnosis and Current Status

Louise Korol is a 46-year-old woman, 18 months post–cerebrovascular accident (CVA), with residual left visual field cut (left homonymous hemianopsia confirmed by neuro-ophthalmologic evaluation). Her upper extremity and lower extremity motor is intact. Her current problems include impaired insight, impulsivity, and distractibility. She failed an on-road driving evaluation 2 months before her referral to the clinic. The driving report describes that the on-road portion had to be abbreviated because of unsafe behaviors and impaired ability to comply with instructions from the evaluator. In her occupational therapy outpatient sessions Louise perseverated on this past driving evaluation, characterizing it as "unfair." She denied having committed any of the errors noted on her report and insisted that "given a fair chance" she could drive "just fine." Louise's husband reports hiding the keys to their car to keep her from driving and expresses fear that Louise will find a way around this intervention.

Intervention

Louise drove an interactive driving simulator. The routes have many active intersections, traffic that approaches from the left, and instances in which Louise would crash if she failed to check the left lane before merging. Louise made numerous errors consistent with her deficits during the simulated drive, with three collisions and numerous narrow avoidances of collision. Louise repeated the driving routes three times, and the errors were consistent each time.

Initially Louise blamed the simulation for her errors, claiming that cars "appeared out of nowhere" or that she had been distracted during the simulation and "that wouldn't happen in real life." With each repetition of the drive she expressed greater surprise at her inability to compensate for her deficit, even when knowing that she was likely to face a potential challenge in that field.

The therapist used the simulator's replay feature to allow Louise to observe her drives, asking her to explain the events as they were occurring and allowing her to recognize and acknowledge her errors. Early excuses were not confronted, but as similar errors recurred, even Louise began to recognize that she should not have the same problem repeatedly. In replay, for example, she was able to see the previously missed car approaching from the left. As the drives were replayed Louise began to acknowledge her errors, at one point exclaiming in surprise, "I really did not see that car."

She left the session amazed, voicing real concern: "I did not see those cars on the left."

Subsequent therapy sessions used driving simulation to improve insight about her field cut. Using a motivational interviewing approach, the DRS asked the client to analyze each driving scenario; being allowed to recognize and acknowledge her own errors, Louise began to appreciate the energy required to pay attention to the left and how easily she could be distracted from this task. Most significantly she stopped complaining to her husband about driving and no longer searched for the keys.

Driving simulation allowed this client to challenge scanning and attention to the left. This practice was placed in the meaningful context of driving, but the therapist was clear that actual driving would involve a complete program of on-road evaluation and training. Driving simulation offered a way to break down the task and gave this client information in a way that she could receive and interpret it. At the end of her simulated driving intervention she recognized her deficits and had made the decision not to drive, but she also was committed toward trying to remediate these deficits with ongoing treatment and held the hope that she might yet return to driving.

CASE STUDY #2: SVEN ANDERSEN

Diagnosis and Current Status

Sven Andersen is a 62-year-old man, 6 weeks post-CVA, with residual right hemiparesis. He is ready for discharge from acute in-patient rehabilitation with recommendation for continued outpatient therapy. Improvement has been steady, and his prognosis is excellent. Sven ambulates with a single-tip cane. His speech is improving, but he remains moderately, receptively, and expressively aphasic. This language barrier interferes with his ability to understand the "abstract and unfamiliar" information that the therapists are imparting to him about his condition, exercises, precautions, and restrictions. Sven lives with his wife. He is tired of therapy and frequently expresses the desire to go home. He believes that he will be "fine" once he gets there.

Intervention

Sven's DRS decides to use the driving simulator as a contextually relevant environment to explore how Sven's current limitations impact function. In an effort to drive the car Sven quickly recognizes that his right foot lacks accurate proprioceptive sense and motor control to effectively manage the gas and brake. He appears surprised each time his body does not do what he wants, exclaiming "amazing" repeatedly during the session.

The DRS uses the simulated drive to emphasize the need for outpatient therapy to improve Sven's physical abilities. Sven enjoys the session enormously, saying that he found it "exciting" and "positive." Although the team sees Sven's improvement as steady and his prognosis as good, Sven feels uncertain and concerned that he will remain dependent in many areas of adult function. His driving simulation experience provided a clear demonstration of his functional deficits but also showed him how improvement in these areas would help meet his personal goals. He left his first session with greater appreciation for his need for continued therapy to address residual deficits. Just as kitchen sessions may help a client observe appropriate precautions when using a stove, simulated driving can help Sven understand and adhere to his doctor's prohibition against driving. Sven looked forward to continuing simulated driving as one part of his outpatient occupational therapy treatments.

DRIVING SIMULATION TECHNOLOGY

Virtual reality is not virtually real. Most low-priced ($25,000 to $50,000) or mid-priced ($75,000 to $100,000) driving simulators have several limitations. Simulations often lack a realistic sense of driving speed,[5-7] and they offer incomplete field of view (FOV), which makes it impossible to assess or practice shoulder checks when merging or changing lanes or to assess or practice parallel parking. The larger, more complex, and more costly simulations that permit these actions are not feasible for clinics. However, there are several choices that can improve the realism and validity of even low-priced and moderately priced driving simulators.

INPUTS

Authors generally agree that face validity is improved when objects that come into direct contact with the

driver are more realistic. Thus a real car seat, steering wheel, turn signal, accelerator, and brake pedal afford greater face validity.[8,9] Although smaller steering wheels or alternative game input devices may accurately demonstrate driving skills, the more an input device differs from an actual car, the less realistic the simulation is likely to be to the client drivers.[10]

Not all realism improves simulation. Many experts speak against a full car cab because of the space and cost required and the increase in simulator sickness associated with its enclosed environment.[11,12]

VISUAL DISPLAY

As noted previously, driving simulators offer varying levels of visual realism. Photographically based simulations have the highest visual realism. CGI systems range from flat cartoon-like images to more realistically detailed and textured images of traffic, roadways, and an urban or rural environment. Although improved graphics present a more realistic visual display, it is unknown how they may affect the face validity of driving simulation and the incidence of simulator sickness.

In interactive CGI driving simulations the environment is flexible, and actions taken by the driver produce a change in the displayed roadway and environmental images. Although the realism of visual images is important, it is more important that the simulation change quickly and accurately and that lags are minimized between a driver's actions and responding changes in the visual display. In the better simulations when a driver acts on the steering, brake, or accelerator, the unfolding visual scene accurately matches the driver's action and the proprioceptive feedback from the accelerator, brake, and steering.

There are two ways to create the computer-based world of interactive CGI driving simulations. In one approach authors create a *mapped simulation*, with roads that can be driven at will. In the other approach the roadway is created as the route is driven. In those *route-based simulations*, regardless of whether a driver turns or fails to turn at an intersection, the roadway that is displayed is the same as originally planned. Thus whether one turns right, left, or goes straight, once the intersection is completed, if the road was intended to be a hilly rural two-lane drive with an oncoming tractor, that is what is displayed.

Mapped and route-based simulations can provide driving challenges, also known as critical events, at specific locations within the simulated environment. For example a car that is stopped on the shoulder of the road may be programmed to merge in front of the client's vehicle without warning. In a mapped simulation a driver must drive the route as planned if he or she is to trigger this challenge. If a driver makes a wrong turn and goes off route, he or she will not encounter the challenging event unless or until he or she returns to the designated location that was programmed to trigger the critical event. In some simulations, once off route, it is easier to stop and redrive the correct route to reach the challenging event. In driving simulations that allow one to drive until one finds the trigger, making a wrong turn may alter the order in which challenging events are experienced. In a route-based simulation a driver can never go off route or get lost during a drive because the identical route is created regardless of his or her turning choices. This means that planned challenges are triggered regardless of whether a driver correctly follows route directions, but the same quality is a limitation when route-based simulations are used to assess or train topographical orientation and route-finding behaviors.

Regardless of whether they are mapped or route based, many CGI driving simulations allow individuals to author their own routes and challenges. In most cases writing these scenarios takes time and requires at least basic computer skills, but some manufacturers are working on creating universally connecting scenario segments that would permit less-skilled individuals to put together a route with greater ease.

FIELD OF VIEW

Field of view is defined as the "out the windshield" view that is presented to the driver and measured in numbers of degrees. The visual world of driving simulation may be displayed several ways. Driving simulation manufacturers offer systems using one or several computer monitors (Figure 10-3), head-mounted display (HMD), one or several plasma screens, and screen pro-

jection (Figure 10-4). Although a wide-view monitor can present an FOV of 60 to 75 degrees, a standard single computer monitor presents a more limited view, offering an FOV of 45 to 60 degrees. In both cases these single screens offer a restricted FOV that oversimplifies cross traffic at intersections and may be unable to adequately represent the realistically simulated driving challenges experienced by clients with

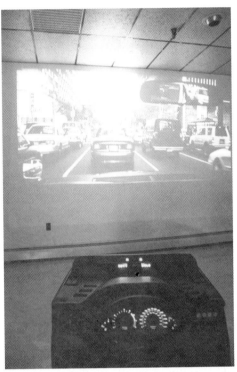

Figure 10-4 Doron Precision System's projected screen system used in an in-patient rehabilitation unit. (Courtesy Doron Precision Systems, Inc., Binghamton, New York.)

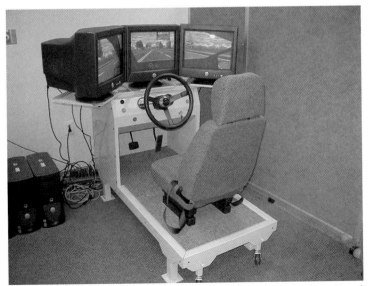

Figure 10-3 STISIM three-monitor system. (Courtesy Systems Technology, Hawthorne, Calif.)

hemispatial neglect or visual field deficits. Screen projections or use of multiple monitors generally provides FOVs ranging from 120 to 180 degrees. Although HMDs offer the potential of 360-degree field of regard (i.e., the total arc that can be seen of a simulated world), their FOV is typically 20 to 40 degrees. Thus the HMD offers the simulated world in narrower wedges, and drivers must turn their heads to see the same forward FOV presented by other display systems. These quick, frequent, side-to-side head motions during driving require simulation updates beyond the system's capacity. As a result, HMDs often produce a noticeable lag or delay between head motion and an updated visual image. This creates a discontinuous visual scene and increases the likelihood of simulation sickness.[13]

Sounds

Most computer-based driving simulations provide auditory cues (such as engine sounds) to increase the realism of the driving experience and to offer feedback on speed to the driver. Fewer simulators allow DRSs to include or exclude crash sounds during collisions, honking horns when a driver is slow or tentative, and sirens when a driver speeds. There are few data indicating which sounds critically improve or impair a simulated driving experience.

Motion

Low- and mid-priced driving simulators tend to be fixed-base systems, providing no motion while driving. Motion bases attempt to mimic the motion cues of driving by moving the simulator cab in response to a driver's inputs. Many experts agree that the current level of technology does not encourage use of these expensive and somewhat mismatched motion bases for clinical driving simulations.

EQUIPMENT SELECTION

As with any costly purchase, driving simulation is a long-term investment, and it is worth gathering information about several systems before making a decision to purchase one over another. DRSs should assess the simulator and experience the simulation firsthand before making the final selection. The DRS should also get to know the length and types of driving scenarios (including critical events) that can be created or provided by the manufacturer of the simulators being evaluated. In addition to the issues addressed previously in this chapter, DRSs should also carefully consider the following factors to enhance their successful integration

of this high-technology modality into their driver evaluation and training tool bag: initial purpose; cost; space; output; troubleshooting, maintenance, and upgrades; and having a "go to" person who can readily address maintenance and other issues that will inevitably arise from time to time.

Intended Purpose

DRSs often find unexpected and inventive ways of using equipment once it becomes familiar. However, to help ensure that one selects the best driving simulation system for a specific clinic or community-based program, it is wise to have a clear idea of the intended populations and the planned uses. For example a less-expensive, noninteractive driving simulator may be suitable for populations with intact insight who are able to interpret symbolic or delayed output, whereas a more costly interactive driving simulator may be more appropriate for populations lacking that insight.

Cost

Commercially available driving simulators range broadly in cost. Many manufacturers offer several styles and types with widely ranging prices, attributes, and abilities. Like most computerized technology, driving simulator prices have decreased over time. This does not mean that they are within the budgets of all programs. At this writing clinically targeted driving simulations range in price from approximately $20,000 to more than $100,000, with higher-priced models sometimes designated as research systems by the manufacturers.

Space

Driving simulation systems require a range of clinic space. Whereas some driving simulators require whole rooms, clinically targeted systems increasingly require less space. A system generally will need floor space to accommodate one or more monitors or projection screens, a driving cab (including driver's seat or chair), one or more computers (generally one computer per screen/monitor), and a control station or monitor with keyboard. Tabletop driving simulators require significantly less space than do simulators that use a mock vehicle but may also offer a less realistic sense of driving. Simulators that use parts of an actual automobile and those that project to a screen require more space than do those using mock-vehicle cabs and computer monitors for displaying the driving scenarios. HMD systems require the least floor space, but the current level of that technology also carries increased risk of simulation sickness.

OUTPUT

Driving simulators can provide vast amounts of data, but making sense of those data may require computer database and statistical skills. DRSs should review samples of a prospective driving simulator's output and explore the system's flexibility for data organization, analysis, and output in hardcopy and electronic formats. Many driving simulators provide a short report of specific driving performance, including numbers of wrong turns, numbers of collisions, tickets issued during the drive (e.g., for failing to stop at stop signs or stop lights), mean lane maintenance, and speed limit violations.

TROUBLESHOOTING, MAINTENANCE, AND UPGRADES

Driving simulations are neither toys nor games. Even when composed of off-the-shelf components, they often need technical, engineering, and computer support personnel to troubleshoot, maintain, repair, and upgrade the simulator's hardware and software so that it stays current with improving technology. Simulator downtime can be expensive and frustrating to clients, therapists, and administrators.

It may help to consider how the institution's personnel resolve basic computer hardware and software problems. If an institution sends out existing computerized devices when they malfunction or purchases replacements rather than repairing devices, it may indicate that current personnel may be unable to support a driving simulation system. Collaborating with a research institution or university on driving simulation projects can help ensure access to a team with the engineering, programming, and other skills needed to keep the simulator in good form. Another option is to pay the manufacturer for maintenance and repair services. If this is the preferred route, the DRS should gather information regarding the costs and the company's record of such service.

Technology changes rapidly, and a center that is contemplating purchasing a driving simulator will especially want to know whether upgrades are included with service costs, how changes in off-the-shelf components could influence the longevity of a driving simulator's utility, and whether the manufacturer is committed to upgrade compatibility. In addition to discussing these issues with the manufacturers, DRSs should consult with several of the driving simulator's current users.

HAVING A "GO TO" PERSON

Many of the currently marketed driving simulation systems were initially developed for use in research environments. Therefore most driving simulators cannot be considered simple "plug in and use" tools. Successful integration of a driving simulator into a clinic's evaluation and treatment repertoire is helped by having one or more "go to" therapists dedicated to understanding the technology, developing "therapist-friendly" protocols and regimens, training peers in driving simulation's use, and educating referral sources regarding driving simulation as a potent assessment and intervention tool. One specified therapist should be designated to serve as the liaison with the driving simulation manufacturer, communicating problems and needs to the support resources responsible for repairs and upgrades.

CASE STUDY #3: CREATIVE FUNDING FOR DRIVING SIMULATION

There are several ways to fund access to driving simulation. Although clinics rarely have the money for such capital purchases, institutional foundations and charities can be excellent sources for funding for purchases of this type of technology. One of this chapter's authors (E.S.D.) originally gained access to a used driving simulation system as a charitable purchase by her institution's foundation. Accessing this older driving simulation allowed her to experiment with the possibilities of driving simulation in her clinical practice and led to her networking with a broad group of people working in driving simulation. Ultimately the network led her to a driving simulation manufacturer experienced in garnering federal funding and interested in examining potential applications of driving simulation technology in a clinical setting. The research project required a multidisciplinary team, creating the opportunity for rehabilitation, manufacturing, and academic settings to work together. She brought her own clinical expertise to a team of university faculty from mechanical engineering and occupational therapy, graduate students in engineering and occupational therapy, and technical experts in simulation and human factors. Collectively the team applied for and received federal grant monies to support their research on the company's driving simulation.

The anticipated consequence of the project was access to driving simulation and development of simulation scenarios and protocols. One unanticipated consequence was the additional attention given to the clinic's new offering. The advanced technology of the driving simulation system generated tours and community requests for additional information about occupational therapy and about driving programs within the community.

SIMULATOR SICKNESS

Simulator sickness is a common problem associated with driving simulation. Simulator sickness (also known as simulator discomfort or simulator adaptation syndrome) is "the generic experience of feeling sick as a result of exposure to computer-generated stimuli"[14] and includes visual and vestibular symptoms that resemble motion sickness.[13]

Although there are anecdotal reports of driving simulation systems with even higher incidence, one expert estimates an incidence of 8% to 10% across driving simulators, decreasing to 5% when all precautions are taken.[15] Neither researchers nor manufacturers commonly report the incidence of simulator sickness associated with the driving simulation.

Simulator sickness occurs when there is a mismatch between anticipated and actual visual, auditory, proprioceptive, and vestibular sensations. Several aspects of driving simulation contribute to this mismatch. Chief among them are the following:

1. Insufficient update rate (simulation frame rate). As noted previously most interactive driving simulations use CGI to create the vehicles, roads, and world in which a drive occurs. If the simulation has an insufficient update rate the simulation becomes less contiguous, and the world becomes chunky rather than smoothly streaming by as one drives.
2. Wide FOV. Wider FOV is associated with higher rates of simulation sickness.[16] Originally it was assumed that this was because a wider FOV was generally associated with wider screens that may have required broader head motions; however, research has not shown a relationship between head motion and simulator sickness. It is now thought that wider FOV may cause greater simulation sickness because wider FOV produces a perceivable flicker in the peripheral visual fields. Faster update and refresh rates are thought to help avoid this flicker and reduce the incidence and severity of sickness in simulations with wider FOVs.[17]

   Ironically, despite their narrower FOV, HMDs produce a higher incidence of simulation sickness than do other display systems. This is primarily ascribed to the lag between head motion and visual update but also may be related to other specific issues related to HMD (e.g., stereoscopic binocular viewing and interpupil distance[18]).
3. Vehicle dynamics. Steering dynamics appear to be especially critical to simulator sickness, affected by the size of deadband width (i.e., the number of degrees that a steering wheel may be rotated before a simulated vehicle turns) and lag between a driver's action, such as turning the steering wheel or applying the brake, and the resulting change in the displayed scene.[18]
4. Visual representation. In simulated driving all objects are presented in equally sharp focus. In real life objects are less clear when they are close or far away, whereas objects in a specific focused depth of view are in focus. In driving simulation we may ". . . receive more information to process per unit-time than . . . (we) would in the real world, given that out-of-focus images may be ignored."[15]

MEASURING SIMULATOR SICKNESS

The Simulator Sickness Questionnaire (SSQ)[19] is the most commonly used assessment for simulation sickness. The questionnaire uses a four-point scale (0 = none, 1 = slight, 2 = moderate, and 3 = severe) to evaluate 16 simulator sickness symptoms. In addition to this score each symptom is weighted across three components of sickness: nausea, oculomotor, and disorientation. Table 10-1 shows the SSQ and grading scale. In a simpler but nonstandard interpretation, some people simply calculate a weighted total score.

Clinics using driving simulation may wish to implement anti–simulation sickness protocols before, during, and after simulation (Box 10-2).

REDUCING SIMULATOR SICKNESS

There are several actions that can help to reduce the incidence and intensity of simulation sickness:

1. Avoid using simulation with at-risk clients. People who report sickness symptoms just before accessing the driving simulator probably should not participate in the driving session. People with a history of frequent motion sickness or postural insecurity also are at higher risk than are those without such a history.[18,21] The data are unclear whether women are more susceptible to simulator sickness than men.[18]
2. Use one or two short (5- to 10-minute) simulated drives before exposing the driver to longer simulations. Simulator sickness decreases significantly by the third closely spaced, short, simulator exposure.[4] These familiarization experiences should be simple, relatively slow drives, with straight roadways progressing to simple curves. Intersections requiring turns should appear only toward the end of the familiarization exposure. There appears to be a buildup of tolerance to simulation. People appear to be less prone to simulation sickness when they have experienced several drives, even if these are separated by several days without any exposure to simulation.

Table 10-1 Simulator Sickness Questionnaire (SSQ) and Scoring

SSQ Symptom	Scoring				Weight		
	0	Slight	Moderate	Severe	Nausea	Oculomotor	Disorientation
General discomfort	0	1	2	3	1 × =	1 × =	0
Fatigue	0	1	2	3	0	1 × =	0
Headache	0	1	2	3	0	1 × =	0
Eyestrain	0	1	2	3	0	1 × =	0
Difficulty focusing	0	1	2	3	0	1 × =	1 × =
Increased salivation	0	1	2	3	1 × =	0	0
Sweating	0	1	2	3	1 × =	0	0
Nausea	0	1	2	3	1 × =	0	1 × =
Difficulty concentrating	0	1	2	3	1 × =	1 × =	0
Fullness of head	0	1	2	3	0	0	1 × =
Blurred vision	0	1	2	3	0	1 × =	1 × =
Dizzy (eyes open)	0	1	2	3	0	0	1 × =
Dizzy (eyes closed)	0	1	2	3	0	0	1 × =
Vertigo*	0	1	2	3	0	0	1 × =
Stomach awareness†	0	1	2	3	1 × =	0	0
Burping	0	1	2	3	1 × =	0	0
Column scores‡					N =	0 =	D =
Total SSQ score§	$(N + 0 + D) \times 3.74 =$						

*Vertigo is experienced as loss of orientation with respect to vertical upright.
†Stomach awareness is usually used to indicate a feeling of discomfort that is just short of nausea.
‡To calculate column scores, insert patient's score for each value and multiply by the given value, and then sum down the columns. In addition, and separate from the mathematics needed to determine the total SSQ, weighted scores for each component can be obtained by multiplying the Nausea column score by 9.54, the Oculomotor column score by 7.58, and the Disorientation score by 13.92.
§Total SSQ score equals the total of the column scores multiplied by 3.74.

| **BOX 10-2** | **Protocol to Reduce Simulation Sickness** |

BEFORE SIMULATION

1. Discuss the early signs of simulation sickness with client, emphasizing the need to break from simulation at first sign. The Simulator Sickness Questionnaire (SSQ) can help guide understanding of the symptoms.
2. Have the driver complete the SSQ, and check to see whether it is above the established high-risk threshold. If high risk, defer using simulation.
3. Provide several additional short drives if driver is in a high-risk group or has higher, but acceptable, SSQ score.
4. Do not allow drivers to drive the simulation on an empty stomach.

DURING SIMULATION

1. Stop simulation at first indication of simulation sickness.
2. Have emeses basin and towels available.
3. Provide water or juice if a driver becomes ill or overheated.
4. Make sure that there is good airflow.

AFTER SIMULATION CARE

1. Studies have linked some nondriving forms of simulation (e.g., flight simulation) to impaired postural stability after simulation.[18-20]
2. To be safest individuals should wait at least 30 minutes after driving simulation before driving on-road.
3. Individuals should practice controlled acceleration and braking several times on their real car before entering traffic.

3. Create a physical environment that feels open.[16] Avoid positioning simulators in corners or other cramped space or using roofed mockups or vehicles.[11,12] Therapists should stand behind the simulator, not to the side where they close in the driver. Keep the room lights low to reduce glare and eyestrain,[15,18] and use a fan to keep the room cool and the air moving during the simulation.

4. Keep computer monitors or projection screens as far from the driver as possible.[15] It is unclear whether this reduces simulation sickness by maintaining an open space or by slightly reducing the FOV.

5. Consider which drivers should wear their eyeglasses. The eyeglasses worn while driving generally correct for impaired far vision. Far vision may be used during projected simulation, but simulations that use computer monitors are more likely to require middle vision. Determine whether a person is better off wearing or not wearing their glasses by having them drive portions of the familiarization simulation with the glasses on and off.

6. Treat early signs of simulation sickness. Ask drivers to tell you as soon as they begin to experience even mild signs of simulation sickness. Simulation sickness does not improve by ignoring early feelings of dizziness, nausea, or fatigue.

7. Consider simulator sickness when you choose a driving simulation. If possible select fixed-base simulations with small steering deadbands and no perceptible lags. Simulation systems should have computers powerful enough to permit update rates ≥ 60 Hz (higher rates are preferred).[15] When motion-based simulations are powerful, fast, and exact, they may reduce simulation sickness, but motion-based systems that slightly mismatch stimuli are more likely to produce simulation sickness than are fixed-base systems that provide no stimuli.[18]

SUMMARY

Occupational therapists and other professionals working as DRSs strive to improve participation through therapeutic use of meaningful experiences.[22] In addition to being a key means of community mobility and community engagement,[23,24] driving is strongly linked to self-identity as a competent adult. Driving simulation can provide rich objective and subjective data for driving evaluation and can serve as a motivating clinical activity to improve insight into driving errors and related deficits that affect not only driving but also other instrumental activities of daily living. Finally, driving simulation can help connect more abstract interventions (such as strengthening, increasing range of motion, or improving cognition) with a goal that has personal significance to the client, thus enhancing motivation and encouraging the client to persevere while he or she travels down the long and often arduous road to rehabilitation and a better quality of life. Although it requires funding, space, and personnel resources, driving simulation offers an opportunity to bring a contextually rich environment into the rehabilitation setting.

REFERENCES

1. Wachtel J: Brief history of driving simulators, *TR News* 179:45, 1995.
2. Brooke MM, Questad KA, Patterson DR, et al: Driving evaluation after traumatic brain injury, *Am J Phys Med Rehabil* 71:177-182, 1992.
3. Korner-Bitensky N, Sofer S, Kaizer F, et al: Assessing ability to drive following an acute neurological event:

are we on the right road? *Can J Occup Ther* 61:141-148, 1994.

4. Watson GS: *Simulator adaptation in a high fidelity driving simulator as a function of scenario intensity and motion cueing*, Paper presented at the Driving Simulation Conference, Paris, France, 1997, ETNA.

5. McLane RC, Wierwille WW: The influence of motion and audio cues on driver performance in an automobile simulator, *Hum Factors* 17:488-501, 1975.

6. Alicandri E, Roberts K, Walker J: A validation study of the DOT/FHWA Highway simulator (HYSIM), NTIS No PB 86-211778, 1986.

7. Martinic TM: *Effectiveness of STISIM simulator in assessing post-brain injury driving ability: a pilot study*, Master's Project, Occupational Therapy Program, University of Minnesota, June 2002.

8. Glaski T, Ehle HT, Williams JB: Off-road driving evaluations for persons with cerebral injury: a factor analytic study of pre-driver and simulator testing, *Am J Occup Ther* 51:352-359, 1997.

9. Reed MP, Green PA: Comparison of driving performance on-road and in a low-cost simulator using a concurrent telephone dialing task, *Ergonomics* 42:1015-1037, 1999.

10. Schiff W, Arnone W, Cross S: Driving assessment with computer-video scenarios: more is sometimes better, *Behavior Research Methods Instruments Computers* 26:192-194, 1994.

11. Hays RT, Singer MJ: *Simulation fidelity in training system design*, New York, 1989, Springer-Verlag.

12. Wachtel J: Are we training operators upside down? *Proceedings of the Ninth Symposium on the Training of Nuclear Facility Personnel*, Oak Ridge, TN, 1991, Oak Ridge National Laboratory, Report No. CONF-9104135.

13. Biocca F: Will simulation sickness slow down the diffusion of virtual environment technology? *Presence* 1:334-343, 1992.

14. Prothero J: University of Washington, Interface Technology Lab 1989. Available at: *www.hitl.washington.edu/publications/r-98-11/node134.html.* Accessed May 28, 2004.

15. Wachtel J: Some brief notes on simulator sickness, Unpublished paper, 2004.

16. Kennedy RS, Lilienthal MG, Berbaum KS, et al: Simulator sickness in US Navy flight simulators, *Aviat Space Environ Med* 60:10-16, 1989.

17. Maxwell CA: Flicker science and the consumer, *Information Display* November:7-10, 1992.

18. Kolansinski EM: *Simulator sickness in virtual environments*, US Army Research Institute Technical Report (Army Project number 20262785A791, Technical report #1027), 1995.

19. Kennedy RS, Lane NE, Berbaum KS, et al: Simulator Sickness Questionnaire: an enhanced method for quantifying simulator sickness, *Int J Aviat Psychol* 3:203-220, 1993.

20. Hamilton KM, Kantor L, Magee LE: Limitations of postural equilibrium tests for examining simulator sickness, *Aviat Space Environ Med* 60:246-251, 1989.

21. Kennedy RS, Fowlkes JE, Berbaum KS, et al: Use of motion sickness history questionnaire for prediction of simulator sickness, *Aviat Space Environ Med* 64:912-920, 1992.

22. American Occupational Therapy Association: Occupational therapy practice framework: domain and process, *Am J Occup Ther* 56:609-639, 2002.

23. Katz R, Golden R, Butter J, et al: Driving safely after brain damage: follow-up of twenty-two patients with matched controls, *Arch Phys Med Rehabil* 71:133-136, 1990.

24. Dobbs BM, Autovich ND, Vanderberghe C: Dementia and driving cessation: an overview of the development of group interventions for clients and caregivers, and preliminary results. *6th National Workshop for Driver Rehabilitation Specialists*, Glenrose Rehabilitation Hospital, Edmonton, Alberta, Canada, May 29, 2004.

Part III

MEASURING AND IMPROVING DRIVING PERFORMANCE

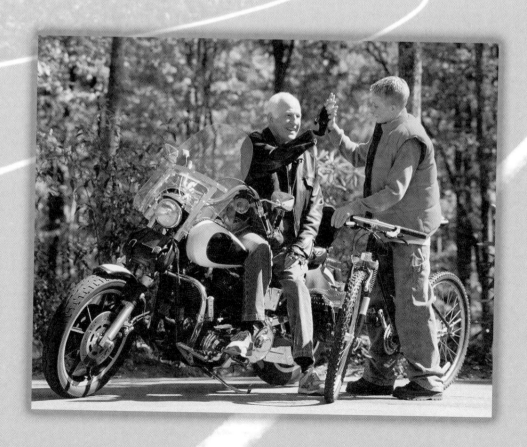

Chapter 11

PREPARING FOR THE ON-ROAD EVALUATION

Jerry Bouman • *Joseph M. Pellerito, Jr.*

KEY TERMS

- Evaluation vehicle
- Functional evaluation
- In-vehicle demonstration

CHAPTER OBJECTIVES

After completing this chapter, the reader will be able to do the following:

- Know the steps the DRS should follow for the on-road evaluation and training.
- Be aware of issues or potential problems with vehicles in order to help clients select appropriate adaptive equipment and vehicles.
- Know what to ask clients when meeting with them for the first time.

SELECTING THE OPTIMAL VEHICLE TYPE AND ADAPTIVE DRIVING EQUIPMENT

Once the predriving clinical evaluation has been completed and the client has been recommended for an on-road evaluation, driver rehabilitation specialists (DRSs) have the opportunity to use their insight and creativity to apply the knowledge they have gained about vehicles, vehicle modifications, and adapted driving aids during the next step in the comprehensive driver rehabilitation evaluation process. That step is the selection of a vehicle and the most appropriate adaptive driving equipment, which is critical to the success of the evaluation. This chapter presents the primary steps a DRS should follow when preparing for the on-road evaluation and training: (1) selecting a vehicle that is the closest to meeting the client's actual needs, (2) adapting the vehicle to help ensure the client's optimal driving performance, and (3) giving the client an opportunity to test drive the mocked-up vehicle on the road. This process has worked well for many DRSs; however, each specialist must develop and continually improve his or her own system for completing this portion of the comprehensive driver rehabilitation evaluation.

Depending on the scope of the DRS's practice and his or her access to vehicles and adaptive driving equipment, the primary aim is to match a client with a vehicle and the adaptive driving equipment that they will need for optimal driver and/or passenger safety. In reality, this may not be possible due to the lack of access to every possible vehicle type that can be modified and the myriad of adaptive devices and vehicle modifications available. However, every DRS should become familiar with a range of vehicles and the general concepts related to making them accessible to people with disabilities or aging-related concerns.

Vehicles are constantly being changed, improved, redesigned, raised, lowered, shortened, lengthened, discontinued, and replaced by new models on a yearly basis. It is difficult to keep up with all of the changes, and it is a real challenge to keep up-to-date with the latest devices and modifications that enhance vehicle access and adapted driving. For example, DRSs recommend, and vehicle modifiers install, steering devices on an original equipment manufactured (OEM) steering wheel to make it easier to control the vehicle with one hand. Proper positioning of the steering device was fairly simple to determine until the introduction of driver-side airbags into the steering wheel. The size of the first airbags almost eliminated the space needed to install the steering devices on steering wheels. Then there was a concern that the steering device would injure the user in the event that the airbag was deployed. Today we know that the airbag can be safely deployed without the steering devices injuring anyone because the device is pushed aside as the airbag inflates. The location of the steering device on the wheel is still limited, however, but DRSs and vehicle modifiers have found creative ways to work around the challenges airbags present and continue using these and other functional devices.

It is imperative for DRSs to figure out ways to stay abreast of important issues such as these so that they can educate their clients about what to look for when selecting a vehicle or adaptive driving equipment. Currently, there are limited ways to become aware of the state-of-the-art vehicles and modification procedures. One of the most important educational activities that a DRSs can do is to regularly attend one of several conferences sponsored by the professional organizations that support driving specialists and vehicle modifiers; that is, the Association of Driver Rehabilitation Specialists (ADED) and the National Mobility Equipment Dealers Association (NMEDA). DRSs should also develop a working relationship with the companies that provide vehicle modifications in any given geographic service area. This helps to ensure that each client will be given the most current and accurate information about vehicles and adaptive driving equipment. One of the most important things for a DRS to do is to ask prospective clients not to purchase a vehicle or adaptive equipment prior to a comprehensive driver rehabilitation evaluation. If a client needs a vehicle, he or she should wait until the evaluation has been completed before making a selection.

THE VEHICLE SELECTION PROCESS

CARS

Most driver rehabilitation programs select a car to use for their behind-the-wheel evaluations because the majority of clients served by these programs are able to get into and out of a car independently. There was a time when a two-door car was the most logical choice for a driver rehabilitation program, so that clients who used wheelchairs could more easily transfer into and out of the vehicle as well as learn to stow a folding wheelchair behind the front seat. Two things have occurred that have made a four-door car the most likely first selection instead: (1) increased use of rigid frame wheelchairs, which can be stowed in two- and four-door cars, and (2) an increase in the numbers of older

clients who don't require any adaptive equipment. These individuals often consider two-door cars to be sporty, and therefore the two-door cars may not be like the cars they were used to driving before an injury, illness, or other concern that has required them to be evaluated by a DRS. If the car is very different from their own vehicle, it can actually have an impact on their willingness to accept the results of the evaluation. Some programs use minivans and sport utility vehicles (SUVs), which have become preferred choices for much of the general public, but the four-door car is probably the most universal vehicle to select as a basic *evaluation vehicle*. For those individuals who are unable to transfer into a car, modified full-size vans or minivans are the most appropriate vehicles.

Two-Door Cars

For many years, the two-door car was the standard evaluation vehicle and was often the preferred vehicle for many clients. Two-door cars offered wider door openings for easier access for transferring from a wheelchair into a car. There was access to the rear seat space that was usually large enough to stow a folding manual wheelchair. Over the years, as cars got smaller, the amount of space available for transfers was reduced. Two-door cars began to include consoles, which can get in the way of wheelchair loading and reduce room for transfers. Individuals who transfer into the car from the passenger's side and slide across the seat to get into the driver's seat are unable to use a two-door car with a console. Cars with center consoles often have the transmission selector in the center as well, and these gear shifters require the driver to push in a button to release an interlock that allows the car to be put out of and back into the park position.

The style of wheelchairs has dramatically changed, too. Individuals who use a wheelchair for mobility and who are capable of transferring independently and manually loading a wheelchair into a car often use a rigid frame wheelchair. These chairs do not fold in the traditional sense. They need to be dismantled, and the frame must be lifted over one's lap and placed on the front passenger seat or over the seat back and placed onto the rear seat. The wheels are removed and also stowed inside the vehicle, either in the front passenger seat area or in the rear seat area.

Four-Door Cars

Four-door cars are more commonly used today in driver rehabilitation programs. Older drivers seem more comfortable with this style of car because they are more likely to have been using this type of car prior to the driver rehabilitation evaluation. Walkers and canes can be stowed in the rear seat area. For individuals who need to use a rigid frame wheelchair, the chair can be dismantled to fit inside the car. With the wheels removed and the back folded down, the chair can be lifted over the lap (with the seat back folded down) and placed in the front seat or rear seat area. The wheels are loaded into the vehicle over the lap and into the front seat area or on or in front of the back seats.

Individuals who use a traditional style wheelchair that folds and is heavier than lightweight rigid models can opt to use an automatic wheelchair loading system that is installed on the roof of the vehicle. This type of device picks up the wheelchair by lifting up on the seat so that the chair is automatically folded and then lifts the folded wheelchair onto the roof of the car and into an enclosed container. This type of device can be used with two-door cars, four-door cars, minivans, SUVs, and pickup trucks. Other devices are available that can stow manual wheelchairs, power wheelchairs, and scooters into a variety of vehicles. These devices are presented in greater detail in Chapters 6, 9, 12, and 17.

MINIVANS AND SPORT UTILITY VEHICLES

Minivans can be used by DRSs for evaluations. The height of the seat, generally at least 30 inches from the ground, will make it very difficult, if not impossible, for most people who use wheelchairs to get into a minivan; however, individuals who can stand to enter may find it an easier vehicle to get in and out of without having to drop down onto the lower seat height of a car that is generally around 20 to 22 inches. SUVs, like pickup trucks, have higher seat heights that require the individual to step up or lift themselves up and onto the seat. This can create a real barrier for entry for any individual with impaired ambulation, strength, standing balance, or any combination of these and other client factors.

WHEELCHAIR-ACCESSIBLE VANS

The use of a car is limited to those individuals who can comfortably and safely get into and out of the car and load a mobility device or ambulation aid independently in the event that they use one. Anyone who uses a mobility device that cannot be safely and independently stowed in a car will generally use a van that has been modified for easier access. There are two types of vehicles that can be modified effectively: (1) the full-size, rear-wheel drive van, and (2) the front-wheel drive minivan.

Full-Size Vans

Ford Motor Company's full-size van has been the favorite vehicle for wheelchair access modification since the early 1970s. The vehicle was roomy and easy to modify, and the floor of the van could be lowered up to 6 inches without significant structural modification to the vehicle. Lowering the floor was necessary to reduce the height of an adult seated in a wheelchair to allow the adult to see out of the van windows. Nearly all of the modifications and equipment created for drivers with disabilities were designed with the Ford van in mind, and this continues to the present day. For individuals who are able to transfer independently, the van can be modified with a special transfer seat in the driver and front passenger seat area. The individual can also remain seated in the wheelchair and ride as a passenger or drive the vehicle. For individuals who are able to transfer independently, the General Motors full-size van can also be modified for wheelchair access.

Front-Wheel-Drive Minivans

In the mid 1980s, the front-wheel-drive minivan, introduced by Chrysler Corporation, was modified for wheelchair access by lowering the floor 10 inches and installing a wheelchair ramp in the side or rear door. Since 2000, a 12-inch lowered floor has been available in a General Motors minivan. The rear entry system is used as a transport vehicle or when a driver is capable of transferring independently out of the wheelchair and into a modified six- or eight-way driver's seat. The side entry system is modified so that the person using a wheelchair can remain seated in the wheelchair and sit in the driver or front passenger seat areas, or transfer into a modified driver or front passenger seat. Because of the popularity of the minivan, nearly all of the adaptive equipment designed for accessible driving is available for this type of vehicle.

PICKUP TRUCKS, SUVs, AND MINIVANS WITH ALTERNATE ACCESS MODIFICATIONS

Since these vehicles are very popular with the general public, there is a demand for them from some members of the disabled community as well. In order to make these vehicles accessible to the individual who uses a wheelchair for mobility, a variety of special seat lifts and wheelchair lifts have been created on a limited basis. Most are not as easy to use as the fully accessible full-size van and minivan, but certain individuals are able to use them successfully. In the event that the client decides to use one of these vehicles, it is strongly recommended that a *functional evaluation* be completed with a demonstration vehicle prior to the purchase and modification of the vehicle to be sure that the individual has the strength, range of motion, and balance to use it safely, as well as to be sure that the client can successfully maneuver the wheelchair into the vehicle.

ADAPTATIONS FOR DRIVING: CAR-BASED EQUIPMENT

When DRSs meet clients for the first time, they should spend time discussing their clients' experiences with driving, the types of vehicles the clients currently own or lease or have used in the past, and the type of vehicle that they expect to use in the future. DRSs should then establish their needs related to transporting mobility equipment and what the clients believe they need in order to be safe and independent as a driver or passenger. Once a DRS has determined that a car is appropriate and the client's goal is to be a driver, the DRS proceeds to an evaluation car. DRSs may select a two-door car for very tall or large clients, or if the larger door will make transfers from a wheelchair easier. DRSs will likely select a four-door car for most other clients, especially older drivers.

Once in the car, the DRS must next consider the client's optimal seating position for safety and comfort. The DRS should be certain that the client is able to see out of the windows and over the dash and reach the foot pedals or hand control, depending on the method of vehicle operation being considered. Upper body stability is important, and for clients who have sustained higher thoracic or cervical level spinal cord injuries (SCIs), a DRS will often need to add an upper body support strap (e.g., chest strap) with Velcro closure to provide this stability. Clients must also be able to reach the floor with their feet, which is another important factor that can contribute to the client's overall stability. For more information on wheeled mobility and seating for optimal driver comfort and safety, see Chapter 9.

Before entering the car, the DRS should have a good idea of the type of driving equipment, if any, the client requires. Set up the vehicle with the appropriate adaptive driving equipment in advance of the on-road evaluation and be sure to demonstrate how the equipment operates by completing a predriving *in-vehicle demonstration*, which entails explaining how each modification works. The next step is to have the client try driving the car with the adaptive equipment within a protected driving area, such as a large parking lot or driving range. Once the DRS has selected and set up all of the equipment necessary to allow the client to independently operate the vehicle, and the equipment trials in a protected area have been completed, the actual on-road evaluation commences.

If the client is able to operate the vehicle without any adaptive equipment, the evaluation will proceed with an evaluation of the client's ability to drive safely in a wide variety of driving environments. If the client requires adaptive equipment to drive, the evaluation proceeds with a gradual increase in traffic and route complexity to complete a baseline of information about the client's potential to drive using adaptive equipment. Training in the use of the adaptive equipment is recommended before the client completes a final driving evaluation to ensure overall safety in all driving environments.

SEATING AND POSITIONING

The following adaptive equipment and recommendations can be used for seating and positioning.

Cushions

For optimum vision out of the vehicle, comfort, and postural support, a variety of cushions can be used to improve seating and positioning. The DRS can communicate with the rehabilitation team member responsible for making recommendations pertaining to the client's seating and positioning needs. If a formal evaluation is required, the DRS should initiate a referral to an occupational therapy or physical therapy seating specialist.

Armrests

There are no commercially available modifications to the OEM armrests for most vehicles. Because the armrests in vehicles are generally poorly positioned (i.e., too low and away from the driver) to provide any benefit such as upper extremity support, it may be necessary to have a custom modification completed in the client's personal vehicle. When steering with one hand is necessary, it is critical to have a properly positioned armrest for the elbow to rest on when the vehicle is moving in a forward direction in order to reduce the driver's fatigue level.

Seat Belt

Modifications to seat belts may be required to help ensure proper fit and function of the vehicle's seat belts. A short extension to the center buckle portion of the belt is available from the auto manufacturer. Customization of the safety belts may be necessary in the client's personal vehicle to help ensure the driver's safety, health, and well-being. See Chapter 17 for more information on wheeled mobility tie-down systems and occupant restraints for improved safety and crash protection.

Airbags

The National Highway Traffic Safety Administration (NHTSA) recommends that the driver maintain a minimum of 10 inches of space between the center of the airbag and the center of the driver's sternum. If the driver needs to sit closer to the steering wheel, the airbag

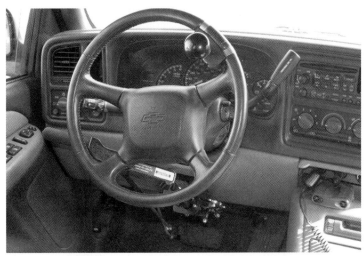

Figure 11-1 Spinner knob steering device.

should be equipped with a shutoff system and a warning light indicating that the airbag has been deactivated. NHTSA also recommends that no one 12 years of age or younger should be seated in a seat equipped with an airbag. If the prospective adult driver is close to the size of a 12-year-old in height or weight, the same concerns should be addressed.[1]

Upper Body Support with Velcro Closure

The upper body support with Velcro closure is for individuals with impaired upper body strength. An upper body support is used for improved postural and lateral support.

STEERING

A steering assist device is generally used when the client has one hand available for steering. It allows full control over the steering wheel during turns, emergency maneuvers, and parking. The steering device can be set up for left hand or right hand use, and its position on the steering wheel is determined by the client's specific needs. Ideally, the steering device is positioned so that the driver can rest his or her elbow on an armrest to reduce fatigue while driving. The steering device is generally attached to the steering wheel with a base that is attached to the wheel with two straps. The device can be easily removed from its base. Thanks to its quick-release design, it also allows alternate drivers to use two hands safely on the steering wheel without interference from the disconnected steering device. Finally, the steering device only works in vehicles equipped with power steering.

Steering Knob

This adapted driving aid requires that the client possesses a fully functional spherical grasp.

Spin Pin

This adapted driving aid (Figure 11-1) features a single upright cushioned post that requires a fully functional cylindrical grasp.

V-Grip

This adapted driving aid (Figure 11-2) is used when the client's hand grip is impaired but retains some function. Additionally, keeping the distal upper extremity (i.e., from the elbow to the hand) in a position that is vertical to the steering wheel may improve the client's comfort and reduce his or her level of fatigue.

Palm Grip

This adapted driving aid (Figure 11-3, *A*) is a flat spinner used when the client's hand grip is impaired but retains some function. Similar to the V-grip, the client may need to maintain his or her distal upper extremity (i.e., from the elbow to the hand) in a position that is

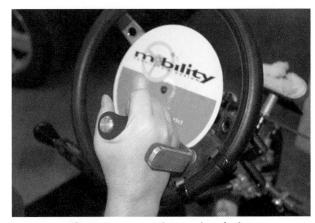

Figure 11-2 V-grip steering device.

vertical to the steering wheel, which may improve the client's comfort and reduce his or her level of fatigue.

Tri-Pin

This adapted driving aid (Figure 11-3, *B*) can be used when the client's hand grip is impaired and retains very little or no residual function. This device captures the client's wrist securely and may need to be modified with a small cap on top of the center pin to make it easier for the client to position his or her hand in place and to prevent the client's hand from pulling away from the adapted driving device while turning the vehicle and during the recovery phase.

Steering Splint

This adapted driving aid is a type of specialized hand splint with Velcro straps that features a post that fits into its base, which is connected to the steering wheel.

Amputee Ring

This adapted driving aid usually features a simple metal ring attached to the steering wheel that can accommodate a prosthetic hook. The size of the opening of the ring may need to be adjusted to accommodate the specific hook used by the client and to help make a more secure and functional client–steering wheel interface.

ACCELERATOR AND BRAKE CONTROLS

This section describes the modifications that can be made to the accelerator and brake controls.

Left Foot Accelerator

This adapted driving aid (Figure 11-4) is a mechanical device that is bolted to the floor on the left side of the brake pedal to allow the left foot to operate the accelerator. A quick-release design is available to allow the

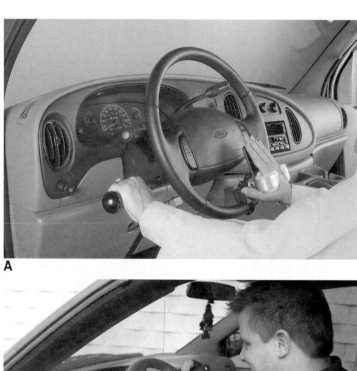

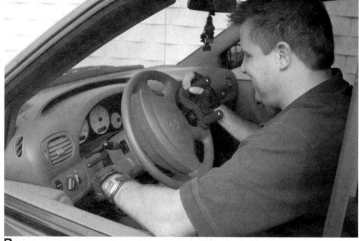

Figure 11-3 **A,** Palm-grip steering device. **B,** Tri-pin steering device.

vehicle to be safely used by an alternate driver who will be using his or her right foot. This device requires that the vehicle be equipped with automatic transmission.

Gas Pedal Block

This adapted driving aid (Figure 11-5) is a metal cover plate that is positioned over the original gas pedal to prevent the client inadvertently making contact with it while using a left foot accelerator with his or her right foot or prosthesis. This device is also available as a component of a left foot accelerator package.

Pedal Extensions

These adapted driving aids (Figure 11-6) are designed for the client whose lower extremities cannot easily reach the OEM gas and brake pedals. The pedal extensions can be used instead of hand controls if the client

is able to access and operate the extensions safely, which allows the client to use two hands for steering. It is important to support the client's feet (i.e., heels) by providing a solid sub floor to reduce fatigue and improve overall control of the vehicle. There are four types of pedal extensions, including the following:

- Short: 2-inch block style extensions
- Medium: 2- to 8-inch extensions
- Long: 8- to 18-inch extensions
- Power: Remote-powered pedals that can be positioned to accommodate the client's particular ergonomic needs

Hand Controls

This adapted driving aid (Figure 11-7) is a mechanical device that is attached under the vehicle's dashboard with a single handle that connects to the accelerator and brake. This device only works in vehicles equipped with power brakes and comes in both left- and right-handed versions.

- Left: Standard setup is designed for left-handed operation. This allows easy access to the turn signal stalk, which is also located on the left side of the steering wheel in most vehicles. This configuration also allows the client to use his or her right hand to access the vehicle's transmission shift lever.
- Right: Nonstandard setup designed for right-handed operation. Generally, this configuration is selected when the client's right hand does not have the range of motion, dexterity, strength, or any combination of these or other client factors that are required for steering. The biggest challenge the DRS faces is determining how the client should operate the shift lever, which may need to be extended toward the left side of the steering wheel to improve access with the left hand.

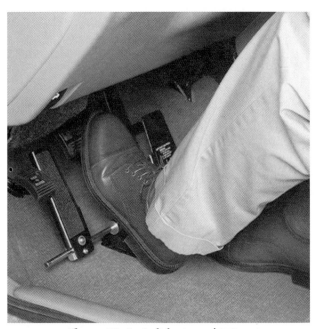

Figure 11-4 Left foot accelerator.

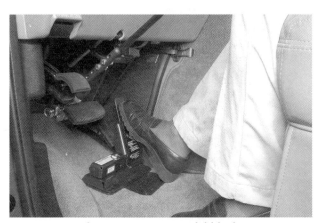

Figure 11-5 Gas pedal block.

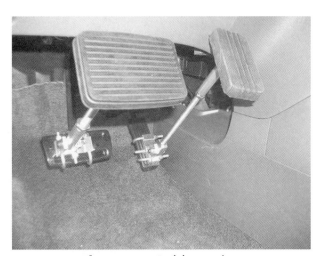

Figure 11-6 Pedal extension.

By and large, four types of hand controls are available to consumers. The types and their primary mechanism for activation are listed as follows:

- Right Angle: Push forward for brake, down for accelerator
- Push Pull: Push forward for brake, pull back for accelerator
- Push/Twist: Push forward for brake, twist handle or lever for accelerator
- Push/Tilt: Push forward for brake, pull/tilt for accelerator

Extensions

This adapted driving aid handle extension/modification may be required to make it easier to maintain hand position or bring the hand control brake handle closer to the driver for enhanced leverage and improved braking.

Pedal Block

This adapted driving aid is a quick-release removable barrier positioned to prevent inadvertent contact with the accelerator pedal and brake pedal as well as preventing the driver's feet from getting caught under the foot pedals when he or she is using hand controls.

Parking Brake

This adapted driving aid is a mechanical extension handle to convert an OEM foot-operated parking brake to one that is hand-operated.

Horn/Dimmer

This adapted driving aid enables remote electrical operation of the horn and/or headlight dimmer that is installed on the handle of the hand control device for improved access and control. Most of today's vehicles use the turn signal stalk to operate the headlight dimmer, which some drivers can operate without modification. The remote device allows easy access to the horn and headlight dimmer for the client who cannot operate them using the OEM turn signal stalk.

Wiper/Washer

This adapted driving aid is installed on the handle of the hand control and provides the client with remote operation of the wiper/washer control and cruise control. Clients with limited finger dexterity are precluded from using these OEM functions because many vehicles require the driver to twist the turn signal stalk in order to operate the wiper/washer and cruise control functions.

Cruise Control

Many vehicles require the user to push a recessed button on the end of the turn signal stalk to activate the cruise control, which precludes most drivers with limited finger function from operating this function.

AUXILIARY (SECONDARY) SYSTEMS

Turn signal, wipers/washers, dimmer, horn, cruise control, ignition, and mirror modifications are all modifications to the auxiliary, or secondary, systems.

Turn Signal

The turn signal stalk, usually located on the left side of the steering wheel, must be accessible to the driver. The most common modification to the turn signal is to attach a mechanical lever that extends the turn signal stalk to the right side of the steering wheel. This allows the turn signal stalk to be activated with the right hand on the right side of the steering wheel. Not all vehicles can be modified with a mechanical extension, so an

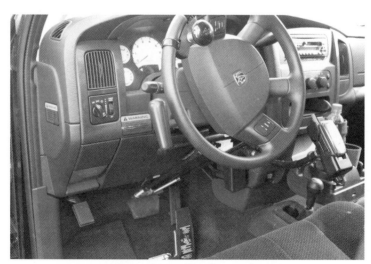

Figure 11-7 Hand controls.

electric turn signal device that allows the turn signals to be activated by the right hand can be installed on the right side of the wheel. It is also possible to locate switches to control the turn signals on the steering wheel, either next to or attached to the steering knob.

Wipers/Washer, Dimmer, Horn, and Cruise Control

In many vehicles, these devices are located on the left side of the steering wheel. In the event that the driver is unable to use his or her left hand, these devices will need to be remotely operated from the right side of the steering wheel. It is also possible to locate the switches that control these devices on the steering wheel, either next to or attached to the steering knob.

Ignition

Modifying the ignition may be required if the client is unable to turn the key due to limited upper extremity and hand function. A wide variety of simple plastic and metal key extensions and adaptors make it easier to hold on to a key, insert it into the ignition, and turn the key with improved leverage. The ignition can also be converted to a fixed or wireless push-button system if use of a modified key is not a viable option.

Mirrors

Convex and multifaceted mirrors may need to be added to the vehicle to assist with blind spot checking for clients with limited neck rotation, trunk rotation, or both.

ADAPTATIONS FOR DRIVING: VAN-BASED EQUIPMENT

A van-based evaluation generally means that there is a need to address the issue of a client being able to access a vehicle while remaining seated in a wheelchair or motorized scooter. The DRS and client should discuss the types of vehicles available (i.e., full-size and mini-vans) plus the wide range of lifts, ramps, lowered floors, raised roofs and doors, and seat modifications available. The client is then introduced to both styles of vans followed by an in-vehicle assessment with the adaptive driving equipment that the client requires.

Seating is first addressed by determining the client's preferred method of transferring into and out of the vehicle, which is affected by whether the client will be transferring from the wheelchair into a modified driver's seat or remaining seated in the wheelchair while driving the vehicle. If the client's ability to transfer is limited, he or she should consider the use of the vehicle as a tool for independence rather than a challenge to overcome obstacles. If it takes an inordinate amount of time and a great deal of the client's available energy to

complete the transfer, the van will likely be a barrier to independence rather than a tool to achieve it. On the other hand, if riding in a wheelchair while driving a van is uncomfortable or causes stress, transferring may be the better option if it can be reasonably accomplished. Once the seating style is selected, the next step is to make sure that the client is securely and safely seated with proper upper body support, including armrests and cushions if required.

The next step is to figure out how the client is going to steer the vehicle. It is prudent to have the client use his or her strongest arm for steering, since it has to do the majority of the work involved in the total driving task. Selecting the best method of operating the gas and brake is next, and positioning the adaptive equipment to allow the client full access to the equipment is a critical part of the preparation for the on-road evaluation. Finally, the selection of an appropriate method for accessing the auxiliary or secondary controls such as ignition, gear shift, and turn signals is made. Since evaluation vans are often set up with higher levels of modified equipment, it may be necessary to have the client try out some of the auxiliary equipment in other vehicles as the training program progresses to be sure that the client's personal vehicle is not modified beyond what is necessary for him or her to achieve the established driver rehabilitation objectives.

Once the evaluation vehicle has been set up as closely as possible to meet the client's particular needs, the DRS should proceed to have the client drive the vehicle with the adaptive equipment in a protected environment such as a large parking lot or driving range. The driving environment is then expanded as much as possible during the initial session to get an accurate view of the client's potential to learn to drive the adapted vehicle under different driving conditions. Training in the use of the adaptive equipment is recommended before the client completes a final driving evaluation to ensure overall safety and optimal performance in all environments.

SEATING AND POSITIONING

These considerations are the same as when exploring adapted driving solutions in a car. Whether the driver is transferring into the driver's seat or remaining seated in a wheelchair, the modifications for seating and positioning need to be properly positioned and easily accessible without requiring assistance for the driver. For more information on seating options and driving, see Chapter 9.

Lowered Floor Systems

There are two reasons that the floor of a van needs to be lowered for most adults who get into the van while remaining seated in a wheelchair (Figure 11-8). First, the average adult sits between 48 and 56 inches tall from the floor to the top of the head when seated in a wheelchair. Because the original door opening of the van is 48 inches, it is usually necessary to increase the amount of headroom at the doorway. Lowering the floor of the van provides the additional room to get many clients through the doorway without difficulty. In some cases of extreme height, it may be necessary to raise the roof and doors and lower the floor to get the necessary head clearance through the doorway. Second, the wheelchair seat is generally at least 6 inches higher than the original driver's seat in a van. If the driver is to remain seated in the wheelchair while driving, the lowered floor is necessary to bring the seat height down so that the client can see out of the windshield.

For full-size vans, there are two options. One is the 6-inch lowered floor, which gives 53 inches of headroom clearance through the doorway. The second is the 9-inch lowered floor, which gives 56 inches of headroom clearance through the doorway. There are two options for minivans, as well. The first is a 10-inch lowered floor, which gives 53 inches of headroom clearance through the doorway. The second is the 12-inch lowered floor, which gives 56 inches of headroom clearance through the doorway.

Six-Way Transfer Seat

The six-way transfer seat (Figure 11-9) is the seat base that is used in both full-size and minivans to allow for easier transfer into the driver's seat. The seat travels back away from the steering wheel, swivels 90 degrees, and can be raised or lowered to the same height of the wheelchair seat.

Empty Wheelchair Securement

While the client is driving the van from the driver's seat, the empty wheelchair needs to be secured to the floor of the van to prevent it from becoming a pro-

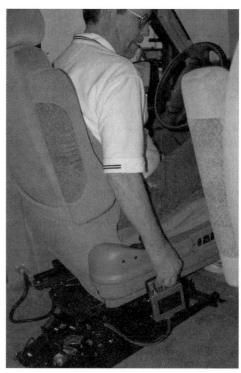

Figure 11-9 Six-way transfer seat.

jectile inside the vehicle in the event of a motor vehicle accident or the client being required to stop abruptly.

Wheelchair Securement and Occupant Protection

If the client is going to drive while seated in a wheelchair, the wheelchair needs to be secured to the floor of the van with an automatic securement system.

Safety Belts

The DRS must assess the client's ability to independently apply and remove lap and shoulder seat belts, as well as review applicable belt wearing laws and the importance of wearing seat belts to help prevent injuries and to improve his or her stability while behind the wheel.

STEERING

The following section describes the modifications that can be made in order to make steering easier for the client in preparation of the on-road evaluation of driving performance.

Modified Effort with Backup

If the client is unable to turn the standard power steering wheel using the adaptive steering devices, the steering effort can be modified, or reduced, by 40% (reduced effort steering) or 70% (minimal effort steering). This problem is most often related to clients who

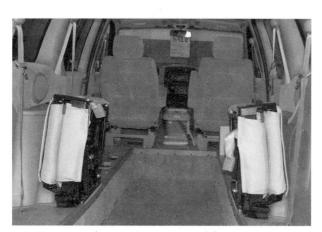

Figure 11-8 Lowered floor.

have sustained spinal cord injuries and have difficulty steering through the 11 o'clock and 2 o'clock positions of the turn. There is a loss of steering road feel or feedback with these types of adaptive driving aids; the more the steering effort is reduced, the greater the loss of this feedback, so it is important to select the steering level that is most appropriate for the client's needs. A backup steering system is always included that automatically provides reserve power to the steering system in the event that the engine fails (e.g., stalls or runs out of gas). When using zero effort steering, a counterbalance should be added to the steering wheel to offset the effect of the weight of the steering device.

Extended Steering Column
When using a full-size van with a 6-inch lowered floor, the steering column needs to be extended to reposition the steering wheel for optimum access. This is generally not required in lowered-floor minivans and in vans with 9-inch lowered floors.

Steering Wheel Size
The size of the steering wheel may be reduced if there is insufficient clearance or for individuals with reduced range of motion. Smaller steering wheels require greater effort and more revolutions of the wheel and are generally combined with modified effort steering for improved safety.

Horizontal Steering Column
This device replaces the original steering column and steering wheel with an articulated column that positions a 10-inch steering disk in a horizontal plane in front of the driver. This adaptation is most commonly used by individuals who have sustained spinal cord injuries and who are unable to turn a regular steering wheel with zero effort steering. This device positions the steering wheel in a gravity-eliminated plane and is used in conjunction with zero effort steering.

Remote Steering
This device replaces the original steering wheel with an alternate steering system. It can be positioned freely for an optimal driving position, thereby allowing for optimum positioning and accessibility for the driver. Depending on the manufacturer, the original steering wheel may or may not be available for alternate drivers. This device is functional for individuals with spinal cord injuries, spinal muscular atrophy, and muscular dystrophy (MD), as well as other clients with significant range of motion or strength limitations.

The 6-inch steering wheel, depending on the manufacturer, requires up to six revolutions of the wheel for full lock-to-lock steering with the following interfaces available to the client:

- Spinner Ball (1-inch, 1.25-inch, 2-inch): Requires grasp
- Swivel Pin: Requires grasp
- Tri-Pin: No grasp required
- Hand Splint (Custom)

In another modification, steering is accomplished by using a single joystick lever. Types of joystick steering devices include a pin, round knob, oval knob, or a custom device.

HAND CONTROLS
Hand controls regulate the brake and accelerator of a motor vehicle and are described in this section, as well as several other adapted driving aids.

Power Parking Brake
This modification provides the client with access to the parking brake and allows for emergency access to a back-up brake system that is separate from the vehicle's hand controls or primary power brakes.

Modified Effort Brakes
This features a modification to the vehicle's braking system to reduce the effort necessary to fully apply the brakes to stop the vehicle. A back-up system is required to provide independent power to the brakes in the event of engine failure. This modification is generally used in conjunction with mechanical hand controls.

Power-Assisted Hand Controls
These devices allow a person with limited strength and range of motion to operate hand controls (accelerator and brake). They are powered by using motors or a pneumatic system to provide the power the client requires to push the foot pedals via the hand controls. The control lever can be positioned for optimum access by the client and is available in the following styles:
- Lever: A simple push/pull lever. Can be set up for forward/backward or side-to-side action.
- Tri-Pin: Similar to the steering tri-pin, but set up in a horizontal plane, capturing the wrist for secure operation. It can be a t-handle (one of several handles designed to match the driver's needs) or a custom device.

Alternative Joystick
This adapted driving aid features a smaller lever with less range of motion and effort required than the one listed above. The device is similar to the joystick control on a wheelchair and is available in the following styles: pin, round knob, oval knob, or custom device.

COMBINED DRIVING CONTROL SYSTEMS

The following section describes vehicle modifications that are combined driving control systems.

Joystick

This adapted driving aid is a single control device that operates the vehicle's steering, accelerator, and brakes. The device looks similar to the joystick control of a power wheelchair and uses electric motors to operate the vehicle's primary controls. This device can be used by clients who have been diagnosed with SCIs, MD, spinal muscular dystrophy, polio, and other disabling conditions.

Mechanical/DSI Unilever

This adapted driving aid is a single control device that operates the vehicle's steering, accelerator, and brakes. This device uses mechanical linkages to the vehicle's original steering, accelerator, and brake controls. It is unique in that it only requires a 180-degree or 270-degree rotation of the steering wheel (or lever) for full lock-to-lock steering. This device can be used by clients who have SCIs, MD, spinal muscular dystrophy, polio, and other disabling conditions.

AUXILIARY SYSTEMS

Modifications to the motor vehicle's auxiliary systems can be made to the full console, primary auxiliary control, voice activation, and mirrors.

Full Console

In some situations, all of the vehicle's auxiliary controls need to be remotely operated by the client (Figure 11-10). This can include some or all of the following functions: ignition, start, lights, dimmer, wipers, wipers/washer, cruise control (i.e., on/set), parking brake, wheelchair securement system release, automatic shifting, fan speeds, turn signals, horn, power windows, and power door locks. The control panel can be located to facilitate optimal accessibility while helping to ensure the safety and well-being of the client, passengers, and others traveling on the road.

Primary Auxiliary Control

Certain devices need to be operated while the vehicle is in motion. These include turn signals, horn, dimmer, wipers/washer, and cruise control. Several devices are available that provide instant one- or two-touch access to all of these devices by using a single switch and multifunction electronic system. The activation switch can be located in a variety of locations (e.g., the handle of the hand controls, near the elbow, in the joystick control, or near the driver's head).

Primary Auxiliary Control/Voice Activation

For (true) one-handed drivers, it may be necessary to add a system that allows the vehicle's gear shift to be operated by use of a voice command. The client can safely control up to 16 devices while the vehicle is in motion by simply uttering preprogrammed voice commands.

Mirrors

Vans have multiple blind spots that are accentuated when the client is seated in a wheelchair or when a wheelchair lift blocks the client's view through the vehicle's side windows. Simple rectangular convex

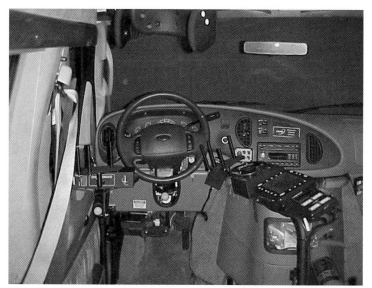

Figure 11-10 Full console.

mirrors (Figure 11-11) located above the exterior mirrors provide assistance in checking these problematic blind spots. Other mirror systems may also be added for clients who present other physical limitations, visual limitations, or both.

SAMPLE CASES

The following are brief case examples of driver rehabilitation evaluations and the recommendations that are often formulated by DRSs. There is a relatively simple case, a more complex one, and a foot steering project that requires some advanced problem solving.

CASE #1

The client presents with a diagnosis of multiple sclerosis (MS). He is currently driving a car without adaptive equipment and reports that he is having difficulty moving his right foot from the gas pedal to the brake without physically lifting the leg with his right hand while controlling the steering wheel with his left hand. He reports that he is having greater difficulty walking and recently purchased a three-wheeled scooter that he keeps at work since he cannot transport it in his car independently. The predriving clinical evaluation revealed that his functioning is within functional limits (WFL) in all areas except lower extremity reaction time, with both lower extremities severely affected.

Vehicle Selection

The client currently owns a car, and his wife owns a minivan. The minivan has a sliding door on the left side for passenger access to the vehicle. The client reported that he is able to get into and out of a minivan and a car independently, and these skills were confirmed during the evaluation.

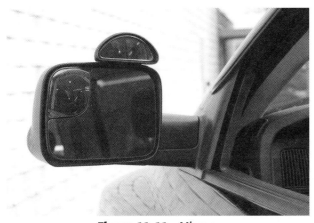

Figure 11-11 Mirrors.

The evaluation vehicle that was selected was a car equipped with hand controls, although a minivan equipped with hand controls would have worked, too. The client was introduced to the operation of the vehicle using hand controls. He was able to operate the hand controls with his left hand without difficulty. He was also able to operate the steering wheel equipped with a steering knob with his right hand without difficulty. While driving the evaluation vehicle with hand controls, he was unintentionally pushing the accelerator pedal with his right foot. A pedal barrier plate was installed to prevent the client's feet from interfering with the foot pedals. There was no concern with upper body stability. An armrest was modified on the right side with extra height to provide support for the right elbow to reduce fatigue.

Recommendations

Hand controls, right angle style, left hand operation, steering knob, parking brake extension, and emergency communication devices were recommended for driving. Behind-the-wheel training and road testing with the license bureau to add hand controls to the client's driver's license as a restriction were also recommended.

It was recommended that the client exchange vehicles (i.e., car for van) with his spouse and install an automatic loading device for the scooter into the left side door of the minivan. As part of the evaluation process, the DRS established the make, model, and weight of the scooter to be sure it was compatible with the scooter loading device. The DRS also made certain that the client was able to open and close the sliding door of the minivan.

An alternate vehicle recommendation was also made. The DRS recommended purchasing a lowered-floor, side-entry minivan and equipping it with a six-way powered transfer seat. This would allow the client to drive the scooter into the van and transfer into the driver's seat while inside the van and out of the elements. Since this is an expensive alternative, the first recommendation seems more appropriate at this time.

CASE #2

The client presents with a diagnosis of a right cerebrovascular accident resulting in left upper and lower extremity paralysis. The client has not driven since the onset of the stroke 6 months ago. He owns a four-door car with automatic transmission and power steering. We selected a four-door car for the evaluation and set up the car with a steering knob on the right side of the steering wheel located at the 2 o'clock position. We also set up a two-button electronic turn signal device on the right side of the wheel near the 2 o'clock position of the steering wheel. The client was able to transfer into and out of the vehicle independently. He stowed his cane in the back seat after getting into the car and was able to apply the seat belt. After a demonstration of the adaptive equipment, he was able to drive the vehicle in a protected area to test the equipment and then proceeded to an on-road evaluation.

Recommendations

For driving, the client was recommended for training in the use of the adaptive equipment, a follow-up evaluation to assure safety, and a road test with the license bureau for adding restrictions requiring the use of a steering knob, automatic transmission, and crossover turn signal extension to the right side.

The addition of a steering knob and turn signal extension on the right side was also recommended. The client was unable to operate the wiper or headlight dimmer in his car because they were located on the left side of the steering wheel. We recommended the use of a four-button remote electric control pod on the right side of the steering wheel to allow him to operate the turn signals, wipers, and headlight dimmer with his right hand.

CASE #3

This 30-year-old client presented with a diagnosis of bilateral upper extremity amputation caused by an electrical accident. No concerns were noted on the clinical evaluation other than the client's inability to use either upper extremity for any functional tasks. The client reported that he was planning to obtain upper extremity myoelectric prostheses, but he was advised that it would not be functional for driving due to the level of the amputations. After meeting the client, we were able to determine that he would need to operate the steering wheel with his left foot in order to return to independent driving. After searching for an evaluation program that had a vehicle equipped with a foot steering system and not finding one nearby, we decided to adapt a van equipped with a high tech steering system for foot steering evaluation and training. A remote electric steering system was adapted with a 10-inch steering plate with a slip-on style shoe attached as a steering spinner. We installed the steering system into the raised sub floor of a lowered floor minivan so that the 10-inch steering plate was in approximately the same place as a commercially available foot steering system would be located. Through careful positioning, the client was able to operate the foot steering system with the left foot and the regular gas and brake control with the right foot. The vehicle was equipped with an electronic auxiliary control system that included voice activation for the gear selector. The master control panel was located for access with the left foot. We set

up a pair of switches by the left side of the driver's head to allow him to activate the voice activation system for gear shift selection and a scanner system for turn signals, horn, dimmer, wiper, and cruise. In the evaluation vehicle, the client was unable to apply the seat belts. Modifications were planned to modify the seat belts in the client's personal vehicle.

Once the vehicle was set up, the client proceeded to drive the evaluation vehicle. He was able to demonstrate an ability to operate the vehicle safely using the adaptive equipment as planned.

Recommendations

The client was asked to complete an on-road training program before completing a road test with the license bureau to obtain a driver's license using the recommended adaptive equipment.

For the vehicle, the client selected a pickup truck that was similar to vehicles he had used in the past. The upright seating of the pickup truck was more comfortable and functional for him than a car. He was able to demonstrate the ability to enter and exit the pickup truck with minimal modifications. The following equipment recommendations were made: a foot steering system with reduced effort steering; electronic auxiliary control system for all auxiliary systems; voice-activated auxiliary control for gear selector and several other functions; and a scanner system for operation of turn signals, horn, dimmer, and wiper. A door kick out opener features a remote activated system to unlatch the driver's door and open it enough to allow the driver to use his foot to open the door all the way. A seat belt system modification to allow hands-free operation of the seat belts and a step-in system were developed. By the time the client's personal vehicle was ready, he had obtained a powered prosthetic arm, and he was able to use it to apply the seat belt independently with a minor modification to the seat belt.

SUMMARY

The process of selecting an appropriate vehicle and adaptive driving equipment to meet the special needs of each client can be an exciting challenge for the DRS. The goal of any comprehensive driver rehabilitation evaluation is to assist the client in becoming truly independent in the operation of a motor vehicle. This means that the DRS must do more than address the client's physical ability to operate a vehicle's steering, gas, and brakes. A comprehensive evaluation involves examining all of the activities related to the client getting into and out of the vehicle, applying the seat belts, being able to see and perceive the interior and exterior environments, maintaining balance and postural support, adjusting the seats, and loading a mobility device as necessary. It is important for DRSs to have a good understanding of the possible variations of vehicle types, vehicle access methods, structural vehicle modifications, and adaptive driving aids. DRSs should impart their knowledge to clients with the aim of helping them make informed decisions about driving, vehicle selection, structural modifications, and adaptive driving equipment; and the in-vehicle predriving assessment is an important step in helping to prepare the client for the on-road evaluation.

REFERENCES

1. U.S. Department of Transportation National Highway Traffic Safety Administration: *Airbags and On-off Switches,* report No. DOT HS 808 629, November 1997. Available at: *http://www/pueblo.gsa.gov/cic_text/cars/airbags/brochure.html. Accessed March 1,* 2005.

Chapter 12

ON-ROAD DRIVER EVALUATION AND TRAINING

KEY TERMS

- Remediation program
- Service delivery model
- Validity
- Reliability
- Programmed observations
- Construct validity
- Content validity
- Face validity
- Criterion validity
- Predictive validity
- Functional deficits
- Tactical driving

CHAPTER OBJECTIVES

After completing this chapter, the reader will be able to do the following:

- Understand the broader issues surrounding driving evaluation to adopt a client-centered approach.
- Know the general principles that should inform on-road evaluations.
- Understand why the driver rehabilitation specialist needs to identify evaluation objectives clearly for each case.
- Know what clues to look for when assessing a client's vision and other client factors when the aim is to determine driver readiness.

SECTION I

On-the-Road Evaluation of Driving Performance

Marilyn Di Stefano • Wendy Macdonald

In this chapter the principles underlying evaluation of driving performance are discussed, and the general procedures that need to be followed for an on-road evaluation are described. Details of on-road performance documentation and reporting are addressed elsewhere in this book (Chapter 14). Here the main focus is on the general requirements to help ensure that evaluation outcomes are reliable and valid in relation to the intended purposes of the evaluation. Evaluation design guidelines to support achievement of these objectives are identified.

The importance of the context in which a driver rehabilitation specialist (DRS) evaluation of driving performance is undertaken is emphasized. Typically on-road evaluations are conducted after an assessment of the client's functional abilities and underlying sensory, cognitive, and motor capacities, as has been discussed in Chapters 5, 6, 7, 13, and 21. However, driver rehabilitation services vary in the extent and precise nature of predriving clinical evaluations, and in some circumstances these may serve only as screening procedures, with many underlying capacities and attributes being evaluated on-road, either implicitly or explicitly. See Chapter 6 for more information on the predriving clinical evaluation.

Even when the clinical assessments that comprise the comprehensive clinical evaluation are broad and detailed in their coverage, they are usually limited in that they cannot adequately predict an individual's complex, multidimensional driving abilities, which depend on the coordinated functioning of many factors including underlying capacities and learned subskills. Relatively simple driving subtasks, such as starting the car and entering a traffic stream in a quiet traffic environment, require coordination of perceptual, cognitive, and motor subskills; multiple subskills underpin the effective performance of functions such as problem solving, reasoning, judgment and planning, and perceptual-cognitive and motor control operations (see Box 1-2). Few off-road or clinical assessment methods that address these composite driver abilities are available and affordable, although advances in computer-based tests and driving simulators may offer this possibility as a valid alternative to on-road testing in the future.[1-3]

In the meantime the on-road evaluation is usually seen as the most satisfactory means of achieving a valid evaluation of driving ability.[4] Even if a totally comprehensive and reliable set of off-road tests were available, the high face validity of an on-road evaluation is likely to ensure that it remains a part of the evaluation procedure for significant numbers of clients (except those cases when driving is contraindicated because of recent seizure activity for example). As discussed in Chapter 6, the decision to undertake an on-road evaluation is usually based on results from previous predriving clinical evaluations, considered within the contexts of the individual client, and the general policies of the driver rehabilitation service provider.[5-7]

WHY—AND THEREFORE WHAT—ARE WE ASSESSING?

The two most common reasons why DRSs evaluate driving performance are to determine whether the client meets defined competency criteria (e.g., whether he or she would be likely to pass a standard license test) and to identify impairment-related deficiencies in driving performance to develop a *remediation program*. Most referrals fall into one or more of the categories depicted in Table 12-1.

The present chapter deals with driver evaluations for all of the purposes shown in Table 12-1, except the last one related to vocational rehabilitation. Within each of these different categories, more specific evaluation goals for each client can be identified. Goals will be influenced by many factors, including the issues that emerge during the preceding clinical evaluation, and by various individual characteristics and driving-related factors. These include the client's:
• Driver's license status and any associated requirements of the licensing jurisdiction

• Specific medical conditions and their possible implications for vehicle modifications, for general remediation requirements, or for more specific driver (re)training
• Age, sociocultural issues, previous driving and instruction history, and any associated implications for on-road safety or driver training needs
• Particular needs or wishes of the individual client concerning his or her future driving
• Know how to optimize the communication process and create a safe environment for the client

Before proceeding to a more detailed examination of the issues involved in evaluating a driver's performance, it may be useful to consider the evaluation process within the context of occupational therapy evaluation of instrumental activities of daily living (IADL) more generally.

AN OCCUPATIONAL THERAPY PERSPECTIVE ON DRIVER EVALUATION

The DRS must observe, document, and interpret client behaviors in relation to evaluation goals. Rogers and Holm[8] have identified a number of key aspects of performance that are important to consider when describing or measuring activities of daily living (ADL) or IADL functioning. These factors are presented in Table 12-2, which highlights the kinds of client-related issues that may be important for DRSs to consider when making decisions about on-road evaluations. Some of these issues are illustrated by the following case example.

Ron is a middle-aged male client who presents for driver evaluation with an incomplete T10-level spinal cord injury sustained 6 months ago. He is able to mobilize (i.e., ambulate) independently with elbow or loft-strand crutches for short distances but frequently uses a manual wheelchair. He fatigues easily and has muscle spasms and bouts of depression. He is married with three high school–aged children, and having no access to financial compensation or other funding, he must pay for his own vehicle modifications and any associated retraining costs. He lives in a small country town where he has managed to remain employed as a salesman in the local furniture store, and his wife works shifts as a nurse's aide at a nursing home in the next town.

During the clinical evaluation he emphasizes the many reasons why he feels that he must continue to drive, including the need to transport his children to after-school activities, to travel to and from work (a round trip of 15 miles into town), and to access local

Table 12-1 **Categories of Driver Evaluation and Rehabilitation Referrals**

General Purposes of Driving	Typical Issues
Evaluation of overall driver competency. May include review of the need for license conditions or restrictions (either their imposition or removal)	Potential deterioration of driving performance, typically indicated by decline in health status or health- or aging-related declines in ADL/IADL functioning Potential improvement of driving performance, typically indicated by progress in rehabilitation program after major trauma or illness (e.g., recovery after a stroke) Formal requirements of a license review system (e.g., age-related mandatory reviews at prescribed intervals)
Equipment-related issues: prescription, trialing, and associated training	Clients typically have physical impairments, including deteriorating medical conditions such as muscular dystrophy or rheumatoid arthritis, in which high-order driving skills are intact but there is a potential need for vehicle modification (e.g., to facilitate ingress/egress, use of primary or secondary vehicle controls, or specialized seating)
Evaluation of a client's potential to learn how to drive	Teenagers with congenital disabilities such as spina bifida, visual impairment, or cerebral palsy who are approaching licensing age may require evaluation to identify their needs/potential for entry-level driver training, needs for previous remediation, or for compensatory measures such as vehicle modifications
Evaluation of abilities for work-related driving	Within a vocational rehabilitation process, clients wishing to resume work-related driving may require evaluation of their ability to operate equipment and vehicles such as forklifts, cranes, tractors, trucks, or buses. Normally their ability to drive an ordinary vehicle would be assessed initially, before more specialized assessments. The latter are beyond the scope of this chapter.

ADL, Activity of daily living; *IADL*, instrumental activity of daily living.
Data from American Occupational Therapy Association: *Position paper on community mobility: driving position paper draft III, May 2004,* Bethesda, in press, American Occupational Therapy Association; Caust S: Driving rehabilitation and new techniques for older drivers, *Technical Aid Disabled J* December:24-25, 1994; Di Stefano M, Macdonald W: *Survey of Australian occupational therapists to determine disabled driver on-road assessment practice,* Paper presented at the World Federation of Occupational Therapists Conference: Sharing a Global Perspective, Montreal, Canada, May 31-June 5, 1998; Hunt LA: A profile of occupational therapists as driving instructors and evaluators for elderly drivers, *IATSS Research* 20:46-47, 1996; Klavora P, Young M, Heslegrave RJ: A review of a major driver rehabilitation centre: a ten-year client profile, *Can J Occup Ther* April:128-134, 2000; School of Occupational Therapy: *Driver assessment and rehabilitation course manual,* Melbourne, Victoria, 2003, La Trobe University; Schold Davis E: Defining OT roles in driving, *OT Practice* January 13:15-18, 2003; Somerville P: Behind the wheel: a safe workplace? *Aust Safety News* August:58-62, 1997; Sprigle S, Morris BO, Nowachek G, et al: Assessment of the evaluation procedures of drivers with disabilities, *Occup Ther J Res* 15:147-164, 1995.

community facilities. Although the majority of his driving is local, undertaken on country roads where traffic density is low and there is no such thing as rush hour, Ron occasionally used to drive on the interstate to visit family and friends in the city.

Ron's future driving independence will undoubtedly be influenced by the motor and sensory limitations in his lower limbs, which are associated with low endurance, pain, and spasm with fatigue. Although he might be more independent if he chose to use hand controls, he would clearly prefer to drive an unmodified vehicle because he wants to minimize changes to his life and avoid being labeled as disabled. Therefore he must be content with driving his own vehicle, which is an older-model, automatic sedan that has no power steering or cruise control.

Table 12-2 **Parameters of Activity Performance**

Parameters	Relevance to Driving	Examples
Value	The importance or significance of the task to the client	Value of driving in relation to life roles such as spouse, father, worker, football coach
Independence	Rating of independence in relation to the task, with or without use of assistive devices, human physical or verbal assistance, modifications to task or environment	Requirement for vehicle modifications, human assistance for transfer in/out of vehicle, or to prompt regarding navigational cues
Safety	Related to the risk of performance failure and/or injury as a result of the person-car-task-environment configuration	Driver disregards intersection priority rules or consistently fails to perform over-the-shoulder checks when changing lanes
Adequacy or efficiency of actions	The ease with which activities can be completed, considering the steps, actions, or process required to achieve driving goals. Includes the following:	
Difficulty	Driver's perceived ease: how easily the task and subtasks are completed	Excessively low or high confidence in performing some driving tasks is likely to affect performance adequacy
Discomfort	Discomfort or pain associated with driving-related tasks or maneuvers, or occurring after driving task completion	Discomfort or pain may be experienced each time a shoulder check is performed
Fatigue	Fatigue or exhaustion may be experienced during or after a trip	Driving endurance may be reduced by high level of required physical or mental effort expenditure
Duration	Time needed to complete task components	Duration of driving tasks may pose a risk to other drivers (e.g., parking maneuvers may take 15 minutes to complete)
Resources available and acceptability of aspects of task performance	Addresses resources available to support driving performance, and the personal, community, and societal acceptability of varying driver competence levels	
Personal experience	The individual's temporal history and overall duration of driving experience	A client may be seeking to resume driving activities after many years of not having driven
Conflict with normal behavioral standards	The individual's driving behavior may fall outside the realm of what is accepted as the normal	Consistently drives at speeds much lower than the speed limit
Personal satisfaction	The individual's contentment with the task performance level achieved	Driver may not be satisfied with a local area license,* or feels embarrassed by existence of vehicle modifications
Resources available	The availability of resources that will support task performance	Inadequate money to pay for vehicle modifications or for specialized instructors to support driver rehabilitation

*A local area license restricts the driver to driving only within his or her own, geographically defined community.
Data from Rogers JC, Holm MB: Section 1: Activities of daily living and instrumental activities of daily living, Chapter 24, Evaluation of areas of occupation. In Crepeau EB, Cohn ES, Boyt Schell BA, editors: *Willard and Spackman's occupational therapy*, ed 10, Philadelphia, 2003, Lippincott Williams & Wilkins, pp. 315-339.

These factors influenced the decision for the DRS to arrange an off-street (i.e., protected parking lot or driving range) assessment with a similar style of vehicle, in which Ron demonstrated that he could manage the vehicle controls adequately. On-road training was then commenced, but it became clear that Ron could not cope with driving in complex driving situations because he needed to allocate significant attention to managing the altered motor functioning of his legs; he also fatigued easily. The DRS and Ron discussed the fact that if he had a more modern vehicle with adapted driving controls he could probably drive farther, whereas with his current vehicle he would have to limit his driving to no more than 15 minutes at a time because of its greater physical demands and his reduced endurance.

Ron placed great value on driving and thought he could be independent in driving his existing car; however, he recognized that his safety and the safety of other road users and anyone riding with him would be compromised if he exceeded these limits. In these circumstances the decision was made to undertake an on-road evaluation just in his local area, on which basis he could be issued with a license that restricted him to driving only in this prescribed geographic area. This would allow Ron to undertake the driving tasks that were most important to him in his own vehicle. Because he displayed a high level of insight and was motivated to comply with this restriction, this was an acceptable outcome of driver rehabilitation. The DRS also requested a 12-month review and explained to Ron that should his situation alter before that time, a reevaluation could occur.

A clear and detailed understanding of the broader issues surrounding driving evaluation, as outlined in Table 12-2, is essential to enable the DRS to adopt a client-centered approach consistent with the existing license review system and within the local service delivery context.

INFLUENCE OF THE SERVICE DELIVERY CONTEXT

Driver evaluation and rehabilitation services operate under a variety of different *service delivery models.* The nature of the particular model is likely to influence the role of the DRS, including whether he or she conducts any on-road evaluations, whether he or she has sole responsibility for such evaluations, the scope of the evaluation, and whether an additional licensing authority test will be required in addition to the DRS evaluation.

As described in Chapter 4,[5,6,9-13] a range of different service delivery scenarios can be identified, including but not limited to the following:

- The occupational therapist working as a DRS works alone to undertake all on-road evaluations and any associated (re)training directly with the client.
- The occupational therapist working as a DRS has responsibility jointly with a driver educator DRS. Together they coordinate who will be responsible for conducting all on-road evaluations and make joint decisions concerning evaluation outcomes, including details of any required on-road driver rehabilitation. They also share the responsibility for designing and implementing any subsequent on-road training programs.
- The occupational therapist has full responsibility of the clinical evaluation; however, on-road evaluations are undertaken and training regimens implemented in collaboration with the driver educator.
- A driver educator who works alone conducts on-road evaluations and training but does so after consulting with the occupational therapy DRS who conducted the clinical evaluation and together they determine how the evaluations and training are to be carried out and how performance data are interpreted and reported to the rest of the treatment team.
- A licensing authority testing officer may assess some clients with impairments that are deemed not to require DRS involvement, or a licensing authority testing officer may assess clients after their involvement in a comprehensive driver rehabilitation evaluation and training program, regardless of the recommendations provided by the DRS.

The variation in service delivery models outlined above is associated with differences in the extent to which evaluation is focused on the client's particular disabilities and rehabilitation needs, relative to emphasis on administering a standardized evaluation of driving performance. The particular approach adopted by any given driver rehabilitation service provider is of course partially determined by the relevant legislative requirements in that jurisdiction.

To illustrate how the different evaluation models influence driver evaluation procedures, consider the case of a driver who has experienced a stroke that has left her with residual functional, cognitive, and motor restrictions. In some U.S. jurisdictions she would meet all formal requirements to resume driving simply by providing a medical report to the licensing authority; no on-road evaluation would necessarily be required.[14] In other jurisdictions, as well as providing a medical report, she may need to be clinically evaluated by a DRS, followed by on-road evaluation and possible retraining. After any prescribed retraining, she may need to be assessed by a DRS or licensing authority tester. Alternatively initial screening conducted by the licensing authority might determine whether a referral to a DRS was required. This wide variation between different jurisdictions and driver rehabilitation services in evaluation requirements and in service delivery more generally has been noted previously.[9,15,16] However, the implications for the nature of on-road evaluation and associated rehabilitation or training services have not always been clearly articulated.

Licensing authorities vary in their policies concerning evaluation of drivers with medical impairments and in whether the outcome of a formal, on-road evaluation administered by a DRS is acceptable in lieu of a licensing authority test. Such differences are likely to influence the degree to which DRSs collaborate with licensing authority assessors and will also affect whether the DRS is required to conduct standardized on-road evaluations. If the licensing authority has primary responsibility for on-road (re)testing, the DRS may be more likely to focus his or her attention on the specific impairment or disability issues that are identified as most likely to impact on driving performance. Such a disability-focused approach is probably only justified when the client has a discrete, musculoskeletal impairment that does not involve other sensory, cognitive, or perceptual functioning (e.g., a limb amputation). In such a scenario the DRS's role is to optimize the match between the driver, the vehicle, and the task, as well as to provide training to maximize skills and safe driving performance in preparation for the client undertaking an on-road test administered by the licensing authority, if necessary, in that jurisdiction. A continuum can be seen from a purely disability approach to on-road evaluation, in which the major focus is on remediation and rehabilitation, through to an approach that is concerned largely with licensing and associated road safety issues. Some different stages along this continuum are identified in Table 12-3.

Most evaluations conducted by DRSs focus to a greater or lesser degree on health-related issues. In Table 12-3 the first evaluation approach is characterized as focusing on one or more specific impairments. In such cases the clinical and on-road evaluations may primarily focus on the presenting impairment and disability issues. In the predriving clinical evaluation screening test implementation may depend on the results of a self-report covering medical history and functional abilities rather than a comprehensive predriving screening procedure. Similarly during the on-road test the DRS may only consider selected aspects of driving performance, as deemed relevant to the identified disability issues. For example a client with reduced upper limb function caused by finger amputations may need to use a steering device, necessitating prescription and trialing of a suitable adaptive driving

aid, with on-road evaluation limited to negotiation of a test route that emphasizes steering requirements. In cases falling into the second category in Table 12-3, the clinical and on-road evaluations are more comprehensive in the coverage of driver functioning, but the approach is still disability focused because the primary aim is to provide the basis for individual diagnosis and future rehabilitation rather than to administer a standard test. Accordingly the standard form of on-road evaluation is still likely to be varied somewhat from client to client in accord with his or her individual characteristics and needs.

These first two approaches to evaluation can be adopted only in jurisdictions where DRS evaluations are separated from the driver licensing system; that is, the licensing authority still requires the driver to pass a formal test after DRS intervention. The DRS may report on disability-related issues to the licensing authority but not on the applicant's ability to meet all licensing requirements. In contrast the third approach identified in Table 12-3, termed the licensing approach, uses a much more standard form of evaluation. This may be seen in jurisdictions where drivers with disabilities who come to the attention of the licensing authority (e.g., via referrals from health practitioners or by police after an accident) may be assessed by license testing officers if their disability is not seen as major or relevant. Older drivers with possible aging-related impairments often fall into this category. They may be required to undertake a standard entry-level evaluation or perhaps a modified "older" or "experienced" driver test administered by a specialist testing officer. With this approach the presence of some impairment is acknowledged, but the main goal of the evaluation is to establish whether the driver is sufficiently competent to retain (or be granted) a license, with or without possible conditions or license restrictions and requirements for periodic review.

The last, combined, evaluation approach shown in Table 12-3, incorporating aspects of the disability-focused and licensing approaches, is intended to accommodate individual driver needs within a broad-based, licensing framework. An example of this approach has operated in the state of Victoria, Australia since the late 1980s. In that jurisdiction occupational therapists with postgraduate training in driver evaluation (OT-DRSs) have been identified within road safety legislation as competent to assess functionally impaired drivers.[17] After initial referral and medical evaluation, OT-DRSs take responsibility for all evaluation and retraining requirements of drivers with significant cognitive or health problems that are likely to affect their driving abilities, working closely with specialist driving instructors. After completion of a standard on-road evaluation, such OT-DRSs submit a formal report

Table 12-3 Some Different DRS Approaches to On-Road Evaluation

Evaluation Approach	Description	Advantages	Possible Disadvantages
Focus on specific impairment	Specialized intervention for clients with a major, specific disability (e.g., orthopedic, visual)	DRS has specialist expertise and refers clients to other specialists for related needs (e.g., equipment or vehicle modifications, specific training); no licensing role	Although a standard approach may be applied to assess specific impairments, broader aspects of driving competence are unlikely to be addressed adequately; this is not a problem provided that the licensing authority fulfills this role
Broader, disability-oriented focus	Focus primarily on broad disability needs, including remediation and rehabilitation	DRS concentrates on a range of disability issues, provided that licensing decisions are made by the licensing authority	Facility-specific evaluations may be used, with individualized approaches consequently limiting reliability and hence equity; DRS may not provide a standardized evaluation of driving competence unless this is a primary objective of the client's driver rehabilitation goals
Licensing approach	Focus on road safety at the community level rather than on individual impairments and needs	All applicants are scored against the same driving competency criteria, which optimizes reliability and equity	Scoring criteria may be unduly harsh (e.g., for older drivers); evaluations are typically not conducted by DRSs and hence may not identify potential risks to road safety that fall beyond standard test criteria
Combined approach	Incorporates focus on client within standard but flexible and multidimensional framework	Optimizes road safety and client well-being; for clients this is likely to be the most "user friendly" approach	The client focus and high involvement of health professionals may make this approach more costly to implement; it also demands a high degree of efficient coordination across multiple agencies and provision of associated resources and infrastructure

DRS, Driver rehabilitation specialist.

containing their licensing recommendations to the licensing authority regarding the client's future driver's license status. Although the authority is not bound to accept such recommendations, it is normal practice to do so; that is, the OT-DRS evaluation functions as a license test.[18]

The challenge with such an approach is to achieve a balance between assisting individuals to maintain their driving independence and maintaining a level of safety for all road users that is acceptable to the wider community. To achieve these objectives, licensing authorities must work in partnership with other stakeholders, including DRSs, to establish and operate referral and specialist evaluation processes that are linked in some way into the licensing review system. Drivers can then be directed to undertake evaluations that are appropriate to their specific requirements. The type of on-road evaluation deemed to be the most suitable for any particular driver will be determined by the referral request, medical opinion, degree of disability, the need for specialist vehicle modifications, previous driving experience, and other factors.[18-21] Those who have cognitive or multiple impairments, which are potentially the highest risk cases, usually require specialist medical and DRS driver evaluation.

The adequacy of an on-road evaluation process needs to be considered in terms of its function within this broader context. However, there are some general principles that should inform any type of on-road (or other) evaluation, as discussed in the following section.

RELIABILITY AND VALIDITY

Testing Versus Evaluation

Evaluations of an individual's ability to perform a particular activity may be conducted in many different ways, depending on the nature of the activity and the purpose of its evaluation. In the case of on-road driving evaluation by a DRS, there are several possible purposes and associated different evaluation approaches as outlined in Table 12-3. When the evaluation outcome may have consequences for the client's driver's license status, it is highly desirable that the on-road evaluation is undertaken using a formal test. If the purpose is primarily related to rehabilitation, with no immediate implications for driver's license status, there may not be any need for the evaluation to be a formal test. For example the DRS may need to ensure that a particular type of vehicle modification is the most appropriate for the driver before undertaking training in its use.

A formal test provides a systematic means by which the assessor manages and controls the data-gathering process using specific procedures to record and analyze the data.[22] Within a rehabilitation context the overall process of evaluating a driver's abilities to manage a motor vehicle is most appropriately defined as one of evaluation, including consideration of the need for adapted vehicle controls and seating. However, to the extent that a licensing or combined approach is adopted, as described previously, the on-road component of the evaluation (or a major part of it) should fulfill the requirements of a valid and reliable test. The remainder of this chapter focuses on the specific, on-road procedures that should be followed to achieve this objective.

Before discussing the particular issues relevant to testing driving abilities, it is worth reviewing some basic concepts that underlie effective performance testing. Friedenberg[22] states that a good test is:

> . . . designed carefully and evaluated empirically to ensure that it generates accurate, useful information. The design phase consists of decisions about test purpose, content, administration, and scoring: the evaluation phase consists of collecting and analysing data from pilot administrations of the test: these data are then used to identify the psychometric properties of the test. (p. 11)

In general terms the steps involved in test development[23-25] encompass the following:
- Defining the primary purpose of the test: how information obtained from the test will be used
- Identifying the specific performance or behavioral constructs that need to be assessed, and defining specific behaviors to represent each construct; this will often require a review of research literature to obtain additional information concerning the types of performance/behavioral constructs relevant to the test
- Identifying the form of test items that should be used, and constructing an initial pool of items related to each test construct
- Designing details of the test procedure to be followed, including pilot testing instructions for testers and test takers
- Pilot testing the procedure and evaluating individual items, making necessary adjustments, and retesting in an iterative fashion before implementing field testing on (preferably) large samples of representative individuals taken from the test-taker population
- Analyzing the statistical properties of the item scores to identify those that are unreliable or redundant, and further refining the number and type of items
- Standardizing the test, which includes further testing with large representative "norming" samples to provide data for establishing estimates of test reliability and validity and associated statistics
- Finalizing all documentation relevant to test administration, scoring, and interpretation

The most critically important steps in this process are the initial ones of defining the purpose of the test, and flowing from this, identifying the key constructs to be tested. For an on-road test of general driving competence (as opposed to a narrower, local area test), a statement of purpose may be written as follows: "The XYZ on-road driving test is designed to identify the impact of individual functional impairments on the performance of experienced drivers who wish to hold an unrestricted driver's license. It is intended for application within urban or suburban road traffic environments."

Often entry-level license tests provide the basis for constructing a test for functionally impaired drivers.[26-29] This may be a reasonable starting point, but a test intended for initial license testing is likely to require significant modification for use in rehabilitation settings because of the likely differences in evaluation goals and driver characteristics. Entry-level tests are applied to driving candidates for three main reasons[30,31]:
- To maintain safety standards by ensuring that certain basic competencies can be demonstrated consistently (i.e., preclude from driving those novice drivers who are not yet safe enough to drive independently)

- To apply a procedure to all applicants that is fair and efficient
- To influence the nature of the practice and formal training undertaken by the applicant

Consistent with the above aims of initial license testing, for which demonstration of only a "minimum set of competencies [is] required, the novice car driver may not be required to perform at the same level as that of an experienced driver" (p. 3).[32] Therefore the unmodified application of an entry-level test to assess the performance of *experienced* but medically impaired drivers is likely to be inadequate, as has been demonstrated by researchers.[21,33]

For DRSs the specific objectives of on-road evaluation will be strongly influenced by the evaluation approach adopted. If the focus is on assessing the effects of a discrete disability, the main goal of on-road evaluation will be different from that when the approach is broader based (see Table 12-2). DRSs need to identify their objectives clearly. Is the intention to determine whether clients can drive as well as comparable unimpaired drivers? And/or is it to establish that clients can drive safely? This is an important issue because of its implications for road safety and equity of test outcomes.

Consider the situation for drivers in their 80s whose medical problems result in them undertaking evaluation by a DRS. Some people of this age probably drive less safely than younger people for a variety of reasons. (It is also likely that they drive much shorter distances; therefore their risk of being involved in a crash is unlikely to be high in absolute terms relative to that of younger people.) If older drivers who have *not* been identified as potentially at risk are not required by the licensing system in their jurisdiction to demonstrate their capacity to drive safely, is it equitable that medically impaired drivers should be required to do so? If the approach to on-road evaluation is disability oriented, it may be more appropriate to expect drivers undergoing rehabilitation simply to drive as well as unimpaired drivers of their own age group (as discussed in later sections). See Chapter 23 for more information on legal and professional ethics in driver rehabilitation.

In circumstances in which alternative forms of transportation are inadequate, the maintenance of people's community mobility for as long as possible is likely to be supported best by a disability-oriented approach, in which evaluation focus is on the possible effects of impairment on driving performance. However, there may be some tensions between this and a licensing approach, in which drivers are expected to demonstrate competence to drive safely. If the latter approach is taken, it is important to maximize equity by using an age-matched criterion group to establish test validity.

REQUIREMENTS FOR RELIABLE ON-ROAD TESTING

Along with *validity*, which is discussed in the following section, *reliability* is arguably the most basic requirement of a test. Validity and reliability are required of any test, not least, so that test outcomes can withstand possible legal challenges if necessary. Reliability is necessary for the results of testing to be equitable. A reliable test produces a consistent outcome, given a consistent level of actual performance by the person being tested, so that test outcome does not vary significantly between individual testers or different testing conditions (unless the latter are deliberately varied to manipulate test difficulty). When a driver's license status may be affected by the test outcome, ensuring that testing is reliable is probably even more important for drivers with disabilities than it is for ordinary license testing because clients with disabilities are likely to be more negatively affected by an inappropriate fail outcome if they have fewer independent mobility choices. McKnight[34] observed that "an inconsistent [entry level] test cannot be fair, and fairness is probably as important to the average citizen as validity" (p. 6).

Research has demonstrated that on-road test outcomes are typically unreliable if they are determined simply by global pass/fail evaluations of driving performance, even when the individuals performing the evaluation are highly experienced license testing officers. For example Vanosdall et al[35] investigated the decision-making processes of experienced driver's license testers in Michigan, who at that time simply gave each candidate driver a pass or fail with no quantitative scoring. They found that for some testers the basis for a fail decision seemed to be a gut feeling associated with perceived risk; often this was strongly influenced by the driver's apparent vehicle-handling skill. Other testers were more influenced by what they perceived as risky actions that made them fearful of being involved in a traffic accident. In contrast to these intuitive examiners, others used a legalistic framework to base their decisions. To them, driver behavior at stop signs, yield signs, and so on was most important; therefore relatively minor violations concerning right-of-way, observance of speed limits, and turning from the wrong lane were the main determinants of their decisions concerning test outcomes. Consistent with these findings, separate studies of the performance of license testers in California and Victoria, Australia found large and consistent differences between experienced testing officers in their scoring patterns and average pass rates, despite their use of formal scoring sheets.[36,37] It was clear that this variation between testers in the types of errors recorded was not associated with differences between test locations or the diversity of applicants. Commenting on the large differences among the pass/fail rates of different examiners in the same testing office, as well as between different offices, McKnight and Stewart[37] stated, "These differences in failure rates resulted primarily from wide differences in the types of driver errors that different examiners reported. It was apparent that examiners tended to have 'pet' errors that they were on the lookout for" (p. 126).

Since that time many studies throughout the world have confirmed that to achieve acceptably reliable on-road testing, the procedure should require testers to observe and record specific aspects of driving performance at predesignated points along a preplanned test route.[15,31,34,38-42] For entry-level tests the only additional aspects of driving performance that are recorded and considered are those entailing potentially hazardous errors that necessitate intervention by the supervising DRS. In a license test such errors are typically grounds for an immediate fail and early termination of the test. In summary researchers have demonstrated that reliable outcomes are only likely to be achieved if the test procedure follows that outlined in Box 12-1.

Based on this research, many license testing jurisdictions have now developed and implemented entry-level license test procedures that comply with these requirements, including the Driving Performance Evaluation adopted by the California Department of Motor Vehicles[21,43] and the Programmed Observation License Assessment (POLA).[44]

The kinds of problems with poor reliability that became evident with ordinary license tests during the 1980s and 1990s were also identified in tests used to assess functionally impaired drivers at that time. This suggests that some DRSs may view on-road evaluation

| **Box 12-1** | **Test Procedure** |

- Follow a standard, predetermined, and clearly documented route
- Score predetermined aspects of behavior at predetermined points along the route, often called programmed observations
- Include directions to the driver that are documented clearly so that on each occasion they are given in the same form and sequence in relation to the same set of driving maneuvers
- Assessment criteria for each required driving maneuver are operationally defined and documented in unambiguous, specific terms
- Follow a closely defined scoring procedure, which typically entails discrete criteria such as present/not present or a quality rating for each specified maneuver (e.g., on a 5-point scale)
- Entails extensive training of testers

in a somewhat similar way to that of experienced license testers before the introduction of highly structured procedures. According to McKnight and Stewart[37] license testers did "... not view the drive test as an objective measure of competency itself but rather [saw] it as a means by which a skillful examiner can judge competency" (p. 62). Consistent with this approach Macdonald et al[45] observed when investigating the predriving clinical evaluation procedures used by some OTs in that era that they tended to view specific tests primarily as a means of eliciting informal behaviors that were useful in forming clinical opinions and judgments rather than as a means of generating quantitative test scores. Such informal approaches to testing clearly reduce reliability. Whether, or to what extent, this constitutes a problem depends on how the information is used.

For research purposes the absence of empirical evidence to establish the reliability of on-road tests conducted as part of a comprehensive driver rehabilitation evaluation has been identified as a weakness in studies in which the on-road test outcome has been used as the criterion against which validity of clinical evaluation methods has been evaluated.[46,47] For clinical purposes, however, the issue of how best to observe and document the performance of drivers who may be functionally impaired is a complex one because of the wider range of behaviors that can be expected as a result of the varying effects of many different types of impairment. Unless the evaluation has a purely licensing focus, it is therefore useful, in addition to recording *programmed observations* of predetermined aspects of performance, to document any observations of unusual or significant aspects of performance, regardless of the particular point along the route at which they occur because these can be strongly indicative of the effects of specific impairments (e.g., issues related to confusion, difficulty following instructions, overly cautious or hesitant, self-distracting or impulsive behaviors, jerky motor actions, and incoordination).[48,49]

Departures from a fully standardized evaluation procedure can also be justified as part of a combined approach to evaluation when the DRS may wish to evaluate the impact on the driving task of specific impairments that are hypothesized to influence driving performance in particular ways. For example if a client needs to use a modified steering system to overcome reduced upper limb function, a standard on-road test may be extended to include additional turns or low-speed maneuvers (e.g., different types of parking, turning into driveways, and "U" turns) to determine whether the operational skills required to use the steering device have been sufficiently well developed.[50]

Nevertheless the need for DRSs to use closely defined programmed observations in on-road evaluations has been clearly recognized. In an article discussing the evaluation of medically impaired drivers, Galski et al[51] noted: "On-road evaluations have been regarded as a direct measure of driving abilities. Unfortunately, these evaluations are often lacking in reliability and objectivity . . ." (p. 709). Similarly Antrim and Engum[52] adopted an unequivocal stance on this issue, asserting: ". . . health care professionals will want to show that they adopted and utilized reliable and valid evaluation techniques . . . . Depending only upon general impressions or intuition in assessing the patient's ability to operate a motor vehicle is no longer reasonable professional conduct." (p. 19)

More recently it was demonstrated that DRS on-road evaluations could be scored with high interrater reliability when standard routes and evaluation procedures were implemented[42,53]; this programmed approach to DRS on-road evaluation has been supported also in a review of published literature by Fox et al.[41] Overall there appears to be widespread acceptance of the desirability of increasing the reliability of on-road evaluations for functionally impaired or older drivers by adopting a programmed observation procedure.

However, the extent to which a fully programmed procedure is either feasible or desirable for such drivers is open to debate. An argument can be made that because the impaired driver population presents a much wider range of performance and behavioral characteristics than is the case with entry-level drivers without a medical impairment, there is a greater need for the test to be adaptable to individual characteristics. It also can be argued that this adaptability is achievable only by relying to some degree on the clinical judgment of individual DRSs. If this approach is taken, in an attempt to enhance validity and individual equity, it must be acknowledged that there will be some reduction in reliability. That is, the potential benefits of enhanced validity will not flow to all clients because greater procedural flexibility will reduce reliability. Because current evaluation methods are less than optimal, some such strategy is probably still necessary when evaluation goals address disability and licensing issues and so fall within the combined category shown in Table 12-3.

An example of a combined approach to on-road evaluation (as per Table 12-3) is provided by the test currently used by OT-DRSs in Victoria, Australia.[10,54] Here the highly programmed entry-level license test (POLA) provided the basis for development of a new test for functionally impaired drivers. In the modified form used by OT-DRSs, test content and scoring system have been modified to enable the DRS to make allowance for what are judged to be an individual's bad habits, such as are frequently demonstrated by experi-

enced drivers. Other such tests include the California Modified Driving Performance Evaluation[21,55] and the Washington University Road Test.[42]

In most cases even the most reliable of current tests would probably benefit by fine-tuning to enhance their criterion validity using research on the kinds of driving errors that best discriminate impaired from nonimpaired drivers and safe from unsafe drivers.* More such research is needed to provide a better evidence base for distinguishing those driving errors that are common even among unimpaired or acceptably safe drivers from those errors that characterize impaired or unsafe drivers. Application of this information to the performance scoring or broader evaluation criteria used in DRS on-road evaluations would greatly enhance their criterion validity. Currently available evidence about different types of driving errors is described in the following section. There is also scope to enhance the reliability of DRS tests by developing more formalized performance criteria related to the effects of different types of impairment, particularly of cognitive functioning, on driving performance.

REQUIREMENTS FOR VALID ON-ROAD TESTING

In developing and implementing a good test, it is important to ensure that it will be valid for its intended purpose. At the very least a driving test should have construct validity and content validity. *Construct validity* requires that the behavioral dimensions, or constructs, that are measured in a test should validly represent those aspects of performance that are most relevant, reflecting key components of the activity, and most importantly being relevant to the evaluation objectives, which may focus on specific impairments, on disability more generally, and on road safety. *Content validity* is secondary to construct validity; it requires that the test incorporate a representative sample of performance components for each construct to be assessed. A test with content validity is likely also to have *face validity*; that is, it will appear to be a valid test. Unfortunately content validity does not guarantee the existence of other forms of validity, and a test with only content validity may not be adequate to achieve its objectives.

In more concrete terms the validity of a test is highly dependent on the way in which driving performance is defined, observed, and documented, which typically includes whether driving errors are observed or whether specific aspects of driving performance are performed adequately or otherwise. In the case of complex and variable activities such as driving, the most

---

*References 10,33,42,48,56-58.

appropriate constructs to test are not obvious because there are many different ways in which driving may be conceptualized and errors defined. Some researchers also argue that, as yet, there is no practical taxonomy of normative driver behavior on which to base such an undertaking.[59-61] However, the conceptual frameworks outlined in Chapter 1 can be used to evaluate the comprehensiveness of the constructs assessed in on-road driver evaluation, as discussed by Macdonald[62] when reviewing the functional abilities needed to drive safely. She argued that on-road evaluation is most useful in evaluating performance at the tactical and operational levels, although in the latter, case evaluation will be more reliable for observable actions related to vehicle control or use of indicators (see Box 1-2). It is more difficult in an on-road test to assess perceptual and cognitive operational skills reliably, although most tests attempt to do this to a limited degree.

In addition to having demonstrable construct and associated content validity, a good test should have *criterion validity*. If the approach to evaluation is disability oriented, criterion validity can be demonstrated by showing that test performance is substantially poorer for a group of impaired drivers representative of the intended test clientele, relative to the performance of a group of comparable, unimpaired drivers. If the evaluation approach is licensing oriented, so that a key requirement is to determine whether clients have sufficient driving competence to maintain road safety, the key, defining characteristic of the reference group should be their risk of crashing (controlling for their level of exposure to risk). In this case criterion validity of the test would be demonstrated by showing that test performance of impaired drivers was substantially worse than that of a comparable group of unimpaired drivers whose crash risk was known to be no worse than average.

In other words, the valid interpretation and evaluation of on-road test performance require normative data from a comparable group of drivers who meet criteria appropriate to the specific test objectives. Without such benchmark data the performance of impaired drivers cannot be validly evaluated with dependable reliability because evaluation must then rely solely on all DRSs sharing and consistently applying an accurate understanding of the nature of normal (unimpaired or safe) performance during test conditions. Available evidence suggests that driver testers (including DRSs) as a group are unlikely to achieve this, as discussed in the previous section, unless they are using an evaluation procedure based on programmed observations. For standard tests of basic visual, perceptual-cognitive, and physical capacities, such as are used in many predriving clinical evaluations, normative data are documented in the professional literature of the areas concerned (i.e.,

optometry, neuropsychology, occupational therapy, and physiotherapy). However, few normative data have been published for tests used by DRSs.[33,63-65]

To achieve criterion validity, DRSs must focus on observing and recording those particular aspects of driving performance that are significantly more frequent among impaired (or high-risk) drivers than among drivers who are unimpaired (and/or, depending on the purposes of testing, who do not have a high crash risk). These kinds of performance errors also need to be given higher weighting within a quantitative scoring system, as has been done by Dobbs et al[33] and others.[21,55] Older drivers are known to have difficulty coping with intersections,[66] where they tend to be overinvolved in accidents.[67-70] Hunt et al[49] found that a group of drivers with early dementia had greater difficulties at intersections, drove more slowly, had more difficulty with lane control, and braked more erratically than an age-matched control group. It is therefore likely that errors related to negotiating intersections will be among those that best discriminate risky older or cognitively impaired drivers from others.

Dobbs et al[33] emphasized the importance of distinguishing different types of errors according to their discriminative power rather than assuming that all errors should be given equal weight when evaluating driver performance. To achieve this, they categorized all errors that presented an immediate crash risk as hazardous; most typically these were errors that caused the supervising driver to intervene or caused other road users to take avoidance actions. These hazardous errors were found to be clearly the most effective in discriminating older drivers with diagnosed cognitive impairments from other drivers. The impaired group also was significantly more likely to make scanning errors (e.g., failure to look back over the shoulder to check for the presence of other traffic before changing lanes) and positioning errors (e.g., failing to maintain an appropriate position within the lane) and were also more likely to be excessively cautious (e.g., extremely low speed for the conditions and failure to accept safe gaps in traffic when negotiating an intersection). Importantly there were types of errors, such as rolling through a stop sign and exceeding the posted speed limit, that did not discriminate between impaired drivers and others.

Di Stefano and Macdonald[54] analyzed the errors of older drivers that had been recorded by specialist licensing authority testers during tests to review their license status. They found that errors requiring intervention by the supervising tester (corresponding to those defined by Dobbs et al[33] as hazardous errors) were the major determinant of whether the driver passed or failed the test; almost all drivers who failed had made at least one such error, and in only 9 of 533 cases did someone fail without an intervention. The kinds of errors that most frequently precipitated supervisor intervention were those associated with intersection negotiation, failure to give right-of-way or poor gap selection when crossing or entering a traffic stream, poor lateral positioning of the vehicle, inappropriate speed (either too fast or too slow for the conditions), and problems with low-speed maneuvers (e.g., reversing and parking). It was found that test outcome (i.e., whether the supervising driver had to intervene) was largely predicted by a score based on some other types of errors recorded at other points during the test, particularly errors related to intersection negotiation and maintenance of appropriate vehicle position and speed, although these findings were constrained by the unequal numbers of errors across different performance categories.

These findings highlight the importance of distinguishing errors that have criterion validity, which should therefore be the focus of DRS evaluation, from other errors that may perhaps indicate poor driving habits but should *not* be interpreted as indicators of either functional impairment or increased risk. Research of this kind is currently emerging. To continue improving the validity of on-road test procedures and scoring systems, much more information is needed about the extent to which driving errors normally vary between people of different ages and driving experience and between groups with different types of medical conditions and functional impairments.

Finally the *predictive validity* of a test should be considered. This is demonstrated when a significant relationship can be shown between on-road test performance and subsequent driving performance. Predictive validity is highly desirable, so that when someone does poorly in a test, this constitutes reliable evidence that his or her future driving in real-world situations is also likely to be poor. However, establishing the predictive validity of driving tests is notoriously difficult for a variety of reasons.[71] Particularly in the case of DRS evaluations, one of the main problems is that the driving-related functional abilities of many clients are likely to vary over time. For example someone diagnosed with a psychiatric condition may be unreliable in complying with his or her required medication regimen, in which case he or she may perform well when tested but sometimes may drive dangerously because of failure to take appropriate medication.[72] Others may be experiencing problems related to arthritis or chronic fatigue, which result in diurnal variation in functional abilities. For people with some chronic neurologic conditions, such as multiple sclerosis, weekly variations in muscle strength, spasms, or endurance may be a common pattern. Such variability raises issues concerning the most valid time of day or week to schedule on-road testing.

It also means that even when the on-road test has been optimally designed and implemented, DRSs will still need to exercise their expert judgment concerning the possible effects of variables that may influence real-world driving behavior in the future. For example in the case of clients with progressively deteriorating medical conditions, the DRS must judge when the client should return for another evaluation.

Few on-road evaluations for functionally impaired drivers have been reported in the literature to meet all of the requirements for reliability and validity as described here.[16,41] In a review of tests for older drivers with cognitive impairments, Withaar et al[16] concluded: "More research is needed to establish the validity of on-road tests and to develop on-road tests with good psychometric qualities" (p. 488). Similarly Ekelman et al[73] reported that at that time in North America there was a lack of consistency in evaluation methods and related performance evaluation criteria between different driver evaluation centers.

EVALUATION LOCATION AND ROUTE DESIGN ISSUES

One of the first decisions to be made regarding in-car evaluation concerns the location of initial observations of the driver controlling the vehicle. Should the first observations be in an off-road area, such as an empty parking lot or similar area, or might an open road environment be appropriate?[74] In making this decision the specific goals of the evaluation need to be considered. For example the goal may be to identify any necessary vehicle modifications and to prescribe these; in this case a parking lot would probably be an appropriate location. Or the primary aim may be to conduct an initial evaluation of training needs before commencement of a series of lessons; the location for this would depend much on the client's previous driving experience, medical condition, and functional abilities as indicated by information from the referral and clinical evaluations. If the purpose is to perform a formal, licensing-oriented test of overall driving competence, then a standard route should be used, although this may present problems in jurisdictions where entry-level license tests do not entail use of such routes. Other relevant factors may include the client's level of anxiety and possible communication issues related to particular impairments (e.g., a client with a hearing impairment may require initial practice using hand signal communications in an off-road environment).

For any type of on-road evaluation, the nature of the road traffic environment and the driving maneuvers required by the particular route that drivers have to negotiate are significant determinants of test validity because they constrain the types of errors that are likely to occur. For example a route that has few intersections will reduce opportunities for right-of-way errors; if there are no multilane sections of road, there will be fewer possibilities for drivers to perform poorly when lane keeping or overtaking. The route selected must enable the DRS to assess whether a specific functional impairment is negatively affecting driving performance. For example if a key issue is the driver's ability to cope with cognitively complex situations, an evaluation on a simple route with few controlled and uncontrolled road intersections and little traffic traveling on intersecting paths will not be valid for this purpose.

Route characteristics are also the primary determinant of overall task difficulty. For example if a particular route presents conditions that are extremely easy (e.g., little traffic and no difficult maneuvers), drivers whose functional abilities differ substantially from each other may all be able to perform equally well. Similarly if a route is difficult, a group of drivers with generally poor but differing abilities may all perform equally poorly. In such cases inappropriate route selection results in the evaluation lacking sensitivity. In a licensing context a high level of sensitivity across a wide spectrum of difficulty is not an important requirement. However, when the major purpose of evaluation is to identify the effects of impairment, lack of sensitivity can be a major disadvantage because it will make it more difficult to track the progress of a driver during the course of his or her rehabilitation program.

For the aforementioned reasons, disability-oriented evaluations require the DRS to have access to a set of test locations or perhaps entirely separate routes that are graded in their difficulty. This grading may occur within a single route, typically starting in a nonde-manding environment with only simple driving maneu-vers and gradually progressing to more demanding environments and performance requirements. Such a graduated route may commence within an off-street area where basic vehicle operational and positioning skills are assessed before progressing to an open road context.[41] Alternatively the route may commence on a quiet street with little traffic (e.g., a residential area with a low speed limit). More difficult sections of the route would include higher speeds, more traffic and other types of road users, and more complex maneu-vers. As a general rule it is best to try to ensure that the more demanding driving maneuvers and environments are not encountered during the first 15 minutes to enable the driver to settle down before dealing with more challenging situations. If the road traffic environ-ment surrounding the driver evaluation center is too complex, it may be necessary to drive to a quiet residential area from which to commence the test.

Use of a graded test route or a graded set of routes, if a series of assessments are to be conducted, serves a number of goals. It allows the DRS to do the following:
- Perform preliminary checks and prerequisite tasks, such as adjusting seating, mirrors, and adaptive devices
- Determine the adequacy of basic vehicle handling skills in a safe environment
- Assess whether the driver can follow instructions
- Develop some rapport with the driver

It also allows the driver to have an opportunity to practice in an undemanding environment so that initial anxiety can subside before progressing to more demanding test requirements.

Within an occupational therapy framework the grad-ing of routes can be viewed as an example of the more general grading of tasks.[75,76] Such grading is a means by which occupational performance requirements of eval-uations and interventions can be either upgraded or downgraded to adjust them to suit the capabilities of individual client and therapy goals. Table 12-4 lists some of the factors relevant to grading test routes and other components of the evaluation procedure.

When drivers are required to undertake testing in a vehicle other than their own, they need to have a rea-sonable opportunity to familiarize themselves with the vehicle and to adapt to its particular operational and handling characteristics. This may be possible in an off-road environment, or the first stage of the route may be designed for this purpose. Usually this will include the practice of certain basic maneuvers, including mov-ing forward, stopping, reversing, turning, and perhaps negotiating stationary hazards.[10,49] A period of famil-iarization is particularly important for drivers undertak-ing the evaluation in a vehicle that is significantly dif-ferent from their own, who are highly anxious, who have had a substantial period away from driving, or who are still becoming accustomed to using seating or vehicle adaptations. Recent research has identified that for an older group of medically impaired drivers the requirement to drive an unfamiliar car during a test procedure imposes additional cognitive demands that may compromise their driving performance and test outcomes.[28]

In evaluating the validity of the route as a whole, the activity demands on a driver negotiating it need to be considered in relation to the particular purpose(s) of the evaluation and to the known characteristics of the driver subpopulation represented by the client, particu-larly his or her age, driving experience, and normal driving patterns. On this basis, for example, it might be decided not to test an older driver in peak-hour traffic or for >1 hour because it was determined during the previous clinical evaluation that he or she only drives

Table 12-4 Grading of Route and Test Characteristics

Variables	Examples of Factors to Consider
Vehicle environment	Type/quality of seat: affects postural demands, fatigue Background noise in vehicle: may affect communication demands, increases stress Extraneous attentional demands, distractions: challenges attentional control and more general executive functioning
Test procedural requirements	Duration of test: affects fatigue Navigational requirements: guided versus self-directed Complexity of maneuvers: number and concurrency of steps in each, associated perceptual and cognitive demands
DRS instructions to driver	Complexity, level of detail (e.g., "turn at second street on the right" versus "turn at next street") Delay between delivery and execution (memory demands) Concurrent demands when instructions are delivered Guided versus self-directed route components
Traffic characteristics	Traffic speed and density, both of which influence time pressure Predictability of travel paths Variety of road users: vehicles, cyclists, pedestrians
Traffic management systems	Level of intersection controls: traffic signals, stop/yield signs, uncontrolled intersections Divided versus undivided roads, number of lanes Complexity of signs/signals: signals including turn arrows Mandatory pavement markings: arrows showing turn lanes Number and variety of information sources: signs overhead, on pavement, and roadsides Rate at which speed zones change, number of other signs
Broader road environment	Extraneous attentional demands, distractions: challenges attentional control and more general executive functioning Urban, suburban, rural environments: affect many aspects including visual clutter, speed zone Consistent bitumen roads versus gravel, unmade roads with potholes

DRS, Driver rehabilitation specialist.

short distances and avoids heavy traffic. Such a decision would be consistent with research indicating that older drivers more generally tend to limit their driving trips to <1 hour during nonpeak driving times.[77,78] Conversely for a younger person with a higher exposure profile (e.g., who drives a lot and in all kinds of conditions), an evaluation in more demanding conditions would probably be essential, although it might be necessary first to review the client's abilities informally during previous training sessions.

In some circumstances, if permitted by local licensing legislation and procedures, it may be desirable for a driver with significant functional impairments to be issued a restricted license that is conditional on him or her driving only in defined areas of the local community or within a specified radius from his or her home. In such cases an on-road evaluation within that local area will be appropriate, despite the reduction in test reliability caused by use of a nonstandard route. This option is warranted in cases in which the functional problems are unlikely to resolve or to improve with rehabilitation. In other instances this alternative form of test may be offered at the outset as part of a licensing review procedure.[21,43]

Local area license tests are becoming increasingly common as an evaluation option within licensing systems that allow for a gradual reduction in licensing privileges, or graduated delicensing.[20,79] However, local area tests are not necessarily linked to restricted licenses, in which case the unrepresentative coverage of different types of driving activities raises significant questions concerning their content and construct validity. (Di Stefano and Macdonald[80] discuss this issue in more detail.) Table 12-5 summarizes some key characteristics and implications of local area evaluation.

SCORING

When the purpose of on-road evaluation is to ascertain the overall quality (usually in relation to safety) of driver performance, a quantitative score has the potential to enhance the reliability and validity of the evaluation. This requires use of a standard route with a programmed observation evaluation procedure, in which defined aspects of driving performance are observed and assessed at predetermined points along the route. For example Hunt et al[42] applied a 3-point scale (0 = evidence of moderate to severe impairment; 1 = evidence of mild impairment; 2 = no evidence of impairment) to assess performance at predetermined locations around a route, relating to left turns, stops, lane maintenance, speed, traffic awareness, merging, concentration, lane changes, traffic signs, comprehension of directions, attention to task, awareness of how driving is affecting others, judgment, and need for intervention by instructor for safety reasons. Scores at predetermined locations generated a maximum possible score of 108. These scores had criterion validity because they were significantly associated with the degree of drivers' cognitive impairment as clinically assessed. Dobbs[33] has also demonstrated the value of a

Table 12-5 **Some Key Characteristics and Implications of Local Area Evaluations**

Local Area Evaluation Characteristics	Implications for Evaluation Quality and Outcome
Not possible to use a standard route with prespecified observations at predetermined locations	Reliability of the test outcome is reduced
The specific route is likely to be determined or strongly influenced by the driver	Sampling of driving performance abilities is unlikely to be comprehensive in its coverage, with a consequent reduction in theoretical construct validity compared with a well-constructed standard route; however, given that the route is representative of the driver's actual driving environment its validity may be deemed adequate, at least for the purpose of a local area license
The driver is familiar with the route	The driver is likely to be less anxious, which enhances validity Cognitive demands of the driving task will be substantially lower, making it more likely that the driver will pass the evaluation Face validity for the driver will be high, which reduces the probability of complaints that it was "too difficult" or that "I never drive on such roads"
Instructions are often in the form of "drive me to your shopping center" or other common destinations	The evaluation is easier in that the driver does not have to cope with the demands of following navigational instructions; conversely the driver must rely on his or her own cognitive abilities for topographic orientation and path selection, which may be more cognitively demanding for people with compromised executive functioning

Data from Di Stefano M, Macdonald W: *Older driver errors on VicRoads "review" tests,* Paper presented at the RS2002: Road Safety, Research and Policing Conference, November 3-5, 2002, Adelaide, Australia; Fox GK, Bowden SC, Smith DS: On-road assessment of driving competence after brain impairment: review of current practice and recommendations for a standardized examination, *Arch Phys Med Rehabil* 79:1288-1296, 1998; Hunt LA, Murphy C, Carr DB, et al: Environmental cueing may affect performance on a road test for drivers with dementia of the Alzheimer type, *Alzheimer Dis Assoc Disord* 11(suppl 1):13-16, 1997; Janke M, Eberhard J: Assessing medically impaired older drivers in a licensing agency setting, *Accid Anal Prevent* 30:347-361, 1998; Janke MK: Assessing older drivers: two studies, *J Safety Res* 32:43-74, 2001; Macdonald WA, Scott T: *Disabled driver test procedures,* Canberra, 1993, Federal Office of Road Safety; Withaar FK, Brouwer WH, Van Zomeren AH: Critical review: fitness to drive in older drivers with cognitive impairment, *J Int Neuropsychol Soc* 6:480-490, 2000.

formal scoring system, particularly one that gives greater weight to those errors that enhance criterion validity most effectively. He commented: "More detailed analyses of the errors, . . . and the conditions of the driving errors may help to further refine the meaning of the errors for the purposes of developing an empirically based scoring scheme" (p. 369).

Dobbs[33] and Di Stefano and Macdonald[10] have emphasized the importance of considering the context in which an error occurs when evaluating its significance within an on-road evaluation. For example a shoulder check error would probably be classified as hazardous if the driver failed to look back over his or her shoulder before changing lanes on a heavily trafficked, multilane freeway, resulting in a vehicle in the adjacent lane having to brake sharply to avoid a collision. In contrast failure to perform a shoulder check error when changing lanes on a freeway when clearly there was no other traffic might still be classified as an error but certainly not as a hazardous one. Similarly rolling through a stop sign needs to be interpreted in relation to the potential for collision with other road users at the time. These authors have also both concluded, based on empirical research, that scoring systems should give the greatest weight to errors that, considering the road traffic context, are clearly hazardous because these are the strongest discriminators of impairment level and risk.

IMPLEMENTING ON-ROAD TESTS

Implementing on-road tests requires the use of consistent procedures, the completion of some critical prerequisites, and following protocols before and after the evaluation.

CONSISTENT PROCEDURES

The importance of using standardized procedural protocols is emphasized in texts discussing general testing and evaluation procedures.[22,81,82] It is important to provide the same instructions to all clients using standard questions in the same sequence and controlling any cuing. Protocols specific to on-road testing requirements have been documented in some licensing guidelines and in OT-DRS professional competency standards.[18,83]

This is necessary within a clinical context to maximize equity and reliability—factors that may be critical when driver evaluation is occurring within medicolegal, licensing, or insurance frameworks. Specific procedures should be documented in a policy and procedures manual that can be referred to by program managers, third-party payers, clients, and any other involved party.

PREREQUISITES FOR ON-ROAD EVALUATION

Some of the procedures that should be followed before any on-road driver evaluation or training session are applicable in virtually all circumstances. These include the need for review of information about the client's medical status and functional abilities, his or her driver's license status, and any issues concerning his or her vehicle (if appropriate), and checking potential issues that may preclude on-road activities, as outlined below.

Medical Status and Prerequisite Functional Abilities

Based on information received from non–driving specialist evaluators, the DRS should confirm that the driver's medical condition is stable, based on compliance with any medication requirements, and that his or her visual functioning is optimal; in some cases this may be based on how recently a specialist review has been performed.

Contraindications to on-road evaluation include the following:
- Medical conditions that clearly do not comply with guidelines for driving, such as inadequate visual fields
- Significant neuropsychological impairments, such as a major deficit in visual-spatial functioning
- Insufficient motor function in limbs that would preclude use of any available vehicle control adaptations
- Lack of insight, such as denying the existence or effects of a major impairment
- Unreliability in complying with a prescribed drug or treatment regimen that is necessary to maintain functional abilities important to driving

A more comprehensive listing of prerequisite driver capacities and attributes is provided in Chapter 1 (see Box 1-2). See also other resources mentioned elsewhere in this text (e.g., American Medical Association and National Highway Traffic Safety Administration,[14] Charlton et al,[84] and the National Older Driver Research and Training Center and University of Florida[85]).

Confirmation of Driver's License Status

To meet normal duty of care requirements and to fulfill obligations to professional indemnity insurers, and perhaps also to a licensing authority, funding body, or employer, the DRS must have a thorough knowledge of current licensing requirements to ensure that relevant procedures have been followed. In particular the DRS must confirm the following:
- The client is legally entitled to drive, whether with supervision or independently
- The license is appropriate to the driver's vehicle
- Any vehicle modifications and/or licensing restrictions are correctly documented

In some jurisdictions a license cancellation or suspension may be waived for the purpose of on-road evaluation or training.[11,18]

Vehicle Status and Suitability

If the client's vehicle is to be used during on-road evaluation or training, the DRS must ensure the following:
- Vehicle registration requirements are satisfied
- Any vehicle adaptations comply with industry or other standards
- Vehicle design characteristics are suitable for the driver, including ingress/egress provisions, seating, controls and displays, transportation and cargo needs, and accommodation of other vehicle occupants
- The vehicle has been adequately maintained in accord with safety requirements

It is usually the DRS who decides which vehicle is going to be used during evaluation and training. For some clients using their own car for any portion of the evaluation or training may be inappropriate if major vehicle modifications are either impractical to install or precluded because of inadequate financial resources. In some jurisdictions vehicle requirements are specified by guidelines and competency standards pertaining to medically impaired driver procedures. For example these may require use of a roadworthy, registered vehicle that displays appropriate license plates with additional signage indicating "Driver Under Instruction" or some such wording. Requirements for the use of seat belts and dual controls may also be specified.[18,83] In practice this may mean that virtually all of the testing and training occurs in vehicles owned by either a DRS or driver rehabilitation program. Exceptions may be made for drivers who need to be tested and trained in their own customized vehicles (e.g., with major modifications such as specialized seating or modified driving controls), but the DRS is likely to be responsible for liaising with the appropriate authorities to help ensure that licensing, professional indemnity, occupational health and safety, and insurance provisions are not compromised by such actions.[50,83]

Preliminary Evaluation of Training or Equipment Needs

When clients are likely to require prescription or training in the use of adapted driving aids (e.g., hand controls) before a formal, on-road evaluation, many DRSs first schedule an informal evaluation in either an off-road or quiet on-road area. This may be necessary to obtain information for use in devising a training program with clearly specified compensatory or remediation goals and time frames or to document requests for financial support from potential funding bodies. When substantial training is required (e.g., for drivers

with combinations of visual, cognitive, and physical limitations), a number of on-road evaluations may be undertaken, the last of which determines the ultimate rehabilitation outcome and perhaps also the consequent license status.

PROTOCOLS IMMEDIATELY BEFORE AND AFTER ON-ROAD EVALUATION*

Before commencement, the DRS should do the following:
- Brief the driver regarding the potential threats to safety that may arise as a result of his or her known impairments.
- Orient the driver to the vehicle, ensuring that vehicle controls and information displays are adjusted appropriately; if the driver does not initiate adjustment of mirrors and seating, prompt and provide assistance before the vehicle is in motion.
- Orient the driver to the evaluation procedures, explaining the nature of instructions that will be given and providing a general description of the route to be followed and its anticipated duration; advise the driver to ask for clarification of any instructions that are inaudible or unclear. For clients with hearing or speech impairments, alternative methods of communication will need to be established and verified as reliable.
- Explain what is required to pass the evaluation (if applicable).
- Explain safety procedures (e.g., that the driver should follow instructions only when safe to do so).
- Assure the driver that the evaluation can be interrupted at any stage and that he or she may request to stop for a break or to terminate the evaluation completely at any point.

After completion the DRS should do the following:
- Provide information orally and in writing, according to the policies and procedures of the driver rehabilitation service and more general professional, and possibly licensing authority, requirements.
- Information given should include feedback about specific performance issues and more general comments.
- Discuss the possible implications (e.g., related to training needs or license status).
- If a DI is also involved, it can be useful to coordinate this aspect of the service delivery so that both individuals contribute to the feedback.
- It is helpful if feedback is immediate (i.e., within 5 to 10 minutes of completing the evaluation), delivered in a way that is meaningful and understood, and

---

*References 7,18,41,50,83,86.

relates to the next stage of the driver rehabilitation process.

- If a detailed checklist that includes route directions has been used for scoring, this will be extremely useful for facilitating discussion regarding specific events that occurred during the evaluation, especially if these were associated with interventions by the supervising DRS or otherwise indicated a significant problem.
- At times it may be appropriate for family or significant others to be present at this stage, particularly if recommendations are likely to require their financial support, emotional support, or both.
- Providing detailed written feedback is particularly important if family members and/or other driving school staff may be involved in future training.

SUMMARY

In this first section the features of DRS on-road evaluation that are necessary to achieve reliable and valid outcomes are summarized. These conclusions are based on theory-based analysis of the nature of driving as a complex perceptual, cognitive, and psychomotor activity and on evidence from empirical research as discussed in previous sections of this chapter. These conclusions also are in accord with documentation of on-road evaluation content and procedural standards that have been developed for Australian OT-DRSs by their professional association, working in conjunction with a licensing authority.[18,83] The section concludes by identifying the outstanding issues that require further research to enable continuing improvement of DRS on-road evaluation practices.

The evaluation guidelines that must be applied to achieve reliable, on-road evaluations of driving performance are clear as summarized in Table 12-6. These guidelines are now being applied by licensing authorities in many jurisdictions around the world and also by some DRSs and driver rehabilitation programs. In the case of DRS evaluations, however, there are some particular challenges for those trying to implement these guidelines. First, there is probably greater interdriver variation in performance characteristics and behaviors among driver rehabilitation clients than there is among the entry-level (general population) drivers assessed by license testers. Second, DRS on-road evaluations are performed for a variety of purposes in many different contexts, which vary between individuals and for an individual who is assessed on several different occasions. These two factors present a more difficult evaluation problem than exists with entry-level license testing, and there may sometimes appear to be a conflict

for DRSs between, on the one hand, the goal of dealing sensitively and effectively with each client and, on the other hand, the goal of ensuring that everyone is evaluated in a reliable way.

The varying purposes of DRS evaluation also have important implications for the validity of evaluation practices. Key questions here are the extent to which the purpose is to assess the impact of disability, aging, or both on driving performance and the safety of driving performance. If the purpose is the latter, safety should be assessed relative to a common standard (e.g., entry-level license test criteria) or relative to a criterion group matched with the driver subgroup represented by the client (e.g., older drivers, young drivers, and drivers with the same type of impairment who have been demonstrated to have a good safety record).

These choices have important implications for how construct validity and criterion validity of the evaluation procedure and evaluation criteria need to be established. These issues need to be clarified to demonstrate that an evaluation of a particular client is valid for its intended purpose. For example the purpose may be to assess an older driver (without any diagnosed medical problems of a kind that presents particular road safety risks) who wishes to retain an unrestricted license with full driving privileges. In this case the driving route used for evaluation should present the full range of normally encountered road traffic conditions, including situations and maneuvers known to pose difficulties for older drivers (e.g., intersections, left-hand turns at intersections, and roundabouts). However, for a driver with possible aging-related impairments who has been experiencing some driving difficulties and is contemplating whether to relinquish his or her license, a more valid choice of evaluation route may be one in the individual's own local area that entails performance of a range of maneuvers representative of those that would normally be required. For example because shopping is a frequent driving trip purpose for older people, inclusion in the route of a car-parking maneuver at a local shopping center would probably be desirable. In this case a local area–only restricted license would probably be the goal. In both of the older driver cases referred to here, the criterion validity of their evaluations should be ensured by evaluating driving performance in terms of evidence-based standards related to the performance of normal older drivers with acceptable safety records. In the case of a younger person with a purely physical impairment and no indication of any particular safety risks, a different form of limited evaluation may be valid if the approach to evaluation is on specific impairment (see Table 12-3), particularly because there is no evidence to suggest that drivers with this type of impairment have a crash risk higher than average for drivers of comparable age and experience. In this case the

Table 12-6 DRS On-Road Evaluation Design Guidelines to Achieve Reliable Outcomes

Evaluation Design Guidelines	Benefits	Related References
Design and document a standard route, including details of maneuvers required at specific evaluation points around the route	Reduces variation between different evaluation conditions Supports greater consistency in DRS evaluation administration—greater reliability within and between evaluators Helps the DRS to become more familiar with route characteristics, reducing DRS task demands and facilitating more consistent and accurate observations	Fox et al,[41] Janke and Hersch,[55] Schneider,[83] School of Occupational Therapy, LaTrobe University,[50] VicRoads,[18] Withaar et al[16]
Detailed documentation of driver performance characteristics to be observed and evaluated at certain points along the standard route; in addition hazardous errors or behaviors indicating impairment, regardless of where they occur	Focuses DRS's attention on key aspects of driver performance, supporting more accurate and reliable observations	Hunt et al,[42] Fox et al,[41] Withaar et al,[16] Odenheimer et al,[53] VicRoads,[44] VicRoads[18]
Operational definitions for performance criteria, including examples of acceptable and nonacceptable behaviors and contextual effects where relevant	Facilitates more consistent application of evaluation criteria, reducing variation between assessors and within individual assessors on different occasions	Fox et al,[41] Janke and Hersch,[55] VicRoads,[44] Withaar et al[16]
Relevant and commonly occurring driving maneuvers observed several times, within a variety of traffic situations	Multiple sampling reduces effects of random variations between performance occasions	Fox et al,[41] Janke and Hersch,[55] LaTrobe University,[50] Siegrist,[31] VicRoads[44]
Two-person evaluation team: a supervising DRS to direct the client around the route and maintain safety, and the other to document and assess observed behaviors	Enables much more accurate observations and documentation and more systematic and detailed evaluation of them	Fox et al,[41] Hunt et al,[42] Schneider,[83] LaTrobe University,[50] VicRoads[18]

DRS, Driver rehabilitation specialist.

evaluation may focus just on the affected aspects of driving performance (e.g., steering performance or use of pedals).

In light of these varying needs to achieve validity, along with the concurrent need to achieve reliability by using standard routes and programmed observation of driver performance, it is evident that there is a need for DRSs and researchers to develop a range of standard routes with different route sections identified as appropriate for different evaluation purposes.

The specific aspects of driving performance that are observed, documented, and evaluated at particular points also need to be given careful consideration by DRSs, with a view to identifying aspects that are not normally of concern to entry-level license testers. For example in some cases it may be desirable to identify and document particular aspects of performance that are indicative of cognitive functioning at the executive level, particularly related to appropriate attention allocation and prioritization of subtasks. For example it has been informally reported that some DRSs engage the driver in conversation on trivial topics at predetermined points along the route to determine how he or she copes and whether he or she allows this activity to interfere with driving performance. Evaluation of this aspect of a driver's functioning may be predictive of his or her ability to adopt safe driving tactics and strategies more generally (see Box 1-2). However, research is needed to investigate and establish the validity and reliability of such procedures.

In view of the emerging evidence of the importance of hazardous errors as an indicator of differences between average drivers and those with significant impairments, it will also be important to develop consistent and reliable methods of identifying and documenting such errors. For example this may require the DRS to document some details of situations in which some types of errors occur because the same error will vary in its significance depending on the particular road traffic context. On a related issue Hunt et al[49] noted the influence of environmental cuing on driver performance, whereby a cognitively impaired driver might perform satisfactorily when ample cues are present but poorly if those cues are absent. For example a driver may respond appropriately to a turn arrow at a signalized intersection when he or she can simply follow the vehicle ahead but fail to understand its significance when there are no such environmental cues. Development of systematic procedures for observing, recording, and interpreting these aspects of performance would enhance the validity and reliability of DRS evaluations that comprise a comprehensive driver rehabilitation evaluation.

Finally it is apparent from the above review of key issues related to the on-road evaluation of driving performance that there is a need for further research to enable improvements to the reliability and validity of currently available methods. Such research is often difficult and time-consuming, but it has the potential to enhance the well-being of drivers with disabilities or aging-related concerns who undergo DRS evaluation in the future and the safety of other road users.

SECTION II
On-Road Evaluation and Visual Functioning

Patrick T. Baker

In addition to the clinical evaluation of visual function, the DRS must evaluate the client's functional vision while on the road. The predriving clinical evaluation by definition occurs in a controlled environment, with more or less optimal conditions, neither of which accurately reflects the dynamic driving environment. Lighting changes, movement, relative speed, road and traffic conditions, and stress all affect the client's vision. The DRS should attempt to evaluate the client's ability to see and perceive the vehicle's interior environment and the external traffic environment and to demonstrate competence while driving in a variety of conditions that can add stress during the driving task.

The DRS should keep in mind that the client may be anxious not only about being tested but also his or her perception of residual ability and deficits, particularly if there are recent changes in the client's visual function. In addition to losing some degree of functional vision, the client may have also lost confidence in his or her ability to drive safely. A person with mild vision loss may be more at risk from being overly cautious and anxious while behind the wheel of a motor vehicle than from the visual deficit itself. The DRS should strive to develop a team- and client-centered approach rather than a scenario that features an anxiety-provoking pass versus fail focus. Although the client may have considerable difficulty driving during the initial on-road evaluation, with training and practice, he or she may improve and eventually resume restricted or unrestricted independent driving. Knowing that the DRS's role includes being a teacher, coach, advocate, and motivator, who can be trusted to provide a thorough evaluation along with clear and concise recommendations, even if the recommendations are not what the client wants to hear; this is as important as the final outcome of the comprehensive driver rehabilitation evaluation.

ASSESSING VISUAL FUNCTION BEFORE GETTING BEHIND THE WHEEL

When working with a client whose predriving deficits may impact his or her ability to drive, the DRS may want to first assess residual functional vision in a controlled environmental setting. The client and instructor may go for a walk in the area, indoors and outside, for example, while the DRS observes the client's visual behaviors. The client may be asked to locate specific objects at various distances, read signs, and describe colors and shapes in a casual and protected environment. Observations of how the client negotiates obstacles and how he or she reacts to curbs and oncoming pedestrians and vehicles should be noted by the DRS. Glare recovery can be determined by observing the client's reaction to entering and exiting a building. The client should be asked to describe the environment in well-lit versus dimly lit settings to assess acuity and contrast sensitivity. Peripheral vision can be functionally assessed by asking the client to describe the range (estimate in degrees) of his or her field of view while fixating on a central object. There are a number of computer driving simulators that either use an on-screen video of actual driving scenarios taken from the driver's point of view or provide a fully interactive virtual world. Some simulators have a mock interior of a vehicle complete with a steering wheel and gas and brake pedals the client uses while negotiating the driving scene, much like a sophisticated video game. Unexpected events programmed into the computer, such as the appearance of a child or animal running into the street, can help the DRS assess the client's reaction time in conditions that could not otherwise be presented in the real-world environment. The DRS should carefully assess whether a driving simulator can effectively be used as an evaluation tool, assist the client in remediating driving performance deficits, or both. See Chapter 10 for more information on driving simulators.

THE ON-ROAD EVALUATION AND VISION

In the vehicle the DRS should note how efficiently the client reads the dashboard instruments, uses mirrors to check blind spots, scans for inanimate and animate objects (e.g., road signs, pedestrians, and other vehicles), recognizes stationary and moving objects at various distances, and observes details that indicate visual acuity. Field of view can be assessed at intersections, especially for vehicles on the left side, and on multilane roads as other vehicles pass on the left side of the evaluation vehicle. The client should detect overhead signs, typically in the right upper quadrant, and traffic lights. Can the client look into the rearview mirror efficiently and return his or her gaze to a specific point in front of the vehicle? Does the client take too long to study what is visible in the rearview or sideview mirrors with the purpose of comprehending what is there? Or does the client focus entirely on what is in front of the vehicle, never or rarely looking at the vehicle's mirrors because he or she is afraid to take his or her eyes off the road? Having the client drive in a westerly direction when the sun is low in the sky in the late afternoon or early evening and negotiate a shady side street may help the DRS to assess the client's contrast sensitivity and the effects of glare. The DRS also can instruct the client to drive into a parking garage, park the vehicle, and then return to the roadway. Night driving and conditions of poor visibility should also be assessed whenever possible if appropriate. Scanning and tracking ability can be evaluated in the vehicle as well. The DRS should

not take his or her eyes off the road to watch the client's eye movements, but using a small mirror strategically located on the dashboard, eye movements can be easily monitored while concurrently enabling the DRS to observe where the client's attention is directed versus where it should be and the vehicle's intended versus actual path of travel.

Visual perceptual skills are critical to the safe operation of a motor vehicle because they represent how the brain integrates the visual information it receives. Figure-ground skills enable the client to distinguish important objects from the environment's background and are an important component of depth perception. Inability to locate the curb, observe a bumper block, or recognize that the distant vehicle stopped in front of the driver is closer than the one in the next lane are cues to figure-ground, contrast, and depth issues. The client with visual closure deficits may not realize that a road sign partially covered by a tree branch is a stop sign or that the rear portion of the vehicle seen in the rearview mirror is a complete automobile that is in the process of passing on the left. Functional visual memory means that the client should be able to recall what he or she has just observed in the rearview mirror once his or her gaze has returned to the forward path of travel. Spatial relation skills provide the driver with the ability to judge relative distances and the speed of moving objects. The DRS needs to be able to anticipate and quickly recognize the visual cues in the environment and observe what the client sees, when he or she sees it, his or her reactions, and whether what is being looked at is the most relevant information required at any particular moment.

REFERRAL AND TREATMENT INTERVENTIONS FOR VISUAL ISSUES AFFECTING DRIVING

Once the clinical and initial on-road evaluation portion of the visual evaluation has been completed, the DRS may determine that there should be additional predriving interventions provided before continuing the on-road evaluation, on-road training, or return to independent driving. The intervention plan may be as simple as initiating a referral to a vision specialist for new or updated corrective lenses. It is not uncommon for an elderly client to remark that his or her glasses just do not work as well as they used to and yet not understand why it would be prudent to undergo a comprehensive driver rehabilitation evaluation after being involved in a recent traffic accident. The vision specialist may evaluate and prescribe prismatic lenses, filters, magnification, or bioptic lenses. Surgery may be appropriate to correct retinal detachment, remove cataracts, or correct misalignment of the eyes. The client may require a referral to an occupational therapist specializing in low vision or an orientation and mobility (O & M) specialist, for example, for training with visual devices while performing ADL, IADL, or both. Another intervention technique to explore is learning eccentric viewing techniques to help maximize the use of the remaining visual fields after the onset of macular degeneration. O & M specialists can provide training related to negotiating the environment using mobility aids to compensate for reduced vision. The therapist may teach scanning and tracking skills with the aim of compensating for a loss of central or peripheral visual field associated with various diagnoses, including glaucoma, retinitis pigmentosa, retinal detachment, and cerebrovascular accident (CVA).

Once appropriate interventions by qualified professionals have been completed and the client can adequately perform other meaningful ADL, further on-road evaluation and training may be appropriate. The DRS should be aware of the visual requirements for the operation of a motor vehicle in his or her particular state and should determine whether the client has the potential to meet those standards. It would be inappropriate to continue the on-road evaluation or training if the client cannot meet these requirements; continuing to provide services may cause the client to have false expectations of beginning or resuming independent driving and could create a possible ethical and legal dilemma when billing for treatment that the DRS suspects will not sufficiently improve the client's skills necessary to drive safely.

Predriving interventions performed by the DRS may include the client practicing tracking and scanning skills while seated in the driver's seat of a parked vehicle. The client can practice scanning the dashboard, locating and viewing the rearview mirrors, and observing and describing traffic movements. Practice should include the development of a routine method of eye movements to incorporate the entire visual field for efficiency and to help ensure that the entire visual field is regularly checked. The client may progress to providing a visual commentary to the DRS while seated in the passenger seat as the DRS drives in a variety of traffic situations, especially situations known to be problematic for the client. The DRS should travel an established route with increasing visual complexity while the client practices scanning and tracking techniques. The use of an established route enables the DRS to anticipate what the client will see and when he or she should see it. The client provides a continual verbal description of what is being visualized and perceived, which enables the DRS to develop a sense of what the client sees and when he or she sees it. The route should include single- and multiple-lane traffic, one-way and four-way stops, yield situations, and multiple-lane intersections. Quiet residential streets provide opportunities to negotiate parked vehicles and potholes and to watch for pedestrians crossing the street. Snow- or leaf-covered streets may be used to observe whether the client can visualize a partially or completely covered curb or centerline. As the DRS drives through a business section of town, the client can be requested to find specific signage, such as a restaurant, and to report any relevant traffic signs, lights, or changing traffic conditions. If the client consistently misses relevant information in a portion of his or her visual field or has a delayed response to moving objects coming into the periphery of the field of view, he or she may not be able to compensate sufficiently to warrant taking a position behind the wheel while on the road.

The DRS should choose routes wisely when beginning the on-road intervention, especially with the client in control of the motor vehicle. Off-road areas, such as a deserted parking lot, or on-road areas, such as a quiet residential street, in addition to choosing a day and time when there is optimal lighting and weather conditions, are important factors that can help ensure the client's best performance. Side streets or residential streets often have no centerline, which provides the DRS with an opportunity to evaluate the client's ability to maintain lane position while using other visual cues, such as the right curb and oncoming traffic. In addition to visual deficits, the client may be overcoming physical deficits, cognitive deficits, or both. High levels of anxiety may affect the client's performance. The DRS needs to be able to weigh whether a poor first performance is the result of anxiety, whether the client's performance will improve with practice, and whether the client's deficits appear to be too difficult to overcome.

ADAPTATIONS TO ENHANCE VISUAL FUNCTION IN THE VEHICLE

Vehicle adaptations designed to improve visual function usually involve installing modified mirrors to improve the client's ability to see the traffic environment. There are a number of styles of wide-angle rearview mirrors that fit over the interior mirror that provide a wide view of the environment behind the vehicle. Additional small mirrors may be placed on the dashboard in the corners where the windshield and dashboard meet. The client should adjust these mirrors to enable a view of the opposite peripheral field. That is, a mirror placed in the right corner may assist the driver when there is a need to check the left side at a four-way intersection. Mirrors used in this way may also assist the client who demonstrates difficulty with head (i.e., cervical) rotation. Most motor vehicles have a blind spot on the left side (i.e., driver's side). As another vehicle passes it is possible that the passing vehicle can leave the field of view of the interior rearview mirror and not be in the field of view of the exterior rearview (side) mirror. The driver, thinking the left lane is clear, initiates changing lanes and begins to move into the left lane, potentially sideswiping the vehicle that has not passed because it was still in the left passing lane. Small convex mirrors placed on the outside rearview mirrors can maximize the field of view along the side of the vehicle, reducing the risk of this problem occurring. The DRS should have an ample supply of various styles of mirrors for the client to experiment with during on-road training. For example some wide-angle interior rearview mirrors distort the field of view such that it may take the client longer to comprehend what he or she sees. The reflection may even be uncomfortable to view because of the distortion. Avoidance protection systems mounted on the front and rear of the vehicle may assist the driver when parking in a garage or parking lot. These devices sound an alarm as the vehicle moves within a certain distance of a stationary or moving obstacle. The DRS should have sunglasses and seating cushions available for the client as needed.

Learning to drive with visual impairment is a difficult task. With a reduced field of view, the driver has to use residual vision to compensate for a deficit and cover a larger portion of the environment. Scanning more frequently to one side means the peripheral field of view to the other side is altered and decreased momentarily until the client scans back to the other side. The driver has to be cognizant of the changing traffic environment; coupled with the need for increased head and eye movements, fatigue may also become a risk factor. The DRS must be confident that the client has the cognitive abilities to fully appreciate the additional burden placed on his or her visual capabilities when compensating for visual loss. Compensation strategies include, but are certainly not limited to, the client using scanning and tracking techniques, using adaptive driving aids, and subscribing to a restricted driving plan, such as only driving during specific times and in specific places to minimize risk to all road users. Many drivers with reduced visual acuity, decreased contrast sensitivity, and difficulty coping with glare self-limit their driving by not driving at night or in other adverse lighting conditions, such as during inclement weather (e.g., fog, thunderstorms, and snowstorms). If the DRS is considering recommending that the client be issued a restricted driver's license, the DRS should seek the client's assurance that he or she will comply with the prescribed restrictions.

The DRS should also be aware of the state laws, regulations, and policies regarding restricted driving times and conditions. Many states make no provision for this type of restriction. For those individuals with more significant visual impairment, bioptic lenses may be a solution. The following section discusses on-road training of clients who drive using bioptic telescopic lens systems.

SECTION III

On-Road Evaluation and Training of Clients Using Bioptic Telescopic Lens Systems

Charles P. Huss

In years past Burg[87-89] attempted to establish a strong correlation between traffic accident records and vision characteristics for driver licensure. Similarly Higgins et al[90] and Wood and Higgins[91] attempted to establish a strong correlation between driving performance and certain vision characteristics. In part, after the traditional research paradigm failed to provide the empirical evidence that would justify any of the existing conservative visual acuity standards for driving, many states began relaxing such standards for obtaining or retaining a driver's license and the privilege that it afforded. There has also been a significant increase during the past 20 years in the number of states that allow the use of special prescription lens systems called bioptics for driving.[92]

The West Virginia Low Vision Driving Study (1985 through 1996), which was conducted at the West Virginia Rehabilitation Center (WVRC), Institute, West Virginia, has served as one of the driving forces in both of these national movements. The West Virginia multiyear study continues to be a model for an increasing number of states that are currently developing and implementing their own formalized programs of low vision driver education training.

This section will provide an overview of other aspects of the West Virginia multiyear research endeavor not addressed in Chapter 6. It includes, but is not limited to, exploring what prompted such efforts and the rationale behind them, initial screening findings, evaluation and training strategies, and the major results and conclusions of this research study. Finally some of this author's past personal experiences as the O & M specialist involved in the daily evaluation and training of prospective bioptic drivers participating in this research study at a rehabilitation center will also be highlighted.

FACTORS INFLUENCING THE INCEPTION OF THE WEST VIRGINIA LOW VISION DRIVING STUDY

In 1975 a National Conference on Telescopic Devices and Driving was organized and conducted by the New York Department of Motor Vehicles for the purposes of educating and assisting state licensing officials nationwide and their medical advisory boards about the issue of licensing wearers of bioptic telescopic lens systems.[93] Such nonstandard prescription optical devices are more commonly known as bioptics. The American Medical Association (AMA) and the American Association of Motor Vehicle Administrators (AAMVA) sponsored the 2-day symposium.

It was reported at this conference that in 1975 there were 20 states involved in licensing bioptic drivers. During the conference, however, there were not sufficient statistical data that correlated an increased risk while driving with such accommodative devices as suspected by some eye doctors and licensing authorities.[94,95] As a result conference participants were reluctant to make specific recommendations to licensing agencies regarding the use of bioptics for driving. However, it was agreed that some general guidelines and suggestions had to be offered until sound data were gathered. A couple of the general suggestions that were documented and have applicability to this chapter section are as follows:

- To determine whether such devices can be safely used in dynamic traffic conditions, states that have the facilities, funds, and qualified personnel to conduct scientific research should select highly motivated bioptic users to take part in a carefully controlled long-range scientific study.
- Have respective state Departments of Motor Vehicles work with the Department of Education or other appropriate agencies to develop driver education and training programs for bioptic lens users.

In 1981 low vision specialists at WVRC began tracking and formulating a list of clients whose visual status fit or was slightly below the visual protocol used in other states that were already licensing bioptic drivers. The effort to track these residents was to determine whether there was a future need for developing formalized low vision driving services at the center for certain West Virginia residents. During the next 2 years, 20 such individuals, referred for standard clinical low vision examination services by state Division of Rehabilitation Services field counselors, were identified

as potential student participants because they met the visual protocol for adapted driving education and training services.

Between 1981 and 1983 three of the clients who were being seen by state Division of Rehabilitation Services field counselors were referred to the center for driver evaluation and training. Referrals were initiated in an effort to determine whether the type and extent of driver education offered at that time would meet the needs of these individuals with low vision. During the next several months, all three individuals were able to receive the driver education and training services, performed satisfactorily, and obtained a driver's license in West Virginia. However, this process required intensive instruction beyond that of standard driver education and training practices.

WEST VIRGINIA LOW VISION DRIVING STUDY

As previously indicated in Chapter 6, shortly after beginning employment as an O & M specialist at the center in 1983, this author was invited to be a part of a multidisciplinary research group. The group was organized to explore and formulate ways of screening, training, and assessing the driving potential of a select group of individuals with visual challenges. The effort would come to be known as the West Virginia Low Vision Driving Study. Other principal team members included an optometrist specializing in low vision, a DRS, a psychologist, an occupational therapy generalist, and an audiologist.[96]

VISION REQUIREMENTS FOR CANDIDATES SELECTED FOR INCLUSION IN STUDY

As indicated in Chapter 6, students with visual deficits who participated in the center's initial 3-year pilot study (1985 to 1988) or identical low vision driver services that followed for the next 7 years (1989 to 1996) were required to meet and maintain the following visual requirements:

- Distance visual acuity between 20/50 and 20/200 inclusive with best standard spectacle or contact lens correction in the better eye
- Visual field of 120 degrees horizontally and 80 degrees vertically or greater in the same eye as used for the visual acuity determination
- 20/40 or better distance visual acuity using distance optical low vision aids prescribed by either a licensed optometrist or ophthalmologist
- No ocular diagnosis or prognosis that was likely to result in significant deterioration of vision below the

protocol levels of visual acuity and visual fields as stated below.

INITIAL SCREENING FINDINGS

Most project participants were novice to the driving task and never imagined that someday they would be given the opportunity to demonstrate their functional competency behind the wheel of an automobile. Because there was no expectation or encouragement from others (e.g., teachers, parents, and friends) early on in life to drive when they reached the licensing age in West Virginia, many of these individuals did not attend to or consider the importance of being cognizant of the actions of the drivers, other motor vehicle operators, or the driving environments outside and inside the motor vehicles while they were passengers. In time these individuals became passive and indifferent to the events happening around them.

Preliminary passenger-in-car and behind-the-wheel evaluation results revealed that most students had problems with the complexity of the driving task. For example a number of project participants illustrated limited or a complete lack of knowledge in the areas of anticipatory (defensive) driving skills, critical objects, or conditions within typical driving environments that influence a driver's speed and lane position, hazard perception skills, basic yielding procedures at intersections, and collision avoidance skills.[96] These findings clearly indicated that operating a motor vehicle involves much more than an up-to-date eye examination and a pair of special adaptive eyewear. These deficits and limitations lend support to the notion that certain people with low vision must participate in and satisfactorily complete an adaptive driver education and training program before their applications for driver licensure should be considered and approved.

INTERVENTION TRAINING STRATEGIES

Forty-seven of those 56 participants who completed the required multidisciplinary screening procedures returned voluntarily and participated in a comprehensive and individualized low vision driver education training program during a 6- to 8-week period.[97] Only two people were scheduled and enrolled in each training class to appropriately address the needs of this potential subgroup of drivers (e.g., working one-on-one in the car) throughout this study.

Students who volunteered to participate in the driver education training phase of this study and who demonstrated driver readiness received 30 to 40 hours of classroom instruction, 40 to 50 hours of passenger-in-car experiences, and an additional 40 to 50 hours of actual on-road driving under the auspices of a state-certified driver education instructor. However, there was sufficient latitude in program length and content if needed for shorter or more competency-based programs of instruction; this was dependent on the respective students' needs or deficits, abilities, previous driving skills and experience, and availability if already employed or commuting to and from the center.[97]

Driver education and training services that were provided as a part of this research project generally were undertaken concurrently using two different types of training instructors on a full- or part-time basis. One of the instructors (this author) was the O & M specialist, and the others were driver educators. The four driver educators who provided services as part of the West Virginia Low Vision Driving Pilot Study (1985 to 1988) and the continuation of services (1989 to 1996) were certified driver rehabilitation specialists (CDRSs). CDRS certification is granted through an international organization known as the Association for Driver Rehabilitation Specialists (ADED), formerly known as the Association for Driver Educators for the Disabled. See Chapter 4 and Appendices C, D, and E for more information on ADED.

By concurrent instruction this author means that a respective student would receive approximately 4 hours of classroom instruction (including 2 hours of self-study), 2 hours of passenger-in-car training, and 2 hours of behind-the-wheel (i.e., on-road) instruction 5 days a week for 6 to 8 weeks by the aforementioned staff who shared teaching responsibilities and collaborated to review each student's progress. One of the benefits of this approach was the immediate reinforcement that students received relative to what was covered in class and the real-life situations experienced in the driving environments. For example after classroom and on-road instruction with their assigned DRS, the respective students would be taken by car as passengers over the same route with their environmental awareness training instructor (this author, the O & M specialist) to review and remediate any problem areas that had arisen during the previous session but could not be addressed at the time by the CDRS (e.g., because of the dynamics of the driving scene at the time of the training session). Such on-site reviews might comprise a review of roadway characteristics, including special emphasis on fixed or other hazards that could affect one's line of sight and subsequent path of travel or speed, presence or absence of other road users, and understanding of the pertinent traffic control devices present (e.g., pavement markings, regulatory road signs, and traffic lights).[97]

The other students in training would alternately receive their passenger-in-car reinforcement before actual on-road instruction. The in-car schedules of the two students who were enrolled would be reversed the next week, pending progress made and competencies demonstrated.

CLASSROOM TRAINING

Daily classroom instruction for the project participants consisted of lectures, audiovisual driver education materials, and discussions that addressed what to expect in passenger-in-car and behind-the-wheel hypothetical scenarios. Specifically all of the students were exposed to the following:

- A 300-question written pretest about driving
- Common vision characteristics for driving
- Anticipatory (or defensive) driving skills
- Using mirrors and the importance of checking blind spots
- An introduction to bioptic telescopic lens systems
- West Virginia road laws (preparation of West Virginia instructional permit test)
- Hazard perception and independent decision-making skills (Doron Corporation's Search, Identify, Predict, Decide, and Execute Process series) with special emphasis on critical object/condition awareness, intersection analysis, collision traps, changing lanes, joining and leaving traffic formations, principles of passing of vehicles, and evaluating expressway dynamics
- Driver efficiency (i.e., "The Featherfoot Program")
- Automobile insurance
- Automobile accident reporting
- Steps involved in changing a tire
- Self-study materials: National Safety Council's defensive driving course, Ford Motor Company (i.e., beginner driver video series), Centurion Corporation (i.e., young adult video series), American Automobile Association (i.e., senior driver video series), and Mottala's Zone Control Driving System (i.e., video series)

During the course of the study, audiovisual materials were presented in a variety of formats, including 16-mm driver education simulation films, carousel slides, filmstrip and audiocassettes, 0.5-inch videos, laser disks, and digital videodisks (DVDs). Instead of standard-sized projection screens or television monitors, materials were projected onto a 6- × 30-foot projection screen within a 40- × 45-foot driver education classroom setting.[96] The staff also found that the use of laser disks and DVDs made a considerable difference when an instructor wished to reinforce a point with low vision students by still framing driving scenes or advancing/reversing the still frame one image at a time, without distortion or apprehension of burning a hole in the film. Film occasionally burned when older 16-mm films were used and projected using a Graflex Insta-Load model 1120 film projector with a wide-angle anamorphic lens.

Although the driver educator and students discussed major points while viewing the education materials on a daily basis throughout the driver-training component of the study, a driving simulator was not used. The decision not to use a driving simulator as a tool for education and training was in part based on where the emphasis of instruction was placed for this group of potential drivers. Preliminary screening results of novice driving candidates and observations gained the first year of the pilot study by the driving instructors also supported the methods and media adopted for the study. The concept or idea was to take what was presented in the controlled classroom setting and immediately apply it to actual driving environments during the driving task. The young, novice, and inexperienced drivers who were found to be in need of remedial classroom instruction beyond what was provided by the project's staff during daytime hours were requested to attend and participate in an ongoing standard driver education class that featured classroom instruction that was provided during the evening hours, 4 nights per week for 8 weeks, at the center.

It is worthwhile to note that after the pilot project was completed in 1988, classroom instruction with low vision clients became a shared or alternating responsibility of the assigned driver educator(s) and the O & M specialist.

ENVIRONMENTAL AWARENESS TRAINING

As previously indicated low vision students were found to need and benefit from intensive instruction provided in a variety of formats and settings on a daily (i.e., Monday through Friday) basis. This one-on-one, passenger-in-car instruction that emphasized environmental awareness was used primarily to reinforce all of the aforementioned principal areas of instruction introduced initially during classroom training with a special emphasis on the following:

- How to address and compensate for known functional vision loss
- Visual search and identification skills
- Space cushion awareness (including checking for blind spots)
- Proper and appropriate use of bioptic telescopic lens systems
- Narrative driving abilities, such as critical object or condition awareness exercises, hazard perception awareness skills, and mirror usage
- Preparation for environmental vision screening (i.e., passenger-in-car evaluation with and without use of bioptic lens system, which was a part of the comprehensive driver testing protocol for each of the project graduates in West Virginia)

Some students were unable to gain big picture awareness of their ever-changing driving environment and experienced considerable difficulty when attempting to detect and decipher detail from the dynamic driving settings with or without their bioptics. In cases in which this occurred, the student was encouraged to return home (i.e., for 6 to 12 months before reapplying for the low vision driving services) and was given a recommendation to observe what other drivers and road users were doing to drive or travel safely.

To help students gain the big picture, the O & M specialist would first isolate out, introduce, and reinforce the location and awareness of larger critical objects one object at a time. Next students practiced detecting and identifying smaller critical objects. Driver education professionals define critical objects as any object or condition that can be predicted to cause drivers to modify their vehicle's speed, lane position, or planned path of travel.[98] Experts stress that all drivers learn how to group these objects or conditions into three general categories: roadway characteristics (i.e., hills, dips in the road, intersections, curves in the road, and bushes/hedges), other road users (e.g., trucks, buses, cars, pedestrians, and animals), and traffic control devices (e.g., pavement markings, road signs, traffic lights, and traffic guards). Using a grouping technique helps to facilitate object recognition and decision making; this affords drivers an increased margin of safety by decreasing the likelihood of a collision in their dynamic driving environments.[96]

ON-ROAD TRAINING

All training students received in-car instruction and reinforcement during approximately 20 to 25 prearranged routes of travel and gained hands-on experience in typical rural, residential, commercial, inner city, and interstate freeway driving environments and in a variety of morning and afternoon/evening traffic, lighting, and roadway conditions. Box 12-2 lists the specific areas of instruction to which students should receive ample exposure.

Students were required to wear their prescription bioptic lens systems starting the first day of the on-road training sessions, even before instruction in the proper and appropriate use of the telescopic portion of the device was introduced. This approach enabled students who had not previously worn standard corrected eyewear to become accustomed to wearing eyewear and to practice viewing through the carrier lens portion of the device because this would be the case scenario for the majority of time during a typical driving task.

Integration of brief and intermittent vertically spotting through the telescopic portion of the bioptic lens system during the driving task was required selectively and minimally at first. The students were then

Box 12-2   On-Road Areas of Instruction

- Proper vehicle maintenance and dashboard controls (i.e., location and function)
- Policing one's vehicle and the initial intended path of travel
- Use of brake, accelerator, steering wheel, gearshift, and mirrors
- Reinforcement of safe space cushion driving skills
- Backing and parking skills (including parking garage or lot exits)
- Separation and compromise skills that involved adjustments in speed, lane position, or both
- Joining and leaving traffic formations (including yielding skills)
- Driving on multiple-lane roadways (including lane changing)
- Sharing the roadway with slower moving vehicles (including knowing when and how to pass)
- Reinforcement of hazard perception and independent decision-making skills using Doron Corporation's Search, Identify, Predict, Decide, and Execute Process (SIPDE)
- How and where to safely change a flat tire

encouraged to use these techniques more frequently as their driving skills developed and improved over time. Such vertical spotting tasks (i.e., ≤0.5 second per fixation) allowed students to decipher distance detail, such as symbols or nomenclature off of road signs; color, such as the red, green, or amber traffic light colors; or the actions or movements of distantly positioned objects or forms, such as a school crossing guard or traffic officer's hand signals, which were first detected within their larger nonmagnified peripheral field(s) of view while driving.[99]

INTERVENTION EVALUATION TECHNIQUES
Nonrated Driving Evaluation
Once confidence and rapport were established between a student and his or her assigned driver educator, nonrated driving evaluation was initiated. The nonrated driving evaluation included the presence of a second driver evaluator in the car, namely, the O & M specialist, who was positioned in the left backseat location. The rationale for initiating the nonstandardized on-road evaluations near the end of week 2 of the on-road training was as follows. Students became accustomed to the presence of more individuals in the car by the second week of training. Their adjustment to the increasing amount of distractions afforded the project's staff an opportunity to determine firsthand the amount of knowledge that a student was able to retain and apply from the classroom and passenger-in-car instruction to

the actual on-road driving experience. The staff also was able to identify performance areas that needed improvement. Finally standardized driver evaluation entailed more independent decision-making skills on the part of the student driver, which will be discussed below.

Rated Driving Evaluation

Once sufficient driving experience, driving skills, and self-confidence were gained in a variety of traffic, roadway, and lighting conditions, students were exposed to a 40-mile, 90-minute on-road evaluation. The on-road evaluation was patterned after and developed by one of the researchers involved in the driver performance measurement (DPM) research conducted by Michigan State University in the 1970s.[100] Like most nonrated evaluation measures, the rated evaluation entailed having at least two trained evaluators in the car and use of multiple accessory mirrors, and was completed in a dual brake–controlled driver education vehicle. However, the objective on-road evaluation/test route used standardized measures in all of the following areas:

- Test route
- Route directions
- Driving task requirements
- Evaluation criteria
- Rating forms and procedures
- Feedback procedures

Because approximately 90% of the students in this project had never driven before and lacked independent decision-making driving abilities, these measures were not introduced or incorporated until the midpoint of the students' training experience. The latter evaluation entailed students driving through rural, residential, business, and inner city settings. It exposed the students to a wide range of driving experiences—some easy, which most drivers are expected to handle without difficulty, and others more complex, which even the best drivers have problems negotiating.

For example a couple of rather simple driving tasks on the complex route required the driver to negotiate a narrow two-lane highway and turn left onto a narrow, curved, hilly, two-lane rural road or to travel on a narrow, two-lane residential street crossing three intersections (the first controlled and the last two uncontrolled). Driving tasks that were a bit more challenging required the driver to approach and cross an uncontrolled multilane urban/suburban street from a narrow two-lane residential side street or to exit a high density, high speed metropolitan interchange (via a weave lane) onto a one-way multilane surface street, executing two lane changes to the left, and then turning left onto a side street.

The topography of West Virginia necessitated a longer DPM test route as described previously than the normal length of 10 to 12 miles. Once introduced these procedures were used on a weekly basis during non–rush hour times of the day (i.e., 9:00 to 10:30 AM or 1:00 to 2:30 PM) until the completion of the program for the purposes described above.[96]

RESULTS AND CONCLUSIONS OF PROJECT EFFORTS

Listed below are some of the major results and conclusions of this 10-year project.

Graduates (20 males, 12 females) whose vision was below the standard legal limits for driving in West Virginia (20/60) demonstrated the ability to drive safely with appropriate low vision aids and training. Eleven graduates presented visual acuity between 20/50 and 20/70, 6 between 20/80 and 20/120, and 15 between 20/140 and 20/200.

Project participants who had never driven had a multitude of needs. They required approximately 1.5 times the number of classroom hours and 3 to 5 times the number of on-road hours of instruction than normally sighted individuals would receive through programs of standard driver education training if driving were to become a reality. Such student drivers found themselves often transitioning through stages from being a passive to active passenger and driver.

The passenger-in-car phase of training, provided separately by a second instructor (an O & M specialist), proved to be extremely beneficial to novice or first-time drivers, especially during the transitional passive to active passenger-in-car phase of training.

Students with low vision were able to learn or gain big picture awareness and more effectively locate critical objects within their ever-changing driving environment, as well as adjust their vehicle's speed and lane position to avoid a collision as needed.

The use of DPM procedures as described and implemented as an important part of this research effort dispelled the notion that an accident- or violation-free driving record is always the reflection of being a safe driver. Drivers can cause accidents that involve other road users without being directly involved in the accidents themselves.

One of the major conclusions from repeated use of DPM procedures with project students was that individuals who completed the low vision driver education and training program at the WVRC satisfactorily performed at a level comparable with their sighted counterparts in terms of basic visual skills and demonstrated above average skills in vehicle handling and ability to react to traffic hazards.

By the end of the training the majority of students demonstrated improvements up to an average passing DPM score. The duration of time between DPM evaluation runs was usually 1 week and allowed learning to take place before a student's next scheduled and graded on-road evaluation.

Despite training the three most common types of driving errors by male and female project participants as revealed by DPM evaluations were the following: failure to check opposite the direction of an intended turn, failure to correctly execute the visual checks and other related driving behaviors on lane changes within a defined short distance of space or time, and failure to demonstrate consistent head and eye scanning at intersections. It is worthwhile to note these findings were almost identical to past Michigan State University DPM research results with normally sighted participants.[100]

Once project staff members were trained as DPM evaluators, they observed that some of the driving tasks previously thought to be too challenging for visually impaired people to attempt were actually not difficult to execute. This was in part because the participants learned to recognize and react to the hazards encountered around them after completing the training regimen.

Another finding is the strong need for formalized programs like the one that existed at WVRC in years past, especially for individuals who are visually challenged and have not prepared themselves conceptually or experientially to understand and perform the driving task.

Of a population sample of 107 individuals who were identified initially as meeting the visual protocol for participation in the study, only 33 of 47 individuals who volunteered to participate in the training aspect of the study were able to satisfactorily complete formalized driver education and training at the center. Despite demonstrating the ability to operate a motor vehicle safely, many project graduates were initially denied access to driver's license testing in West Virginia by the state's driver licensing authority because of their known low visual acuity status and use of bioptic lenses. More than 50% of the project graduates were required to participate in internal DMV administrative appeal hearings to be afforded the opportunity to undergo driver testing. Eventually 32 of 33 participants were granted restricted driver's licenses.

As of February 2003, 27 of these graduates were still residing and driving in West Virginia. Twenty-five were still working full-time. The two graduates who are not working but still residing in West Virginia are in their 80s and only drive sparingly on an as-needed basis (e.g., in emergencies). The five other graduates have since moved out of state, work full-time, and continue to enjoy their driving privileges. The sole graduate of the program who was denied access to driver testing elected not to return to the center for additional driver education and training as recommended by West Virginia driver licensing authorities. He is now a college graduate, is working full-time, and drives a scooter back and forth from his home and nearby place of employment in West Virginia.

Other results describing in detail the accrued driving records of project graduates are published in other articles and materials by Huss.[97]

Since the completion of the West Virginia Low Vision Driving Study, at least 12 states (Connecticut, Georgia, Kentucky, Iowa, Indiana, Michigan, Mississippi, Ohio, Oregon, Tennessee, Virginia, and Washington) have passed or have pending legislation that will permit restrictive driving privileges to people with visual acuity levels down to and including 20/200 on a case-by-case basis.

Since 1986 staff at WVRC have provided short-term in-services at the center to 101 professionals, representative of 15 states and 1 Canadian province that have expressed interest in developing similar formalized programs of low vision driver education and training. Former West Virginia project staff members trained on site approximately 130 other professionals who have been or remain involved in other states' bioptic driver education training and testing programs. The latter includes professionals from Kentucky, Maryland, Ohio, Oregon, Virginia, and West Virginia.

In 2001, along with several committed professionals and consumers with low vision, this author contributed to the development and formation of a nonprofit international organization known as the Bioptic Driving Network, Inc. Its web site, which is devoted to bioptic driving issues and concerns, is free to the public and is located at *www.biopticdriving.org.*

Currently 47 states permit some individuals with vision that is below the normal legal limits to obtain or maintain restrictive driving privileges. Moreover, 34 states allow select individuals with low vision to use bioptics for visual assistance during the driving task after an evaluation of the driver's capabilities has been conducted.

FUTURE CONSIDERATIONS AND NEEDS

This chapter provided an overview of collaborative efforts between professionals from different yet related disciplines who volunteered to work with individuals with low vision who wished to explore driving. The information, disseminated nationally as a result of the West Virginia Low Vision Driving Study, was the third and final objective of the study and has been ongoing since 1986. Almost every state in the United States is permitting restricted driving privileges on a case-by-case basis, and two-thirds of states recognize the benefits that can be derived from allowing the use of bioptics by individuals who have received the appropriate training.

Box 12-3	Ideas for Consideration and Future Research

- Curriculum development and lesson plans for predriver readiness and awareness skills (at the very latest for preadolescence candidates)
- Curriculum development and lesson plans for novice versus experienced motor vehicle operators (whose onset of visual impairment is later in life)
- Ongoing short-term staff training seminars for professionals interested in working with people with low vision who want to obtain or retain their driving privileges (coursework extensions and practice on existing professional preparation, training, programs)
- State-funded and -regulated formalized programs of bioptic driver education, training, and evaluation
- Standardized driver testing measures, including passenger-in-car and on-road testing for bioptic users
- National symposium on bioptic driving to update the states' driver licensing agencies and medical advisory boards about advances in bioptic technology, formalized bioptic driver evaluation and training practices, benefits of standardized passenger-in-car and on-the-road driver testing measures, and accrued driving records of trained versus nontrained bioptic drivers

What additional recommendations can be made in this area to enhance the employability and independence of other people with low vision wanting to drive in the future? Box 12-3 lists some ideas for consideration and future research.

SECTION IV

On-Road Evaluation and Training of Clients with Hearing Impairments

Marilyn Di Stefano

In Chapter 6 we considered the clinical evaluation issues relevant to individuals with hearing loss. In this section we will address the specific factors relevant to hearing loss and on-road evaluation and on-road driver training.

DIFFICULTIES EXPERIENCED WHILE DRIVING

Auditory system impairments may be manifested in different ways depending on the individual's health profile, age, onset of his or her health condition(s), and the nature and degree of the *functional deficit(s)* that are present.[101,102] The direct impact of any such impairment on the driving task will vary depending on many factors, including previous driving history and experience. Hearing impairments do impact on functional status[103] and have been implicated as a risk factor for motor vehicle accidents in groups of older drivers.[104]

The following discussion will refer to auditory system dysfunction related to hearing loss. Other associated difficulties, such as speech and language deficits because of cognitive challenges, are often complex, requiring the DRS performing the on-road driving evaluation to work collaboratively with other health care team members, including occupational therapists who are working as generalists, medical specialists, neuropsychologists, audiologists, and speech-language pathologists. These problems, which often involve a perceptual-cognitive component, are beyond the scope of this section and will not be discussed further.

Table 12-7 presents auditory system impairments that impact on driving with examples of behaviors that may be exhibited by clients with hearing loss during a clinical evaluation or on-road evaluation or training session.

The nature of the driving task and the driving environment will influence whether hearing deficits become evident and problematic for driving. More demanding driving environments (e.g., high vehicle density while traveling at high speeds or unpredictable pedestrian traffic in high density traffic) pose different challenges for accommodating a hearing loss. It will be important for certain clients (e.g., novice drivers learning to drive or older drivers with a recently acquired hearing loss) to be gradually exposed to more complex driving environments during their driving rehabilitation or alternative community mobility program so that they gain insight into the impact of various driving demands and develop suitable coping strategies and skills.

OPTIMIZE THE COMMUNICATION PROCESS AND CREATE AN ENVIRONMENT THAT FACILITATES NEW LEARNING

When a client with a significant hearing loss presents for driver evaluation or community mobility services, it is important to create a suitable environment that helps the client to feel at ease with acknowledging his or her hearing impairment and implementing alternative ways of communicating. If a hearing loss is noted in any referral documentation, it may be useful to seek further information from the client, the referrer, or the client's family. In this way the DRS can be prepared to use the most appropriate communication method with the

Table 12-7   **Auditory System Impairments Impacting on Driving**

Symptom or Condition Related to Impairment of the Auditory System	Examples of Impairments and Their Impact on the Driver and Driving Performance
Difficulty hearing speech environments	Frequently asks for instructions to be repeated, does not hear well in noisy driving environments
Tinnitus (the experience of hearing sounds/noises not originating from the external environment)	Condition interferes with being able to hear sounds from inside/outside the car May fatigue faster, experience headaches, and/or have low concentration span
An imbalance in hearing abilities between the two ears	Difficulty localizing sounds (e.g., the client can hear the siren of an ambulance but does not know from which direction the vehicle is approaching)
Cannot hear certain high frequencies	May not be aware of auditory feedback systems or alarms related to the vehicle controls (e.g., cannot hear a vehicle's indicator "clicks" or reminder chime to fasten a seat belt)
Cannot hear certain low frequencies	Cannot hear whether the engine is running and needs to check visually to ensure that the vehicle's ignition system is working properly Cannot hear if the air conditioning or heater fan is operational
Profound deafness	Requires alternative forms of communication No auditory sensory input is received, and the client may fatigue more easily because he or she must rely entirely on other senses to compensate for the hearing loss

client in the first face-to-face meeting. Developing a positive rapport with clients who are hearing impaired will help them to feel more confident with using alternatives to speech and will optimize the conditions necessary for engaging in dialogue that can help to facilitate new learning.

The following general principles summarize key factors that will assist with the implementation of either a clinical evaluation or on-road training program. Unless otherwise stated the following discussion will refer to the client with a hearing impairment as the client or driver and to the DRS delivering the evaluation or training as the speaker, trainer, or simply the DRS.

ENCOURAGE AN OPEN APPROACH TO THE ISSUE OF HEARING LOSS

Clients with a hearing loss need to feel comfortable discussing their limitations and how they cope with them. Creating an atmosphere of openness and willingness to

face challenges is important. DRSs should ask the client to explain what works best for him or her, and regularly asking for feedback regarding one's communication skills is a good place for a DRS to start. If a DRS has little or no experience working with individuals with hearing impairments, he or she should review the literature, seek the advice of trusted colleagues, and most importantly ask the client about his or her preferred method of communication.

DISCUSS WHICH COMMUNICATION STRATEGIES WORK BEST FOR THE CLIENT

Different clients will have varying needs. For some individuals with a hearing loss, it may be sufficient for a DRS to increase the volume of his or her voice when speaking; however, with others it may be necessary to use a special amplification device in the car, implement speech reading or hand or sign language, or use a combination of these or other strategies.

Lip or Speech Reading and Sign Language

The older term lip reading has now been expanded to the term speech reading, which refers to the speaker's ability to communicate using their face and body and to use the information provided by the language and the situation or context.[105]

To optimize speech reading, the following general factors[106-110] should be considered:

- The speaker should ensure that he or she has the client's full attention.
- It may assist the client with a hearing impairment if the speaker makes an effort to speak more distinctly, clearly, and slowly, while keeping hands away from his or her face. The speaker's body also should be orientated toward the listener.
- Use body language, gestures, and visual cues to augment the spoken word.
- Ensure adequate light so that the hearing-impaired client can clearly see the speaker's face.
- Environmental distractions should be minimized.
- Try to be calm and relaxed to help the client not to become anxious.
- Confirm that the client is wearing his or her hearing aid(s) and/or glasses when applicable to optimize his or her sensory abilities.
- Speech reading relies on the speech reader to fill in the gaps, and sometimes it is easy to make errors. For this reason it may be important to monitor the client's confidence to seek clarification, especially with clients who may be shy or reluctant to acknowledge that they have a disability.
- The client should be alert and focused on the driving task; the DRS should be aware that speech reading can be fatiguing. It may be better to schedule appointments in the morning or at other times of the day when the client is well rested.
- DRSs should plan for additional time to accommodate alternative communication methods, especially initially.

Using Alternatives to Speech in a Vehicle

If speech reading is to be used for on-road driver evaluation or training, implementation requires careful planning. The primary concern is that speech reading requires a client with a hearing impairment to look at the speaker, and in a dynamic driving context this can be distracting and even dangerous because the client's and DRS's eyes are not focused on the road ahead of the vehicle.

One way of addressing this problem is to provide opportunities for closed-circuit or off-road evaluation and training initially. This will allow the client and DRS to establish and refine alternative communication methods and vehicle-handling skills in a much safer and controlled environment, in which it is possible to maneuver the training vehicle without having to be concerned with a potentially dangerous traffic environment.

When it is suitable to move to an open on-road context, there may be an initial requirement for frequent pulling off the road to the curb, so that the client can face the speaker and be fully engaged in the communication process without having to be concerned with negotiating traffic. Choosing an appropriate driving route and low-density traffic environment is important. For example a quiet residential street with little through traffic during nonpeak hours may be suitable. As the client's skills improve and the communication process becomes more reliable and consistent, the client can be gradually exposed to increasingly more complex driving maneuvers and traffic conditions.

In some situations it may be best to use a combination of speech reading and sign language. The client could teach the trainer a series of hand signals that convey key commands, such as stop, go, slow, fast, pull to the curb, turn left, turn right, first street, second street, and so forth. If the client is used to using sign language, he or she will be able to identify and demonstrate the signs that are meaningful. It may help the trainer to write these down, practice them, and at least initially have a prompt sheet handy in the motor vehicle to refer to from time to time as needed.

Some general principles regarding the use of speech reading or sign language in the vehicle when instructing or giving feedback include the following[110,111]:

- Carefully grade the evaluation or training program so that easier, more achievable tasks are attempted first, which will help to consolidate communication and driving-related skills and a gradual increase in the client's confidence level
- A written plan for training, including measurable goals and performance criteria, will assist with tracking a client's progress and documenting his or her on-road driving performance
- Provide encouragement and constructive criticism when either is warranted
- Provide feedback verbally or via alternative communication such as sign language
- Provide written feedback to the client after the driving session has been completed to reinforce learning
- Use visual aids, such as diagrams and scale model cars, to assist with reviewing different driving responses during hypothetical driving scenarios
- Observe and talk about the driving environment to reinforce learning (e.g., observe and discuss how other drivers perform particular driving maneuvers in varied settings and in different circumstances)

- Confirm that hearing-impaired clients understand complex ideas by asking them to explain what they have learned; communication is necessary to discern their comprehension level
- The presence of a family member or significant other who is willing to work with the client once the training session has concluded may help to reinforce the client's understanding outside the formal on-road training sessions

If the client has some residual hearing, then it is important to keep the following in mind:

- Reduce any background noise
- Avoid the use of fans, and close the vehicle's windows whenever possible
- Confirm that the client is wearing his or her hearing aid(s), and encourage him or her to carry spare batteries in case they are needed during an on-road training session

COMPENSATION STRATEGIES FOR INDIVIDUALS WITH HEARING LOSS

The best way for clients to make up for hearing loss while driving is to optimize their other senses to compensate for the lack of sensory information available through the hearing modality. This is why it is so vital in the clinical evaluation to confirm optimal function of alternate sensory abilities. These must provide all the sensory information from the immediate environment within the car and the external driving environment to enable safe and consistent driving performance.

Clients must rely primarily on visual and sensorimotor feedback systems (e.g., proprioception, kinesthesia, and tactile sensation) to effectively interpret and respond to a vehicle's interior displays and controls. Vehicle designers are increasingly developing systems that feature sounds and digitized or recorded speech to alert clients to the status of various control and safety systems. Numerous vehicle functions include auditory feedback (e.g., a series of clicks, beeps, or warning tones) and visual feedback that features illuminated displays on the dashboard (e.g., indicator operation and cruise control, as well as key, light, and seat belt reminder systems). When a client is deaf or hard of hearing he or she will need to check vehicle function status visually; for example a client can check the vehicle's indicators by either looking at the indicator displays or symbols on the dashboard or checking the actual position of the indicator levers.

It may be appropriate to investigate the possibility of amplifying the volume of existing auditory feedback systems if clients have some residual hearing. In other instances the client may be able to compensate for the lack of hearing by obtaining feedback regarding certain vehicle functions (e.g., engine ignition and operation of climate control functions) via vibration, touch, or temperature senses. Whether these options can be used will depend on the specific characteristics of the vehicle being driven and the integrity of the client's other sensory systems.

Clients with hearing loss must be cognizant of the need to frequently visually check the environment around their vehicles. Optimizing awareness of blind spots can often be accomplished by visually scanning the environment using adapted interior and exterior mirrors that expand the client's field of view. Because the visual sensory system plays such an important role in maintaining optimal visual surveillance of the external driving environment, it is crucial that the client is positioned correctly within the driver's compartment. Correct seat height, backrest position, postural support, seat angle, and adjustment of the steering wheel will facilitate optimal positioning of the client. Moreover minimizing the use of stickers on windshields and tags (e.g., parking or handicapped placards) hanging from rearview mirrors and avoiding obstructions close to windows (e.g., items on the rear parcel shelf) are also worthwhile safety considerations.

It also may be worthwhile to consider training in defensive driving techniques to assist with negotiating complex driving environments in which the client with a hearing loss may be particularly at a disadvantage. Many defensive driving strategies build on the concepts related to hazard perception and situational awareness. Clients are educated and trained to assess the immediate external driving environment and what is further ahead along their travel path, so that they can adjust the vehicle's speed and plan their driving movements accordingly. There is an emphasis in defensive driving approaches on anticipating (and learning to accommodate or negotiate) the behaviors of other drivers and road users. Anticipating what other road users may or may not do can help to ensure that suitable *tactical driving* decisions are made with sufficient time to avoid potentially hazardous and even deadly situations.

Performing tasks that are extraneous to driving usually are not warranted because they place an additional psychomotor load on drivers. Drivers must maintain a high level of vigilance with regard to visual awareness to efficiently interpret and respond to the dynamic driving environment. That is, any task that is distracting and requires additional visual and cognitive demands could decrease safe driving performance. Minimizing distractions is important for all road users, and clients with major hearing loss are no different. There are numerous ways that drivers can easily become distracted, including the following examples: communication tasks, such as using a cellular phone or other electronic device for text messaging; navigational tasks, such as attempting to read a map or computer-generated directions, responding to a frustrated copilot, or using a global positioning system (GPS) while discussing with a passenger issues related to topographic orientation; and drivers who demonstrate high-risk behavior when they perform ADL in their cars, such as shaving, applying makeup, and eating a quick meal from a fast food restaurant. These are just a few of the ways in which drivers become distracted and increase the likelihood of a traffic accident. Of course these tasks are always best undertaken before getting into a vehicle or after a driver has pulled his or her vehicle over to the curb and is not interacting with other road users.

Clients with hearing impairments must also address the communication methods that enable interaction between road users and vehicle support personnel, such as gas station attendants and auto mechanics. For example drivers typically communicate with each other by using indicators such as brake lights, turn signals, hazard lights, gestures, and maneuvering the vehicle itself, to name a few. There are occasions when using the vehicle's horn is necessary to alert other road users of one's location, when road users have committed a driving error that could impact their safety or the safety of others, or to alert others when there is a hazard on the roadway. Clients with hearing impairments may not hear when other drivers use their horns; therefore they may need to strategize ways to contend with drivers who may become frustrated and demonstrate aggressive driving behaviors. Finally communication strategies need to be identified and practiced during simulated scenarios, which should include, but are certainly not limited to, purchasing gasoline, interacting with automobile mechanics, dealing with other road users in a situation in which an exchange of personal information is required such as a motor vehicle accident, and communicating with police officers and emergency medical professionals.

COMMUNICATION METHODS USED IN DYNAMIC DRIVING ENVIRONMENTS

As previously noted it is essential to ascertain the client's degree of hearing impairment and his or her preferred communication method before commencing with the clinical evaluation or on-road evaluation. It also is important that the client has taken the necessary steps to optimize his or her hearing before participating in the on-road evaluation or training. If severe or profound hearing loss requires the DRS and client to use alternative communication methods such as speech

reading or sign language, the DRS may require specialized training to learn particular communication techniques. Trial testing the selected communication method before it is implemented in a more demanding and dangerous on-road situation is advised.

IMPLEMENTING THE ON-ROAD EVALUATION

Many driver rehabilitation programs rely on standard driving routes as the basis for on-road evaluation protocols. This approach helps to optimize equity, reliability, and validity of testing procedures.[16,41] Implementing such a test, which usually relies on the client following verbal instructions given by the DRS, poses some unique and interesting challenges for clients with hearing impairments and DRSs.

If the standard route is located in a geographic area that is unfamiliar to the client, a combination of sign language symbols together with predetermined locations along the driving route that allow clients to pull over to the curb can be used to allow the DRS to communicate the next set of route instructions to the client. Referencing a street directory for topographic orientation would facilitate the curb-side communication session. Such an approach to evaluation relies on well-coordinated, nonspeech communication skills between the DRS and client, a high level of driving skill proficiency, intact short-term memory, and sufficient confidence. If these conditions are not met, it may be difficult to implement an equitable, consistent, and valid testing procedure.

DRSs may opt to review the standard travel routes with their clients before the on-road evaluation to reinforce the program's general expectations, requirements, and travel routes. This would of course contravene usual testing criteria because it could be argued that the client has the advantage of practicing and is being trained to pass the test rather than pass the criteria for the test. Another option might be for the DRS and client to plan an alternative route together in a familiar area that would meet all the evaluation route criteria (e.g., negotiating a certain number of complex intersections, completing a parking maneuver, and a freeway entry and exit). It also would be important to ensure that the test route adequately, but not unfairly, exposes clients to situations that might elicit the compensatory strategies that they have learned to use to overcome the functional implications of their hearing loss. For example it may be important to see how the client negotiates the following:

- A busy strip mall shopping area or car park where there are pedestrians and other road users (e.g., cyclists, adults and children, and animals)

- Roadways where there is industrial traffic (e.g., trucks, vans, and cars) that creates background noise or blocks a client's view of the broader traffic environment
- Complex intersections that are visually demanding (e.g., intersections that contain numerous traffic signs that require expeditious interpretation and response, automatic traffic signals that place time demands on a client's decision making, and increased numbers of pedestrians and other more vulnerable road users)
- Railway crossings or negotiation of shared roadways with other vehicles (e.g., trams and buses)

Some degree of flexibility with testing procedures may be warranted to balance the requirements to meet test criteria and adequate communication without unduly increasing the client's performance anxiety and creating an unsafe testing situation.

The DRS can tailor the demands of the on-road driving evaluation to meet the requirements of the driver evaluation program and the relevant licensing authority. As discussed in other sections, some clients are required to pass a specialist test with a certified assessor and a licensing authority test. In such cases usually the driving assessor has prime responsibility to report on the impact of any health-related functional limitations on driving, whereas the licensing authority determines whether the applicant can meet the criteria for licensure. The assessor may be required to comment on the need for license conditions and restrictions, such as vehicle adaptations and limiting driving within a specified geographic area or during a specific time frame.

LICENSING ISSUES

The implications of hearing loss on the driving task must be considered within the context of clients' health and medical status, their work and lifestyle, the geographic location where they live, and other relevant factors. License conditions for clients with health conditions, medical impairments, and functional limitations will depend on what the respective licensing authority in the client's geographic location permits and what can be effectively implemented and monitored. DRSs recommend license restrictions with the aim of assisting clients to accommodate their hearing loss and its impact on driving. Driving restrictions are generally implemented to optimize clients' visual surveillance of the driving environment. For example the client may be permitted to drive only if the vehicle meets one or more of the following criteria:

- A minimum of two external mirrors (i.e., one on each side of the vehicle)

- An additional internal mirror that is positioned to show a view of the blind spot on the driver's side of the vehicle
- Additional convex or fisheye mirrors to expand and enhance the vehicle's rear and side views

Depending on the client's other issues, in some instances it also may be appropriate to recommend that a profoundly hearing-impaired client not drive certain vehicles. This may apply to large trucks, vans, or types of four-wheel drive vehicles that have the driver positioned well above the roadway and do not allow for adequate visual surveillance to the side or rear of the vehicle without special provisions. For other hearing-impaired clients, it also may be problematic to tow a boat, caravan, horse float, or trailer. Such vehicles usually require drivers to modify their driving techniques (e.g., merging, overtaking, parking, accelerating, and stopping) and to implement more complex driving skills over and above the well-learned, routine skills they rely on to drive a standard-sized vehicle. Therefore clients driving such vehicles must cope with additional cognitive and sensory or motor requirements over and above the elevated information-processing demands associated with trying to compensate for a lack of sensory information from the hearing modality. DRSs must evaluate clients' capabilities on a case-by-case basis. As mentioned in other sections, some licensing jurisdictions place restrictions on individuals with hearing impairments who seek a commercial license, depending on the degree of loss and vehicle adaptations.[112]

In some jurisdictions DRSs may also be required to make recommendations to licensing authorities regarding the need for medical, paramedical, or on-road test reviews. The need for formally implemented systems to ensure clients have such checks will depend on the nature of their impairments, their age, any intervening factors that may influence their functional abilities, and the requirements of the licensing jurisdictions.[113]

SELF-REGULATION OF DRIVING

Although not all clients with hearing impairment report that they regulate their driving,[114] some groups of drivers (e.g., older drivers) do consciously reduce the demands associated with driving. They do this by managing their exposure to driving tasks as demonstrated by their choices regarding when, where, and how they drive.[115-117] Some examples of self-regulation of driving strategies, which can be applicable to clients with hearing impairments, include the following:

- Mapping out the route ahead of time to reduce the complexity of the travel path (e.g., reducing the number of turns required, avoiding complex intersections, and staying on streets versus using freeways)

- Traveling with passengers who can assist with navigational tasks if required while acknowledging the potentially distracting effect of having passengers acting as copilots
- Avoiding driving during times of likely traffic congestion
- Avoiding driving at night or during inclement weather

Considering the specific issues related to the detrimental effect of background noise or not being able to hear sounds from the external driving environment, the following strategies also may be relevant:

- Avoiding travel routes with noisy industrial traffic
- Avoiding travel routes with unpredictable and heavy pedestrian traffic
- Driving when alert, and avoiding getting behind the wheel when fatigued
- Avoiding driving when taking over-the-counter medications, prescription medications, or both that can cause drowsiness and decrease reaction time
- Avoiding the use of radios, compact disk players, cellular phones, and other devices that can be distracting

All these techniques can help clients process critical information and important cues within the driving environment with greater efficiency, thereby leaving them with sufficient cognitive resources, such as attention and problem solving, to compensate for their hearing loss. Other strategies relevant to maintaining driving independence, which may be applicable to this client group, are discussed further in other sections.

CASE STUDY

Sarah had profound bilateral hearing loss associated with her premature birth. She could not benefit from hearing aids and used a combination of speech and sign language to communicate. Sarah was completing her high school education in a mainstream school and sought to keep up with her peers by learning how to drive. She enjoyed a variety of passive teenage interests (e.g., movies, computer games, and playing cards) but did not participate in sports because she lacked upper and lower extremity coordination. Sarah had managed to obtain her written learner's permit and approached the local driving school for lessons. The instructor tried to manage the communication requirements in a few closed-circuit training sessions but did not feel adequately qualified to continue with her driver education. He subsequently referred Sarah to a DRS for a comprehensive driver rehabilitation evaluation that included a clinical evaluation and an on-road driver evaluation. A medical evaluation and completion of the licensing authority's medical report form and an up-to-date review of her communication needs by a speech and language pathologist were prerequisites for entry into the driver rehabilitation program.

The DRS met with Sarah and her parents as part of the clinical evaluation to clarify what the driving goals were and to ascertain the level of family support. The consensus was to aim for Sarah to initially obtain a local area license if possible. The clinical evaluation process helped the driver rehabilitation team to determine that Sarah lacked basic knowledge of the rules of the road and traffic laws, had reduced visual acuity that was previously undetected, had slowed reaction time, and had reduced upper and lower extremity coordination and endurance. The DRS initiated a referral to a vision specialist to address Sarah's apparent need for glasses and to an occupational therapy generalist for a remedial program aimed at improving her motor deficits. Sarah and her parents also worked on improving her knowledge of road laws and rules, as well as undertaking twice-weekly commentary drives with Sarah as a passenger as a means of increasing her general awareness of driving skills and defensive driving techniques.

Three months later a clinical reevaluation highlighted sufficient improvement to enable an on-road evaluation and on-road training. The DRS had also in the interim period undertaken some training to learn techniques relevant to speech and sign language. A number of driving lessons were undertaken in a closed-circuit environment to consolidate basic vehicle handling and compensatory driving techniques. Sarah's father always sat in during each formal lesson because he was supervising additional sessions at home to reinforce key learning strategies. Training in traffic was based on a graded program with an emphasis on developing situational awareness and compensatory visual scanning skills. Sarah and her father agreed that Sarah would maintain a logbook to record the frequency, duration, and nature of each training session that was reviewed to reinforce learning. After sufficient training had occurred, Sarah undertook a driver's license test to enable her to gain a restricted area license. Although legally able to drive independently, Sarah and her parents agreed that one of her parents should accompany her for the first month of her probationary driving period to help ensure that she remembered her driving techniques and to help boost her confidence. A telephone review of her driving situation was scheduled every other month for the first 6 months of her licensure. It was agreed that Sarah and her parents would discuss the issue of local area versus open license status with the DRS after she had held her license for 1 year without being involved in a motor vehicle accident or receiving a traffic citation (e.g., speeding ticket).

SUMMARY

Clients with hearing loss who are seeking driver evaluation and rehabilitation services have special needs that must be readily identified and addressed by DRSs. Clients' needs and driving outcomes will be influenced by the onset, nature, and severity of their hearing impairment and by their preferred communication method(s), driving experience, and other related factors. DRSs must assess how other client factors will impact on driving and community mobility during the clinical evaluation and the on-road evaluation or on-road training. DRSs also should collaborate with therapy specialists to ensure that their clients receive specialist services whenever it is deemed appropriate by the driver rehabilitation team. The intervention strategies subscribed to are influenced by a client-centered approach, the expertise and professional training of the DRS, the driver rehabilitation team's philosophy about evaluation and intervention, the client's priorities for goal attainment, and the requirements of the respective state licensing authority.

REFERENCES

1. Galski T, Ehle HT, Williams JB: Off-road driving evaluations for persons with cerebral injury: a factor analytic study of predriver and simulator testing, *Am J Occup Ther* 51:352-359, 1997.
2. Lee HC, Cameron D, Lee AH: Assessing the driving performance of older adult drivers: on-road versus simulated driving, *Accid Anal Prevent* 35:797-803, 2003.
3. Lee HC, Lee AH, Cameron D, et al: Using a driving simulator to identify older drivers at inflated risk of motor vehicle crashes, *J Safety Res* 34:453-459, 2003.
4. Messinger-Rapport B: How to assess and counsel the older driver, *Cleve Clin J Med* 69:184-192, 2002.
5. Fenton S, Kraft W, Marks E: Section II: therapeutic driving and community mobility, Chapter 24, Evaluation of areas of occupation. In Crepeau EB, Cohn ES, Boyt Schell BA, editors: *Willard and Spackman's occupational therapy*, Philadelphia, 2003, Lippincott Williams & Wilkins, pp. 340-341.
6. Hunt LA: A profile of occupational therapists as driving instructors and evaluators for elderly drivers, *IATSS Res* 20:46-47, 1996.
7. Lewis SC: Driving and the older adult. In Lewis SC, editor: *Elder care in occupational therapy*, New York, 2003, Slack, pp 311-321.
8. Rogers JC, Holm MB: Section 1: Activities of daily living and instrumental activities of daily living, Chapter 24, Evaluation of areas of occupation. In Crepeau EB, Cohn ES, Boyt Schell BA, editors: *Willard and Spackman's occupational therapy*, ed 10, Philadelphia, 2003, Lippincott Williams & Wilkins, pp 315-339.
9. Di Stefano M, Macdonald W: *Survey of Australian occupational therapists to determine disabled driver on-road assessment practice*, Paper presented at the World Federation of Occupational Therapists Conference: Sharing a Global Perspective, May 31-June 5, 1998, Montreal, Canada.
10. Di Stefano M, Macdonald W: Assessment of older drivers: relationships among on-road errors, medical conditions and test outcome, *J Safety Res* 34:415-429, 2003.
11. Klavora P, Young M, Heslegrave RJ: A review of a major driver rehabilitation centre: a ten-year client profile, *Can J Occup Ther* April:128-134, 2000.
12. School of Occupational Therapy: *Driver assessment and rehabilitation course manual*, Melbourne, Victoria, 2003, La Trobe University.
13. Schold Davis E: Defining OT roles in driving, *OT Practice* January 13:15-18, 2003.
14. American Medical Association and National Highway Traffic Safety Administration: *Physician's guide to assessing and counseling older drivers*, 2003. Available at: http://www.ama-assn.org/ama/pub/category/10791.html. Accessed September 2, 2003.
15. Macdonald WA, Scott T: *Disabled driver test procedures*, Canberra, 1993, Federal Office of Road Safety.
16. Withaar FK, Brouwer WH, Van Zomeren AH: Critical review: fitness to drive in older drivers with cognitive impairment, *J Int Neuropsychol Soc* 6:480-490, 2000.
17. Victorian State Government: *Road safety act 27 and road safety procedures regulations*, 1988.
18. VicRoads: *Resources and guidelines for OT driving assessors*, Melbourne, 2000, Roads Corporation.
19. National Highway Traffic Safety Administration, U.S. Department of Transportation: *Safe mobility for older people notebook*, 1999. Available at: *http://www.nhtsa.dot.gov/people/injury/olddrive/safe/*. Accessed September 6, 2004.
20. Fildes B, Pronk N, Langford J, et al: *Model licence re-assessment procedure for older and disabled drivers* (Report to Austroads no. AP-R 176/00), Melbourne, Victoria, 2000, Monash University Accident Research Centre.
21. Janke M, Eberhard J: Assessing medically impaired older drivers in a licensing agency setting, *Accid Anal Prevent* 30:347-361, 1998.
22. Friedenberg L: *Psychological testing: design, analysis and use*, Boston, 1995, Allyn & Bacon.
23. Anastasi A, Urbina S: *Psychological testing*, ed 7, Upper Saddle River, NJ, 1997, Prentice Hall.
24. Crocker L, Algina J: *Introduction to classical and modern test theory*, New York, 1986, Holt, Rinehart and Winston.
25. Ramsay MC, Reynolds CR: Development of a scientific test: a practical guide. In Goldstein G, Hersen M, editors: *Handbook of psychological assessment*, Amsterdam, 2000, Pergamon.
26. Cushman LA: Cognitive capacity and concurrent driving performance in older drivers, *IATSS Res* 20:38-45, 1996.
27. Heikkila V-M, Turrka J, Korpelainen J, et al: Decreased driving ability in people with Parkinson's disease, *J Neurol Neurosurg Psychiatry* 64:325-330, 1998.
28. Lundberg C, Hakamies-Blomqvist L: Driving tests with older patients: effect of unfamiliar versus familiar vehicle, *Transportation Res Part* 6:163-173, 2003.

29. Mazer BL, Korner-Bitensky N, Sofer S: Predicting ability to drive after stroke, *Arch Phys Med Rehabil* 79:743-749, 1998.

30. Macdonald W: *Driving competencies for learner drivers* (No. RUB 97/98-13), Melbourne, Victoria, 1998, VicRoads.

31. Siegrist SE: *Driver training, testing and licensing: towards theory-based management of young drivers' injury risk in road traffic. Results of EU-Project GADGET, Work Package 3.* (bfu Report no. 1/99/500). Berne, 1999, Accident Prevention bfu Human Research Department, Swiss Council.

32. Austroads: *Novice car driver competency specification AP-121/95*, Sydney, 1995, Austroads.

33. Dobbs A, Heller R, Schopflocker D: A comparative approach to identify unsafe older drivers, *Accid Anal Prevent* 30:363-370, 1998.

34. McKnight AJ: The validity and reliability of road test scoring by means of programmed versus extemporaneous observations, *J Traffic Educ* 36:6-9, 1989.

35. Vanosdall FE, Rudisill MD: The new Michigan driver performance test, *Proceedings of the American Association for Automotive Medicine*, Louisville, October 1979.

36. Fabre J, Christie R, Frank L: *Victorian car drive test evaluation: report RN/88/3*, Melbourne, Victoria, 1988, Road Traffic Authority.

37. McKnight AJ, Stewart MA: *Development of competency based driver license testing system* (contract no. 88-424), 1990, California Department of Motor Vehicles.

38. Jones MH: Safe performance curriculum: performance measures development. Final report, Los Angeles, 1978, University of Southern California.

39. McPherson K, McKnight AJ: *Automobile driver on-road performance test, Volume I: final report* (Publication no. DOT-HS-806-207), Washington, DC, 1981, National Highway Traffic Safety Administration.

40. Christie R: *Driver licensing requirements and performance standards including driver and rider training*, Melbourne, Australia, 2000, National Road Transport Commission.

41. Fox GK, Bowden SC, Smith DS: On-road assessment of driving competence after brain impairment: review of current practice and recommendations for a standardized examination, *Arch Phys Med Rehabil* 79:1288-1296, 1998.

42. Hunt LA, Murphy C, Carr DB, et al: Reliability of the Washington University Road Test: a performance-based assessment for drivers with dementia of the Alzheimer type, *Arch Neurol* 54:707-712, 1997.

43. Janke MK: Assessing older drivers: two studies, *J Safety Res* 32:43-74, 2001.

44. VicRoads: *Pola Criteria: version 3.01, December 1999*, Melbourne, 1999, Roads Corporation.

45. Macdonald WA, Griffith J, Gregory S, et al: *Performance capacity evaluation of head-injured drivers: an investigation of the validity of some off-road tests*, Proceedings of the 28th Annual Conference of the Ergonomics Society of Australia, Melbourne, Australia, 1992, pp. 92-99.

46. Gouvier WD, Maxfield MW, Schweitzer JR, et al: Psychometric prediction of driving performance among the disabled, *Arch Phys Med Rehabil* 70:745-750, 1989.

47. Korteling JE, Kaptein NA: Neuropsychological driving, fitness tests for brain-damaged subjects, *Arch Phys Med Rehabil* 77:138-146, 1996.

48. Di Stefano M, Macdonald W: *Driver errors on OT tests: implications for on road testing procedures*, Paper presented at the OT Australia 22nd National Conference and Exhibition, Melbourne, Australia, 2003.

49. Hunt LA, Murphy C, Carr DB, et al: Environmental cueing may affect performance on a road test for drivers with dementia of the Alzheimer type, *Alzheimer Dis Assoc Disord* 11(suppl 1):13-16, 1997.

50. School of Occupational Therapy, LaTrobe University: *Driver education and rehabilitation course manual for occupational therapists*, Melbourne, 2003, School of Occupational Therapy, La Trobe University.

51. Galski T, Enle HT, Bruno RL: An assessment of measures to predict the outcome of driving evaluations in patients with cerebral damage, *Am J Occup Ther* 44:709-713, 1990.

52. Antrim JM, Engum ES: The driving dilemma and the law: patients' striving for independence vs public safety, *Cogn Rehabil* March/April:16-19, 1989.

53. Odenheimer GL, Beaudet M, Jette AM, et al: Performance based driving evaluation of the elderly driver: safety, reliability and validity, *J Gerontol Med Sci* 49:M153-M159, 1994.

54. Di Stefano M, Macdonald W: *Driving instructor interventions during on-road tests of functionally impaired drivers: implications for test criteria*, Proceedings of the 2003 Road Safety Research, Policing and Education Conference, Sydney, Australia, 2003, pp. 70-77.

55. Janke MK, Hersch SW: *Assessing the older driver: pilot studies* (no. RSS-97-172), Sacramento, 1997, California Department of Motor Vehicles Research and Development Branch.

56. McKnight AJ, McKnight AS: Multivariate analysis of age related driver ability and performance deficits, *Accid Anal Prevent* 31:445-454, 1999.

57. Staplin L, Gish KW, Decina L, et al: *Intersection negotiation problems of older drivers: volume 1: final technical report* (Final Technical Report, October 1993-September 1997. no. 1446/FR), Washington, DC, 1998, Office of Research and Traffic Records, National Highway Traffic Safety Administration.

58. Staplin L, Gish KW, Decina L, et al: *Intersection negotiation problems of older drivers: volume II: background synthesis on age and intersection driving difficulties* (No. contract DTNH22-93-C-05237), Washington, DC, 1998, Office of Research and Traffic Records, National Highway Traffic Safety Administration.

59. Groeger JA, Rothengatter JA: Traffic psychology and behaviour, *Transportation Res Part F* 1:1-9, 1998.

60. Groeger JA: *Understanding driving: applying cognitive psychology to a complex everyday task*, East Sussex, 2000, Psychology Press.

61. Rothengatter T: Errors and violations as factors in accident causation. In Rothengatter T, Carbonell Vaya E, editors: *Traffic and transport psychology: theory and application*, Amsterdam, 1997, Pergamon, pp. 59-64.

62. Macdonald W: *Functional abilities needed to drive safely*. Paper presented at the Proceedings of the International Conference on Aging, Disability and Independence, Washington, DC, 2004. Available at: *http://icadi.phhp.ufl.edu/2003/ppt/macdonald1.ppt. Accessed October 30, 2004.*

63. Engum ES, Lambert W: Restandardisation of the cognitive behavioural driver's inventory, *Cogn Rehabil* 8:20-27, 1990.
64. Sivak M, Olson PL, Kewman DG, et al: Driving and perceptual/cognitive skills: behavioural consequences of brain damage, *Arch Phys Med Rehabil* 62:476-483, 1981.
65. Van Zomeren AH, Wrouwer WH, Rothengatter JA, et al: Fitness to drive a car after recovery from severe head injury, *Arch Phys Med Rehabil* 69:90-96, 1988.
66. Daigneault G, Joly P, Frigon J-Y: Executive functions in the evaluation of accident risk of older drivers, *J Clin Exp Neuropsychol* 24:221-238, 2002.
67. Fildes B: *Safety of older drivers: strategy for future research and management initiatives* (General Report, 1997, No. 118), Melbourne, Victoria, 1997, Monash University: Monash University Accident Research Centre.
68. Hakamies-Blomqvist L: Fatal accidents of older drivers, *Accid Anal Prevent* 25:19-27, 1993.
69. Preusser DF, Williams AF, Ferguson SA, et al: Fatal crash risk for older drivers at intersections, *Accid Anal Prevent* 30:151-159, 1998.
70. Ryan GA, Legge M, Rosman D: Age related changes in drivers' crash risk and crash type, *Accid Anal Prevent* 30:379-387, 1998.
71. Macdonald WA: *Driving performance measures and licence tests: a literature review* (Federal Office of Road Safety Report CR57), Victoria, 1987, Road Traffic Authority.
72. Harris M: Psychiatric conditions with relevance to fitness to drive, *Adv Psychiatr Treatment* 6:261-269, 2000.
73. Ekelman BA, Mitchell S, O'Dell-Rossi P: Driving and older adults. In Bonder BR, Wagner MB, editors: *Functional performance in older adults*, ed 2, Philadelphia, 2001, FA Davis Company, pp. 448-472.
74. Jacobs K: OTs in the driver's seat: occupational therapy provides an ideal background for driver rehabilitation specialists, *Rehab Manag* February/March:126-127, 1994.
75. Holm MB, Rogers JC, James AB: Treatment of occupational performance areas: treatment of activities of daily living. In Neistadt ME, Blesedell Crepeau E, editors: *Willard and Spackman's occupational therapy*, ed 9, Philadelphia, 1998, Lippincott, pp. 323-363.
76. Watson DE: *Task analysis: an occupational performance approach*, Bethesda, 1997, American Occupational Therapy Association.
77. Frith WJ: *Engineering for safe mobility for older land transport users*, Paper presented at the Road Safety Committee of the Victorian Government, Mobility and Safety of Older People Conference, Sheraton Towers, Melbourne, Australia, 2002.
78. Hildebrand ED, Hutchinson BG: *An activity based travel needs model for the elderly*, Proceedings of the Transportation Research Board 78th Annual Meeting, Washington, DC, January 10-14, 1999.
79. Eberhard J: Safe mobility for senior citizens, *IATSS Res* 20:29-37, 1996.
80. Di Stefano M, Macdonald W: *Older driver errors on VicRoads "review" tests*, Paper presented at the RS2002: Road Safety, Research and Policing Conference, Adelaide, Australia, November 3-5, 2002.
81. Dittmar SS, Gresham GE: *Functional assessment and outcome measures for the rehabilitation health professional*, Gaithersburg, MD, 1997, Aspen.
82. Goldstein G, Hersen M: *Handbook of psychological assessment*, Amsterdam, 2000, Pergamon.
83. Schneider C: *Competency standards for occupational therapy driver assessors*, Melbourne, 1998, OT Australia, Victoria.
84. Charlton J, Koppel S, O'Hare M, et al: *Influence of chronic illness on crash involvement of motor vehicle drivers* (Literature review no. 213), Melbourne, 2004, Monash University Accident Research Centre.
85. National Older Driver Research and Training Center and University of Florida: *Summary report international older driver consensus conference*, 2003. Available at: *http://driving.phhp.ufl.edu/ publications/CC%20Summary%20Final%2008-19-04.pdf*. Accessed August 29, 2004.
86. Kalina TD: Starting a driver rehabilitation program, *WORK J Prevent Assess Rehabil* 8:229-238, 1997.
87. Burg A: An investigation of some relationships between dynamic visual acuity, static visual acuity and driving record, *Int Library Arch Museum Optometry* (Report 64-18), 1964.
88. Burg A: Some preliminary findings concerning the relation between vision and driving performance, *J Am Optom Assoc* 38:372-377, 1967.
89. Burg A: Vision test scores and driving record: additional findings, *Int Library Arch Museum Optometry* (Report 68-27), 1968.
90. Higgins KE, Wood E, Tait A: Closed road driving performance: effect of degradation of visual acuity. In *Vision science and its applications, vol 1, OSA Technical Digest Series* (78-81), Washington, DC, 1996, Optical Society of America.
91. Wood JM, Higgins KE: How well does high contrast acuity predict driving performance? *Ophthalmology* 104:997-1003, 1999.
92. Peli E, Peli D: *Driving with confidence: a practical guide to driving with low vision*, Singapore, 2002, World Scientific Publishing Co, p 123.
93. National Conference on Telescopic Devices and Driving: Report on 1975 New York Telescopic Lens System and Driver Licensing Workshop, Washington, DC, 1975, Safety Management Institute.
94. Fonda G: Bioptic telescopic spectacles for driving a motor vehicle, *Arch Ophthalmol* 92:348-349, 1974.
95. Kenney A: Field loss vs. central magnification: telescopes and the driving risk, *Arch Ophthalmol* 92:273, 1974.
96. Huss CP: Model approach—low vision driver's training and assessment, *J Vision Rehabil* 2:31-44, 1988.
97. Huss CP: Training the low vision driver. In Stuen C, Arditi A, Horowitz A, et al, editors: *Vision '99: vision rehabilitation: assessment, intervention and outcomes*, New York, 2000, Swets & Zeitlinger Publishers b.v., pp. 264-267.
98. Doron Precision Systems, Inc: *Driver educational audio visual programs*, Binghamton, NY, 1985, Doron.
99. Huss CP: *Driving with bioptic telescopic lens systems*. Paper presentation at the Eye and the Auto International Forum, Auburn Hills, MI, 2001, Daimler Chrysler Technology Center.
100. Forbes TW, Nolan O, et al: Driver performance measurement based on dynamic driver behavior

patterns in rural, urban, suburban and freeway traffic, *Accid Anal Prevent* 7:257-280, 1975.

101. Ballantyne J: Deafness: types and clinical characteristics. In Ballantyne J, Martin MC, Martin A, editors: *Deafness*, ed 5, London, 1993, Whurr Publishers Ltd., pp. 62-65.

102. Doyle J: Forms of hearing difficulty. In Doyle J, Bench J, Day N, et al, editors: *Practical audiology for speech-language therapists*, London, 1998, Whurr Publishers, pp. 32-57.

103. Keller BK, Morton JL, Thomas VS, et al: The effect of visual and hearing impairments on functional status, *J Am Geriatr Soc* 47:1319-1325, 1999.

104. Ivers RQ, Mitchell P, Cumming RG: Sensory impairment and driving: the Blue Mountains eye study, *Am J Public Health* 89:85-87, 1999.

105. VicDeaf HEAR Service: Lip reading/speech reading, 1999. Available at: *http://www.vicdeaf.com.au/informationResources*. Accessed June 16, 2004.

106. Davis P: *Listen up! Overcoming hearing loss*, Woollahra, Australia, 1996, Gore and Osment Publications.

107. Fozard JL, Gordon-Salant S: Changes in vision and hearing with aging. In Birren JE, Warner Schaie K, Abeles RP, et al, editors: *Handbook of the psychology of aging*, ed 5, San Diego, 2001, Academic Press.

108. National Institute on Deafness and Other Communication Disorders: *Statistics about hearing disorders, ear infections and deafness*, Bethesda, MD, 2004, National Institute on Deafness and Other Communication Disorders. Available at: *http://www.nidcd.nih.gov/index.asp*. Accessed June 16, 2004.

109. Shimon DA: *Coping with hearing loss and hearing aids*, San Diego, 1992, Singular Publishing Group, Inc.

110. VicDeaf HEAR Service: Understanding Hearing Loss, 2002. Available at: *http://www.vicdeaf.com.au/informationResources*. Accessed June 16, 2004.

111. Fisk AD, Rogers WAE: *Handbook of human factors and the older adult*, San Diego, 1997, Academic Press.

112. AustRoads: *Assessing fitness to drive: for commercial and private vehicle drivers: medical standards for licensing and clinical management guidelines*, ed 3, Sydney, 2003, AustRoads Inc.

113. VicRoads: *Resources and guidelines for OT driving assessors*, Melbourne, 1998, VicRoads.

114. Stutts JC: Do older drivers with visual and cognitive impairments drive less? *J Am Geriatr Soc* 46:854-861, 1998.

115. Charlton J, Oxley J, Fildes B, et al: *Self regulatory behaviour of older drivers*. Paper presented at the Regain the Momentum: Road Safety Research, Policing and Education Conference, Melbourne, November 2001.

116. Hakamies-Blomqvist L: Older drivers' accident risk: conceptual and methodological issues, *Accid Anal Prevent* 30:293-297, 1998.

117. Harris AE: *Safety and mobility of older drivers living in rural Victoria* (Report no. PP 98/1), Melbourne, 1998, Royal Automobile Club of Victoria.

Chapter 13

ADVANCED STRATEGIES FOR ON-ROAD DRIVER REHABILITATION AND TRAINING

Marilyn Di Stefano • Wendy Macdonald

KEY TERMS

- Remediation
- Compensation
- Advocacy
- Negative transfer

CHAPTER OBJECTIVES

After completing this chapter, the reader will be able to do the following:

- Be familiar with the key issues that should be considered when devising and implementing a driver rehabilitation and training program.
- Know which strategies are appropriate in different situations.
- Understand the factors that are required for effective implementation of a driver rehabilitation and training program.

After some form of initial on-road driving evaluation, as discussed in Chapter 12, on-road training is often an important component of the rehabilitation process. Driver rehabilitation interventions need to be designed and implemented in light of the specific needs of the client, often tempered by the availability of resources. An understanding of client needs is usually derived from the initial referral documentation; interviews with the client, family, or caregivers; results from predriving clinical evaluations; and from any in-vehicle or on-road evaluations of driving performance. At times the results

of further specialist reviews may also be required to gain a more thorough understanding of the client's impairments and consequent driving and alternative community mobility–related needs. All such information can be useful for a driver rehabilitation specialist (DRS), who is responsible for planning a driver rehabilitation and training program.

This chapter describes some of the key issues that should be considered when devising and implementing such programs. Different types of driver rehabilitation interventions are considered within the general categories of *remediation*, *compensation*, and *advocacy* in relation to varying client goals and characteristics. Throughout the chapter emphasis has been placed on issues relevant to on-road training rather than on interventions with more specific remediation or advocacy functions. After identifying prerequisites to on-road training, the factors that must be considered in planning and documenting a training program are reviewed, followed by discussion of requirements for effective implementation, monitoring, and evaluation of the program. The chapter concludes with a review of research evaluating the effectiveness of driver rehabilitation and training interventions.

The phrase *driver rehabilitation and training* refers here to interventions that are intended to improve the client's driving skills and safety. This component of the overall driver service offered to clients is seen as distinct from the clinical and on-road driver evaluation components, although it is important for it to be closely coordinated with assessment procedures and integrated within the overall rehabilitation process.

According to the report from a recent International Older Driver Consensus Conference,[1] "rehabilitation is a blending of compensatory and remediation strategies to facilitate skill improvements and strategies to help individuals to compensate for their limitations" (p. 7).

Consistent with this the DRS who is responsible for formulating a driving rehabilitation program for a particular client has to determine the optimal blend of remediation, compensation, and advocacy interventions that will be most beneficial for that individual.

REMEDIATION, COMPENSATION, AND ADVOCACY INTERVENTIONS

Remediation, compensation, and advocacy are types of driver rehabilitation interventions that need to be considered when assessing a client's goals.

REMEDIATION

Remedial interventions are those intended to improve driving performance by enhancing one or more of the driver's basic capacities, associated functional abilities, or more general behavioral characteristics. In driver rehabilitation, remediation commonly focuses on musculoskeletal, sensory, or cognitive abilities or sociocultural characteristics, such as habits, values, or behavioral roles.[2] Examples of remedial interventions include programs to improve hand or upper limb strength or to improve the client's management of his or her own stress or anger. Driving simulators or computer-based programs may be used to develop or retrain more driving-specific skills, such as visual scanning or foot or upper limb coordination.[1,3] See Chapter 10 for more information on driving simulators.

COMPENSATION

Compensatory approaches to rehabilitation entail interventions to help the client cope with continuing impairments by either adopting different performance tactics or strategies or modifying environmental factors, including the nature of tools or equipment used, the environment in which the activity is performed, or aspects of the activity itself.[2] Many drivers with some degree of impairment are known to use compensatory strategies such as limiting the nature and amount of their driving, including avoidance of driving at night, during inclement weather, or during times when traffic is heavy.[4,5] More specific compensatory techniques related to environmental factors include selection of vehicle parking locations to avoid more difficult parking maneuvers, purchase of a vehicle that is easier to drive (e.g., smaller and with more automated controls), and using customized seating or modified vehicle controls.[6]

Strategies that are applied at the level of individual task performance include compensation for a deficit in one body part by using an alternative limb or body part to perform a particular function; for example turn indicators may be mounted on the headrest and operated by head movements rather than by using a hand to operate conventional indicator controls located adjacent to the steering wheel. Similarly hand-operated controls mounted on or near the steering wheel may substitute for conventional foot-operated brake and accelerator controls. Examples of more general compensatory performance strategies are provided by drivers with reduced visual fields who learn to compensate for this impairment by greater use of head and eye movements[7] and by drivers with limited neck range of motion who use movement of the whole trunk rather than just neck movements to maintain adequate visual search and mirror-scanning behaviors.

ADVOCACY

In addition to strategies adopted by the client, the DRS may sometimes be able to adopt an advocacy role on behalf of clients when their driving is limited by factors outside of their own control but is able to be influenced by the DRS. For example this may be possible in relation to parking opportunities, driver licensing issues, access to suitable services and benefits, or issues of more general importance at a community level, such as road design characteristics or the provision of transportation services.[8-11]

CASE STUDY

This example illustrates some of the ways in which remediation, compensation, and advocacy approaches may be applicable in a particular case.

Sue had a closed head injury and damaged her cervical vertebrae as a result of a motor vehicle accident. As a result her visual fields and neck mobility were impaired, and she also had high levels of anxiety in relation to motor vehicle travel, regardless of whether she was a passenger or contemplating a return to driving. Sue was referred for driver rehabilitation because she wished to resume her previous driving-related activities to improve her independence and to fulfill her parenting and job roles. After relevant clinical screening and referral to specialist health practitioners to quantify her medical impairments, a DRS may adopt the following strategies.

Remediation

Sue may be referred to a physiotherapist (physical therapist) to improve her neck mobility and endurance and to a psychologist for counseling and a driving desensitization program.

Compensation

A range of techniques to compensate for her reduced visual field and any remaining impairment to neck mobility could be suggested. For example Sue may apply additional mirrors to her vehicle to reduce the impact of her visual field deficits and her difficulty with performing shoulder checks.[1] She also may use a parking aid (e.g., device that communicates the proximity to the nearest object by a series of beeps) to assist with slow-speed maneuvers such as negotiating her driveway, and she may also choose to position her vehicle to drive in and out of parking spots rather than undertake 90-degree or reverse (i.e., parallel) parking procedures.

Advocacy

If Sue needed support in making a formal request to her employer for a parking position that would enable her to drive in and out, the DRS might intercede on her behalf or take whatever other actions would be most appropriate in this situation.

Many factors can influence whether remediation, compensation, advocacy, or combinations of these approaches are best for any particular client. These include the nature of the health issue (e.g., chronic or deteriorating); whether there is potential for remediation to achieve functional improvements; performance variability or stability related to factors such as the medication regimen, degree of physical endurance, or pain management; and the availability of resources to support the rehabilitation process, including funding.

CLIENT GOALS AND RELATED CHARACTERISTICS

The nature of an appropriate driver rehabilitation and training program will vary according to client goals and related characteristics. In this section some of the main categories of clients are described, along with examples of typical remediation or compensatory strategies. It can be seen that these differing categories of clients reflect the variety of referral purposes summarized in Table 12-1.

LEARNING TO DRIVE

A young person with major physical, cognitive, or behavioral limitations who has not previously driven may require specialized instruction before a formal evaluation of his or her capacity to become a licensed driver. Specific remediation before driving and on-road training in compensatory strategies may have the potential to improve future driving performance and independence.

LEARNING TO COMPENSATE FOR A FUNCTIONAL IMPAIRMENT

An injury or illness that has resulted in a major functional limitation may require a driver to modify or adapt some components of his or her previously developed driving skills. In these circumstances rehabilitation training typically involves compensatory strategies. For example a driver may need to perform more active and wide-ranging visual scanning and perhaps also use additional mirrors if he or she has lost functional vision in one eye, or to a lesser degree if he or she has a major hearing loss. The impact of sensory limitations, such as reduced proprioception and kinesthesia, may be controlled in some instances by the compensatory use of visual feedback in monitoring and adjusting posture and motor function in some limbs. In the case of drivers with limited physical endurance who become fatigued or with circulatory problems who have particular requirements for pressure care, necessary strategies are likely to include driving only short distances and taking more frequent breaks during longer drives.

Compensation for cognitive impairments may also be feasible to some degree. The impact of reduced memory or planning abilities on driving to unfamiliar places may be addressed by careful route planning before the trip, including the preparation of step-by-step written instructions. If the ability to share attention between different activities is impaired, consideration could be given to compensatory strategies such as driving only during off-peak times, avoiding complex intersections, and minimizing in-vehicle distractions by not carrying multiple passengers or using a cellular phone. Approaches such as these fall into the "Strategic" level of the Gadget matrix of driving behavior described in Chapter 1.

LEARNING TO USE ADAPTED VEHICLE CONTROLS OR OTHER DEVICES

To resume driving after a major injury or illness, some clients must learn to use a modified vehicle. For example it may be necessary to learn to use a different type of turn indicator control or to use a hand-operated accelerator or brake, additional mirrors, cruise control, or parking aids. When previously learned patterns of driving performance have to be modified to incorporate use of such assistive devices, some unlearning of previously existing cognitive and motor skills is required, which needs to be considered. This issue is discussed further in a later section of this chapter. Chapter 11, which covers adaptive equipment and vehicle configuration, discusses the range of devices available for such purposes.

---

[1]Looking back over the shoulder to observe any traffic to the side and rear of the vehicle, often in the driver's blind spot, is referred to as a making a shoulder check.

ENHANCEMENT OF GENERAL DRIVING COMPETENCE

There are many circumstances in which a driver's previously learned skills could benefit from on-road training and specialist advice. This may be the case for clients who have not driven for a substantial period or whose confidence in their own driving ability has been significantly reduced by life events. Many older drivers in particular become concerned by the possibility that aging-related deterioration in some of their functional abilities may have rendered them unsafe.

In such circumstances it is important that the DRS, when conducting an on-road evaluation of the client's driving performance before training, is able to discriminate acceptable bad habits that are typical of most experienced drivers from those that may justify a training intervention. In many cases such behaviors can only be evaluated within the specific contexts of their occurrence; the importance of this issue was also discussed in Chapter 12. For example rolling over a stop line, failing to check back over the shoulder before changing lanes, or traveling a bit faster than the speed limit are common behaviors that in some circumstances are of little concern. A key issue is whether, in a variety of different road traffic conditions, the driver demonstrates a reliable capacity to adapt his or her behavior according to the conditions. For example failing to come to a complete stop at a stop sign may be acceptable in a quiet residential area with no vehicular or pedestrian traffic, but the same behavior in a busy shopping area when stopping at a pedestrian crossing could have dire consequences. When a driver fails to show such discernment, the possibility of some impairment in the capacities and attributes that underpin competent driving performance needs to be considered (see Box 1-2). The problem also may be caused by overloading of the driver's limited attentional resources (Figure 1-3) by the demands of executing the compensatory strategies required to cope with a physical impairment (e.g., motor coordination limitations or postural instability). The DRS may decide to recommend an on-road training intervention if no such underlying problem is evident but the driver consistently demonstrates unsafe habits. In this case a few driving lessons with an experienced DRS may be beneficial.

Sometimes training may be useful in helping clients to revise and update their knowledge of road law and road craft.[12] For example an older driver may have had difficulty keeping up-to-date with road system changes with resultant problems in correctly interpreting variable speed signs or in negotiating roundabouts or some complex, uncontrolled intersections. Road law knowledge related to intersections is of particular concern because older drivers are known to have difficulty negotiating intersections[13,14] and are more likely than others to be involved in intersection accidents, although attentional overloading is more often suggested as a causal factor.[15-18]

In other instances the primary purpose of a training intervention may be to address an unjustified lack of confidence that is detracting from the client's community mobility. This could be associated with a lack of recent driving experience, a recent adverse event, or simply the need to adapt to a new vehicle or an unfamiliar, more demanding driving environment. In these cases a refresher course of training may be required, with the DRS guiding the process of revising basic skills, road law knowledge, and road craft and proceeding at a pace determined by the driver.

BEHAVIORAL PROGRAMS

A training program with a behavioral rather than a skills emphasis (i.e., focusing on issues at levels 1 and 2 in Table 1-4) is sometimes required in cases in which broader psychological or mental health issues may influence the driver's behavior. This is particularly likely for drivers who have sustained a major closed head injury[19] or who have a psychiatric condition[20] that may impact on executive functioning.

Such programs commonly combine off- and on-road interventions. For example a driver without any specific physical or cognitive impairment may be referred for driver rehabilitation because of extreme driving-related anxiety associated with the irrational belief that he or she will be involved in another crash if he or she drives again. This fear prevents the person from resuming driving after having been injured in an accident. In such a situation a desensitization program may be planned, entailing clinical sessions with a psychologist in combination with a graded, in-vehicle program of driving that involves off- and on-road sessions. With guided assistance the client could be helped to develop a range of coping strategies and to implement these within progressively more demanding driving situations. Similarly a driver whose impairment relates to extreme distractibility may have predriving sessions with a neuropsychologist to learn attentional control strategies that he or she can later implement during simulator or on-road training with a DRS.

PREREQUISITES TO ON-ROAD TRAINING

To be eligible to participate in on-road training under the supervision of a DRS, a client must meet certain prerequisite criteria. Adequate financial resources or other factors such as driver licensing limitations may preclude participation, and in some instances the opportunities for participation may be hampered by limited program availability. Some of the more common considerations when reviewing the feasibility of on-road driver training for a particular client include the following.

SATISFY DRIVER LICENSING REQUIREMENTS

The client requires appropriate driver licensing status to participate in on-road driver training. In some cases a license may have been suspended for medical, legal, or administrative reasons. In other instances license conditions or restrictions may limit driving privileges. In all cases the DRS should check that the client could meet the prerequisite license conditions that will allow him or her to engage in on-road training programs.

HAVE ADEQUATE KNOWLEDGE OF ROAD SYSTEMS AND NECESSARY CAPACITIES AND ATTRIBUTES

To benefit from driver training interventions, clients require basic knowledge of road law and road craft and a minimum set of capacities related to sensory, perceptual, cognitive, physical, psychomotor, and executive functioning[1] (see also Box 1-2 and Table 1-4). Without such basic prerequisites the client may have inadequate ability to absorb, retain, and demonstrate skills.

Adequate insight and motivation to benefit from training are particularly important driver attributes that play an important role in any rehabilitation intervention.[1,21] Can clients appreciate their deficits and how they impact on driving-related tasks? Do they exhibit sufficient interest and application to support the behavioral change that is the goal of training? The client's attitudes toward driving more generally may also need to be considered, especially in the case of novice drivers, those with an intellectual disability, or for persons who have significant behavioral or cognitive difficulties.[12] Table 1-4 describes key driver competencies and examples of associated risk factors that may be relevant when considering training interventions.

PREVIOUS REMEDIATION TO OPTIMIZE MEDICAL STATUS

Is there significant potential for the client's current medical condition or functional abilities to be improved? Are basic capacities intact, or can they be enhanced? For example does a client with impaired eyesight or hearing consistently use corrective lenses or hearing devices? If motor function is not optimal, is it better to postpone specific training while the client engages in a remediation program to improve functional abilities first?

OPTIMAL TIME FOR TRAINING

Issues relevant to timing within a wider rehabilitation process are important, especially for clients with multiple problems who may be receiving active treatment. Questions to consider include the following: Is the client still within a period of medical stabilization or recovery such that it is not yet clear whether functional abilities will be adequate? Are other treatments or health interventions currently being implemented, which may be associated with an unstable health status or fluctuations in endurance, motor or sensory function, or cognitive state?

Sometimes clients present for driver evaluation and rehabilitation while they are still recovering from a major illness, accident, or health event. They may not be ready for retraining despite having undertaken an on-road evaluation.[22] Of course discussions early within a client's recovery or adaptation process may be important to provide an overview of the overall driver rehabilitation service and to introduce appropriate goals. This is especially the case for clients with major disabilities who undertake long periods of rehabilitation (e.g., those with spinal cord or major closed head injuries) and for those with deteriorating neurologic conditions (e.g., multiple sclerosis, Parkinson's disease, and dementia). Often the initial information about driver evaluation and rehabilitation may be provided by other treating health practitioners (e.g., occupational therapy generalists) before the client meets with a DRS. In all such cases it will probably be important for the DRS to liaise closely with the treating medical and health care team in developing functional goals and associated timelines that are realistic and in communicating with the client and family members or caregivers regarding these issues.

FUNDING

Funding issues can play a major role in the timing and extent of driver rehabilitation, particularly for clients who require extensive vehicle modifications or retraining interventions. Often the client's insurance or injury compensation status will determine available funding sources. For clients who have no insurance and no recourse to compensation, some alternative organizations that may be approached for financial support may include government rehabilitation agencies, charities, or community-based service organizations (see Chapter 15 for more information on funding and related issues).

FAMILY SUPPORT

Family support in undertaking a rehabilitation program can be important.[12] For young novice drivers in particular the funding of professional driving lessons and vehicle modifications may require commitment of their family's financial resources, and family support is also likely to be crucial if they are to have supervised driving practice in addition to formal, on-road training with a professional instructor. For older people the support of a spouse or other family members also can have an important influence on rehabilitation program outcomes.[23]

PLANNING AND DOCUMENTING TRAINING REQUIREMENTS

All rehabilitation interventions should be carefully planned in light of each client's short- and long-term needs and goals. It also is important that adequate details of the rehabilitation and training interventions are documented, including services provided by other team members and third parties. This information is important to enable service monitoring, quality assurance, and evaluation; to facilitate communications between team members and others; to enable data collection of such information for ongoing and future research; and to ensure that medicolegal requirements are met.

Because the processes of planning and documenting service delivery are closely connected, they are addressed together in this section. In the following section the content of information that may be documented for a range of different purposes is discussed, including the possible content of formal file notes, client progress reports, and requests for funding. Chapter 14 includes some discussion of general documentation requirements for in-vehicle training, including client history, training recommendations, and follow-up.

DESCRIPTION OF THE SPECIFIC IMPAIRMENT AND ITS EFFECT ON DRIVER PERFORMANCE

This information should be consistent with referral details and with the findings of the clinical evaluation and the initial on-road test if this has taken place. It may be useful to ensure that terminology conforms to that of the International Classification of Functioning, Disability, and Health (ICF) classifications, including terms referring to body functions, structures, and impairments, activities and participation, and environmental and personal factors.[24] See Chapter 1 for more information on the ICF. For example:

> Mr. Y. has a flaccid left upper limb as a result of a hemiparesis associated with a stroke. This has resulted in a nonfunctional left upper limb, which limits his ability to manage vehicle operational tasks. He therefore is unable to control the vehicle's gear lever and steering wheel and is consequently unable to drive a vehicle with standard controls. As a result Mr. Y. requires a vehicle with automatic transmission and a steering wheel aid (e.g., spinner knob).

INTERVENTION GOALS

Documentation should include a clear statement of intervention goals using behavioral terms that specify the expected functional outcomes and using conventional "if . . . then" phrasing. For example:

> . . . as a result of x [*number*] prescribed lessons, Mr. Y. should be able to use his right upper limb to operate a spinner knob steering wheel attachment and thus to perform all steering activities required for normal driving (e.g., traveling straight, making right and left turns, reversing, and performing all types of parking and other low-speed maneuvers, including negotiating entry to a garage).

A statement of anticipated functional outcomes may be the following:

> As a result of this intervention and provided that his vehicle is fitted with a suitable steering device, Mr. Y. is expected to be competent to operate a medium-sized sedan as a fully independent driver, and by this means to access his place of employment and other places as necessary to maintain his independent community mobility.

If rehabilitation interventions are extensive, it may be important to list subgoals or prerequisites to enable the major, long-term goals to be met. This may be the case for remediation strategies addressing specific impairments, which constitute prerequisite requirements for on-road driver training.

EXPECTED FREQUENCY AND DURATION OF INTERVENTIONS

Regardless of whether the interventions are on-road driving lessons or clinical remediation sessions with a health professional, the planned frequency and overall time frame of the intervention should be specified. For example this could be described as six, 1-hour periods of specialist driving instruction at weekly intervals. The expected date by which the intervention will be concluded may also be specified to assist with follow-up requirements, such as a review of the intervention effectiveness. Such reviews are important so that the intervention process is regularly monitored to track progress, which is likely to be appreciated by the client, funding bodies, and service providers.

PROVIDERS, COSTS, AND FUNDING SOURCES

The specific individuals or bodies responsible for rehabilitation service provision should be nominated in the documentation, along with an unambiguous statement of costs and details of the funding organization, to assist with clarifying financial responsibility.

AGREEMENTS WITH THE CLIENT, FAMILY, CAREGIVER, AND FUNDING BODY

Creating formal agreements between parties regarding aspects of a driver rehabilitation program may be a requirement of employer, rehabilitation, or funding bodies. Commonly such agreements will document the roles and responsibilities of the DRS, client, family, and other service providers. Learning and intervention contracts are used extensively in educational, vocational, and therapy settings. Such documentation can be an important component of the driver rehabilitation process; it can help to establish clear expectations regarding outcomes and to confirm commitments to mutually agreed goals.

IMPLEMENTATION OF EFFECTIVE ON-ROAD DRIVER TRAINING

The effective implementation of a driver rehabilitation and training program requires consideration of many factors. Some key implementation issues are outlined here.

SUITABLE PERSONNEL

Only appropriately trained professionals should have responsibility for formulating, implementing, monitoring, and evaluating such programs. It is therefore likely to be necessary for several people with differing areas of specialization to work together in a multidisciplinary team to address the variety of issues that can affect the driving independence of each client. All driver rehabilitation and training interventions must be based on adequate knowledge of the client's health and an understanding of its potential effects on functional characteristics and driving performance. Because team members are likely to vary in the extent of their health training, it is important to ensure that there is always an appropriate match between the nature of the service provided and the competencies of the particular service provider.

CLIENT CHARACTERISTICS

The content of the training program must be appropriate to the individual characteristics of each client, considering factors such as the client's specific impairments, the amount and nature of his or her previous driving experience, the client's age, and any other factors that affect his or her capacity to benefit from training. For example many older people have never had formal driver training, and they may therefore require more detailed explanations of some aspects of their program. In other instances cultural or social issues can affect the driver's interactions with instructors or other health providers. Women in some cultures may request or be permitted by other family members to undertake instruction only with a female DRS; conversely some men may have difficulty in accepting guidance from female instructors.

Some aspects of a client's perceptual or cognitive functioning can be particularly important; for example a previous neuropsychological assessment might have identified particular difficulties in processing auditory information. In such a case the DRS should maximize use of information presented visually with minimal reliance on instruction via auditory information.[25,26]

The extent of a client's previous driving experience is a key variable because it may influence the required extent of required new learning and the time that may be required for the learning to occur. If a driver has to modify a previously learned skill as part of a compensatory approach to overcoming functional deficits, it may well take longer to learn than in the case of a novice driver who has to develop that skill without any previous learning. This is because of the possible effects of *negative transfer*, whereby components of the old skill interfere with similar but different components of the new one.[27,28] For example when drivers must adapt to driving on the opposite side of the road when traveling abroad, more attentional resources must be directed to recalling the new spatial schemata required for safe driving in these circumstances as compared with learning to drive on this side of the road for the first time.

Of course the superior skills of drivers with greater driving familiarity provide many advantages, particularly because considerable experience is required to develop the perceptual and cognitive skills that underlie good situation awareness and hazard perception. For example recent research by Whelan et al[29] comparing novice and experienced drivers in terms of these aspects of performance demonstrated:

> . . . in relation to situation awareness . . . novices are less accurate in remembering the number of lanes and whether a lane was occupied by a car. Furthermore, novices' ability to remember the location of vehicles is more affected by distraction than [is the case with] experienced drivers. (p. 37)

Clearly it is important for DRSs to consider such deficiencies in drivers who have not yet had the years of experience that are necessary for the full development of all aspects of driving skill.

ENVIRONMENTS

Choices concerning the environments in which interventions are conducted should take careful account of the intended goals; that is, whether the approach to driver rehabilitation is to address a specific impairment or a broader set of disability-related issues, to ensure driver licensing status, or some combination of these approaches (see Table 12-3). As discussed in Chapter 12, the road traffic environments selected for driver evaluations and training should be graded in their complexity, with more demanding environments used only when the driver is likely to be able to cope, considering variables such as traffic density and speeds, complexity of driving maneuvers, and the additional cognitive demands associated with interpreting and complying with traffic management systems and associated time pressures.[12,30,31]

Off-road environments, such as large car parking areas or a closed-circuit driving range if available, are likely to be appropriate when drivers are initially familiarizing themselves with new vehicle modifications or are being given a lot of instruction or feedback related to basic vehicle control, perhaps including the learning of new compensatory strategies. The generally static nature of these environments allows for a lot of flexibility in vehicle movements, including frequent stopping and starting to facilitate the provision of immediate and detailed feedback, which may not be possible if training is taking place along a busy road or high-speed freeway. If available, driving simulators may also be used as a controlled environment within a training program, particularly to support the development of specific visuospatial, motor, sensory, or cognitive skills relevant to driving (see Chapter 10 for further details).

Training on open roads should occur only when the behaviors entailed in the control of vehicle operations are being performed with adequate reliability and safety and at an automatized level sufficient to leave enough spare mental capacity to support the driver's performance at a tactical level, as required to interact safely with other road users (see Box 1-2). Depending on the goals of the intervention, training environments may eventually include the road, traffic, and other environmental features and conditions that the particular client is likely to encounter in everyday situations relevant to his or her lifestyle. For some drivers this may include negotiating uncontrolled train crossings, driving on gravel roads, using car ferries, negotiating thoroughfares shared by trams, driving through snow, using multilane highways, and so on.

Training may be conducted in either a program's vehicle or the driver's own car. It is important to consider the difficulties that a driver may have in transferring skills between his or her own vehicle and that of the DRS if required. However, the ability to operate a range of different vehicles may be an important requirement within an employment or family context for some clients. In instances in which there are major

vehicle modifications (e.g., electronic controls or joystick steering), it is often advisable to use the driver's car, considering also the DRS's insurance requirements and any licensing authority guidelines.[32] In some instances it may be a requirement that dual controls are installed initially for training purposes and then removed once driver independence, training, formal testing, and licensing are complete.

INSTRUCTIONAL STRATEGIES

The general method and particular procedures used to deliver a training program will influence how well the driver is able to use the available information. The timing and distribution of training sessions and any associated practice sessions should consider impairment-related variables, such as limited endurance and the weather and other environmental factors. For example it may be better for people with arthritis to undertake lessons in the afternoon when their joints are more mobile; for those with chronic pain, however, it may be best to be active in the morning when they are less fatigued. Duration of sessions may also be a consideration, with some clients preferring sessions of ≤30 minutes rather than routine 45- or 60-minute lessons. In both cases the timing would also need to consider traffic levels and associated driving demands. The heat may adversely affect clients with multiple sclerosis and those with certain levels of spinal cord injuries; it may therefore be advisable to postpone lessons when the temperature is likely to exceed the client's comfort zone or to schedule sessions earlier in the day to maximize the client's comfort and his or her learning ability.

Instructional methods should be tailored to the driving experience and age of the client because this will influence the nature of the DRS–client relationship. For example novice drivers may see instructors as experts, whereas older, experienced drivers may view them more as peers. In the latter scenario it is important for the instructor to acknowledge the older person's good attributes and skills and perhaps refer to skill retraining as skill enhancement rather than new learning. Of course feedback to all clients regarding errors should be delivered in a nonjudgmental rather than punitive way.[26] At times communication methods have to be modified or altered because of impairments related to hearing or speech. In such cases an individually focused instructional strategy is clearly necessary. See Chapters 6 and 12 related to hearing loss.

Effective training requires that the trainee have an adequate understanding of the specific behaviors and performance characteristics that are required. To this end, a variety of different communication aids may be useful, in addition to conventional written and orally presented information. These may include various diagrams or photographs, and it can be useful to use model cars to describe vehicle maneuvers and travel paths.[25]

The provision of feedback information can also be critically important as a means of facilitating learning and hence to the success of a training intervention.[27,28,33] Feedback can be provided while performance is ongoing to help in shaping the driver's performance toward the desired goal. Positive feedback about overall performance quality is also likely to be helpful at the end of each training segment to assist in maintaining the learner's motivation.

DRSs making decisions concerning when to give feedback and how much to give should consider the amount of spare attentional capacity that the driver is likely to have available to process the feedback information at any given point. This will vary according to the complexity of the driving maneuver being undertaken, the environmental demands, and with individual driver factors. For clients whose information-processing abilities are impaired, immediate and repeated feedback may be particularly important, but the nature of their impairment makes this particularly difficult to achieve because such people will also be easily overloaded by having to divide their attention between information from their environment that is centrally important to maintaining driving performance and the extraneous feedback information being given by a DRS. For these reasons training drivers to perform overtaking maneuvers, for example, may be achieved more effectively and safely on a section of highway where there are frequent opportunities to stop the vehicle while giving instructions and feedback rather than in locations where stopping is not permitted or impractical for other reasons.

Instructions can be graded in accord with the client's abilities in parallel to the grading of road traffic environments. Initially it may be necessary to provide a lot of direction, step-by-step instruction, and ongoing prompting or cuing either verbally or with hand gestures. As skill levels improve the DRS can reduce the amount of such support. The degree of instruction, cuing, or feedback required has been found to be a good indicator of novice driver skill level.[27]

If the client is able to drive independently or under the supervision of a family member or caregiver, prescribing homework tasks can be useful. In this case it is important that the behaviors to be practiced are clearly documented in an easily understandable way—again making use of diagrams as appropriate. The details specified should include particular task sequences and procedures related to target behaviors and related road traffic conditions. This documentation will serve as a memory aid and as the basis for revision before the next session. The use of logbooks to document driving practice is increasingly being recognized as a valuable means of facilitating novice driver skill development.[34,35]

There is evidence indicating that informal practice (e.g., with family) may be a more effective means of developing driving skill than lessons from a professional instructor for novice drivers.[36,37]

If family members or others are involved in supervising the client's driving practice, they may also be useful participants in providing feedback to facilitate the acquisition of target behaviors. The involvement of others in this way is potentially useful, but it demands detailed and accurate communication between them and the DRS to ensure that everyone is working consistently toward the same goals.

LIAISON, MONITORING, AND LICENSING AUTHORITY REQUIREMENTS

The DRS is responsible for maintaining communications (verbal, face to face, and written) with the client and his or her family and with other members of the rehabilitation team. The DRS also plays a central role in coordinating and monitoring client progress within the overall driver rehabilitation process and may also be responsible for communications with funding bodies or with the driver licensing authorities. These requirements are considered in Chapters 4, 15, 26, and Appendix B.

DECIDING WHEN TO STOP DRIVER REHABILITATION

Sometimes despite having met the basic prerequisites for commencement of on-road training or a related intervention, clients may fail to make adequate progress toward achieving the competencies required for safe and independent driving (with or without adaptive devices or compensatory strategies). In such cases a range of factors may have contributed to this outcome. For example a fluctuating or unstable medical condition or a rigorous medical treatment regimen can interfere with someone's capacity for new learning. Some clients also may be expending significant energy in coping with grief or with interpersonal difficulties associated with their illness or injury, leaving them with inadequate personal resources to invest in their driving performance.

DRS responses to these situations should be determined on a case-by-case basis. Sometimes postponing the client's participation in the program until a more suitable time will be appropriate. In others cases using a different training modality such as a driving simulator may be appropriate. Some clients may need to acknowledge that they cannot continue driving and must now look at other ways to maintain their community mobility and other goals that have previously depended on their driving. The DRS should be able to provide substantial assistance in this process (as discussed in Chapters 5, 7, 21, and 22 and Appendices G and H).

In all cases in which rehabilitation goals have not been met, it is important to ensure that all relevant parties are made aware of the circumstances and that adequate supports are instituted to assist the client to deal with any consequent problems. Sometimes referral to support agencies for further counseling or exploration of other mobility options will be required.

EVIDENCE OF THE EFFECTIVENESS OF DRIVER REHABILITATION AND TRAINING INTERVENTIONS

Driver evaluation and rehabilitation for functionally impaired clients have been available in many countries for a number of years, with articles describing such programs published in a variety of journals, newsletters, and conference proceedings during this time.[12,22,38-46] Information about suitable vehicle adaptations and rehabilitation interventions for specific diagnostic groups is also available in occupational therapy and rehabilitation literature; for example Murray-Leslie described a variety of interventions and discussed the special needs of drivers with neurologic, congenital, and musculoskeletal conditions.[47] The driving evaluation requirements of older persons have also been documented,[48,49] and a detailed discussion of driving-related functional issues and evaluation requirements for this population is provided by Ekelman et al.[50]

However, there are few peer-reviewed, published studies relevant to driver training and rehabilitation techniques of either a descriptive or experimental nature. It appears that information concerning the effectiveness of driver rehabilitation clinical practice has tended to be shared more informally, primarily via study groups, professional development training, and conferences. This is not altogether surprising because, although driver rehabilitation has advanced considerably,[51] it is still a relatively young field of endeavor, characterized by context-related variable service delivery models.[52,53]

Remediation interventions aimed at addressing perceptual-cognitive deficits are used in various driver rehabilitation programs, and some of these have been evaluated more rigorously. After an initial pilot project that examined useful field of view (UFOV) retraining in clients who had experienced a stroke,[54] Mazer et al[55] proceeded to a larger study in which they compared a traditional computer-based visual-perceptual retraining program with a UFOV training intervention that focused on selective and divided attention and visual processing speed. This randomized, controlled trial involving 84 participants entailed use of a number of outcome measures, including clinical evaluations and on-road driving evaluation. After training there were no significant differences between the groups on any of the clinical (i.e., predriving) measures, but participants with a right-sided lesion who undertook UFOV training were almost twice as likely to pass the on-road test. To some extent this result supports the positive findings of a review of literature examining the effectiveness of cognitive rehabilitation for people with stroke or traumatic brain injury,[56] but the researchers concluded that a larger study was needed to evaluate such a conclusion more rigorously.

Educational interventions aimed at assisting clients to understand their functional limitations and inform them of effective self-regulation are often incorporated within driver rehabilitation programs.[57] A study undertaken by Stalvey and Owsley[6] investigated the efficacy of a theory-based Knowledge Enhances Your Safety (KEYS) curriculum delivered to a group of drivers aged ≥60 years who were designated as at risk because of a history of visual acuity or visual processing deficits and who had experienced at least one crash in the preceding year and had a relatively high level of driving exposure. The experimental design involved 365 participants who were randomly assigned to either a control group or an experimental group, and all participants received a visual assessment and related visual counseling. The experimental group also received two, one-on-one educational sessions 1 month apart. These sessions were intended to assist clients to understand their visual functional limitations and to inform them of driving situations in which older drivers are overrepresented in crashes. It was hypothesized that such information would support more effective self-regulation of their exposure to such situations. The evaluation, for which results have been published, was based on a questionnaire completed by participants initially and then 6 months postintervention. Results indicated that participants were more likely to acknowledge functional limitations and suggested that they would be more likely to avoid challenging driving situations and to reduce their overall driving exposure (trips per week). As yet, no data are available concerning any impact on crash risk.[6,58]

Although such research is making an important contribution to the body of knowledge regarding driver rehabilitation, there is a great need for much more research to establish the value of different types of possible interventions for drivers with health-related functional limitations.[8] In the meantime it is particularly important that all DRSs should review the theoretical rationale of their programs and any available evidence concerning the potential benefits of specific interventions.

Overall it is clear that, as in many medical and rehabilitation spheres, there is a paucity of empirical evidence that is directly and specifically relevant to particular interventions. Nevertheless a recent international consensus meeting of professionals involved in this area agreed on a set of recommendations related to driver evaluation, remediation, and counseling regarding alternative means of maintaining mobility.[1] This material has been referred to in this and the previous chapter as appropriate.

SUMMARY

This chapter has provided an overview of some key factors relevant to devising and implementing a driver rehabilitation and training program. Although driver rehabilitation services have been available for a long time, relatively little has been documented about the specific nature of the individual programs offered. The content of this chapter represents current knowledge and best practice. However, there is a severe lack of generally available empirical evidence to demonstrate the effectiveness of particular types of intervention for specific purposes. The challenge now is to build on professional experience by undertaking research that will provide an evidence base to further refine and guide driver rehabilitation and community mobility practice.

REFERENCES

1. National Older Driver Research and Training Center, University of Florida: *Summary report international older driver consensus conference*, 2003. Available at: *http://driving.phhp.ufl.edu/publications/CC%20Summary%20Final%2008-19-04.pdf*. Accessed August 29, 2004.
2. McColl MA: Therapeutic processes to change occupation. In McColl MA, Pollock N, Law M, et al, editors: *Theoretical basis of occupational therapy*, ed 2, Thorofare, NJ, 2003, Slack Incorporated, pp. 179-182.
3. Underwood M: The older driver: clinical assessment and injury prevention, *Arch Int Med* 152:735-740, 1992.
4. Charlton J, Oxley J, Fildes B, et al: *Self regulatory behaviour of older drivers* [Abstract], Regain the Momentum: Road Safety Research, Policing and Education Conference, Melbourne, Australia, 2001, p. 22.
5. Gallo JJ, Rebok GW, Lesikar SE: The driving habits of adults aged 60 years and older, *J Am Geriatr Soc* 47:335-341, 1999.
6. Stalvey B, Owsley C: The development and efficacy of a theory-based educational curriculum to promote self-regulation among high-risk older drivers, *Health Promotion Pract* 4:109-119, 2003.
7. Strano MC: Effects of visual deficits on ability to drive in traumatically brain-injured population, *J Head Trauma Rehabil* 4:35-43, 1989.
8. Fildes B, Pronk N, Langford J, et al: *Model licence reassessment procedure for older and disabled drivers* (Report to Austroads no. AP-R 176/00), Melbourne, Victoria, 2000, Monash University Accident Research Centre.
9. Harris AE: *Safety and mobility of older drivers living in rural Victoria* (Report number PP 98/1), Melbourne, 1998, Royal Automobile Club of Victoria.
10. Staplin L, Lococo K, Byington S, et al: *Older driver highway design handbook* (No. FHWA-RD-97-135), Washington, DC, 1998, Federal Highway Administration.
11. The Road Information Program: *Designing roadways to safely accommodate the increasingly mobile older driver: a plan to allow older Americans to maintain their independence*, 2003. Available at: *http://www.tripnet.org/OlderDrivers2003Study.PDF*. Accessed July 28, 2003.
12. Jones R, Gidders H, Croft D: Assessment and training of brain-damaged drivers, *Am J Occup Ther* 37:754-760, 1983.
13. Daigneault G, Joly P, Frigon J: Previous convictions or accidents and the risk of subsequent accidents of older drivers, *Accid Anal Prevent* 34:257-261, 2002.
14. Staplin L, Gish KW, Decina L, et al: *Intersection negotiation problems of older drivers: Volume 1: final technical report* (October 1993-September 1997, no. 1446/FR), Washington, DC, 1998, Office of Research and Traffic Records, National Highway Traffic Safety Administration.
15. Fildes B: *Safety of older drivers: strategy for future research and management initiatives* (General Report no. 118), Melbourne, Victoria, 1997, Monash University Accident Research Centre.
16. Hakamies-Blomqvist L: Fatal accidents of older drivers, *Accid Anal Prevent* 25:19-27, 1993.
17. Preusser DF, Williams AF, Ferguson SA, et al: Fatal crash risk for older drivers at intersections, *Accid Anal Prevent* 30:151-159, 1998.
18. Ryan GA, Legge M, Rosman D: Age related changes in drivers' crash risk and crash type, *Accid Anal Prevent* 30:379-387, 1998.
19. Fisk GD, Schneider JJ, Novack TA: Driving following traumatic brain injury: prevalence, exposure, advice and evaluations, *Brain Inj* 12:683-695, 1998.
20. Harris M: Psychiatric conditions with relevance to fitness to drive, *Adv Psychiatr Treat* 6:261-269, 2000.
21. Lewis SC: Driving and the older adult. In Lewis SC, editor: *Elder care in occupational therapy*, New York, 2003, Slack, pp. 311-321.
22. Klavora P, Young M, Heslegrave RJ: A review of a major driver rehabilitation centre: a ten-year client profile, *Can J Occup Ther* April:128-134, 2000.
23. Corcoran MA: Occupational therapy intervention for persons with dementia and their families, *AOTA Continuing Education Article* CE1-CE7, 2002. Available at: *http://www.aota.org/nonmembers/area3/docs/intervdementia.pdf* Accessed December 8, 2004.

24. World Health Organization: *ICF international classification of functioning, disability and health,* Geneva, 2001, World Health Organization.

25. Di Stefano M, Lovell R: *Teaching older drivers: a handbook for driving instructors,* Melbourne, Victoria, 2001, LaTrobe University.

26. Hunt L: Evaluation and retraining programs for older drivers, *Clin Geriatr Med* 9:439-447, 1993.

27. Groeger JA: *Understanding driving: applying cognitive psychology to a complex everyday task,* East Sussex, 2000, Psychology Press.

28. Proctor RW, Van Zandt T: *Human factors in simple and complex systems,* Boston, 1994, Allyn and Bacon.

29. Whelan M, Senserrick T, Groeger JA, et al: *Learner driver experience project* (No. 221), Melbourne, 2004, Monash University Accident Research Centre.

30. Clark M, Hecker J, Cleland E, et al: *Dementia and driving* (No. T99/0574), Canberra, ACT, 2000, Australian Transport Safety Bureau.

31. Galski T, Ehle HT, Williams JB: Estimates of driving abilities and skills in different conditions, *Am J Occup Ther* 52:268-275, 1998.

32. VicRoads: *Resources and guidelines for OT driving assessors,* Melbourne, 2000, VicRoads.

33. Wickens CD, Gordon SE, Liu Y, et al: *An introduction to human factors engineering,* ed 2, Upper Saddle River, NJ, 2004, Pearson Education International.

34. Christie R: *Driver licensing requirements and performance standards including driver and rider training,* Melbourne, Australia, 2000, National Road Transport Commission.

35. Christie R: *The effectiveness of driver training: a review of the literature* (Report no. 01/03), Melbourne, 2001, Royal Automobile Club of Victoria.

36. Groeger JA, Brady SJ: *Road safety research report no. 42: differential effects of formal and informal driver training,* London, 2004, Department for Transport.

37. Matthew DR, Simpson HM: *Effectiveness and role of driver education and training in a graduated licensing system,* Ontario, Canada, 1996, The Traffic Injury Research Foundation of Canada.

38. Beatson CJ: Transport technology: New Zealand perspectives, *WORK J Prevent Assess Rehabil* 8:271-280, 1997.

39. Caust S: Clinical perspectives: occupational therapy driver assessment course—a report by a course participant, *Aust J Occup Ther* 35:181-185, 1988.

40. Di Stefano M: *Assessment and retraining of drivers with a functional impairment,* Proceedings of the Specialised Transport Conference, Melbourne, Australia, 1994, pp. 46-51.

41. Di Stefano M, Macdonald W: *On the road again: the complexity of assessing the functionally impaired driver.* Paper presented at the Ergonomics and Safety—the total package: International Workplace Health and Safety Conference and the thirty-third Ergonomics Society of Australia Conference, 1997, Gold Coast, Queensland.

42. Galski T, Bruno RL, Ehle HT: Prediction of behind-the-wheel driving performance in patients with cerebral brain damage: a discriminant function analysis, *Am J Occup Ther* 47:391-396, 1993.

43. Jacobs K: OTs in the driver's seat: occupational therapy provides an ideal background for driver rehabilitation specialists, *Rehab Manag* February/March:126-127, 1994.

44. Kalina TD: Starting a driver rehabilitation program, *WORK J Prevent Assess Rehabil* 8:229-238, 1997.

45. Korner-Bitensky N, Sofer S, Kaizer F, et al: Assessing ability to drive following an acute neurological event: are we on the right road? *Can J Occup Ther* 61: 141-148, 1994.

46. Schold Davis E: Defining OT roles in driving, *OT Practice* 13:15-18, 2003.

47. Murray-Leslie C: Driving independently. In Goodwill CJ, Chamberlain MA, Evans C, editors: *Rehabilitation of the physically disabled adult,* ed 2, Cheltenham, UK, 1997, Stanley Thornes, pp. 709-726.

48. Hunt LA: A profile of occupational therapists as driving instructors and evaluators for elderly drivers, *IATSS Res* 20:46-47, 1996.

49. Pierce S: On the road again? OT and the older driver, *OT Practice* 3:30-32, 1998.

50. Ekelman BA, Mitchell S, O'Dell-Rossi P: Driving and older adults. In Bonder BR, Wagner MB, editors: *Functional performance in older adults,* ed 2, Philadelphia, 2001, FA Davis Company, pp. 448-472.

51. Gianutsos R: Driving and visual information processing in cognitively at risk and older individuals. In Gentile M, editor: *Functional visual behavior: a therapist's guide to evaluation and treatment options,* Bethesda, MD, 1997, American Occupational Therapy Association, pp. 321-342.

52. British Psychological Society: *Fitness to drive and cognition: a document of the multi-disciplinary working party on acquired neuropsychological deficits and fitness to drive 1999* (Working Party Report), Leicester, 2001, The British Psychological Society.

53. Springle S, Morris B, Nowachek G, et al: Assessment of the evaluation procedures of drivers with disabilities, *Occup Ther J Res* 15:147-164, 1995.

54. Mazer BL, Sofer S, Korner Bitensky N, et al: Use of the UFOV to evaluate and retrain visual attention skills in clients with stroke: a pilot study, *Am J Occup Ther* 55:552-557, 2001.

55. Mazer BL, Sofer S, Korner Bitensky N, et al: Effectiveness of a visual attention retraining program on the driving performance of clients with stroke, *Arch Phys Med Rehabil* 84:541-550, 2003.

56. Cicerone KD, Dahlberg C, Kalmar K, et al. Evidence-based cognitive rehabilitation: recommendations for clinical practice, *Arch Phys Med Rehabil* 81:1596-1615, 2000.

57. Gourley M: Driver rehabilitation: a growing practice area for OTs, *OT Practice* 25:15-20, 2002.

58. Owsley C, Stalvey BT, Phillips JM: The efficacy of an educational intervention in promoting self-regulation among high-risk older drivers, *Accid Anal Prevent* 35:393-400, 2003.

Part IV

DOCUMENTATION AND FUNDING

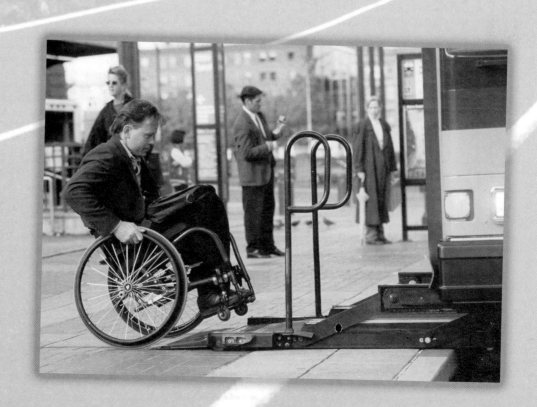

Chapter 14

DOCUMENTING DRIVER REHABILITATION SERVICES AND OUTCOMES

Michael K. Shipp • Ann B. Havard

KEY TERMS

- Clinical evaluation
- On-road evaluation
- Off-road assessment

CHAPTER OBJECTIVES

After completing this chapter, the reader will be able to do the following:

- Be familiar with the four basic parts of the driver rehabilitation evaluation report.
- Understand the five steps in interpreting evaluation results.

Driver evaluation and rehabilitation documentation that is thorough, clear, concise, and standardized is an important component of any reputable driver rehabilitation program. There is an old saying that health care providers and those entities responsible for reimbursing services rendered are familiar with: "If it is not documented, then it did not happen!"

In this chapter we will examine the assessments that are combined to create the comprehensive driver rehabilitation evaluation and standards of practice for documenting services rendered, including the following:

- Documenting the *clinical evaluation*
- Documenting the driver's performance during the *on-road evaluation*
- Interpreting evaluation results and making recommendations that identify a preferred vehicle type,

adapted driving aids, and structural modifications to the vehicle
- Preparing specifications for the recommended vehicle modifications and adapted driving aids

Figure 14-1 shows a sample driver rehabilitation evaluation report; driver rehabilitation specialists (DRSs) should refer to it from time to time to reinforce some of the concepts discussed in this chapter. This chapter also explores documenting on-road and off-road training plans and performance outcomes. DRSs should keep in mind when they are documenting a client's functional status, intervention outcomes, or both that others will need to be able to read and comprehend the report. Individuals that have a vested interest in the client's well-being, such as the professional driver rehabilitation team members, the client's caregivers, and the client himself or herself, are most likely to access the driver rehabilitation report at some point in time to review the documented driver evaluation and training outcomes. See Box 14-1 for a nonexhaustive list of the other professionals who often read what DRSs have documented about a client's driving and community mobility status.

It is also important to point out that the DRS is included in this list because he or she will undoubtedly be required to review his or her own documentation in the short or long term.

Documentation must be clear and concise to help ensure accurate recall of a client's performance, especially after many days, weeks, months, or even years. In the documentation process another important consideration is to institute a policy that requires the use of a protocol for report writing. When setting up or revamping an existing driver rehabilitation program, the DRS should work with the other driver rehabilitation team members to establish policies and procedures that will

CENTER FOR BIOMEDICAL ENGINEERING
and REHABILITATION SCIENCE
Louisiana Tech University

Driver Rehabilitation Program

Driver Evaluation Report
(Suggested Format)

NAME: DOB: DOE:
DRIVER LICENSE NUMBER: EXP: RESTR:
AGE: EVALUATOR(S):

REFERRAL INFORMATION:

- referral source
- type and nature of disability (primary and secondary)
- date of onset; cause
- current medications and effects

GENERAL OBSERVATIONS:

- client's attitude/state of mind
- ambulatory/mobility aids

SUMMARY:

- general statement of test results
- statement regarding vehicle type
- statement regarding adaptive equipment

_____

Ann B. Havard, LOTR, CDRS   Date
Certified Driver Rehabilitation Specialist
Driver Rehabilitation Program Manager

Michael K. Shipp, M.Ed., CDRS
Certified Driver Rehabilitation Specialist

RECOMMENDATIONS:

1   Driving Status
2   Further Diagnosis
3   Driver Improvement Course (classroom)
4   Vehicle selection
5   Vehicle modification specifications
6   Behind-the-Wheel Training
7   Report to driver license agency

NOTES:

Where applicable, equipment should meet or exceed the requirements established by the United States Department of Transportation, Department of Veterans Affairs, Louisiana Rehabilitation Services, Society of Automotive Engineers, and the National Mobility Equipment Dealers Association.

These recommendations should be considered valid for one year from the date of evaluation. Beyond that time, a re-evaluation of the client may be necessary.

Any changes in the client's medical status, wheelchair and seating system, vehicle, and/or other items that might have an affect on the personal transportation needs of the client should be reported to the evaluators for review and possible changes in recommendations and specifications.

These recommendations have been developed based upon the education and experience of the evaluation team and the client's experience in using the assessment equipment available at the Louisiana Tech University Center for Rehabilitation Science and Biomedical Engineering.

The results and recommendations included in this report are based on the client's performance during the period of the evaluation and should not be relied on as absolute predictors of future performance.

The conclusions reached and the recommendations made in this report are based, in part, upon the medical information available at the time this report was written. If subsequent to the issuance of this report, the client's medical status changes in such a manner that may compromise the client's abilities as a driver, this report can no longer be relied upon as valid.

Any questions regarding this report should be directed to:

Ann B. Havard, LOTR, CDRS
Driver Rehabilitation Program Manager
Louisiana Tech University
P.O. Box 3185
Ruston, LA 71272
(318) 257-4562

TEST RESULTS AND OBSERVATIONS:

VISION:

HEARING:

RANGE OF MOTION:

STRENGTH:

REACTION TIME:

TRANSFERS:

VISUAL-PERCEPTION:

COGNITION:

DRIVER KNOWLEDGE:

ON-ROAD PERFORMANCE EVALUATION:

VEHICLE INSPECTION:

VEHICLE SELECTION RECOMMENDATIONS:

Figure 14-1 Driver evaluation report form. (Courtesy Louisiana Tech University, Ruston, LA.)

guide the report-writing process. There should be little if any deviation from the established protocol. The protocol will also help DRSs to recognize the key components that should be included in any driver rehabilitation report, provide a uniform look and feel for all reports generated, improve interrater reliability, and expedite reimbursement for driver rehabilitation services.

THE DRIVER REHABILITATION REPORT: FOUR BASIC PARTS

As stated previously there are four parts that comprise a comprehensive driver rehabilitation evaluation report:
• Documenting the clinical evaluation
• Documenting the on-road evaluation

- Clients
- Client's caregiver(s)
- Occupational therapy generalists
- Driver educators
- Therapists who provide specialty services other than driver rehabilitation (e.g., an occupational therapist specializing in wheeled mobility and seating or low vision)
- Funding agency representatives (e.g., vocational rehabilitation counselors and workers' compensation officials)
- Case managers
- Insurance claims adjustors
- Physicians outside of the driver rehabilitation team
- Psychologists/neuropsychologists
- Driver licensing and relicensing agency personnel
- Attorneys
- Primary driver rehabilitation specialists (DRSs)
- DRSs who are not assigned to the case in question but are sought out for their expert opinion or advice

- Interpreting evaluation results and making recommendations for education and training
- Preparing vehicle modification specifications and overseeing the client-vehicle fitting

The following section of this chapter will discuss each of these parts in more detail.

DOCUMENTING THE CLINICAL EVALUATION

Documenting the clinical evaluation begins with obtaining client information that is pertinent to driving and community mobility. Clinical areas should be assessed as well.

Client Information

DRSs should begin documenting the clinical evaluation by eliciting some basic demographic information on the client, such as name, address, telephone number, date of birth, driver's license numbers, and any past or current driver's license restrictions. The DRS also should document the contact information that indicates who referred the client and who will be paying for the requested services. The DRS or any other professional working with the client can retrieve this information from the medical record. A brief summary of the primary disability, secondary disabilities (if applicable), the cause (i.e., the etiology of the injury or illness), and the date of onset should be included. This information is especially important because it will help

to establish whether the client has reached his or her maximum level of functioning and expectations for the near and long term. For example a client who has sustained a spinal cord injury (SCI) resulting in a complete T12 injury presents a fairly static clinical picture versus a client diagnosed with amyotrophic lateral sclerosis (ALS), who presents a much more dynamic clinical picture and different long-term prognosis.

An exhaustive list of the medications that the client is taking and any existing or potential side effects from these drugs should be recorded, especially if the drugs can impair driving. The list should include both prescription and over-the-counter medications. See Chapter 8 for more information on medications and driving. If a DRS suspects that medications are causing a decrease in the client's level of alertness, visual acuity, cognition, perception, or any aspect of driving performance, this information must be thoroughly documented and immediately conveyed to the client and other pertinent driver rehabilitation team members (e.g., physiatrist and case manager). General observations about the client are also noted, including his or her willingness to participate in the driver rehabilitation processes and his or her personal mobility status. The report should state whether the client is currently using an ambulation aid or aids, such as braces, canes, crutches, or a walker. If the client is a wheelchair user, the DRS should document the make and model and the seating system used (e.g., a Quickie 626 power wheelchair with a ROHO high-profile seat cushion and an Invacare personal back). This information is important to note for the mobility equipment dealer (i.e., vehicle modifier), especially if the client is driving from his or her wheelchair. See Chapter 9 for more information on the impact of positioning and mobility devices on driving.

The Clinical Evaluation

During the clinical evaluation, several areas should be thoroughly assessed. They include vision, visual perception, hearing, range of motion, functional strength and endurance, sensation, reaction time, transfers, cognition, and the driver's overall knowledge of the rules of the road. The comprehensive driver rehabilitation evaluation report should provide summaries of each one of these areas.

Visual Acuity and Perception

A DRS should record the results of the visual acuity testing and document whether the client was wearing eyeglasses or contact lenses during the evaluation. Any abnormalities in the client's visual acuity are noted along with a description of how these impairments could potentially affect driving performance. Visual-perceptual strengths and deficits are also noted in the report. This portion of the report provides valuable information as to how visual-perceptual deficits could potentially affect the on-road portion of the evaluation. For example if a client is having significant difficulty with depth perception, this deficit could influence how closely he or she follows other vehicles or maneuvers the vehicle in tight situations, such as maneuvering a vehicle in a busy parking lot. See Chapters 6, 12, and 21 for more information on vision and driving.

Hearing

The client's ability to hear and a description of the make and model of the client's hearing aid or aids are documented. The client's ability to hear and discern meaningful environmental sounds versus noise can significantly affect a client's driving performance and should be a part of the on-road (i.e., in-vehicle) evaluation and training activities. See Chapters 6 and 12 for more information on hearing and driving.

Active Range of Motion and Muscle Tone

Measurements of active range of motion (AROM) are recorded, especially if significant deficits are noted in either one or both upper and/or lower extremities. Active movement that is assessed to be within normal limits (WNLs) should also be documented in the report. If abnormal tone is present and could potentially affect the client's ability to drive, the DRS should document its severity and potential functional implications. See Chapters 6 and 12 for more information on AROM and driving.

Functional Strength, Sensation, Endurance, and Skin Integrity

Functional upper and lower extremity strength, sensation, endurance, and skin integrity (e.g., presence of a pressure sore located at the client's left ischial tuberosity could potentially make sitting in a vehicle contraindicated until the pressure sore has healed) should also be noted. This information helps to justify the medical necessity of adapted driving equipment, structural vehicle modifications, and ongoing driver rehabilitation. The results documented in this portion of the evaluation also can provide a rationale for why a client is unable to use an extremity (or extremities) to drive secondary to the deficits observed and noted in range of motion, sensation, strength, endurance, or skin integrity. See Chapters 6 and 12 for more information on assessing functional strength, sensation, endurance, and skin integrity and how these factors can impact driving outcomes.

Brake Reaction Time Test

The results of the brake reaction time tests are recorded in seconds and can provide valuable information for

DRSs who provide on-road training. If decreased brake reaction time is noted, the client will be required to make adjustments in his or her driving habits and patterns (e.g., increase the following distance or limit driving to daylight hours or familiar environments and travel routes). A stronger emphasis also needs to be placed on the client's visual scanning techniques during the training phase of the driver rehabilitation program.

Transfers

The client's preferred method of transferring is another factor that is critical to document because it is one of the key variables that helps determine what type of vehicle will best meet the client's needs. Once the client's primary ambulation or wheeled mobility aid is determined, the DRS must identify the most efficient and safest method for the client to access the vehicle and stow (i.e., secure) his or her mobility aid. For example if a client is able to transfer into and out of a wheelchair but is unable to disassemble and transfer the manual wheelchair into a car, the DRS will need to recommend a van equipped with a ramp or lift and a six- or eight-way adjustable driver's seat. The vehicle modifier also needs this information to properly install the recommended adaptive equipment that pertains to transferring and securing a mobility aid. See Chapters 5, 9, 11, 12, 13, and 17 for more information on seating, transfers, selecting the optimal vehicle type, and tie-down systems for drivers and passengers.

Cognitive Testing

The results of cognitive testing are important when trying to assess the client's mental fitness for driving. If the overall outcome associated with the cognitive assessment is positive, this information provides the evaluator and driver rehabilitation team with another reason why driving may be a viable pursuit. Conversely if cognitive deficits are noted, the client may be precluded from driving. Identifying cognitive deficits may provide the client, the caregiver(s), the physician, the referring agency, and other interested parties with the rationale as to why driving is no longer an appropriate goal. See Chapters 7 and 21 and Appendices G and H for more information on neuropsychology and driving, driving cessation, and counseling the client who is no longer able to drive.

Driver Knowledge

It is necessary to note the client's knowledge of the rules of the road. The client's baseline knowledge is greatly influenced by his or her level of driving experience and will determine whether further instruction is required.

DOCUMENTING A CLIENT'S DRIVING PERFORMANCE

Assessing an individual's driving performance may occur in two environments, including off road (i.e., driving range or protected area such as a private parking lot) or on road. These two terms are preferred over "behind the wheel," which does not clarify whether the evaluation or training occurred off or on road.

Off-Road Driving Assessment

If individuals will be using adaptive driving equipment for the first time, they are inexperienced drivers, or both, the initial assessment could occur in an off-road area if possible. The area should be free of stationary objects (i.e., unintended obstacles), distractions, and vehicular and pedestrian traffic. A minimum area for setting up an off-road driving range for assessing a client while he or she is behind the wheel of a motor vehicle is approximately 200 by 400 feet (i.e., 61×122 m). This will allow the client to practice basic driving range exercises and driving maneuvers while receiving feedback from the DRS.

When conducting an *off-road assessment*, the DRS should observe, evaluate, and document the following performance components whenever they are applicable:

- The client's ability to safely transfer into and out of the driver's position within the vehicle
- The need for adaptive driving equipment
- The client's brake reaction time
- The effects of vehicle dynamics

Ability to Transfer

The ability to transfer involves several factors in addition to the ability to get into and out of the driver's position. These include the following questions:

- Is the client's medical condition stable? For an individual with a progressive disability, consideration should be given to how long independent transfers are feasible. Conversely if an individual has a new injury and has not yet completed the rehabilitation process, he or she may have the potential to transfer in the future. The evaluation may need to be delayed until the individual's medical condition and recovery trajectory can be determined.
- Can the client lock and unlock the vehicle's doors, hatch, and trunk? The client must be able to handle the keys or remote entry system and lock and unlock the vehicle's doors, hatch, and trunk.
- Can the client open and close the vehicle's doors, hatch, and trunk? The individual must be able to independently operate the vehicle's door handles with or without adaptive devices. In cases in which vans are being considered, the client's ability to operate power door openers, wheelchair lift controls, or scooter loaders should be observed and noted.

- Can the client perform transfers into and out of the vehicle safely and within a reasonable amount of time? Individuals must be able to transfer independently to and from their wheelchair or scooter and vehicle seat and can be performed with or without a transfer aid, such as a sliding board. The transfer should not require an exorbitant amount of time or energy that could lead to exhaustion and diminished driving safety. The total number of transfers a client is required to perform per day should also be considered when trying to decide on the most appropriate recommendations.
- Can the client store and retrieve his or her wheeled mobility device or ambulation aid? Individuals should be able to independently store and retrieve their wheelchair, scooter, or ambulation aid. This can be done in a variety of ways, which may include folding and transferring the wheelchair into and out of the vehicle by taking it apart and transferring the components into the vehicle. Clients may also opt to use one of the many wheelchair or scooter loading devices commercially available and compatible with a variety of cars, trucks, and vans.

Adaptive Driving Equipment Needs

Before evaluating the client off or on road, the DRS should determine the client's specific adaptive driving equipment needs. A vehicle set up with the necessary adaptive driving equipment and other vehicle modifications will help to ensure that a client can safely access the evaluation vehicle and achieve his or her optimal driving performance. See Chapter 11 for more information on setting up a vehicle before performing an on-road evaluation. The client's performance should be observed, and any necessary changes or adjustments should be made in response to the documented driving performance.

DRSs should use a comprehensive checklist to document the client's equipment and vehicle modification needs. The checklist should parallel the format that a DRS uses when documenting recommendations for vehicle modifications. Sample checklists for sedans, pickup trucks, sport utility vehicles, and vans (i.e., full sized and minivans) are included in Figures 14-2 and 14-3. It is also beneficial to take digital images of how a client's vehicle is set up with the client seated in the driver's position. Detailed notes should be taken that explain how adaptive driving equipment is positioned. This is a good practice because these notes are extremely helpful to the mobility equipment dealer (i.e., vehicle modifier). Written documentation can also be augmented by digital images that record the specific types and position of adaptive driving aids and structural vehicle modifications. Digital images provide the DRS with an effective memory aid and can be stored electronically and in hardcopy formats for later retrieval if necessary.

SEDAN/PICKUP TRUCK/SUV MODIFICATION CHECKLIST

Consumer: _____ DOE: _____

Type of Conversion: Driver: _____ transfer _____ ambulatory
Passenger: _____ transfer _____ ambulatory

Vehicle: Year _____ Make _____ Model _____

Evaluator(s):
Mobility Equipment Dealers:
(Indicate which approved mobility equipment dealers [minimum of three] have been selected by the consumer for obtaining price quotations)

1. _____   3. _____

2. _____   4. _____

NOTE: Complete and attach a Vehicle Information Form, Wheelchair Data Form and/or Torso Support Form where applicable

* * * * * * *

I   VEHICLE ENTRY

A _____ Transfer Seat
_____ Driver*   _____ Passenger*
_____ Step/running board*
_____ Transfer assist
_____ overhead bar/strap   _____ transfer board
_____ Grab handle
_____ A-pillar _____ Driver side* _____ Pass. Side*
_____ Overhead _____ Driver Side* _____ Pass. Side*
*Make/model

B _____ Door handle assist device*
*Make/model

NOTES:

II   DRIVER POSITION

A _____ Occupant Protection   _____ Seat belt extension
_____ Air bag On/Off switch*
_____ Disconnect air bag system*
B _____ Seat Cushion
_____ Wheelchair cushion* _____ Custom fabricated
(Attach notes and dimensions)
C _____ Other
*Make/model

NOTES:

III   STEERING SYSTEM

A   Steering effort:
_____ Standard OEM power effort _____ Low effort (20-24 ounce)*
_____ Maximum reduced effort (4 - 6 ounce)* _____ Emergency backup system*
*Make/Model

B   Steering column:
_____ Standard wheel _____ Reduced size wheel* _____ Inches
*Make/Model

C   Steering Device: _____ spinner knob* _____ tri-pin* _____ V-grip*
_____ flat spinner* _____ amputee ring* _____ Other*
*Make/model

D _____ Other

NOTES:

IV   BRAKE/ACCELERATOR SYSTEM

A   Braking effort:
_____ Standard OEM power brakes _____ Low effort (11 ft. pounds)
_____ Maximum reduced effort (7 ft. pounds) _____ Emergency backup
B   Hand Controls:
Mechanical:
_____ Push/right-angle* _____ Push/Rock* _____ Push/pull*
_____ Push-twist* _____ Other*
_____ Quad grip handle
Mounted for: _____ Left hand use _____ Right hand use
*Make/model

C _____ Pedal Guard*
_____ Brake & Accelerator _____ Brake Only _____ Accelerator Only
*Make/Model

D _____ Left foot accelerator*
*Make/model

E _____ Pedal extensions*
_____ Both _____ Brake only _____ Accelerator only
Length: _____ Brake pedal _____ "
_____ Accelerator pedal _____ "
*Make/model

F _____ Other

NOTES:

V   SECONDARY CONTROLS

Mode A: Items to be operable by the driver while the vehicle is in motion

A Horn	_____ OEM	_____ Remote* Location
B Dimmer	_____ OEM	_____ Remote* Location
C Turn Signals	_____ OEM	_____ Remote* Location
D Wiper	_____ OEM	_____ Remote* Location
E Washer	_____ OEM	_____ Remote* Location
F Cruise "SET"	_____ OEM	_____ Remote* Location
G Cruise "ON"	_____ OEM	_____ Remote* Location
Remote Panel(s)	*Make/Model Position	

NOTES:

Mode B: Items to be operable while brake is activated (i.e. with steering hand)

A Parking brake _____ OEM _____ Extension lever*
_____ Power* Switch location
*Make/model

B Ignition _____ OEM _____ Key holder*
_____ Keyless* Switch location
*Make/model

C Gear selector _____ OEM _____ Extension lever* _____ Power system*
*Make/model _____

NOTES:

Mode C: Other secondary controls (to remain OEM unless otherwise noted)

_____ HVAC system	Modification
_____ Rear Heat/Air fan	Modification
_____ Power windows	Modification
_____ Power door locks	Modification
_____ Power mirrors	Modification
_____ Headlight/parking lights	Modification
_____ Interior lights	Modification
_____ Flasher	Modification
_____ Rear Wiper/Wash	Modification
_____ Rear Defrost	Modification
_____ Other	Modification
_____	Modification

NOTES:

VI   MISCELLANEOUS

A   Torso support (attach torso support order form)
_____ Driver seat mounted* _____ Passenger seat mounted
*Make/model

B   Electrical System
_____ Battery protection system* _____ Power backup*
*Make/model

C _____ Rear hazard detector*
*Make/model

D _____ Mirrors
_____ Convex blind spot mirrors on both exterior mirrors
_____ Panoramic view mirror on windshield mounted rear view mirror
D _____ Dual instructor brake
E _____ Suspension modifications*
*Make/model

F _____ Other

NOTES:

Figure 14-2 Sedan and pickup truck checklist. (Courtesy Louisiana Tech University, Ruston, LA.)

VII WHEELCHAIR/SCOOTER TRANSPORT

A Vehicle interior
____ Rear*   ____ Passenger side*   ____ Driver side*
____ Trunk*   ____ Truck bed*   ____ Other*
*Make/Model

B Vehicle exterior
____ Car top carrier*
____ Driver side   ____ Passenger side
____ Trailer   ____ Bumper/hitch mounted*
*Make/model

NOTES:

Figure 14-2   cont'd

Driver Rehabilitation Program
Center for Biomedical Engineering and Rehabilitation Science

Ann B. Havard, LOTR, CDRS   Michael K. Shipp, M.Ed., CDRS

VAN MODIFICATION CHECKLIST

Consumer: _____ DOE: _____

Type of Conversion: Driver: ____ transfer ____ wheelchair occupant ____ ambulatory
                    Passenger: ____ wheelchair occupant ____ transfer ____ ambulatory
Vehicle: Year ____ Make ____ Model ____

Evaluator(s):
Mobility Equipment Dealers:
(Indicate which approved mobility equipment dealers [minimum of three] have been selected by the consumer for obtaining price quotations)

1. _____   3. _____

2. _____   4. _____

NOTE: Complete and attach a Vehicle Information Form, Wheelchair Data Form and/or Torso Support Form where applicable

* * * * * * *

I   VEHICLE ENTRY

A Power door operator: ____ Side/swing   ____ Side/sliding
                        ____ Rear/swing   ____ Front/driver
B Door/Lift Control   ____ Keyless-magnetic   ____ Third station/driver area
                        ____ Electronic Remote ____ Attendant control
C Wheelchair lift: ____ Fully Automatic platform*
                        ____ Side Entry
                        ____ Extension ____ Inches
                        ____ Rotary*
                        ____ Front Post
                        ____ Rear Post
                        ____ Under Vehicle (UVL)*
                        *Make/Model

D Door Opening: ____ Raised roof system
                 ____ Fiberglass top painted to match vehicle exterior
                 ____ Minimum interior head room ____ Inches
                 ____ Roof support structure
                 ____ Maximum insulation
                 ____ Head liner
                 ____ Raised door opening ____ Inches

E Lowered Floor Modification
   Full-size van:
                 ____ Driver   ____ Passenger (center only)
                 ____ 4" ____ 6" ____ "   ____ 4" ____ 6" ____ "
                 ____ Aft-axle fuel system mod. ____ Aft-axle fuel system mod.

   Lowered Floor Mini Van Conversion:
                 ____ Fully automatic ____ 10" ____ 8"
                 ____ Fold out ramp   ____ Slide out ramp
                 ____ Removable front passenger seat
                 ____ Kneel system
                 ____ Rear Heat/Air up charge
                 *Make/Model

F Other: ____ Entry lighting
          ____ Transfer Seat
               ____ Driver*   ____ Passenger*
          ____ Step/running board*
          ____ Grab handle
               ____ A-pillar   ____ Driver side* ____ Pass. Side*
               ____ Overhead   ____ Driver Side* ____ Pass. Side*
          *Make/model

NOTES:

II   DRIVER POSITION

A ____ Removable driver seat w/rearward lockdown
B ____ Power pan
        ____ Inches   ____ Switch location
C ____ Automatic wheelchair driver tie-down*
        ____ Front stabilizer ____ Switch location
        *Make/model

D ____ Occupant Protection ____ Wheelchair-mounted lap belt
                             ____ Add-on retractable shoulder harness
                             ____ Add-on non-retractable shoulder harness
                             ____ Center stanchion with one receptacle
                             ____ Center stanchion with two receptacles
                             ____ Extra seat belt receptacles
                                  ____ Driver side ____ Right ____ Left
                                  ____ Passenger side ____ Right ____ Left
                             ____ 3 point OEM lap/shoulder belts
                             ____ Supplemental Restraint System Modifications
                                  ____ Air Bag On/Off Switch
                                       ____ Driver ____ Passenger
                                       ____ Both
                                  ____ Disconnect Air Bag System
E ____ Power seat base   ____ 6-way   ____ Delco after market power seat base
                           ____ 4-way
F ____ Hinged foot plate to allow for use of standard pedals
G ____ Transfer assist
        ____ overhead bar/strap ____ transfer board
H ____ Head Rest
        ____ Power   ____ Wheelchair-Mounted
I ____ Other

NOTES:

III STEERING SYSTEM

A Steering effort:
   ____ Standard OEM power effort ____ Low effort (20-24 ounce)*
   ____ Maximum reduced effort (4 - 6 ounce)* ____ Emergency backup system*
   *Make/Model

B Steering column:
   ____ Standard wheel   ____ Reduced size wheel* ____ Inches
   ____ Remote steering*   ____ Right ____ Left
   *Make/Model

C Steering Device: ____ spinner knob* ____ tri-pin* ____ V-grip*
                    ____ flat spinner* ____ amputee ring* ____ Other*
   *Make/model

D Other

NOTES:

IV   BRAKE/ACCELERATOR SYSTEM

A Braking effort:
   ____ Standard OEM power brakes ____ Low effort (11 ft. pounds)
   ____ Maximum reduced effort (7 ft. pounds) ____ Emergency backup

B Hand Controls:
   Mechanical:
   ____ Push/right-angle* ____ Push/Rock* ____ Push/pull*
   ____ Push-twist* ____ Other* ____
   ____ Quad grip handle
   Mounted for: ____ Left hand use ____ Right hand use
   *Make/model

   Powered Control Systems:

   Control Motion:
   ____ Push-gas/Pull-Brake ____ Push-brake/Pull-gas
   ____ Outward - gas/Inward-Brake
   Control handle interface

NOTES:

Figure 14-3   Vehicle modification checklist. (Courtesy Louisiana Tech University, Ruston, LA.)

Continued

____ Lever ____ T-handle ____ Tri-pin
____ Tri-pin w/linear platform ____ Dual lever
____ Other
Mounted for: ____ Left hand use ____ Right hand use
*Make/model

C ____ Pedal Guard*
____ Brake & Accelerator ____ Brake Only ____Accelerator Only
*Make/Model

D ____ Left foot accelerator*
E ____ Pedal extensions*
____Both ____Brake only ____Accelerator only
Length: ____ Brake pedal ____ "
____ Accelerator pedal ____ "
*Make/model

F ____ Other

NOTES:

V SECONDARY CONTROLS
Mode A: Items to be operable by the driver while the vehicle is in motion
A Horn ____ OEM ____ Remote* Location ____
B Dimmer____ OEM ____ Remote* Location ____
C Turn Signals ____ OEM ____ Remote* Location ____
D Wiper ____ OEM ____ Remote* Location ____
E Washer____ OEM ____ Remote* Location ____
F Cruise "SET" ____ OEM ____ Remote* Location ____
G Cruise "ON" ____ OEM ____ Remote* Location ____
Remote Panel(s)* Make/Model
Location

NOTES:

Mode B: Items to be operable while brake is activated (i.e. with steering hand)
A Parking brake ____ OEM ____ Extension lever*
____ Power* Switch location____
*Make/model

B Ignition ____ OEM ____ Key holder*
____ Keyless* Switch location ____
*Make/model

C Gear selector ____ OEM ____ Extension lever* ____ Power system*
*Make/model

NOTES:

Mode C: Other secondary controls (to remain OEM unless otherwise noted)
____ HVAC system Modification ____
____ Rear Heat/Air fan Modification ____
____ Power windows Modification ____
____ Power door locks Modification ____

____ Power mirrors Modification ____
____ Headlight/parking lights Modification ____
____ Interior lights Modification ____
____ Flasher Modification ____
____ Rear Wiper/Wash Modification ____
____ Rear Defrost Modification ____
____ Other Modification ____
_____ Modification ____

NOTES:

VI MISCELLANEOUS
A Passenger position (occupied wheelchair)
____ Wheelchair tie-down ____ Automatic* ____ Four point*
____ Occupant protection ____ lap/shoulder belts*
*Make/model

B Unoccupied wheelchair/scooter
____ Tie-down*
*Make/model
Location

C Torso support (attach torso support order form)
____ Wheelchair-mounted* ____ Driver seat mounted*
*Make/model

D Electrical System
____ Battery protection system* ____ Power backup*
*Make/model

E ____ Rear hazard detector*
*Make/model

F ____ Dual instructor brake
G ____ Suspension modifications*
*Make/model
H ____ Other

NOTES:

VII WHEELCHAIR/SCOOTER TRANSPORT
A Vehicle interior
____ Rear* ____ Passenger side* ____ Driver side*
____ Trunk* ____ Truck bed* ____ Other*
*Make/Model

B Vehicle exterior
____ Car top carrier*
____ Driver side ____ Passenger side
____ Trailer*
____ Bumper/hitch mounted*
*Make/model

NOTES:

Figure 14-3 cont'd

Reaction Time

It is a good idea for the DRS to check the individual's reaction time in an evaluation vehicle. This is one of the on-road assessments that clients often perceive as pertinent to real-life, on-road driving. This view is in sharp contrast with the reaction time test that is performed in a clinical environment, which is often perceived by clients as less relevant than the reaction time test that is performed in the "real world." The dynamic conditions on the road will allow the DRS to observe how the vehicle's motion and other dynamic environmental factors (e.g., distractions, traffic, lighting, weather) that are not present during the clinical evaluation will affect the client's reaction time. The DRS should expect a client's responses to be slightly slower on the road versus an indoor evaluation setting.

Effects of Vehicle Dynamics

The effects of vehicle dynamics can only be determined while driving or riding in a vehicle that is moving while on the road. The following factors should be assessed whenever applicable:

- Sitting balance: An individual with a physical disability may have decreased sitting balance that can affect driving even during routine vehicular maneuvers, such as stopping and starting or changing lanes.
- Trunk control: For individuals with impaired or absent trunk muscle strength and endurance, their ability to maintain control of a vehicle may be affected while performing turning, starting, or stopping maneuvers. For example if a hand control is being used, only one hand is available for steering because the other hand is required for controlling the brake and accelerator.

A combination of minimal or absent lower extremity or trunk muscle strength and endurance and the inability to hold a steering wheel with both hands may create problems with maintaining control of the vehicle. Torso supports and belts can be added directly to the wheelchair or the vehicle seat to compensate for this problem.

- Use of extremities: For persons with higher-level disabilities, control of their arms also may be affected by the dynamics of the vehicle. The client's upper extremities may need to be supported with armrests or other types of positioning devices. See Chapter 9 for more information on seating and driving.

On-Road Driving Evaluation

The evaluation of on-road driving performance is critical to the DRS's ability to make appropriate recommendations pertaining to an individual's driving status, structural modifications to the vehicle, and adaptive driving aids. In rare instances DRSs recommend that a client cease driving based on clinical evaluation results; however, a DRS should never recommend that an individual operate a vehicle until a comprehensive driver rehabilitation evaluation, including an on-road evaluation, has been completed. Results of a well-documented on-road driving evaluation will also increase the client's acceptance of the evaluation results and recommendations. DRSs should keep in mind that their reports will most likely be read by clients, family members, physicians, driver's license agency personnel, third-party funding sources, insurance company representatives, lawyers, and others. Recommendations based on an evaluation that included observation of a client's on-road driving performance will go a long way in establishing credibility and face validity, as well as acceptance of the documented status and subsequent recommendations.

In conjunction with using the results of the clinical evaluation, an on-road performance evaluation also provides valuable information that influences the DRS's decision-making process. Specifically, reviewing evaluation results that are clear and concise may assist with determining and planning the following:

- Follow-up activities: The results of the on-road evaluation will help the DRS develop a list of follow-up activities, including referring the client for a specialty evaluation such as a vision examination or wheeled mobility and seating evaluation, general therapy services, or a driver improvement course.
- Compensatory strategies: Based on a DRS's observation of the client's on-road performance, the DRS should determine a series of compensatory strategies to improve driving performance. These strategies will assist in determining on- and/or off-road instruction activities.
- Amount of on-road training: In all cases in which significant driving performance deficits exist or when a client is inexperienced in using adaptive driving equipment, on-road training should be provided while on the road. The DRS can estimate the amount of time required based on the deficits noted and compensatory strategies being recommended. An estimate of on-road training time and rationale may be required by a third-party funding source before training can commence.

When to Conduct an On-Road Evaluation

In rare cases DRSs will find that behind-the-wheel activities while on the road are not appropriate for some clients. The DRS should develop a policy for determining if and when to assess a client while off or on road. If a DRS is concerned about safety for any reason that can be clearly articulated, the on-road evaluation should not be conducted. This decision may be based on how the DRS interprets the clinical evaluation results or other observations, such as the client's interpersonal communication, general mood and disposition (i.e., state of mind), and physical health (e.g., the client reported that he or she has had seizure activity within the past several months). The DRS should always keep in mind that operating a motor vehicle not only has safety implications for the client and DRS but can also impact the safety and well-being of other roadway users. The DRS may have to recommend that the client cease driving and help him or her to pursue alternative transportation (i.e., alternative community mobility) options.

Documenting the On-Road Evaluation

After a client has acquired sufficient vehicle control skills or is an experienced driver who does not require the use of adapted driving aids, an on-road evaluation of driving performance is conducted, and the results are documented. Some initial considerations when documenting the results of the on-road driving evaluation include the importance of using a standardized rating system that features a simple scoring procedure that can help improve interrater reliability and testing validity:

- Standardized rating system: The rating system should be developed and used for every assessment conducted within a given program. A performance rating checklist and standardized documentation procedures will foster greater reliability (i.e., DRSs will rate a client's performance with greater consistency) and overall validity of the assessments conducted.
- Interrater reliability: This concept is used to validate a DRS's ratings of a client's driving performance. An experienced DRS should work with his or her colleague who is new to the field of driver rehabilitation to determine an acceptable level of agreement when

rating driving performance and determining subsequent recommendations. In other words, two DRSs should be able to observe an individual's performance, document similar ratings of driving performance, and agree on the basic recommendations that address an individual's driving status and needs.

• Simple scoring procedure: A simple scoring procedure should be developed for the on-road evaluation. This procedure will increase scoring reliability, facilitate greater accuracy in the interpretation of evaluation results, and improve interrater reliability.

The On-Road Evaluation Form

The on-road evaluation should include specific performance categories that are meant to determine the individual's ability to demonstrate competency with performing a variety of driving tasks. These tasks include observation, communication, speed adjustment, vehicle positioning, time and space judgment, and vehicle response.

Observation relates to the client's ability to observe important visual cues in the driving environment. Some specific items that DRSs may want to include in the on-road evaluation are listed in Box 14-2.

Other items relate to how well the individual is able to communicate with other highway users by using turn signals, horn, and emergency flashers. Box 14-3 includes some specific items DRSs may want to include in their checklists.

The performance category of speed adjustment indicates how well the client observes and adjusts to changes in roadway and traffic conditions and situations. Box 14-4 includes checklist items.

Vehicle positioning relates to how well the driver positions the vehicle before, during, and after maneuvers, such as turns, exits, and entrances. It also relates to positioning the automobile in relationship to other vehicles and roadway users. Some checklist items are included in Box 14-5.

Time and space judgment relates to the consumer's ability to determine and control the space around his or her vehicle. Box 14-6 lists some items the DRS may wish to include to help ensure there are adequate adjustments.

Vehicle response relates to the client's ability to demonstrate appropriate control of vehicle speed and direction in various driving environments. Items included in this category are listed in Box 14-7.

In addition to a checklist with performance items, the evaluation form should include some identifying information, such as the client's name, evaluator(s), date(s) of evaluation, starting and ending time(s), road condition(s), and weather conditions at the time of the evaluation(s).

A summary page that includes space for the DRS's comments also should be included on the form. This space can be used to note specific items of concern that

Box 14-2	**Visual Cue Checklist for the On-Road Evaluation**

• Demonstrates proper use of mirrors
• Demonstrates proper techniques for checking blind spots
• Demonstrates proper intersection checks
• Observes changes in roadway surfaces and configurations
• Observes traffic control devices
• Observes cues from other road users
• Demonstrates proper visual scanning techniques
• Identifies potential and real hazards

Box 14-4	**Speed Adjustment Checklist for the On-Road Evaluation**

• Adjusts vehicle's speed in response to changing environmental conditions
• Makes appropriate adjustments when approaching and passing through a busy intersection
• Makes adjustments when being overtaken by or passing another vehicle
• Adjusts for railroad crossings and bridges
• Observes maximum and minimum posted speed limits
• Adjusts to roadway surfaces and configurations
• Adjusts to traffic patterns and flow

Box 14-3	**Communication Checklist for the On-Road Evaluation**

• Demonstrates appropriate turn signal use
• Signals far enough in advance
• Uses the vehicle's horn appropriately
• Demonstrates proper headlight use
• Demonstrates proper emergency flasher use
• Understands and can demonstrate proper arm signals for turns and stopping

Box 14-5	**Vehicle Positioning Checklist for the On-Road Evaluation**

• Demonstrates proper vehicle positioning before, during, and after turns
• Avoids positioning his or her own vehicle in the blind spots of other roadway users
• Maintains an appropriate following distance
• Yields the right of way when appropriate or required to help ensure optimal safety
• Maintains adequate lateral space cushions

Box 14-6	Time and Space Judgment Checklist for the On-road Evaluation

- Negotiating intersections
- Turning
- Lane changes
- Passing
- Backing up
- Parking
- Following another vehicle
- Merging

Box 14-7	Vehicle Response Checklist for the On-road Evaluation

- Demonstrates adequate brake control
- Demonstrates adequate accelerator control
- Demonstrates adequate steering control
- Responds appropriately to traffic signs, signals, and markings
- Operates the vehicle smoothly and efficiently

the DRS will use to develop recommendations and follow-up strategies. The form should also include some disclaimers, such as the following:

> The on-road performance evaluation should be administered and interpreted only by a properly trained driver rehabilitation specialist. Moreover, the results of this evaluation should be viewed as an indication of the driver's functional driving ability at the time of the evaluation, and NOT as a comprehensive measure of driving potential or predictor of future performance.

A sample on-road performance evaluation form is included in Figure 14-4.

VEHICLE INSPECTIONS

When a client owns a vehicle that is being considered for vehicle modifications, it should be thoroughly inspected by a knowledgeable DRS or engineer (e.g., rehabilitation or mechanical engineer). The inspection is conducted to evaluate the vehicle's condition (e.g., structural integrity), dependability, and overall potential to serve as the client's primary means of mobility. In all cases in which a used vehicle is being considered, the vehicle should be inspected before the modifications.

Premodification Vehicle Inspections
The formal vehicle inspection should be conducted by a qualified DRS, mobility equipment dealer, or certified

automotive mechanic. The DRS and mobility equipment dealer are involved in the inspection process because they are knowledgeable about the kinds of vehicle modifications that are required to address the client's specific needs. The inspector should also be knowledgeable of any applicable guidelines or standards, such as the U.S. Department of Transportation's Federal Motor Vehicle Safety Standards (FMVSS), the National Mobility Equipment Dealers Association (NMEDA) guidelines, the Department of Veterans Affairs (VA) Standards, and applicable state rehabilitation services agency guidelines.

Vehicle inspection documentation should include the following specific information:
- Vehicle description
- Vehicle make, model, and year
- Vehicle identification number (VIN)
- Registered vehicle owner(s)
- Actual mileage
- Inspection validation
- License plate number validation tabs
- Factory equipment, including steering, brakes, HVAC system (i.e., heater, vent, air conditioner), power equipment (e.g., door locks, windows, and mirrors), number and type of doors and hatches, and seating
- After-market equipment and modifications, including custom conversions, electronics, trailer hitch, and mobility options, such as a wheelchair/scooter lift, adaptive driving equipment, and seating system
- Condition of vehicle, including tires, brakes, steering, suspension, engine, transmission, electrical, body and upholstery, and test drive
- Recommendations, including answers to the following questions: Is the vehicle safe to operate? Is the vehicle type appropriate for the proposed modifications? What is the estimated remaining useful vehicle life? Does the vehicle meet applicable funding agency guidelines?

A sample premodification vehicle inspection form is included in Figure 14-5.

INTERPRETING EVALUATION RESULTS AND MAKING RECOMMENDATIONS

Once the on-road evaluation has been completed, the DRS should review the results of the clinical and the on-road evaluations. Each client demonstrates different abilities and deficits during the various parts of the overall comprehensive driver rehabilitation evaluation; therefore the DRS's next task should be to interpret the evaluation results in advance of generating recommendations.

Interpreting Evaluation Results
Interpreting the evaluation results is an important first step before making definitive recommendations

Figure 14-4 On-road performance test form. (Courtesy Louisiana Tech University, Ruston, LA.)

because the proper analysis of the evaluation results will lead the DRS to generate recommendations that are efficacious, relevant, and cost-effective. Interpretation of the evaluation results should include (1) comparing and relating the clinical evaluation results and the on-road observations, (2) determining the nature and extent of the noted deficits, (3) identifying critical problems and challenges that impede driving performance, (4) considering potential solutions, and (5) considering the client's driving environment, including inside and outside of the motor vehicle.

Before the DRS documents his or her recommendations, he or she should review the results of the on-road evaluation to determine whether they correlate with

Driver Rehabilitation Program
Center for Biomedical Engineering and Rehabilitation Science
Ann B. Havard, LOTR, CDRS   Michael K. Shipp, M.Ed., CDRS

PRE- MODIFICATION VEHICLE INSPECTION FORM

Note: Form is to be completed by a qualified automotive mechanic, mobility equipment technician, rehabilitation engineer, or driver rehabilitation specialist.

Client's Name _____ Date _____
Registered Owner of Vehicle _____
Relationship to Client _____

DESCRIPTION OF VEHICLE

Year _____ Make _____ Model _____
Vehicle Identification Number (V.I.N.) _____
Mileage (Actual) _____ License Plate Number _____ State _____
Valid Inspection Sticker _____ Yes _____ No Expiration Date _____

FACTORY EQUIPMENT

Please check the factory equipment included on this vehicle.

_____ Power Steering	_____ Automatic Transmission
_____ Power Brakes - Disc	_____ Manual Transmission
_____ Power Brakes - ABS	_____ Sliding Side Door - Driver Side
_____ Air Conditioner	_____ Sliding Side Door - Passenger Side
_____ Rear Air Conditioner	_____ Swing Side Doors
_____ Power Windows	_____ Trailer Towing Package
_____ Power Door Locks	_____ Load Leveling Suspension
_____ Power Driver Seat	_____ Heavy Duty Suspension
_____ Speed (Cruise) Control	_____ Hand Parking Brake
_____ Tilt Steering	_____ Foot Parking Brake
_____ Power Exterior Mirrors	_____ Split Bench Seat
_____ Other (please list)	

AFTER-MARKET EQUIPMENT & MODIFICATIONS

Please list any additional items (custom conversion, raised roof, wheelchair lift, etc.).

VEHICLE CONDITION

Item	Condition			Comments
	Excel	Good Fair	Poor	
Tires	~	~~	~	
Brakes	~	~~	~	
Steering System	~	~~	~	
Suspension System	~	~~	~	
Engine	~	~~	~	
Transmission	~	~~	~	
Air Conditioning	~	~~	~	
Electrical System	~	~~	~	
Body	~	~~	~	
Upholstery	~	~~	~	
Cooling System	~	~~	~	
Test Drive	~	~~	~	
Overall Condition	~	~~	~	

In your opinion, is this vehicle safe to operate? _____ Yes _____ No
Is this vehicle suitable for the modifications for this consumer? _____ Yes _____ No _____ N/A
Estimate the remaining useful life of this vehicle _____ Years _____ Miles
Meets funding agency guidelines?   _____ Yes _____ No _____ N/A
Additional Comments:
Inspector:
Address:
Phone:

_____   _____
Signature   Date
Please Return Form to: Driver Rehabilitation Program
                                      Louisiana Tech University
                                      711 S. Vienna
                                      Ruston, LA 71270

Figure 14-5 Premodification vehicle inspection. (Courtesy Louisiana Tech University, Ruston, LA.)

the results of the clinical evaluation. For example a client's driving performance that indicates difficulty with determining appropriate following distances may be related to a deficit in depth perception found during the clinical vision or visual perception testing.

After deficient performance areas have been identified, the DRS should determine the possible etiology of the deficits. A problem may be because of a particular disability (e.g., someone with a traumatic brain injury may have cognitive processing problems that decrease his or her ability to make quick and accurate decisions). The client may also have deficits related to premorbid driving behaviors (e.g., poor driving habits such as speeding). A driver who does not perform blind spot checks or use turn signals when changing lanes is a common example. Another reason that driving deficits are observed may be because of a client's limited driving experience. People with limited time behind the wheel are usually new drivers or individuals who have not driven in a number of years. These clients initially should not be expected to perform basic vehicle control skills with the precision of an experienced driver.

The DRS next should identify the critical problems and challenges that can have a significant impact on the client's ability to drive safely. These deficits are generally related to cognitive or visual perceptual aspects of driving. As previously noted the extent of these problems will vary with each client. The DRS must use his or her clinical reasoning skills to accurately assess the subtle performance nuances in addition to the more apparent deficits that are impacting the client's overall driving performance and potential to be a safe driver.

The DRS should begin considering potential solutions once any critical problems have been identified. Consultation with other health care professionals may be required to further clarify the type and extent of these deficits and possible solutions. For example if an individual with a stroke has homonymous hemianopsia resulting in a visual field deficit, he or she may be referred to a rehabilitation optometrist and an occupational therapist specializing in low vision. This is a critical step that must occur before documenting the final recommendations because the client's status may change or not be accurately assessed.

The final step in this process is to consider the client's driving environment inside and outside the motor vehicle. Although every client should be evaluated using the same on-road performance test route, the normal driving environment will vary with each individual. Some clients will be from small, rural communities where the surroundings require relatively little cognitive activity while driving when compared with clients who live in highly populated metropolitan areas with a wide variety of urban and suburban roadway and traffic situations that demand increased cognitive loads. To illustrate this point consider a scenario in which two clients demonstrate the same level of proficiency during an on-road evaluation. However, one of the clients lives in a smaller community set within a pastoral environment and therefore is able to drive safely considering the reduced environmental challenges. Conversely the other client lives in a large city and is required to adhere to specific driving restrictions or cease driving altogether because of the high cognitive load required to drive in the busy urban environment from which he or she came.

Documenting Driver Rehabilitation Recommendations

Once the DRS has thoroughly reviewed the information gathered during the predriving and on-road evaluations, solutions should be identified and recommendations documented. There are seven main categories to consider when formulating and documenting driver rehabilitation recommendations: (1) the client's driving status, (2) further specialized evaluations, (3) the need for driver improvement courses, (4) vehicle selection, (5) vehicle modifications, (6) on-road training needs, and (7) driver licensing or relicensing issues. The DRS should document his or her recommendations that reflect the sequential order listed here.

Driving Status

The most important thing that clients usually want to know is whether they are going to be able to drive. In most cases there are three possible recommendations that address the client's driving status:

1. The client may drive without restrictions.
2. The client may drive with restrictions.
3. The client must cease driving and work with the DRS to identify dependable alternative transportation options.

DRSs are responsible to stay abreast of the specific driver restrictions that can be placed on a client's license and applicable policies and laws that govern licensing and relicensing procedures in each respective state. DRSs must also be aware of the procedures and laws that govern how to report drivers who should not drive because of safety considerations. See Appendix A for more information on state driver licensing requirements and reporting laws.

Further Specialized Evaluations

The client may need a more specific evaluation by a health care professional specializing in a particular area. These may include visual, medical, or psychological specialists. Services provided by specialists can help to shed light on the client's status and provide additional interventions designed to address a specific deficit or set of deficits. In writing these recommendations, the DRS should be specific about requesting an evaluation that is related to driving. For example when referring a client to a neuropsychologist, the DRS must make sure that the neuropsychologist understands that the evaluation has been requested to help determine the client's

fitness for driving. The neuropsychologist will modify his or her approach by providing the client with a series of standardized tests that assess cognitive processing skills that are more closely related to the driving task versus conducting an entire battery of neuropsychological standardized assessments. The former is more likely to result in recommendations that are related to driving and augment the comprehensive driver rehabilitation evaluation. See Chapter 7 for more information on neuropsychological testing and determining a client's fitness to drive.

Need for Driver Improvement Courses

Whenever a DRS documents a deficit identified during the driver evaluation process, he or she should provide a recommendation for remediation. A common recommendation is for the client to participate in a driver improvement course. This recommendation is especially relevant for those clients who are new drivers and have not completed a driver education course recently, those who have not driven for an extended period (i.e., several months to years), and those who do not exhibit adequate knowledge of the rules of the road or basic knowledge of the driving task.

Driver improvement courses are available from several sources, are 4 to 8 hours in length, and consist of didactic classroom instruction. Classroom instruction topics include general rules of the road, proper driving procedures, collision avoidance, time and space management, and awareness about the effects of drugs and alcohol on driving. There are also driver improvement programs that have been developed for older drivers that emphasize mature driver issues and strategies to continue driving safely. The National Safety Council, the American Automobile Association (AAA), and the American Association of Retired Persons (AARP) have developed driver improvement courses that are available in or near most communities throughout the United States. These courses are well established and are often accepted by automobile insurance carriers for a discount on insurance. Information regarding these courses is included in Box 14-8. See Chapter 1 and Appendices F, G, and H for information on the effectiveness of driver improvement courses and programs in the United States designed to address driving-related issues, including driving cessation.

Vehicle Selection

If a client does not have a vehicle available for modification or an existing vehicle will not accommodate the necessary modifications, the DRS should assist the client in determining the most appropriate type of vehicle that could best meet his or her particular driving needs. Factors that should be considered when providing a client with vehicle options include the following:

Box 14-8	Traffic Safety Resources: Driver Improvement Programs

AAA: American Automobile Association
1000 AAA Drive, MS 33
Heathrow, FL 32746
407-444-7960
www.aaapublicaffairs.com

Managing Visibility, Time and Space
Safe Driving for Mature Operators
AARP
601 E Street, NW
Washington, DC 20049
888-667-2277
www.aarp.org

55 Alive Driver Safety Program
National Safety Council
1121 Spring Lake Drive
Itaska, IL 60143
630-285-1121
Fax: 630-285-1315
www.nsc.org

Defensive Driving Course
Coaching the Mature Driver
Smith System Driver Improvement Institute
2201 Brookhollow Plaza Drive, Suite 200
Arlington, TX 76006
800-777-7648
www.smith-system.com

- Structural modifications (e.g., raised roof, raised doors, lowered floor, and rear versus side-entry lifts)
- Primary control modifications (e.g., steering, braking, and accelerator)
- Secondary control modifications (e.g., ignition, turn signals, horn, and climate control)
- Wheelchair/scooter transport (e.g., trailer hitch capacity and trunk/door dimensions)

The combination of these factors may limit the vehicle options that are available for the client. The DRS should provide a list of specific vehicle chassis options and standard equipment versus options available for each model. As the need for advanced levels of adaptive driving controls increases, combined with a client's need to use a wheelchair for vehicle entry, the vehicle options that are available generally decrease. The DRS and client should also feel free to consult with a mobility equipment dealer (i.e., vehicle modifier) for guidance when making a vehicle selection. If a third-party funding source will be involved in the purchase of a vehicle, vehicle modifications, or adaptive driving equipment, the DRS and the consumer should be knowledgeable of the funding source's guidelines and policies related to accessing and using available funds.

Vehicle Modifications

Once the client's vehicle selection has been determined, documented, reviewed, and approved by the applicable driver rehabilitation team members (e.g., DRS, client, case manager, and insurance claims adjustor), the DRS should prepare the client's vehicle modification plan, which includes detailed specifications that address the structural modifications and adaptive driving controls that are necessary to meet the client's mobility needs. A detailed vehicle modification plan will enable the

vehicle modifier to provide the funding source or client with accurate price estimates and a timeline for fittings and completion of the vehicle modifications.

When a DRS is considering potential vehicle modifications and associated specifications, it is imperative that the client is involved in the decision-making process. Moreover the DRS and client should also keep the following issues and considerations in mind:

- Informed choice: Clients should have access to information regarding the product choices available that address their needs. Vendors should be willing to inform a client about a product or products, such as cost, durability, and function, even if they are not a distributor for the product or products in question.
- Vendor products: Clients need to know what products are available from reputable driver rehabilitation vendors.
- Cost estimate: A cost estimate should be provided to the client that is easy to read and itemizes the associated costs for procurement, taxes, shipping, and labor, such as setup, fitting costs, and delivery.
- Safety concerns: Any safety concerns about using a product should be thoroughly discussed with the client. For example changing to a smaller steering wheel that requires the vehicle modifier to disconnect the air bag system may create viable health- and safety-related concerns for the client and must be addressed before the modification is initiated.

A sample document for vehicle modification specifications is included in Figure 14-6.

On-Road Training

Behind-the-wheel training while on the road should be considered for all clients receiving driver rehabilitation services. DRSs should make every effort to help clients improve driving skills and knowledge that have been

Driver Rehabilitation Program
Center for Biomedical Engineering and Rehabilitation Science

Ann B. Havard, LOTR, CDRS   Michael K. Shipp, M.Ed., CDRS

VEHICLE MODIFICATION SPECIFICATIONS
(Suggested Format)

Date:
Date of Evaluation:
Consumer: Name
           Address
           Telephone
Evaluators:
Type of Conversion:
              (See attached wheelchair data form)
Vehicle Description:
              (see attached Vehicle Information Form)

IMPORTANT NOTES TO VENDORS:
Allowable substitution of functionally equivalent products
List specific substitute items
Unusual items or information

Louisiana Tech University
711 South Vienna   Ruston, LA 71270   318 257-4562   318 255-4175 FAX

I   VEHICLE ENTRY

Items included:

Automatic Door Operators	Entry Control Systems
Wheelchair Lift	Raised Roof
Raised Door(s)	Lowered Floor Conversion
Entry Lighting	Automatic Ramp System
Rear Fuel System Relocation	

II   DRIVER POSITION

Items Included:

Power Pan	Power Transfer Seat
Wheelchair Tie-down	Head Rest
Seat Modifications	
Removable Driver Seat	

III   STEERING SYSTEM

Items Included:

Reduced Effort Steering w/backup	Steering Extensions
Reduced Size Wheel	Steering Device
Air Bag Modification	Remote Steering System
Joystick Driving System	Horizontal Steering

IV   BRAKE/ACCELERATOR SYSTEM

Items Included:

Reduced Effort Brakes w/backup	Mechanical Hand Controls
Pedal Extensions	Servo Controls
Left Foot Accelerator	Pedal Block (protector)

V   SECONDARY CONTROLS

Items Included:

Mode A - to be operated while the vehicle is in motion

High Beam Selector	Turn Signals
Horn	Cruise "SET"
Windshield Washer/Momentary Wipe	

Mode B - to be operable while maintaining control of the vehicle brake function

Ignition/Starter	Gear Selector

Mode C - to be operable while the vehicle is stationary

HVAC	Door Locks
Cruise "ON" and "OFF"	Parking Brake
Hazard Flasher	Rear Accessories
Mirrors	Light Controls
Power Seat	Window Regulator

VI   MISCELLANEOUS

Items Included:
  Wheelchair Tie-down for Unoccupied Wheelchair
  Occupant Protection System (passenger)
  Torso Restraint
  Dual Battery/Back up Power Supply
  Rear Suspension Modification
  Communication System
  Auxiliary Air Conditioner
  Dual Instructor Brake
  Audible Alerting Devices
  Wheelchair/scooter Hoists

VII   TRANSPORTATION and TRAVEL

Items Included:
  The vendor will be responsible for pickup of the vehicle from the client's residence, including fuel costs.
  The vehicle will be transported via commercial carrier from the consumer's residence to the mobility equipment dealer's location.

VIII   FITTINGS

Items Included:
  Intermediate fittings
  Final fittings
  Except when noted otherwise, final fittings, inspections and delivery of the vehicle will occur at the vendor location. Cost will be the responsibility of the client or third party payer.

IX   ON-ROAD TRAINING

  Due to the nature of some vehicle modifications and the potential for needing to make adjustments, the initial training session(s) should be conducted from the dealer's location.

X   WARRANTIES:

  The vendor will be responsible for meeting manufacturer and funding agency warranty requirements.
  The consumer will be responsible for the cost of transporting the vehicle to and from the service location.

XI   MAINTENANCE AND SERVICE

  The consumer will be responsible for following the maintenance and service schedules for the adaptive equipment and vehicle modifications.
  The consumer will be responsible for the cost of transporting the vehicle to and from the service location.

XII   ESTIMATES

Cost
  Estimates should be provided according to funding agency requirements.
  Time of completion
  Time required for completion for the modifications _____ the mobility dealer has received a purchase order

XIII   MOBILITY EQUIPMENT DEALERS

  A list of mobility equipment dealers meeting the funding source's guidelines is attached.
  The consumer should select a vendor according to funding agency guidelines.

XIV   NOTES

Where applicable, equipment should meet or exceed the requirements established by the Department of Veterans' Affairs, Louisiana Rehabilitation Services, Society of Automotive Engineers, and the National Mobility Equipment Dealers Association.

These recommendations should be considered valid for one year from the date of evaluation. Beyond that time, a re-evaluation of the client may be necessary.

These recommendations have been developed based upon the education and experience of the evaluation team and the client's experience

Figure 14-6   Vehicle modification specifications format. (Courtesy Louisiana Tech University, Ruston, LA.)

Figure 14-6 cont'd

identified as deficient during the comprehensive driver rehabilitation evaluation. Training should be recommended in all of the following cases:

- When the client is a new driver
- When the client has not driven for several months or longer
- When the client demonstrates deficits related to driving procedures and knowledge
- When the client is in need of learning compensatory driving strategies

Driver instruction and training should be provided by a DRS with an appropriate endorsement or experience working with clients with disabilities or aging-related concerns while on the road. In some jurisdictions the authority that controls driver licensing and relicensing requires and offers specialty certification for DRSs to legally provide driver rehabilitation services and provides consumers and health care professionals with a list of qualified DRSs who provide driving instruction.

In cases in which a DRS only provides the clinical evaluation, he or she should prepare a comprehensive training plan that will be used by the DRS who will provide the on-road driver training. Training plans should include the following information:

- Client history: This part of the document should include information about the client's diagnosis or diagnoses, current driving status and history, mobility status, and summaries of the clinical and on-road evaluation results. The DRS should provide copies of the evaluation report to other driver rehabilitation team members, such as the client and the client's case manager.
- Goals and training regimen: The DRS and client should formulate short- and long-term goals that reflect desired driver training outcomes once the on-road driver training sessions have been completed. The DRS should also provide general recommendations for enhancing the client's driving skills. Detailed recommendations should highlight compensatory strategies that address the client's specific deficits and needs. Finally DRSs should also estimate the total number of hours they expect will be

required for training and the duration and frequency of each session to achieve the established goals. In many states there are limits placed on the number of hours of on-road instruction that can be provided per day for any given client, and DRSs must be aware of (and adhere to) their respective state's guidelines.

- Follow-up recommendations: The DRS should provide a list of recommendations for short- and long-term follow-up review that feature the specific action steps needed to be taken after the training sessions have been completed. The recommendations will most likely pertain to initiating the required steps for licensure or relicensure and requesting a report from the DRS who provided the on-road training.

A sample on-road training plan format is included in Figure 14-7.

Driver Licensing or Relicensing Agencies

It is critical for DRSs to become familiar with the driver licensing agency policies and procedures in their respective jurisdictions where driver rehabilitation services are provided to clients and their caregivers. Each agency often has different rules and regulations regarding licensure and relicensure procedures for people with disabilities or the elderly population. DRSs must be able to make appropriate recommendations for their clients regarding initial licensure or relicensure, the medical review, testing or retesting, and restrictions and endorsements.

It is also important for DRSs to establish a good working relationship with the examiners who are employed by driver licensing agencies in their service delivery areas. By providing assistance to each other, the DRS and license examiner teams can better serve clients and address their specific licensing needs.

In most jurisdictions clients are responsible for reporting to their local licensing agency any condition or conditions that may affect their ability to operate a motor vehicle. In most cases clients and their caregivers are unaware of this requirement or do not wish to compromise their driving status, so they prefer not to say anything. Clients are not likely to address this sensitive issue until after they have recovered from their illness or

Driver Rehabilitation Program
Center for Biomedical Engineering and Rehabilitation Science

Ann B. Havard, LOTR, CDRS   Michael K. Shipp, M.Ed., CDRS

ON-ROAD TRAINING PLAN

DATE:
D.O.E.

CONSUMER:

DRIVER LICENSE #:   EXPIR: RESTR:
EVALUATOR(S):
TRAINING VEHICLE:
(See Attached Specifications)

CONSUMER HISTORY:

MOBILITY STATUS:

CLINICAL ASSESSMENT RESULTS:

IN-VEHICLE ASSESSMENT RESULTS:

TRAINING RECOMMENDATIONS

TRAINING TIME: Maximum Hours: Per Session:_____ Per Day:

GENERAL:

SPECIFIC:

FOLLOW-UP RECOMMENDATIONS

Michael K. Shipp, M.Ed., CDRS   Date
Certified Driver Rehabilitation Specialist

Louisiana Tech University

711 South Vienna   Ruston, LA 71270

Figure 14-7 On-road training plan model. (Courtesy Louisiana Tech University, Ruston, LA.)

injury. Therefore recommending that a client report to his or her local driver licensing authority should be routinely included in the driver rehabilitation evaluation report. The client should also be made aware of any applicable restrictions placed on his or her driver's license because of specific deficits or needs identified during the evaluation process. Many states require that a specific restriction be placed on a client's license for using an adapted driving control, such as hand controls. The consumer should be informed that it might not be legal to operate a vehicle without proper adaptive driving equipment.

DRSs should possess knowledge of the requirements as they apply to specific clients, including the following:
• Basic requirements for licensing and relicensing: The DRS should be knowledgeable of the basic licensing requirements and processes, including age, graduated licensing, prelicense requirements, vision testing, knowledge of the rules of the road, on-road performance standards, initial licensing and renewal procedures, and available testing accommodations, including translation services and alternative formats (e.g., a proctor can read the test questions in English or some other preferred language and use pictures to convey the test's content).

• Medical requirements: Anyone wishing to drive in the United States must be in compliance with the medical requirements that are mandated by each state's licensing agencies. Medical requirements include clients meeting minimum standards for visual acuity and not having experienced neurologic (e.g., recent seizure activity or loss of consciousness), orthopedic, or cardiac deficits within a specified period that would otherwise prevent clients from driving. The licensing agencies also can provide the mandatory requirements for physician involvement in their respective states.
• Driver licenses and restrictions: Each licensing authority has its own system for establishing and enforcing restrictions placed on a driver's license. Restrictions enable people with disabilities, elderly persons, and others a means to drive under specified conditions. Most restrictions are categorized as follows:
  • Sensory: These include restrictions that address decreased vision or hearing; for example deficits that require the client to use corrective lenses, hearing aids, or adapted mirrors.
  • Factory equipment: These restrictions relate to motor vehicle factory options, such as requiring a person to drive a vehicle that has an automatic transmission, power steering, or mechanical turn signals.
  • Adaptive equipment: This category involves requiring people to use items such as a hand control, left foot accelerator, or an adapted steering device.
  • Time of day: Some individuals benefit from a time-of-day restriction. These restrictions may include daylight driving only or driving only at specified times of the day when traffic may be lighter.
  • Driving radius: Some people can benefit a great deal from limiting their driving to a specified radius near their home, school, and place of employment. This strategy often enables clients to continue driving to essential locations in a familiar area and maintain some degree of community participation that is essential for quality of life.
  • Limited speeds or roadways: Examples of restrictions in this category include limiting an individual to driving at speeds ≤45 mph or not driving on expressways.
  • Medical restrictions: These restrictions generally apply to situations such as wearing a prosthesis or requiring periodic medical reviews because a client has been diagnosed with a progressive disability.

In addition to being aware of the various state mandated licensing restrictions, DRSs should be aware of the procedures for reporting unsafe drivers and sharing driver rehabilitation evaluation reports and other pertinent information with licensing agency authorities.

PREPARING VEHICLE MODIFICATION SPECIFICATIONS

When documenting vehicle modification specifications, it is important to know who will be reading and processing the report. The specifications should provide sufficient detail so that purchasers and vehicle modifiers have a clear understanding of the modification and equipment a DRS is recommending for a client. In the following sections information that should be included in a document that features specifications for recommended vehicle modifications is presented.

General Information
Identifying Information
This section should include information such as the date that the recommended modifications were documented, date(s) and types of driver rehabilitation evaluations completed, the name or names of the DRSs who performed the evaluations, and the client's name and contact information.

Type of Vehicle Conversion
This portion of the document should describe the way in which the client will be driving or riding as a passenger in the vehicle. As a driver the client may be able to ambulate independently without an ambulation aid, ambulate using a walking aid, transfer from a wheelchair or scooter into and out of the vehicle, or access the vehicle and drive from a wheelchair. As a passenger the client may ride in the vehicle while seated in a wheelchair or transfer from a wheelchair or scooter into the vehicle's original equipment manufacturer (OEM) passenger's seat. See Chapters 5 and 9 for more information on issues pertaining to vehicle accessibility, stowing an ambulation aid in a vehicle, and the impact wheeled mobility devices can have on driving.

Vehicle Description
The vehicle modification specifications should include the following information about the vehicle when applicable: date of premodification inspection (in the case of a used vehicle); registered owner(s); make, model, year, mileage, and VIN; existing factory options and packages; after-market modifications and equipment (e.g., custom interiors, running boards, and entertainment equipment); and mobility modifications and equipment (e.g., lowered floor conversion, wheelchair lift, wheelchair tie-down system, and adaptive driving equipment).

Vehicle Modification Specifications
The specific plan for modifying a vehicle may be divided into categories that will assist the vehicle modifiers and other driver rehabilitation team members to

understand the rationale supporting each specific recommendation. Suggested categories include vehicle entry, driver position, steering system, brake/accelerator system, secondary controls, and miscellaneous.

Vehicle Entry
This includes such items as wheelchair lifts, power door operators, lowered floor modifications, raised roofs and doors, and entry controls.

Driver Position
The next factor to consider is how the driver will be positioned and secured in the vehicle with the aim to maximize safety, independence, and comfort when accessing primary and secondary driving controls and ensuring a clear line of sight. Items in this category include the power pan, wheelchair tie-down system, occupant restraint and protection systems, transfer seat, and seating modifications.

Steering System
Steering system modification options include reduced effort steering, emergency back-up systems, joystick driving systems, remote or horizontal steering, air bag modifications, and other steering devices, such as a spinner knob installed on the steering wheel (e.g., at the 6 or 2 o'clock position).

Brake/Accelerator System
Modifications in this category include mechanical hand controls, left foot accelerators, pedal extensions, pedal guards/blocks, and powered control systems.

Secondary Controls
This category includes a myriad of modification options. When documenting these items the DRS should categorize them according to the client's functional use of the controls. A suggested method for grouping these modifications is to organize them according to the vehicle's status. For example the Society of Automotive Engineers (SAE) in their Recommended Practice on Secondary Controls (J2388) uses the following definitions:
- Mode A: These controls are accessible to a driver while the vehicle is in operating mode, such as braking, steering, and accelerator; for example the cruise control "set" function, headlight beam selector, horn, turn signal, and windshield washer.
- Mode B: These controls are operable by the driver while maintaining control of the vehicle's brake function when the vehicle is not in motion; for example vehicle startup or restart that is necessitated by a stalled engine requiring access to the gear shift selector and ignition/starter.
- Mode C: These controls are accessible by the driver when the vehicle is temporarily stationary or parked;

for example cruise control "on" and "off" function, hazard flashers, mirrors, power seat, windshield wipers, door locks, HVAC, parking brake, rear accessories, and window regulator.

Miscellaneous

This heading may be used to include such items as vehicle modifications that enable wheelchair or scooter transportation, instructor brakes, wheelchair tie-down systems, suspension system upgrades, power back-up systems, torso supports, and audible alerting devices.

Other Considerations

After providing an exhaustive list of recommended vehicle modifications and adaptive driving equipment necessary to address the client's specific driving needs, the DRS should include several other sections to provide further information and clarification for anyone reading the document. Some of these categories may include, but are certainly not limited to, the following: (1) transportation and travel, (2) client-vehicle fittings, (3) on-road training, (4) warranties, (5) maintenance and services, (6) estimates, (7) qualified mobility dealers, (8) documentation and note writing, and (9) attachments.

Transportation and Travel

This section includes content that describes the current location of the vehicle and who is responsible for pickup and delivery. The method of transport is also specified; for example it may read "transport via common carrier" or "to be driven to the vendor location."

Client-Vehicle Fittings

Information should be provided regarding the type and number of fittings necessary, the location of the fittings (normally at the vendor's place of business), and participants who should be present.

On-Road Training

To help ensure that the vehicle modifier is available to make necessary adjustments to the vehicle or adapted driving equipment, the initial training sessions may need to be close to the vendor's location.

Warranties

Vendors should be responsible for honoring the manufacturer's warranty and the funding agency's expectations and requirements. Vehicle modifiers should also provide all of the necessary information and training to educate the client about the applicable warranties and responsibilities of the manufacturer, vehicle modifier, and client; for example the client may be responsible for the cost of transporting the vehicle to and from the vehicle modifier's facility for routine maintenance and repairs.

Maintenance and Service

The vehicle modifier is responsible for providing all maintenance and service information to the client. The client should be responsible for following the maintenance and service schedules for the adaptive driving equipment, vehicle modifications, and OEM chassis. The client is usually responsible for the cost of transporting the vehicle to and from the service facility.

Estimates

When applicable the report should include an estimate of the costs for completing the recommended vehicle modifications and installing the adaptive driving equipment. A timeline that estimates the date for the completion of the vehicle modifications should also be included. The DRS should have already contacted the vehicle modifier to confirm the anticipated timeline before providing the client and other driver rehabilitation team members an estimated vehicle completion date.

Locating Qualified Mobility Equipment Dealers

DRSs should refer their clients to reputable mobility equipment dealers who are qualified to perform recommended vehicle modifications and install adapted driving equipment. A list of qualified vendors may be obtained from a funding agency, such as the Department of VA, rehabilitation services, or NMEDA Quality Assurance Program where available. In cases in which FMVSS will be affected, the vehicle modifier should also be registered with the National Highway Traffic Safety Administration's (NHTSA's) vehicle modifier database.

Notes

This section includes information regarding the following items:
- Allowable substitutions for functionally equivalent products.
- Expiration of the documented recommendations: This is especially important when a client has been diagnosed with a progressive disability.
- Applicable standards and guidelines should be followed and can be ascertained from the appropriate organizations, including SAE, NMEDA, Association for Driver Rehabilitation Specialists (ADED), American Occupational Therapy Association (AOTA), NHTSA, VA, and other funding agencies.
- Disclaimer statements regarding evaluation conditions, equipment availability, and evaluator training should be included to reduce the DRS's and driver rehabilitation program's liability.
- The location of the driver rehabilitation program and the DRS's contact information, including address, telephone and facsimile numbers, e-mail address, and cellular phone number, if available.

Attachments

Attachments can provide important information that can clarify the report's content. Attachments may include information and specific data pertaining to the client's vehicle, wheeled mobility device or ambulation aid, torso support ordering information, and diagrams that help to clarify the DRS's recommendations and thoughts about equipment placement and fabrication. A sample format for vehicle modification specifications is shown in Figure 14-6.

SUMMARY

There are many steps involved in developing professionally prepared documentation for comprehensive driver rehabilitation evaluation and on-road training outcomes. One of the most important steps a program can take to help ensure that its DRSs produce well-prepared documentation is to establish a protocol (i.e., policy and procedure) for report writing. It is important that a program's administrators periodically assess adherence to the protocol by all members of the driver rehabilitation team. This chapter also provided a template and suggestions for content that can be used for generating a driver rehabilitation documentation protocol.

Chapter 15

FUNDING FOR DRIVER REHABILITATION SERVICES AND EQUIPMENT

Karen Monaco • Joseph M. Pellerito, Jr.

KEY TERMS

- Vocational rehabilitation
- Managed care
- Current procedural terminology (CPT) codes
- Documentation

CHAPTER OBJECTIVES

After completing this chapter, the reader will be able to do the following:

- Identify the sources of funding for driver rehabilitation equipment and services.
- Understand the restrictions of each type of funding.
- Recognize the advantages and disadvantages of insurance reimbursement.
- Explain the importance of documentation.

There are financial costs associated with securing or maintaining the privilege to operate a motor vehicle in the United States and elsewhere around the world. Costs vary and are impacted by a number of factors, not the least of which is a client's driver rehabilitation and community mobility goals. Irrespective of whether a client or a funding entity pays for driver rehabilitation services and equipment, the greatest costs are incurred when a new or used car, van, or truck is purchased and then modified by a vehicle modifier according to the driver rehabilitation specialist's (DRS's) recommendations. Additional costs are incurred when a client insures a vehicle, fills it with gasoline or charges its bat-

teries (or both if the client is driving a hybrid vehicle), pays for routine maintenance, has unexpected repairs performed as necessary, and, of course, pays for driver rehabilitation services, including a comprehensive driver rehabilitation evaluation and training program.

When driver rehabilitation services, equipment, or both are warranted, either the client or some other funding source must incur the associated costs. In some cases the funding source or sources are specified and viable. Funding is granted by a limited number of entities that generally include the following:

- State vocational rehabilitation (VR) services
- Automotive insurance companies
- Workers' compensation

In other instances the client must either pay out of pocket or devise a strategy to secure funding, such as working with organizations with a philanthropic mission (e.g., United Way), borrowing money from friends and family members, securing a bank loan, or some combination of these and other procurement strategies.

Advances in the field of driver rehabilitation have helped to increase the likelihood that people with severe disabilities and elderly persons can safely drive motor vehicles, assuming they have access to the levels of funding required to pay for structural modifications and installation of adaptive driving equipment. Funding is often the key that enables clients to take advantage of the positive changes that are occurring within the field of driver rehabilitation. Some examples of the changes in the field include but are certainly not limited to the following:

- Advances in sophisticated electronic technology have made primary and secondary controls increasingly accessible to people with disabilities.
- The adoption of universal design principles by engineers who design cars, vans, and trucks has made vehicles more user friendly right off the assembly line.

- Some motor vehicles have become much safer thanks in part to components designed to enhance driver and passenger safety, such as side curtain air bags, as well as the more traditional front air bags, seat belts, and crumple zones.
- Improvements have been made in traffic safety thanks to research that is guiding the design of the external environment. See Chapters 16 and 19 for more information on universal design and traffic safety.
- An increase in the number of vehicles that can be modified by a vehicle modifier has resulted in more choices for the consumer.
- Professional organizations have revised their standards of practice, which has helped to improve the effectiveness of evaluation and training services rendered by DRSs and the vehicle modification techniques used by vehicle modifiers. Key professional organizations that are involved in monitoring and enhancing the standards of practice include the Association of Driver Rehabilitation Specialists (ADED), the American Occupational Therapy Association (AOTA), the National Mobility Equipment Dealer's Association (NMEDA), and the National Highway Traffic Safety Administration (NHTSA).

The obstacle to these developments is that driver rehabilitation services and equipment are inaccessible to a large percentage of prospective clients in need because they lack the necessary financial resources. That is why practice patterns are changing and DRSs are spending more time helping clients and caregivers identify alternative funding sources in addition to the traditional services, such as conducting clinical evaluations and providing on-road rehabilitation and training. The process is often delayed because it is not unusual for a client who has participated in the clinical and on-road evaluations to defer on-road driver training until a funding source that pays for vehicle modifications, including adaptive driving equipment, has been identified and the required funds have been secured. This approach is usually subscribed to by DRSs and their clients because of the expenses associated with purchasing and modifying a vehicle.

The best time to resume driver rehabilitation and training is at the same time financial resources become available, and the DRS can assist the client with selecting and purchasing a vehicle and consult with the mobility equipment dealer to complete the prescribed vehicle modifications. This approach is not ideal because of the delay in the client achieving driving independence or optimal passenger safety; however, in many cases the DRS and client have no other choice. A prescription for adaptive driving equipment and structural vehicle modifications is generally considered to be valid for 1 year from the date that it is written, except in those instances when the client has been diagnosed with a condition that will cause a rapid or moderate decline in his or her health and overall functional status. After 1 year has passed, a comprehensive driver rehabilitation reevaluation of the client's driving status may be necessary, along with a repeated course of on-road driver training. Driving needs may change in 1 year, and driving equipment technology is constantly evolving and improving; either of these situations could invalidate previous recommendations for adapted driving. It is an unfortunate scenario for anyone (e.g., a young person with a disability) to have to postpone this long-anticipated rite of passage, not because the technology is not available to make him or her as independent as his or her able-bodied peers, but simply because of a lack of available funding.

In other cases the client may be eligible for the traditional funding sources identified earlier in this chapter. In either case DRSs and clients will share a sense of accomplishment and relief once driver training has been completed and the client receives his or her license to drive a motor vehicle.

FUNDING SOURCES

The most widely used funding sources for driver rehabilitation services and equipment (e.g., the comprehensive driver rehabilitation evaluation, driver training, adaptive driving equipment, and vehicle modifications) are state vocational and rehabilitation agencies and workers' compensation agencies. *Vocational rehabilitation* services are often used to assess a client's work-related capacity and to enable a person to drive to and from work. Workers' compensation agency representatives become involved when a person sustains a work-related injury that affects safe motor vehicle operation. When an individual does not qualify for either workers' compensation or VR services, identifying a combination of funding sources may be required to cover the driver rehabilitation expenses that will be incurred.

Once again traditional funding sources may include, but are not limited to, state agencies that address the needs of disabled consumers (e.g., state funded commissions for the blind), national organizations that advocate for people with specific disabilities or elderly persons (e.g., Multiple Sclerosis Society, Arthritis Foundation, and American Association of Retired Persons [AARP]), the Department of Veterans Affairs, public school systems, charitable organizations (e.g., Kiwanis, Knights of Columbus, Optimist, and Rotary clubs), vehicle manufacturers, and health insurance carriers, to name a few. Availability of funding varies from state to state and is impacted by strict eligibility criteria.

VOCATIONAL REHABILITATION FUNDING

VR services were first provided to clients in 1920, and the benefits have grown exponentially since that time. It is estimated that the federal government spends >$1 billion each year to provide VR services to individuals who meet the eligibility requirements.[1] VR monies may be used for part or all of the following driver rehabilitation services and equipment:

- Predriving clinical evaluations
- On- and off-road driver training
- Structural modifications to the vehicle
- Adaptive driving equipment
- Driving cessation planning
- Exploring alternatives to driving that enable community mobility

Eligibility for VR services should always be considered before providing driver rehabilitation services for clients with disabilities and elderly persons who would like to return to work or seek employment. Needless to say, DRSs should explore funding sources that can help to minimize or eliminate the client's costs whenever possible.

In keeping with the central goal of VR, many clients are not eligible for driver rehabilitation services until employment has been secured. In other states driver rehabilitation may be provided while the client is pursuing educational objectives related to prospective or actual future employment opportunities or simply to eliminate one of the barriers to becoming gainfully employed.

A written authorization must be obtained from the client's vocational counselor before driver rehabilitation services can be initiated. Reimbursement may be flexible or fixed and may include mileage and travel time; however, restrictions may be set for the amount of training time and radius of travel. A bidding process is usually involved in awarding the vehicle modification contract, with consideration given to vendor location and client preference. Limitations may be required on the age and mileage of the vehicle to be modified. Some VR agencies will only pay for vehicle modifications after the completion of the driver training program, including the successful completion of the state licensing road test. Adaptive driving equipment may be guaranteed for a specified period, after which time it must be replaced with new driving aids; however, VR may or may not provide funding for updated driving equipment and subsequent driver training. Other state agencies may work in conjunction with state VR services to provide comprehensive reimbursement for driver rehabilitation services and equipment. In South Carolina, for example, county boards of disabilities and special needs work alone or in tandem with the state VR service providers to pay for services rendered by DRSs. Other state agencies may serve as resource centers to assist clients and caregivers to identify a potential funding source.

WORKERS' COMPENSATION

"Workers' compensation programs are government-sponsored and employer-financed systems for compensating employees who incur an injury or illness in connection with their employment. . . . Benefits provided under workers' compensation laws include medical care, disability payments, rehabilitation services, survivor benefits, and funeral expenses."[2] Workers' compensation laws became effective in every state in 1948 as a means of "avoiding litigation over industrial accidents by equating a specific injury with a particular amount of compensation."[1]

Driver rehabilitation services, which may encompass vehicle modifications for the client as either a passenger or driver, may be provided under workers' compensation. The cost of acquiring and modifying a new vehicle may be covered when the client's transportation needs require an adapted vehicle. DRSs must receive authorization from the client's case manager, with a written guarantee for the itemized costs to guard against cost reductions based on the Medicare fee schedule or other state fee schedules. Submitting an invoice rather than a claim form also helps to ensure a guaranteed rate for services rendered. Documentation supporting the provider's fee structure is required, especially when fees exceed the payer's fee schedule allowance, and should reflect the service provider's customary charges and nature of the services provided. Reimbursement for travel time and mileage may also be included in the cost of conducting a comprehensive driver rehabilitation evaluation and developing and implementing a personalized on-road training regimen.

DEPARTMENT OF VETERANS AFFAIRS

Driver rehabilitation services are provided through the Veterans Administration (VA) for service-connected and non–service-connected veterans who served in a branch of the U.S. military. The VA Medical Centers employ DRSs with various educational backgrounds including occupational therapy, among others. DRSs provide comprehensive driver rehabilitation evaluations and develop and implement on-road training programs for veterans with disabilities. Adaptive driving equipment and vehicle modifications are paid for once the bidding process has taken place among qualified, VA-approved mobility equipment dealers (i.e., vehicle modifiers). The VA has established strict guidelines for the vehicle modification process, which must be followed by the driver rehabilitation team members including the DRS and vehicle modifiers.

NATIONAL ORGANIZATIONS FOR PEOPLE WITH DISABILITIES

Funding for adaptive driving equipment may be obtained from national organizations for the disabled. For example the Georgia chapter of the National Multiple Sclerosis Society has funded hand controls and other mechanical adaptive driving devices for its members. With a greater understanding of the need for evaluation and training in the therapeutic use of adaptive driving equipment, national service organizations also have been persuaded to provide funding for the services rendered by DRSs as well.

PUBLIC SCHOOL SYSTEMS

In 1975 the Individuals with Disabilities Education Act (IDEA) was passed by Congress to ensure that all children with disabilities in need of special education are provided an appropriate education at public expense in the least restrictive environment.[3] When driver's education is provided in a school system appropriate accommodations must be made for students with special needs using specialized instruction and/or adaptive driving equipment. The student must often be enrolled in the school's driver education program to qualify for funding for adaptive driving services and equipment. School systems may contract with DRSs to provide evaluation and training when those resources do not exist within the school district. Fees for travel may be included in the cost of driver rehabilitation.

MOBILITY ASSISTANCE REBATES

Most major vehicle manufacturers offer rebates up to $1000 toward the cost of vehicle modifications and adaptive driving equipment on new vehicles. Ford, Chrysler, General Motors, Saturn, Toyota, Volkswagen, and Audi currently offer mobility assistance rebates. Applications for rebates are provided through the individual vehicle dealerships. See section VI of the Adapted Driving Decision Guide on the CD-ROM provided with this book for more information on mobility assistance rebates.

PASS PLAN FOR VEHICLE PURCHASE

Individuals who receive supplemental security income (SSI) through the Social Security Administration may qualify for a plan for achieving self-support (PASS) to purchase a vehicle. The PASS program allows income and other financial resources to be set aside for a specified time for a work goal without affecting SSI payment amount or eligibility.[4] Using the PASS program can enable an individual to make lower monthly payments for a longer period, which otherwise would make a vehicle purchase cost-prohibitive. Using the PASS plan also could enable an individual to qualify for SSI. Applications must be approved according to specific eligibility criteria.

VEHICLE INSURANCE

When the cost of adaptive driving equipment and vehicle modifications exceeds the cost of the vehicle, it is especially important to insure the total package for damages or loss. Some insurance companies specialize in providing policies for adaptive equipped vehicles, with unique provisions for covering the cost of driver training courses and new adaptive driving equipment. Insurance companies should not discriminate when providing coverage for drivers with disabilities. The only cost difference should be reflected in the costs associated with insuring the client's adaptive driving equipment and vehicle modifications.

Vehicle insurance companies may also refer their customers for driver rehabilitation evaluations to determine potential for resuming driving after illness, injury, or the identification of aging-related deficits. Certification as a safe driver may be reassuring enough to the insurance company for the company to pay for the driver evaluation when it is performed at the company's request, even if no modifications are needed.

HEALTH CARE PLANS AND REIMBURSEMENT

The continually increasing health care costs can be attributed to general inflation, population increase, medical inflation, and new technologies.[5] This is despite the growth of health care through the involvement of the federal government in Medicaid and Medicare programs (one-fourth of all health care costs) and increasing involvement of private employers (one-third of all health care costs).[5] Spiraling health care costs have resulted in a lack of insurance coverage for 43 million Americans in 2003.

Managed care came about as a means to balance the delivery and financing of health care services. Managed care plans are created with incentives for enrollees to purchase services within established networks. The types of managed care plans include preferred provider organizations (PPOs) and health maintenance organizations (HMOs), both generally offered through employer group insurance plans. Civilian Health and Medical Program of the Uniformed Services (CHAMPUS), Medicare, and Medicaid are government-funded programs.

Preferred Provider Organizations

PPOs offer discounted fee schedules for health care providers in exchange for a guaranteed number of customers, who receive lower out-of-pocket expenses for services with a co-payment. Disincentives in the forms of higher deductibles and co-payments are applied for going outside of the approved network. Service providers can bill the PPO even if they are not a member of the network but may receive a lower rate of reimbursement for out-of-network services. The client will have a larger portion to pay when seeking services outside of his or her assigned network.

Health Maintenance Organizations

HMOs set fixed, prepaid, per-member fees with providers. Delivery of health care services is restricted through the primary care physician, who acts as a gatekeeper for referral to all other health care services. All care provided by the HMO must be approved by the primary care physician. Authorization is often required for all services. HMO plans that offer point-of-service provisions allow for out-of-network visits, although higher deductibles and co-payments are applied. Authorization for driver rehabilitation services is often denied but can still be billed to the HMO and appealed if denied on review.

CHAMPUS

CHAMPUS is provided to military personnel and their family members. Providers must be enrolled in the CHAMPUS program to receive reimbursement, which is based on the Medicare fee schedule. Tricare is an enhancement of CHAMPUS and is offered through the Department of Defense for military families and retirees. Active duty personnel automatically receive Tricare benefits.

Medicare

Congress established Medicare in 1966 as a federally funded medical assistance program for Americans aged ≥65 years and for people with disabilities who are indigent. In light of the estimation that the number of older drivers will double in 20 years, DRSs and other driver rehabilitation professionals will undoubtedly look to Medicare for reimbursement of services.

Medicare Part A is managed by an insurance intermediary that oversees payment for services provided to recipients receiving services at inpatient hospitals, skilled nursing facilities, home health, and hospice care facilities. Medicare Part B is managed by an insurance carrier that oversees reimbursement for outpatient hospitalization and services provided by physicians, independent practitioners, and other professional service providers. Providers must enroll if billing other third-party payers for the same services, but they do have the option of enrolling as assigned (paid directly by Medicare) or nonassigned (paid by the customer). Medicare providers are required to submit claims for services regardless of whether they accept assignment. Medicare reimburses 80% of approved charges following the Medicare fee schedule, which sets rates for *current procedural terminology (CPT) codes* used in billing for services. Outpatient (Part B) services are limited to $1500 annually.

Medicaid

Medicaid came into legal existence with the passage of Title XIX of the Social Security Act in 1965 and was designed to serve the poor and people with disabilities. Medicaid is managed at the state level, although the federal government provides funding. Each state program determines what medical services are covered and establishes payment amounts for each service.[6] For example Georgia Medicaid reimburses more than twice the amount for outpatient occupational therapy services as South Carolina Medicaid. Medicaid is always the payer of last resort. Enrollment in state Medicaid programs is optional, although once enrolled providers agree to accept the Medicaid rate of reimbursement and cannot bill the customer for the services rendered. Providers must enroll in each state where services are provided. Each state offers different programs of enrollment, such as Children's Intervention Services, Independent Care Waiver Program, and Mental Retardation Waiver Program. To enroll as a provider, the state's Medicaid program often requires written documentation to support the role of driver rehabilitation within the broader context of occupational therapy practice.

ISSUES IN HEALTH CARE REIMBURSEMENT

To date health care plans have been significantly underutilized as a funding source for driver rehabilitation services. Changes in the health care structure and the evolution of managed care have made it more difficult to determine health plan benefit coverage. Faced with increased paperwork and the possibility of denial for services, some programs opt for the less complicated approach of simply charging a fee for service. Charging clients for services benefits service providers because they are not required to fill out paperwork that is required for billing purposes and because they can set the service rates at whatever levels are deemed necessary and appropriate. The disadvantage to the consumer is the lack of affordable services, which also impacts the revenue sources and customer base for service providers. The inherent disadvantages of using insurance reimbursement to pay for driver rehabilitation services include time-consuming paperwork for filing claims and submitting documentation and the frequent inability to negotiate rates. Advantages include increased payer sources, patient advocacy, and professional recognition. The remainder of this chapter will focus on health care reimbursement from the perspective of the occupational therapist in private practice specializing in driver rehabilitation.

DOCUMENTATION

Documentation for driver rehabilitation services should include a current (30 days) physician referral written for an occupational therapy evaluation and treatment of driving skills. An HMO referral is needed to obtain authorization from the physician for individuals enrolled in HMOs. Medical history and age-related factors may impact current level of functioning. Driving history and recent motor vehicle record reflect past occupation in safe motor vehicle operation. Documentation must show how treatment has led to the client's ability to resume safe motor vehicle operation.

Detailing the importance of driving is critical in substantiating the role of driving as an instrumental activity of daily living (IADL). The need to drive is reinforced when specific errands and destinations are enumerated: driving to the grocery store, shopping centers, bank, drug store, church, medical and therapy appointments, and so on. "Driving is an essential activity of daily living in today's society, playing a pivotal role in personal independence, employment, and aging."[7]

CPT codes most often used in billing for occupational therapy driver evaluation and training include 97535 (self-care, training with adaptive driving equipment) and 97537 (community reentry). Physicians and nonphysicians who are state licensed to perform the services billed may use CPT codes. Insurance carriers and commissioners have specific reporting and reimbursement policies pertaining to services provided by non–state-licensed health care professionals.[8] Claim forms are submitted on the universally accepted CMS-1500 form (Figure 15-1). The top half of the form provides client information, and the bottom half includes provider information. Medicaid and Medicare provider enrollment workshops offer training on the process of completing claim forms.

COVERED SERVICES AND EXCLUSIONS

Health benefits should be verified before billing for services. With the policyholder's identification number and date of birth, coverage for occupational therapy services can be verified. Plan type, deductible, and number of visits per calendar year can also be identified. The health plan booklet further details coverage, definitions, exclusions, and limitations. Most plan booklets are broad in scope, and none of them specifically exclude driver rehabilitation. It is not unusual for occupational therapy to be denied as "not a covered service" when provided for driver rehabilitation despite the fact that occupational therapy is a covered service. Supportive documentation is needed to educate the medical review team on how driver rehabilitation fits within the scope of occupational therapy practice and how the services provided meet the coverage parameters for delivery of occupational therapy in the health benefit plan. When an occupational therapist provides driver rehabilitation services within the scope of occupational therapy practice, it cannot be excluded from occupational therapy services. When occupational therapy is a covered service of a health benefit contract, driver rehabilitation should be included as a covered service when provided by an occupational therapist.

Medicare guidelines for outpatient occupational therapy allow for service delivery when provided in either leased office space or the patient's home. Coverage for on-road evaluations can be justified by documenting that the vehicle has been leased or purchased and modified with adaptive driving equipment for the specific purpose of providing driver rehabilitation services. For the therapy services to be covered, they must relate directly and specifically to the treatment plan initiated by the physician; established by the physician, therapist, or both; be viewed as reasonable and medically necessary; and with an expectation of improved function in the client within a reasonable period. Before enrolling as a Medicare provider, the provider relations representative in the region should be contacted. The representative can direct the prospective provider to the proper source for information about coverage issues. The medical director of the regional Medicare office is usually responsible for determining what medical services are covered. Professional documentation that supports the inclusion of driver rehabilitation, on-road evaluation in particular, within the scope of occupational therapy practice can be provided from texts used in occupational therapy curricula, *Occupational Therapy: Practice Skills for Physical Dysfunction* and *Occupational Therapy in Physical Dysfunction*. Information that specifically refers to driving as an IADL can be provided from these resources. AOTA's series *Occupational Therapy Practice Guidelines for Adults with Traumatic Brain Injury* and *Occupational Therapy for Adults with Stroke* not only include coding information for driving, but they also state that comprehensive occupational therapy driving

PLEASE
DO NOT
STAPLE
IN THIS
AREA

CARRIER

| PICA | | | HEALTH INSURANCE CLAIM FORM | PICA |

HEALTH INSURANCE CLAIM FORM

| 1. MEDICARE   MEDICAID   CHAMPUS   CHAMPVA   GROUP HEALTH PLAN   FECA BLK LUNG   OTHER | 1a. INSURED'S I.D. NUMBER   (FOR PROGRAM IN ITEM 1) |
| (Medicare #)   (Medicaid #)   (Sponsor's SSN)   (VA File #)   (SSN or ID)   (SSN)   (ID) | |

| 2. PATIENT'S NAME (Last Name, First Name, Middle Initial) | 3. PATIENT'S BIRTH DATE   MM   DD   YY   SEX   M   F | 4. INSURED'S NAME (Last Name, First Name, Middle Initial) |

| 5. PATIENT'S ADDRESS (No., Street) | 6. PATIENT RELATIONSHIP TO INSURED   Self   Spouse   Child   Other | 7. INSURED'S ADDRESS (No., Street) |

| CITY   STATE | 8. PATIENT STATUS   Single   Married   Other | CITY   STATE |

| ZIP CODE   TELEPHONE (Include Area Code)   (   ) | Employed   Full-Time Student   Part-Time Student | ZIP CODE   TELEPHONE (INCLUDE AREA CODE)   (   ) |

| 9. OTHER INSURED'S NAME (Last Name, First Name, Middle Initial) | 10. IS PATIENT'S CONDITION RELATED TO: | 11. INSURED'S POLICY GROUP OR FECA NUMBER |

| a. OTHER INSURED'S POLICY OR GROUP NUMBER | a. EMPLOYMENT? (CURRENT OR PREVIOUS)   YES   NO | a. INSURED'S DATE OF BIRTH   MM   DD   YY   SEX   M   F |

| b. OTHER INSURED'S DATE OF BIRTH   MM   DD   YY   SEX   M   F | b. AUTO ACCIDENT?   PLACE (State)   YES   NO | b. EMPLOYER'S NAME OR SCHOOL NAME |

| c. EMPLOYER'S NAME OR SCHOOL NAME | c. OTHER ACCIDENT?   YES   NO | c. INSURANCE PLAN NAME OR PROGRAM NAME |

| d. INSURANCE PLAN NAME OR PROGRAM NAME | 10d. RESERVED FOR LOCAL USE | d. IS THERE ANOTHER HEALTH BENEFIT PLAN?   YES   NO   If yes, return to and complete item 9 a-d. |

READ BACK OF FORM BEFORE COMPLETING & SIGNING THIS FORM.

| 12. PATIENT'S OR AUTHORIZED PERSON'S SIGNATURE I authorize the release of any medical or other information necessary to process this claim. I also request payment of government benefits either to myself or to the party who accepts assignment below. | 13. INSURED'S OR AUTHORIZED PERSON'S SIGNATURE I authorize payment of medical benefits to the undersigned physician or supplier for services described below. |
| SIGNED   DATE | SIGNED |

PATIENT AND INSURED INFORMATION

| 14. DATE OF CURRENT: MM   DD   YY   ILLNESS (First symptom) OR   INJURY (Accident) OR   PREGNANCY(LMP) | 15. IF PATIENT HAS HAD SAME OR SIMILAR ILLNESS.   GIVE FIRST DATE   MM   DD   YY | 16. DATES PATIENT UNABLE TO WORK IN CURRENT OCCUPATION   MM   DD   YY   MM   DD   YY   FROM   TO |

| 17. NAME OF REFERRING PHYSICIAN OR OTHER SOURCE | 17a. I.D. NUMBER OF REFERRING PHYSICIAN | 18. HOSPITALIZATION DATES RELATED TO CURRENT SERVICES   MM   DD   YY   MM   DD   YY   FROM   TO |

| 19. RESERVED FOR LOCAL USE | 20. OUTSIDE LAB?   YES   NO $ CHARGES |

| 21. DIAGNOSIS OR NATURE OF ILLNESS OR INJURY. (RELATE ITEMS 1,2,3 OR 4 TO ITEM 24E BY LINE)   1. L___.___   2. L___.___   3. L___.___   4. L___.___ | 22. MEDICAID RESUBMISSION   CODE   ORIGINAL REF. NO. |
| | 23. PRIOR AUTHORIZATION NUMBER |

24. A DATE(S) OF SERVICE From To MM DD YY MM DD YY	B Place of Service	C Type of Service	D PROCEDURES, SERVICES, OR SUPPLIES (Explain Unusual Circumstances) CPT/HCPCS MODIFIER	E DIAGNOSIS CODE	F $ CHARGES	G DAYS OR UNITS	H EPSDT Family Plan	I EMG	J COB	K RESERVED FOR LOCAL USE
1										
2										
3										
4										
5										
6										

| 25. FEDERAL TAX I.D. NUMBER   SSN EIN | 26. PATIENT'S ACCOUNT NO. | 27. ACCEPT ASSIGNMENT?   (For govt. claims, see back)   YES   NO | 28. TOTAL CHARGE $ | 29. AMOUNT PAID $ | 30. BALANCE DUE $ |

| 31. SIGNATURE OF PHYSICIAN OR SUPPLIER   INCLUDING DEGREES OR CREDENTIALS   (I certify that the statements on the reverse   apply to this bill and are made a part thereof.)   SIGNED   DATE | 32. NAME AND ADDRESS OF FACILITY WHERE SERVICES WERE   RENDERED (If other than home or office) | 33. PHYSICIAN'S, SUPPLIER'S BILLING NAME, ADDRESS, ZIP CODE   & PHONE #   PIN#   GRP# |

PHYSICIAN OR SUPPLIER INFORMATION

(APPROVED BY AMA COUNCIL ON MEDICAL SERVICE 8/88)   **PLEASE PRINT OR TYPE**   APPROVED OMB-0938-0008 FORM CMS-1500 (12/90),   FORM RRB-1500,
APPROVED OMB-1215-0055 FORM OWCP-1500,   APPROVED OMB-0720-0001 (CHAMPUS)

Figure 15-1   CMS-1500 form. *(From www.cms.hhs.gov/providers/edi/cms1500.pdf)*

programs include clinical and on-road evaluation and training.

OUT-OF-NETWORK PROVIDERS

The private practitioner specializing in driver rehabilitation is more than likely not a member of the network of participating providers in commercial insurance plans. In this case documentation must be supplied to support the need to go out of network when driver rehabilitation services cannot be provided in the plan's network of service providers. If, for example, the closest participating provider is located outside a reasonable geographic radius, the customer may be justified in going out of network to receive services, and the out-of-network provider should be paid at the in-network rate.

MEDICAL NECESSITY

Health benefit plans list criteria for determining medical necessity, which include that services meet the following conditions:

1. Services are prescribed by a physician
2. Services are in accordance with current practice trends and accepted medical practices
3. Services are provided in the least costly setting
4. Services are rendered for an appropriate duration and frequency
5. Services are appropriate or consistent with the client's symptoms or diagnosis
6. Services are not provided primarily for convenience
7. Services do not entail educational or vocational training
8. Services are not custodial care

Criteria for medical necessity of treatment under Medicare guidelines also include that services require a skilled therapist and the client demonstrate a significant improvement in condition as a result of the approved intervention. A waiver of liability (Figure 15-2) should be signed by the client and maintained in the client's file whenever Medicare denial is anticipated. Medicare denials based on medical necessity must be appealed within 6 months. The process varies for assigned versus nonassigned providers and for Part A providers versus Part B providers.

Figure 15-2 Medicare waiver of liability.

MEDICARE WAIVER OF LIABILITY

Medicare will only pay for services that it determines to be reasonable and necessary under section 1862(a)(1) of the Medicare law. If a particular service, although it would otherwise be covered, is not reasonable and necessary under Medicare program standards, Medicare will deny payment for that service. I believe that, in your case, Medicare is likely to deny payment for:

Outpatient Occupational Therapy Driver Rehabilitation

for the following reason(s):_____

_____

Please read and sign the following statement:

"I have been informed by my therapist that he/she believes that, in my case, Medicare is likely to deny payment for the service(s) identified above, for the reason(s) stated. If Medicare denies payment, I agree to be personally and fully responsible for payment."

Signed: _____

Dated: _____

CLAIMS APPEAL PROCESS

An explanation of benefits (EOB) should be questioned when services are denied. Clarification with the insurance carrier may reveal that services were denied as not covered because they were determined to be "not medically necessary." It is important that the provider (i.e., DRS) speak the same language as the insurance company because an effective claims appeal must specifically address the basis of the denial. It is not unusual for a claim to be repeatedly denied with a different reason for denial provided each time.

The health plan booklet should be consulted to verify exclusions and coverage limitations. Deadlines for appeal should be followed with a reason for delay provided when appropriate. The question of who can make the appeal should be determined at the outset. Sometimes the provider can only appeal after obtaining written permission from the client. Telephone calls should be documented and may need to be included in the documentation for the appeal process. At each level of the appeal all previous documentation should be included so that the medical review board has a complete history of the case under review.

The Medicare Part B appeals process starts at the review level and can move to a fair hearing at the next level, with the final step at the administrative law judge (ALJ) hearing. Proper timing and reimbursement request limits do apply at each level of appeal. "Approximately two out of three Part B decisions are reversed at the first level of appeal."[6] Unfortunately many providers believe otherwise and are unwilling to undertake what they view as a difficult, if not impossible, task. Medicare provides guidelines and information on appealing denials. Medicare has even created forms to use to request a review or a hearing, although they are not required for requesting an appeal. Similar cases may be grouped together for a hearing when the denial is essentially the same for all of the claims. The following excerpt was taken from a successful appeal for a claim that was denied as a "non-medical service":

> In her denial letter, KN, claims specialist, erroneously lumped occupational therapy under other specifically excluded, non-medical services. These general exclusions are listed on page nine of the plan booklet to which I refer. Page sixteen lists occupational therapy under "Other Medical Benefits" and specifically states conditions, which this provider met, for payment. Please explain how a covered service, one that is paid for by the subscriber, and considered a medical benefit, can be excluded and alternately considered a non-medical service. The plan does not list specific services that are covered or not covered under the scope of occupational therapy. Therefore, I have every reason to expect payment for occupational therapy services.[9]

This next excerpt was taken from a successful appeal for a claim denied as "educational" and not covered:

During E's initial rehabilitation for her spinal cord injury, she received a lot of educational instruction from her therapists. E had to learn how to do everything all over again, in a different way, because of the impact her diagnosis had on her activities of daily living. From learning how to bathe and dress her lower-body, to learning how to safely transfer out of bed into a wheelchair, to learning how to maneuver a wheelchair, to learning how to stretch her paralyzed legs to maintain flexibility and prevent muscle contractures, to learning how to perform bladder and bowel care, to learning how to strengthen her upper-body to compensate for the paralysis in her lower-body, to learning how to appropriately use her adaptive equipment, etc. E's rehabilitation therapies could not have been adequately provided without educational instruction. It would be unfair to single out adaptive driving as an educational service when the role of an occupational therapist includes therapeutic instruction in a variety of activities, which include adaptive techniques as well as adaptive equipment. Driver rehabilitation is just one activity of daily living addressed under the scope of occupational therapy practice. The services I provided to E included therapeutic instruction in the use of adaptive driving equipment. E already knew how to drive. I did not provide conventional instruction in motor vehicle operation, as a driver educator would. My job as an occupational therapist and a driver rehabilitation specialist was to ensure that E was capable of operating adaptive driving equipment in a safe, independent manner. My goal was to restore E to her prior level of independent functioning.[10]

This last example was taken from a successful appeal for a claim denied as a "convenience":

> There is nothing convenient about not being able to operate a motor vehicle with standard driving controls. There is nothing convenient about not being able to teach your son how to drive a car without first obtaining a professional evaluation to determine whether your son needs adaptive driving equipment. There is nothing convenient about having to buy and install adaptive driving equipment in your vehicle in order to be able to operate it. . . . How can it be so convenient for an insurance company to blatantly deny an individual's bodily injuries that require all of the above in order to accomplish a necessary activity of daily living that the rest of us conveniently take for granted? . . . The need to drive on a daily basis is not a convenience, it is a necessity. To state otherwise is simply not true. To expect an individual with even less mobility skills than someone like myself who can walk and run without the use of adaptive aids, and still must depend on her vehicle to get to the doctor, grocery store, drug store, library, job, church, and anywhere else I need to go—this without a doubt is discrimination of the worst kind! There was no way B's parents could sidestep my services in order to assist B in his need to learn to operate a motor vehicle. B's parents did not have the knowledge base or the expertise to evaluate their son's physical abilities and limitations in order to determine whether he needed adaptive driving equipment. They did not have the resources to identify what type of assistive driving aids would be most appropriate for their son. They did the most logical, prudent thing they should have done.[11]

How does reimbursement from health insurance plans affect the field of driver rehabilitation, including DRSs, from other educational disciplines? At the very least it is a first step in getting more recognition for the field of driver rehabilitation. Currently medical professionals only use CPT codes in billing for services.

As the value of driver rehabilitation services gains increased recognition, the role of the DRS in the provision of services could be expanded to include reimbursement. The increasing population of older drivers and drivers with disabilities of all ages in need of driver rehabilitation services will help to ensure DRSs' continuing role in assisting people with safe driving and adaptive community mobility issues. It is up to the collective membership of professional organizations, such as ADED and the American Occupational Therapy Association (AOTA), to advocate for reimbursement in the interest of making driver rehabilitation and community mobility services available and affordable for anyone who needs them.

REFERENCES

1. Berkowitz E: *Disabled policy*, New York, 1987, Cambridge University Press.
2. Bruyere SM: Disability non-discrimination in the employment process: the role testing professionals. In Ekstrom RB, Smith DK, editors: *Assessing individuals with disabilities*, Washington, DC, 2002, American Psychological Association.
3. Individuals with Disabilities Act (IDEA), 1994, 20 U.S.C. 1400 et.seq.
4. *2003 Red Book*, Social Security Administration, SSA Pub. No. 64-030, ICN 436900, January 2003, p 41.
5. Weinstein M: *Guide to teaching managed care*, Bethesda, 1999, American Occupational Therapy Association.
6. Fordney MT: *Insurance handbook for the medical office*, Philadelphia, 2002, WB Saunders.
7. Lillie SM: Driving with a physical dysfunction. In Pedretti LW, editor: *Occupational therapy practice skill for physical dysfunction*, St. Louis, 1996, Mosby.
8. American Medical Association: *CPT-IS coding questions,* Chicago.
9. Monaco K: Personal communication, July 28, 1998.
10. Monaco K: Personal communication, April 18, 1999.
11. Monaco K: Personal communication, June 1, 1999.

Part V

ENVIRONMENTAL FACTORS IMPACTING DRIVERS, PASSENGERS, AND PEDESTRIANS

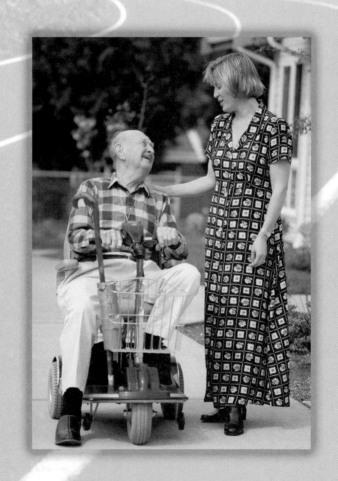

Chapter **16**

UNIVERSAL DESIGN AND THE AUTOMOBILE

R. Darin Ellis • Gary Leonard Talbot

KEY TERMS

- Universal design
- Society of Automotive Engineers (SAE)
- International Organization for Standardization (ISO)
- Original equipment manufacturer (OEM)
- Adapted vehicles
- Shared potential benefits
- Assistive technology
- Ergonomic design
- X-by-wire architecture
- Telematics
- Anthropometrics
- Reach envelope

CHAPTER OBJECTIVES

After completing this chapter, the reader will be able to do the following:

- Identify design considerations for people with disabilities and aging-related concerns.
- Understand the importance of universal design principles and how they are applied to the motor vehicle design process.
- Consider the potential benefits to continuing innovation in automotive design.

This chapter proposes that the principles of *universal design*, which has made a large impact in areas such as

architecture and telecommunications, can be successfully applied to the auto design process. Our premise is twofold: (1) many design innovations that are aimed at a sought-after market sector (e.g., suburban minivan drivers) can have positive consequences for people with disabilities and others; and (2) there are instances in which, all other things being equal, a design choice can be made that will lead to greater vehicle access for everyone including people with disabilities and aging-related concerns. With phrases such as "mass customization" being bandied about in the marketplace, it is time to concentrate on a broader view of design, design choices, and customer needs. Universal design concepts that incorporate the needs of a broad segment of the population can be extremely important and helpful for drivers and passengers ranging from seniors experiencing limitations for the first time to people with disabilities attempting to regain or maintain their independence and quality of life.

TRADITIONAL VEHICLE ARCHITECTURE

If we first step back and look at where standard vehicle design practices came from and for whom the requirements focused on for input, we would better understand the limitations of many current motor vehicles. In the 1950s when many current design practices began developing into standard approaches, the country was in the midst of producing the baby boomer generation. As a result the typical consumer group profile was a young family in their middle 30s with two or more children. This was an accurate model given the demographic breakdown of our society in the United States at that time. The *Society of Automotive Engineers (SAE)* design requirements were developed after focusing

345

on this new emerging population of baby boomers to determine how to best meet their needs and wants with regard to driving. However, the requirements did not factor in the impact of including a more diverse population model that also considered seniors experiencing aging-related challenges, well elderly persons, and people with disabilities. Focusing on a mere segment of the total population was considered appropriate at that time because most people did not subscribe to the notion that all groups, irrespective of the group's size, should be considered when developing design standards (or much of anything else for that matter). This issue was compounded by the fact that people with disabilities were often overlooked as a viable consumer group because of diminished life expectancy and a fundamental lack of advocacy for equal access to goods and services. Much of the efforts to raise the public's awareness of disability and aging-related issues had, for the most part, not yet been undertaken. As a result the engineering community did not include a more diverse population when it developed the SAE and *International Organization for Standardization (ISO)* standards relevant to human body dimensions in the vehicle cockpit.

Therefore vehicles that were designed using the specifications and practices (Table 16-1) placed drivers and occupants in the best location possible for driving the motor vehicle or riding as a passenger as long as they were a part of the baby boomer group. Little thought was given to how the wants or needs of the baby boomer population would change as a function of time. In the 1950s people with mobility-limiting disabilities also did not have as many opportunities to remain active and independent because of cumbersome (i.e., large and heavy) personal mobility equipment and inflexible vehicle designs. Things like removable seats, larger door openings, and sliding doors were not mainstream design solutions at that time. Traditional vehicle architectures also were developed around what the manufacturer could build and what the customer would accept. By and large, the customer at that time was young, active, able bodied, and able to get in and out of a vehicle with relative ease, comfort, and safety.

DEMOGRAPHICS AND THE DOMESTIC MARKET

When considering the potential impact of universal design in the automotive design process, it is instructive to first consider the consumer population and the size and nature of the automotive market. Results from Census 2000 found that 49.7 million people* have some sort of long-term disabling condition. Other

Table 16-1 SAE and ISO Standards Relevant to Human Body Dimensions in the Vehicle Cockpit

Standard	Description
SAE J941	Motor vehicle drivers' eye locations
SAE J1052	Motor vehicle drivers and passengers' head position
SAE J826	Devices for use in defining and measuring seating accommodation
SAE J1516	Accommodation tool reference point
SAE J1517	Driver-selected seat position
SAE J1100	Motor vehicle dimensions
ISO 6549	H-point machine
ISO 4131	Vehicle dimensions

SAE, Society of Automotive Engineers; *ISO*, International Organization for Standardization.

estimates place the number at >54 million. These numbers indicate that the disabled population represents approximately 20% of the civilian noninstitutionalized population, or one of every five people. Looking more closely at the population aged >65 years, >40% of the population indicated they had some sort of disability.[1]

Recent estimates[2] place the number of wheelchair users at approximately 1.7 million, including approximately 150,000 motorized wheelchair users. This group is relatively small when considered in light of the overall U.S. population and when compared with the size of the domestic motor vehicle market of approximately 16 million vehicles manufactured per year.[3] The size of the minivan market is approximately

---

*Those under the age of 5, in an institution (e.g., prison, nursing home, mental health care facility), and in the military were not considered in the Waldrop and Stern[1] analysis.

1 million vehicles per year[4] or approximately 7% of the total light vehicle sales. The combination of an apparent need for large vehicle design modifications and a relatively small market has resulted in mobility equipment dealers providing vehicle modification services for drivers and passengers. (See Chapters 4 and 11 for more information on the role of the vehicle modifier.) Personal transportation is incredibly important to people with disabilities, aging-related concerns, or both, but the market forces do not exist to create wholesale change in the mainstream auto design process.

LEVERAGING SHARED BENEFITS WITH OTHER CONSUMERS

Given the demographics of both disabilities and the motor vehicle market, as well as the inertia of traditional design practices, it perhaps is understandable why *original equipment manufacturer (OEM)* design innovation in a market-driven economy seems to be making a rather limited impact on the accessibility of personal transportation for people with disabilities and elderly persons. There is little hope in the near future for OEM-designed, mass-produced *adapted vehicles*. However, the advancement of a shared customer vision by people with disabilities and other consumer groups with *shared potential benefits*, combined with smart application by the OEMs of the principles of universal design, offers great promise.

Shared potential benefits are a vehicle feature (e.g., powered sliding passenger door on minivans) that is designed for one consumer group (e.g., suburban soccer moms) but can have great benefits for another. By breaking down the use of a vehicle into goals and behaviors (e.g., ingress/egress, controls, operation) and comparing across consumer groups, we can identify opportunities for design innovation with a much broader impact. Instances of this phenomenon occurring have already been recognized by industry observers; for example Walker[5] observed that the Toyota Scion, a vehicle designed explicitly for consumers in their 20s (the Generation Y market), also has been received favorably by older consumers because of features such as a high seat height and a versatile interior, including fold-flat front passenger seats.

There are potential shared benefits between people with disabilities and many other more highly targeted consumer groups. For example consider the senior population. Older adults are an increasing proportion of the overall population, a significant and sought-after segment of the vehicle market, and a group that presents particular design challenges. In terms of demo-

graphics a recent report[6] found that the older adult population (aged >65 years) in the United States reached nearly 36 million in 2002. By 2020 as many as one in three Americans will be aged >50 years, representing a growth of >82%. Approximately one in eight people (12%) in the United States is aged >65 years. Older people also are expected to live longer; remaining life expectancy for 65-year-old persons is 18 years (one-half are expected to live past age 83 years). By the year 2030 the older population will reach >70 million. The median net worth of households headed by someone aged >65 years is two times greater than that of the overall population.

Approximately one-half of new vehicles are purchased by someone aged >40 years. The older adult vehicle consumer makes up a disproportionate share of the upscale and luxury vehicle market. For example the average age of the Buick Park Avenue buyer is 68 years.[7] This is an important consideration when planning future vehicle options; a several hundred dollar option is much more likely to be accepted on a vehicle with a large purchase price.

The OEMs have begun to recognize the power of this market segment and the specific design considerations that should be taken into account when designing for older adults. For example Ford Motor Company developed a suit to sensitize designers to issues that are important to older adults: their Third Age Suit (Figure 16-1) simulated limitations in areas such as vision, touch, and range of motion. Recommendations that arose from using the suit led to the implementation of design features in the 1999 Ford Focus.[8] The scientific community has also recognized the parallels between the older adults and the general populace and the potential impact of design decisions on both populations. For example in a study of vehicle ingress and egress, Petzall[9] found that a sample of healthy older adults and a sample of wheelchair users had trouble with particular vehicle characteristics, such as a high door sill height.

UNIVERSAL DESIGN

Better design for people with disabilities or aging-related concerns can be better design for everyone universally. The initial use of the term universal design in the United States is generally credited to Mace.[10] Universal design is an approach to the practice of creating environments, tools, and products so that they are inherently maximally inclusive. Table 16-2 presents seven principles of universal design.[11] The most visible successes of the universal design movement to date include the redesign of public buildings to enhance access and ease of use[12] and the redesign of access to

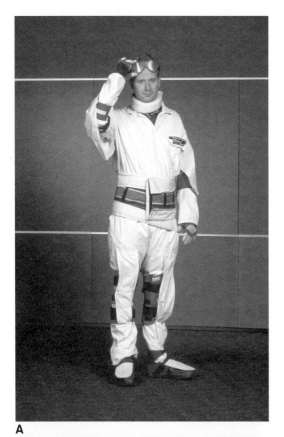

A

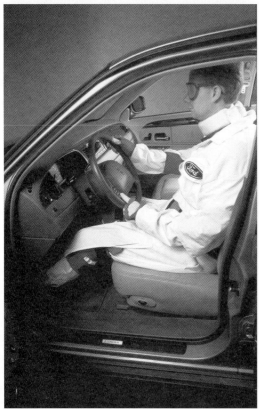

B

Figure 16-1 **A** and **B,** The Ford Motor Company
Third Age suit. (Courtesy Ford Motor Company, Dearborn, MI.)

telecommunications technology and information technology.[13]

The universal design approach stands in contrast to, but also complements, the traditional approaches of accommodation through *assistive technology* (which focuses on the unique fit between a specific individual and his or her tools and the environment) and *ergonomic design* (which aims to create products that are suitable for the vast majority, typically 95%, of the population). As previously discussed the approach of accommodation through assistive technology is by definition ad hoc and idiosyncratic. Solutions designed with this approach are limited in generality and thus limited in the scope of their potential impact. Ergonomic approaches also have limitations. Consider the 50th percentile fallacy; that is, by designing for the "average-sized" person, one actually excludes the majority of the population. In a study of 4063 men who were measured for 10 body dimensions, <8% of average men (the middle 30% in this case) were average with respect to two measurements and <2% were average for four measurements.[14] Vanderheiden[15] notes a similar phenomenon with respect to the ergonomic principle of accommodating 95% of the population; there are no tools available to predict that a product can or cannot be used by 95% of the population. Using these data we can predict that a particular dimension will be accommodated, but because people on the threshold of one dimension may or may not fall into the distribution for the next dimension, the number of people who would be accommodated by a 95th percentile design can be markedly smaller than one might expect. Also note that most ergonomic databases used for design purposes do not include disabled populations when describing the distribution of the characteristic of interest.

Although there appears to be no concerted effort across the OEM community to understand and promote the principles of universal design, there are nonetheless good examples of what the principles can affect. What follows are some case examples of what can be considered good universal design, whether or not they were intended as such. Each example is presented from the perspective of one or more of the universal design principles, and potential benefits from the perspective of the general population and people with disabilities have been included.

CASE EXAMPLE: AUTOMATIC TRANSMISSION SHIFTER INTERLOCK

Automatic transmissions are required by regulatory authorities to have safety interlocks that prevent unintended engagement of the transmission. Historically

Table 16-2 The Principles of Universal Design

Principle	Definition	Guidelines
Equitable use	The design is useful and marketable to people with diverse abilities	Provide the same means for all users: identical whenever possible; equivalent when not Avoid segregating or stigmatizing any users Provisions for privacy, security, and safety should be equally available to all users Make the design appealing to all users
Flexibility in use	The design accommodates a wide range of individual preferences and abilities	Provide choice in methods of use Accommodate right- or left-handed access and use Facilitate the user's accuracy and precision Provide adaptability to the user's pace
Simple and intuitive	Use of the design is easy to understand, regardless of the user's experience, knowledge, language skills, or current concentration level	Eliminate unnecessary complexity Be consistent with user expectations and intuition Accommodate a wide range of literacy and language skills Arrange information consistent with its importance Provide effective prompting and feedback during and after completion
Perceptible information	The design communicates necessary information effectively to the user, regardless of ambient conditions or the user's sensory abilities	Use different modes (pictorial, verbal, tactile) for redundant presentation of essential information Provide adequate contrast between essential information and its surroundings Maximize "legibility" of essential information Differentiate elements in ways that can be described (i.e., make it easy to give instructions or directions) Provide compatibility with a variety of techniques or devices used by people with sensory limitations
Tolerance for error	The design minimizes hazards and the adverse consequences of accidental or unintended actions	Arrange elements to minimize hazards and errors: most used elements, most accessible; hazardous elements eliminated, isolated, or shielded Provide warnings of hazards and errors Provide fail-safe features Discourage unconscious action in tasks that require vigilance
Low physical effort	The design can be used efficiently and comfortably and with a minimum of fatigue	Allow user to maintain a neutral body position Use reasonable operating forces Minimize repetitive actions Minimize sustained physical effort
Size and space for approach and use	Appropriate size and space are provided for approach, reach, manipulation, and use, regardless of user's body size, posture, or mobility	Provide a clear line of sight to important elements for any seated or standing user Make reach to all components comfortable for any seated or standing user Accommodate variations in hand and grip size Provide adequate space for the use of assistive devices or personal assistance

Data from Connell BR, Jones M, Mace R, et al: Principles of universal design, version 2.0, Raleigh, NC, 1997, North Carolina State University, The Center for Universal Design. Available at: http://www.design.ncsu.edu/cud/univ_design/principles/udprinciples.htm.

there has been some aspect of the control itself, such as a thumb button that must be depressed, to keep the shifter from inadvertently slipping into the wrong position. More recently a brake interlock has been required; it is impossible to get the car's transmission out of park without pressing the brake pedal. The brake interlock has the potential to make the thumb button on most console-mounted shifter controls redundant. Among other vehicles the Chrysler Crossfire transmission now has no such button, relying on the brake interlock instead (Figure 16-2).

Consider this from the perspective of people with disabilities or elderly persons with decreased upper extremity and hand function. For a person who needs right hand–mounted hand controls, getting the car out of park would require holding the brake lever with his or her right hand and reaching across with his or her left hand to manipulate the hand controls. Or consider a person who has experienced a stroke and has weakness because of hemiparesis or a person with severe rheumatoid arthritis; he or she may be able reach the control adequately but not possess the fine motor strength and coordination to operate the thumb button effectively. Having this feature adapted by a vehicle modifier is possible but costly.

Now consider the buttonless shifter that relies on the brake interlock. Not only is this easier to operate for people with many types of disabilities and elderly

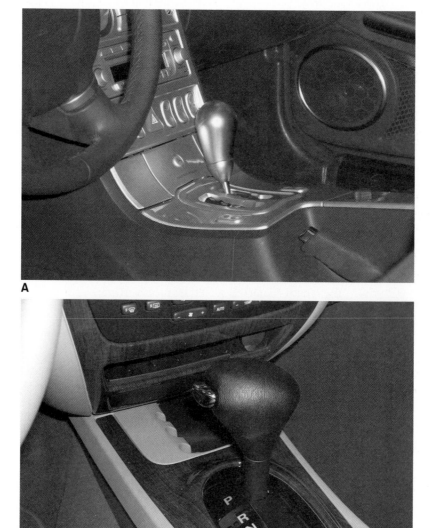

Figure 16-2 Automatic transmission shifters that **(A)** can be operated without a thumb button and **(B)** require a thumb-press for operation. (Copyright 2004, R. Darin Ellis.)

persons with aging-related concerns, such as generalized weakness, but also there is a universal benefit to all users in terms of simplified operation. Further there is a potential for reduced cost in all vehicles. Finally in addition to the simplified operation and reduced cost, there is a large cost avoidance for vehicles that would need to be modified with a powered after-market option by a vehicle modifier.

CASE EXAMPLE: B-PILLAR–FREE BODY ARCHITECTURE

Another major change in vehicle architecture is enabling easier access to people with disabilities: a vehicle architecture that has no support pillar between the front and rear doors (i.e., the B-pillar). This feature has been applied to concept cars presented at auto shows, including the Chrysler Citadel and the Lear Trans G (Figure 16-3), and to production vehicles such as the Saturn ION Quad Coupe and the GMC Colorado truck (Figure 16-4). Combined with fold-flat seating this feature adds considerable flexibility in terms of using the space inside the vehicle's cab. As can be seen from Figure 16-4, however, there is a considerable benefit that accrues to wheelchair users. With vehicles that use this architecture, it is much easier to transfer into the vehicle and stow a folding wheelchair than with the traditional motor vehicle architecture.

CASE EXAMPLE: FOLD-FLAT SEATING

Fold-flat seating has become a popular feature in many vehicles, such as the Ford Freestar and Toyota Matrix.

In the typical application this feature eases cargo hauling by folding the back of the seat flat onto the seat pan. In the 2005 model year manufacturers began introducing seating in their minivans in which seats fold flat all the way into the floor (such as the Ford Freestar; Figure 16-5). The Chrysler version of this feature, Stow-n-Go, has perhaps the greatest potential because it includes both the rear and middle rows of seats. For the general population this has obvious benefits in terms of cargo hauling and flexibly using the space inside the vehicle. There are obvious benefits to people with disabilities and elderly persons. First there is a considerable reduction in the force required to remove the seats. Removing a standard seat (which can weigh >50 lb) from a minivan is a difficult (if not nearly impossible) task for most people to accomplish on their own. This feature has the added benefit of opening up the middle of the minivan where the second row of seats normally resides, allowing the possibility of wheelchair or motorized scooter users to flexibly use that space (which would of course require some additional vehicle modifications such as a proper wheelchair tie-down system). Finally, and most significantly, is the fact that this feature is a major architectural change to the vehicle underbody that costs consumers and other entities that finance such changes at least $400 million annually.[16] The mobility equipment dealer community has created extensions to lower the vehicle floor for some time, but this is the first time such an undertaking has found a mass market. There is great promise in the future for people with disabilities, elderly persons, and their caregivers benefiting from such vehicle architectural flexibility.

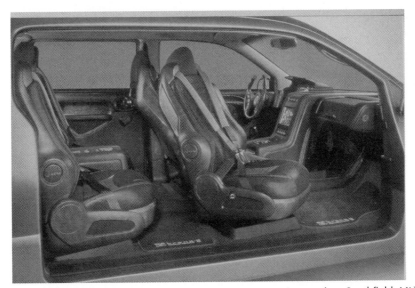

Figure 16-3 Lear Trans G concept car. (Courtesy Lear Corporation, Southfield, MI.)

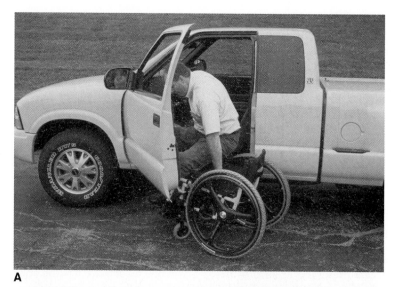

A

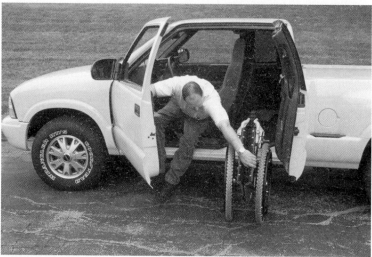

B

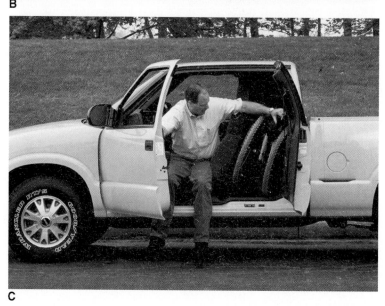

C

Figure 16-4   **A** to **C,** Transferring into a vehicle with B-pillar–free design. (Courtesy General Motors, Detroit, MI.)

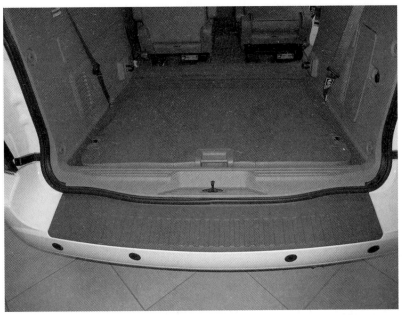

Figure 16-5 Automakers are producing cars with seats that fold flat to stow under the floor. (Copyright 2004, R. Darin Ellis.)

FUTURE TECHNOLOGY

Continuing innovation in automotive design can lead to an enormous potential benefit for people with disabilities or aging-related challenges. For example an electronic throttle control (i.e., gas pedal) is used today by many OEMs for improved throttle response and emission control. With this implementation there is no mechanical coupling from the throttle pedal to the engine. Rather the pedal's position is detected by a sensor and is translated to a digital controller via wires that connect each component. Given that the connection to the digital throttle controller is simply a set of wires, then it follows naturally that the wires can be connected to a surrogate device that could function as a pedal but not necessarily physically look or operate like one. The second author of this chapter in U.S. Patent 6,672,281 B1 captured this idea (Figure 16-6). New technology can be plugged in for alternative interfaces; it will soon be much more possible to configure vehicle controls to meet almost any conceivable need regarding driver input to the vehicle. Instead of a gas pedal a driver will be able to easily plug in a joystick or whatever input device could serve him or her best.

This bridge technology can be enormously beneficial as vehicle design moves from existing technology and architecture to the *X-by-wire architecture* (e.g., steer by wire and brake by wire) of the future. Concept cars such as the GM Autonomy and technology platforms such as the FlexRay data communication proto-

col are already exploring the general benefits of this technology, such as reduced overall vehicle weight and improved reliability. As this technology is implemented the same benefit seen in throttle control flexibility will accrue to people with disabilities, elderly persons, and others for driving tasks such as steering and braking. Although this will not make the car truly universal in terms of access, it will get us most of the way there, drastically reducing the cost of modifying a vehicle and at the same time gaining general benefits for the automakers.

Another area for which future technology holds great promise is that of *telematics*. Telematics is the general umbrella under which fall all computer and communication-related technologies intended for the vehicle's occupants. These include applications such as voice communications (e.g., cell phones and GM's OnStar), in-vehicle navigation (e.g., BMW's iDrive), crash avoidance, and driver vision enhancement. Fortunately there is a strong movement of universal design practitioners already working in the area of accessibility and human-computer interaction (e.g., http://trace.wisc.edu), and manufacturers have recognized the need to provide accessibility options with telematics devices. For example GM's OnStar comes with a teletypewriter (TTY) option for hearing impaired users. (For more information on the OnStar system refer to http://www.gm.com/company/gmability/safety/news_issues/releases/onstar_tty_072604.html.)

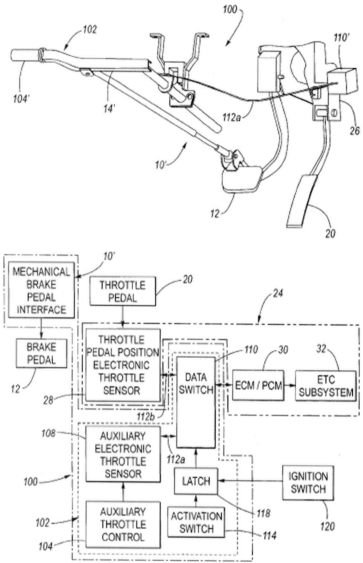

Figure 16-6   U.S. Patent 6,672,281 B1 depicting flexible input to auto throttle controller, showing an auxiliary control throttle (denoted item 104) connected to an auxiliary throttle sensor (denoted item 108).

DISABILITY-AWARE DESIGN TOOLS

This chapter has focused on principles and examples of universal design that have been and will be beneficial to people with disabilities, to elderly persons, and to a broader segment of the population when properly applied. There are also some recent advances in design tools that will further impact and improve the design of automobiles for people with disabilities[17] and others. One such area is *anthropometrics*, or the study of human dimensions.

Anthropometric data are critical to the automotive design task and are incorporated implicitly and explic-

itly in the ergonomics-related standards shown in Table 16-1. On initial consideration it may be counterintuitive to think that a separate or specially developed set of anthropometric data is required to be more inclusive toward people with disabilities or aging-related concerns. For example there is no reason to believe that a dimension like shoulder-to-fingertip length would vary between a sample of people with spinal cord injury–related disabilities and a general sample of the same overall population. As pointed out by Steinfeld et al[18] simple physical anthropometry alone is not an adequate tool for design among any population. In addition to simple physical dimensions, key parameters such as posture and strength play a role in dimensional variance.

For example consider a functional anthropometric characteristic such as *reach envelope* (i.e., the space in which a person can touch, grasp, or move objects with his or her hands). How far one can reach while seated, for example, depends on numerous factors including, but not limited to, the person's static and dynamic sitting balance; head, neck, trunk, and upper extremity motor control; cognition and visual perception; and stability of his or her base of support. A person with paraplegia and a person with full use of his or her legs will have different capabilities in terms of bracing and counterbalancing their body during a reach operation.[19]

SUMMARY

Universal design will succeed if designers and consumers with a wide variety of needs look for opportunities to share the benefit of design innovations. Design innovations such as those discussed in this chapter are good examples of universal design for several reasons. First they make the use of a vehicle more equitable; that is, vehicle features are not designed "for the handicapped" or "for the elderly" and thus are not stigmatizing. Second the design features increase the flexibility of the vehicle and decrease the physical effort required for simple tasks such as ingress and egress. The same benefits that assist the relatively small population of people with disabilities can readily be shown to improve accessibility for older adults experiencing a loss of function associated with aging. Universal design holds great promise for application to automotive engineering, and a large segment of the population will undoubtedly benefit from its implementation.

REFERENCES

1. Waldrop J, Stern SM: *Disability status: 2000* (No. C2KBR-17), Washington DC, 2000, United States Department of Commerce, US Census Bureau.
2. Kaye HS, Kang T, LaPlante MP: *Wheelchair use in the United States* (No. 23), Washington DC, 2002, United States Department of Education, National Institute on Disability and Rehabilitation Research.
3. AIADA: *Auto sales pace well above 2003's levels.* Available at: *http://www.aiada.org/article.asp?id=11435.* Accessed May 21, 2004.
4. Connelly M: Minivans poised to bounce back, *Automotive News* 53, 2003.
5. Walker M: *Scion designed for Gen Y, appeals to older groups also.* Available at: *http://www.motortrend.com/features/news/112_news47/.* Accessed May 24, 2004.
6. Administration on Aging: *A profile of older Americans: 2003.* Available at: *http://www.aoa.gov/prof/Statistics/profile/2003/2003profile.pdf.* Accessed May 21, 2004.
7. Mateja J, Popely R: *Buick uncovers its younger side.* Available at: *www.charleston.net/stories/030704/aut_07lacrosse.shtml.* Accessed May 24, 2004.
8. DiMartino C: *Freedom on four wheels.* Available at: *http://arthritis.org/resources/travel/Car_Guide/.* Accessed May 24, 2004.
9. Petzall J: The design of entrances of taxis for elderly and disabled passengers: an experimental study, *Applied Ergonomics* 26:343-352, 1995.
10. Mace R: *Universal design: barrier-free environments for everyone,* Los Angeles, 1985, Designers West.
11. Connell BR, Jones M, Mace R, et al: *Principles of universal design,* version 2.0, Raleigh, NC, 1997, North Carolina State University, The Center for Universal Design. Available at: *http://www.design.ncsu.edu/cud/univ_design/principles/udprinciples.htm.* Accessed March 1, 2005.
12. Christophersen J: *Universal design: 17 ways of thinking and teaching,* Oslo, Norway, 2002, Husbanken/The Norwegian State Housing Bank.
13. Vanderheiden GC: Universal design and assistive technology in communication and information technologies: alternatives or complements? *Assistive Technology* 10:29-36, 1998.
14. Cushman WH, Rosenberg DJ: *Human factors in product design,* Amsterdam, 1991, Elsevier.
15. Vanderheiden GC: Thirty-something (million): Should they be exceptions? *Hum Factors* 32:383-396, 1990.
16. Kelly K, Priddle A: *Stow'n Go.* Available at: *http://waw.wardsauto.com/ar/auto_stow_go/index.htm.* Accessed May 25, 2004.
17. Feathers DJ: *Digital human modeling and measurement considerations for wheeled mobility device users, SAE Technical Report 2004-01-2135,* Proceedings of the Digital Human Modeling for Design and Engineering Symposium, Rochester, MI, June 15-17, 2004, Oakland University.
18. Steinfeld E, Lenker J, Paquet V: *The anthropometrics of disability: an international workshop,* Buffalo, NY, 2001, RERC-UD. Available at: *http://www.ap.buffalo.edu/rercud.* Accessed March 1, 2005.
19. Parkinson MP, Reed MP, Chaffin DB: *Balance maintenance during seated reaches of people with spinal cord injury, SAE Technical Report 2004-01-2138,* Proceedings of the Digital Human Modeling for Design and Engineering Symposium, Rochester, MI, June 15-17, 2004, Oakland University.

Chapter 17

WHEELED MOBILITY TIEDOWN SYSTEMS AND OCCUPANT RESTRAINTS FOR SAFETY AND CRASH PROTECTION

Lawrence W. Schneider • Miriam Ashley Manary

KEY TERMS

- Anthropomorphic test devices (ATDs)
- Crash test dummies
- Voluntary standards
- Wheelchair tiedown and occupant restraint system (WTORS)
- Transit wheelchairs
- Wheelchair-seated occupants

CHAPTER OBJECTIVES

After completing this chapter, the reader will be able to do the following:

- Determine the most effective way to reduce injury to wheelchair-seated occupants in motor vehicle crashes.
- Understand the three guiding principles for voluntary equipment standards.
- Understand the three primary elements to the basic principles of occupant protection.
- Know the issues in transportation safety of wheelchair-seated occupants that are being addressed by ongoing research and future standard development.

REDUCING INJURY RISK: RESTRAINT TECHNOLOGIES AND SEAT BELTS

During the past 40 years research in injury biomechanics has significantly increased our understanding of the causes of serious and fatal injuries to drivers and passengers involved in motor vehicle crashes. Data on human impact response and injury tolerance from biomechanical testing have been used to develop improved *anthropomorphic test devices (ATDs)*, more commonly known as *crash test dummies*, and sophisticated computer models that simulate human response and injury under crash conditions. In conjunction with these advances in injury research and injury assessment tools, there have been significant improvements in motor vehicle transportation safety for drivers and passengers who use the vehicle manufacturer's seats and restraint systems. Much of this is the result of Federal Motor Vehicle Safety Standards (FMVSS) that require vehicles and manufacturer-installed restraint systems to comply with minimum crashworthiness and occupant protection design and performance requirements based on these injury assessment technologies. However, there has also been a significant increase in consumer crash test programs, which impose additional and often higher test and performance requirements than federal regulations. Examples are the five-star ratings of the National Highway Traffic Safety Administration's (NHTSA) New Car Assessment Program and the Insurance Institute for Highway Safety's offset-frontal crash tests that are frequently reported and published in the media.

However, although our understanding of human response and injury to crash environments has grown considerably in recent decades, and tools for assessing vehicle and restraint system performance have become increasingly accurate and sophisticated, the fundamental fact remains that the primary cause of disabling and life-threatening injuries to occupants involved in motor vehicle crashes is contact of the occupant's body with the vehicle interior or with objects external to the vehicle. The most effective way to reduce the risk of injury to occupants in motor vehicle crashes is to prevent or minimize occupant contact with the vehicle interior and with objects outside of the vehicle. This requires that occupants are provided with and use effective occupant restraint systems that will keep them seated in the vehicle and allow them to "ride down" the vehicle crash with minimal or no contact with vehicle interior components.

For drivers and passengers using the manufacturer-installed seats, effective occupant restraint is accomplished by three-point belt restraints, consisting of a pelvic or lap belt and a diagonal shoulder and chest belt, which are now required by federal safety standards in front- and rear-seating positions of all passenger vehicles. For small children and infants, there is a wide range of forward-facing and rearward-facing child restraint systems that offer a high level of protection in all types of vehicle crashes. For larger children up to 80 lb (36 kg), belt-positioning booster seats that route the vehicle three-point belt to fit the child's body are strongly encouraged and have become much more common in recent years.

Belt restraint systems and child safety seats are especially effective in frontal crashes, which account for more than one-half of all serious and fatal injuries. For adult front-seat occupants, additional frontal crash protection is now provided by steering wheel– and dashboard-mounted airbags, also known as supplementary inflatable restraints (SIRs). However, seat belts also offer substantial protection in rollover crashes by minimizing the chance of disabling and fatal injuries caused by ejection or partial ejection, as well as in impacts to the side of the vehicle opposite to where the occupant is seated (referred to as far-side impacts) and in rear impacts.

Therefore, in addition to significant improvements in vehicle crashworthiness and occupant restraint technology, it is not surprising that a large proportion of reductions in injury risk have resulted from increased use of seat belt restraint systems and the implementation of three-point belts in the rear seats and in the front seats of passenger vehicles. In large part, the increases in seat belt usage rates are the result of state laws that impose fines for failing to use the seat belt or restrain children and infants in child safety seats.

However, it is also because of a general increase in public awareness about motor vehicle safety resulting from increased media coverage and because of government education programs such as "Click It or Ticket."[1]

OCCUPANTS SEATED IN WHEELCHAIRS: THE SAFETY PROBLEM AND THE NEED FOR VOLUNTARY STANDARDS

During the same period that significant reductions in injury risk for people who use the manufacturer-installed seats and restraint systems have been made through improved restraint technologies and increased seat belt usage, an increasing number of persons with physical disabilities have been traveling in motor vehicles seated in their wheelchairs, which puts them at high risk of serious injury in the event of a vehicle collision and even in the event of a sudden and unexpected vehicle maneuver. The Education for All Handicapped Children Act of 1976, which was renamed the Individuals with Disabilities Education Act (IDEA) in 1997,[2] and the Americans with Disabilities Act of 1990[3] have done much to make school and public transportation available to wheelchair users; however, they have done relatively little to ensure these travelers a reasonable level of crash protection.

In large part, the increased risk of injury to wheelchair-seated occupants is because people in wheelchairs are not able to benefit from the manufacturer-installed, federally regulated belt restraint systems but rather must use after-market restraints that are not required to comply with federal safety standards. However, an equally important part of the wheelchair user safety problem is the wide range of wheelchair types and models that can weigh >250 lb and that have not been designed or tested for occupancy and crashworthiness in motor vehicles. In many cases, these wheelchairs cannot be effectively secured and they will not provide effective seat and seatback support for the wheelchair user during crash conditions, both of which are necessary for seat belts to be effective (Figure 17-1). For these reasons it is generally recommended that wheelchair users transfer from their wheelchairs to the vehicle seats whenever this is feasible. In so doing adults can use the federally regulated occupant restraint systems,[4-6] including three-point belts and airbags, installed by the vehicle manufacturer, and children can use child safety seats that are in compliance with FMVSS 213 *Child Restraint Systems*.[7] The wheelchair can then be stored and secured separately in the vehicle.

There are of course thousands of wheelchair users for whom transferring is not practical because of their

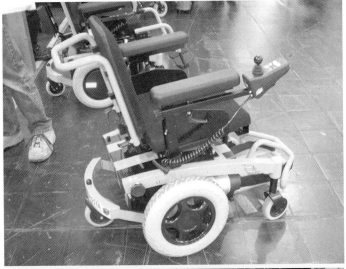

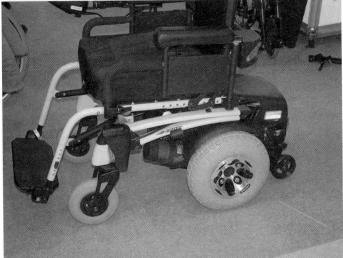

Figure 17-1 Examples of typical wheelchairs for which it is difficult to find suitable tiedown points on the wheelchair frame.

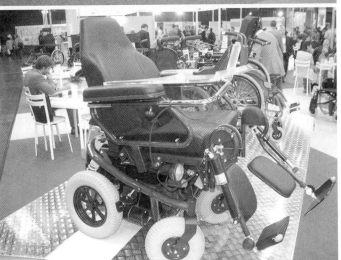

physical condition and level of disability. In these cases the wheelchair becomes the vehicle seat, and an after-market *wheelchair tiedown and occupant restraint system* (WTORS) is needed to secure the wheelchair and protect the wheelchair user during crash conditions.

On recognizing the transportation safety problem for wheelchair-seated travelers and the fact that government legislation to address safety concerns for wheelchair-seated riders was unlikely, national and international efforts were initiated in the mid-1980s to develop voluntary equipment standards. In the United States these efforts began with the formation of the Restraint Systems Task Group of the Society of Automotive Engineers' Adaptive Devices Subcommittee (SAE ADSC), whereas internationally they were initiated in a working group of an International Standards Organization (ISO) wheelchair standards subcommittee (SC1 of ISO TC173). The initial standards were aimed at providing wheelchair users with WTORS that offer a comparable level of occupant restraint and crash protection as that available to occupants who use the manufacturer-installed and federally regulated belt restraint systems. After more than a decade of work, this activity culminated with publication of the SAE Recommended Practice J2249 *Wheelchair Tiedowns and Occupant Restraint Systems for Use in Motor Vehicles*,[8] which was subsequently followed by a similar international standard, ISO 10542, Parts 1 and 2.[9]

As the WTORS standards were nearing completion, it became apparent to the members of these standard development groups that the vehicle seat is an important and integral part of an effective occupant restraint system and that a significant portion of the occupant protection problem for wheelchair-seated occupants lies in the wide range of manual and powered wheelchairs that have been designed without any consideration for their use as seats in motor vehicles. Thus the development of volunteer standards for WTORS led to significant improvements in these after-market products, leaving the wheelchair as the weakest part of the occupant protection "system." Therefore in the mid-1990s efforts were largely directed toward development of the first wheelchair standards to address issues and features of wheelchairs relative to their use as seats in motor vehicles. In the United States this effort moved from the SAE ADSC to a subcommittee of the Standards Committee on Wheelchairs, known as the RESNA Subcommittee on Wheelchairs and Transportation, or SOWHAT. (RESNA was formerly known as the Rehabilitation Engineering Society of North America but is now the Rehabilitation Engineering & Assistive Technology Society of North America.) The result was the completion of Section 19 of American National Standards Institute (ANSI)/RESNA Wheelchair Standards/Volume 1,

Wheelchairs for Use as Seats in Motor Vehicles, in May 2000. Wheelchairs that comply with this new standard are referred to as *transit wheelchairs* or wheelchairs equipped with the transit option, or simply as WC/19 wheelchairs.

The remainder of this chapter reviews progress that has been made on the development and implementation of voluntary standards for WTORS and transit wheelchairs. The guiding principles behind the initial versions of these standards and the key requirements set forth in the standards are reviewed in terms of basic principles of occupant protection. Sources for additional information on these standards and products that have been designed and tested to comply with the design and performance criteria are also provided, along with a review of future standards that will further improve motor vehicle safety for wheelchair users.

GUIDING PRINCIPLES FOR VOLUNTARY EQUIPMENT STANDARDS

The initial versions of voluntary standards for WTORS and transit wheelchairs are based on three general principles. First it was desired to provide wheelchair users with products that adhere to basic principles of occupant crash protection. Second it was desired to provide wheelchair users with the opportunity to use equipment that is comparable in crash performance with manufacturer-installed seats and belt restraints that comply with federal safety standards. Third it was desired to qualify WTORS and wheelchairs for use in all types and sizes of motor vehicles. The following sections describe more specifically how these principles have been incorporated into requirements and test methods of the standards.

ADHERE TO BASIC PRINCIPLES OF OCCUPANT PROTECTION

There are three primary elements to the basic principles of occupant protection. These include (1) occupant orientation in the vehicle, (2) independent anchorage and securement of the vehicle seat, and (3) providing upper and lower torso restraint using belt-type restraints that apply forces to the skeletal parts of the body.

Orient Occupants Facing Forward

Although some of the most important advances in automotive safety have been with regard to frontal crash protection, these types of crashes continue to be the leading cause of disabling and fatal injuries.[10] This statistic is the reason that frontal crash protection has historically been the highest priority in the NHTSA's rulemaking in the form of FMVSS 208 *Occupant Crash Protection*,[4] and it is the basis for the requirement of FMVSS 222 *School Bus Seating Crash Protection*[11] that all school bus seats be forward facing.

Unfortunately for reasons of convenience and efficiency, it has been common practice for wheelchair-seated passengers to travel facing sideways with the wheelchair backed up to the vehicle sidewall (Figure 17-2), especially in public and school transportation. However, facing sideways is the least safe orientation for any occupant during a frontal crash. The belt restraints cannot effectively control movement of side-facing occupants in frontal crashes, which results in injurious twisting and bending of the body into and over the wheelchair armrest (Figure 17-3).

Thus the first basic principle in providing safer transportation is to face wheelchair-seated occupants forward in the vehicle. After initially exempting students in wheelchairs from the safety provisions provided for other students on school buses and identifying them as facing at an angle of ≥45 degrees to the longitudinal axis of the vehicle, the NHTSA modified FMVSS 222 *School Bus Seating and Crash Protection* in 1992 by requiring that all bus manufac-turer–installed wheelchair stations provide only for forward-facing seating as it does for students who use the original equipment manufacturer (OEM) school bus seats. In a similar manner SAE J2249 and WC/19 address only WTORS and wheelchairs that are intended for installation and use when oriented facing forward in the vehicle.

Secure the Wheelchair Independently from the Occupant

A basic principle of occupant protection in frontal crashes is to not allow the mass of the vehicle seat to add to the forces applied to the occupant during a crash. This is particularly important for the person seated in a wheelchair because the wheelchair mass is often ≥200 lb, and the tolerance to impact loading is likely to be lower for wheelchair users than for people with full function and mobility. Adhering to this principle requires that the wheelchair mass is effectively secured or anchored to the vehicle so that there is minimal forward movement relative to the vehicle interior during a frontal crash and that this securement is provided in a manner that is independent of the occupant restraint system. That is, a belt used to provide restraint for the occupant must not provide restraint or even partial restraint for the wheelchair.

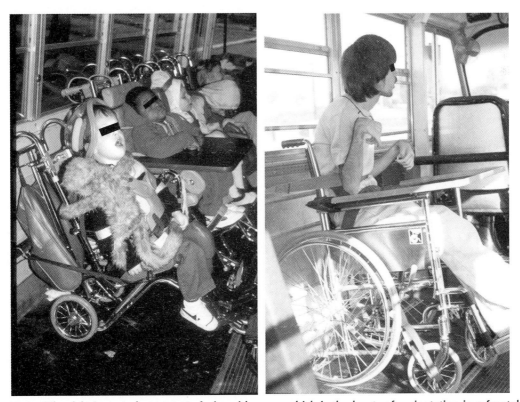

Figure 17-2 Wheelchair-seated occupants facing sideways, which is the least safe orientation in a frontal crash.

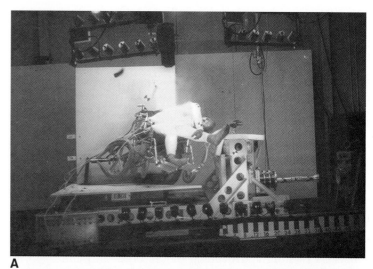

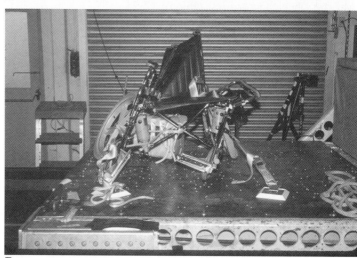

Figure 17-3 **A,** Side view of a side-facing wheelchair and anthropomorphic test device (ATD) during a frontal impact test. **B,** Side-facing wheelchair after a frontal impact test.

Use Properly Positioned Upper and Lower Torso Belt Restraints

Because the primary purpose of an occupant protection system is to prevent or minimize contact of the occupant's body with vehicle interior components and other occupants, upper and lower torso belts are needed to minimize knee, chest, and head excursions in frontal crashes and to keep the occupant inside the vehicle in rollover crashes. The use of a shoulder belt with a pelvic or lap belt also reduces the tendency for the occupant to "submarine" under the lap belt in a frontal crash, which can result in injurious forces being applied to the more vulnerable organs of the soft abdomen rather than to the pelvic bone. In this regard an important principle of occupant protection that has often been ignored with the wheelchair-seated motor vehicle occupant is to apply restraint forces to the bony regions of the body and not to the soft tissue regions, such as the abdomen. Thus every effort should be made to position the lap belt as low as possible over the pelvic bone and near the thigh and abdominal junction of the seated occupant. Movement of the lap belt onto the abdomen during a frontal collision is further minimized if the angle of the lap belt is between 45 and 75 degrees to the vertical, whereas more horizontal belt angles increase the likelihood of the lap belt moving up onto the soft and vulnerable abdomen.

As with lap belts the effectiveness of shoulder belts depends on the belt being in contact with the occupant's shoulder and chest before impact loading with minimal or no slack in the belt. This reduces the forces applied to the occupant by the belt and allows the occupant a maximum amount of ride-down time during the vehicle deceleration. The shoulder belt of a three-point seat belt should be anchored behind and slightly above the top of the shoulder so that it passes over the center of the clavicle. It should cross diagonally across the center of the chest and connect to the lap belt near the hip of the occupant rather than near the midline of the body so that it does not pull the lap belt up onto the soft abdomen when belt tension develops during impact loading.

PROVIDE EQUIPMENT COMPARABLE IN PERFORMANCE WITH MANUFACTURER-INSTALLED EQUIPMENT

The essence of this principle is that WTORS and wheelchairs must be dynamically tested. Whereas static strength testing can be used by manufacturers to perform preliminary evaluations of tiedown/restraint assemblies and components, dynamic testing using articulated ATDs to represent the occupant and a surrogate wheelchair (SWC) to represent a typical wheelchair mass is required to load the equipment and its components similar to the way it would be loaded in real world crashes. Not only do interactions between belt webbing and hardware, such as locking mechanisms, cause webbing failures at significantly lower dynamic forces than static or quasistatically applied forces, but also the loading and timing of loading produced on belt restraints, tiedowns, and seats during real world crashes are complex and cannot be effectively represented by static testing.

Because the full vehicle crash testing required by FMVSS 208 is expensive, dynamic testing of WTORS and wheelchairs is performed on an impact sled in a manner similar to federal testing of child restraint systems in FMVSS 213. The equipment to be tested is set up on the test sled with a rigid platform and sidewall structure for anchoring tiedowns and restraints, thereby simulating structural anchor points in vehicles (Figure 17-4). As with child restraint testing, the test is conducted without other vehicle interior components for the ATD to interact with and therefore constitutes primarily a dynamic strength test of the equipment.

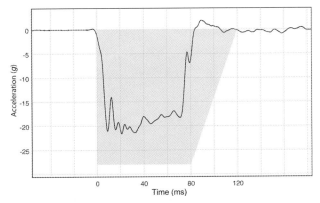

Figure 17-4 A 30-mph, 20-*g* deceleration corridor specified for frontal crash testing of wheelchair tiedown and occupant restraint system (WTORS) and wheelchairs, with typical deceleration pulse of the University of Michigan Transportation Research Institute (UMTRI) impact sled.

PROVIDE EQUIPMENT THAT CAN BE USED IN ALL TYPES OF VEHICLES

This principle is based on the concern that WTORS manufacturers cannot reliably control the types of vehicles in which their products are installed. Therefore it follows that WTORSs must be tested at crash levels that ensure their suitability for use in all types of motor vehicles. Similarly wheelchairs are likely to be used for seating in a wide range of vehicles, from city buses to private and paratransit vans and minivans.

Implementation of this principle requires that WTORS and wheelchairs be tested at crash severities that are appropriate for smaller van-sized vehicles that are more likely to be involved in severe frontal crashes. Because FMVSS 208 has historically required frontal barrier crash tests of passenger vehicles to be conducted at 30 mph, this is the level of sled impact testing required for WTORS and wheelchair standards. Following the example of FMVSS 213, the deceleration pulse must fit within a time-history corridor designed around an average deceleration of 20 *g*. Unlike the FMVSS 213 corridor, the corridor for sled testing of WTORSs and wheelchairs (see Figure 17-4) with a typical deceleration pulse from the University of Michigan Transportation Research Institute's (UMTRI) impact sled allows a relatively wide range of pulse shapes to accommodate deceleration pulses of different impact sleds.

KEY REQUIREMENTS OF WTORS AND TRANSIT WHEELCHAIR STANDARDS

WHEELCHAIR TIEDOWN AND OCCUPANT RESTRAINT SYSTEMS

As previously noted requirements for WTORS are currently set forth in SAE J2249, although this recommended practice is currently being updated and will be republished as Section 18 of Volume 4 of ANSI/RESNA wheelchair standards, along with ANSI/RESNA WC/19 and other standards related to transportation safety of wheelchair-seated occupants. WTORSs that comply with SAE J2249 or WC/18 can use various methods for wheelchair securement but must include a belt-type occupant restraint system that includes a pelvic belt and an upper torso belt consisting either of a diagonal shoulder belt or a dual shoulder harness. One of the most common wheelchair securement systems for use by passengers of private and public vehicles is the four-point strap-type tiedown system (Figure 17-5). The primary advantage of this system is

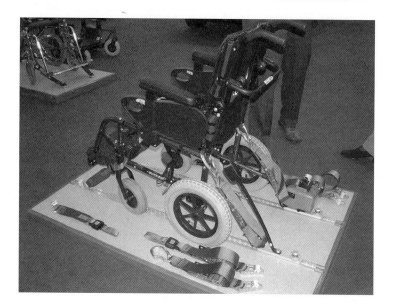

Figure 17-5 Wheelchair secured by a four-point strap-type tiedown—today's universal wheelchair securement system.

that it can be used with a wide range of wheelchair types and models (i.e., it is the most universal tiedown system). The disadvantage of the four-point tiedown is that it requires the manual placement of four tiedown straps on the wheelchair by someone other than the wheelchair user.

The second most common type of wheelchair securement system is a docking-type tiedown, whereby components on the wheelchair engage with a docking station mounted to the vehicle floor when the wheelchair is moved into position in the vehicle. The advantages of the docking-type tiedown are that it is quick, does not require manual effort, and allows the wheelchair user to secure and release his or her wheelchair. The primary disadvantages are higher cost and the need to attach tiedown and securement adapters to the wheelchair that provide wheelchair components that will engage with the docking station mounted in the vehicle. Because of the latter, docking-type securement is not currently practical in public transportation, but it is necessary for wheelchair-seated drivers who want to operate a vehicle independently.

In addition to numerous design requirements intended to ensure that the WTORS and its components are designed to comply with basic principles of occupant protection and sound engineering criteria, SAE J2249 requires dynamic sled testing of the WTORS at 30 mph and 20 g using an 85-kg (187-lb) SWC to load the tiedown system and a 175-lb ATD that is representative of a mid-sized U.S. man in size and mass. Figure 17-6, A, illustrates the SWC and ATD setup on an impact sled before testing a WTORS that uses a four-point strap-type tiedown, and Figure 17-6, B, illustrates a peak-of-action video frame from one test. Successful WTORS performance requires that the

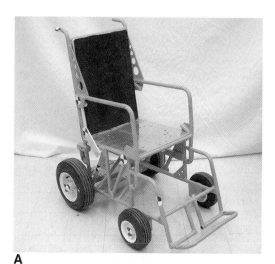

A

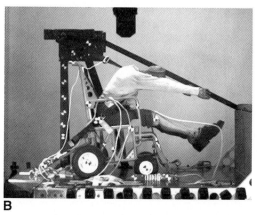

B

Figure 17-6 A, Surrogate wheelchair used for dynamic testing of WTORS. **B,** Surrogate wheelchair loaded with a mid-sized male anthropomorphic test device (ATD) on the University of Michigan Transportation Research Institute (UMTRI) sled before test of wheelchair tiedown and occupant restraint system (WTORS) with four-point strap-type tiedown.

peak excursions of the ATD and SWC remain below established limits and that there be no evidence of failure in any WTORS components.

Today there are several commercial WTORSs with four-point strap-type tiedowns that comply with SAE J2259. Whereas early four-point tiedowns used manual tensioning mechanisms, such as over-the-center cam buckles or ratcheted webbing spools, most four-point tiedowns now incorporate manual- and automatic-locking retractor anchorages and hook-type end fittings (Figure 17-7) that allow easier and faster wheelchair securement.

By comparison there are relatively few docking-type wheelchair securement systems that comply with SAE J2249. The most common docking securement system is called EZ Lock by Constantine, Inc. (Baton Rouge, LA) (Figure 17-8). Primary wheelchair securement is achieved with a single bolt located near the center of the wheelchair that extends down from add-on hardware attached to the wheelchair's lower frame. The bolt engages with a docking station when the wheelchair user moves forward into the driver position, and a front stabilizer provides resistance to wheelchair pitching and rotation.

Creative Controls, Inc. (Troy, MI) offers a second type of docking securement system used by wheelchair-seated drivers. The system requires the addition of rectangular brackets to the lower sections of the wheelchair side frames (Figure 17-9). After the driver moves into position, a front horizontal securement bar

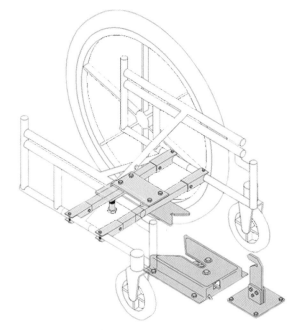

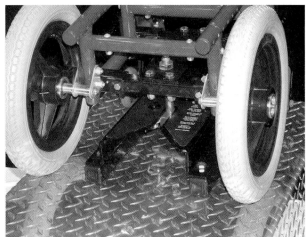

Figure 17-8 EZ Lock docking tiedown by Constantine, Inc., commonly used to secure driver wheelchairs. (Courtesy Constantine, Inc.)

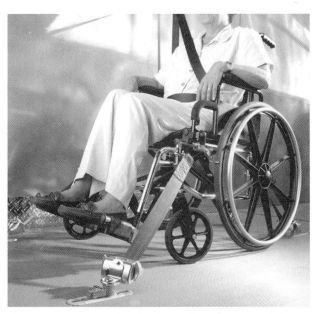

Figure 17-7 Example of a four-point strap-type tiedown using retractor-type anchorages.

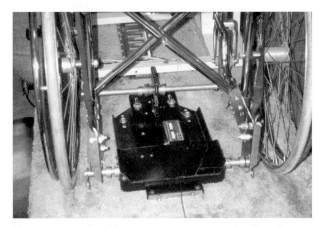

Figure 17-9 Docking securement system by Creative Controls, Inc.

is grabbed by jaws of a motorized docking station. This moves the front of the wheelchair forward and up and causes the rear horizontal securement bar to engage with the primary securement mechanism at the back of the docking station.

Although these docking-type wheelchair securement systems often provide for the use of a crash-tested lap belt that is anchored to the wheelchair tiedown adapter, wheelchair seated drivers usually use some type of vehicle-anchored seat belt consisting of a modified three-point belt, or simply a two-point floor-to-B-pillar shoulder belt that is suspended in position as the driver rolls forward into the driver space (Figure 17-10). Although these types of seat belts offer some level of restraint and protection in frontal crashes, they are not as effective as three-point belts designed for use by people seated in manufacturer-installed automotive seats. In large part, this is because the belts are often held away from making good contact with the driver's body by wheelchair components such as armrests. In addition, the two-point shoulder belt or a three-point belt with the junction between the shoulder and lap portions of the belt located well below the driver's hip are more likely to cause injurious loading of the upper-right portion of the abdomen, which can cause serious liver injuries.

TRANSIT WHEELCHAIRS

Section 19 of ANSI/RESNA Wheelchair Standards Volume 1, better known as WC/19, is the first U.S. wheelchair standard to set forth design and performance requirements for wheelchairs relative to their use as seats in motor vehicles. The primary goal is to improve the effectiveness of occupant restraint systems by (1) making sure that the wheelchair is effectively and independently secured and does not add to belt restraint load on the occupant, and (2) making sure that the wheelchair provides effective seat and seatback support during frontal crashes so that belt restraints remain properly positioned on the occupant during impact loading.

Because of the need for compatibility between the method of wheelchair securement provided in the vehicle and the means for securement provided on wheelchairs, the standard requires all transit wheelchairs to include four securement points of specified geometry fastened rigidly to or designed into the wheelchair

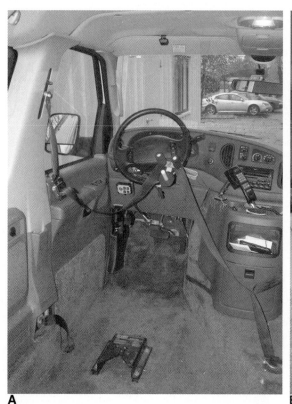 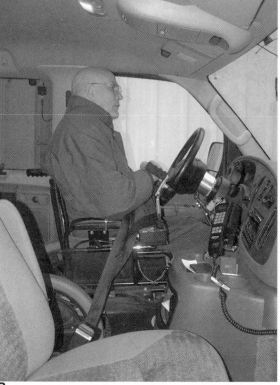

A   B

Figure 17-10 Typical seat belt used by wheelchair-seated driver. **A,** Belt is suspended in place prior to entry of wheelchair user. **B,** View from right side showing low location of lap/shoulder belt junction and poor placement of lap belt in front of wheelchair armrests.

Continued

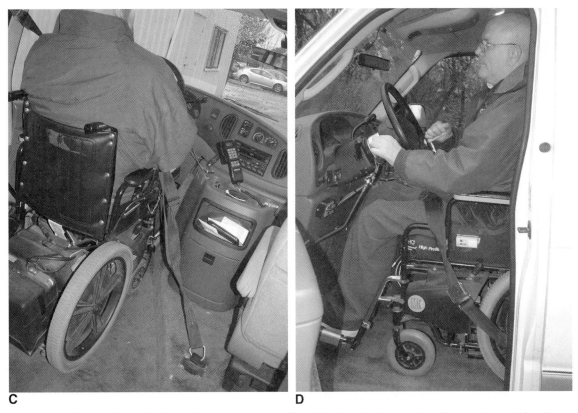

Figure 17-10 cont'd **C,** View of inboard floor anchorage of lap/shoulder belt considerably away from side of wheelchair. **D,** View from left side showing poor placement of lap belt forward of wheelchair armrest and considerable slack in belt.

frame so that the wheelchair can be secured using a four-point strap-type tiedown. Each securement point must have a slot-type opening for strap or hook attachment of the tiedown assembly (Figure 17-11). Each securement point must also be located so that it can be easily reached by a hook-type end fitting of a tiedown strap from one side of the wheelchair, and it must be designated by an anchor/hook symbol. Thus WC/19 not only addresses the effectiveness of wheelchair securement, but also it improves the ease with which wheelchairs can be secured using today's universal four-point, strap-type tiedown system.

In addition to requiring that the wheelchair seating system provide effective support for an appropriate size ATD representative of the upper size range of the wheelchair during the 30-mph frontal crash test, WC/19 addresses the effective use of belt restraints in two different ways. First it requires that wheelchair manufacturers provide the wheelchair user with the option of purchasing and using a wheelchair-anchored pelvic belt that has been designed for use as an occupant restraint and crash tested in the 30-mph, 20-g sled impact test. This pelvic belt must include a standard pin-bushing interface for connecting to a wheelchair-anchored shoulder belt. Second the standard requires

that wheelchairs are rated (A = excellent, B = good, and C = poor) for the ease of properly using and positioning a vehicle-anchored three-point belt on the wheelchair user and that these ratings are disclosed in manufacturer presale literature.

Whereas frontal impact tests of WTORSs use an SWC to load the wheelchair tiedown system, frontal impact tests of wheelchairs are conducted using a surrogate four-point strap-type wheelchair tiedown to secure the wheelchair. This surrogate WTORS (SWTORS) is strong enough to withstand the forces generated by wheelchairs >300 lb in a 30-mph impact test, and the rear anchorages are instrumented to measure the tiedown forces in the event of failure of the wheelchair securement points.

Figure 17-12 shows a peak-of-action sideview photo of a wheelchair during frontal impact testing. During and after testing the wheelchair is evaluated by measuring peak forward excursions of the ATD's head and knee and the wheelchair seating system and peak rearward excursion of the ATD's head. The latter, along with a requirement that the ATD torso is in an upright posture at the end of the test, provides a measure of seatback integrity during ATD rebound. The strength and support offered by the wheelchair frame and seat

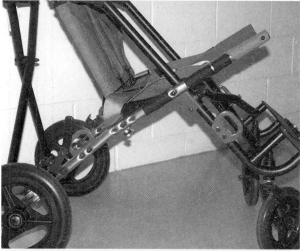

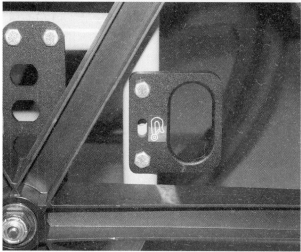

Figure 17-11 WC/19 securement points on transit wheelchairs.

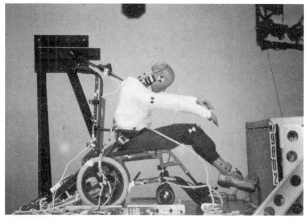

Figure 17-12 Peak-of-action photo of wheelchair and mid-sized adult male anthropomorphic test device (ATD) during a 30-mph sled impact test.

also are evaluated by examining the wheelchair for any signs of failure of primary structural components, including the four securement points, and by checking to make sure that the ATD's pelvis (i.e., hip joints) did not drop >20% from its pretest height.

LABELING AND INFORMATION REQUIREMENTS

In addition to establishing design and performance requirements for WTORSs and transit wheelchairs, both standards require product labeling and specify requirements for manufacturer instructions to installers and users. Major components of WTORS are to be labeled as being in compliance with SAE J2249, which also implies that the belt restraint assemblies are in compliance with selected parts of FMVSS 209 *Seat Belt Assemblies*[8] and FMVSS 210 *Seat Belt Assembly Anchorages*.[9] Similarly a permanent label is required on the frame of transit wheelchairs and on any crash-tested wheelchair-anchored belt restraints to indicate compliance with ANSI/RESNA WC/19. Any wheelchair-anchored belt intended only for postural support also must be labeled as not for use as a restraint in a motor vehicle. Manufacturer instructions must indicate proper installation procedures for different installation scenarios, such as attaching anchorage hardware to sheet metal floors versus structural members of vehicles, appropriate locations of seat belt anchorages to achieve proper fit to the wheelchair occupant, and instructions for maintenance and replacement of worn parts.

IMPLEMENTATION OF STANDARDS AND DEALING WITH NONTRANSIT WHEELCHAIRS

The standards that have been developed for WTORSs and transit wheelchairs to date are aimed at providing frontal crash protection for forward-facing wheelchair occupants in a wide range of vehicles. Because these are voluntary standards their effectiveness depends on manufacturers and consumers understanding and acknowledging the importance to transportation safety of using products that comply with the standards, where the consumer includes transportation providers and vehicle modifiers and wheelchair users.

It is of course also important for equipment that complies with these standards to be properly used regularly. This requires that wheelchair users, drivers and attendants of public transit vehicles, and personal caregivers are properly trained, especially with regard to the proper use and placement of four-point strap-type tiedowns and three-point belt restraints. Toward this end SAE J2249 requires WTORS manufacturers to provide a durable placard with proper usage instructions, including how to release a wheelchair from a tiedown and an occupant from a belt restraint in the event of an emergency or power failure, with each WTORS for mounting and display at each wheelchair station.

Securing wheelchairs with four-point strap-type tiedowns is of course greatly facilitated and most effective when the occupant is seated in a transit wheelchair that complies with WC/19. However, although an increasing number of makes and models of wheelchairs are being offered with the transit option, it will be many years before the majority of wheelchairs in use are provided with four crash-tested securement points. In the meantime transportation providers, caregivers, and wheelchair users need to determine and permanently mark (colored plastic tie wraps can be used for this purpose) the strongest accessible attachment points on the front and back of the wheelchair frame for attaching tiedown hooks and straps. For some power-based wheelchairs with plastic shrouds covering the wheelchair frame, establishing suitable attachment points may require removing part of the shroud to expose the structural frame. However, for some power-based wheelchairs, the cross-section or design of the structural frame will not allow attachment of hook-type or even strap-type tiedown end fittings. In these cases hook-on attachment points can usually be created by attaching loops of webbing designed for this purpose, such as the Secure Loops by Safe Haven, Inc. (New Haven, Los Angeles, CA) or the loops by Sure-Lok, Inc. (Branchburg, NJ; Figure 17-13).

FUTURE STANDARDS

The existing voluntary standards for WTORSs and transit wheelchairs provide the basis for significantly improving the level of crash protection for wheelchair users who are not able to transfer to the vehicle seat and use manufacturer-installed restraint systems. Although the focus to date has been only on frontal crash protection, the enhanced wheelchair securement and occupant restraint offered by use of WTORSs and wheelchairs that comply with these standards will also significantly improve occupant protection in other types of crashes, including vehicle rollovers, impacts to the opposite side of the vehicle to where the wheelchair user is seated, and rear impacts. Even so, efforts are currently underway to develop additional design and performance requirements that will improve protection for wheelchair users in side and rear impacts. The latter will include requirements for improved performance of wheelchair seatbacks and the provision of rear head

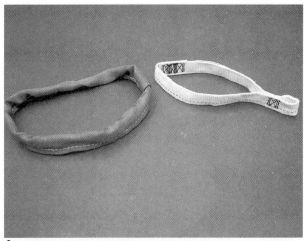

A

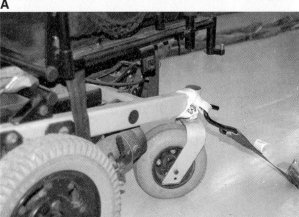

B

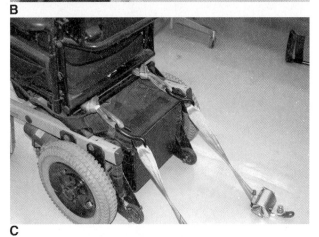

C

Figure 17-13 **A,** Webbing loops by Sure-Lok (left) and Safe Haven (right) used to provide add-on securement points for nontransit wheelchairs. **B,** Safe Haven secure loop attached to front of power wheelchair frame. **C,** Sure-Lok loops attached to back of wheelchair frame.

restraints, as well as design requirements for vehicle-installed back and head supports.

It should also be noted that the WC/19 applies only to complete wheelchairs with a base frame and seating system. However, it is common for wheelchairs to be prescribed with specialized seating systems that are purchased separately from the wheelchair base. The same seating system also is often used on different wheelchair bases. For these reasons a new standard is being developed that will allow the design and crashworthiness of wheelchair seating systems to be evaluated independent of commercial wheelchair bases by conducting a frontal crash test similar to that of ANSI/RESNA WC/19 with the wheelchair seating system installed on a SWC base (Figure 17-14). As with a complete wheelchair test, the ability of the seat and seatback to support an appropriate size ATD and the retention of the seat and seatback are evaluated during and after the test.

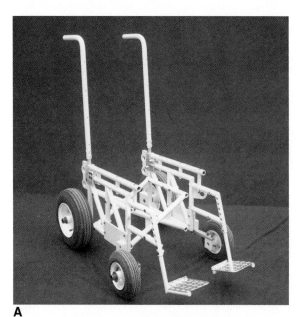

A

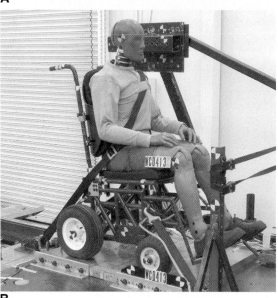

B

Figure 17-14 **A,** Surrogate wheelchair base on which wheelchair seating systems are installed for frontal impact testing. **B,** Surrogate wheelchair base with seating system and mid-size male anthropomorphic test device (ATD) installed ready for testing on UMTRI sled.

Two additional aspects of future standards include the development of design and performance requirements for WTORSs intended only for use on larger vehicles for which 30-mph crash conditions are rare, and the specification of securement point geometry on wheelchairs that would allow docking-type securement in public transit vehicles. The latter concept is analogous to the standard size ball on a trailer hitch that allows a wide range of trailers to be towed by the same vehicle. The idea is for the frames of wheelchairs to include a securement structure of specified size and location that will mate with a docking tie-down device in the vehicle designed to engage with structures on the wheelchair meeting these geometric specifications, regardless of the type of wheelchair. The long-term goal is to replace the current manual universal four-point, strap-type wheelchair securement system with a universal docking method of wheelchair securement that is easier and quicker and that the wheelchair user can operate.

This method of universal wheelchair securement would be particularly beneficial and most readily achievable in larger public and school transportation vehicles, in which the need for rapid wheelchair securement is greatest and the expected crash conditions and securement forces are relatively low.[12] The current universal docking interface geometry (UDIG) consists of two vertical bars of specified cross-section, height, and lateral spacing located at the rearmost structural point on the wheelchair (Figure 17-15, *A*) in a prototype form on a manual wheelchair (Figure 17-15, *B*).

With regard to WTORSs designed and intended only for lower crash performance on larger vehicles, it will be recalled that one of the three guiding principles to the initial WTORS standard was for the equipment to be usable in all vehicles, thereby requiring that it be tested to worst-case frontal crash conditions of 30 mph and 20 *g*. Now that this standard has been in place for several years, the operational needs of large intracity and intercity buses with regard to the transportation of wheelchair-seated travelers have become an important priority. In particular the time and effort required to secure and release wheelchairs using a four-point strap-type tiedown that complies with the high-*g* requirements of SAE J2249 present problems in maintaining bus schedules, and frequent use of this system by drivers of public transit vehicles can be a source of driver injury. Although increased availability and use of transit wheelchairs should greatly decrease the time and effort involved in using the four-point tiedown, alternative methods for wheelchair securement that do not require modifications of wheelchairs may be possible if vehicle-specific, low-*g* impact conditions are established for WTORSs intended and clearly labeled only for use in these larger vehicles.

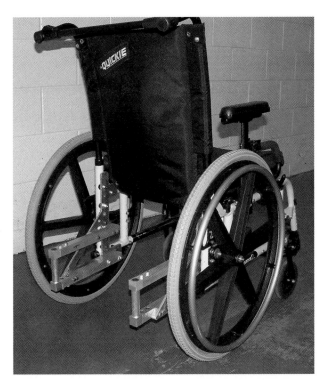

Figure 17-15 Prototype wheelchair tiedown adapter based on proposed universal docking interface geometry (UDIG) installed on a standard manual wheelchair. Docking-type tiedown device in vehicle engages with the rear posts of UDIG when wheelchair user backs into wheelchair station.

SUMMARY

For thousands of wheelchair users who are not able to transfer to the vehicle seat when traveling in public and private motor vehicles, after-market WTORSs are needed to secure the wheelchair and to provide crashworthiness restraint for the wheelchair-seated occupant. In the absence of adequate government safety standards, voluntary standards have been developed to establish design and performance requirements for WTORSs and transit wheelchairs.

The requirements and test methods set forth in the initial versions of these standards apply to complete WTORSs and wheelchairs intended for use in all types of motor vehicles and are aimed at providing a comparable level of frontal crash protection as that offered by manufacturer-installed seats and seat belts that must comply with FMVSS. The standards require that wheelchairs and WTORSs be evaluated in nominally worst-case frontal-crash conditions using a 30-mph, 20-g sled impact test. The transit wheelchair standard, commonly known as WC/19, also requires that wheelchairs provide four easily accessible and crash-tested

securement points so that they can be effectively and more easily tied down using one of the many available and commonly used four-point strap-type tie-down systems that comply with SAE J2249. Transit wheelchairs can also be designed or retrofitted with tiedown adapters for securement by other methods, such as an EZ Lock docking station, which is commonly used by wheelchair-seated drivers who need to be able to secure and release their wheelchair without an assistant or caregiver.

The effectiveness of these voluntary standards depends largely on consumer demand for crash-tested products, where the consumer includes transit providers, family members and caregivers, and wheelchair users. WTORS manufacturers have a responsibility to ensure that their products comply with the requirements of these standards, but the heart of the problem and the key to providing safer transportation for wheelchair users lies with the design and performance of wheelchairs. Therefore it is critical that wheelchair manufacturers and third-party payers recognize that one of the foreseeable uses of a wheelchair is as a seat in a motor vehicle and that the safety of a wheelchair-seated occupant depends on the wheelchair's ability to be effectively secured and to provide effective support for the user during a vehicle collision.

Future voluntary standards are now under development to provide improved protection for wheelchair-seated occupants in rear and side impacts and to provide a method for evaluating the crashworthiness of wheelchair seating systems independent of the different wheelchair bases on which the seating system may be installed. The potential for using docking-type securement systems on public transit vehicles is also under development through specification of docking-type attachment points on wheelchairs with UDIG. Finally the development of a standard for WTORSs intended only for use in larger, low-g public transit vehicles has become a high priority so that a reasonable level of wheelchair securement can be achieved in a manner that is more acceptable to the operational needs and constraints of these vehicles.

REFERENCES

1. Safety Belt Use in 2003—Demographic Statistic, 2004, National Center of Statistic and Analysis Report No. DOT HS 809 729.
2. Individuals with Disabilities Education Act of 1997 (PL 105-17, 4 June 1997), 111 United States Statutes at Large, Washington, DC, 1997, Government Printing Office, pp 37-157.
3. Americans with Disabilities Act of 1990 (PL 101-336, 26 July 1990), 104 United States Statutes at Large,

Washington, DC, 1990, Government Printing Office, pp 327-378.

4. Code of Federal Regulations, Title 49, Transportation, Part 571.208, *Occupant crash protection*, Washington, DC, 2003, National Archives and Records Service, Office of the Federal Register.

5. Code of Federal Regulations, Title 49, Transportation, Part 571.209, *Seat belt assemblies*, Washington, DC, 1999, National Archives and Records Service, Office of the Federal Register.

6. Code of Federal Regulations, Title 49, Transportation, Part 571.210, *Seat belt assembly anchorages*, Washington, DC, 1998, National Archives and Records Service, Office of the Federal Register.

7. Code of Federal Regulations, Title 49, Transportation, Part 571.213; Child restraint systems. Washington, DC, 2003 National Archives and Records Service, Office of the Federal Register.

8. Society of Automotive Engineers: *Recommended practice J2249 wheelchair tiedown and occupant restraint systems for use in motor vehicles, SAE handbook,* Society of Automotive Engineers, 1999, Warrendale, PA.

9. International Standards Organization: *10542 Technical systems and aids for disabled or handicapped persons, wheelchair tiedown and occupant-restraint systems,* Geneva, 2001, International Standards Organization.

10. National Highway Traffic Safety Administration, *Traffic Safety Facts 2002: A compilation of motor vehicle crash data from the fatality analysis reporting system and the general estimates system,* Washington, DC, 2004, U.S. Department of Transportation.

11. Code of Federal Regulations, Title 49, Transportation, Part 571.222, *School bus seating and crashworthiness,* Washington, DC, 1998, National Archives and Records Service, Office of the Federal Register.

12. van Roosmalen L, Reeves S, Hobson DA: *Effect of universal docking interface geometry (UDIG) placement on wheelchair and occupant kinematics,* Proceedings of the Annual RESNA Conference, Atlanta, GA, June 2003.

Chapter 18

IN-VEHICLE INTELLIGENT TRANSPORT SYSTEMS

Marilyn Di Stefano • Wendy Macdonald

KEY TERMS

- In-vehicle intelligent transport systems (IITSs)
- Intelligent transport systems (ITSs)
- Primary safety
- Secondary safety
- Tertiary safety
- Interface
- Executive functions
- Driver underload
- Client-centered model
- Remediation
- Compensation

CHAPTER OBJECTIVES

After completing this chapter, the reader will be able to do the following:

- Understand the importance of intelligent transport systems.
- Understand why a driver rehabilitation specialist must analyze and evaluate the quality of the match between a particular in-vehicle intelligent transport system interface and each driver's needs, coping capacities, and limitations as a driver.
- Understand the importance of efficient user interface design.

- Evaluate the needs of a client, and make recommendations regarding products, devices, or services that are designed to assist him or her in meeting specific short- and long-term goals.

This chapter focuses on the current and possible future uses of *in-vehicle intelligent transport systems (IITSs)*. It commences with a review of the different types of systems that are being developed and their potential impact, positive and negative, on road safety. IITS interface design principles that have been developed to maximize system usability and safety are outlined. Some key issues are illustrated by a detailed analysis of driver interactions with a particular IITS—a cruise control system (CCS). Some possible effects of the types of functional impairment and environmental factors that are typical of various client groups are then considered, along with associated prescription issues. Finally impending future developments are reviewed in terms of their implications for future professional practice among driver rehabilitation specialists (DRSs).

IMPACT OF TECHNOLOGY ON THE DRIVING TASK

The design of vehicles used by ordinary drivers on our roads and highways continues to be significantly affected by technologic developments, with the latest vehicle models usually boasting new features that are often supported by complex, computer-based systems. Some of these developments may make the driving task easier and safer, but every driver will not automatically realize such benefits. To achieve optimal safety there must be a good match between the demands that a driver must cope with and his or her individual coping capacities and limitations. Driving task demands are strongly influenced by many factors, including the road traffic environment and design of the vehicle and its various subsystems, including vehicle-based *intelligent transport systems (ITSs)*. The application of general physical and cognitive ergonomic design principles can achieve a good match with system users—in this case drivers—but research to support the effective implementation of these principles is failing to keep pace with the rate at which such systems are being designed and developed.[1-3]

Even when a design is safe for most drivers, it could present risks for people with physical or cognitive impairments, depending on the nature of the system in relation to the particular impairments. Therefore it is essential that occupational therapists working as DRSs and others who have a responsibility to advise functionally impaired people about their driving should recognize the potential impact of new technology on driving safety.[4]

VEHICLE-BASED INTELLIGENT TRANSPORT SYSTEMS

ITSs have been defined as systems that entail the application of "advanced information processing, communications, sensing, and computer control technologies to the driver–vehicle–highway infrastructure system" (p. 1).[5] ITSs may be intended to enhance travel efficiency, safety, energy conservation, or provide more general economic benefits. They encompass out-of-vehicle systems, such as those presenting real-time information about traffic conditions ahead and the in-vehicle systems with which this chapter is concerned.

This chapter is concerned only with IITSs. IITSs can be categorized according to the way they may affect road safety.[4,6] This chapter is primarily concerned with IITSs that are intended to enhance *primary safety*, that is, the probability of crash involvement. These systems can be subdivided into those that influence the probability of a crash via their effects on the driver's capacity to cope with demands and those influencing it via their effects on driving task demands. The intended functions of some other types of systems are unrelated to safety, but they can nevertheless affect the probability of a crash, positively or negatively, when used by drivers. There are also IITSs that are intended to reduce harm during a crash (*secondary safety*) or to minimize the extent of harm by maximizing postcrash support (*tertiary safety*). Such systems make an extremely

important contribution to road safety but are less likely to be of concern for DRSs and will not be considered further in this chapter. Table 18-1 shows examples of IITSs[5,7-14] within each of these categories.

IITSs in categories 1 and 2 in Table 18-1 are intended to reduce crash risk, but in many cases their use requires the active involvement of drivers, including the allocation of some of their limited attentional resources. As discussed in Chapter 1 and in this chapter, performance of an attentionally demanding task carries with it the risk of errors, which for a driver may increase his or her crash risk. Therefore it is important that such systems are designed and evaluated to ensure that the attentional costs of using them do not increase a driver's crash risk to an extent that neutralizes or outweighs the system's intended safety benefits. Driver interactions with these systems vary considerably in their nature and extent, ranging from the occasional need to identify and respond to a simple auditory and/or visual signal to perceiving and interpreting complex visual displays and, on this basis, making driving-related decisions under some time pressure.[8,15]

These are the types of IITSs that are the primary focus of this chapter. It is essential that DRSs analyze and evaluate the quality of the match between a particular IITS interface and each driver's needs, coping capacities, and limitations as a driver. IITSs designed specifically for use by drivers with impairments secondary to a disability or the aging process are excluded from consideration here because these are addressed in Chapter 11, which presents information on adaptive equipment and vehicle configuration. (Also see Chapter 16, which addresses universal design and the automobile, and Chapter 19 on designing the external environment for traffic safety, which covers some non-vehicle types of ITSs.)

IITS INTERFACE DESIGN

The degree to which an individual can safely use a particular IITS is highly dependent on the quality of its *interface* design. An interface displays information to a driver about the current state of the system; for example the speedometer conveys information about current vehicle speed. Some interfaces also incorporate controls through which the driver can modify the system state; for example buttons or dials on the car radio are typically used to tune into a particular radio station or modify the volume setting. In evaluating the likelihood of a driver benefiting from IITS technology, DRSs must assess the demands of using a particular system's displays and controls in relation to the demands of other driving task elements and in relation to the driver's particular needs, limitations, and capacities. The

Table 18-1 **Examples of Some IITSs, Categorized According to Their Intended or Predicted Effects on Safety**

Primary or Secondary Safety	Categories
IITSs TARGETING PRIMARY SAFETY	
Modify driving task demands	1. Support the acquisition of more or improved task-related information (e.g., night vision systems, navigation systems, tire pressure diagnostics) 2. Intended to reduce vehicle control demands (e.g., antilock brake systems, cruise/speed control, parking aids, collision avoidance systems)
Modify driver capacity to cope with driving task demands	3. Warn or exclude drivers whose current state is unsafe or unlawful because of license status or excessive levels of alcohol, other drugs, or fatigue (e.g., electronic licensing, vehicle interlock, fatigue monitoring) 4. Increase comfort, reduce cumulative fatigue but may also decrease alertness (e.g., electronic adjustment of seats to maximize comfort) 5. Maintain alertness although with potential to distract attention from driving (e.g., entertainment systems: radio, CD and DVD players) 6. Present major risk of distraction; use while driving may therefore be illegal (e.g., communication systems: mobile phones, pagers, CB radios, e-mail, fax, Internet)
IITSs TARGETING SECONDARY OR TERTIARY SAFETY	7. Secondary safety (e.g., intelligent seat belts, air bags adjust to individuals) 8. Tertiary safety (e.g., emergency Mayday or call for help systems)

general nature of displays and controls is discussed next, followed by a more detailed analysis of driver interactions with a particular IITS—a CCS.

Displays and controls in vehicles can take many forms. For example the information displayed may be quantitative, such as the vehicle's speed displayed on a speedometer, or qualitative, as in a color-coded display of engine oil pressure that indicates whether remedial action is needed.[16] Most in-vehicle displays rely primarily on visual information, although the auditory modality may also be used, especially for warnings or alarms. Typical vehicle controls include on/off switches, push buttons, dials with either discrete or continuous settings, pedals, or steering wheels. Manipulating the vehicle's controls usually requires some form of motor input from the user, but voice input is increasingly being used as a means of communicating with devices. For example the driver may operate secondary vehicle functions, such as climate control and radios, by oral instructions directed at a microphone. Auditory displays in the form of spoken information or beeps are also being used to communicate with the driver, such as in some route guidance systems. In the CCS analyzed later in this chapter, the controls include push buttons mounted on the vehicle's steering wheel that operate in conjunction with

the vehicle's normal speed controls (i.e., accelerator and brake pedals). The only display that is specific to the CCS is an indicator light mounted on the dashboard that indicates whether the system is on or off; in some vehicles the current cruise control speed setting also is displayed here. Use of the CCS also entails observation of vehicle speed as displayed on the speedometer.

IITS interface design has the potential to enhance or impede a driver's use of it, to an extent that can significantly affect road safety. Drivers need to be able to use IITS interfaces quickly, accurately, and with minimal attention to avoid negatively affecting the driver's performance of other, possibly more important, elements of the driving task. Currently ITS design is still in a developmental phase, and related design standards are still undergoing development. Current international standards include In-vehicle Visual Presentation of Transport Information and Control Systems (ISO 150008:2003), Symbols and Tell-Tales for Controls (ISO 2575:2003), and Assessment of the Suitability of Transport Information and Control Systems for Use While Driving (ISO 17287:2003).[17] Thus far, however, few publications have addressed the specific needs of people with disabilities or aging-related concerns in relation to ITS design.[5,18,19] A detailed discussion of interface design principles is beyond the scope of this chapter, but some of the key issues relevant to IITS are presented here.

Considering the design of the whole driver workstation within which IITSs must be incorporated, Woodson et al[20] state that it should "...be laid out so that all the driver's visual and manipulative tasks can be performed as easily and efficiently as possible," and that controls and displays should "...be designed so that they will provide the necessary input and output for proper vehicle control and also will not be confusing and cause the driver to make errors or take his or her attention away from the external information needed to cope with traffic" (p. 76). These basic ergonomic principles apply also at the level of an individual IITS.[16,21] However, according to Newell and Gregor,[22] the application of such principles is not always evident and "The vast majority of human interfaces seem to have been designed on the basis of an 'average user' with little or no account being taken of the range of abilities, which are presented by the human race" (p. 818).

A general framework that is useful for evaluating the adequacy of a particular IITS is provided in Figure 1-3, showing the information processing involved in driving a car. Only a subset of the environmental information impinging on the driver's sensory organs is perceived; of this the driver will become consciously aware of a much smaller subset. This is because there is effectively a narrowing in the information-processing channel at the point of conscious awareness because of our limited amount of attentional resources. Inadequate attentional resources, such that the driver is overloaded by the amount of information needing to be processed and reductions in *executive functions*, have been identified as significant causes of errors and hence of increased crash risk.[24,25] Therefore it is important that displays and controls are designed to minimize the demands for the driver to pay attention while interacting with them. It is also important that the form of information displays minimizes the risk of errors caused by misinterpretation and that the form of controls minimizes the risk of errors caused by motor difficulties when using them or accidental operation.

Some important questions to consider are the following:

- What type and amount of information are actually required by the driver for effective task performance? The level of detail and precision of displayed information should not be more than is required.
- How important and urgent is the information? Will it be unexpected and therefore have to be conspicuous to attract the driver's attention, or will the driver be searching for it? Is it presented via the most appropriate sensory modality(ies)?

- How clearly is the intended message conveyed? How well understood are the words, symbols, or other forms of information coding that are used?
- Will the driver need to use the information immediately, or will it have to be retained in memory for a minute or so? Would information feedback after the driver's response be helpful or a potential distraction?
- Will the required forms of response be experienced as natural, being compatible with the driver's expectations based on past experience, and with performance of other components of the driving task?

Depending on the answers to the above questions, the kind of design details that need to be evaluated relate to the following:

- Location of the displays and controls within the vehicle and in relation to each other
- The information's conspicuity (i.e., attention-getting potential) and discriminability (e.g., legibility and audibility) during all likely environmental conditions; many details of the interface design affect these factors
- Suitability of required motor responses, taking account of reach distances/angles, the limb used, and postural requirements
- Choice of control type (e.g., push button, toggle switch, rotary selector, joystick, knob, lever, crank, and handwheel)
- Specific control characteristics (e.g., required force, speed inertia, feel, sensitivity, and control gain)
- Need for provision of protection against inadvertent operation (e.g., by location and guarding)

The British Transport Research Laboratories have devised a checklist specifically for assessing ITS safety and usability, which addresses many of the issues listed above.[7] They identified the following characteristics of a well-designed ITS, which are listed in Box 18-1.

For more details on design issues such as those listed thus far in this chapter, a number of useful references are available, such as Bridger,[25] Helander

---

BOX 18-1	**Characteristics of a Well-Designed ITS**

Visual displays designed to reduce glare
Limited amount of visual information
Shallow menu structures
Information consistent with the road network
Controls that provide tactile feedback
Limited requirements for information input from the user via controls
Limited number of functions assigned to a control

Data from Brook-Carter N: Driver information systems, The Ergonomist June:3, 2003.

et al,[26] Noyes,[27] Pauzie,[28] Rogers,[29] Sanders and McCormick,[16] Steenbekkers and Beijsterveldt,[30] Van Cott and Kinkade,[31] and Woodson et al.[20]

Much of the available information about interface design is concerned with features that affect the sensory or motor demands on the driver. Although both of these are important, attentional demands are the primary issue in a road safety context.[32] This is demonstrated by evidence of the effects on crash risk of using a cellular phone while driving a motor vehicle. Early research on the possible risks of drivers' cellular phone use focused on the manipulative requirements of their use. However, more recent research has demonstrated that, regardless of whether it is a hands-free phone, the attentional demands of phone use are the main cause of an associated deterioration in driving performance and elevated crash risk.[33-37] A recent Australian review[2] of the implications of IITS use for road safety concluded that:

In view of the disturbing findings of increased crash risk associated with mobile phone use ... and its implication that crash risk is increased by an activity as apparently undemanding as carrying out a phone conversation, it seems likely that the introduction of equipment which supports complex activities unrelated to the driving task is also likely to result in increased crash risk. Perhaps one of the key roles for ITS safety products in the future is to compensate for these increasing demands on the driver's processing capacity." (p. 12)

ANALYZING THE DEMANDS OF IITS: A CRUISE CONTROL SYSTEM

Various versions of CCSs have been available in domestic vehicles for a number of years. They provide a good example of IITSs that automate part of the driver's task—in this case the maintenance of a constant vehicle speed. Contrary to popular perceptions, it cannot be assumed that automation of part of a task will necessarily reduce demands on the person responsible for the overall task performance or that it will improve safety.[38] The extent to which an automated subsystem achieves these outcomes is highly dependent on the design of its user interface, as previously outlined.

To illustrate the nature of user interactions with an IITS, Table 18-2 presents an analysis of the processes involved in adjusting and maintaining vehicle speed in accord with environmental requirements, with and without the use of a CCS. This analysis uses the information-processing framework presented in Chapter 1 of this book (Figure 1-3) to identify the various kinds of sensory, perceptual, cognitive, or motor response demands that the system user (in this case the driver) may experience. When conditions allow maintenance of

a fairly constant speed for extended periods, typically at or close to the legal limit, use of a CCS may enhance safety by preventing the vehicle speed from exceeding the posted limit. In such circumstances its use certainly reduces demands on the driver because it removes the need to monitor the vehicle's speed and adjust the brake and accelerator pedal pressures so that the speed limit is not exceeded.

However, the situation is different when the task of resetting the CCS speed is reviewed (see Table 18-2: subtask C, option 2, step 1). This task requires careful coordination of three actions simultaneously: monitoring the speedometer, maintaining thumb pressure on the CCS reset button, and controlling foot pressure on the accelerator. Importantly these demands are all additional to the ongoing demands of maintaining vehicle position in relation to the roadway and other road users and of maintaining more general situational awareness, including topographic orientation. That is, the driver must continue to monitor the road environment and movements of other road users, comply with road signs and laws, and ensure that the vehicle's speed and lateral position are always appropriate to changing conditions. It seems highly likely that drivers with impaired cognitive functioning would have difficulty in maintaining safety while trying to cope with this complex set of demands. They may have insufficient spare attentional capacity to continue monitoring changing events in the road traffic environment, and their information-processing rate may be too slow. They also may not be able to maintain appropriate executive control of their attention allocation strategy to multitask with sufficiently rapid transfers of attention between different subtasks, resulting in excessively long periods of attentional focus on the CCS.

Table 18-2 shows that the demands of making the transition to a different speed setting of the CCS (option 2 in subtasks B and C) are considerably greater than those experienced by drivers who are not using a CCS (option 1 in subtasks B and C). For any driver the decision to use a CCS on a particular trip or for parts of a trip should be based on consideration of the probable road traffic conditions. If these are likely to require fairly frequent resetting of CCS speed, its use is unwarranted.

The problems that may be experienced by some drivers in resetting CCS speed are primarily the result of a driver being cognitively overloaded by the task of using a CCS. Other problems may arise because of *driver underload*, which is most likely to occur during conditions that seem ideal for CCS use; that is, when long periods of driving at or close to the speed limit can be expected. If the CCS performs the subtask of speed maintenance and the road traffic environment is monotonous, the resultant low level of task demands

Table 18-2   Analysis of Task Demands Related to Adjusting and Maintaining Vehicle Speed

Allocate Attentional Resources; Maintain Executive Control;
NB: Demand for Attention Varies Between Task Components and with Individual Capacity/Skill

Task Components	Main Sensory Processes	Perceptual Processes	Cognitive Processing (Comprehension and Situational Awareness)	Cognitive Processing (Decision Making and Response Selection)	Response Execution
ADJUST SPEED IN RESPONSE TO SPEED CONTROL SIGN AND ENVIRONMENTAL REQUIREMENTS (REQUIREMENTS ARE SAME WITH/WITHOUT CCS USE)					
Notice speed limit sign requiring reduction in vehicle speed	*Visual sensory system registers visual stimuli from sign*	*Detect and recognize the sign* *Perceive feedback as foot moves to brake pedal location*	Correctly interpret sign message in relation to current road/traffic environment *Aware of foot/pedal locations*	Decide to slow down *Identify necessary motor responses*	*Initiate motor response for braking: move foot to brake pedal*
Depress brake to slow down	*Proprioceptive and kinesthetic feedback from foot and leg* *Visual feedback from environmental stimuli*	*Initially perceive feedback from foot contact with brake pedal* *Perceive deceleration rate in relation to brake pressure* Perceive changing vehicle position relative to surroundings Perceive other relevant elements of surroundings	*Aware of brake pedal position* *Aware of deceleration rate* Aware of changing vehicle position relative to road environment and other vehicles *Aware of links between above*	*Control brake pedal pressure level in relation to situation awareness* Also control steering wheel position to maintain desired lateral positioning of vehicle	*Depress brake pedal as required* *Move steering wheel as required*
ACHIEVE TARGET SPEED Option 1: *not using CCS*	*Visual stimuli from speedometer display* *Visual stimuli from road/traffic environment* *Proprioceptive*	Perceive current vehicle speed in relation to target speed Perceive spatial relationships between own and surrounding vehicles and roadway	Aware of speed approaching target Aware of changing vehicle position in relation to road environment and other vehicles Aware of need (if any) to accommodate changing roadway and traffic conditions	*Select brake and accelerator pedal control actions to adjust pressures in relation to situation awareness* *Select steering wheel control actions to positions to maintain desired*	*Move foot between brake and accelerator and depress them as required* *Move steering wheel as required* Maintain visual monitoring

Subtask	Stimuli	Perception	Awareness	Decision/thought processes	Behaviors
Option 2: using CCS	and kinesthetic feedback from foot and leg	Perceive other relevant elements of surroundings *Perceive feedback from foot contact with pedals*	*Aware of feedback from pedal actions*	*lateral positioning of vehicle* *Direct visual monitoring behaviors*	Same as above, plus: *More careful visual monitoring of road/traffic conditions to support decision regarding commencement of next subtask*
	Same as above	Same as above, plus: More careful perception of speedometer to identify vehicle speed accurately (required for following subtask using CCS)	Same as above, plus: Aware when target speed has been *precisely* achieved	Same as above, plus: *Select appropriate time to commence following subtask, relative to awareness of road/traffic situation*	
MAINTAIN SPEED Option 1: *not* using CCS	*Visual stimuli from speedometer display (occasional)* *Visual stimuli from road/traffic environment* *Proprioceptive and kinesthetic feedback from foot and leg*	Perceive spatial relationships between own and surrounding vehicles and roadway, and other relevant elements of surroundings Perceive current vehicle speed in relation to speed limit and traffic conditions	Aware of changing vehicle position in relation to road environment and other vehicles Aware of need (if any) to accommodate changing roadway and traffic conditions Aware that speed may need adjustment up or down	*Direct visual monitoring behaviors Select brake and accelerator pedal control actions to adjust pressures in relation to situation awareness* *Select steering wheel control actions to positions to maintain desired lateral positioning of vehicle*	Maintain visual observations *Move foot between brake and accelerator and depress them as required* *Move steering wheel as required*
Option 2: using CCS 1. Reset cruise control to lower speed	Visual stimuli from CCS dashboard display Tactile/proprioceptive stimuli from CCS controls on steering wheel Visual stimuli from speedometer *Proprioceptive*	Perceive that CCS is "on" Perceive that thumb is located correctly to activate CCS reset button Perceive that current speedometer reading is the desired target speed Perceive feedback	Aware of any discrepancy between target and actual speed Aware that thumb ready to reset CCS Aware that foot ready to maintain accelerator pedal pressure to maintain desired speed for few seconds to "lock in" the target speed setting	Decide when to activate reset actions, in context of overall situation awareness Select coordinated thumb and foot movements to reset CCS Decide when to remove foot from accelerator Decide whether to interrupt reset procedure	Move thumb to CCS control on steering wheel Maintain pressure on accelerator Remove foot from accelerator when CCS reset

Continued

Table 18-2 Analysis of Task Demands Related to Adjusting and Maintaining Vehicle Speed—cont'd

Allocate Attentional Resources; Maintain Executive Control;
NB: Demand for Attention Varies Between Task Components and with Individual Capacity/Skill

Task Components	Main Sensory Processes	Perceptual Processes	Cognitive Processing (Comprehension and Situational Awareness)	Cognitive Processing (Decision Making and Response Selection)	Response Execution
	and kinesthetic feedback from foot and leg	from accelerator Perceive spatial relationships between own and surrounding vehicles and roadway, and other relevant elements of surroundings	Aware of changing vehicle position in relation to road environment and other vehicles Aware of need (if any) to accommodate changing roadway and traffic conditions	to respond to changing roadway or traffic conditions	
2. Maintain speed	*Visual stimuli from road/traffic environment*	Perceive spatial relationships between own and surrounding vehicles and roadway, and other relevant elements of surroundings Perceive current vehicle speed in relation to speed limits, road/traffic conditions	Aware of changing vehicle position in relation to road environment and other vehicles Aware of need (if any) to override CCS to accommodate changing roadway and traffic conditions Aware that speed may need adjustment up or down	*Select steering wheel control actions to positions to maintain desired lateral positioning of vehicle Direct visual monitoring behaviors*	Maintain visual monitoring Other control actions if required

will probably leave the driver with a considerable amount of spare attentional resource. Unless the driver is able to direct this resource to some other, optional subtask, such as talking with a passenger or listening to the radio, he or she may start to feel drowsy and, if fatigued, will be at greater risk of falling asleep. On a long road that is not visually stimulating, it may be safer for a driver who is likely to experience difficulty in remaining alert, whether because of fatigue or some other reason, to control vehicle speed manually because the additional demands of this subtask could help to avoid sleepiness.

It is important to note that the amount of attention demanded by a task such as resetting the CCS will vary with the driver's experience and skill in using it, as well as with the ergonomic quality of its interface design. In terms of the Skills-Rules-Knowledge (SRK) model described in Chapter 1, a driver who is practiced in CCS use can be expected to perform many of these subtasks at skill- and rule-based levels. Such tasks have consistently mapped relationships between input information and associated responses.[39] They are indicated by use of italics in Table 18-2. In contrast a new user will be performing all subtasks involving the CCS at a knowledge-based level, which is much more demanding of attention. If a driver inexperienced in CCS use is also inexperienced as a driver or has some degree of functional impairment (particularly of a cognitive nature), then use of such an IITS may not be feasible, at least not without a carefully planned period of training and extended practice during safe conditions (e.g., an off-street driving range or an underused roadway that is familiar to the driver). Issues related to different categories of prospective IITS users are discussed later in this chapter.

A different kind of safety problem that may affect drivers using CCS for long periods stems from the freedom that drivers are afforded when using a CCS to position their feet at some distance from the accelerator and brake pedals because they are not continuously controlling the vehicle's speed. There is a potential for problems to arise because when people have to sit for extended periods they tend to vary their posture, adopting various positions to the extent that is possible within the confines of their vehicle. Such postural fidgeting is a natural and largely unconscious response that serves to maintain blood flow. Therefore drivers using CCS may sit with their legs crossed or tucked in close to the seat—postures that would substantially hamper their use of the brake (or accelerator) if an emergency suddenly arose. Such a risk would be exacerbated if the driver had impaired muscle control and endurance and perhaps associated proprioceptive and kinesthetic dysfunction—conditions that initially would make use of a CCS particularly attractive.

ENVIRONMENTAL CONDITIONS

When assessing whether a driver will be able to use a particular IITS safely and effectively, the DRS should consider the nature of the environments in which it might be used. Aspects of the internal vehicle environment and the external road traffic environment can be important influences on the performance of all drivers, with or without the use of IITSs. However, drivers with particular impairments will be more prone to some of these problems, and the additional demands of using some IITSs may increase the negative impact of their impairments on driving performance.

INTERNAL VEHICLE ENVIRONMENT

In the internal vehicle environment there are two factors affecting sensory reception or perception of information. The effectiveness of IITS visual information displays can be significantly affected by lighting conditions within the vehicle (particularly light sources that may cause reflections); this may be a particular problem in the case of head-up displays on or beyond the vehicle windshield and particularly at night. In the case of IITSs that display auditory information, noise levels within the vehicle (e.g., from passengers) could be a problem.

Cognitive and attentional factors are also present in the internal vehicle environment. Drivers who are likely to experience difficulties in focusing and allocating their attention appropriately are likely to perform more poorly if there are significant distractions within the vehicle (e.g., from passengers, the radio or other communication devices extraneous to the driving task, or from physical discomfort induced by poor seating). The driver's level of attentional resources will vary with his or her physiologic and psychological arousal, which is likely to be lower if the internal vehicle climate is too hot.

Finally there is a factor that affects vehicle control. It is important that the vehicle's cabin design (including adjustability of the seat and perhaps other controls such as the steering wheel) is set up so that reaching and operating all controls requires minimal attention and physical effort.

ROAD TRAFFIC ENVIRONMENT

Factors affecting sensory reception or perception of information are important in the road traffic environment. The impact of a driver's visual impairments on driving performance is likely to be greater when the quality of visual information is degraded, such as low light levels (e.g., dawn, dusk, night time), glare from the sun or at night from the headlights of other vehicles, or because of fog, rain, or snow.

The impact on driving performance of a driver's cognitive impairments will be greater when road and traffic conditions are more demanding. Demanding road conditions can include multiple or confusing road signs; limited forward visibility because of horizontal or vertical road curvature; poor or inconsistent quality of the road surface; limited lateral visibility at intersections because of obstacles, such as vegetation, buildings, or stationary vehicles; multilane highways without a median strip separating opposing traffic; frequent speed zone changes; and uncontrolled intersections. Demanding traffic conditions can include the following: high traffic volume; high and/or variable speeds; high rate of maneuvering (e.g., lane changing); wide variety of other road users, including large trucks, cyclists, pedestrians, and others; and a noisy environment within the vehicle, outside the vehicle, or both.

Factors affecting vehicle control are also present in the road traffic environment. In some circumstances (particularly vehicle/driver combinations), vehicle control demands may be significantly increased by steep or winding roads or by having to negotiate particularly narrow clearances (e.g., between vehicles or along narrow roads).

IDENTIFYING INDIVIDUAL CLIENT REQUIREMENTS AND RELEVANT CONTEXTUAL FACTORS

Some general questions that should be considered when evaluating an individual's needs and other characteristics in relation to his or her possible use of an IITS include the following:
- Does the system have a potential benefit for this person? How may it affect his or her safety when driving?
- Does the driver need to obtain and use information from the IITS while also controlling the vehicle? If so, how appropriate is the means by which information is displayed? Are there possible alternative ways by which the driver may obtain this information? How appropriate are the IITS controls? Are there alternative means by which the driver may interact with them?
- To what extent can the driver determine the timing of his or her interaction with the IITS? If this is to some degree dependent on his or her own decision, is he or she likely to have insight into the most appropriate times to choose?
- Will the driver be able to manage any additional attentional demands of using the IITS?

- Will his or her attentional resources be affected by having to perform other subtasks or by distractions?

Most DRSs adopt an individually customized approach to assessing a driver's need for and ability to benefit from ITS technology. Early in this process it will often be important to consider high-level issues[40]; the Gadget Matrix[41] referred to in Chapter 1 provides a suitable framework within which to undertake this task. At the highest level of the matrix are the individual's goals for life and skills for living; these are concerned with the broad personal and social contextual issues that can affect CCS use. Factors at this level are linked to life roles, such as worker, family chauffeur, or retiree, which may significantly influence the client's ability and willingness to plan when, where, and how often he or she will use the IITS (if the IITS is not always in use). Individual personality, previous learning, social conditioning, and general lifestyle may also influence the nature and extent of IITS use. A particularly relevant factor at this level is the individual's general propensity for risk taking, which can be seen as a function of personal and social contextual influences.

Consideration of such factors would be relevant, for example, when weighing the potential benefits and risks for a given client that might result from using an IITS such as a CCS. It would be important to consider how frequently he or she drives on long roads where the speed limit is consistent. Other relevant issues to consider would be whether there are likely to be major distractions within the vehicle, such as from children or several passengers. For some people lifestyle factors that entail towing a large trailer or boat, for example, might need to be considered because under these circumstances the speed at which a CCS is set would need to allow for longer braking distances. IITSs that support parking and reversing also would be nonoperational when towing.

Sometimes the decision to use a particular IITS may involve a trade-off between competing client goals and needs. For example communication devices such as cellular phones provide a convenient means for the driver (and potentially other vehicle occupants who do not own one of their own) to communicate with family, friends, work colleagues, and emergency service personnel if necessary. For drivers who may be heavily dependent on assistance in the event of a medical emergency, the availability of this helpline may be a critical need rather than simply a convenient resource. Conversely availability of a cellular phone in the car presents the risk of it being used while driving for purposes that are far from life preserving. For unimpaired drivers cellular phone use has been demonstrated to significantly increase crash risk, as previously noted in this chapter. For drivers with reduced attentional capacity, a slow rate of information processing, or an impaired ability to divide attention appropriately between concurrent tasks, the risks of such behavior will be considerably greater. This issue is evidently a difficult one for drivers to appreciate because there is evidence suggesting that many drivers are not aware that simply talking on a phone is negatively affecting aspects of their driving performance such as brake response time.[42] This highlights the key importance of the extent to which a driver has insight into the effects of his or her impairment on driving performance.

IITS ISSUES RELEVANT TO DIFFERENT CLIENT GROUPS

In this section the characteristics of key client groups are considered in relation to the kind of problems that can arise in their possible IITS use. The most easily identified and managed issues are also those that often appear to present the least threat to road safety (i.e., specific motor impairments and some [particularly nonvisual] sensory impairments). As outlined in Chapter 1, research evidence of the impact of common medical conditions on crash risk is far from definitive. However, available evidence suggests that people with the following conditions have an elevated crash risk: dementia, epilepsy, multiple sclerosis, psychiatric disorders (particularly schizophrenia), sleep apnea, alcohol abuse, and cataracts.[43] Remarkable for their absence from this list are conditions of a purely motor nature, such as arthritis and orthopedic conditions. Although the visual impairment associated with cataracts has been clearly shown to be a risk factor, this is the only medical condition involving substantial sensory impairment to have been thus identified. Some studies have reported significant but usually low correlations between impaired vision and crash risk, whereas other studies have failed to show such a link. Overall the evidence is clear that cognitive impairments present the largest risk to safety. Therefore it is the cognitive demands of using an IITS, as well as visual requirements where these exist, that should be of greatest concern to the DRS and researchers examining this issue. We will now examine cognitive issues that are relevant for specific driver groups: inexperienced drivers (relative to experienced ones), age of drivers, drivers with aging-related cognitive impairment, and drivers with visual/perceptual impairment.

DRIVER EXPERIENCE

One of the major determinants of a driver's capacity to cope with the cognitive demands of driving is the extent of his or her experience as a driver. A useful framework for reviewing the interacting effects of

driver experience and cognitive task demands is the SRK model described in Chapter 1.[44,45] With increasing experience driving becomes automatized to the maximum extent that is possible in light of the degree of consistent mapping between incoming information and resultant responses (i.e., the extent to which the same response always follows a particular incoming stimulus). With a complex activity such as driving a vehicle in traffic, full automatization of vehicle control skills typically requires a period of many months or even years, depending on the total amount of time spent driving. The automatization of perceptual and cognitive elements of driving skills is manifested in the development of highly detailed cognitive schemata and more specific mental models that represent the driver's understanding, knowledge, and associated expectancies about driving. These schemata enable an experienced driver to read the road traffic environment more easily and accurately than a novice driver and on this basis to make good driving-related decisions with greater ease and efficiency. Experienced drivers therefore have more spare attentional capacity that can be devoted to additional activities such as learning to use an IITS. In contrast novice drivers typically have few, if any, attentional resources available for additional subtasks and are less able to allocate their available attention appropriately. This is one reason why some licensing jurisdictions limit the rights of newly licensed drivers to carry passengers who may constitute a risky distraction from driving.

DRIVER AGE

Among adults many sensory, cognitive, and physical capacities tend to decline with increasing age.[46] Mean levels of muscular strength, range of movement, cardiovascular capacity, and aerobic power all tend to decrease in time. More importantly in the present context, older adults typically perform cognitive and psychomotor tasks more slowly than younger people, and their decline in information-processing capacity is most strongly evident when tasks are more complex and their attention must be divided between concurrent activities, particularly when they are under some stress. Working under time constraints is therefore more difficult for older people than for younger ones.[46-48] However, older people are typically highly experienced drivers and therefore can often compensate to some degree for the probable deterioration in many of their underlying capacities. For example highly developed perceptual and cognitive skills that enable the early identification of potentially hazardous situations are likely to compensate at least to some degree for slower decision times, thus enabling many older drivers to respond appropriately and with sufficient time to maintain safety. There also is great variation between individuals at any given age, and it is important to note that the extent of this variation increases with age, so that the difference between the strongest and the weakest, for example, or between the fastest and the slowest is greater among a group of older people than among younger people. Variation is caused by differences in factors, such as general health, fitness levels, medication intake, and genetic makeup.

Nevertheless learning new skills may take longer for some older people. Older drivers may find it more challenging to make the required changes in their driving behavior to incorporate the use of IITSs compared with their younger counterparts.[49] Learning to use IITSs also may be more difficult for those who have had little previous exposure to such technology because their mental models of how such devices are likely to operate will be less detailed and accurate and possibly even counterproductive. In such situations older people often have lower self-confidence and perhaps a resistance to new learning. It has been noted, however, that the perceived utility of an IITS will influence an older driver's motivation to learn to use the device.[50]

Older people are more likely to take prescription medications,[51,52] the side effects of which may influence their capacity to use IITSs, particularly during the learning phase. For example drugs that can influence arousal levels, reaction or movement time, or visual functioning would be of particular concern. In other cases medication management may not be optimal, for example, when managing muscle spasms, motor coordination, or pain. Some older clients also have multiple health and disability issues. In such cases the client may need to be referred for medical review and perhaps a comprehensive driver rehabilitation evaluation to identify specific factors that may impact on safe, efficient, and consistent use of IITSs. The factors of greatest concern are those related to undetected cognitive impairment, which is more likely among the oldest old.[53-55]

DRIVERS WITH SPECIFIC COGNITIVE IMPAIRMENTS

Individuals with cognitive impairment require careful evaluation regardless of the impairment's etiology. If there are known or suspected deficits of memory, attention, judgment, problem solving, or any other areas of executive functioning, learning to use previously unfamiliar IITSs will probably be inappropriate until the ability to drive safely during reasonably nondemanding conditions has been established. In some cases, such as

in those with progressive neurologic conditions, learning to use an IITS may not be possible unless treatment is available to retard or arrest cognitive decline. Although cognitive rehabilitation has been shown to be helpful for persons with stroke or traumatic brain injury (TBI),[56] more research is required to identify which intervention strategies are the most relevant for the (re)habilitation of cognitive functioning that is related to specific driving skills. As yet there is little published research evidence to guide practitioners in this area of practice, although recent studies show some promise.[57,58]

Some cognitive impairment is manifested in behavioral management problems, such as decreased insight, poor impulse control, or distractibility. In such cases the use of IITSs may be inadvisable and it may even be necessary to consider disabling or removing a communication or entertainment device from a vehicle, particularly as evidence accumulates to demonstrate the potential for these systems to increase crash risk.[33,36,37,59]

DRIVERS WITH VISUAL/PERCEPTUAL IMPAIRMENTS

Despite widespread acceptance of the need for appropriately qualified professionals to ascertain the visual health and functional status of prospective drivers,[60,61] research continues to show that large numbers of drivers have less than optimal vision.[62] Use of many IITSs requires good visual functioning, particularly when the driver is required to move his or her visual fixation point back and forth between the dashboard and the external environment, as demonstrated in the CCS task analysis in Table 18-2. This relies on several important aspects of visual function, including eye coordination, accommodation, and contrast sensitivity. It also demands rapid shifting of attention between different subtasks—an ability that is among those that decline with increasing age.[49,63] See Chapters 6, 12, and 21 and Appendix A for more information on vision and driving.

It may sometimes be feasible to use IITSs that rely on other sensory modalities to display information (e.g., auditory reminder tones), although there is some research evidence that voice-controlled systems may impose relatively high attentional demands. For example Lee et al[64] found that there was a 30% increase in reaction time when a speech-based system was used. He concluded that "...speech-based systems may pose cognitive demands that could undermine driving safety" and "a speech-based interface is not a panacea that eliminates the potential distraction of in-vehicle computers" (p. 639). Improvement of IITS interface designs to facilitate their use by drivers with suboptimal visual functioning is therefore highly desirable.

CASE STUDY

Peter is a 20-year-old apprentice carpenter who sustained a head injury and an incomplete spinal cord injury as a result of a motor vehicle accident in which he was a driver. It has been 12 months since his accident, and he has undertaken extended periods of inpatient and outpatient rehabilitation. Peter is able to ambulate independently, although he still has some difficulty with balance, muscle strength, and endurance with his lower limbs, especially if fatigued. He also experiences some limitations with executive functions, such as divided attention and problem solving. His driver rehabilitation program has commenced, and once his driving status is confirmed, he will start a graduated return-to-work trial in a furniture factory as a carpenter's assistant. Peter lives about a half-hour's drive from the regional town where the main entertainment and recreational facilities are located and where his work trial will be based. The transport route is mostly open highway with a speed limit of 70 mph. Peter has undertaken three graded, on-road assessments (increasing in duration and complexity) with an occupational therapist working as a DRS, as well as a number of driving lessons with a driver educator. During the course of his rehabilitation, the use of in-vehicle communication and entertainment systems and the availability of cruise control in his vehicle have been discussed. Peter has insight into his limitations, and he is aware of his increased difficulties when fatigued or in the company of peers. After consulting with the driver educator, the occupational therapist providing driver rehabilitation services has made the following recommendations regarding his driving privileges:

- Area-restricted license to 45 mph and avoid freeway driving, which is sufficient to drive to and from his home from the regional center
- No use of a cellular phone, CB radio, or personal computer while driving
- Limited use of the CCS in his car; specifically, use of the vehicle's CCS is permissible only when driving on the stretch of road between home and town where there is an open highway with no intersections and a consistent speed limit
- No use of other interactive ITSs (e.g., navigational devices)
- No passengers other than adult family members

A review of his driving status is to take place within 6 months.

PRESCRIPTION ISSUES: CHOOSING THE CORRECT IITS TO MEET INDIVIDUAL NEEDS

Many health care practitioners evaluate the needs of their clients and make recommendations regarding products, devices, or services that are designed to assist them in meeting specific short- and long-term goals. For occupational therapy generalists and specialists, a *client-centered model* is often applied, in which the clients are actively involved in the evaluation and decision making.[65] (See Chapters 1 and 5 for more information on the client-centered approach.) A high level of client involvement is likely to increase their engagement in the process and their motivation to use the prescribed devices. As previously mentioned an activity analysis is an important component of the evaluation.[40] This will help to identify the most appropriate design criteria for a particular IITS, and so to achieve the best possible match between the user, the task, and the environment. At present the limited range of add-on IITSs available may limit the possible recommendations, but this problem is likely to decrease over time. A few years ago, for example, in-vehicle navigational devices were only available in late-model vehicles, but now they are available for purchase off the shelf as turnkey solutions that can be installed in just about any brand of motor vehicle. It will probably not be long before many more options will be available from which to choose, which will make it even more important to ensure that the decision-making processes used to arrive at recommendations are client-centered, transparent, objective, and founded on valid and reliable evidence whenever possible. A number of other factors are relevant to the decision-making process, and a brief overview of these will help illuminate some of the key issues.

COMPENSATION VERSUS REMEDIATION

The evaluation process that is used to identify a client's strengths and weaknesses, to then to address his or her existing or anticipated driving-related needs, should identify whether a compensation approach, remediation approach, or some combination of the two will be the most suitable means of assisting the client to meet his or her short- and long-term goals related to driving and alternate modes of transportation that enable community mobility.

Remediation is generally directed at aspects of the client's abilities or other characteristics relevant to a particular activity. This may involve, for example, working to modify his or her physical strength, range of motion, thoughts, values, or life roles. Conversely *compensation* attempts to address difficulties in occupational performance by modifying how the person performs the task or by modifying the task itself or the environment in which it is performed.[66] In the case of an individual with reduced visual abilities, for example, compensatory strategies may include avoiding driving at night, during adverse weather conditions, and in unfamiliar areas.

It is useful to consider the application of both approaches when evaluating an IITS, for example, a CCS. In this case remediation of the client's lower limb function by activities designed to strengthen muscles and improve coordination may be appropriate. From a compensation perspective a CCS may be useful to compensate for the client's lack of endurance and susceptibility to fatigue, which would otherwise severely limit his or her ability to undertake long trips. The type of intervention approach used may be influenced by whether the driver already has access to a CCS, by whether recovery from an illness or injury has stabilized, and perhaps by whether funding support needs to be sought.

TRIALING AND TRAINING NEEDS

When IITSs are being considered as a possible means of compensating for an individual's reduced functioning, it is important to trial the use of the device if possible. This will become even more important as the range of available IITS devices increases because different models of functionally similar IITSs may have dissimilar design features. Training in the use of a particular IITS is likely to be essential to optimize safe and independent use. Taking the time to carefully read instruction manuals and to experiment with the available functions will help the DRS identify whether the IITS can be customized to suit a particular driver's needs. Instructions may need to be translated, modified, or simplified to meet a client's individual requirements. Safety issues, such as ongoing maintenance requirements and troubleshooting and management of the IITS functions when the system is not working, are crucial to understand and address.

MAINTENANCE OF IITS

The maintenance of particular IITS systems is an important consideration for any prospective user. Most obviously there needs to be easily available and user-friendly information about when and how often maintenance should occur. It also is important to consider the expertise required and the costs involved, particularly for drivers residing in rural or remote areas or who may have limited financial resources. In the case of IITSs that remove control over some vehicle functions from the driver, a more

critical concern relates to the level of impact that a malfunctioning IITS may have on the vehicle's functioning and safety. For example the DRS should ask whether there are automatic backup systems and whether the driver might need to take remedial action of some kind. These issues will become increasingly important with the emergence of more sophisticated IITSs that automate and simplify more of the core driving functions, such as intelligent speed adaptation, vision enhancement systems, and automatic lane-keeping systems.

ITS AND FUTURE CHALLENGES

Growth in computer and microchip technology is creating more and more options for ITSs, and it is likely that the distinction between in-vehicle systems (the focus of this chapter) and ITSs based in the external (i.e., road) environment will become increasingly blurred. Systems that are already operational within some road systems or available as features within late-model vehicles include the following:

- Advanced traffic management systems that assist with managing and coordinating traffic congestion; for example variable speed signs on major roads that inform drivers of optimal speeds to minimize stop-start driving (based on current traffic densities and signal timing), variable message signs on freeways, and parking guidance signs.
- Advanced traveler information systems that provide drivers with accessible information via in-vehicle units regarding traffic conditions, parking, speed limits, topographic orientation, and routes. Drivers are thus better informed to make decisions concerning travel routes and time or an optimal mode of transportation.
- Infrared night-vision systems, which are in-vehicle displays that allow the driver to view enhanced depictions of the driving environment ahead of the vehicle.
- Adaptive or intelligent CCSs that incorporate a mechanism whereby the vehicle monitors the following distance behind the lead vehicle and alerts the driver with an auditory or visual display or automatically slows the vehicle as the distance between the vehicles narrows.
- Voice recognition systems, which are likely to be increasingly used in interfaces for IITSs such as navigation, climate control, and entertainment systems.[11,13]

Systems that are currently under development, being trialed, or in the early stages of implementation include the following:

- Fully automated highways that interact with IITSs and guide the vehicle along a designated route and at certain times take full control of the vehicle from the driver.

- Collision avoidance systems, which are roadway systems that monitor and control the travel paths of multiple vehicles along a predetermined route.
- Driver drowsiness detectors that monitor the driver's eye movements, blink rate, or both as an indicator of the imminence of sleep onset and that warn the driver or slow the vehicle to avoid a collision.
- Pocket personal computers or mobile phones with the capacity to provide drivers with route navigation, parking, weather, and traffic information.
- IITSs that supply the driver with real-time traffic information, such as the speed limit, hazard warnings, and weather conditions.

The latter systems may offer drivers with special needs a broader range of options to support their driving performance. For example real-time traffic information systems have the potential to provide drivers with information earlier than is available via conventional road signs by using alternative sensory modalities and enhanced displays that can retain and repeat information if required.[11,13,14,68] However, to maximize their potential value and to ensure that road safety is not threatened, it will be essential that cognitive ergonomics knowledge is applied to their design.[11,13,17,69] Achievement of this will require system developers and manufacturers to work collaboratively within multidisciplinary teams that include occupational therapists and human factors specialists, conducting research that examines the needs of all types of potential users, including those of drivers with disabilities, aging-related concerns, or both.

SUMMARY

As the numbers and variety of IITSs increase, they seem likely to present increasing challenges to DRSs, for whom the key requirement is to match client needs and abilities to the characteristics of particular systems. Currently this is difficult because there is considerable doubt about how well some of them have been tested before their commercial release.[70,71] Moreover there is not yet a large body of research literature to support the newly emerging design standards,[32] and there is some concern about the possible long-term effects of using IITSs on driver behavior and crash risk.[5]

In this context DRS recommendations concerning IITS use need to be cautious, particularly with clients who have cognitive or behavioral impairments. This may be difficult when family members or the clients themselves see the IITS as a potential means of achieving their goal of driving independence without under-standing the possible risks. There are no easy rules to guide DRSs who need to decide when to include IITSs in their evaluation and training regimens.

Decisions should be made on a case-by-case basis, involving the client or caregiver whenever possible. However, recommendations must also be well founded on the DRS's expert and detailed analysis, in accord with professional duty of care obligations to the client and the wider community. Depending on state licensing authority requirements and legislation, recommendation of license conditions (i.e., restrictions) may sometimes be advisable, either to make driving conditional on use of a particular IITS or to preclude use of some systems. (See Chapters 7, 21, and 23 and Appendix H for more information on ethics, driving cessation, and counseling the older driver who is no longer able to drive. See also Appendix A for more information on reporting laws and Appendix I for more information on the legal responsibilities of physicians and other health care personnel.)

From medicolegal and professional practice perspectives, practitioners have a responsibility to use current IITS standards and to maintain their professional knowledge and skills in relation to new research and developments pertinent to driver rehabilitation service delivery, including the use of IITSs by people with disabilities and elderly persons. More pragmatically, funding bodies will be looking for empirical evidence to justify expenditure on IITSs. Already they are asking for evidence to justify how a particular IITS could improve an individual's safety, health, independence, well-being, and community participation. DRSs and others in this field have a professional obligation to be active but critical consumers of leading-edge research in the rapidly emerging area of IITSs.

REFERENCES

1. Australian Transport Safety Bureau: *Road safety in Australia: a publication commemorating World Health Day 2004*, Canberra, ACT, 2004, Australian Transport Safety Bureau.
2. Austroads: *The implications of intelligent transport systems for road safety* (no. AP-134/99), Sydney, 1999, Austroads.
3. Raymond P, Knoblauch R, Nitzburg M: *Older road user research plan*, Washington, DC, 2001, National Highway Traffic Safety Administration, U.S. Department of Transportation.
4. Di Stefano M, Macdonald W: Intelligent transport systems and occupational therapy practice, *Occup Ther Internat* 10:56-74, 2003.
5. Regan MA, Oxley JA, Godley S, et al: *Intelligent transport systems: safety and human factors issues* (Literature Review), Victoria, Australia, 2002, Royal Automobile Club of Victoria Limited.

6. Haddon W Jr, Suchman EA, Klein D: *Accident research: methods and approaches*, New York, 1964, Harper & Row.

7. Brook-Carter N: Driver information systems, *The Ergonomist* June:3, 2003.

8. Cairney P, Green F: *The implications of intelligent transport systems for road safety*, Melbourne, Australia, 1999, Australian Road Research Board.

9. Harris A: *Alcohol Ignition Interlock Programs—RACV Survey* (No. PP 99/02), Melbourne, Australia, 1999, Royal Automobile Club of Victoria.

10. Intelligent Transportation Society of America: Delivering the future of transportation: the national intelligent transportation systems program plan: a ten year vision, 2002. Available at: *http://www.its.dot.gov/*. Accessed July 30, 2002.

11. PIARC Committee on Intelligent Transport: *ITS Handbook 2000: recommendations from the World Road Association (PIARC)*, Boston, 1999, Artech House.

12. Regan MA: A sign of the future: intelligent transport systems. In Castro C, Horberry T, editors: *The human factors of transport signs*, pp 213-224, Boca Raton, FL, 2004, CRC Press.

13. Regan MA: A sign of the future II: human factors. In Castro C, Horberry T, editors: *The human factors of transport signs*, pp 225-238, Boca Raton, FL, 2004, CRC Press.

14. Whelan R: *Smart highways, smart cars*, Boston, 1995, Artech House.

15. Schieber F: *Beyond TRB 218: A select summary of developments in the field of transportation and aging since 1988* (No. Version 1.01), Vermillion, South Dakota, 1999, University of South Dakota.

16. Sanders JS, McCormick EJ: *Human factors in engineering and design*, ed 7, New York, 1993, McGraw Hill.

17. Abram F: Safe driving, *ISO Focus: The Magazine of the International Organization for Standardization* March:7-10, 2004.

18. Hakamies-Blomqvist L, Peters BJ: Recent European research on older drivers, *Accident Analysis Prevention* 32:601-607, 2000.

19. Molnar LJ, Eby DW, Miller LL: *Promising approaches for enhancing elderly mobility* (UMTRI Report no. 2003-24), Ann Arbor, MI, 2003, University of Michigan Transportation Research Institute.

20. Woodson WE, Tillman B, Tillman P: *Human factors design handbook*, ed 2, New York, 1992, McGraw-Hill.

21. Prabhu PV, Prabhu GV: Human error and user-interface design. In Helander M, Landauer TK, Prabhu P, editors: *Handbook of human-computer interaction*, pp 489-501, New York, 1997, Elsevier.

22. Newell AF, Gregor P: Human computer interfaces for people with disabilities. In Helander M, Landauer TK, Prabhu P, editors: *Handbook of human-computer interaction*, ed 2, pp 813-824, New York, 1997, Elsevier Science.

23. Daigneault G, Joly P, Frigon J-Y: Executive functions in the evaluation of accident risk of older drivers, *J Clin Experiment Neuropsychol* 24:221-238, 2002.

24. Parker D, McDonald L, Rabbitt P, et al: Elderly drivers and their accidents: the aging driver questionnaire, *Accident Analysis Prevent* 32:751-759, 2000.

25. Bridger RS: *Introduction to ergonomics*, ed 2, New York, 2003, Taylor and Francis.

26. Helander M, Landauer TK, Prabhu GV: *Handbook of human-computer interaction*, ed 2, New York, 1997, Elsevier.

27. Noyes J: *Designing for humans*, New York, 2001, Taylor and Francis.

28. Pauzie A: In-vehicle communication systems: the safety aspect, *Inj Prevent* 8(suppl IV):26-29, 2002.

29. Rogers WAE: *Designing for an aging population: ten years of human factors/ergonomics research*, Santa Monica, CA, 1997, Human Factors and Ergonomics Society.

30. Steenbekkers LPA, Beijsterveldt CEM: *Design relevant characteristics of aging users: backgrounds and guidelines for product innovation*, Delft, 1998, Delft University Press.

31. Van Cott HP, Kinkade RG: *Human engineering guide to equipment design*, rev. ed, Washington, DC, 1972, U.S. Government Printing Office.

32. Rupp G: Ergonomics in the driving seat, *ISO Focus: The Magazine International Organization Standardization* March:11-15, 2004.

33. Harbluk JL, Noy YI: *The impact of cognitive distraction on driver visual behaviour and vehicle control*, Montreal, Canada, 2002, Transport Canada-Road Safety.

34. Laberge-Nadeau C, Maag U, Ballavance F, et al: Wireless telephones and the risk of road crashes, *Accident Analysis Prevent* 35:649-660, 2003.

35. Matthews R, Legg S, Charlton S: The effect of cell phone type on drivers' subjective workload during concurrent driving and conversing, *Accident Analysis Prevent* 857:1-7, 2002.

36. Patten CJD, Kircher A, Ostlund J, et al: Using mobile telephones: cognitive workload and attention resource allocation, *Accident Analysis Prevent* 36:341-350, 2004.

37. Strayer DL, Johnston WA: Driven to distraction: dual-task studies of simulated driving and conversing on a cellular telephone, *Psychol Sci* 12:462-466, 2001.

38. Parasuraman R, Mouloua M, editors: *Automation and human performance: theory and applications*, Mahwah, NJ, 1996, Lawrence Erlbaum.

39. Strayer DL, Kramer AF: Aging and Skill acquisition: learning-performance distinctions, *Psychol Aging* 9(4):589-605, 1994.

40. Crepeau EB: Analyzing occupation and activity: a way of thinking about occupational performance. In Crepeau EB, Cohn ES, Boyt Schell BA, editors: *Willard and Spackman's occupational therapy*, ed 10, pp 189-198, Philadelphia, 2003, Lippincott, Williams & Wilkins.

41. Hatakka M, Keskinen E, Gregersen NP, et al: Theories and aims of educational and training measures. In Siegrist SE, editor: *Driver training, testing and licensing—towards theory-based management of young drivers' injury risk in road traffic*, pp 13-44, Berne, Switzerland, 1999, Human Research Department, Swiss Council for Accident Prevention bfu.

42. Lesch MF, Hancock PA: Driving performance during concurrent cell-phone use: are drivers aware of their performance decrements? *Accident Analysis Prevent* 36:471-480, 2004.

43. Charlton J, Koppel S, O'Hare M, et al: *Influence of chronic illness on crash involvement of motor vehicle drivers* (Literature review No. 213), Melbourne, 2004, Monash University Accident Research Centre.

44. Rasmussen J, Pejtersen A, Goodstein LP: *Cognitive systems engineering*, New York, 1994, Wiley.
45. Rasmussen J, Jensen A: Mental procedures in real-life tasks: a case-study of electronic trouble shooting, *Ergonomics* 17:293-307, 1974.
46. Comcare: *Productive and safe workplaces for an ageing workforce: implementing organisational renewal, mature-aged workers in the Australian Public Service*, Canberra, 2003, Commonwealth of Australia. Available at: *http://www.apsc.gov.au/publications03/maturecomcare.pdf. Accessed January 18,* 2005.
47. Bolstad CA, Hess TM: Situation awareness and aging. In Endsley MR, Garland DJ, editors: *Situation awareness, analysis and measurement*, pp 277-301, Mahwah, NJ, 2000, Lawrence Erlbaum Associates.
48. Fisk AD, Rogers WAE: *Handbook of human factors and the older adult*, San Diego, 1997, Academic Press.
49. Eby DW, Kostyniuk LP: Maintaining older driver mobility and well-being with traveler information systems, *Transportation Quart* 52:45-53, 1998.
50. Oxley PR: Elderly drivers and safety when using IT Systems, *IATSS Res* 20:102-110, 1996.
51. Darzins P, Hull M: Older road users: issues for general practitioners, *Aust Fam Physician* 28:663-667, 1999.
52. Roller L, Gowan J: Drugs and driving, *Current Therapeutics* February:65-71, 2001.
53. Black SA, Rush RD: Cognitive and functional decline in adults aged 75 and older, *J Am Geriatr Soc* 50:1978-1986, 2002.
54. Brayne C, Spiegelhalter DJ, Dufouil C, et al: Estimating the true extent of cognitive decline in the old old, *J Am Geriatr Soc* 47:1283-1288, 1999.
55. Collie A: *Cognitive decline and mild cognitive impairment in older individuals: issues, methods of identification and neuropsychological characterisation*, Unpublished PhD dissertation, Melbourne, 2001, LaTrobe University.
56. Cicerone KD, Dahlberg C, Kalmar K, et al: Evidence-based cognitive rehabilitation: recommendations for clinical practice, *Arch Phys Med Rehabil* 81:1596-1615, 2000.
57. Ball K, Berch DB, Helmers KF, et al: Effects of cognitive training interventions with older adults: a randomized controlled trial, *JAMA* 288:2271-2281, 2002.
58. Mazer BL, Sofer S, Korner Bitensky N, et al: Effectiveness of a visual attention retraining program on the driving performance of clients with stroke, *Arch Phys Med Rehabil* 84:541-550, 2003.
59. Hancock PA, Lesch M, Simmons L: The distraction effects of phone use during a crucial driving maneuver, *Accident Analysis Prevent* 862:1-14, 2002.
60. American Medical Association and National Highway Traffic Safety Administration: Physician's guide to assessing and counseling older drivers, 2003. Available at *http://www.ama-assn.org/ama/pub/category/10791.html*. Accessed September 2, 2003.
61. Austroads: *Assessing fitness to drive: for commercial and private vehicle drivers: medical standards for licensing and clinical management guidelines*, ed 3, Sydney, 2003, Austroads Incorporated.
62. Keeffe JE, Jin CF, Weigh LM, et al: Vision impairment and older drivers: who's driving? *Br J Ophthalmol* 86:1118-1121, 2002.
63. Mourant RR, Tsai F-J, Al-Shihabi T, et al: Measuring divided-attention capability of young and older drivers, *Transportation Res Record 1779* Paper no. 01-2239:40-45, 2001.
64. Lee JD, Caven B, Haake S, et al: Speech-based interaction with in-vehicle computers: the effect of speech-based e-mail on drivers' attention to the roadway, *Hum Factors* 43:631-640, 2001.
65. Law M, Baum BM: Measurement in occupational therapy. In Law M, Baum BM, Dunn W, editors: *Measuring occupational performance: supporting best practice in occupational therapy*, pp 1-19, Thorofare, NJ, 2001, Slack Incorporated.
66. McColl MA: Therapeutic processes to change occupation. In McColl MA, Pollock N, Law M, editors: *Theoretical basis of occupational therapy*, ed 2, pp 179-182, Thorofare, NJ, 2003, Slack Incorporated.
67. Reference deleted in pages.
68. U.S. Department of Transportation: *Report to Congress on the National Highway Traffic Safety Administration ITS Program*, Washington, DC, 1997, National Highway Traffic Safety Administration, U.S. Department of Transportation.
69. Hancock PA, Parasuraman R, Byrne EA: Driver-centered issues in advanced automation for motor vehicles. In Parasuraman R, Mouloua M, editors: *Automation and human performance: theory and application*, pp 337-364, Mahwah, NJ, 1996, Lawrence Erlbaum Associates.
70. Stamatiadis J: ITS and human factors for the older driver: the U.S. experience, *Transportation Quart* 52:91-101, 1998.
71. McKnight AJ: Too old to drive? *Issues Sci Technol* 17:63-69, 2000.

Chapter 19

DESIGNING THE EXTERNAL ENVIRONMENT FOR TRAFFIC SAFETY

Tapan K. Datta

KEY TERMS

- PIEV time
- Reaction time
- Risk assessment
- Risk
- Pure risk
- Speculative risk
- Reaction time
- Expectancy
- Hazards
- Stopping sight distance
- Coding
- Chunking
- Traffic control devices
- Traffic signals

CHAPTER OBJECTIVES

After completing this chapter, the reader will be able to do the following:

- Understand the relationships between the driver, physical environment, and vehicle to design and develop an effective driver rehabilitation program.
- Understand the primary performance components related to the driving task to successfully incorporate human factors into traffic control strategies.
- Understand why highway environmental issues are critical for safe driving and community mobility.

Highway transportation has three basic elements: the driver, the physical environment, and the vehicle. These elements must function as a system to achieve safe and efficient transportation of goods and people. The linkages between these three basic elements of transportation are real. Recent innovations in vehicle safety and operations, such as automated in-vehicle laser detection of front- and rear-end obstructions and antiskid traction systems, have improved vehicle safety significantly. A driver's ability to safely operate a vehicle is influenced by the vehicle's operating characteristics and the laws and regulations of the surrounding community. A sudden breakdown of the vehicle or a deficiency in the highway infrastructure or traffic control system may cause the basic system to fail, thus causing an accident. Sometimes driver error or misjudgment also plays a major role in causing traffic accidents. Understanding these relationships is essential for designing and developing an effective driver rehabilitation program.

Driver education and training programs in the United States provide lessons in the basic "dos and don'ts" of vehicle operation. Programs also include some lessons recognizing and understanding the functions of basic regulatory traffic control devices. However, a closer examination of the highway environment in detail and its impact on vehicle operation and safety is often lacking. Experience is required for new drivers to become familiar with many critically important highway infrastructure and traffic control–related issues.

Driver rehabilitation programs are generally designed for drivers who have either temporary or permanent physical, cognitive, or psychosocial challenges because of accidents, illnesses, aging-related concerns, or a combination of these and other factors. These drivers must have a complete and detailed understanding of the highway environment and an ability to recognize and understand risks related to driving to help ensure driver, passenger, and pedestrian safety while on the road. The comprehensive driver rehabilitation evaluation and training programs should also be extensive enough to allow drivers to identify and assess potential risks while driving in various highway environments under a myriad of potential conditions.

HIGHWAY-DRIVER-VEHICLE RELATIONSHIP

Highway and road users, including drivers, pedestrians, cyclists, and others are the basic elements of the highway transportation system. To achieve safety and efficiency in this environment, the following must be provided:
- A well-designed highway facility that promotes safety and efficiency that can handle the travel demand
- A vehicle that is in good working condition and can perform well on demand under a variety of environmental situations
- Road users who are able to identify hazards caused by deficiencies related to infrastructure or traffic control, unexpected actions by other road users, and other unforeseen environmental conditions. The road users must then be able to make appropriate decisions in a timely manner so as to take action to avoid hazardous consequences

Failure in any one of these elements can result in operational inefficiencies and traffic collisions.

The safety and operational characteristics of vehicles are generally well designed to avoid or withstand traffic accidents when operators take appropriate actions. Auto manufacturers have made great strides in equipping the vehicles with safety features (e.g., air bags; front-, four-, and all-wheel drives; and antilock braking systems). However, because the driver is a major part of the system, human limitations and, in particular, behavior must be examined carefully to develop strategies that can begin to foster driver, passenger, and pedestrian safety.

Human error is at least a contributing factor (if not the primary reason) in most motor vehicle crashes (Table 19-1). Most of the vehicle safety features rely on

a driver's appropriate reaction to threatening external stimuli. Human reaction involves a series of events closely related to various human factors, including the following:
- Perception that involves seeing and making sense of stimuli in the internal (i.e., inside the vehicle) and external (outside the vehicle) environments
- Intellection that involves recognizing and identifying (i.e., assign meaning to) external stimuli
- Emotion that involves a decision-making process that results in an appropriate course of action, such as stopping, swerving, merging, or blowing the horn
- Volition that involves the execution of the decision made in the previous subtask, emotion

The total time required for completing an assessment of these four subtasks (i.e., perception, intellection, emotion, and volition [PIEV]) often varies from person to person. The total time from seeing and becoming aware of some kind of internal or external stimuli to actually executing a response is called *PIEV time*, commonly known as *reaction time*. The length of PIEV time demonstrated by a particular driver is a function of a variety of factors:
- Training of driving tasks
- Experience
- Age
- Familiarity with the internal and external environments

This is why racecar drivers have low PIEV times and older drivers typically have high PIEV times. It is important to note that most of the highway infrastructure is designed for a minimum PIEV time of 2.5 seconds. Therefore anyone who has a PIEV time of ≤2.5 seconds can successfully negotiate any number of specific highway environments.

A person in a rehabilitation program may have some temporary physical, cognitive, or psychosocial challenges that impact his or her PIEV time. Tests must be done to identify the actual PIEV time for each individual before a customized driver rehabilitation or community mobility program can be developed and implemented by a driver rehabilitation specialist (DRS).

The factors that impact total PIEV time are listed in Box 19-1. These factors are critical for competent driving, and understanding them is essential when developing a driver rehabilitation program.

Visual acuity is of great importance to the driver. It provides information about the highway, such as roadway characteristics, topographic orientation, speed limit, special roadway conditions (e.g., traffic volume, detours, and an icy bridge), roadside features and hazards, and traffic control–related information, to name a few. Seeing such highway-related characteristics enables a driver to understand the potential effects highway elements can have on reducing a driver's overall PIEV time for any given stimulus.

Visual acuity relates to the field of clearest vision, which is generally a 3- to 5-degree cone of vision. However, a 10- to 12-degree cone of vision also provides drivers with fairly clear vision and assists them to recognize and interpret essential environmental stimuli necessary for safe and efficient driving. See Chapters 6, 12, and 21 and Appendix A for more information on vision and driving.

Peripheral vision relates to a field of view in which a driver can see objects, although not clearly and without color perception. Normal drivers have 120 to 180 degrees of peripheral vision. Recognition of the presence

Table 19-1   **Driver Involvement Rates per 100,000 Licensed Drivers by Age, Gender, and Crash Severity**

Age (Years)	Male		Female		Total	
	Licensed Drivers	Crash Involvement Rate per 100,000 Licensed Drivers	Licensed Drivers	Crash Involvement Rate per 100,000 Licensed Drivers	Licensed Drivers	Crash Involvement Rate per 100,000 Licensed Drivers
DRIVERS IN FATAL CRASHES IN YEAR 2002						
<16	228	*	108	*	336	*
16-20	5,696	89.04	2,386	39.27	8,082	64.80
21-24	4,855	71.54	1,430	21.83	6,285	47.12
25-34	8,698	47.11	2,718	15.31	11,416	31.52
35-44	8,086	38.87	2,809	13.69	10,896	26.37
45-54	6,309	33.78	2,208	11.75	8,517	22.73
55-64	3,793	30.30	1,270	10.14	5,063	20.22
65-69	1,144	26.89	438	10.22	1,582	18.53
>69	3,159	33.09	1,529	14.80	4,689	23.59
Unknown	166	*	15	*	937	*
Total	**42,134**	**43.23**	**14,911**	**15.40**	**57,803†**	**29.75**

Continued

Table 19-1   Driver Involvement Rates per 100,000 Licensed Drivers by Age, Gender, and Crash Severity—cont'd

Age (Years)	Male		Female		Total	
	Licensed Drivers	Crash Involvement Rate per 100,000 Licensed Drivers	Licensed Drivers	Crash Involvement Rate per 100,000 Licensed Drivers	Licensed Drivers	Crash Involvement Rate per 100,000 Licensed Drivers
DRIVERS IN INJURY CRASHES IN YEAR 2002						
<16	22,000	*	7,000	*	29,000	*
16-20	314,000	4,910	253,000	4,172	568,000	4,551
21-24	247,000	3,636	155,000	2,361	401,000	3,010
25-34	413,000	2,235	316,000	1,781	729,000	2,012
35-44	398,000	1,911	309,000	1,507	707,000	1,710
45-54	292,000	1,565	218,000	1,163	511,000	1,363
55-64	171,000	1,367	121,000	967	292,000	1,167
65-69	47,000	1,103	34,000	800	81,000	951
>69	119,000	1,245	74,000	716	193,000	970
Total	2,023,000	2,075	1,487,000	1,537	3,511,000	1,807

Table 19-1 Driver Involvement Rates per 100,000 Licensed Drivers by Age, Gender, and Crash Severity—cont'd

Age (Years)	Male		Female		Total	
	Licensed Drivers	Crash Involvement Rate per 100,000 Licensed Drivers	Licensed Drivers	Crash Involvement Rate per 100,000 Licensed Drivers	Licensed Drivers	Crash Involvement Rate per 100,000 Licensed Drivers
DRIVERS IN INJURY CRASHES IN YEAR 2002						
<16	125,000	*	46,000	*	172,000	*
16-20	1,025,000	16,025	772,000	12,705	1,797,000	14,409
21-24	774,000	11,411	511,000	7,803	1,286,000	9,639
25-34	1,381,000	7,477	947,000	5,336	2,328,000	6,428
35-44	1,293,000	6,215	929,000	4,525	2,222,000	5,376
45-54	976,000	5,224	673,000	3,580	1,648,000	4,399
55-64	539,000	4,304	342,000	2,734	881,000	3,519
65-69	154,000	3,621	98,000	2,289	252,000	2,953
>69	336,000	3,525	223,000	2,163	560,000	2,817
Unknown	‡	*	‡	*	1,000	*
Total	**6,603,000**	**6,776**	**4,541,000**	**4,690**	**11,147,000**	**5,737**

* Not applicable.
†Includes 758 drivers of unknown gender.
‡Less than 500.
Data from Licensed Drivers—Federal Highway Administration, Traffic Crash Rates: USDOT—Traffic Safety Facts 2002 and 2002 Motor Vehicle Crash Data from Fatal Analysis Reporting System (FARS) and General Estimate System (GES).

BOX 19-1	**Factors That Impact Total PIEV Time**

Visual acuity
Peripheral vision
Depth perception
Sensitivity to glare
Color discrimination
Hearing
Reaction time
Effects of fatigue
Distractions
Pedestrian factors

of any object in the peripheral field of view allows a driver to be proactive; for example a driver may move his or her head to see an object more clearly before determining whether it is an actual or potential threat. Drivers who have a peripheral vision of ≤40 degrees are known to have tunnel vision and often require professional assistance to determine the etiology and explore potential interventions.

Depth perception relates to a person's ability to estimate distance and speed. Proper depth perception allows a driver to maintain safe headway. Decreased depth perception is often the cause of rear-end traffic crashes.

Sensitivity to glare (i.e., glare vision and increased recovery time) becomes a safety issue when driving in a westerly direction as the sun is setting and especially during early evening driving. The effect of high-intensity lights on a driver's eyes from a vehicle coming from the opposite direction often causes a temporary inability to recognize the normal driving environmental stimuli. This condition often extends from 2 to 3 seconds. Any driving actions that are required during or just after this period often are inaccurate and can lead to a traffic accident. Such glare effects also occur when a driver enters a lighted tunnel from a dark highway. The factors associated with glare vision and decreased recovery are often related to increased age. Older people generally have poorer night vision capabilities and require a longer recovery time than younger to middle-aged people.

Color discrimination is an important factor because most traffic signs and pavement markings are color coded, and color recognition often helps to facilitate timely and error-free driver actions and reactions. However, a significant percentage of the driving population is color-blind. Therefore being able to assess a subject's ability to discern color characteristics is an essential component for developing an effective driver rehabilitation program.

Hearing is essential for recognizing and understanding warning sounds that may be associated with impending danger. Hearing deficiencies among drivers may be alleviated by the use of a hearing aid or aids or other intervention strategies designed to improve hearing. Clients may not recognize that their hearing is decreased in one or both ears and often require testing by a hearing specialist to be diagnosed and treated. Because hearing loss is often associated with the aging process, DRSs should expect that many of their clients could present hearing-related issues and require professional assistance, without which the conditions can go undetected. See Chapters 6, 12, and 13 for more information on hearing and driving.

The time required for various driver actions to be taken to maintain safety is an important factor to understand when designing an effective driver rehabilitation program. Driver response (PIEV) time is a function of the number of choices and the complexity of judgment required to make decisions and react to environmental stimuli. PIEV time in controlled laboratory conditions varies between 0.2 and 1.5 seconds. However, in real driving situations drivers often face multiple choices depending on various highway and environmental conditions, which in turn can increase the time it takes to react to external stimuli. Some of the factors a driver considers before selecting an action during real driving situations are as follows:

- The vehicle's speed when the external stimuli are perceived
- The distance to the next vehicle and the level of traffic congestion
- Environmental conditions, such as the weather, time of day, and topography
- The severity of consequences for driving errors
- The type of highway situations and traffic control infrastructure
- The vehicle's design and functional capabilities

Therefore the total reaction time during real-world situations is greater than the times determined in laboratory experiments. The design of the highway and traffic control infrastructure requires an assessment of PIEV time. The American Association of State Highway and Transportation Officials (AASHTO) recommends using a PIEV time of 2.5 seconds as a common standard to be followed in the design of highway systems.[1]

Effects of fatigue on driver performance still raise more issues that must be considered in the design of highway and traffic control systems. Past research has shown the impact of driver fatigue on driving performance; however, understanding to what extent different levels of driver fatigue can impact total reaction time and the associated negative consequences is not well established. Therefore it is understandable that highway safety professionals recommend people avoid driving when they are tired. In recent years various innovative measures, such as rumble strips on the shoulders along highways, are meant to arouse sleepy and fatigued drivers and prevent them from veering off the roadway. Vehicle designers are also testing audible warning systems related to head positioning of drivers who are fatigued and momentarily fall asleep (briefly "nodding off") while behind the wheel of an automobile.

Distractions in the vehicle or in the visual field often cause drivers to take incorrect or delayed actions in response to external stimuli. Some of the issues related to distractions include the following:

- Music or other radio programs played in the vehicle. Certain types and levels of music can be helpful to driving operations; however, for others music or talk radio can be a potentially dangerous distraction.
- Intersections with high pedestrian movement
- Visual clutter in the driving environment. For example drivers must process much more visual and auditory stimuli while driving on a busy urban highway or street versus traveling on a country road through a rural setting.
- Other distractions, such as bright lights, neon signs, sirens, and drivers "honking" their vehicles' horns

The effect of such distractions is often more critical during nighttime driving, especially among elderly drivers. The effect of aging on night vision is well established in the literature[2]; therefore impaired night vision is another important factor to consider when determining the magnitude of a client's training and need for driving restrictions. See Chapters 6, 12, 13, and 21 for more information on evaluating and developing intervention strategies that compensate for impaired night vision.

Pedestrian factors, especially in the urban driving environment, are critical to the safety and well-being of all road users. Drivers often have to predict pedestrian actions to avoid accidents. Therefore rehabilitation and training programs targeted for drivers with physical or cognitive challenges must consider pedestrian factors in the driving environment.

Safe operation of a motor vehicle is a function of all three elements: highway, vehicle, and drivers. The vehicle and highway infrastructure characteristics generally remain unaltered and fairly constant within a particular location. Clients who are prospective candidates for driver rehabilitation must meet applicable local, state, and federal laws to help ensure an optimal level of safety while on the road. See Appendix A for more information on state driver licensing requirements and reporting laws. Therefore understanding the factors that can impact driving performance is critical.

It is important to note that highway infrastructure and traffic control systems are designed for "average" drivers and will probably continue to be designed in this way for the foreseeable future. Vehicles are also built to most effectively accommodate drivers who fall within a narrow range for height and weight. Although the highway infrastructure and vehicles are built with safety in mind, a driver must meet a minimum level of competency to help ensure his or her safety and the well-being of his or her passengers, other roadway users, and pedestrians. See Chapter 16 for more information on universal design and the automobile.

RISK ASSESSMENT

Drivers continuously assess possible consequences of actions they may take when selecting their speed and route while driving. The appropriateness of *risk assessment* in challenging conditions often determines driving outcomes. *Risk* is defined as the variation in the possible outcomes in a given situation. To measure the variation that exists in nature, one would have to know the underlying probability distribution and how to assess the variation inherent in that distribution. For example a gambler skilled in probability theory may be able to calculate precisely the probability of each hand of cards that may be dealt in a game of 21. That is, the gambler has an exact picture of the underlying probability distribution and can initiate his or her response based on what he or she predicts will likely occur. However, because he or she does not know which cards will be dealt next, there are risks because there are many possible outcomes. During real-life driving conditions, however, drivers do not know the precise probability distribution of possible outcomes, and the probabilities of various risks associated with driving must be estimated. See Chapter 1 for more information on measuring driver crash risk within a systems framework.

Situations that require a driver's assessment of risk may be classified as a pure or a speculative risk assessment. A *pure risk* exists when there is a chance of loss but no chance of gain. For example the owner of an automobile faces a pure risk when involved in an automobile collision. If a collision occurs, the owner does not gain. A *speculative risk* exists when there is a chance of gain and a chance of loss. Nondriving examples of speculative risk include casino gambling, horse racing, and various lotteries. A driver faces a speculative risk when traveling >15 mph above the posted speed limit. The driver will reach his or her destination sooner than if he or she was obeying the law; however, he or she also risks getting a traffic ticket that could result in a fine and an increase in insurance premiums. Pure risks are always distasteful, but speculative risks have some attractive features.

The driver training programs used in the United States are generally brief, and in some instances they do not adequately prepare prospective drivers. Student drivers are largely trained to acquire an acceptable level of skills and are given driving licenses with minimal driving experience during trained supervision. Therefore driver judgment of potential risks in the driving environment is primarily intuitive versus being grounded in knowledge of the driving task. For example a driver who knows what causes hydroplaning on a wet road and the actions that are necessary to prevent such incidences will assess the risk of driving in wet weather conditions much higher than an inexperienced driver who may not even consider the potential negative consequences of hydroplaning. Consequently the inexperienced driver in this example will most likely assess such a risk at a lower level than the informed driver. In-depth knowledge of traffic accident causation makes a driver assess the risks of driving at a much higher level compared with those who do not possess such knowledge.

DRIVER EXPECTANCY AND HIGHWAY FACTORS THAT CONSTITUTE HAZARDS

Drivers look for clues about environmental conditions from a variety of sources, including the roadway itself; traffic control features such as signs, signals, and pavement markings; and the environment at large, to make the necessary decisions that are often required for safe and efficient driving.

To successfully incorporate human factors into traffic control strategies one must understand the primary performance components related to the driving task. Driving includes the following three performance levels: control, guidance, and navigation.

The control function includes all activities involved in the driver's interaction with the vehicle and its controls and visual displays. These tasks range from relatively simple interactions, such as steering and maintaining a reasonable travel speed for passenger vehicles, to relatively complex activities, such as driving a tractor-trailer with multiple gears and clutches. A driver receives information (i.e., feedback) from the "feel" of the vehicle, from its displays, and from the physical environment (e.g., the roadway). Competent drivers continually make small adjustments to maintain vehicle control, and most of the control functions become intuitive with driving experience.

At the guidance level the driver's main function involves the maintenance of a safe speed and proper path relative to the roadway, roadside environment, and the most dynamic feature—traffic. The guidance function involves the use of judgment, estimation, and

prediction within an environment that is constantly changing. Guidance-level decisions are translated into adjusting one's speed and maneuvering the vehicle to alter its path in response to the roadway, geometric features, traffic, and the broader environment.

The navigation level of the driving task includes activities in which trips are planned and routes are selected. This plan is followed during the actual trip. Pretrip information sources include maps and destination directions obtained from the Internet. In-trip information sources include landmarks and route guidance signs. Navigational activities are generally cognitive in nature.

The following is a discussion of the concepts and principles related to information display techniques that should be considered in highway design and engineering to allow drivers to achieve desirable levels of performance in the control, guidance, and navigation functions.

DRIVER INFORMATION

One of the keys to successful driving is efficient information gathering and processing. This is relatively easy when drivers are only performing one activity at any given time. However, driving usually requires performing several activities related to various levels (control, guidance, and navigation). At any instant drivers generally receive information from multiple sources, establish priorities relative to the available information, make decisions, and perform controlled actions and reactions with various time constraints.

Drivers use sensory perception and cognition to collect, receive, and process information. They hear horns, sirens, and radio broadcasts; they feel road surface textures, raised pavement markers, and vehicle vibrations; they sense acceleration; and they see signs, vehicles, and the roadway. However, although most senses are used in driving, as much as 90% of all information is received visually.

Visually Displayed Information

Although it is not possible to identify and describe all of the pertinent visual reception factors, the following are vision-related issues that require consideration:

- Visually displayed information must be seen and attended to.
- The visual information source must be within the driver's field of view and "cone of clear vision" while the vehicle is in motion and stationary.
- Drivers must have the capability (e.g., visual acuity and color vision) to receive the information.
- Information displayed in the internal (i.e., inside of the vehicle) or external driving environments must be properly designed (e.g., brightness, color, size, shape,

and contrast) and positioned to help facilitate accurate recognition of the pertinent information so that there is sufficient time for the driver to perform the requisite maneuver(s), for example, to avoid a crash or maintain the correct travel route.

- Highway designers have a responsibility to ensure that all necessary information is adequately displayed on the roadways. Drivers are also responsible for receiving the information and taking appropriate actions to help ensure safety for themselves and other road users.

Information Handling

Driving entails an "information-decision-action" function. Drivers receive information from a number of different sources and combine current information and the knowledge gained from past experiences to make decisions about which actions to perform. While driving they may have to perform many actions at the same time that often have overlapping information needs. To satisfy these needs, drivers must search the environment, receive and process pertinent information, make decisions expeditiously, and take action (i.e., act or react to perform the necessary vehicle control function or functions).

People can only handle one source of visual information at a time. Given their need to process various displays and views simultaneously while driving, they respond by seeing a little bit of information at a time from several information sources and assign meaning to that constructed reality. Drivers integrate various activities and maintain an appreciation of an external driving environment that is dynamic and constantly changing by sampling information in short glances and shifting attention from source to source. Drivers also must rely on judgment, estimation, prediction, and memory to fill in the gaps and to eliminate lower priority information.

Memory

Drivers filter incoming information and transfer the most relevant and important information to their short-term memory for storage, rapid access, and retrieval. If the information that is in a driver's short-term memory is not relevant, reinforced, repeated, and processed, it is usually forgotten. Each short-term memory lasts from 30 seconds to 2 minutes, with a span of approximately five to nine information sources. Important information sources may be transferred to long-term memory, which has no limitations on the amount of information it can store or on the time frame for retrieval at some future time.

Reaction Time

Reaction time is the time between the receipt of information, information processing, and an action or reac-

tion initiated by the driver. Actions are often in the form of braking, changing the path or direction of the vehicle, and changing the vehicle's operating speed. It varies from driver to driver and is a function of the complexity of the information presented. Complex decisions take longer than simple ones, as do decisions in which the driver's expectancies are violated.

Expectancy

Through their experiences, all drivers develop some internal prediction capabilities of situations; these are often referred to as expectancies. When highway situations meet such expectancies, people perform the driving task safely and efficiently. *Expectancy* relates to a driver's readiness to respond successfully to situations, events, and information. It influences the speed and accuracy with which drivers process information and is a major factor that influences vehicle design, operation, and traffic control strategies. Aspects of the highway system that agree with commonly held expectancies also facilitate the driving function. Violated expectancies can lead to longer reaction times, confusion, inappropriate responses, and errors that can ultimately lead to traffic accidents.

Expectancies related to control functions pertain to vehicle handling and responsiveness. Expectancies related to guidance function involve highway design, traffic operations, hazards, and traffic control devices. Navigation expectancies affect pretrip and in-transit phases and relate to route, service, and guide signs. Most drivers develop some expectancies for highway driving situations based on their lifetime of experience in driving. Such expectancies are called a priori expectancy. These expectancies are long term and often become a habit. Drivers also form some site-specific expectancies while driving in specific environments. These expectancies are short term and are often site specific. They are called ad hoc expectancies.

Drivers do not remember crossing a political jurisdiction and associated differences in highway infrastructure design and traffic control. Therefore to achieve optimal safety and efficiency, all infrastructure and traffic control features for highways must be consistent and standardized as much as possible.

Priority of Information

Drivers continuously receive information from the highway environment (such as from traffic control devices) and prioritize it internally. They retain important information and use it in performing the driving task. The driver prioritization process addresses the relative importance of information, between levels of performance and within a given level, when information competes for attention or when performance of one function precludes attention to additional information.

Priority is assigned based on a driver recognizing the potential result of not attending to one piece of information and its relative importance.

Control function has the highest priority, followed by guidance and navigation. Losing control of a vehicle can be catastrophic and therefore is the highest or first priority for any driver, followed by the second highest priority, which is tracking the road, and the least important priority, getting lost because lacking topographic orientation potentially leads to the least catastrophic outcome. Similarly when two or more activities during driving compete for the driver's limited cognitive and physical capital (e.g., hazard avoidance and maintaining desired speed), the function with either the greatest undesirable consequences or the closest proximity becomes the higher priority.

Hazards

Any object, condition, or situation is considered a hazard when it is not successfully responded to as a result of driver failure or highway system failure. Unintended system inefficiencies are noncatastrophic failures that do not result in an accident, such as erratic maneuvers, confused or lost drivers, or traffic conflicts. Accidents are a result of catastrophic system failures.

Hazards can be classified as fixed or moving object hazards. Trees, light poles, and sign supports are fixed objects, whereas pedestrians, animals, and vehicles en route are moving objects. Potholes and lane drops and horizontal and vertical curves are examples of highway condition hazards. A combination of object and condition hazards is called a situation hazard and may be transitory, such as a stopped queue over a crest vertical curve, like during rain or fog (e.g., a slippery-when-wet curve in the rain).

Hazards avoidance depends on a driver's ability to know in advance that a hazard exists, recognize and identify a hazard as he or she is approaching it, be able to ascertain whether the hazard is a threat, visualize (or be given) an appropriate avoidance strategy, and perform the maneuvers that are required to avoid the hazard. Hazard avoidance is a continual feedback process, and its functions include the following:

- Detection and recognition: Depending on the type of hazard, visibility, conspicuousness, priority, expectancy, and visual clutter, the time required to recognize and detect the hazard varies. It is relatively easy to detect and recognize common hazards, such as trees and vehicles, whereas others, such as potholes and traffic signals that are inoperative, may be difficult to detect and recognize.
- Hazard avoidance maneuvers: Maneuvers to achieve avoidance of a hazard can vary from stopping to swerving the vehicle abruptly to avoid a pedestrian or to steer around a stationary obstacle, such as a disabled vehicle.

- Use of positive guidance to mitigate hazard avoidance problems: Positive guidance can assist drivers when they are experiencing problems with any aspect of the hazard avoidance process. This assistance could vary from making a hazard more visible by painting, lighting, or "flagging" it with a hazard marker, installing advance warning signs, and making the driver aware of what to do, such as assigning a right-of-way with a traffic signal.

Sight Distance

Because drivers overwhelmingly rely on their vision for driving and demonstrate lengthy reaction times when making complex decisions, they must have adequate forward sight distance. Adequate sight distance is necessary to provide enough time for drivers to collect information, process it, perform the necessary control functions, factor in vehicle response time, and evaluate the appropriateness of the response through a feedback process. In applying the positive guidance procedure, two types of sight distances are used—stopping sight distance and decision sight distance.

Stopping Sight Distance

AASHTO defines *stopping sight distance* as "the sum of two distances: (1) the distance traversed by the vehicle from the instant the driver sights an object necessitating a stop to the instant the brakes are applied; and (2) the distance needed to stop the vehicle from the instant brake application begins. These are referred to as brake reaction distance and braking distance, respectively."[1]

Stopping sight distance can be calculated using the following equation:

$$\text{Stopping sight distance} = d = 1.47Vt + 1.075 \frac{V^2}{a}$$

where:
V = Design speed in mph
t = Reaction time in seconds, nominally assumed as 2.5 seconds
a = Deceleration rate in ft/sec/sec, generally assumed as 11.2 ft/sec/sec

The equation for stopping sight distance changes when there is either an up or down highway surface grade. In such instances the following equation is applicable for computing stopping sight distance:

$$d = 1.47Vt + \frac{V^2}{30(a/g \pm G)}$$

where:
g = Acceleration caused by gravity = 32.2 ft/sec/sec
G = Percent of grade of the highway

Decision Sight Distance

There are various situations in which the stopping sight distance does not allow enough time for an appropriate response. This happens when there are complex or multiple decisions to be made, when vision is not clear, when expectancies are violated, or when stopping is an inappropriate hazard avoidance maneuver. Extended sight distance is needed to allow drivers the necessary time to detect, recognize, and respond to hazards in these cases. Extra time is necessary to allow for a margin for error if a hazard is not detected or recognized right away or if information is not present, improperly located, or not readily understood. Decision sight distance provides a longer sight distance and therefore more time.

The distance at which a driver can detect a hazard in an environment of visual noise or clutter, recognize it or its threat, select a speed and path that is appropriate, and perform the necessary avoidance maneuver safely and efficiently is called decision sight distance. Decision sight distance is used to ascertain the adequacy of forward sight distance to a hazard or to position highway information when there is not enough sight distance.

Specific Information Display Techniques

The techniques discussed in this section may be used to display information in an optimal manner so that drivers will receive and process the information in a timely manner to help ensure safe and efficient travel on the roadways.

Spreading

By distributing the information to a longer stretch of a roadway, the chance for overload is reduced, especially in high processing demand locations. This is accomplished by moving lower priority information sources either upstream or downstream. For example consider the highway work zone scenario presented in Figure 19-1, which shows various sources of information and a potential situation for driver overload. Nine pieces of information are given to the motorists through 19 traffic signs on a 1.5-mile stretch of road. In addition to the traffic signs, channelizing devices and pavement markings are provided to assist drivers through a no-passing zone and a lane transition area. By plotting the influence areas of the information sources, 12 cues of information are given to the drivers, which is excessive considering the short distance. This scenario presents a complex and demanding driving situation. There are too many visual cues provided that often overlap and may not provide a driver adequate time and distance to respond accordingly and make the appropriate action. By spreading the information over a distance of 2.8 miles (versus 1.5 miles), as shown in Figure 19-2,

and by strategically providing additional cues positioned in strategic locations, the amount of information at any given time can be reduced, thus avoiding potential information overload and reducing the likelihood of a traffic accident.

Coding and Chunking

Drivers have to observe, read, and understand written or displayed information (known as *coding*) and then act on the information they have absorbed in real time, sometimes with extreme time constraints. Coding sets forth the information into symbols that drivers are aware of and understand because of their previous experience and acquired knowledge. Thus coding assists drivers in increasing their capacity to handle and reduce their reaction time to information observed in the form of shapes, colors, or numbers. The merging of two or more codes into larger units (e.g., multiple symbol signs, interstate route numbers and shields, and color coding) is called *chunking*, and it minimizes a driver's reaction time. Codes and chunks must be known or learned by the driver, and their application must be uniformly applied on the highway system for drivers to quickly understand them and minimize their reaction time.

Repetition

Most drivers have a short-term memory span, basically 30 seconds to 2 minutes, and if a period of time longer than that elapses between observing information and acting on that information, they have a tendency to forget.

Redundancy

Redundancy is defined as the same information being shown on at least one or more carriers that use a minimum of two or more display techniques. An example would be the stop sign, which exhibits its message by color, shape, and terminology. Redundancy helps to minimize uncertainty and increase the number of drivers able to absorb the information. The stop sign is a good example because someone not well versed in the English language can still understand the sign because of its distinct color and shape.

Navigation Information Presentation Aids

There are many situations in which navigation-level problems exist by themselves or in combination with guidance-level problems despite the fact that the primary focus of positive guidance is on the performance of the guidance level. This procedure is applicable to the entire highway information system, including direction finding and route guidance functions. Navigation problems must be resolved before the problems of a site can be solved.

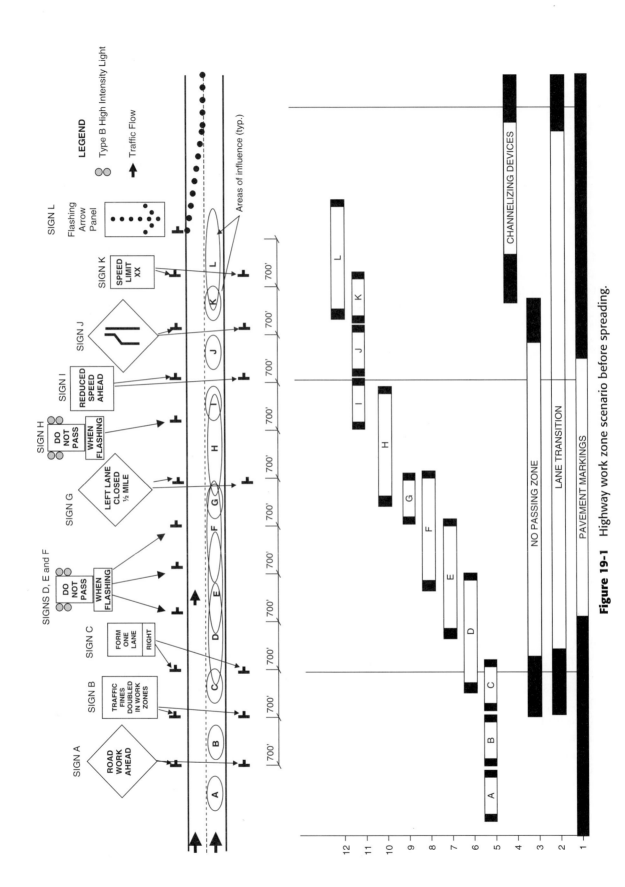

Figure 19-1 Highway work zone scenario before spreading.

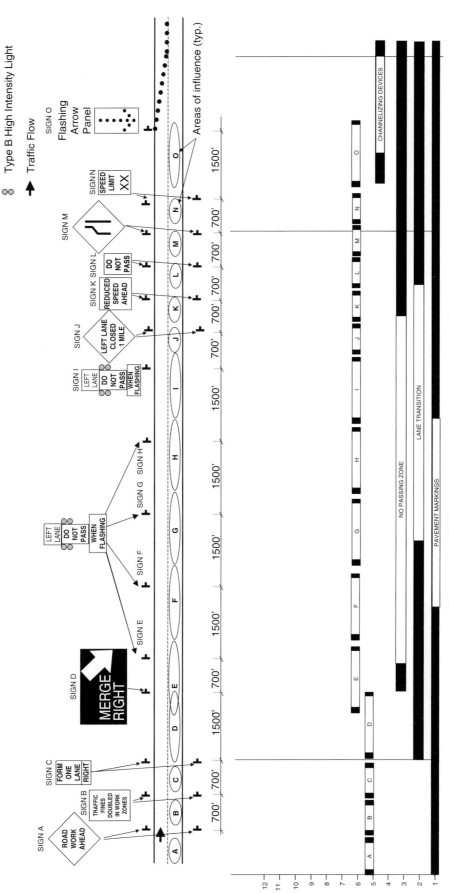

Figure 19-2 Highway work zone scenario after spreading.

At the navigation level there are many aids, such as the following:

- Urban street and arterial signs are placed mid-block to assist drivers in locating streets after dark or in situations involving driving at higher speeds.
- Placement of overhead signs where trucks and other larger vehicles may block drivers' line of sight.
- Placement of route guidance signs larger than normal at choice locations to assist drivers.
- Transmission of information to the driver of a vehicle through the use of Highway Advisory Radio (HAR).
- Real-time signs on which messages can be changed to make drivers aware of road problems and in turn assist in the management of traffic congestion problems.
- Some examples of navigation aids include Intelligent Vehicle and Highway System (IVHS) technology and chevron signs at severe curves:
  - IVHS: Drivers are continuously provided with navigation, guidance, and control information through on-board information displays. However, the main source of driver information continues to be more traditional aids to navigation, such as maps and verbal directions, along with the highway information system. See Chapter 18 for more information on in-vehicle intelligent transport systems.
  - Chevron signs at severe curves: Delineation at severe curve sections of highways has been an ongoing challenge for highway designers. Negotiating such curves at higher than recommended speeds often results in drivers losing control and being forced to take evasive actions. During the nighttime it becomes even more dangerous because drivers are constantly looking for visual cues to be able to choose the appropriate speed and path. The installation of chevron signs following the curvature of the highway provides drivers with the necessary cues to negotiate the curve without any hazardous incidents occurring.

Consistency of Highway Signage

Drivers' expectations are generally formed over time. As they encounter various highway situations and corresponding traffic control devices (including special delineation treatments), their expectations are reinforced. When drivers face such special circumstances in the future, they will expect similar or the same special delineation treatments. Thus consistency in treating similar situations with a consistent treatment is essential to preserve driver expectancies and maximize road user safety. Consistency of treatment leads to a safer and more efficient highway system.

HIGHWAY INFRASTRUCTURE

Highway infrastructure characteristics and their condition have a profound effect on safety. Although motorists drive on the part of the highway that is paved, the entire highway cross-section, including the shoulders, sidewalks, curbs, and guardrails, often influences vehicle operations directly or indirectly.

The design of each highway cross-section element depends on its intended use. Roadways with higher design volumes and speeds require more lanes, flatter grades, and gentler curves than those with lower volumes and slower design speeds. For the former type of facility, consideration also should be given to wider shoulders and medians, separate turning lanes, and control of access.

The highway cross-section is made up of elements that can be classified into three broad groups:

- The highway: Surface, width, cross slope, and number of travel lanes
- Road margins: Shoulders, sidewalks, curbs, guardrails, and ditches
- Traffic separators: The median and median barriers

The right-of-way is the width of land owned by a public agency (e.g., state, county, and city) for the sole purpose of providing the public highway, including the elements of road margin and the traffic separators.

The highway surfaces are classified into three general categories: high, intermediate, and low. The magnitude of traffic volume, the availability of the pavement materials, the cost, and the extent and cost of maintenance determine the category of roadway surface.

Because of high traffic volumes and a higher percentage of commercial vehicles, a smooth riding surface with good all-weather skid-resistant properties is required. The surface should be constructed to retain these qualities with a minimum of maintenance. A smooth surface of this kind offers little frictional resistance to the flow of surface water and may be designed with appropriate cross slopes. Conversely low-type rough surfaces must be crowned enough to drain the surface water.

The color of the pavements often influences traffic operations and safety. Light-colored pavements have better nighttime visibility than darker-colored pavements with either headlight or streetlight illumination. The lighter pavements generally have higher reflective qualities and also provide a better contrast for dark-colored obstacles or objects on the pavement surface.

The following components of the roadway cross-section are critical to safety design.

LANE WIDTHS

Lane widths have a significant influence on safety and driving comfort. Ten- to 12-foot lane widths are standard, and the tendency is to use the larger value with the continued upward trend in traffic volumes, vehicle speed, and widths of trucks. Lane widths narrower than 12 feet can adversely affect capacity. However, recent studies indicate that the wider the lane width, the higher the speed of travel. At higher speeds driver control deteriorates, and sometimes such high-speed travel leads to severe traffic accidents. Thus the designs that improve capacity may not be ideal for achieving safety.

CROSS SLOPES

All roads and highways have a high point in the middle and slope downward toward both sides to facilitate drainage. The downward cross slope may be a plane or curved section or a combination of both. Curved cross slopes usually are parabolic. On divided highways each one-way pavement may be crowned separately.

Because the majority of highways are on a tangent, the rate of cross slope is an important element in highway design. The cross slope rates should be as low as possible for comfortable vehicle operation; however, they must be sufficiently high for proper drainage. Where two or more lanes are inclined in the same direction on multilane pavements, each successive lane outward from the crown line should preferably have an increased slope. The lane adjacent to the crown line should be pitched at the normal minimum slope, and on each successive lane outward the rate should be increased by $\frac{1}{16}$ in/ft. Normal cross slopes vary from a minimum of $\frac{1}{8}$ in/ft on high-type pavement surfaces to $\frac{1}{4}$ in/ft for the low type of pavements.

SHOULDERS

Shoulders are provided to accommodate stopped vehicles for emergency use and for lateral support of the pavement. The type of highway, traffic volume, speed of traffic, traffic composition, and type of terrain determine the need for shoulders. Shoulders may vary from a minimum width of 4 feet to a desirable width of 12 feet for heavily traveled and high-speed roads.

An important element of shoulder design is its cross-section. Normally shoulders are sloped to drain water away from the pavement. Shoulders must be sloped sufficiently to remove surface water from the pavement; however, the slope should not be too steep as to create a hazard for motorists.

SIDEWALKS AND CURBS

In urban and suburban areas sidewalks are considered to be an integral part of the street system. However, sidewalks are needed for the safety of the pedestrian in many rural areas. Sidewalks are typically provided near schools, local businesses, industrial plants, and other areas where foot traffic is necessary. Recently many urban areas are promoting pedestrian-friendly communities called "walkable communities," where the sidewalks are wider and well landscaped and the roads are designed for lower speeds. Such designs also use narrower roadways, and consequently the motorists drive slower. The presence of pedestrians along such roads creates a sense of heightened risk among the drivers, which results in more cautious driving and thus creating a safer environment. See Chapter 22 for more information on urban planning and alternatives to driving.

Curbs are generally used in urban and suburban roads to control drainage, prevent vehicles from leaving the pavement, present an appearance of a limited driving space, and separate the vehicle path from the spaces that are commonly used by pedestrians. In rural areas many highways do not use a curb at the edge of pavements. There are two general types of curbs: barrier and mountable. Barrier curbs are relatively high and steep faced and are designed to prevent vehicles from leaving the pavement. They range from 6 to 12 inches in height. Barrier curbs that are used on bridges and around piers can be as high as 20 inches, and they often have two steps.

In urban and suburban roadways the curb height is kept between 6 and 8 inches. Recent explosion of the use of sports utility vehicles (SUVs) and pickup trucks in everyday life requires revisiting the basic definition of 6-inch curbs as barrier curbs. SUVs and pickup trucks have larger wheels and can easily mount a 6-inch curb. Mountable curbs have flat, sloping faces and are designed so that vehicles can ride over them without a jolt. Mountable curbs are used primarily on medians and urban freeway pavement edges with concrete shoulders.

DESIGN ELEMENTS OF ROADWAYS

There are various design elements for highways that impact safety and efficiency of traffic flow. These are mainly related to the design of the horizontal and vertical alignment of the roads. Some specific design elements addressed in the following section include superelevation at curves, circular curves, spiral easement curves, crest and sag vertical curves, and their relation to stopping and passing sight distances.

Horizontal Alignment

The horizontal alignment of a highway often consists of a series of tangent sections connected by circular curves. It is good practice to use transitional or spiral curves between tangents and circular curves. Alignment must be consistent; sudden changes from straight sections to sharp curves and long tangents followed by sharp curves must be avoided to reduce the likelihood of a driver going off the pavement surface. The compound, broken-back curves and reverse curves should not be used unless suitable transitions are provided between them. Long, small-degree curves are preferable at all times because they are pleasing in appearance and pose minimal hazard to motorists. In highway design all such geometric elements should be used as necessary to provide a safe, continuous operation at the desired speed. In the design of highway curves it is necessary to establish the proper relationship between the design speed and the curvature and their relationship to superelevation. These follow the laws of mechanics; however, the actual values used in highway design depend on practical limits and empirically determined factors.

Superelevation at Curves

Superelevation at curves is required to balance the tendency of vehicles to slide away from the center of the desired vehicle path or to overturn because of centrifugal force. Centrifugal force acts above the roadway surface through the center of gravity of a vehicle and creates an overturning movement about the points of contact between the outer wheels and the pavement. Opposing the overturning tendency of a vehicle in motion is the stabilizing moment created by the weight of the vehicle acting downward through the center of gravity. Overturning can occur only when the overturning moment exceeds the stabilizing moment. Modern passenger cars have low centers of gravity, and consequently the overturning moment is relatively small. As a result vehicles in this scenario will slide sidewise rather than overturn. Trucks and SUVs have higher centers of gravity and therefore create relatively large overturning moments, and they often overturn before they slide.

On a flat, circular curve the frictional force between the pavement and the tires allows a vehicle to resist sliding. When a curved section of a highway uses superelevation, the tendency of sliding and overturning can be completely eliminated if friction is negated by superelevating sufficiently so that the component of weight and the centrifugal force parallel to the roadway surface are equal. Figure 19-3 shows the relationship of forces when a vehicle travels through a superelevated curve.

To resist sliding and overturning (neglecting friction), W_h must equal C_h. Thus:

$$W \sin \theta = \frac{WV^2}{gR} \cos \theta$$

Dividing both sides by $W \cos \theta$ gives:

$$\tan \theta = \frac{V^2}{gR}$$

But $\tan \theta = e$, so:

$$e = \frac{V^2}{gR}$$

where:
W = Weight of vehicle, in pounds
θ = Angle of pavement slope
V = Speed of the vehicle, in ft/sec
e = Superelevation = tan θ
F = Side friction factor
F = fW cos θ, where f is the coefficient of friction
g = Acceleration caused by gravity, 32.2 ft/sec²
R = Radius of curve, in feet

Changing the unit of measurement for *V* from ft/sec to mph, the following equation can be obtained:

$$e = \frac{V^2}{15R}$$

When a vehicle travels at a speed greater than the speed at which the superelevation balances all centrifugal

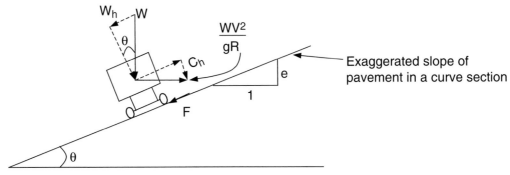

Figure 19-3 Various forces acting in a vehicle while traveling around a curve.

force, the additional balancing force that is necessary to keep the vehicle in the proper path must be generated from the friction. Considering friction and superelevation, the resistance to sliding and overturning can be calculated from the following equations:

$$e + f = \frac{V^2}{15R}$$

or

$$e = \frac{V^2}{15R} - f$$

Drivers become uncomfortable at higher values of side friction when slipping starts because it is difficult to keep the vehicle under control. AASHTO standards recommend side friction factors as shown in Table 19-2.

In a curved section of a highway, when a vehicle is traveling slower than the designated speed, the centrifugal force is reduced, and there is a tendency of the vehicle to slide toward the low point of the incline. For stationary vehicles there is no centrifugal force, and to prevent sliding down the incline, the coefficient of side friction must be equal to the superelevation. Because highways are used in all weather conditions, maximum superelevation must never exceed the minimum coefficient of friction during the worst weather conditions. Maximum superelevation recommended by AASHTO is 0.12 ft/ft. If snow and ice conditions prevail, this maximum is often reduced to 0.08 ft/ft. On icy surfaces the coefficient of side friction may be ≤0.05; therefore vehicle operators must take skid-prevention measures, or road maintenance crews must clear the icing condition on the pavement surface. In recent practice superelevation up to 0.16 ft/ft has proved satisfactory on freeway ramps at interchanges.

Circular Curves

Either the radius or the degree of curve describes circular curves. The degree of curve is the central angle subtended by a 100-foot length of curve. Degree of curve is inversely proportional to the radius, and their relationship is expressed as follows:

$$D = \frac{5729.58}{R}$$

where:
D = Degree of curve
R = Radius of curve, in feet

The standard design parameters for curvature are related to superelevation and side friction factors. The relationship for superelevation can be expressed in terms of the radius or the degree of curve by rearranging the equation for resistance t sliding and overturning, which gives

$$R = \frac{V^2}{15(e + f)}$$

Note that the resulting equation is the same equation as cited previously.

Substituting the value for R given above,

$$D = \frac{85,950(e + f)}{V^2}$$

For the maximum degree of curve allowed by AASHTO standards, superelevation and coefficient of side friction are set at the maximum values. For flatter curves the superelevation and side friction may be reduced. AASHTO standards make no specific recommendations in this regard, and current practice varies among agencies. Many agencies recommend that curves sharper than 1 degree should be superelevated.

Spiral Easement Curves

These curves are provided to form a smooth transition between a tangent and a curved section of a highway because no superelevation is required on tangents and full superelevation is required at a circular curve. The use of spiral easement curves ensures the safety of the vehicle and the comfort of its occupants at high operating speeds. This transition is often accomplished by the use of a spiral curve. The effect of the

---

Table 19-2 **Maximum Safe Side Friction Factors (where e = 0.12 ft/ft)**

Design speed (mph)	30	40	50	60	70	80
Maximum safe side friction factors	0.16	0.15	0.14	0.13	0.12	0.11

spiral easement curve is to gradually change the radius from infinity at the tangent section to the radius of the circular curve, so that the centrifugal force develops gradually when driving. By careful application of superelevation along the spiral, a gradual application of centrifugal force can be achieved.

The minimum length of easement curves recommended by AASHTO is

$$L_S = 1.6 \frac{V^3}{R}$$

where:

L_S = Length of easement curve, in feet
V = Speed, in mph
R = Radius of circular curve, in feet

Easement curves are not used for roadway sections of 1 degree and flatter circular curves. AASHTO standards for the interstate freeway system recommend that curves sharper than 2 degrees have spiral transitions. Easement curves should be used to separate reverse and compound curves (i.e., where degrees of curvature differ by >5 degrees).

Vertical Alignment

The longitudinal grade line is shown on a profile taken along the centerline of the highway that may consist of a series of straight lines connected by parabolic vertical curves. In establishing this grade line, road designers attempt to keep earthwork (i.e., cut and fill) to the minimum, consistent with meeting sight distance and other design requirements. In mountainous terrain the grade may be set to balance excavation against fill. In flat or level terrain the grade will be approximately parallel to the ground surface but sufficiently above it to allow surface drainage. In all conditions smooth, flowing grade lines should be the goal of the highway designer. When two grade lines have a difference of ≥0.5%, a vertical curve is used for proper transition.

Vertical curves are used to achieve gradual changes between tangent grades and any of the crest or sag curves shown in Figure 19-4. Vertical curves should be simple in application and should result in a design that is safe and comfortable for traffic operation, as well as allowing adequate drainage. The provision of sufficient sight distances for the design speed controls the design features. The vertical curves should be designed to provide adequate stopping sight distances. Wherever practical, more liberal stopping sight distances should be used. Additional sight distance should also be provided at decision points.

For driver comfort the rate of change of grade should be kept within tolerable limits. This consideration is critical in sag vertical curves in which gravita-

tional and vertical centripetal forces act in opposite directions. A long curve has a more pleasing appearance than a short one; short vertical curves may give the appearance of a sudden break in the profile.

Drainage of curbed roadways on sag vertical curves (type III in Figure 19-4) should retain a grade of not less than 0.5% or in some instances 0.30% percent for the outer edge of the roadway.

Crest Vertical Curves

The length of crest vertical curves based on sight distance criteria is satisfactory from the standpoint of safety, comfort, and appearance. An exception may be at decision areas, such as sight distance to ramp exit gores, where longer lengths are necessary.

Figure 19-5 illustrates the parameters used in determining the length of a parabolic crest vertical curve needed to provide adequate sight distance. The equations for calculating the length of a crest vertical curve in terms of algebraic difference in grade and sight distance are as follows:

When S is less than L,

$$L = \frac{|A|S^2}{200(\sqrt{h_1} + \sqrt{h_2})^2}$$

When S is greater than L,

$$L = 2S - \frac{200(\sqrt{h_1} + \sqrt{h_2})^2}{|A|}$$

where:

L = Length of vertical curve, in feet
S = Sight distance, in feet
A = Algebraic difference in grades, in percent
h_1 = Height of eye above roadway surface, in feet
h_2 = Height of object above roadway surface, in feet

When the eye height of the driver (3.5 feet) and the height of the object (2.0 feet) are used for calculating stopping sight distance, the equations become:

When S is less than L,

$$L = \frac{|A|S^2}{2158}$$

When S is greater than L,

$$L = 2S - \frac{2158}{|A|}$$

Design values of crest vertical curves for passing sight distance are different from those for stopping sight distance because of the different sight distance and object height criteria. The general equations for calculating the

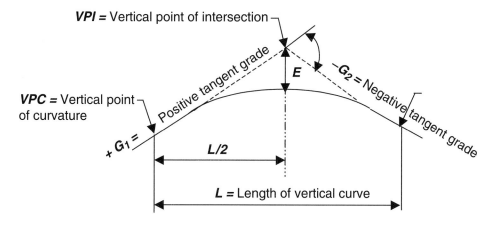

Type I

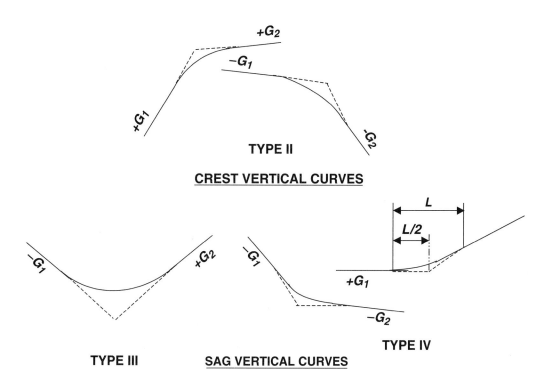

G_1 and G_2 = Tangent grades in percent

A = Algebraic difference in grade

L = Length of vertical curve

E = External distance from VPI to the middle of curve

Figure 19-4 Types of vertical curves.

Stopping Sight Distance

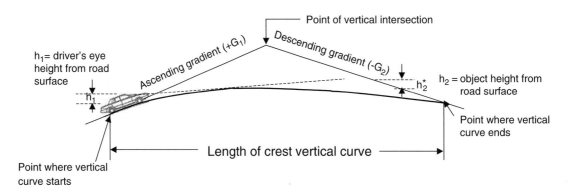

*h_2 represents the height of the object above road level

Passing Sight Distance

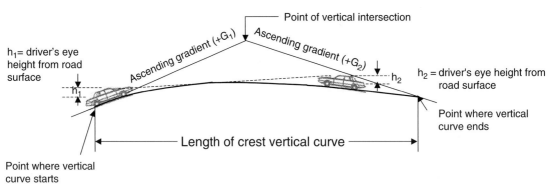

Here, one of the drivers is passing another driver in the vertical curve.

Figure 19-5   Parameters used in determining the length of a crest vertical curve for adequate sight distance.

length of a crest vertical curve are also used in calculating the passing sight distance; however, the drivers' eye height of 3.5 feet is used for both of the vehicles (see Figure 19-5).

When S is less than L,

$$L = \frac{|A|S^2}{2800}$$

When S is greater than L,

$$L = 2S - \frac{2800}{|A|}$$

The minimum passing sight distances for various design speeds are shown in Table 19-3.

Crest vertical curves generally are designed to provide adequate passing sight distance because of the high cost of cuts and difficulty of fitting the resulting long vertical curves to the terrain, particularly for high-speed roads. Ordinarily passing sight distance is provided only at locations where combinations of alignment and profile do not need the use of crest vertical curves.

Stopping Sight Distance. For general use in the design of a horizontal curve, the sight line is a chord of the curve, and the stopping sight distance is measured

Table 19-3 Design Controls for Crest Vertical Curves Based on Passing Sight Distance

Rate of Vertical Design Speed (mph)	Passing Sight Distance (ft)	Curvature, K* design
20	710	180
25	900	289
30	1090	424
35	1280	585
40	1470	772
45	1625	943
50	1835	1203
55	1985	1407
60	2135	1628
65	2285	1865
70	2480	2197
75	2580	2377
80	2680	2565

*Rate of vertical curvature, K, is the length of curve per percent algebraic difference in intersecting grades (A). K = L/A.

along the centerline of the inside lane around the curve.

The middle ordinate values are calculated from geometry for the several dimensions, as indicated in Figure 19-6 and in the following equation. The equation applies only to circular curves that are longer than the sight distance.

$$M = R\left(1 - \frac{\cos 28.65 S}{R}\right)$$

where:

S = Sight distance
R = Radius of the circular curve
M = Middle ordinate

In some instances retaining walls (e.g., concrete median barriers on the inside of curves) may cause sight obstructions and should be checked for stopping sight distance. When stopping sight distance is insufficient because a railing or a longitudinal barrier causes a sight obstruction, alternative designs should be considered

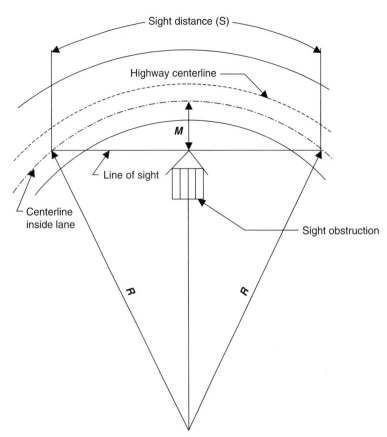

Figure 19-6 Various components for determining horizontal sight distance.

for safety. The alternatives are to (1) increase the offset to the obstruction; (2) increase the radius; or (3) reduce the design speed.

Passing Sight Distance. For two-lane roads the minimum passing sight distance is generally higher. To conform to those greater sight distance requirements, clear sight areas on the inside of curves should be provided. The previous equation is directly applicable to passing sight distance but is of limited practical value except on long curves.

Passing sight distance is measured between the eye heights of two drivers as 3.5 feet. For many cut sections, design for passing sight distance should only be limited to tangents and flat curves. Even in level terrain, provision of passing sight distance would need a clear area inside each curve that might extend beyond the normal right-of-way line. When passing sight distance is not available for geometric reasons, it should be posted as a no-passing zone.

Sag Vertical Curves. At least four different criteria for establishing lengths of sag vertical curves are used. They are (1) headlight sight distance, (2) passenger comfort, (3) drainage control, and (4) general appearance.

Headlight sight distances are used by some agencies, and AASHTO recommendations are based on this. When a vehicle traverses a sag vertical curve at night, the portion of highway lighted ahead depends on the position of the headlights and the direction of the light beam. A headlight height of 2 feet and a 1-degree upward divergence of the light beam from the longitudinal axis of the vehicle are commonly assumed. The upward spread of the light beam above the 1-degree divergence angle provides some additional visibility length of roadways. The following equations show the relationships between light beam distance (S), length of the vertical curve (L), and difference in grades (A) using S as the distance between the vehicle and point where the 1-degree upward angle of the light beam intersects the roadway surface:

When S is less than L,

$$L = \frac{|A|S^2}{200[2.0 + S(\tan \beta)]}$$

or

$$L = \frac{|A|S^2}{400 + 3.5S}$$

When S is greater than L,

$$L = 2S - \frac{200[2.0 + S(\tan \beta)]}{|A|}$$

or

$$L = 2S - \frac{400 + 3.5S}{|A|}$$

where:

L = Length of vertical curve, in feet
S = Light beam distance, in feet
A = Algebraic difference in grades, in percent
β = Beam angle, approximately 1 degree

For overall safety on highways, a sag vertical curve should be long enough that the light beam distance is nearly the same as the stopping sight distance. The effect on passenger comfort caused by the change in vertical direction of motion is higher on sag than on crest vertical curves because gravitational and centripetal forces are working in the opposite directions. Comfort caused by change in vertical direction is not readily measurable. Past attempts of such measurements have led to the conclusion that riding is comfortable on sag vertical curves when the centripetal acceleration is ≤1 ft/s². The general expression for such a criterion is:

$$L = \frac{|A| V^2}{46.5}$$

where:

L = Length of vertical curve, in feet
A = Algebraic difference in grades, in percent
V = Design speed, in mph

Considerations of all these issues are important for designing a highway environment to achieve safety.

TRAFFIC CONTROL DEVICES

Traffic control devices are a part of the highway infrastructure and assist drivers in understanding the driving environment for safe and efficient operation. Their purpose is to ensure highway safety by providing for orderly and predictable movement of all road users through the highway infrastructure. Traffic control devices include traffic signs, pavement markings, and traffic signals. To be effective a traffic control device must fulfill a need, command attention, convey a clear and simple message, command the respect of road users, and give adequate time for proper interpretation and response.

To ensure that traffic control devices, when applied, follow the noted criteria, a national committee under the leadership of the Federal Highway Administration (FHWA), U.S. Department of Transportation (DOT) produces the Manual of Uniform Traffic Control Devices (MUTCD).[2] It recommends that engineers consider the following five factors:

- Design: The traffic control device should be designed with a combination of size, color, and shape that will convey a clear message and command the respect and attention of the driver.
- Placement: The device should be located within the cone of vision of the driver and must be seen at a time that provides an adequate response time at a normal speed of travel.
- Operation: The device should be used in a consistent and uniform manner.
- Maintenance: The device must be regularly maintained to ensure that the legibility and reflectivity are maintained.
- Uniformity: To facilitate the recognition and understanding of traffic control devices by drivers, similar devices should be used at locations with similar traffic and geometric characteristics.

In addition to these considerations, engineers must avoid using control devices that conflict with one another. It is imperative that the traffic control devices complement each other in transmitting the required message to the driver.

TRAFFIC SIGNS

The functions of traffic signs are to provide regulations, warnings, and guidance information to all road users. Signs are classified into three broad categories: (1) regulatory signs, (2) warning signs, and (3) guide signs.

Regulatory signs are used to inform drivers of traffic laws and regulations at specific roadway locations (e.g., intersections). Road users must observe such signs because failure to do so can lead to a traffic citation. Some examples of regulatory signs include stop signs, speed limit signs, no turn on red signs, and no parking signs. Warning signs call attention to conditions on or adjacent to a highway or street that require caution on the part of the driver. They are essential at locations identified to have hidden or visible hazards. Guide signs show route designations, directions, distances, services, and points of interest, as well as provide other geographic, recreational, or cultural information.

Traffic signs typically are passive control devices, with the exception of changeable message signs (CMSs). Even with CMSs the message generally remains constant for a reasonable period to allow motorists to comprehend and take necessary actions. Therefore signs are permanent devices, presenting permanent messages until taken down or replaced.

It is desirable to establish an order of priority for sign installation. This is especially critical where space is limited and when there is a demand for several different signs. Overloading motorists with too much information can cause improper driver actions and impact safety. Some information is more important than others. Regulatory and warning signs whose locations generally are critical should be displayed first rather than the guide signs. Less important information and supplementary information should be moved to less critical locations or deleted.

A highway traffic sign must be legible to all drivers so that it can be understood in time to permit a proper response. This requires high visibility, lettering or symbols of adequate size, and a short legend for instant recognition and quick comprehension by a driver approaching a sign at a high speed. Standard colors and shapes are essential so that the various groups of traffic signs are promptly recognized. Simplicity and uniformity in design, placement, and application are essential to achieve efficiency and safety in traffic operations.

Design

Uniformity in design includes shape, color, dimensions, legends, and illumination or reflectorization. MUTCD contains many typical standard signs approved for use on streets and highways. Design details of these and other approved signs are available to state and local highway and traffic agencies, sign manufacturers, and the FHWA. Most standard symbols are oriented facing left; however, this does not preclude the use of mirror images of these symbols where the reverse orientation may better convey the required message to the driver. Standardization of these designs does not preclude further improvement by minor changes in the proportion of symbols, width of borders, or layout of word messages, but all shapes and colors must follow the standards included in the MUTCD.

Standard sign shapes include rectangles, octagons, triangles, diamonds, and circles. Sign shapes are typically reserved for specific signs, such as the octagon for a stop sign, an equilateral triangle with one point downward for yield signs, a round shape for advance warning of a railroad crossing, a diamond shape for warning signs, a rectangle ordinarily with the longer dimension vertical for most regulatory signs, and a rectangle ordinarily with the longer dimension horizontal for guide signs. Other shapes are reserved for special purposes, such as the shield type of signs that are used for highway routes and the crossbuck used for railroad crossings.

Specific colors are used on signs to portray certain meanings. For example white and red are used for stop signs. Red is also used in multiway supplemental plates, "do not enter" messages, and wrong way signs. Red is also used as a legend color for yield signs, parking prohibition signs, and the circular outline and diagonal bar prohibitory symbol. Black and white are used on one-way signs, certain weigh station signs, and night speed limit signs as specified in MUTCD. Black is used as a message on white, yellow, and orange background. White is used as the background for route markers, guide signs, and regulatory signs, except stop signs, and for the legend on brown, green, blue, black, and red signs. Orange is used as a background color for construction and maintenance signs and must not be used for any other signs. Yellow is used as a background color for warning signs. Brown is used as a background color for guide and information signs related to points of recreational or cultural interest. Green is used as a background color for guide signs and mileposts. Blue is used as a background color for information signs related to motorist services.

Standard wordings must be used for signs. Word messages are typically brief with letterings that are large enough to provide the necessary legibility distance. Proper sign lettering is in uppercase letters based on standard approved alphabets. The designated alphabet has relatively wide spacing between letters, which improves legibility.

Signs generally are located on the right side of the roadway, where the driver is used to looking for them. In certain instances overhead signs are provided on wide expressways or where space is not available at the roadside. Signs located any other place are considered to be supplementary signs, such as on median islands and on the left shoulder of the road. Signs should be located so that they do not obscure each other and are not hidden from view by other roadside elements, parked vehicles, and trees. Signs requiring different action by the driver must be spaced far enough apart for the required decisions to be made safely. Spacing should be determined in units of time as determined by the expected vehicle approach speed.

Examples of standard sign placements for some typical signs are shown in Figure 19-7.

PAVEMENT MARKINGS

Pavement markings include all lines, patterns, and words used on the pavement to regulate, warn, guide, and help to ensure safety for the motorist. They are used to control the lateral position of vehicles on the roadway and to delineate the pavement edge and obstructions near or adjacent to the pavement. Pavement markings have specific functions in the roadway network. They are used to supplement regulatory or warning signs and to easily convey regulations, warnings, and information without diverting the driver's attention from the roadway. Pavement markings

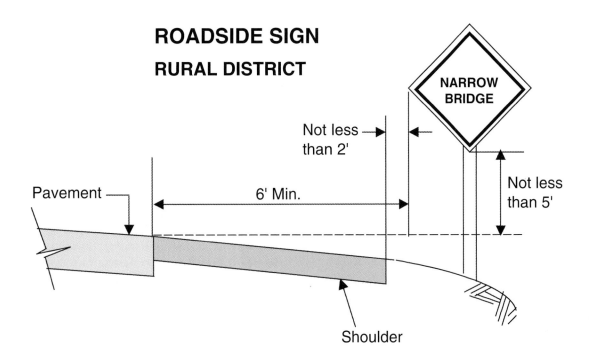

ROADSIDE SIGN
RURAL DISTRICT

NARROW BRIDGE

Pavement

Not less than 2'

6' Min.

Not less than 5'

Shoulder

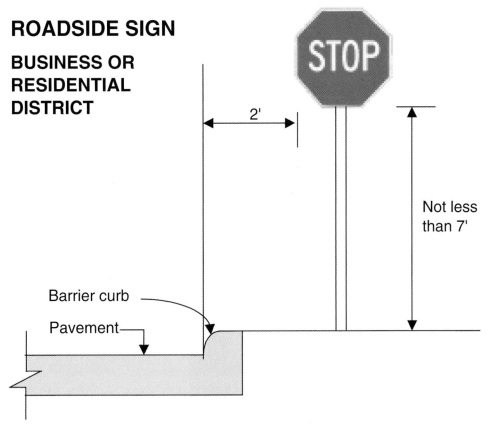

ROADSIDE SIGN
BUSINESS OR RESIDENTIAL DISTRICT

STOP

2'

Not less than 7'

Barrier curb

Pavement

Figure 19-7 Standard sign placements for some typical signs.

must be recognizable and understandable. To achieve this, a uniform system of markings is used on the roadways. Motorists should encounter the same type of markings wherever they travel; these markings should convey the same meaning regardless of the environment in which they are installed.

The visibility of pavement markings may be sensitive to weather and road conditions. For example they may be entirely covered by snow or are not clearly visible when wet or partially covered by dirt or oil. As a result pavement markings require routine maintenance and replacement to ensure their effectiveness.

Pavement markings consist of three colors (i.e., yellow, white, and red), and each color has specific meanings. The MUTCD specifies the use of yellow to separate opposing directions of traffic, white to separate flows in the same direction, and red to delineate a roadway as out of bounds by the motorists. Black pavement markings may also be used as an outline for white pavement markings on light pavements to increase the contrast.

The type of line being solid or broken also has specific meaning, especially in combination with the marking colors. A broken line generally is permissive in character and may be crossed at the discretion of the driver. Solid lines are restrictive in character and may not be crossed. For example the centerlines on two-lane highways consist of a broken yellow line where passing is permitted and a solid yellow line where it is prohibited. When passing in only one direction is permitted, a solid yellow line and a broken yellow line (on the side where passing is permitted) are used. A solid white line indicates a line separating traffic in the same direction and shall not be crossed (e.g., the solid white lines used for exclusive turn lanes).

The width of a line generally indicates emphasis of the desired message. A normal width longitudinal pavement marking is from 4 to 6 inches wide. Double lines consist of two normal width lines separated by a recognizable gap. Line segments and gaps, usually in the ratio of 3:5, form broken lines. On rural highways the length of each line segment is 15 feet with a gap of 25 feet.

Longitudinal pavement markings are intended for specific uses, including the separation of traffic flows in the opposing directions, the separation of traffic flows in the same direction, and the delineation of roadways that are not to be used. The following examples illustrate the use of longitudinal pavement markings as stated in the MUTCD. A normal broken white line is most commonly used to delineate lane lines of a multi-lane roadway. A normal broken yellow line is most commonly used to delineate a centerline of a two-lane, two-way roadway where passing is permitted. A normal solid white line is most often used to delineate left- or right-turn lanes at intersections where lane changing is

not permitted. A double line consisting of a normal broken yellow line and a normal solid yellow line indicates a separation between the traffic flows in the opposite directions where passing with care is permitted for traffic adjacent to the broken line and is prohibited for traffic adjacent to the solid line (one-direction no-passing marking). A double solid yellow line delineates the separation between travel paths in opposite directions where passing is prohibited in both directions of travel. A solid yellow line delineates the left edge of a travel path.

Traverse markings are typically white and include shoulder markings, word and symbol markings, stop lines, crosswalk lines, and parking space markings. Traverse median markings are yellow. Markings visible only to traffic proceeding in the wrong direction on a one-way street may be red. Examples of common pavement markings used in delineation are shown in Figure 19-8.

Because of the shallow viewing angle, it is necessary that transverse lines be proportioned to give visibility equal to that of longitudinal lines. Pavement marking letters, numerals, and symbols are consistent, and standards included in MUTCD must be followed.

TRAFFIC SIGNALS

All power-operated devices (except signs) for regulating, directing, or warning motorists or pedestrians are called *traffic signals*. When traffic signals are installed at locations where warranted, they provide temporal separation between the conflicting traffic movements and can provide safe and efficient traffic movement.

Traffic signals offer the most positive form of control of all traffic control devices. A traffic signal relays a message to the motorists of what to do (i.e., stop or go) at an intersection. Signals are useful in providing relief to congested situations where no other control device is adequate. The alternating assignment of right-of-way to specific directions of travel can eliminate most, or all, conflicting movements in the intersection area. By alternately assigning right-of-way to various traffic movements, signals provide for orderly movement of heavy or conflicting flows. They often interrupt the major direction of traffic flow to permit the crossing of minor movements that otherwise could not have moved safely through an intersection.

Traffic signal indications are red, yellow, and green and may have circular or arrow signals, and each has specific meanings. A green signal indication informs motorists to proceed through the intersection. A yellow signal indication warns motorists that the green signal is being terminated and that a red indication will be displayed immediately thereafter. A red signal indication instructs motorists to stop at a clearly marked stop line

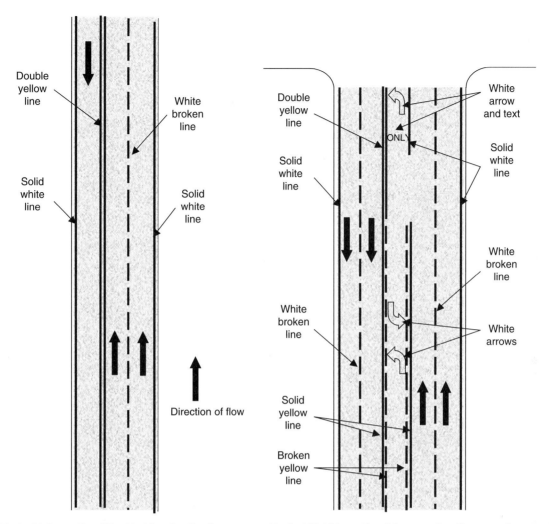

Typical 3-Lane, Two-Way Marking Application   Typical Multi-Lane Road Segment Leading to an Intersection

Figure 19-8 Examples of common pavement markings used in delineation.

(or before entering the intersection if a stop line is not provided) and to remain stopped until an indication to proceed is displayed through a green signal.

Proper design and use of signs, pavement markings, and traffic signals are an essential part of highway infrastructure design. In many instances designing and installing a well-designed traffic control system can alleviate hazards caused by minor geometric deficiencies.

SUMMARY

Understanding the basic principles of design for highway infrastructure, traffic control, and human behavioral characteristics is essential for developing and practicing a successful driver rehabilitation and com-

munity mobility program. Basic driver training programs rely on only minimal knowledge and some practice before the participants are considered eligible and worthy of receiving driving permits. However, the candidates for a driver rehabilitation program need extensive background knowledge to influence their decision-making processes. Unfortunately physical or psychosocial challenges experienced by some driver rehabilitation candidates must be provided with remedial training to the extent that safe driver action becomes a natural reaction to the external stimuli provided by the dynamic driving environment.

The highway environmental issues are critical for safe driving. Understanding the relationship between the highway, driver, and vehicle is crucial to appreciate the myriad of tasks associated with driving, especially for drivers who may experience temporary or permanent physical, cognitive, or psychosocial impairments.

BOX 19-2	Key Good Driving Practices

- Drive at or slightly under the posted speed limit, provided the environmental, highway, and traffic conditions permit.
- Maintaining a safe distance with the lead vehicle is essential to avoid accidents.
- Operate a vehicle that is in good condition, especially the brakes, traction devices, and antilock brake systems.
- Be mindful of the environment, including vehicles in front and on the sides.
- Observe all traffic control devices.
- Observe all driving rules and regulations.
- Know the capability of one's vehicle, and select a safe speed and path accordingly.

For safe travel many elements are needed, including a well-designed highway, a vehicle in reasonably good condition, and a driver who is well trained and knowledgeable of the negative consequences of violating elements of good driving practices. Box 19-2 lists some of the key good driving practices.

DRSs working within a driver rehabilitation program must consider the highway design issues, such as horizontal and vertical alignments, sight distance, shoulders and curbs, and traffic control devices to provide effective driver rehabilitation evaluations and training. They must also consider driver issues such as human factors and limitations and deficiencies, which often lead to traffic accidents and injuries. To design and provide effective driver rehabilitation and community mobility services, it is essential to use the materials presented in this chapter and, if necessary, to refer to other resources.

REFERENCES

1. American Association of State Highway and Transportation Officials: *A policy on geometric design of highways and streets*, ed 4, Washington, DC, 2001, AASHTO.
2. Federal Highway Administration. *Manual on Uniform Traffic Control Devices for Streets and Highways*, 2003 Edition. US Department of Transportation, Washington, D.C., 2003.
3. Pignataro LJ: *Traffic Engineering Theory and Practice.* Prentice-Hall, Inc., Englewood Cliffs, New Jersey, 1973.
4. Post TJ, Robertson HD, Price HE: *A Users' Guide to Positive Guidance*. Publication DOT-FH-11-8864. FHWA, U.S. Department of Transportation, 1977.

Chapter 20

DRIVER REHABILITATION FOR RECREATION AND LEISURE

Bethany Broadwell • Susan Popek-Boeve

KEY TERMS

- **Adaptations**
- **Recreational activities**
- **Leisure pursuits**
- **Flow**

CHAPTER OBJECTIVES

After completing this chapter, the reader will be able to do the following:

- **Understand how adaptations made to vehicles used to engage in recreational activities can enhance a person's quality of life.**
- **Know the range of vehicles to which adaptations could be made.**
- **Know what types of adaptations can be made to enhance motor vehicle usability.**

In the rehabilitation process professional caregivers strive to assist individuals with disabilities or aging-related challenges to discover their innate and fundamental ability to push to excel in the midst of what are often monumental challenges. A period of reflection and self-evaluation often follows the initial shock and grieving process most individuals experience after experiencing a traumatic injury or confronting a serious health condition. "What am I going to do with the rest of my life?" "What can I do independently?" "What goals should I set for myself?" These questions naturally reflect concerns about activities of daily living

(ADL), returning to home, work, or school and avocational issues such as changes in socialization, recreation, and leisure. Ultimately the aim of rehabilitation is to support individuals in their quest to develop a renewed sense of self-efficacy in the management of all of their occupational pursuits, whether work oriented or leisure based. This chapter focuses specifically on leisure time occupations and the *adaptations* available for the range of vehicles used to engage in *recreational activities* and *leisure pursuits.*

The Latin translation of leisure (*licere*) is literally "to be free." The Latin translation of recreation (*recreatie*) is "to refresh or restore." Freedom, refreshment, and restoration are all requisite components for experiencing a satisfying lifestyle. Adaptations that allow individuals with physical disabilities to drive recreational vehicles have opened up a new avenue of restoration after injury. Importantly these modifications allow the person with a disability to experience freedom not only as a passenger but also by driving a vehicle for practical purposes and recreation.

Driving adaptations for recreational vehicles, including race cars, all-terrain vehicles (ATVs), recreational vehicles (RVs), sleds, golf carts, boats, and airplanes, offer individuals with disabilities or aging-related concerns an opportunity to experience true *flow*. According to Csikszentmih, flow occurs when an individual has a loss of ego and self-consciousness, engages in self-forgetfulness and transcendence of individuality, while simultaneously retaining control of his or her actions and of the environment.[1] Taking the wheel, whether driving a motor vehicle on a Sunday afternoon, flying over the clouds at hundreds of miles per hour, or racing on a sunny day, provides individuals with opportunities to begin the true rehabilitation of experiencing life to its fullest.

ADAPTED RACE CARS

Technologic developments in this specialized field of sport driving can benefit driver rehabilitation efforts in competitive and noncompetitive contexts. The case of Ray Paprota of Birmingham, Alabama illustrates the nearly infinite possibilities of driver rehabilitation, specifically in the area of automotive racing, by using specially adapted vehicles and equipment. Paprota sustained a complete spinal cord injury at the T10 level while driving behind the wheel of what he called "a sweet black and red Z/28." The accident occurred 1 week before his twenty-second birthday in May 1984. Today the owner/driver of Pioneer Racing Incorporated holds the distinction of being the first person with paraplegia to compete in a National Association for Stock Car Auto Racing (NASCAR) touring event.[2] Evolving into a race car driver is an experience that Paprota described as an almost natural progression. He and his two younger brothers had always been competitive; after Paprota's injury he reported that it was difficult convincing racing officials that he could still compete despite his disability. Eventually he did return to racing. "It is incredibly satisfying to hop from my wheelchair into my race car and become just another race car driver," Paprota said. He considers himself fortunate that the Rehabilitation Center in New Jersey encouraged him to drive as soon as possible after his injury. Now he is able to take cars around the track in excess of 170 mph as a professional race car driver, but it took determination and perseverance to reach his goal.

For 2 years after becoming interested in racing, Paprota and his team struggled to design hand controls that NASCAR would approve. "NASCAR is big business and they tend to move slow and resist change," he said. "We were doing something no one had ever attempted to do before and they just wanted to test our tenacity and be sure we were for real. In racing, nothing is handed to you. You earn every inch of racetrack," Paprota added. "It takes that same spirit to transition successfully from a hospital bed to a productive life with a spinal cord injury."[2]

To compete in the NASCAR Dash Series, racers drive mid-sized stock cars. They are hand-built, tube-framed race cars with handmade steel bodies strictly for racing. Paprota's team races a Mercury Cougar on the short tracks and a Pontiac Sunfire, which is more aerodynamic, on the super speedways. His everyday vehicle now is a 2003 Dakota pickup truck. He also drives a 1993 General Motors Corporation Typhoon with all-wheel drive and a 600-horsepower turbo-charged engine, a 1993 Ford Mustang, and a few Legends Series race cars. He uses off-the-shelf, right-angle hand controls to adapt his vehicles for driving and maneuverability.

Paprota's suggestion for others with disabilities who want to get involved with racing or hot rods is to first network with people in the sport. "The street scene is cool because all you need is a nice Friday or Saturday night and a big parking lot; the cars just start to multiply. Park one rod and before you know it you have a hangout." Racing takes more work, requiring trips to a local short track or drag strip, getting a pit pass, and exploring the scene. Paprota states that he wants to continue to make it easier to transition from driving to racing. "I would like to be an owner and groom a young kid with a disability from a go-cart to a Cup car."[2]

ADAPTED MOTORCYCLES

Millions of people own motorcycles and prefer the experience of traveling in an open-air vehicle. Adapted motorcycles are becoming more commonplace throughout the world and afford individuals with disabilities the opportunity to pursue this adventurous recreational experience.

Ron Uesseler, President and owner of Ecstasy Cycles Corporation in Jeffersonville, Indiana, believes the company he has headed since 1997 meets the needs of customers with disabilities better than any other company, making three-wheeled motorcycles ("trikes") accessible for people with disabilities. According to Uesseler the most frequently requested item for motorcycles has been the relocation of the rear brake pedal for those with a weak or missing right leg. Uesseler stated: "As more people are finding out how well these units can be matched to special needs, there has been a significant widening to the scope and frequency of alterations we are making."[3]

Currently a number of adaptations are available for motorcycles (Box 20-1).

BOX 20-1	Adaptations Available for Motorcycles

Lowered running boards for easier mounting
Push-button shifting for automatic transmission
Power-assisted brakes
Handlebars with front and rear hand brake controls
Special seat belts
Flip-up armrests
Special seating
Mounts for wheelchairs
Relocation of the shifter and parking brake
Lowered center console
Relocation of foot brake
Front throttle to supplement the hand throttle

ALL-TERRAIN VEHICLES

Some people with disabilities may prefer driver rehabilitation that also includes working on developing skills necessary to use ATVs rather than stay within the confines of staying within city streets and highways. Todd Macke, age 31 years, of Decatur, Illinois is convinced that learning to drive an ATV helped him develop coordination and to better contend with being diagnosed with cerebral palsy that affects his legs, hands, and speech. Driving ATVs gives people with disabilities "a stable machine that can go through or over any terrain, thus giving them an opportunity to explore areas they might not be able to go on foot or wheelchair."[4] Macke learned fundamental ATV riding skills on a 1980 Honda ATC70 three-wheeler that had a top speed of approximately 30 mph. He explained, "Before my father turned me loose on my first ride, he showed me how to make the ATC70 go, but he also showed me what made it stop, which is the most important part."[4] As he gained experience he began racing in monster truck shows. "Riding in competition events got my fuels burning for more," Macke said, "because I was actually able to compete against people without disabilities and be competitive with them."[4] Macke participated in national races across the country and was interviewed and filmed with the 1986 Honda TRX250R for an ATV movie, "Air Force." He went on to win a Triple Crown National Championship in 1998 for the 250D class.

Learning to straddle the seat, sit up straight, control the throttle with his thumb, and navigate turns by leaning to one side to avoid falling off were all challenges when Macke originally began riding approximately 25 years ago. Macke has his sights set on future goals revolving around ATVs. To give others with disabilities the thrill of riding, the ATV enthusiast said he would like to open a school with their needs in mind. His mission would be "to explore ATVs as an option to enhance their life and coordination skills, to help them enjoy the outdoors and guide them to push themselves to try something new and exciting."[4]

Box 20-2 lists a variety of ATVs available.

RECREATIONAL VEHICLES

Accessible RVs (i.e., motor homes) provide individuals with disabilities an opportunity to travel long distances with many of the comforts of home. "Traveling in a motor home helps to ease anxieties brought on by certain unknown elements that can make travel unpleasant," stated Sheila Davis, spokesperson for Winnebago Industries, headquartered in Forest City, Iowa.[5] The vehicle, she pointed out, can actually make life easier

BOX 20-2	Available All-Terrain Vehicles

Honda ACT110 (three-wheeler)
Honda ATC250 SX (three-wheeler)
Yamaha Banshee YF350 (four-wheeler)
Suzuki QuadRacer 250 (four-wheeler)
Honda TRX250R (four-wheeler)
Honda TRX500R (four-wheeler)
Honda 400EX (race quad)
2004 Yamaha YFZ450 (race quad)
2004 Honda TRX450R (race quad)

than traveling by car or airplane and staying in hotels because people can be assured of details like whether the bathroom is accessible or the hallways are wide enough for maneuvering. "An accessible motor home allows you to take everything you need with you instead of having to pack and repack a suitcase each day," Davis added. "A motor home provides the opportunity literally to take your home and all its familiar comforts with you wherever you go."[5]

Two common adaptations that Winnebago Industries can install for persons with disabilities are hand-operated driving controls and a power seat base for the driver cab seat to assist with transfers in and out of the driving position.[5] A reduced-effort steering control is another adaptation mentioned by Bob Helvie, owner of Starship Custom Vehicles in northern Indiana. "For the most part, we design the complete vehicle to meet our client's requirements."[6]

Bathrooms can be made accessible by raising the height of the toilet or repositioning the toilet for easier transfers and adding assist bars in strategic locations. Some may find a roll-in style shower with a flat floor helpful, combined with a shower chair or bench. An adjustable-height showerhead, assist bars, and a single-control faucet are other available shower options.[5] A "roll-under"-style lavatory sink with a single-control faucet and lowered mirror or cabinet can assist with personal grooming. Adjustable beds can be installed in the RV, as well as equipment to facilitate easier transfers. Wardrobe closets can be made with a lowered garment rod and door pulls to assist with grasp. Easy-care vinyl flooring works well in high-traffic areas. Kitchen cabinets are another feature that can be lowered or modified to provide clearance for a person using a wheelchair or scooter.

Keith and Cathy Dewald of AuGres, Michigan purchased a 2004 model year Sightseer Winnebago 33' in September 2003. Keith has a spinal cord injury at the C6/7 level and a tracheotomy as a result of a March 2000, work-related accident. "Since my husband's accident 4 years ago, we had been unable to do any overnight expeditions until we purchased our RV," said Cathy. "The RV allows us accessibility to all supplies, clothes, food, (and) equipment that is needed. Our purchase was not based on the premise that we wanted to go camping, but that we wanted to be able to travel again."[7] In addition to trips close to home, the couple, with the assistance of a care attendant, took 1 month to travel from Michigan to Las Vegas and back.

Some of the Winnebago's features may need modifying after receipt of the RV, but the accessibility issues have for the most part been resolved, Cathy explained. Significant planning and discussions about Winnebago's Ability Equipped vehicles took place during the customization process. According to Davis, "Most customers who purchase a Winnebago Industries Ability Equipped motor home will choose to have the majority of the adaptations for their motor home completed here at the factory, though the order for the motor home is always placed through an authorized Winnebago Industries dealer. Nearly all of our motor homes can be adapted for people with disabilities."[5] As an additional customer service, she said, some dealerships offer courses in motor home driving skills. In the early stages of purchasing an RV, however, learning the fundamentals is important. Davis suggested, "Gathering useful information regarding the motor home lifestyle is a good start."

GOLF CARTS

The Model Tee single-riding golf cart was developed by USA Golf Products, Inc. and according to the inventor, Patrick Yates, is based on years of researching the needs and potential solutions for golfers with disabilities.[8] For safety and security the golf cart has a wide and long wheel base. Its mechanical power steering makes it possible for people to operate with one hand. Drivers can flip a selector switch to activate the right or left throttle for use with the dominant hand. The electromagnetic brake is released when the throttle is applied. Golfers can carry their golf bag on the right or left side for low center of gravity, easy-to-reach clubs, and visibility. The seat rotates 360 degrees, locks in 35 positions, and has a rotating function during the swing. A footrest also rotates with the seat; therefore people with paralysis do not have to lift and drag their legs. A locking handle for the seat rotation can be put in the open position until the player is ready to address the ball. A special spring suspension gives a smooth ride for medium and heavier bumps. Four-belt systems are available to players who need upper body support. Storage is substantial, too, with places under the seat, two pockets on the firewall, two cup holders, two ball holders, and dashboard space for eight golf tees.

SoloRider Management LLC also offers an adapted single-rider golf cart called the AteeA. The developers' goal with this model was to create a drive system with emphasis on safety.[9] The car has a ground clearance that enables it to navigate 6-inch curbs and other barriers without high centering. It has hand controls for braking and acceleration that can be operated by either the left or right hand. "The car is designed to allow easy access to controls, clubs, and assistance devices such as canes or crutches," said Tom Durbin, Vice President of Sales. The AteeA's soft automotive suspension system provides a cushioned ride. Its seat swivels 360 degrees to allow golfers to make their swing and to have easy accessibility. The seat can position people with paralysis in a standing stance for golfing. The car has transfer bars, chest belts, and seat belts. All of these features are standard on the vehicle.

The Model Tee and the AteeA are designed to have the appearance of an ordinary golf cart that would appeal to any golfer. They are also built to preserve the golf course landscape. "Single-rider golf carts are part of creating accessibility, and golf course owners and operators are beginning to recognize their responsibilities and are investigating the issues," said Durbin. He also stated: "Some golf courses are acquiring single-rider golf carts and creating access to their physical golf facilities. There is more progress every day."[9]

NONMOTORIZED SNOW SLEDS

The Arctic Shark, designed by Robert Gibbons, President of Gibbons Fiberglass & Aluminum Boat Repair in Bismarck, North Dakota, is a nonmotorized sled designed for individuals with disabilities. Gibbons modified a Polk sled, including adding skis with a concave edge to grip the snow. He built on a cockpit, a roll bar, and a bumper. A windshield, additional foot room, a taller roll bar, and improved braking were also eventually added. A guide may stand behind the Arctic Shark rider to apply the brakes if assistance is needed. A double-sled version of the Arctic Shark is also available that allows the guide to sit next to the rider. Both passengers then have steering and brake controls. The sled is capable of reaching speeds as fast as 100 mph. The Arctic Shark has been tested and operated extensively by participants in the Rapid City, South Dakota Ski for Light program.

BOATS

Combining the great outdoors with relaxation and water are all components of sailing and boating. With new adaptive designs that allow not only for access to the boats but also opportunities to skipper and drive, an individual with a disability may choose to be either captain or a passenger on the open water. These adaptations allow for experts and novices alike to own or rent an adapted boat. There are a number of recreational therapy and community programs designed to teach individuals with disabilities how to sail, race, or improve their watercraft skills. Sailing is an activity that can be done for pure pleasure or the thrill of competition, and the opportunities continue to grow. Sailing moved quickly from a demonstration sport at the 1996 Atlanta Paralympics to a medal sport at the 2000 Sydney Paralympics.

Sailing for individuals with disabilities is becoming more common and more accessible in many countries throughout the world. Organizations such as the International Handicap Sailing Committee (IHSC), the U.S. Sailing Association/Sailors with Special Needs Committee, and the International Foundation for Disabled Sailors are just a few of the resources available for those interested in participating.

Adaptive Adventures is an organization that works with a variety of adaptive organizations around the United States and touts the motto, "Sailing is a metaphor for the celebration of life." Their effort is to help ensure that opportunities exist for people with disabilities to sail safely while experiencing "adventure and freedom-building mobility, self-confidence, and pride through achievement."[10] One program that provides opportunities for adaptive sailing across the United States is the Broad Reach Adaptive Sailing Program. The mission of this program is "to provide the environment, instruction, and support for individuals with special needs to experience the thrills of sailing."[10] Box 20-3 lists some of the equipment available to boating enthusiasts.

PLANES

Helen Keller, who overcame blindness, deafness, and an early inability to speak or communicate, once

---

BOX 20-3	**Equipment for Sailing**

ACCESS DINGHIES
Using a dinghy is an excellent way to begin sailing. The access dinghy is available in two sizes. The Access 2.3 is 2.3 m long, 1.2 m wide, weighs 36 to 48 kg, and has a 15-kg ballasting centerboard, depending on the particular configuration. Lifts for marine vessels, including powerboats, sailboats, fishing boats, and private boats, are difficult to capsize. They can be steered with a joystick and can be outfitted with electric servo-line controls. The Access 3.0 is a newer model and features a similar hull design but is longer and boasts greater stability. It can be sailed with the main sail alone by one person or with the main sail and jib by two people.

FREEDOM INDEPENDENCE
The Freedom 20, built by Catalina Yachts, features the unique Freedom unstayed mast system. At 20'6" it is one of the larger boats used for adaptive sailing. The Independence cockpit is equipped with two pivoting seats for helmsmen and one crew person. The specially designed seats are counterweighted beneath the cockpit. Two wheelchairs may be accommodated in the cabin, and there is adequate room for sails and gear.

MARTIN 16: AN "ACCESSIBLE KEELBOAT"
Built for recreation and racing, the Martin 16 may be sailed solo or with a passenger.
  Martin Yachts states: "The stability of the keep makes it a very safe boat for people with severe disabilities. The high lift keel makes trailer launching simple from any ramp and can be easily rigged and sailed by one person. Stability and adjustable seating, as well as specialized control

systems, make the Martin 16 ideal for sailors with mobility impairments. The Martin 16 offers optional automated systems for steering, sail sheeting, and the bilge pumping."

RACING BOATS
The Norlin Mark III is a racing boat. The 2.4-m class is a widely raced one-design keelboat, especially popular in Europe. It is stable and easily controlled. Norlin's version of the 2.4 sailed in the single-handed class at the 2000 Paralympics in Sydney. It is a small boat, just 13.8 feet, with a beam (i.e., width) of 2'8" and a draft of 3'3" (i.e., how much of the boat is under water).

BOAT RAMPS
Motorboats, speedboats, and pontoon boats are usually driven using one or two hands. Just as adapted driving controls have enabled people with disabilities to drive cars and trucks, hand controls on boats can now be tailored to meet individual needs, making a variety of boats accessible as well.[11] However, before an individual can drive a boat, access to the boat is necessary. Boat ramps that allow easy access are becoming more common at state parks throughout the United States. Adapted Engineering Ltd. produces a variety of wheelchair-accessible yachts. This company has designed the Mobilift, which has an adjustable lifting height, which can be important especially for areas affected by tides and undetermined bridging distances. Other options include nonslip metal docks with multiple landings that allow boaters with disabilities and others to easily board their boats regardless of the level of the tide.

observed, "One can never consent to creep when one feels an impulse to soar." This is especially true for those persons with disabilities who really want to fly.

There are a variety of resources involving travel by airplane for individuals with disabilities.[12] There is also the technology available to allow those individuals to pilot an airplane if desired. The International Wheelchair Aviators (IWA), a worldwide organization of disabled and able-bodied pilots, states that a person with a disability in good health and able to counter his or her disability with quick reflexes or a suitable alternative control can probably fly an airplane. Flying does not require great strength but does demand good headwork. Pilots who are able-bodied use rudders with their feet. With hand controls added, individuals with spinal cord injuries or lower limb amputations are also able to pilot an airplane. There also are a variety of hand controls and adaptive equipment available for individuals with limited use of their hands.

IWA was originally the Southern California Wheelchair Aviators, established in 1971. The original founders were four pilots with paraplegia who wanted to promote flying for people with spinal cord injuries. Several hundred pilots with paraplegia, quadriplegia, and amputations have successfully flown and become certified through the Federal Aviation Association to date.[13] According to the IWA, pilots with disabilities are flying a variety of airplanes, including Ercoupe; Cessna models 152, 172, 182, 210, and 337; Cardinal; Cutlass; and Piper Cherokee 140.[13] There are portable and permanent hand controls available to pilot the airplanes.

Freedom's Wings International is a nonprofit organization offering qualified persons with disabilities opportunities to fly specially adapted sailplanes. "Soaring" involves airplanes that fly without engines. This type of flying is good for individuals who have limited or no experience at piloting. There are adaptations that can be made for grip, and the pilot travels in a semireclining position; therefore limited trunk stability may not pose a problem. The Soaring Society of America offers information on airplanes and adaptations, as well as training sites. The first step for piloting any plane begins with research and sound planning.

SUMMARY

Mark Twain once wrote, "Twenty years from now you will be more disappointed by the things you didn't do than by the ones you did. So throw off the bowlines, Sail away from the safe harbor. Catch the trade winds in your sails. Explore. Dream." Twain's insight is just as relevant today as it was when he first conveyed this important notion more than a century ago. Driving for recreation and leisure has been a meaningful activity for millions of people in the United States and around the world. Advances in technology, including adapted driving controls and enhanced methods for providing accessibility to modified cars, planes, boats, and other RVs, have enabled many people with disabilities to fully participate in driving for recreation and leisure. Taking the time to pursue leisure interests results in positive consequences for just about everyone, including people with disabilities and their caregivers, and should be considered when performing a comprehensive driver rehabilitation evaluation.

REFERENCES

1. Csikszentmih M: *The psychology of optimal experience*, ed 1, New York, 1990, Harper & Row.
2. Personal communication, Ray Paprota, 2004.
3. Personal communication, Ron Uesseler, 2004.
4. Personal communication, Todd Macke, 2004.
5. Personal communication, Sheila Davis, 2004.
6. Personal communication, Bob Helvie, 2004.
7. Personal communication, Cathy Dewald, 2004.
8. Personal communication, Patrick Yates, 2004.
9. Personal communication, Tom Durbin, 2004.
10. *http://www.adaptiveadventures.org*
11. Winnick JP: *Adapted physical education and sport*, ed 3, 2000.
12. Corbet B, Dobbs J, Bonin B: *Spinal network: the total wheelchair resource book*, ed 3, Santa Monica, CA, 2002, Nine Lives Press, Inc.
13. *http://www.wheelchairaviators.org/info.html*

Chapter 21

DRIVING CESSATION AND ALTERNATIVE COMMUNITY MOBILITY

*David W. Eby • Lisa J. Molnar • Joseph M. Pellerito, Jr.**

KEY TERMS

- Driving reduction
- Driving cessation
- Accommodation
- Dark adaptation
- Static visual acuity
- Dynamic visual acuity
- Visual field
- Space perception
- Motion perception
- Divided attention
- Selective attention
- Spatial cognition
- Simple reaction time
- Choice reaction time
- Supplemental transportation programs (STPs)
- Mobility management

*We thank Linda A. Miller and Jonathon M. Vivoda for comments on this chapter. Portions of this chapter were adapted from previous research reports (Eby DW, Trombley D, Molnar LJ, et al: *The assessment of older driver's capabilities: a review of the literature*, Report No. UMTRI-98-24, Ann Arbor, Mich, 1998, University of Michigan Transportation Research Institute; Molnar LJ, Eby DW, Miller LL: *Promising approaches to enhancing elderly mobility*, Report No. UMTRI-2003-14, Ann Arbor, Mich, 2003, University of Michigan Transportation Research Institute.)

CHAPTER OBJECTIVES

After completing this chapter, the reader will be able to do the following:

- Be familiar with the various medical conditions and aging factors that affect safe driving abilities to best approach cessation of driving.
- Know the strategies that a driver rehabilitation specialist can use to help a client maintain safe driving abilities.
- Know the options available to a client for education and training in safe driving, including driver refresher courses.
- Understand the challenges of persuading older drivers to recognize deficits in their driving-related abilities.
- Be familiar with the behavioral models for understanding the process of driving cessation.

The issue of older driver safety continues to be an important research topic despite increasing attention during the past decade. It is clear that people are living longer than in the past. In the United States the proportion of people aged ≥65 years has increased from <10% in 1950 to approximately 13% currently. By 2050 the percentage of the U.S. population aged >65 years is projected to reach nearly 20%.[1] In terms of absolute numbers those aged 65 years will increase from approximately 35 million currently to approximately 70 million in 30 years.[1] As described by Hakamies-Bloomqvist,[2] it is less clear whether older drivers are at a higher risk of being involved in a motor vehicle crash than younger drivers because the typical measures of exposure (i.e., population, licensed drivers, and vehicle-miles traveled) are either potentially biased or difficult to determine accurately. However, there is strong evidence that for a crash of given dimensions, older drivers are more likely to be injured than younger drivers, presumably because of increased frailty.[3] As such, older drivers are likely to be overrepresented in fatal and serious crashes.[4,5]

Older drivers as a group tend to be involved in different types of crashes than younger drivers. For example drivers aged >65 years, especially those aged >75 years, have more vehicle-to-vehicle collisions, more intersection crashes, and fewer alcohol-involved crashes.[2,4,6,7] Such findings are consistent with what is known about older driver behavior. Older drivers tend to adjust their driving to reduce the demands of the driving task[8,9]; that is, they travel slower and choose times, roads, and routes that make them feel safest. Such findings suggest that unlike crashes among younger drivers, older driver crashes do not result from risk taking or careless driving but rather from age-related declines in driving abilities.

Although there are many benefits to an aging population, one challenge faced by society generally and gerontologic researchers particularly is how elderly persons can maintain safe mobility. As abilities decline and driving becomes more difficult, increasing numbers of older people will begin the process of *driving reduction* and ultimately *driving cessation*. For many older people giving up a driver's license has grave psychological consequences; the action represents not only a significant loss of mobility and independence but also it is a marker for entering the last stage of life.

The purpose of this chapter is to describe what is known about the process of driving reduction and cessation, including the factors found to affect safe driving, strategies for maintaining safe driving for as long as possible, the role of the driver rehabilitation specialist (DRS) in the process, models to help understand the process, and alternatives for maintaining mobility once a person has given up driving.

MEDICAL CONDITIONS AFFECTING SAFE DRIVING ABILITIES

A particularly controversial issue in driver rehabilitation and community mobility involves how to determine a person's fitness to drive when he or she has one or more medical conditions. The issue is complicated for several reasons: the same medical diagnosis can lead to different effects and magnitudes of impairment in different people; treated medical conditions can improve driving ability; medications that effec-

tively treat a condition can also lead to side effects that adversely affect driving ability; and multiple medical conditions and medication usage can have a wide range of effects on driving ability. The research to date that has attempted to relate measures of unsafe driving (such as crashes) to abilities thought to be important to safe driving also has met with only moderate success. With these issues in mind, we present brief summaries of the research comparing the more common medical conditions and driving ability (as measured generally by crash risk).

HEART DISEASE

Coronary heart disease (CHD) is relatively uncommon for young people but is the leading cause of death among U.S. individuals aged ≥65 years.[10] Although CHD is a chronic and progressive condition, slightly >40% of deaths from CHD occur suddenly.[11] However, the incidence of death from this condition while driving is thought to be low because drivers experiencing a heart attack are generally able to stop their vehicles before crashing.[12,13] An examination of studies relating CHD and crashes showed that CHD did not increase the risk of a crash and may have even reduced the risk.[14] However, these findings do not indicate that those with CHD are safer drivers. Most likely the reduced risk of crash is related to changes in driving behavior, such as less driving or driving during safer conditions. Thus there does not seem to be a serious problem with heart disease and driving safety among older drivers because those with heart disease self-restrict their driving activities.

SLEEP APNEA

Sleep apnea is characterized by snoring, breath cessations, sleep disturbances, and daytime drowsiness.[15] The condition has been shown to affect various abilities related to safe driving, such as forced choice and delayed reaction times, decreased vigilance and attentive abilities, impaired cognitive functioning, and psychomotor difficulties.[16-19] One obvious concern of apnea is drowsiness while driving. Studies have found that up to 54% of people with untreated apnea report falling asleep while driving and having drowsiness-related "near crashes" or actual crashes compared with only 7% of matched control drivers.[20-22] Drivers with untreated apnea also perform significantly worse than matched control subjects on simulated driving tests,[15,23,24] are overrepresented in single-vehicle but not multiple-vehicle crashes,[15] and have significantly more at-fault crashes and traffic citations than drivers without apnea.[25]

CARDIAC ARRHYTHMIA

Cardiac arrhythmia, or simply arrhythmia, is an irregular rhythm of the heart not occurring during a heart attack or as a result of drug toxicity or electrolyte imbalance.[26] The condition itself does not negatively affect driving ability, but the treatment can have serious consequences. A common treatment for the condition is a pacemaker or implantable cardioverter-defibrillator (ICD). ICDs are used to manage arrhythmia by delivering a high-energy electric shock to the heart to restore proper rhythm. This shock can sometimes result in loss of consciousness (syncope) or temporary impairment of movement.[12,27] The incidence of loss of consciousness after shock delivery can be as high as 9% in those with ICDs.[27] To complicate matters, it is hard to know how a patient will be affected; there are no clinical predictors for loss of consciousness or paralysis related to arrhythmia, and even a patient's history of these side effects or their absence does not predict future occurrences.[27] Thus it is difficult to determine whether patients with ICD-treated arrhythmia should drive. However, recent research suggests that well-treated arrhythmia should not preclude a person from driving.[28]

SYNCOPE

Syncope can result from a variety of causes, including a sudden decrease in blood pressure, a neurologic pathology, or an increase in blood sugar.[29] It occurs most frequently in older persons, with an incidence of approximately 3% among those aged ≥65 years.[30-32] In approximately 40% of cases of syncope no cause can be found.[33-35] The chance that a person who has had a previous episode of syncope will eventually faint while driving is low (0.33% per driver-year). The risk of syncope causing a crash or injury is even lower.[36] There is little agreement about whether syncopal people should drive, with guidelines ranging from complete driving cessation of 1 to 3 months after a single episode of syncope, to driving cessation for 1 year, to complete cessation after multiple episodes of syncope.[26,36,37]

STROKE

Stroke, or cerebrovascular accident (CVA), becomes more likely as a person ages. The prevalence rates for those aged ≥65 years are as much as 10 times higher than the overall population prevalence rate.[38] The physical effects of a stroke depend largely on the location in the brain where the stroke occurred, but these effects can include partial or incomplete paralysis, impaired visuospatial abilities, agnosias, aphasia, attention deficits, impaired recognition ability, reduced numerical ability, and emotional disruptions.[39] As with other medical conditions, there are no universally accepted criteria for assessing fitness to drive after a stroke. However, because the effects of CVAs are individual, DRSs, occupational therapy generalists, and other health care professionals should help patients after stroke in making decisions about their driving capability, including when it is prudent to reduce driving or cease driving altogether.

DIABETES MELLITUS

Diabetes is classified into two types: type 1 (insulin-dependent) and type 2 (non–insulin-dependent). Five percent to 10% of all people diagnosed with diabetes have type 1 diabetes, and the remaining people have type 2 diabetes.[40] The prevalence of diabetes in the U.S. population ranges from 2% to 6%[40-42] and is more likely in older adulthood.[41-43] Diabetes causes a variety of vascular problems that can lead to various health conditions, including heart attacks, visual deficits, and loss of feeling in the extremities, which can in turn directly affect the ability to drive safely. Insulin and other medications used to control diabetes can also adversely affect driving abilities. Studies relating crash risk and diabetes have yielded inconsistent results.[14] However, patients found to have an increased crash risk tend to be those with type 1 diabetes, suggesting that more careful medical screening is needed for this type of diabetes to help ensure safe driving.

EPILEPSY

Epilepsy is a chronic neurologic condition characterized by abnormal electrical activity in the brain, resulting in seizures. Seizures can range from dramatic grand mal seizures to subtle seizures that lead to adverse changes in cognition or consciousness. Although the cause of epilepsy is unknown in approximately 75% of cases, risk factors include vascular disease, head trauma, congenital factors, central nervous system (CNS) infections, and neoplasms.[44] Epilepsy is relatively common in the United States, with prevalence estimated at 5 to 7 per 1000 persons in the general population and slightly lower in the older adult population.[45] Typical treatment involves drug therapy; however, surgery can be used in severe cases. The main risk of epilepsy for driving is that the occurrence of a seizure can cause loss of consciousness and motor control. Because seizures often occur without warning, drivers may not have enough time to safely stop their vehicle. This potential for crashes is supported by studies that have found an increased risk of crashes and injury among drivers with epilepsy.[46-48]

Dementia/Alzheimer's Disease

Dementia/Alzheimer's (DA) disease is characterized by intellectual deterioration in an adult, severe enough to interfere with occupational or social performance.[49] This condition occurs almost exclusively in the older adult population. DA can be caused by a variety of medical conditions, including stroke, hypothyroidism, acquired brain injuries, brain tumors, carbon monoxide poisoning, and alcoholism.[50,51] Because of variation in how DA is diagnosed, prevalence estimates range from 4% to 16% of the older adult population.[52-55] Three severity stages of DA have been indexed by the Clinical Dementia Rating Scale: early, middle, and late.[56] Progression usually spans an average of 8 years from the time symptoms first appear, although DA has been known to last as long as 25 years.

Despite, and perhaps because of, the cognitive declines caused by DA, many afflicted people continue to drive. Studies show that up to 45% of patients with DA still drive,[57-59] and the majority of these people drive alone.[59] Evidence shows that people with DA do not change their behaviors after a crash.[59] Thus DA has severe consequences for safe driving, and therefore it is not surprising that people with DA tend to have an elevated crash risk.[60] In one study DA drivers had 263.2 crashes per 1 million vehicle-miles of travel compared with 14.3 crashes per 1 million vehicle-miles of travel for older adult control subjects, an 18-fold increase in crash risk.[61] Drachman and Swearer[62] found that of 83 drivers with DA, 26% had crashes while driving after diagnosis. During the same period, only 8% of 83 matched control subjects had crashes. Because of the serious crash risk posed by drivers with DA and their inability to self-monitor and restrict driving, research efforts have focused on driving behaviors that may indicate DA. Studies have shown several driving problems associated with DA, including getting lost while driving, even in familiar areas[53,59,63]; vehicle speed control difficulties,[64] particularly driving consistently below posted speed limits[59]; failure to signal lane changes[64,65]; failure to check blind spots before lane changes[65]; failure to maintain lateral lane position[64]; running stop signs[54]; and failure to recognize and obey traffic signs.[53,54,65-67] As DA progresses these errors appear to become more frequent.[68]

Parkinson's Disease

Parkinson's disease (PD) is a disorder that affects nerve cells in the area of the brain that controls coordinated movement. PD usually affects people aged >50 years but can also affect younger people. The psychomotor symptoms of PD include tremors, muscle rigidity, difficulty walking, and problems with balance and coordination.[69] PD also causes cognitive impairment, including memory deficits; slowed information processing; decreased, sustained, and divided attention abilities; and decreased visuospatial awareness.[70] The disorder is progressive, with symptoms gradually worsening during the course of many years. PD is not curable, but the symptoms can be controlled to some degree by surgery, occupational and physical therapy, and medications. One adverse side effect of the medications is drowsiness. Because of the progressive nature of PD, drivers with this disorder will need to give up driving at some point but may have difficulty knowing when that time has arrived.[71] Research in the United Kingdom comparing cognitive and physical deficits of drivers with PD with on-road driving performance found that cognitive abilities were not associated with fitness to drive but that physical declines were.[70] These findings suggest that assessment of movement ability in drivers with PD is probably sufficient to determine fitness to drive.

Multiple Sclerosis

Multiple sclerosis (MS) is a disease of the CNS characterized by inflammation of seemingly random parts of the brain and spinal cord. Because of the random nature of the disease, no two people have the same set of symptoms. MS has the potential to affect nearly all functioning of the body, depending on where the inflammation is in the CNS. Symptoms can include numbness, tingling, weakness, paralysis, spasms, blindness, blurred or double vision, loss of balance, fatigue, depression, short-term memory deficits, decreased information processing speed, and many other types of cognitive dysfunction.[72] Clearly many of these symptoms affect safe driving. Studies in Europe have found that drivers with MS have higher numbers of traffic citations and crashes than matched healthy drivers.[73-75] Determining fitness to drive is difficult for people with MS. Although impairments of psychomotor ability are of obvious importance,[76] research has shown that emotional problems and cognitive deficits are also important factors to consider.[74,75]

AGING FACTORS AFFECTING SAFE DRIVING ABILITIES

There are many factors related to aging that affect one's safe driving abilities. These include vision, cognition, and psychomotor function.

Vision

Anatomic changes, eye movements, sensitivity to light, dark adaptation, visual acuity, spatial contrast sensitivity, visual field, space perception, and motion perception can all change in ways that affect one's driving abilities.

Anatomic Changes

The organs for visual perception include the eyes and brain. Aging can adversely affect the function of these organs, leading to greater difficulty seeing while driving. As reviewed by several authors,[77-80] the amount of light reaching the retina (retinal illuminance) is markedly decreased in older adults. This seems to occur for two reasons. First the maximum diameter of the pupil decreases with increasing age[81,82]; the smaller the pupil, the less available light that can enter the eye. In dim illumination conditions it has been shown that the average pupil diameter of 20-year-old persons is approximately 7 mm compared with only 4 mm for 80-year-old persons.[81] A second reason for decreased retinal illuminance in older individuals is an increase in the absorption of light that enters the eye.[83-86] When light enters the eye it passes through several relatively transparent structures and media, including the cornea, aqueous humor, crystalline lens, and vitreous humor. Increases in opacity in any of these ocular structures will increase the amount of light that is absorbed, thereby decreasing the amount of light reaching the light-sensitive retina. With increasing age a corneal grayish-yellow ring begins to develop in approximately 75% of the population[86]; corneal opacity slightly increases[83,87]; crystalline lens opacity increases[84,85,88,89]; and the formation of condensations in the vitreous, known as floaters, increases.[77] Collectively the decreased diameter of the pupil and increased absorption of light by ocular structures reduce the amount of light reaching the older adult retina to approximately one-third the light reaching the retina of a 21-year-old person.[90] Thus during nighttime driving, an older driver requires brighter lights than a young driver to see well.

When light enters the eye it bends as it passes through the cornea and crystalline lens.[91] The amount of bending can be controlled by changing the shape of the crystalline lens to focus an image on the retina. Objects that are closer require greater focusing to be clearly seen than objects that are far away. This process, called *accommodation*, is disrupted by age-related declines in the ability to change the shape of the lens in a condition known as presbyopia.[77] It has been shown that by about age 65 years, the crystalline lens has lost most of its ability to accommodate.[92] Thus older individuals have difficulty clearly seeing objects that are nearby, such as a vehicle dashboard. Presbyopic individuals are generally prescribed corrective lenses (bifocals or trifocals) that help them accommodate to the near distances.[78] However, the near correction is usually set for reading distance (approximately 40 cm), whereas motor vehicle controls are typically >40 cm away, leading to potential difficulty in reading dashboard displays.

Eye Movements

The ability to resolve fine spatial detail is not uniform across the retina. A small region in the retinal center, known as the fovea, is densely packed with special cells (cone photoreceptors) that have the greatest ability to resolve fine spatial detail.[93] When we look directly at an object, the image of the object falls on the fovea. As such our ability to see fine detail is partially dependent on eye movement ability to keep an object centered on the fovea. There is evidence of age-related declines in eye movement ability. Studies have found that older adults have an increased latency for saccadic eye movement (short duration and high velocity movements); that is, it takes older adults longer to start a saccadic movement than it takes younger adults.[94-97] It also appears that older adult saccadic movement velocity is slower than that of younger adults.[94,95,97] Older adults also tend to require more saccadic eye movements than younger adults to fixate an image on the fovea.[98] Collectively these results suggest that it would take older adults longer to locate objects in the visual scene, and in fact this has been found.[97] The accuracy of saccadic eye movements does not seem to be affected by age.[97] Pursuit eye movements (long duration and slow velocity movements) also show age-related declines. When compared with young adults, older adults show significantly slower pursuit velocities and decreased latencies for onset of pursuit movements.[98,99] Sharpe and Sylvester[99] discovered that young people could accurately track targets moving at velocities up to 30 degrees/sec, whereas older adults could only accurately track targets up to a velocity of 10 degrees/sec. Thus older drivers would have more difficulty than younger drivers resolving the details of objects that are in motion. The resulting decline in dynamic visual acuity is discussed later in this chapter.

In addition to its effects on saccadic and pursuit eye movements, aging also restricts the maximum extent of gaze without head movement.[100-102] Chamberlain found that the maximum extent of upward gaze for the 75- to 84-year-old age group was less than half the maximum extent found in the 5- to 14-year-old age group. Similar results have been obtained for downward gaze extent.[102] There do not appear to be any age differences for left or right eye movement extents. These results show that older drivers may have to initiate head movements to read the dashboard after looking at the road, whereas younger drivers only need to move their eyes.

Sensitivity to Light

In a darkened environment, such as a car at night, dim lights may be difficult to see. The dimmest light that a person can see, some percentage of time (usually one-half of the time), is called his or her sensitivity to light.[103] There is good evidence showing that visual sensitivity decreases dramatically with age. Sensitivity to light is typically studied after being in a darkened environment for approximately 30 minutes. In these conditions it has been shown that sensitivity decreases with age; that is, the older the individual, the brighter the light must be to be seen.[104-107] In one study[107] the sensitivity of 20-year-old persons was 200 times greater than the sensitivity of 80-year-old persons.

Dark Adaptation

When going from a bright to a dark environment, such as walking into a darkened movie theater or driving into a mountain tunnel, it is at first difficult to see dim lights. Then after a few minutes, dim lights become easier to see. This process of increasing sensitivity to light with increasing length of time in the dark is known as *dark adaptation*.[103] Findings are inconclusive with respect to the rate at which the eyes adapt to the dark, with some studies showing that the rate is slower for older people than for young people[104,105,107-109] and others finding no age differences.[104,109] However, a related issue, glare recovery time, has been shown to increase with age.[110] Glare occurs when light enters the eye in such a way as to temporarily disrupt vision.[77] In nighttime driving glare occurs, for example, when a passing car's headlights shine into a driver's eyes. Brancato[110] found that the time required for glare recovery was approximately 9 seconds for 65-year-old persons compared with approximately 2 seconds for 15-year-old persons. Other work has shown that the debilitating effects of glare are greater for older drivers.[111] In a test of ability to see an object, Wolf[111] found that after a glare stimulus, older adults required the object to be significantly brighter than younger people to be seen. The 75- to 80-year-old age group needed the object to be 50 to 70 times brighter to be reliably seen than the 5- to 15-year-old age group. Thus drivers who are aged ≥65 years would have greater difficulty seeing after having headlights flashed in their eyes and would take longer to recover from the glare than younger drivers.

Visual Acuity

Acuity is the ability to perceive spatial detail, such as a road sign, at a given distance.[112] It is clear that *static*

visual acuity (when objects and the driver are not moving) begins to decline from normal levels at approximately ages 40 to 50 years[79] and continues to decline through at least age 90 years. Combining the results of several studies, Verriest[113] found that acuity decreases from approximately 20/20 for 50-year-old persons (acuity is better than normal in the younger age groups) to approximately 20/60 in 90-year-old persons. Thus as a person ages, spatial details, such as letters, have to be increased in size to be seen at the same distance as when he or she was younger. For persons of all ages, static acuity improves when the overall stimulus illumination is increased and the contrast between the stimulus and background is increased.[77] A related type of acuity is *dynamic visual acuity*, that is, the ability to resolve fine detail when there is relative motion between the stimulus and the observer, as in a driver in a moving vehicle reading a traffic sign.[114] Dynamic visual acuity has been shown to decline with age in much the same way as static visual acuity.[114-117] However, the decline tends to start at an earlier age and tends to be steeper than the decline in static visual acuity. Burg[114] found that when compared with 20-year-old persons, dynamic visual acuity of 70-year-old persons had declined by approximately 60%.

Spatial Contrast Sensitivity

Spatial contrast sensitivity refers to the amount of difference between light and dark parts of a pattern of a certain size required for an individual to detect the pattern.[79] The size of the pattern is often defined by spatial frequency and contrast sensitivity and is typically studied using gratings that vary sinusoidally in luminance. Low frequency gratings have few changes in luminance contrast (cycles) for a given size, whereas high frequency gratings have many. For a given cycle the smallest difference between the maximum and minimum luminance that people can reliably detect can be directly converted to their contrast sensitivity for that spatial pattern. Spatial contrast sensitivity is affected by aging. Older adults with healthy, normal eyes show a marked decline in contrast sensitivity for high frequency gratings,[118-122] with notable declines for people aged >60 years starting at frequencies of 2 cycles/degree visual angle. Measures of contrast sensitivity may be a predictor of driving problems for the older driver.[80] There appears to be some relationship between contrast sensitivity and crash risk in older drivers, although the relationship has not been well established. Schieber et al[122] found that age-related declines in contrast sensitivity are related to increased frequency and magnitude of self-reported vision and driving problems. Their results indicate that this relationship may have been related to increased difficulty in seeing unexpected vehicles in the peripheral visual field, reading dim dashboard display panels, seeing through windshields, and reading signs at a distance.

Visual Field

The *visual field* is the "extent of visual space over which vision is possible with the eyes held in a fixed position"[123] (p. 499). The larger the visual field, the more a person can see without moving his or her eyes. There is clear evidence that shrinkage in the size of the visual field leads to an increase in crash risk (see Schieber[80] for a review of this literature). Vision performance in the periphery of the visual field (peripheral vision) is poorer for older adults than for young adults.[124-126] Studies have shown that shrinkage of the visual field with age is much more pronounced when the person performs a distracting task or distracting stimuli are presented with the target.[127-130] Thus when attentional demands are placed on an older person, the size of the visual field that can be used (the useful field of view [UFOV]) is reduced. Ball et al[127] found that the UFOV in an older adult can be reduced to one-third that of a young adult. Several studies have documented that the size of the UFOV is sensitive and specific in predicting older driver crashes.[131-135] Interestingly Ball et al[127] have shown that the size of the UFOV can be enlarged through training.

Space Perception

The ability to perceive the relative distances of objects and the absolute distance from an object to the observer is known as *space perception*. The ability to accurately perceive space allows a driver to know how much distance is between his or her car and the car ahead or the amount of space in a traffic gap for merging with or crossing a traffic stream. Given the frequency with which older drivers are involved in intersection crashes[136] and left turn crashes,[137] one may suspect that older drivers have deficient perception of space. Unfortunately few studies have investigated the effect of aging on space perception. Only one type of space perception, stereopsis, has received much research attention. Stereopsis is a source of depth information that uses the retinal images from both eyes to determine depth and distance relationships.[93,138] The general finding in the literature indicates that stereopsis, as measured by either a stereoscope or a random-dot stereogram, declines significantly with age in people aged >40 years.[139-142] However, because of methodological and reporting problems, these studies are not conclusive.[79] Thus it is not known how space perception is affected by aging.

Motion Perception

Objects in the environment, such as cars, people, birds, or trees, are frequently changing their location from one place to another or changing their shape. The ability to perceive these changes is known as *motion perception*. Because driving creates and takes place in a dynamic environment, adequate motion perception is critical to safe and efficient driving. Studies have shown that certain kinds of motion perception may decline with age and that sensitivity to motion (i.e., the ability to detect small motions) may be lower in older individuals than in young adults, with older people requiring more motion than young people to see motion.[143-145] However, other work has suggested no age-related decline or that the decline in motion sensitivity may be restricted to older women.[144,146,147] Older drivers may also have greater difficulty perceiving motion in depth, an important process involved in drivers' knowing the change in position of their vehicle relative to the vehicle in front of them. Hills[148] found that the ability to detect the movement of two lights moving away from each other (as would happen perceptually with two taillights as a driver approached) declined after approximately age 60 years, especially during simulated night driving conditions. Although Hills[148] interpreted these findings as a decline in sensitivity to angular displacement, subjects most likely perceived the stimuli as moving in depth rather than moving apart. Other studies have shown that the ability to detect and accurately perceive the motion of an object in depth declines with age.[149,150] Older drivers also have greater difficulty than young adults detecting the relative speeds of objects but are more accurate at judging the absolute speed of a vehicle.[151,152] Collectively these results suggest that older drivers may not perceive critical, motion-defined traffic situations as quickly as younger drivers and would therefore have less time to react.

COGNITION

Cognitive ability includes the following: attention, memory, problem solving, and spatial cognition. Aging can affect these abilities and result in unsafe driving abilities.

Attention

Attention has been described as a process of concentrating a limited cognitive resource to facilitate perception or mental activity.[153-155] Thus good attentional abilities are required for safe driving. Two types of attention are reviewed here: divided and selective.

Divided attention occurs when a person monitors two or more stimulus sources simultaneously or performs two tasks simultaneously.[156] Driving situations in which divided attention is required are numerous. Crash statistics and observational studies suggest that older drivers are particularly hindered by situations that require divided attention (e.g., turning left at an intersection and perceiving relevant traffic signs).[157-159] Although divided attention ability is poor for people of all ages,[160] older adults show a significantly decreased ability to divide attention when compared with young and middle-aged adults.[161,162] These age differences were shown using laboratory tests and may be more pronounced in actual traffic situations. Greater problems with divided attention for older drivers may be expected in real-life traffic situations because the laboratory tests do not include an active visual search for information at unpredictable locations; this type of visual search is especially age sensitive.[161] To assess divided attention ability in actual traffic conditions, Crook et al[163] developed a test requiring older drivers to drive and to monitor weather and traffic reports played on a radio. Significant declines were found for the oldest age groups on driving performance and recall of weather and traffic reports when drivers had to pay attention to both tasks at the same time. This suggests that the ability to simultaneously attend to more than one stimulus or task is poorer for older drivers than for drivers in younger age groups.

Selective attention is the ability to ignore irrelevant stimuli while focusing attention on relevant stimuli or tasks.[156,164] To drive effectively people must be able to ignore the hundreds of sensations impinging on their perceptual systems and focus their attention on the control of the vehicle, the dashboard information, and the movement of nearby vehicles. They must also be able to quickly shift their attention among several important stimuli, a task called attention switching.[164] Numerous studies have found an inverse relationship between traffic crashes and selective attention ability.[157,158,165-167] It is also fairly clear that selective attention and attention switching abilities are poorer for older adults than for younger ones.[156,168,169] In a review of several studies Parasuraman[156] concluded that poor selective attention can lead to an elevated crash rate. He also suggested that attention switching, rather than selective attention per se, might be most predictive of crash risk, particularly in older drivers.

Memory

Memory is the mental process whereby people store their knowledge and experiences. Because it is the process that allows drivers to recall traffic laws and driving skills, to be able to predict traffic situations, and to determine their location, good memory ability is essential to safe and efficient driving. Older people report more problems with their memory than younger people.[170,171] Studies controlling for declining health have found that people aged >60 years perform more poorly on memory tasks than younger people.[172-177] The reason for the decline in memory performance is not well understood.[178] Two types of memory processes are particularly important in driving: short-term and long-term memory.

Short-term memory (STM) is used to conduct ongoing cognitive activities and is sometimes called working memory.[179] Short-term memory is the conscious part of memory where thinking takes place[180] and is therefore critical for driving. The capacity of STM is limited[181]; that is, only a certain amount of information can be considered simultaneously. Numerous studies, using several different STM tasks, have shown that older adult performance is worse than that of young adults.[162,182-184] These results suggest that some decline in memory ability for older people comes from a reduction in the capacity of STM or in the ability to effectively organize information.[185,186]

Information in STM also has a limited duration.[187] If a person is prevented from rehearsing the information in STM, that information will be forgotten. Typically the duration of STM is determined using the Brown-Peterson task, that is, by showing a person a stimulus that does not exceed STM capacity, like the letters *HKP*, and then asking him or her to recall the letters after waiting for a variable period of time.[188] Rehearsal is prevented by having the person perform some other mental task, like counting backward, during the waiting period. STM duration is determined by how accurately a person can recall information after the various waiting periods. Schonfield[189] has shown that older peoples' performance on the Brown-Peterson task is poorer than the performance of young adults, with significant forgetting occurring after only 6 seconds.

There also seem to be age-related differences in the speed with which people can access the information in STM. Processing speed is studied using the Sternberg task.[190] In this task a subject is shown a set of items to be remembered, such as digits. On different trials the number of items in the set varies. On each trial the subject is asked whether a target item is contained in the set. The time it takes for the subject to respond correctly (i.e., reaction time), as a function of the number of items in the set, is taken as the speed at which a person can process information in STM. Older people in the Sternberg task have significantly longer reaction times than young people.[191-193] STM processing speed for older people is generally about one-half the speed of young adults.[185] The speed at which information is processed may play an important role in crash risk because information about potential traffic hazards must be thought about rapidly to avoid dangerous situations.[177] Significant correlations have been found between "hesitancy" in decision making and crash rates among people aged >60 years[177,194] and between lack of "thoroughness" in decision making and crash risk.[195] Thus the age-related decline in processing speed may show up on the road as slow driving, hesitant driving, and unexpected maneuvers, all of which probably combine to increase the crash risk of older drivers.

Long-term memory (LTM) stores peoples' experiences and knowledge. All of the things that we know, and all that we are, are stored in LTM. It appears that the capacity of LTM is unlimited, or at least large,[196] and that it is possible for information to remain in LTM for a lifetime[197] regardless of age. There also does not seem to be much age difference in how fast information in LTM is searched.[198] However, studies suggest that older people have more difficulty than young adults transmitting information to LTM.[199-202] That is, older people have more difficulty forming new LTMs than younger people. With changing road and vehicle characteristics, it is not surprising that drivers aged ≥65 years report having more difficulty driving now than in the past.[203] The ability to accurately retrieve information from LTM also seems to decline with age. Several studies have shown that when compared with younger people, older people have greater difficulty with recalling information from LTM.[204-208] Thus even healthy older drivers may have greater difficulty than young people remembering what to do in certain driving situations and recalling driving laws, leading to increased crash risk.

Problem Solving

The most complex cognitive activity that people engage in is problem solving, including decision making. Finding accurate and efficient solutions to problems is paramount to the task of driving. Older adults generally believe that their problem-solving ability improves with age.[209] However, there is strong empirical evidence that problem-solving ability decreases with increasing age, with the quality of problem solutions decreasing after age 40 to 50 years.[210-212] As reviewed in Kausler,[185] age-related declines in problem-solving ability have been found for numerous tasks, including number problems,[213] the water jug problem,[214] the 20 questions paradigm,[215] and reasoning.[216] Thus it appears that general problem-solving ability begins to decline after age 40 to 50 years, but the relationship between this decline and driving ability or traffic crash experience has yet to be determined.

Spatial Cognition

Spatial cognition refers to the ability and knowledge to think about the arrangement of objects in space, including one's position relative to the environment.[155] Spatial cognition is used frequently in driving and may be related to the safe and efficient operation of a motor vehicle. Spatial abilities are used when drivers attempt to find their way across town and in solving other spatial problems. There is consistent evidence that spatial

cognition ability declines with increasing age.[185,217] Studies of mental rotation speed[218] (i.e., the speed at which a person can rotate imagined images of objects in a mental rotation experiment) have shown that older adults are slower at rotating images than young adults.[219-222] In a study by Gaylord and Marsh,[221] older adults were approximately two times slower at mental rotation than young adults. In addition to slowed mental rotation times, some studies have shown that the accuracy of rotation declines with increasing age.[221,223] Aubrey et al[224] found that older adults have greater difficulty than young adults in understanding and using "you-are-here" maps like those found in shopping malls. Salthouse[182] found that when compared with young adults, older adults had greater difficulty solving problems that required them to mentally integrate a series of lines to determine what they would look like if combined, called a synthesis problem. Collectively these results suggest that older drivers take longer and have more difficulty performing tasks that require spatial thinking, which could lead to detrimental effects on traffic safety. However, the link between spatial cognition ability and driving performance has not been empirically determined.

Other abilities mediated by spatial cognition are cognitive mapping and way finding. Although the two abilities are highly related, cognitive mapping refers to the ability to accurately represent a spatial environment mentally,[155] and way finding refers to the ability to navigate efficiently in an environment. Cognitive mapping ability has been shown to decrease with increasing age. Older people are also less able than younger people to create detailed and organized mental maps of their neighborhoods, even when they have lived in their neighborhood an average of 18 years,[225] and to have more difficulty and be less accurate than young adults in remembering and recalling landmark locations in a simulated simple environment.[226] Navigation ability has also been shown to decline with increasing age, with older drivers reporting more difficulty navigating and finding locations than when they were younger[203] and exhibiting less navigational accuracy than young adults.[227]

PSYCHOMOTOR FUNCTION

Psychomotor function refers to the coordinated and controlled ability to move and orient parts of the body.[228] Good psychomotor function is critical to safe driving. Psychomotor abilities tend to decline with increasing age. This section reviews the effects of age on the speed at which movements are initiated and completed (reaction time), the range of motion that is possible (flexibility), the accuracy of movements (coordination), and the forces required to execute the movement (strength).

Reaction Time

There are two types of reaction time that are important for good driving performance: simple and choice. *Simple reaction time* involves a driver making one response to a single stimulus. *Choice reaction time* involves a person distinguishing among two or more stimuli and possibly having one or more responses to make.[229] Both types of reaction times clearly increase with age. There is also a greater difference between young and older adults for choice reaction time than for simple reaction time[229]; that is, as task demands increase, older adults take increasingly longer to respond than young adults. The age difference in reaction time is particularly relevant for the complicated tasks and decisions that must be made quickly while driving. Mihal and Barrett[157] found that as choice reaction time increased, so did motor vehicle crash involvement. The same relationship was not found for simple reaction time. Ranney and Pulling[167] found that slower choice reaction time among drivers aged >74 years had a strong association with overall driving performance and measures related to vehicle control. However, correlations between measures of reaction time and crash history were weak.

Flexibility

Joints and muscles have a physiologically determined range through which they can move. As drivers age, physiologic changes occur in the musculoskeletal system that can affect driving ability. It has been found that older adults with less joint flexibility exhibited poorer on-road driving ability than those with wider ranges of motion.[230] Joint flexibility changes as a precursor to various forms of arthritis and other health conditions. Muscle strength also decreases by age 55 years, and musculature may be tighter because of decreases in active stretching from heavy manual labor, sports, or stretching exercises that occur with age.[231] A common age-related decline in flexibility has to do with head rotation.[232] Restrictions in range of neck motion can impede an older driver's ability to scan to the rear, back up, and turn the head to observe blind spots.[14,232] Reverse parking can be difficult when drivers are unable to look over their shoulders.[233] In a survey of 446 older drivers, 21% said it was "somewhat difficult" to turn their heads and look to the rear when driving or backing.[234] Most drivers in a study by Bulstrode[233] reported that the original interior rearview and near-side exterior door mirrors did not compensate for their limited neck mobility.

Coordination

Psychomotor behavior involves not only adequate flexibility and reaction time but also precision of movement or coordination. Older adults have less accuracy

in movement than younger adults.[235-238] Szafran[237] had young and older people move their hand sideways for a set distance. The magnitude of hand movement error was approximately one-third greater for those subjects who were aged 50 to 69 years than for younger people. A discrete task like that in the hand movement study may not be related to continuous tasks like driving, in which motoric actions are continuously altered based on sensory feedback.[185] Studies have shown that the accuracy of continuous movements showed an even greater decline with age than did discrete movements.[239-241] As an example Ruch[239] had young and older adult subjects try to keep a stylus directly pointed at a spot on a disk; when the stylus pointed at the spot, the disk rotated. Thus the task was to keep the disk rotating, and the precision measure was the number of disk rotations in 30 seconds. Ruch's results showed that the mean number of rotations for people in the 60- to 82-year-old age group was 82% of the mean for people in younger age groups. Thus it is clear that the precision of discrete and continuous movements decreases after approximately 60 years of age. The influence of these age-related deficits on driving performance and crash involvement has not been established.

Strength

Physical strength is of obvious necessity for safely operating a vehicle, particularly hand, shoulder, and leg strength. One clear effect of aging is a decrease of muscle strength. After approximately age 40 years muscle strength begins to decline, with a 25% decrease by age 65 years.[242,243] Loss of strength continues with increasing age and eventually impedes activities of daily living. The relationship between crashes and decreased muscle strength has not received adequate research attention. However, studies using surrogate measures of strength, such as walking speed, have found that those drivers who walk more slowly have more safety-related errors while driving[244] and are more likely to be in adverse traffic events.[245,246] Fortunately muscle strength can be increased in a short period through a proper weight training regimen.[247]

THE ROLE OF THE DRS IN THE DRIVING CESSATION PROCESS

Clearly the process of driving reduction and cessation is complex. Changes in driving abilities can occur for a variety of reasons and can be unrecognized by the driver. Others, such as family, friends, or medical professionals, may have important information regarding the driver's abilities and history, but they may not know how this information relates to safe driving or how to express their concerns to the driver. The occupational therapist (OT) trained in driver evaluation and rehabilitation plays a critical role in the driving reduction and cessation process. The American Occupational Therapy Association[248] discusses seven roles of the OT to help drivers remain driving for as long as they can safely do so (Box 21-1).

STRATEGIES FOR MAINTAINING SAFE DRIVING

The DRS should be able to use several different strategies to help the client maintain safe driving abilities. These are discussed below.

ASSESSMENT

Making informed decisions about whether and how older drivers can continue to drive safely in the future requires accurate and timely information about the changes in driving-related abilities the drivers are currently experiencing and how these changes are affecting their driving. There are many ways in which this information can be ascertained. Licensing agencies have a unique opportunity to screen for fitness to drive because older drivers, like everyone else in the driving population, must go through a license renewal process. The general process of license renewal varies from state to state in terms of the length of the renewal cycle,

requirements for in-person renewal, and requirements for vision testing.[249] Fourteen states require accelerated renewal for older drivers, and nearly one-half of states have special provisions requiring older drivers to renew in person, undergo vision screening, or both.[249] Even with these provisions, however, it may be several years before older drivers have to appear at a licensing agency to renew their license. Thus licensing agencies also rely on review of driver history records and referrals from health professionals (e.g., physicians, DRSs, OT and physical therapy generalists, social workers, and vision specialists), law enforcement officers, courts, and families and friends of older drivers to alert them to situations in which an individual's driving fitness may be in question.[250] Provisions vary from state to state; the majority of states do not require reporting but rather encourage it or at least do not prohibit it.[251] Close to one-half of the states provide some type of protection from liability for physicians, and a fewer number offer legal protection or anonymity (see Chapter 7 for more information on assessing driver fitness and Appendix A for information about state licensing and reporting laws).

Within the licensing agency itself, there are several potential mechanisms for screening older drivers for fitness to drive, including visual inspection of drivers' appearance or demeanor when they first come to the counter, asking them questions about their health and medication use, reviewing their driving history, and conducting screening tests for visual, cognitive, or

---

BOX 21-1	Seven Roles of the OT to Help Drivers Remain Driving

1. *Evaluate*: Occupational therapists (OTs) can administer a battery of tests to assess a person's vision, cognition, and movement abilities to determine whether there are any deficits that could affect safe driving. This evaluation can help to determine whether an on-road assessment is necessary and, if so, which type of assessment.
2. *Assess*: OTs can conduct an on-road driving assessment. This assessment allows the OT to determine how certain deficits affect driving and to determine whether there are other problems with driving that were not detected during the predriving assessment (evaluation). The driving assessment can be useful for determining how best to help the driver continue driving by suggesting areas in which remediation or vehicle modification may be possible.
3. *Train*: OTs can provide appropriate training that can improve a driver's abilities. For example a person with limited neck movements can be trained on the safe use of mirrors.

4. *Modify*: OTs can provide recommendations for appropriate vehicle modifications or adaptive equipment to improve safe driving. OTs should also provide the necessary hands-on training with this equipment.
5. *Help*: If the evaluation and assessment indicate that the person should stop driving, the OT can help the person identify and use alternate forms of transportation so that his or her community mobility needs can still be met.
6. *Consult*: OTs can consult with family, friends, and medical personnel about the individual. This consultation can be useful for helping to understand the person's ability to drive and to help ensure that the person is able to continue participating in activities that give meaning to his or her life.
7. *Assist*: An important component of an OT's job is to assist the older adult who is no longer able to drive in maintaining a high level of health, safety, and well-being. This assistance can include counseling, identifying meaningful activities that do not require driving, or providing appropriate information sources for the older adult.

psychomotor deficits that may impair driving.[13,246,250] Results of these initial screening activities are best used to determine whether more in-depth evaluation of fitness to drive is necessary. Based on the final outcome of these various screening and assessment activities, the licensing agency has several choices: it can allow the person to keep his or her license, refuse to renew the license, or suspend, revoke, or restrict the license (e.g., prohibit night driving, require additional mirrors on the vehicle, and restrict driving to specific places or limited radius from the driver's home), or shorten the renewal cycle.[249] In making these choices licensing agencies consider each individual's abilities and circumstances and the options available for driving compensation or remediation, as well as rely on the advice of their state medical advisory board if one is in place.

Meaningful assessment of older drivers by professionals and others in the community is clearly important for an effective referral system for licensing agencies. At the same time efforts to assess older drivers' abilities by people outside the licensing agency—particularly physicians, DRSs, and other health care professionals, as well as family and friends, and perhaps most importantly older drivers themselves—play an important role well beyond that of providing referral information to licensing agencies.[251-253] Many older drivers may be willing to take immediate action to voluntarily restrict or even stop their driving based on the advice of trusted professionals or others in their lives. Physicians are uniquely positioned to assess driving-related problems as part of more general medical treatment and care. To the extent that declines in abilities are identified early, opportunities for compensation or remedial action can be recommended and facilitated (e.g., vehicle adaptations, driver training, modified drug therapy regimens, or fitness training). Other health professionals, such as OTs, can also help older drivers, once declines have been identified, by assessing whether a return to driving is possible through training and rehabilitation and by determining what specific remedial activities should be undertaken.

Self-assessment can also be a useful tool by providing cognitively capable older drivers with information about driving-related declines so that they can make more informed decisions about driving and by facilitating discussions between older drivers and their families about driving-related concerns.[253,254] Because self-assessment can be done privately with the results remaining confidential, it may be less threatening than other types of assessment and something older drivers would be willing to do earlier in the aging process and to repeat over time. Clearly older drivers must be honest in their responses and willing to follow through on suggested courses of action for the process to be of real benefit.

Each type of assessment carries with it different requirements and is associated with different strengths and weaknesses. Having available several types of assessments that can be done in different settings can serve to complement the screening and assessment process that goes on in licensing agencies and can contribute to a more comprehensive, multifaceted approach for identifying older drivers who may be at risk.

Screening and assessment efforts need to focus on the age-related abilities that affect driving. Many changes occur to people as they age, but not all of them compromise people's ability to drive safely. Whereas research efforts during the past several years have focused on identifying those age-related deficits most important for safe driving, findings need to be translated into practical, consistent, and up-to-date guidelines for physicians and others about what should be assessed and how it should be done. These guidelines should also address the specific medical conditions that adversely affect fitness to drive and the specific driving problems that may result from them. There also should be training opportunities available for using the guidelines.

LICENSING AGENCY SCREENING AND PHYSICIAN REPORTING

The ability of licensing agencies to screen and assess older drivers can be enhanced in several ways.[255] First legislation can be encouraged in states that currently do not require accelerated or in-person renewal for older drivers so that there are more opportunities for direct contact between licensing agencies and older drivers. Second appropriate referrals from physicians and others in the community can be encouraged or required, particularly because they are of such importance in bringing older drivers with impairment to the attention of licensing agencies. Physicians may be reluctant to report patients because of uncertainty about whether they represent a clear risk to public safety or because of fears of legal ramifications or the potential to undermine the physician-patient relationship. Recommendations for improving the ability of physicians to identify potential problems and for making physician involvement more effective include having clear and publicized information available on the role of physicians; their legal responsibilities for reporting, who to report to, and what happens once a referral is made; what to look for that may signal problems with driving; and where to refer patients for further evaluation.[256] Third there is an opportunity for medical review boards to become more active in supporting licensing decisions regarding older drivers. Many states have relatively inactive medical review boards, and some states lack them altogether. Making medical review boards more effective may require adding members with expertise in aging and driving and garnering more state support. Strong medical review boards can play an important role not only in assisting licensing agencies directly but also in helping to educate and train physicians and other health professionals. Fourth licensing agency examiners need guidelines that can help them decide when further evaluation is called for, who can provide it, and, in the event that remediation is necessary, what options are available. Finally there are many practical considerations that affect the successful implementation of screening and assessment efforts in licensing agencies; screening procedures need to be valid and yet require minimal additional time, space, and resources.

OTHER TYPES OF ASSESSMENT

Incentives may be effective in getting older drivers to voluntarily participate in assessment and follow-up remediation activities. For example legislation has been passed in a number of states that requires automobile insurance companies to provide discounts to people who have completed assessment and training classes.[257] The effectiveness of self-assessment can be enhanced in several ways.[253,258] Like assessment in general, self-assessment tools must be based on what is known about age-related declines and how they affect driving. Tools must be easy to use and understand and provide concrete information about what older drivers can do to compensate for or overcome declining abilities, where to go for further evaluation, and how to plan for continued mobility when driving is no longer possible. Feedback should be individualized; that is, it should be linked to the identified problems of individual users. Because self-assessment is especially useful for early detection of problems, it must be targeted and made available to appropriate groups of older drivers who are cognitively capable of completing a self-assessment tool and are able to benefit from its feedback.

EDUCATION AND TRAINING

The aging process affects everyone in one way or another, and most older drivers will eventually be faced with questions about their ability to continue to drive safely. How they answer these questions, and whether they are willing to consider them, depends to a great extent on the information available to them about age-related declines in abilities that can affect driving, strategies for compensating for or overcoming these declines, and how to plan for a time when driving is no longer possible. For those older drivers who come to

the attention of licensing agencies or have impairments that require medical intervention, answers may be forced on them (e.g., having their license revoked). However, many older drivers will, at least initially, have to wrestle with these issues on their own or with help from their families. Thus the availability of sound education and training can be essential to enhancing elderly community mobility.

Whereas many older drivers do recognize their declining abilities and take steps to adjust their driving, others are unaware of the changes they are experiencing and the implications of these changes for safe driving. Thus one focus of many education programs is simply to increase older drivers' awareness and knowledge about these issues. Other programs combine education with some type of training to help older drivers compensate for or when possible to overcome age-related declines. For example driver refresher courses use classroom instruction to reinforce older drivers' existing driving skills and knowledge and to teach them about new traffic laws and practices for defensive driving. National programs of this type include 55 Alive/Mature Driving sponsored by the American Association of Retired Persons (AARP), Safe Driving for Mature Operators sponsored by the AAA, and Coaching Mature Drivers sponsored by the National Safety Council (NSC).[259,260] On-road driver training programs for older drivers focus on enhancing driving skills by providing opportunities for behind-the-wheel practice. Programs of this type include the Driving School Association of the Americas, the Driver Skill Enhancement Program, and on-road add-ons to some of the AAA driving refresher courses. Although little is known about the impact of driver refresher courses and on-road driver training on actual crash risk, these efforts appear to at the very least help older drivers overcome problems related to lack of knowledge and thus are of some value in enhancing elderly community mobility.

Various types of fitness-training programs seek to help older drivers overcome declines in psychomotor abilities that have been found to be amenable to remediation (e.g., shoulder flexibility and trunk rotation). Improving range of motion can help older drivers do a better job of scanning the rear, backing up, and turning their head to check blind spots while they are driving.[261] There have also been efforts to train older drivers to overcome some deficits in attention and information processing (e.g., relative to UFOV), although these are still under study.[127]

Effective education and training efforts must build on what is known about age-related declines, how they affect driving, and what can realistically be done to address the declines. In the case of declines that cannot be reversed, this may mean simply increasing knowledge and personal awareness so that older drivers can make informed decisions about how to recognize declines and how to reduce or stop their driving if safe driving is no longer possible. In the case of declines that can be overcome, it may mean teaching older people to do new things or to do things in a different way (e.g., learning to do stretching and strengthening exercises or learning to use an adapted driving aid such as a spinner knob). In many cases the focus of training is not so much on individual declines but rather on general driving skills that need to be improved because of lack of knowledge about new traffic laws or safe driving practices (e.g., stopping distances on wet versus dry pavement). In these cases the goal of training is to provide the necessary information and practice opportunities to improve driving skills.

Regardless of the program's focus, older drivers must not only be made aware of the program but also believe that they can benefit from it. Because many older drivers are unwilling or unable to recognize deficits in their driving-related abilities, self-assessment is often a useful first step in getting people to take action about their driving habits. The challenge for self-assessment efforts and education and training efforts is to get people to participate, and that means that programs must be effectively marketed. One successful approach for doing this has been to apply the principles of consumer marketing to the promotion of health and safety behavior, a practice called social marketing.[262]

Programs must also be accessible to the elderly population they are trying to serve. One way of making programs accessible is to offer them through existing programs or organizations that are known to and used by elderly persons. For example, fitness-training programs can be developed and delivered through existing community or senior centers, recreation centers, public health departments, housing authorities, and religious institutions.

Effective education and training efforts consider what is known about how people learn, especially older adults. In classroom learning the physical environment is known to be important; room size and seating arrangements should be responsive to potential vision and hearing deficits of participants. Legibility of written and visual materials is important. Other general learning principles also apply to elderly persons, for example providing opportunities for interactive learning and for learning inside and outside the classroom, finding ways to make the learning as interesting and understandable as possible, and making participants feel like they have some control over their learning. Finally important information should be presented in a variety of ways so that older drivers can retain it.

VEHICLE ADAPTATIONS AND INTELLIGENT TRANSPORT SYSTEMS

Vehicle adaptations and advanced technology provide an opportunity for older drivers to compensate for some age-related abilities that can lead to unsafe driving, such as reduced strength, flexibility, range of motion, and vision-related deficits.[263,264] Vehicle adaptations help drivers with disabilities or aging-related concerns to do things like get in and out of the car, fasten and unfasten their safety belt, and exert control in operating the car (e.g., steer, accelerate, brake, and use control levers).[265] Although vehicle designs can be altered or adapted by automobile manufacturers to make driving easier, more comfortable, and safer (e.g., by modifying door height and width, seat positioning and adjustability, and dashboard controls), the focus of this section is on adaptive driving aids that can be added to cars after they have reached the market. Common types of adaptive equipment include hand controls, spinner knobs, signal switches, and spot mirrors.[264,266]

In addition to vehicle adaptations, advanced technology systems for vehicles have the potential to increase the safety and mobility of older drivers.[267] Intelligent transportation systems (ITSs) combine advances in wireless communication technologies, automotive electronics, computing, and global positioning systems. The most promising ITSs for older drivers appear to include route guidance, emergency vehicle location and response, vision enhancement systems, adaptive cruise control, and collision warning systems.[268] For example drivers who have difficulty seeing at night could benefit from a vision enhancement system that extends a driver's visibility range by detecting and displaying upcoming objects on a "head-up" display.[268] The U.S. Department of Transportation has supported a number of projects to develop design guidelines for various ITS applications that consider the needs and preferences of system users. Most of the guidelines published from these efforts have focused on the general population and do not specifically address the unique needs of drivers with disabilities or aging-related concerns. See Chapter 18 for more information on ITSs.

Effective use of adaptive equipment requires not only selecting the right equipment, installing it, and checking it for fit, but also receiving training on how to use it and having an opportunity to practice with it in low-risk conditions.[269] OTs who specialize in driver rehabilitation can be helpful in making recommendations for adaptive driving aids as part of their assessment of the impact of functional impairments, such as decreased shoulder range of motion caused by arthritis, fracture, stroke, or PD, on driving. Older drivers not working with an OT may be able to get advice from a rehabilitation agency or hospital about how to contact a DRS who conducts comprehensive driver rehabilitation evaluations to identify and recommend an appropriate vehicle type and adaptive driving equipment that enable optimal driving performance. DRSs also facilitate the procurement, acquisition, and installation of adapted driving equipment by assisting older drivers in locating reputable mobility equipment dealers (vehicle modifiers) who perform these services with expertise. Finally DRSs can design and implement the necessary off- or on-road training regimen to address a driver's deficits and community mobility goals.

Successful ITS applications, particularly for older drivers, need to be affordable, relatively easy to use, and work to enhance safe driving rather than produce additional driver distractions that may increase crash risk. One way to promote affordability is to develop systems that are flexible enough to benefit drivers of all ages yet are still able to help older drivers compensate for decreased abilities. The general idea that what works for elderly people will also benefit other drivers is the basis of many successful approaches discussed in this chapter. However, in the area of ITSs the impacts on driver safety and community mobility, especially for older drivers, are still not well understood. Early research suggests that older drivers appear to have more trouble learning to use some ITS applications, such as in-vehicle navigation systems, than younger drivers and find them less functional.[270] Although older drivers compensate to some degree for the increases in attention demanded by the systems, they also still seem to make more safety-related errors than younger drivers.[270] To achieve widespread use of ITSs by older drivers, future ITS applications will need to be carefully designed to ensure that safety is enhanced rather than reduced. Effective training also will need to be available to help older drivers learn how to use the systems and to overcome any fears they may have about the technology.

USING BEHAVIORAL MODELS TO UNDERSTAND DRIVING CESSATION

During the past several years driving behavior has increasingly become linked to more general health behavior, and the issue of driving safety is now considered very much a public health issue. Within this framework stopping driving when it can no longer be done safely can be thought of as adopting a health-protective behavior, whereas continuing to drive beyond the time it can be done safely can be thought of as engaging in an unhealthy behavior not unlike other risky health behaviors, such as smoking cigarettes. Thus it makes sense to examine some of the behavioral models that have been developed to explain and influence various health-related behaviors as a way to better understand the process of driving cessation. Of the many theories and models commonly found in the health literature (e.g., health belief model, social cognitive theory, and theory of reasoned behavior[271]), three of the more promising models for understanding the process of driving cessation are the Stages of Change (or Transtheoretical) Model, the Stress and Coping Model, and the Precaution Adoption Process Model (PAPM).

THE STAGES OF CHANGE, OR TRANSTHEORETICAL, MODEL

The Stages of Change, or Transtheoretical, Model was developed by Prochaska and DiClemente[272,273] and incorporates processes and principles of change from different theories of intervention, thus the name transtheoretical. According to the model, health behavior change involves progress through six stages, including precontemplation, contemplation, preparation, action, maintenance, and termination. As described by Prochaska and Velicer,[274] precontemplation is the stage in which people do not intend to take action in the next 6 months; contemplation is the stage in which people do intend to change within the next 6 months; preparation is the stage in which people intend to take action in the next month; action is the stage in which people have made overt modifications in their lifestyles within the past 6 months; maintenance is the stage in which people are working to prevent relapse, but they do not apply change processes as frequently as do people in the action stage; and termination is the stage in which people are fully certain they will not return to their old behavior.

The model also identifies 10 processes of change, described as covert and overt activities, that people use to progress through the stages. The model assumes that people use different processes of change in different stages of change, implying that people will respond to and benefit from stage-tailored interventions to move them from early to later stages.[275] The processes of change, their descriptions, examples related to smoking cessation (the behavior the model was developed to address), and interventions that may facilitate the processes are presented in Table 21-1.

In addition to stages and processes of change, key constructs of the model include decisional balance, self-efficacy, and temptation.[274] Decisional balance refers to people's relative weighting of the pros and cons of changing. According to the model the balance between the pros and cons varies depending on which stages

Table 21-1 Processes of Change

Process of Change	Description	Examples for Smoking Cessation	Facilitating Interventions
Consciousness raising	Seeking new information and understanding of the causes, consequences, and cures for the behavior in question	I look for information related to smoking	Feedback, education, confrontation, interpretation, bibliotherapy, media campaigns
Dramatic relief	Emotional experiences associated with change	Warnings about health hazards of smoking move me emotionally	Role playing, grieving, personal testimonials, media campaigns
Self-reevaluation	Cognitive and emotional assessments of one's self-image with and without the behavior	My depending on cigarettes makes me feel disappointed in myself	Value clarification, health role models, imagery
Environmental reevaluation	Cognitive and emotional assessments of how the behavior affects the physical and social environments	I stop to think that smoking is polluting the environment	Empathy training, documentaries, family interventions
Self-liberation	Choice and commitment to change, including the belief that change is possible	I tell myself I am able to quit smoking if I want to	Public testimonials, multiple rather than single choices
Social liberation	Awareness, availability, and acceptance of alternative behaviors in society	I notice that public places have sections set aside for nonsmokers	Advocacy, empowerment procedures, appropriate policies
Contingency management	Focusing on consequences (usually rewards) for taking steps to change	I am rewarded by others if I do not smoke	Contingency contracts, reinforcements, positive self-statements, group recognition
Counterconditioning	Finding alternative behaviors to substitute for the behavior	I do something else instead of smoking when I need to relax	Relaxation as substitute for stress, assertion as substitute for peer pressure
Stimulus control	Removing cues for unhealthy behaviors and adding prompts for healthier alternatives	I remove things from my place of work that remind me of smoking	Avoidance, environmental reengineering, self-help groups
Helping relationships	Using support from others during attempts to change	I have someone who listens when I need to talk about my smoking	Rapport building, counselor calls, buddy systems

Adapted from Gorely T, Gordon S: An examination of the transtheoretical model and exercise behavior in older adults, *J Sport Exerc Psychol* 17:312-324, 1995; Prochaska JO, Velicer WF: The transtheoretical model of health behavior, *Am J Health Promotion* 12:38-48, 1997; Prochaska JO, Velicer WF, Guadagnali E, et al: Patterns of change: dynamic typology applied to smoking cessation, *Multivariate Behav Res* 26:83-107, 1991.

people are in.[276] People in precontemplation judge the pros of the problem behavior as outweighing the cons, whereas people in action and maintenance judge the cons as outweighing the pros. Self-efficacy refers to the situation-specific confidence people have that they can cope with high-risk situations without relapsing to their unhealthy or high-risk habits. Temptation refers to the intensity of urges to engage in specific habits when confronted with difficult situations.

The Stages of Change Model has been applied to or expanded for a wide range of health and mental health behaviors, including smoking,[277-279] alcohol and substance abuse,[280] AIDS prevention,[281] exercise and physical fitness,[282-288] fruit and vegetable consumption,[275] anxiety and panic disorders, delinquency, eating disorders and obesity, high-fat diets, mammography screening, medication compliance, unplanned pregnancy prevention, radon testing, sedentary lifestyles, and sun exposure, as well as for physicians practicing preventive medicine. Collectively these studies provide support for the idea of stages of change and processes of change.

The pattern of change in decisional balance (i.e., the pros and cons of change) across the stages also has been found to be consistent in 12 behaviors (smoking cessation, quitting cocaine, weight control, high-fat diets, adolescent delinquency, safer sex, condom use, sunscreen use, radon gas exposure, exercise acquisition, mammography screening, and physician's preventive practices with smokers).[276] For all 12 behaviors people in the precontemplation stage evaluated the cons of making a healthy behavior change as higher than the pros. The opposite was true for people in the action stage. Prochaska et al[276] concluded that for the majority of problems, the balance between the pros and cons was clearly reversed before the action occurred. In a related study Prochaska[289] found that progression from precontemplation to action required approximately a 1 SD increase in the pros of a health behavior change and a 0.5 SD decrease in the cons of a health behavior change. In his view such large effects would require some combination of individual change processes and public health policies.

Findings from Herrick et al[290] support those of Prochaska and his colleagues. The authors examined differences in decisional balance and self-efficacy across four health behaviors (exercise, protection from sun exposure, smoking, and dietary fat consumption) and found pros scores to be generally higher for subjects during the action and maintenance stages than during the precontemplation stage; cons scores were significantly lower in the action stage than in the contemplation stage. Self-efficacy scores also generally increased from the precontemplation stage to the maintenance stage. The authors concluded that the best method for changing health behaviors might be to systematically increase the self-efficacy and pros of a health behavior during the early stages of change and to focus on decreasing the cons of the health behavior later.

There has been some question about the extent to which the Stages of Change Model can be applied to the behavior of older adults.[291] Among the identified limitations of the model are the difficulty of accurately assessing people's stages in general and the difficulty of clearly determining what the implications are for helping older people change even if their stages can be accurately assessed. More importantly the model may not be easily adaptable to older driver behaviors related to self-restriction and cessation of driving. Unlike the behaviors that have been previously studied within this framework, driving is not, on its face, an unhealthy or risky health behavior. It only becomes a behavior that warrants change when other factors come into play, such as declining abilities or health that can adversely affect driving performance. Because many of these factors cannot be controlled or overcome, it may be productive to focus on how drivers cope with these declines, as well as their readiness to make changes in response to these declines.

THE STRESS AND COPING MODEL

Although conceptualizations of stress and coping have come from a number of diverse fields of study, a cognitive-behavioral model appears to be most relevant to health behavior change.[292] The Transactional Model of Stress and Coping[293] provides a framework for evaluating the processes of coping with stressful events. According to the model,[292] stressful experiences represent person-environment transactions in which the effects of an external stressor are mediated by a person's appraisal of the stressor and the coping resources available to the person. When faced with a stressor, a person evaluates the potential threat or harm (primary appraisal) and his or her ability to alter the situation and manage negative emotional reactions (secondary appraisal). Coping efforts are then undertaken to deal with the stressor.

These coping efforts or strategies can be characterized as either problem focused (directed at changing the stressful situation) or emotion focused (directed at changing the way one thinks or feels about it). There appears to be strong evidence that people use multiple strategies when coping with major life events or ongoing strains and that stressors appraised as more serious elicit greater numbers of coping responses.[294] Situations that are appraised as controllable or for which more information is needed also are generally more likely to result in problem-focused coping, whereas situations that have to be accepted or in which people have to hold back from acting are more likely to result in emotion-focused coping.[295]

The choice and effectiveness of coping efforts are influenced not only by the nature of the stressor but also by the styles of coping on which people draw to deal with the stressor.[294] These coping styles or resources represent relatively stable social and personal characteristics (e.g., sense of optimism and locus of control), unlike coping efforts or strategies, which are situation specific, changing in response to primary and secondary appraisals. One possible coping resource that has been largely ignored in the literature is money, despite evidence that people often draw on their financial resources when coping with a variety of problems.[294] Key concepts of the Transactional Stress and Coping Model are presented in Table 21-2.

There appears to be some overlap between the Stages of Change Model and the Transactional Stress and Coping Model. There particularly are similarities between the coping strategies in the transactional model and the change processes in the transtheoretical model.[292] For example the change process of self-evaluation, which involves assessing and in some cases altering how one feels about a problem, is similar to emotion-focused coping strategies, such as reappraisal. Other change processes, such as stimulus control and counterconditioning, can be thought of as problem-focused coping strategies.

Thoits[294] reviewed the literature on stress, coping, and social support to determine what is known with some certainty. She found strong support for the following: (1) the experience of negative major life events and chronic difficulties increases the likelihood of psychological problems and physical illness; (2) a sense of personal control over life circumstances reduces psychological symptoms directly and buffers the psycho-

Table 21-2   Transactional Model of Stress and Coping

Concept	Definition	Application
Primary appraisal	Evaluation of the significance of a stressor or threatening event (e.g., perceived susceptibility or severity, personal relevance, personal responsibility)	Perceptions of an event as threatening can cause distress. If an event is perceived as positive, benign, or irrelevant, little negative threat is felt.
Secondary appraisal	Evaluation of the controllability of the stressor in a person's coping resources (e.g., perceived ability to change situation or manage one's emotional reactions, expectations about effectiveness of coping resources, such as self-efficacy)	Perception of one's ability to change the situation, manage one's emotional reaction, or cope effectively can lead to successful coping and adaptation.
Coping efforts	Actual strategies used to mediate primary and secondary appraisals	
Problem-focused	Strategies directed at changing a stressful situation	Active coping, problem solving, and information seeking may be used.
Emotion-focused	Strategies directed at changing the way one thinks or feels about a stressful situation	Venting feelings, avoidance, denial, and seeking social support may be used.
Outcomes of coping (adaptation)	Emotional well-being, functional status, health behaviors	Coping strategies may result in short-term and long-term positive or negative adaptation.
Dispositional coping styles or resources	Generalized ways of behaving that can affect a person's emotional or functional reaction to a stressor; relatively stable across time and situations	

Table 21-2 **Transactional Model of Stress and Coping—cont'd**

Concept	Definition	Application
Optimism	Tendency to have generalized positive expectancies for outcomes	Optimists may experience fewer symptoms or faster recovery from illness.
Information seeking	Attentional styles that are vigilant (monitoring) versus those that involve avoidance (blunting)	Monitoring may increase distress and arousal; it may also increase active coping. Blunting may mute excessive worry but may reduce adherence.
Locus of control	Generalized belief about one's ability to control events (sense of control or mastery over life)	Internal locus of control can lead to more active coping and increased adherence.

Adapted from Lerman C, Glanz K: Stress, coping, and health behavior. In Glanz K, Lewis FM, Rimer BK, editors: *Health behavior and health education: theory, research, and practice*, San Francisco, 1997, Jossey-Bass Publishers.

logical effects of negative events and chronic strains; (3) social integration decreases the likelihood of morbidity and mortality; and (4) perceived emotional support decreases psychological symptoms directly and buffers the physical and psychological impacts of negative events and chronic strains. There also is evidence that the simplest and most powerful measure of social support has to do with whether a person has an intimate, confiding relationship (usually with a spouse or significant other, although friends or relatives can also serve in this role but less effectively). Having such a confidant can significantly reduce the effects of stress experiences on physical and psychological outcomes.

Thoits[294] found qualified support for sex differences in coping with stress, with some indication that men are more likely to report controlling their emotions, accepting the problem, not thinking about the situation, and engaging in problem-solving efforts, whereas women are more likely to report seeking social support, distracting themselves, letting out their feelings, and turning to prayer. As Thoits noted, however, other studies have yielded different results. Porter and Stone[296] found that men and women report differences in the content of the stressful events they experience but not in the way they appraise them or in the coping strategies they use to handle them. Folkman and Lazarus[295] found no sex differences in emotion-focused coping but reported that men use more problem-focused coping than women in situations that cannot be changed. They concluded that men might persist in problem-focused coping longer than women before deciding that nothing can be done.

These latter findings may help explain why older male drivers studied in focus groups are apparently less likely than older female drivers to acknowledge or express acceptance of the eventual need to self-restrict or stop driving.[297] Unfortunately most research on stress and coping has either excluded older people or included them in mixed-age adult samples without analyzing results for older adults separately[298]; thus it is difficult to generalize findings to older adults, let alone drivers.

Findings from studies that have targeted older adults suggest that coping and adjustment may be different for younger and older adults. For example one such study found that of several factors previously identified as coping resources for young and middle-aged people (i.e., presence of a confidant, social network involvement, being married, feelings of self-esteem and confidence, high occupational status, and income), only income served the same role for older adults.[299] Some factors also acted as coping inhibitors for older adults, intensifying the negative effects of life changes. The idea that coping resources may make people more vulnerable has been advanced by others as well.[300]

THE PRECAUTION ADOPTION PROCESS MODEL

The PAPM[301] contains elements from the Stages of Change and the Stress and Coping models that seem applicable to driving reduction and cessation behavior. The PAPM identifies seven stages during which an individual comes to adopt a precaution (i.e., a protective behavior): (1) the individual is unaware of the problem; (2) the individual is aware of the problem but not necessarily engaged by it; (3) the individual is engaged by the problem and is considering his or her response; (4) the individual decides not to take action (at which point the process ends, at least for the time being); (5) the individual decides to adopt the precaution; (6) the individual initiates the precaution; and (7) the behavior is maintained over time.[302] According to the PAPM, the decision to take a precaution (moving from stage 3 to 5) is significantly influenced by perceptions of personal vulnerability, whereas moving from stage 5 to 6 is influenced by situational obstacles.

Like the Stages of Change Model, the PAPM postulates that people go through a series of stages with regard to health behavior change, that people in different stages have different needs, and that stages have a temporal order. One distinguishing aspect of the PAPM approach is the need for an individual to recognize the possibility of a problem before contemplation of any action can take place. This fits well with the observation-based speculation that the recognition or anticipation of problems with driving ability may be a key factor in the driving reduction and cessation process.[303] Thus the PAPM may provide a better framework than other models for understanding the driving reduction and cessation process by treating it as an iterative process that includes decisions about compensatory behaviors that occur throughout the driving reduction process and the ultimate decision to stop driving.

Unfortunately there has been virtually no empirical work examining the applicability of the PAPM for driving cessation. Kostyniuk et al[303] tested a single assumption of PAPM—that individuals must be aware of a problem and recognize their own vulnerability before they can consider protective behaviors—to determine how well it fit older drivers' decision making about reducing and stopping driving. Using data from a telephone survey of >1000 older drivers and former drivers in Michigan, the researchers found that the degree to which drivers reported anticipating problems with their driving abilities in the future helped predict where they fit in the process of driving reduction and cessation. There is clearly an opportunity to study older drivers over time, using a PAPM approach, not only to better understand the process of driving cessation but also to identify opportunities for tailoring interventions for promoting safe driving based on where drivers fit in the driving reduction and cessation process.

ALTERNATIVE TRANSPORTATION OR ALTERNATIVE COMMUNITY MOBILITY

Whereas many older drivers are able to compensate for declines in age-related abilities and continue to drive safely for some time, others stop driving, often suddenly, because of health conditions, medical problems, being involved in a crash, being reported by a physician or other health care worker, or just recognizing that they are no longer safe drivers. People who are no longer able to drive must still be able to meet their transportation needs to retain their community mobility and hence quality of life. This can be especially challenging for older drivers because of the increasing trend for people wanting to age in place. By staying in their own homes (particularly in rural and suburban areas) they may have fewer transportation resources available to them than if they sought out more transportation-friendly retirement areas.[304,305]

EXISTING ALTERNATIVE TRANSPORTATION OPTIONS

Unfortunately few people plan for the time when they will no longer be able to drive. When the time comes they often rely on friends and relatives to drive them. However, for many older drivers the availability and willingness of family and friends have become increasingly constrained by trends toward smaller family size, higher divorce rates, and more women in the workplace.[305] However, there are a number of alternative transportation options, including traditional public transportation or transit (e.g., buses), paratransit and shared rides, private transit (hired drivers), and specialized transit (e.g., volunteer services, business shuttles, and hospital or other organization/agency-based transit services).[306] The extent to which these services are available varies from community to community. There is also considerable variation among the various services in terms of how aware people are of the services, how difficult the services are to use, and how much they cost.

Public transit is usually provided "on a repetitive, fixed-schedule basis along a specified route with vehicles stopping to pick up and deliver passengers to specific locations, with each route serving the same origins and destinations"[307] (p. 33). Although public transportation is the most traditional form of alternative transportation, it is not available for much of the population; more than one-third of U.S. households do not have public bus service within 2 miles of their homes, and in rural areas more than three-quarters of the population lack these services. When public transportation is available, older people often do not use it; public transportation accounts for <3% of trips made by older people.[308] To some extent this is because many of the same deficits in abilities that are problematic for driving also discourage the use of public bus services. Older people particularly may have difficulty walking to the bus stop, waiting for the bus to arrive, climbing aboard, standing if no seats are available, and knowing when to get off at their stop. Other reasons for not using public transportation include safety concerns, lack of knowledge regarding use, inability to pay the costs, being fearful of getting lost, and inconvenience.[306]

Other alternative transportation options have emerged that seek to overcome some of the barriers posed by public transportation. Among them is paratransit, a service with "flexible routing and scheduling of relatively small vehicles, including taxi cabs, to provide door-to-door, curb-to-curb or point-to-point transportation at the user's demand"[307] (p. 33). Although paratransit or shared ride services provide flexible route options, they may not be available when needed or may require scheduling well in advance. Private transit is also available in many communities but can be rather costly.[306]

A common form of specialized transit services are volunteer ride programs that use private cars and other vehicles and are operated by private resources or volunteer drivers.[307] Because of most people's lifelong reliance on cars and lack of experience with public transportation, volunteer ride programs may be particularly appealing to older people because they retain many of the characteristics of private car travel.[309] Such programs may also be more affordable than public transportation, although they tend to have restricted hours and requirements for advanced scheduling. A broad array of volunteer ride and other types of community-based programs have emerged throughout the country that are often referred to as *supplemental transportation programs (STPs)*.[306,310] STPs are formal or informal community-based transportation programs for older people that are generally more flexible than traditional transportation alternatives and highly responsive to individual needs. They are intended to complement traditional public transit and paratransit in communities by reaching out to elderly residents (especially those aged ≥85 years) with special community mobility needs.

ASSESSING AND IMPROVING ALTERNATIVE TRANSPORTATION

A widely used measure of the effectiveness of a transportation service is the extent to which it is available, accessible, acceptable, adaptable, and affordable.[306,310-312] First and foremost transportation must be available, and this means not just that it exists but that it is in operation when and where people need it. Accessibility has to do with whether people can get to and physically use the service. For public transportation buses, for example, this means being able to get to the bus stop, having a safe and comfortable place to wait for the bus, being able to enter and exit the bus, and having the

necessary information to plan and complete a bus trip. Acceptability has to do with how well the service meets the personal standards of users relative to such things as cleanliness of the vehicle, safety of the waiting area if there is one, and politeness of the driver and other riders. Adaptability has to do with whether the service is flexible enough to be responsive to the special needs of individual users, such as accommodating a person in a wheeled mobility device or someone needing to make multiple stops on the same trip. Affordability has to do with whether the costs are within reach of users and whether there are options for reducing out-of-pocket expenses through such things as discounts, vouchers, or coupons.

Improving the availability, accessibility, acceptability, adaptability, and affordability of alternative transportation services can go a long way toward enhancing the mobility of older people. In the case of public transportation, for example, this may mean expanding hours of service, improving schedule reliability, making it easier for older drivers to enter and exit the bus by reducing physical barriers such as steps, having more seats reserved for older riders, and calling out the name of stops.[311,312] Public transit agencies can also provide better information for trip planning and trip taking using advanced technologies to generate real-time arrival and departure information. They also can partner with other community agencies to better serve the specialized needs of elderly people.

Focusing on individual transportation services to make sure they are responsive to the needs of older people is an important part of enhancing mobility. However, alternative transportation options collectively are often fragmented and uncoordinated in communities. Therefore it is also important to view individual transportation services within a given community as part of a system and to determine where there may be gaps and where there may be opportunities for improved coordination and collaboration. Communities, working in concert with state and federal agencies, have an opportunity to forge alternative transportation systems comprising different types of transportation services at different prices that best meet unique community needs. It is this type of approach, rather than the "one size fits all" approach, that has the most promise for enhancing the mobility of not just elderly persons but of people with disabilities and all other community residents.[311]

Although this is no simple task, it must begin at the local level, with community agencies taking the lead in identifying goals for community-wide mobility and for the provision of comprehensive transportation services for elderly persons.[305] Communities can then reach out to state and federal agencies like the Departments of Transportation and Health and Human Services, which are able to fund comprehensive programs that provide transportation services for elderly persons. Some communities may find that their needs will be best served by a broader regional approach to transportation planning. Opportunities for increased coordination and collaboration at the local level include forming alliances between public transportation agencies and nontraditional partners, such as social service agencies, community-based organizations, volunteer groups, and businesses, and more informal cooperation and information sharing among agencies.[307] A more general practice that can foster coordination and collaboration among alternative transportation services is the use of *mobility management*. Mobility management, as used here, should not be confused with the concept of a personal community mobility manager—someone who serves as a one-stop resource for older drivers (e.g., through a telephone hotline) to provide information on all aspects of maintaining community mobility. A small but growing number of local transportation agencies have become mobility managers; that is, they go beyond the traditional mission of transit by brokering, facilitating, encouraging, coordinating, and managing traditional and nontraditional (e.g., volunteer and community-based) services to expand the array of alternative transportation options available to the community.[313] Some do this directly; some work in collaboration with other organizations; and some rely extensively on contracting. DRSs are also uniquely positioned to serve the public in this capacity. Regardless of the approach used, effective mobility management requires viewing the alternative transportation system as a whole. Thus although the focus of community mobility management is on the entire community and not just on the elderly population, older people can derive much benefit from a more coordinated transportation system.

SUMMARY

This chapter has briefly reviewed the research and issues related to driving reduction and cessation, including the factors that affect safe driving abilities, the role of the DRS in the process, strategies for maintaining safe driving, models that help to understand driving cessation, and options for maintaining community mobility once elderly persons have stopped driving. One theme of this chapter, as well as of this book, is that transportation is a basic human need. People must be able to get around not only to satisfy other basic needs but also to engage in those activities that make life worthwhile, such as visiting friends and family. Maintaining safe and effective mobility is the greatest challenge for those involved in the driving cessation process.

A second theme is that the driving cessation process is unique for each individual. This is because people naturally vary in their ability to drive safely, the effects of medical conditions and medications on driving abilities can vary widely, the community resources that are available will depend on where the person lives, and people vary in the level of resources that are personally available to them, such as finances and family. In part because of this uniqueness, researchers have had difficulty developing adequate driving cessation models, assessment instruments, and guidelines. Thus effective navigation through the driving cessation process largely depends on the knowledge and abilities of DRSs.

A third theme is that information relevant to a person's ability to drive safely can and should come from a variety of sources. The family, medical personnel, the driver, assessment instruments, and impressions of the DRS all provide a unique and important perspective on how safely the person can drive and how remediation can be provided to keep the person mobile. For the DRS it is important to keep in mind the inherent biases presented by each perspective. For example a spouse who depends on the driver to provide transportation may present a more positive picture of the driver than another family member who is more removed from the situation.

Although researchers have made great progress understanding driving reduction and cessation in the past 15 years, there is still much more to learn and develop. For example few assessment instruments exist that can adequately predict future crash involvement. Development of these instruments is a critical aspect of maintaining safe driving. Modeling the driving cessation process is also important. Having a model that can help predict where the person currently fits in the process is helpful for developing interventions to successfully transition drivers from driving to nondriving. Finally the most important but least advanced research area is the development of effective alternative transportation or alternative community mobility options. If accessible, acceptable, adaptable, and affordable alternate transportation options were available, most of the issues surrounding the reduction and cessation of driving would be ameliorated.

REFERENCES

1. U.S. Department of Commerce: *An aging world: 2001*, Washington, DC, 2001, National Academy Press.
2. Hakamies-Bloomqvist L: Safety of older persons in traffic. In *Transportation in an aging society: a decade of experience*, Washington, DC, 2004, Transportation Research Board, pp. 22-35.
3. Evans L: *Traffic safety and the driver*, New York, 1991, John Wiley.

4. Hauer E: The safety of older persons at intersections. In *Special Report 218: transportation in an aging society: improving mobility and safety for older persons, vol 2*, Washington, DC, 1988, Transportation Research Board.
5. Maycock G: *The safety of older car users in the European Union*, Basingstoke, UK, 1997, Foundation for Road Safety Research.
6. Dulisse B: Older drivers and risk to other road users, *Accid Anal Prevent* 25:19-27, 1997.
7. Hakamies-Bloomqvist L: Aging and fatal accidents in male and female drivers, *J Gerontol Social Sci* 49:S286-S289, 1994.
8. Gallo JJ, Rebok GW, Lesiker SE: The driving habits of adults aged 60 years and older, *J Am Geriatr Soc* 47:335-341, 1999.
9. Kostyniuk LP, Shope JT, Molnar LJ: *Reduction and cessation of driving among older drivers in Michigan: final report*, Report no. UMTRI-2000-06, Ann Arbor, MI, 2000, University of Michigan Transportation Research Institute.
10. Centers for Disease Control and Prevention: *Preventing heart disease and stroke: addressing the nation's leading killers, 2004*, Washington, DC, 2004, CDC.
11. Kannel WB, Gagnon DR, Cupples LA: Epidemiology of sudden coronary death: population at risk, *Can J Cardiol* 6:439-444, 1990.
12. Epstein AE, Miles WM, Benditt DG, et al: Personal and public safety issues related to arrhythmias that may affect consciousness: implications for regulation and physician recommendations, *Circulation* 94:1147-1166, 1996.
13. Janke MK: Assessing older drivers: two studies, *J Safety Res* 32:43-74, 2001.
14. Janke MK: *Age-related disabilities that may impair driving and their assessment: a literature review* (Report no. RSS-94-156), Sacramento, CA, 1994, California Department of Motor Vehicles.
15. Haraldsson PO, Carenfelt C, Tingvall C: Sleep apnea syndrome symptoms and automobile driving in a general population, *J Clin Epidemiol* 45:821-825, 1992.
16. Bedard M, Montplaisir J, Richer F, et al: Nocturnal hypoxemia as a determinant of vigilance impairment in sleep apnea syndrome, *Chest* 100:367-371, 1991.
17. Findley LJ, Barth JT, Powers DC, et al: Cognitive impairment in patients with obstructive sleep apnea and associated hypoxemia, *Chest* 90:686-690, 1986.
18. Greenberg G, Watson R, Depula D: Neuropsychological dysfunction in sleep apnea, *Sleep* 10:254-262, 1987.
19. Kales A, Caldwell AB, Cadieux RJ, et al: Severe obstructive sleep apnea-II: associated psychopathology and psychosocial consequences, *J Chronic Dis* 38:427-434, 1985.
20. Engleman G, Asgari-Jirhandeh N, McLeod A, et al: Self-reported use of CPAP and benefits of CPAP therapy, *Chest* 109:1470-1476, 1996.
21. Guilleminault C, Van den Hoed J, Mitler M: Clinical overview of the sleep apnea syndrome. In Guilleminault C, Dement W, editors: *Sleep apnea syndrome*, New York, 1978, AR Liss.
22. Gonzalez-Rothi R, Foresman G, Block A: Do patients with sleep apnea die in their sleep? *Chest* 94:531-538, 1988.
23. Findley LJ, Fabrizio MJ, Knight H, et al: Driving simulator performance in patients with sleep apnea, *Am Rev Respir Dis* 140:529-530, 1989.
24. George CFP, Boudreau AC, Smiley A: Simulated driving performance in patients with obstructive sleep apnea, *Am J Respir Crit Care Med* 154:175-181, 1996.
25. Findley LJ, Unverzagt ME, Suratt PM: Automobile accidents involving patients with obstructive sleep apnea, *Am Rev Respir Dis* 138:337-340, 1988.
26. Canadian Cardiovascular Society: Assessment of the cardiac patient for fitness to drive: 1996 update, *Can J Cardiol* 12:1164-1170, 1996.
27. Kou WH, Calkins H, Lewis RR, et al: Incidence of loss of consciousness during automatic implantable cardioverter-defibrillator shocks, *Ann Intern Med* 115:942-945, 1991.
28. Bleakley JF, Akiyama T: Driving and arrhythmias: implications of new data, *Card Electrophysiol Rev* 7:77–79, 2003.
29. Rehm CG, Ross SE: Syncope as etiology of road crashes involving elderly drivers, *Am Surg* 61:1006-1008, 1995.
30. Bonema JD, Maddens ME: Syncope in elderly patients: why their risk is higher, *Postgrad Med* 91:129-144, 1992.
31. Kapoor WN: Syncope in older persons, *J Am Geriatr Soc* 42:426-436, 1994.
32. Savage DD, Corwin L, McGee DL, et al: Epidemiological features of isolated syncope: the Framingham study, *Stroke* 16:626-629, 1985.
33. Kapoor WN, Karpf M, Wieand S, et al: A prospective evaluation and follow-up of patients with syncope, *N Engl J Med* 309:197-204, 1983.
34. Spudis EV, Penry JK, Gibson P: Driving impairment caused by episodic brain dysfunction: restrictions for epilepsy and syncope, *Arch Neurol* 43:558-564, 1986.
35. Kapoor WN, Hammill SC, Gersh BJ: Diagnosis and natural history of syncope and the role of invasive electrophysiologic testing, *Am J Cardiol* 63:730-734, 1989.
36. Sheldon R, Koshman ML: Can patients with neuromediated syncope safely drive motor vehicles? *Am J Cardiol* 75:955-956, 1995.
37. Decter BM, Goldner B, Cohen TJ: Vasovagal syncope as a cause of motor vehicle accidents, *Am Heart J* 127:1619-1621, 1994.
38. Kurtzke JF: Epidemiology of cerebrovascular disease. In McDowell F, Caplan LR, editors: *Cerebrovascular survey report for the national institutes of neurological and communicative disorders and stroke, revised.* Rochester, MN, 1985, Whiting Press.
39. Lings S, Jensen PB: Driving after stroke: a controlled laboratory investigation, *Int Disabil Stud* 13:74-82, 1991.
40. Centers for Disease Control and Prevention: *National diabetes fact sheet*, Atlanta, 1997, National Center for Chronic Disease Prevention and Health Promotion.
41. Davidson MB: *Diabetes mellitus: diagnosis and treatment*, ed 3, New York, 1991, Churchill Livingstone.
42. Hu PS, Young JR, Lu A: *Highway crash rates and age-related driver limitations: literature review and evaluation of data bases*, Oak Ridge, TN, 1993, Oak Ridge National Laboratory.

43. Hansotia P: Seizure disorders, diabetes mellitus, and cerebrovascular disease: considerations for older drivers, *Clin Geriatr Med* 9:323-339, 1993.

44. Hauser WA, Kurland LT: The epidemiology of epilepsy in Rochester, Minnesota, 1935 through 1967, *Epilepsia* 16:1-66, 1975.

45. Centers for Disease Control and Prevention: Prevalence of self-reported epilepsy: United States, 1986-1990, *MMWR Morb Mortal Wkly Rep* 43:810-811, 817-818, 1994.

46. Hansotia P, Broste S: The effect of epilepsy and diabetes mellitus on the risk of automobile accidents, *N Engl J Med* 324:22-26, 1991.

47. Popkin CL, Waller PF: Epilepsy and driving in North Carolina: an exploratory study, *Accid Anal Prevent* 21:389-393, 1989.

48. Taylor J, Chadwick D, Johnson T: Risk of accidents in drivers with epilepsy, *J Neurol Neurosurg Psychiatry* 60:621-627, 1996.

49. McKhann G, Drachman D, Folstein MF, et al: Clinical diagnosis of Alzheimer's disease: report of the NINCDS-ADRDA work group, *Neurology* 34:939-944, 1984.

50. Haase GR: Diseases presenting as dementia. In Wells CE, editor: *Dementia*, ed 2, Philadelphia, 1977, FA Davis.

51. Katzman R: Alzheimer's disease: advances and opportunities, *J Am Geriatr Soc* 35:69-73, 1987.

52. Terry RD, Katzman R: Senile dementia of the Alzheimer type, *Ann Neurol* 14:497-506, 1983.

53. Adler G, Rottunda SJ, Dusken MW: The driver with dementia, *Am J Geriatr Psychiatr* 4:110-120, 1996.

54. Cushman LA: *The impact of cognitive decline and dementia on driving in older adults*, Washington, DC, 1992, AAA Foundation for Traffic Safety.

55. Evans DA, Funkenstein HH, Albert MS, et al: Prevalence of Alzheimer's disease in a community population of older persons: higher than previously reported, *JAMA* 262:2551-2556, 1989.

56. Hughes CP, Berg L, Danziger WL, et al: A new clinical scale for the staging of dementia, *Br J Psychiatry* 140:556-572, 1982.

57. Carr DB, Jackson T, Alguire P: Characteristics of an elderly driving population referred to a geriatric assessment center, *J Am Geriatr Soc* 38:1145-1150, 1990.

58. Logsdon RG, Teri L, Larson EB: Driving and Alzheimer's disease, *J Gen Intern Med* 7:583-588, 1992.

59. Lucas-Blaustein MJ, Filipp L, Dungan C, et al: Driving in patients with dementia, *J Am Geriatr Soc* 36:1087-1092, 1988.

60. Reger MA, Welsh RK, Watson GS, et al: The relationship between neuropsychological functioning and driving ability in dementia: a meta-analysis, *Neuropsychology* 18:85-93, 2004.

61. Dubinsky RM, Williamson A, Gray CS, et al: Driving in Alzheimer's disease, *J Am Geriatr Soc* 40:1112-1116, 1992.

62. Drachman DA, Swearer JM: Driving and Alzheimer's disease: the risk of crashes, *Neurology* 43:2448-2456, 1993.

63. Underwood M: The older driver: clinical assessment and injury prevention, *Arch Intern Med* 152:735-740, 1992.

64. Odenheimer GL, Beaudet M, Gette AM, et al: Performance-based driving evaluation of the elderly driver: safety, reliability and validity, *J Gerontol Med Sci* 49:153-159, 1994.

65. Hunt LA, Morris JC, Edwards D, et al: Driving performance in persons with mild senile dementia of the Alzheimer type, *J Am Geriatr Soc* 41:747-753, 1993.

66. Hunt LA: Dementia and road test performance. Proceedings of *Strategic Highway Research Program and Traffic Safety on Two Continents*, Gothenburg, Sweden, 1991.

67. Mitchell RK, Castleden CM, Fanthome Y: Driving, Alzheimer's disease and ageing: a potential cognitive screening device for all elderly drivers, *Int J Geriatr Psychiatr* 10:865-869, 1995.

68. Fox GK, Bowden SC, Bashford GM, et al: Alzheimer's disease and driving: prediction and assessment of driving performance, *J Am Geriatr Soc* 45:949-953, 1997.

69. Mayo Clinic Staff: *Parkinson's disease*, 2004. Available at: *http://www.mayoclinic.com/invoke.cfm?id=DS00295*. Accessed October 2004.

70. Radford KA, Lincoln NB, Lennox G: The effects of cognitive abilities on driving in people with Parkinson's disease, *Disabil Rehabil* 26:65-70, 2004.

71. Campbell MK, Bush TL, Hale WE: Medical conditions associated with driving cessation in community-dwelling ambulatory elders, *J Gerontol* 45:S230-S234, 1993.

72. Jones P: *All about multiple sclerosis*, 2004. Available at: *http://www.mult-sclerosis.org/.m*. Accessed October 2004.

73. Knecht J: The multiple sclerosis patient as a driver [in German], *J Suisse De Medecine* 107:373-378, 1977.

74. Schanke AK, Grismo J, Sundet K: Multiple sclerosis and prerequisites for driver's license: a retrospective study of 33 patients with multiple sclerosis assessed at Sunnaas hospital [in Norwegian], *Tidsskrift Den Norske Laegeforening* 115:1349-1352, 1995.

75. Schultheis MT, Garay E, DeLuca J: The influence of cognitive impairment on driving performance in multiple sclerosis, *Neurology* 56:1089-1094, 2001.

76. Goodwill CJ: Mobility for the disabled patient, *Int Rehabil Med* 6:1, 1984.

77. Corso JF: *Aging sensory systems and perception*, New York, 1981, Praeger.

78. Owsley C, Ball K: Assessing visual function in the older driver, *Clin Geriatr Med* 9:389-401, 1993.

79. Owsley C, Sloane ME: Vision and aging. In Bolter F, Grafman J, editors: *Handbook of neuropsychology, vol 4*, Amsterdam, 1990, Elsevier.

80. Schieber F: *Recent developments in vision, aging, and driving: 1988-1994* (Report no. UMTRI-94-26), Ann Arbor, MI, 1994, The University of Michigan Transportation Research Institute.

81. Lowenfeld IE: Pupillary changes related to age. In Thompson HS, editor: *Topics in neuro-ophthalmology*, Baltimore, 1979, Williams and Wilkins.

82. Weale RA: The ageing eye. In *Scientific basis of medicine: annual reviews*, London, 1971, Athlone Press.

83. Boettner EA, Wolter JR: Transmission of the ocular media, *Invest Ophthalmol Vis Sci* 1:776-783, 1962.

84. Said FS, Weale RA: The variation with age of the spectral transmissivity of the living human crystalline lens, *Gerontologia* 3:213-231, 1959.

85. Sarks SH: The aging eye, *Med J Aust* 2:602-604, 1975.

86. Stocker FW, Moore LW Jr: Detecting changes in the cornea that come with age, *Geriatrics* 30:57-69, 1975.
87. Block MG, Rosenblum WM: MTF measurements on the human lens, *J Optical Soc Am* 4:7, 1987.
88. Coren S, Girgus JS: Density of human lens pigment: in vivo measure over an extended age range, *Vision Res* 12:343-346, 1972.
89. Spector A: Aging of the lens and cataract formation. In Sekular R, Kline DW, Dismukes K, editors: *Aging and human visual functions*, New York, 1982, Alan Liss.
90. Weale RA: *A biography of the eye*, London, 1982, HK Lewis.
91. Westheimer G: The eye as an optical instrument. In Boff KR, Kaufman L, Thomas JP, editors: *Handbook of perception and human performance, vol I: Sensory processes and perception*, New York, 1986, John Wiley and Sons.
92. Hofstetter HW: A longitudinal study of amplitude changes in presbyopia, *Am J Optom* 42:3-8, 1965.
93. Matlin MW, Foley HJ: *Sensation and perception*, Needham Heights, MA, 1992, Allyn and Bacon.
94. Abel LA, Troost BT, Dell'Osso LF: The effects of age on normal saccadic characteristics and their variability, *Vision Res* 23:33-37, 1983.
95. Spooner JW, Sakala SM, Baloh RW: Effect of aging on eye tracking, *Arch Neurol* 37:575-576, 1980.
96. Wacker J, Busser A, Lachenmayr J: Influence of stimulus size and contrast on the temporal patterns of saccadic eye movements: implications for road traffic, *German J Ophthalmol* 2:246-250, 1983.
97. Warabi T, Kase M, Kato T: Effect of aging on the accuracy of visually guided saccadic eye movement, *Ann Neurol* 16:449-454, 1984.
98. Lapidot MB: Does the brain age uniformly? Evidence from effects of smooth pursuit eye movements on verbal and visual tasks, *J Gerontol* 42:P329-P331, 1987.
99. Sharpe JA, Sylvester TO: Effects of age on horizontal smooth pursuit, *Invest Ophthalmol Vis Sci* 17:465-468, 1978.
100. Chamberlain W: Restriction of upward gaze with advancing age, *Trans Am Ophthalmol Soc* 68:234-244, 1970.
101. Chamberlain W: Restriction of upward gaze with advancing age, *Am J Ophthalmol* 71:341-346, 1971.
102. Huaman AG, Sharpe JA: Vertical saccades in senescence, *Invest Ophthalmol Vis Sci* 34:2588-2595, 1993.
103. Hood DC, Finkelstein MA: Sensitivity to light. In Boff KR, Kaufman L, Thomas JP, editors: *Handbook of perception and human performance, volume I: Sensory processes and perception*, New York, 1986, John Wiley and Sons.
104. Birren JE, Shock NW: Age changes in rate and level of dark adaptation, *J Appl Psychol* 26:407-411, 1950.
105. Domey RG, McFarland RA, Chadwick E: Dark adaptation of a function of time II: a derivation, *J Gerontol* 15:267-279, 1960.
106. McFarland RA, Fischer MB: Alterations in dark adaptation as a function of age, *J Gerontol* 10:424-428, 1955.
107. McFarland RA, Domey RG, Warren AB, et al: Dark adaptation of a function of age: a statistical analysis, *J Gerontol* 15:149-154, 1960.
108. McFarland RA: The sensory and perceptual processes in aging. In Schaie KW, editor: *Theory and methods of research in aging*, Morgantown, WV, 1968, West Virginia University Press.
109. Eisner A, Fleming SA, Klein ML, et al: Sensitivity in older eyes with good acuity: cross-sectional norms, *Invest Ophthalmol Vis Sci* 28:1824-1831, 1987.
110. Brancato R: Il tempo di recupero in seguito ad abbagliamento in funzione dell'età, *Atti della "Fondazione Georgio Ronchi"* 24:585-588, 1969.
111. Wolf E: Glare and age, *Arch Ophthalmol* 64:502-514, 1960.
112. Olzak LA, Thomas JP: Seeing spatial patterns. In Boff KR, Kaufman L, Thomas JP, editors: *Handbook of perception and human performance, vol I: Sensory processes and perception*, New York, 1986, John Wiley and Sons.
113. Verriest G: L'influence de l'age sur les fonctions visuelles de l'homme, *Bull de l'Acàdemie Royale de Mèdecine Belgique* 11:264-265, 1971.
114. Burg A: Visual acuity as measured by dynamic and static tests, *J Appl Psychol* 50:460-466, 1966.
115. Burg A, Hurlbert S: Dynamic visual acuity as related to age, sex, and static acuity, *J Appl Psychol* 45:111-116, 1961.
116. Heron A, Chown SM: *Age and function*, London, 1967, Churchill.
117. Long GM, Crambert RF: The nature and basis of age-related changes in dynamic visual acuity, *Psychol Aging* 5:138-143, 1989.
118. Derefeldt G, Lennerstrand G, Lundh B: Age variation in normal human contrast sensitivity, *Acta Ophthalmol* 57:679-690, 1979.
119. Kline D, Schieber F, Abusamra LC, et al: Age, the eye, and the visual channels: contrast sensitivity and response speed, *J Gerontol* 38:211-216, 1983.
120. Madden DJ, Greene HA: From retina to response: contrast sensitivity and memory retrieval during visual word recognition, *Exp Aging Res* 13:15-21, 1987.
121. Owsley C, Sekuler R, Siemsen D: Contrast sensitivity throughout adulthood, *Vision Res* 23:689-699, 1983.
122. Schieber F, Kline DW, Kline TJB, et al: *The relationship between contrast sensitivity and the visual problems of older drivers* (SAE Technical Paper no. 920613), Warrendale, PA, 1992, Society of Automotive Engineers, Inc.
123. Sekuler R, Blake R: *Perception*, New York, 1985, Alfred A. Knopf, Inc.
124. Burg A: Lateral visual field as related to age and sex, *J Appl Psychol* 52:10-15, 1968.
125. Crassini B, Brown B, Bowman K: Age related changes in contrast sensitivity in the central and peripheral retina, *Perception* 17:315-332, 1988.
126. Wolf E: Studies on the shrinkage of the visual field with age, *Transport Res Record* 164:1967.
127. Ball K, Beard BL, Roenker DL, et al: Age and visual search: expanding the useful field of view, *J Optical Soc Am* 5:2210-2219, 1988.
128. Sekuler R, Ball K: Visual localization: age and practice, *J Optical Soc Am* 3:864-867, 1986.
129. Scialfa CT, Kline DW, Lyman BJ: Age differences in target identification as a function of retinal location and noise level: examination of the useful field of view, *Psychol Aging* 2:14-19, 1987.
130. Triesman AM, Gelade G: A feature integration theory of attention, *Cogn Psychol* 12:97-136, 1980.

131. Ball K: Attentional problems and older drivers, *Alzheimer Dis Assoc Disord* 11:42-47, 1997.

132. Ball K, Owsley C, Sloane ME, et al: Visual attention problems as a predictor of vehicle crashes in older drivers, *Invest Ophthalmol Vis Sci* 34:3110-3123, 1993.

133. Ball K, Owsley C: Identifying correlates of accident involvement for the older driver, *Hum Factors* 33:583-595, 1991.

134. Ball K, Rebok G: Evaluating the driving ability of older adults, *J Appl Gerontol* 13:20-38, 1994.

135. Owsley C, Ball K, Sloane ME, et al: Visual/cognitive correlates of vehicle accidents in older drivers, *Psychol Aging* 6:403-415, 1991.

136. Vivano DC, Culver CC, Evans L, et al: Involvement of older drivers in multi-vehicle side impact crashes. In *Proceedings of the 12th International Technical Conference of Experimental Safety Vehicles,* Washington, DC, 1989, National Highway Traffic Safety Administration, pp. 699-705.

137. National Highway Traffic Safety Administration: *Addressing the safety issues related to younger and older drivers: a report to Congress,* Report no. DOT HS 807-957, Washington, DC, 1993, U.S. Department of Transportation.

138. Arditi A: Binocular vision. In Boff KR, Kaufman L, Thomas JP, editors: *Handbook of perception and human performance, vol I: Sensory processes and perception,* New York, 1986, John Wiley and Sons.

139. Hoffman CS, Price AC, Garrett ES, et al: Effect of age and brain damage on depth perception, *Perceptual Motor Skills* 9:283-286, 1959.

140. Jani SN: The age factor in stereopsis screening, *Am J Optom* 43:653-657, 1966.

141. Bell MD, Wolf E, Bernholz CD: Depth perception as a function of age, *Aging Hum Develop* 3:77-81, 1972.

142. Hofstetter HW, Bertsch JD: Does stereopsis change with age? *Am J Optom Physiol Opt* 53:664-667, 1976.

143. Ball K, Sekuler R: Improving visual perception in older observers, *J Gerontol* 41:176-182, 1986.

144. Schieber F, Hiris E, White J, et al: Assessing age-differences in motion perception using simple oscillatory displacement versus random dot cinematography, *Invest Ophthalmol Vis Sci* 31(suppl):355, 1990.

145. Trick GL, Silverman SE: Visual sensitivity to motion: age-related changes and deficits in senile dementia of the Alzheimer type, *Neurology* 41:1437-1440, 1991.

146. Brown B, Bowman KJ: Sensitivity to changes in size and velocity in young and elderly observers, *Perception* 16:41-47, 1987.

147. Gilmore GC, Wenk H, Naylor LA, et al: Motion perception and aging, *Psychol Aging* 7:654-660, 1992.

148. Hills BL: *Some studies of movement perception, age and accidents,* Supplementary Report no. TTRL-137UC, Crowthorne, UK, 1975, Transport and Road Research Laboratory.

149. Shinar D: *Driver visual limitation diagnosis and treatment,* Report no. DOT-HS-803-260, Washington, DC, 1977, U.S. Department of Transportation.

150. Schiff W, Oldak R, Shah V: Aging persons' estimates of vehicular motion, *Psychol Aging* 7:518-525, 1992.

151. Hills BL: Vision, visibility, and perception in driving, *Perception* 9:183-216, 1980.

152. Scialfa CT, Guzy LT, Leibowitz HW, et al: Age differences in estimating vehicle velocity, *Psychol Aging* 6:60-66, 1991.

153. Anderson JR: *Cognitive psychology and its implications,* New York, 1985, Freeman and Company.

154. Bernstein DA, Roy EJ, Srull TK, et al: *Psychology,* ed 2, Boston, 1991, Houghton Mifflin Company.

155. Matlin MW: *Cognition,* ed 2, Fort Worth, TX, 1989, Holt, Rinehart and Winston, Inc.

156. Parasuraman R: Attention and driving performance in Alzheimer's dementia. Proceedings of the Conference, *Strategic highway research program and traffic safety on two continents,* Gothenburg, Sweden, 1991.

157. Mihal WL, Barrett GV: Individual differences in perceptual information processing and their relation to automobile accident involvement, *J Appl Psychol* 6:229-233, 1976.

158. Kahneman D: *Attention and effort,* Englewood Cliffs, NJ, 1973, Prentice-Hall.

159. van Wolffelaar PC, Brouwer WH, Rothengatter JA: Older drivers handling road traffic informatics: divided attention in a dynamic driving simulator. Proceedings of the Conference, *Strategic highway research program and traffic safety on two continents,* Gothenburg, Sweden, 1991.

160. Sexton MA, Geffen G: Development of three strategies of attention in dichotic monitoring, *Dev Psychol* 15:299-310, 1979.

161. Ponds RWHM, Brouwer WH, van Wolffelaar PC: Age differences in divided attention in a simulated driving task, *J Gerontol* 43:151-156, 1988.

162. Salthouse TA, Mitchell DR, Skovronek E, et al: Effects of adult age and working memory on reasoning and spatial ability, *J Exp Psychol Learn Mem Cogn* 15:507-516, 1989.

163. Crook TH, West RL, Larrabee GJ: The driving-reaction time test: assessing age declines in dual-task performance, *Dev Neuropsychol* 9:31-39, 1993.

164. Parasuraman R: Vigilance, monitoring, and search. In Boff KR, Kaufman L, Thomas JP, editors: *Handbook of perception and human performance, vol II: Cognitive processes and performance,* New York, 1986, John Wiley and Sons.

165. Barrett GV, Mihal WL, Panek PE, et al: Information-processing skills predictive of accident involvement for younger and older commercial drivers, *Industr Gerontol* 4:173-182, 1977.

166. Avolio BJ, Kroeck KG, Panek PE: Individual differences in information-processing ability as a predictor of motor vehicle accidents, *Hum Factors* 27:577-587, 1985.

167. Ranney TA, Pulling NH: *Relation of individual differences in information-processing ability to driving performance,* Proceedings of the Human Factors Society, 33rd Annual Meeting. Santa Monica, CA, 1989, Human Factors Society.

168. Rabbitt P: An age-decrement in the ability to ignore irrelevant information, *J Gerontol* 20:233-238, 1965.

169. Nebes RD, Madden DJ: Different patterns of cognitive slowing produced by Alzheimer's disease and normal aging, *Psychol Aging* 3:102-104, 1988.

170. Cutler SJ, Grams AE: Correlates of self-reported everyday memory problems, *J Gerontol Social Sci* 43:82-90, 1988.
171. Ryan EB: Beliefs about memory changes across the adult lifespan, *J Gerontol Psychol Sci* 47:41-46, 1992.
172. Bahrick HP: Memory for older people. In Harris JE, Morris PE, editors: *Everyday memory, actions and absentmindedness*, New York, 1984, Academic Press.
173. Hultsch DF, Hammer M, Small BJ: Age differences in cognitive performance in later life: relationships to self-reported health and activity style, *J Gerontol Psycholog Sci* 48:1-11, 1993.
174. Maylor EA: Recognizing and naming tunes: memory impairment in the elderly, *J Gerontol Psychol Sci* 46:207-217, 1991.
175. Perlmutter M, Nyquist L: Relationships between self-reported physical and mental health and intelligence performance across adulthood, *J Gerontol Psychol Sci* 45:145-155, 1990.
176. Rabbitt P: Inner-city decay? Age changes in structure and process in recall of familiar topographical information. In Poon LW, Rubin DC, Wilson BA, editors: *Everyday cognition in adulthood and late life*, Cambridge, MA, 1989, Cambridge University Press.
177. West RL, Crook TH, Barron KL: Everyday memory performance across the life-span: effects of age and noncognitive individual differences, *Psychol Aging* 7:72-82, 1992.
178. Light LL: Memory and aging. In Bjork EL, Bjork RA, editors: *Memory*, New York, 1996, Academic Press.
179. Baddeley AD: The fractionation of human memory, *Psychol Med* 14:259-264, 1984.
180. Siegler RS: *Children's thinking*, ed 2, Englewood Cliff, NJ, 1991, Prentice Hall.
181. Miller GA: The magic number seven plus or minus two: some limits on our capacity for processing information, *Psychol Rev* 63:81-97, 1956.
182. Salthouse TA: Adult age differences in integrative spatial ability, *Psychol Aging* 2:254-260, 1987.
183. Salthouse TA: Working memory as a processing resource in cognitive aging, *Dev Rev* 10:101-124, 1990.
184. Salthouse TA, Skovronek E: Within-context assessment of age differences in working memory, *J Gerontol Psychol Sci* 47:110-120, 1992.
185. Kausler DH: *Experimental psychology, cognition, and human aging*, New York, 1991, Springer-Verlag.
186. Taub HA: Coding for short-term memory as a function of age, *J Genetic Psychol* 125:309-314, 1974.
187. Brown JA: Some tests of the decay theory of immediate memory, *Q J Exp Psychol* 10:12-21, 1958.
188. Peterson LR, Peterson MJ: Short-term retention of individual verbal items, *J Exp Psychol* 58:495-512, 1959.
189. Schonfield AED: *In search of early memories*, Paper presented at the International Congress of Gerontology, Washington, DC, 1969.
190. Sternberg S: High-speed scanning in human memory, *Science* 153:652-654, 1966.
191. Anders TR, Fozard JL, Lillyquist TD: Effects of age upon retrieval from short-term memory, *Dev Psychol* 6:214-217, 1972.
192. Cerella J: Information processing rates in the elderly, *Psychol Bull* 98:67-83, 1985.
193. Eriksen CW, Hamlin RM, Daye C: Aging adults and rate of memory scan, *Bull Psychonomic Soc* 1:259-260, 1973.
194. French DJ, West RJ, Elander J, et al: Decision-making style, driving style, and self-reported involvement in road traffic accidents, *Ergonomics* 36:627-644, 1993.
195. Reason J, Manstead ASR, Stradling SG, et al: *The social and cognitive determinants of aberrant driving behavior*, Crowthorne, UK, 1991, UK Transport Research Laboratory.
196. Tulving E: Recall and recognition of semantically encoded words, *J Exp Psychol* 102:778-787, 1974.
197. Bahrick HP, Bahrick PO, Wittlinger RP: Fifty years of memory for names and faces: a cross-sectional approach, *J Exp Psychol* 104:54-75, 1975.
198. Thomas JC, Waugh NC, Fozard JL: Age and familiarity in memory scanning, *J Gerontol* 33:528-533, 1978.
199. Arenberg D: The effects of input condition on free recall in young and old adults, *J Gerontol* 31:551-555, 1976.
200. Craik FIM: Two components in free recall, *J Verbal Learn Verbal Behav* 7:996-1004, 1968.
201. Parkinson SR, Lindholm JM, Inman VW: An analysis of age differences in immediate recall, *J Gerontol* 37:425-431, 1982.
202. Salthouse TA: Age and memory: strategies for localizing the loss. In Poon LW, Fozard JL, Cermak LS, et al, editors: *New directions in memory and aging: proceedings of the George A. Talland memorial conference*, Hillsdale, NJ, 1980, Lawrence Erlbaum Associates.
203. Kostyniuk LP, Streff FM, Eby DW: *The older driver and navigation assistance systems* (Report no. UMTRI-94-47), Ann Arbor, MI, 1997, The University of Michigan Transportation Research Institute.
204. Holland CA, Rabbitt PMA: Aging memory: use versus impairment, *Br J Psychol* 82:29-38, 1991.
205. Kausler DH, Puckett JM: Adult age differences in recognition memory for a nonsemantic attribute, *Exp Aging Res* 6:349-355, 1980.
206. Kausler DH, Puckett JM: Adult age differences in memory for modality attributes, *Exp Aging Res* 7:117-125, 1981.
207. Kausler DH: Automaticity of encoding and episodic memory processes. In Lovelace EA, editor: *Aging and cognition: mental processes, self-awareness, and interventions*, Amsterdam, 1990, Elsevier.
208. Light LL, La Voie D, Valencia-Laver D, et al: Direct and indirect measures for memory modality in young and older adults, *J Exp Psychol Learn Mem Cogn* 18:1284-1297, 1992.
209. Williams SA, Denney NW, Schadler M: Elderly adults' perception of their own cognitive development during adult years, *Int J Aging Hum Dev* 16:147-158, 1983.
210. Denney NW, Palmer M: Adult age differences on traditional and practical problem-solving measures, *J Gerontol* 36:323-328, 1981.
211. Denney NW, Pearce KA: A developmental study of practical problem solving in adults, *Psychol Aging* 4:438-442, 1989.
212. Denney NW, Pearce KA, Palmer M: A developmental study of adults' performance on traditional and

practical problem-solving tasks, *Exp Aging Res* 8:115-118, 1982.

213. Wright RE: Aging, divided attention, and processing capacity, *J Gerontol* 37:76-79, 1981.

214. Heglin H: Problem solving set in different age groups, *J Gerontol* 11:310-317, 1956.

215. Denney NW, Denney DR: Modeling effects on the questioning strategies of the elderly, *Dev Psychol* 10:458, 1974.

216. Cornelius SW, Caspi A: Everyday problem solving in adulthood and old age, *Psychol Aging* 2:144-153, 1987.

217. Ogden JA: Spatial abilities and deficits in aging and age-related disorders. In Boller F, Grafman J, editors: *Handbook of neuropsychology*, New York, 1990, Elsevier.

218. Shepard RN, Metzler J: Mental rotation of three-dimensional objects, *Science* 171:701-703, 1971.

219. Berg CA, Hertzog C, Hunt E: Age differences in the speed of mental rotation, *Dev Psychol* 18:95-107, 1982.

220. Cerella J, Poon LW, Fozard JL: Mental rotation and age reconsidered, *J Gerontol* 38:447-454, 1981.

221. Gaylord SA, Marsh GR: Age differences in the speed of a spatial cognitive process, *J Gerontol* 30:674-678, 1975.

222. Jacewicz MM, Hartley AA: Rotation of mental images by young and old college students: effects of familiarity, *J Gerontol* 34:396-403, 1979.

223. Herman JF, Bruce PR: Adults' mental rotation of spatial information: effects of age, sex, and cerebral laterality, *Exp Aging Res* 9:83-85, 1983.

224. Aubrey JB, Li KZ, Dobbs AR: Age differences in the interpretation of misaligned "you-are-here" maps, *J Gerontol Psychol Sci* 49:P29-P31, 1994.

225. Walsh DA, Krauss IK, Regnier VA: Spatial ability, environmental knowledge, and environmental use: the elderly. In Libon L, Patterson A, Newcombe NI, editors: *Spatial representation and behavior across the life span*, New York, 1981, Academic Press.

226. Ohta RJ: Spatial orientation in the elderly: the current status of understanding. In Pick HL, Acredelo LP, editors: *Spatial orientation: theory, research, and application*, New York, 1983, Plenum Press.

227. Wochinger K, Boehm-Davis D: *The effects of age, spatial ability, and navigational information on navigational performance* (Report no. FHWA-RD-95-166), Washington, DC, 1995, U.S. Department of Transportation.

228. Kelso JAS: *Human motor behavior, an introduction*, Hillsdale, NJ, 1982, Lawrence Erlbaum Associates.

229. Marottoli RA, Drickamer MA: Psychomotor mobility and the elderly driver, *Clin Geriatr Med* 9:403-411, 1993.

230. McPherson K, Michael J, Ostrow A, et al: *Physical fitness and the aging driver. Phase I*, Washington, DC, 1988, AAA Foundation for Traffic Safety.

231. States JD: Musculo-skeletal system impairment related to safety and comfort of drivers 55+. In Malfetti JW, editor: *Proceedings of the older driver colloquium*, Falls Church, VA, 1985, AAA Foundation for Traffic Safety.

232. Malfetti JW: *Needs and problems of older drivers: survey results and recommendations*, Falls Church, VA, 1985, AAA Foundation for Traffic Safety.

233. Bulstrode SJ: Car mirrors for drivers with restricted neck mobility, *Int Disabil Stud* 9:180-181, 1987.

234. Yee D: A survey of the traffic safety needs and problems of drivers age 55 and over. In Malfetti JW, editor: *Needs and problems of older drivers: survey results and recommendations*, Falls Church, VA, 1985, AAA Foundation for Traffic Safety.

235. Anshel MH: Effect of aging on acquisition and short-term retention of a motor skill, *Perceptual Motor Skills* 47:993-994, 1978.

236. Marshall PH, Elias JW, Wright J: Age related factors in motor error detection and correction, *Exp Aging Res* 11:201-206, 1985.

237. Szafran J: *Some experiments on motor performance in relation to aging*, 1953, Unpublished Thesis, Cambridge University.

238. Welford AT: Psychomotor performance, *Ann Rev Gerontol Geriatr* 4:237, 1959.

239. Ruch PL: The differentiative effects of age upon human learning, *J Gen Psychol* 11:261-286, 1934.

240. Snoddy GS: Learning and stability, *J Appl Psychol* 10:1-36, 1926.

241. Wright BM, Paine RB: Effects of aging on sex differences in psychomotor reminiscence and tracking proficiency, *J Gerontol* 40:179-184, 1985.

242. Petrofsky JS, Lind AR: Aging, isometric strength and endurance, and cardiovascular responses to static effort, *J Appl Psychol* 1:91-95, 1975.

243. Shepard RJ: Aging and exercise. In Fahey TD, editor: *Encyclopedia of sport medicine and science*, 1998. Available at: http:\\sportsci.org. Accessed February 11, 2005.

244. Eby DW, Molnar LJ: Older drivers: validating a self-assessment instrument with clinical measures and actual driving, *Gerontology* 41:370, 2001.

245. Marottoli RA, Cooney LM, Wagner DR, et al: Predictors of automobile crashes and moving violations among elderly drivers, *Ann Intern Med* 121:842-846, 1994.

246. Staplin L, Gish KW, Wagner EK: MaryPODS revisited: updated crash analysis and implications for screening program implementation, *J Safety Res* 34:389-397, 2003.

247. Fiatarone MA, Marks EC, Ryan ND, et al: High intensity strength training in nonagenarians: effects on skeletal muscles, *JAMA* 263:3029-3034, 1990.

248. American Occupational Therapy Association: *Keeping older drivers safe on the road*, Bethesda, MD, 2004, AOTA.

249. Insurance Institute for Highway Safety: *U.S. drivers licensing renewal procedures for older drivers, as of June 2003*. Available at:*http://www.highwaysafety.org/safety_facts/state_laws/older_drivers.htm*. Accessed November 5, 2004.

250. Staplin L, Lococo KH, Stewart J, et al: *Safe mobility for older people: notebook*. Report no. DOT HS 808 853, Washington, DC, 1999, National Highway Traffic Safety Administration.

251. Wang CC: *Physicians guide to assessing and counseling older drivers* [electronic version], Chicago, 2003, American Medical Association.

252. Carr DB: The older adult driver, *Am Fam Physician* 61:141-146, 2000.

253. Eby DW, Molnar LJ, Shope JT, et al: Improving older driver knowledge and awareness through self-assessment: the Driving Decisions Workbook, *J Safety Res* 34:371-381, 2003.

254. Eby DW, Shope JT, Molnar LJ, et al: *Improvement of older driver safety through self-evaluation: the development of a self-evaluation instrument* (Report no. UMTRI-2000-04), Ann Arbor, MI, 2000, University of Michigan Transportation Research Institute.

255. CH2MHILL: *Guidance for implementation of the AASHTO strategic highway safety plan: a guide for addressing crashes involving older drivers, 2000.* Available at: *http://www.ch2m.com/nchrp/old_drvr/assets/ODguide.pdf.* Accessed March 4, 2003.

256. Marottoli RA: The physician's role in the assessment of older drivers, *Am Fam Physician* 61:39-42, 2000.

257. American Association of Retired Persons: *Auto insurance discounts for AARP driver safety program graduates*, 2004. Available at: *http://www.aarp.org/life/drive/driveprogram/Articles/a2004-06-07-insurancediscounts.html#mandatory.* Accessed November 10, 2004.

258. Elsworth J: *Older driver, wiser drivers: about the Wiser Driver Program*, 2002. Available at: *http://www.saferoads2002.com/papers/Elsworth,J.pdf.* Accessed March 30, 2003.

259. American Association of Retired Persons: *55 alive/mature driver safety program*, Washington, DC, 1998, AARP.

260. National Safety Council: *State certified programs*, 2004. Available at: http://www.nsc.org/training/programs.htm. Accessed November 10, 2004.

261. Ostrow AC, Shaffron P, McPherson K: The effects of a joint range-of-motion physical fitness training program on the automobile driving skills of older adults, *J Safety Res* 23:207-219, 1992.

262. American Association of Motor Vehicle Administrators: *Aging drivers: getting around safe and sound*, 2003. Available at: http://www.aamva.org/drivers/drv_AgingDriversGettingAround.asp. Accessed June 25, 2003.

263. Mollenhauer MA, Dingus TA, Hulse MC: *The potential for advanced vehicle systems to increase mobility of elderly drivers*, Iowa City, IA, 1995, University of Iowa.

264. Mitchell CGB: *The potential of intelligent transportation systems to increase accessibility to transport for elderly and disabled people*, Report no. TP 12926E, Montreal, Quebec, 1997, Transportation Development Centre.

265. Shaheen S, Niemeier D: *Integrating vehicle design and human factors: minimizing elderly driving constraints*, Report no. UCD-ITS-REP-01-06, Davis, CA, 2001, Institute of Transportation Studies, UC Davis.

266. Koppa R: Automotive adaptive equipment and vehicle modifications. In *Transportation in an aging society: a decade of experience*, Washington, DC, 2004, Transportation Research Board, pp. 227-235.

267. Caird JK: In-vehicle intelligent transportation systems: safety and mobility of older drivers. In *Transportation in an aging society: a decade of experience*, Washington, DC, 2004, Transportation Research Board, pp. 236-255.

268. Caird JK, Chugh JS, Wilcox S, et al: *A design guideline and evaluation framework to determine the relative safety of in-vehicle intelligent transportation systems for older drivers*, Report no. TP 13349E, Montreal, 1998, Transportation Development Centre.

269. National Highway Traffic Safety Administration: *Adapting motor vehicles for people with disabilities* [brochure], Washington, DC, 2001, U.S. Department of Transportation.

270. Dingus T, Hulse MC, Mollnehauer MA, et al: Effects of age, system experience, and navigation technique on driving with an advanced traveler information system, *Hum Factors* 39:177-179, 1997.

271. Glanz K, Lewis FM, Rimer BK: Linking theory, research, and practice. In Glanz K, Lewis FM, Rimer BK, editors: *Health behavior and health education: theory, research, and practice*, San Francisco, 1997, Jossey-Bass Publishers.

272. Prochaska JO, DiClemente CC: Stages and processes of self change in smoking: towards an integrative model of change, *J Consult Clin Psychol* 51:390-395, 1983.

273. Prochaska JO, DiClemente CC: Common processes of self change in smoking, weight control, and psychological distress. In Shiffman S, Willis TA, editors: *Coping and substance abuse*, San Diego, 1985, Academic Press.

274. Prochaska JO, Velicer WF: The transtheoretical model of health behavior, *Am J Health Promotion* 12:38-48, 1997.

275. Brug J, Glanz K, Kok G: The relationship between self-efficacy, attitudes, intake compared to others, consumption, and stages of change related to fruit and vegetables, *Am J Health Promotion* 12:25-30, 1997.

276. Prochaska JO, Velicer WF, Rossi JS, et al: Stages of change and decisional balance for 12 problem behaviors, *Health Psychol* 13:39-46, 1994.

277. Prochaska JO, Velicer WF, Guadagnali E, et al: Patterns of change: dynamic typology applied to smoking cessation, *Multivariate Behav Res* 26:83-107, 1991.

278. Ruggiero L, Redding C, Rossi JS, et al: A stage-matched smoking cessation program for pregnant smokers, *Am J Health Promotion* 12:31-33, 1997.

279. Unger JB: Stages of change of smoking cessation: relationships with other health behaviors, *Am J Prevent Med* 12:134-138, 1996.

280. Werch CE: Expanding the stages of change: a program matched to the stages of alcohol acquisition, *Am J Health Promotion* 12:34-37, 1997.

281. Jamner MS, Wolitski RJ, Corby NH: Impact of a longitudinal community HIV intervention targeting injecting drug users' stage of change for condom and bleach use, *Am J Health Promotion* 12:15-24, 1997.

282. Cardinal BJ: Construct validity of stages of change for exercise behavior, *Am J Health Promotion* 12:68-74, 1997.

283. Courneya KS: Perceived severity of the consequences of physical inactivity across the stages of change in older adults, *J Sport Exerc Psychol* 17:447-457, 1995.

284. Courneya KS: Understanding readiness for regular physical activity in older individuals: an application of the theory of planned behavior, *Health Psychol* 14:80-87, 1995.

285. Lee C: Attitudes, knowledge, and stages of change: a survey of exercise patterns in older Australian women, *Health Psychol* 12:476-480, 1993.

286. Gorely T, Gordon S: An examination of the transtheoretical model and exercise behavior in older adults, *J Sport Exerc Psychol* 17:312-324, 1995.

287. Marcus BH, Banspach SW, Lefevre RC, et al: Using the stages of change model to increase the adoption of physical activity among community participants, *Am J Health Promotion* 6:424-429, 1992.

288. Reed GR, Velicer WF, Prochaska JO, et al: What makes a good staging algorithm: examples from regular exercise, *Am J Health Promotion* 12:57-66, 1997.

289. Prochaska JO: Strong and weak principles for progressing from precontemplation to action on the basis of twelve problem behaviors, *Health Psychol* 13:47-51, 1994.

290. Herrick AB, Stone WJ, Mettler MM: Stages of change, decisional balance, and self-efficacy across four health behaviors in a worksite environment, *Am J Health Promotion* 12:49-56, 1997.

291. Haber D: Strategies to promote the health of older people: an alternative to readiness stages, *Fam Commun Health* 19:1-10, 1996.

292. Lerman C, Glanz K: Stress, coping, and health behavior. In Glanz K, Lewis FM, Rimer BK, editors: *Health behavior and health education: theory, research, and practice*, San Francisco, 1997, Jossey-Bass Publishers.

293. Lazarus RS, Folkman S: *Stress, appraisal, and coping*, New York, 1984, Springer Publishing, Inc.

294. Thoits PA: Stress, coping, and social support processes: where are we? What next? *J Health Soc Behav* extra issue:53-79, 1995.

295. Folkman S, Lazarus RS: An analysis of coping in a middle-aged community sample, *J Health Soc Behav* 21:219-239, 1980.

296. Porter LS, Stone AA: Are there really gender differences in coping? A reconsideration of previous data and results from a daily study, *J Soc Clin Psychol* 14:184-202, 1995.

297. Kostyniuk LP, Trombley DA, Shope JT: *The process of reduction and cessation of driving among older drivers: a review of the literature*, Report no. UMTRI-98-23, Ann Arbor, MI, 1998, The University of Michigan Transportation Research Institute.

298. Landreville P, Dube M, Lalande G, et al: Appraisal, coping, and depressive symptoms in older adults with reduced mobility, *J Soc Behav Pers* 9:269-286, 1994.

299. Simons RL, West GE: Life changes, coping resources, and health among the elderly, *Int J Aging Hum Dev* 20:173-189, 1985.

300. Wortman CB, Silver RC: Reconsidering assumptions about coping with loss: an overview of current research. In Montada L, Filipp S-H, Lerner ML, editors: *Life crises and experiences of loss in adulthood*, Hillsdale, NJ, 1992, Lawrence Erlbaum.

301. Weinstein ND: The precaution adoption process, *Health Psychol* 7:355-386, 1988.

302. Weinstein ND, Rothman AJ, Sutton SR: Stage theories of health behavior: conceptual and methodological issues, *Health Psychol* 17:290-299, 1998.

303. Kostyniuk LP, Shope JT, Molnar LJ: Driving reduction/cessation among older drivers: toward a behavioral framework. In Hensher B, editor: *Travel behaviour research, the leading edge*, Amsterdam, 2001, Pergamon Press.

304. Coughlin JF, Lacombe A: Ten myths about transportation for the elderly, *Transport Q* 51:91-100, 1997.

305. U.S. Department of Transportation: *Improving transportation for a maturing society*, Report DOT-P10-07-01, Washington, DC, 1997, Office of the Assistant Secretary for Transportation Policy.

306. Beverly Foundation: *Innovations for seniors: public and community transit services respond to special needs*, Pasadena, CA, 2004, The Beverly Foundation.

307. Bruff JT, Evans J: *Elderly mobility and safety: the Michigan approach final plan of action*, 1999. Available at: *http://www.semcog.org/Products/pdfs/eldmob_final.pdf*. Accessed March 24, 2003.

308. Federal Highway Administration: *1995 nationwide personal transportation survey data files*, Report no. FHWA PL-97-034, Washington DC, 1997, U.S. Department of Transportation.

309. Kostyniuk LP, Shope JT: Driving and alternatives: older drivers in Michigan, *J Safety Res* 34:407-414, 2003.

310. Beverly Foundation: *Supplemental transportation programs for seniors*, 2001. Available at: *http://www.seniordrivers.org/research/stp.pdf*. Accessed March 11, 2003.

311. Burkhardt JE, McGavock AT, Nelson CA: *Improving public transit options for older persons, vol 1: handbook* [electronic version] (Report no. 82), Washington, DC, 2002, Transportation Research Board.

312. Burkhardt JE, McGavock AT, Nelson CA, et al: *Improving public transit options for older persons, vol 2: final report* [electronic version] (Report no. 82), Washington, DC, 2002, Transportation Research Board.

313. Murray G, Koffman D, Chambers C, et al: *Strategies to assist local transportation agencies in becoming mobility managers* (TCRP Report no. 21), 1997. Available at: *http://gulliver.trb.org/publications/tcrp/tcrp_rpt_21-a.pdf*. Accessed March 16, 2005.

Chapter 22

URBAN PLANNING FOR EFFICIENT COMMUNITY MOBILITY

Kevin Borsay • Mark Nickita

KEY TERMS

- Single-use zoning
- Housing density
- Mixed-use zoning
- Neighborhood

CHAPTER OBJECTIVES

After completing this chapter, the reader will be able to do the following:

- Understand how the physical design of different communities affects one's daily life and impacts mobility choices.
- Understand the difference between suburban and urban living and how it applies to the client's driving needs.
- Recognize options specific to the client's community mobility needs.

URBAN DESIGN

The physical design of a community intimately affects our daily lives. It is intricately woven into our daily activities. It affects everything we do: from how we live, to how we get around, to how we interact with our fellow citizens. The design of a community not only influences these activities but also determines how we go about them.

More specifically the mobility choices that are available to the general population are largely determined by the physical design of the communities we live in. Communities are designed with physical characteristics that directly restrict or enhance personal mobility choices. These characteristics range from the presence of sidewalks, to the distances between buildings, to the availability of diverse alternative transportation options, all of which greatly affect the amount of time and expense people spend getting to and from their destinations. However, for people with disabilities, elderly persons, and individuals who care for them, the expenditure of time and money that is required to access reliable community mobility is well beyond their means.

Driving an automobile is the universally available transportation option in North America. But is driving the best choice for cost-effective, reliable, accessible, and safe community mobility? Driving is an expensive and dangerous undertaking. Automobile ownership is costly on many levels. First it costs its owner a great deal monetarily each year to own and operate. A car not only must be purchased but also maintained, repaired, kept filled with fuel and other critical fluids, licensed, insured, and housed. Even more importantly driving also has proven to be an extraordinarily dangerous activity. According to the National Highway Transportation and Safety Administration,[1] >40,000 Americans are killed in automobile accidents every year, and another 250,000 people are seriously injured. Even with the continuous introduction of automobile safety features, such as front air bags, side air bags, antilock brakes, crumple zones, and many others, the yearly death and injury toll from motor vehicle crashes remains high.

The physical structure of a community will determine the number of mobility options that residents have available to them beyond the automobile. A community's physical structure includes the proximity of its amenities and transportation infrastructure to residences and businesses. Communities that offer a number of mobility options, from which people can choose, can greatly enhance or detract from the ease, safety, and quality of living.

Communities can be categorized based on their physical design characteristics. The three types of communities that constitute most metropolitan living, work, and social arrangements in North America are as follows:

- Suburban
- Urban
- Some combination of the two

SUBURBAN CHARACTERISTICS

Suburban communities exist outside the periphery of larger cities and most often exhibit physical characteristics that greatly differ from urban neighborhoods. The major common physical characteristic that these communities exhibit is that they are designed specifically and almost exclusively for automobile use. Wide roads, large distances between structures, and the lack of pedestrian and transit infrastructure are common visual cues that indicate such areas. The majority of suburban communities in North America were founded and built in the second half of the twentieth century. This was a time when government officials, urban planners, architects, and developers broke away from traditional town and neighborhood planning methods and developed concepts that were at the time considered modern. The automobile was seen as the wave of the future for personal mobility, and the post–World War II period in the United States saw a rush to fully embrace and exclusively promote its use when planning and building new communities. Laws and building codes across the country were enacted that promoted this philosophy. Tax structures and government funding mechanisms were created to subsidize it, and ultimately, from the desire to create automobile-centric communities, the 1950s planning concept that evolved and became entrenched across the suburban United States was that of single-use zoning.

Single-Use Zoning

Single-use zoning legally mandates a separation of most community uses, including all residential, retail, and office activities. During community planning stages, uses are isolated and grouped by similarity. Retail stores are separated from residential areas. Office uses are often separated from retail and residential areas, and so on. For example a restaurant, pharmacy, or grocery market may be prohibited from being too close to a residential area. This legally mandated separation has led to the building of countless suburban communities where residents are often disconnected and isolated

from one another and unable to meet their daily needs. The result of single-use zoning is that in most cases residents and visitors are forced to depend on an automobile for community mobility.

Single-use residential and commercial suburban structures are generally constructed without efficiently using land and often have an excessive amount of space between them. Commercial and retail establishments in suburban communities are generally set far from the road where access is difficult or dangerous without an automobile.

Residential areas are often created in a physical form commonly referred to as subdivisions. Housing in these areas tends to be single family in nature and one or two stories in height. Large open spaces generally separate the houses from each other and from the street. A sidewalk may or may not exist, and the street itself tends to be wider than necessary to accommodate subdivision needs. These subdivisions tend to be physically isolated from other subdivisions. Housing units in subdivisions also are most often located a great distance from any type of amenity, including retail stores, banks, pharmacies, restaurants, parks, schools, and religious and cultural institutions. An automobile generally is required to access the main road and to accomplish almost all daily errands.

Commercial areas, along with any amenities that they may offer, are generally placed far from the residents who use them and are designed so that access without an automobile is difficult. Commercial areas are dominated by large, unsightly surface parking lots that are created to accommodate extreme parking capacities that rarely if ever occur. These parking lots are generally the first view one sees when visiting a suburban retail store or commercial establishment, which further isolates it from its surrounding community.

Suburban Housing Density

Another constraint on the proximity of suburban commercial amenities is their direct relation to suburban housing density. *Housing density* is defined as the number of residential dwellings per acre. Suburban housing tends to be at low densities, sometimes as low as one residential unit per acre. Commercial amenities, such as retail stores, directly depend on the number of nearby residential dwellings. Developers will often count "rooftops" (dwelling units) to justify the need for a certain type of establishment, such as a produce market or hardware store. The lower the housing densities, the farther the distance between amenities. The higher the residential densities, the closer the amenities are together.

Auto-centric Communities

The common theme one will find for suburban, subdivision-based communities is that an automobile is required for every need, from commuting to work, to visiting friends, to buying a quart of milk or a loaf of bread. These auto-centric communities offer almost no alternative to driving. The many communities that lack sidewalks force residents without automobile access to walk in the street. They also lack full integration with a comprehensive transit system, such as buses, streetcars, subways, or rail lines. Although sometimes serviced by a public bus system, service is usually extremely limited with vast distances between transit stops. Their excessively wide roads with fast moving motor vehicles are difficult and dangerous for pedestrians to cross. By virtue of their physical design, these communities isolate and divide residents, severely limit driver alternatives, and prevent or restrict almost all nonautomobile-centered activities. For example a senior citizen who does not drive and is living in a subdivision has almost no hope of getting to the grocery store or pharmacy without a personal driver or access to a costly private transportation service.

The physical design of a subdivision can lead to not only physical isolation but also the emotional isolation of its residents. Because of the excessive distances between houses, lack of sidewalks and public spaces, and many other reasons caused by the design of their single-use environment, there are few places for casual public interaction. With few public opportunities for informal meetings and interaction, it is difficult to nurture a sense of community with others. Many times residents know only the person living in the housing unit on either side of their own. This can leave many residents, especially those who do not have a personal driver or access to private transportation or an automobile—namely, the young and the elderly populations or people with disabilities—feeling increasingly isolated and alone. By default they are reduced to the status of second-class citizens. Often isolated and stranded in a single-family housing unit subdivision, far from amenities and a robust social life, they must rely on others for accessibility to the outside world. In need of the constant assistance of a personal driver or chauffeur service to maintain social ties and their personal freedom, independence to come and go as they choose is virtually nonexistent. Even those with automobile access are most likely to travel to and from every destination inside their car, van, or truck, isolated from casual public contact.

Unfortunately for many, subdivisions, by the nature of how they are planned and constructed, isolate and discriminate against many segments of the population. Automobile ownership in these areas is mandatory to be a full participant in community life. Without access to automobiles, residents are often left isolated and therefore denied opportunities to achieve full community participation.

The Costs of Owning an Automobile
The burden of automobile ownership can be extreme in suburban communities. The annual cost of owning, maintaining, and insuring a vehicle is a great expense for a large part of the U.S. population. A suburban lifestyle often mandates automobile ownership for full participation in the community, and therefore its owner is responsible for all of the expenses that go along with it.

URBAN CHARACTERISTICS
Urban communities are the historic population and business centers that exist throughout the United States. These areas are generally found in larger cities and often offer a wide range of amenities and community mobility options. Because the built environment is by design intended to be compact (i.e., dense), these neighborhoods or districts generally have a variety of housing types, amenities, and transportation options close by. For example a resident can walk out the front door of his or her residence and be within 1200 feet or a 5-minute walk to access parks, schools, restaurants, libraries, and a constellation of other public and private spaces, not to mention other humans. Possessing the ability to access places that enable social interaction and access to needed services and commodities allows for daily needs to be met. Groceries, general shopping, restaurants, pharmacies, and various transportation and mobility options are close by, and connecting with friends and relatives or attending work, school, leisure, or religious activities is easily achieved.

Mixed-Use Zoning
Historically urban communities have used the traditional planning concept of *mixed-use zoning*. This permits and encourages a mixed use of activities in a designated district, block, or even one building. This allows for residential, retail, and office activities to coexist within a more compressed area. For example a restaurant or grocery store can be directly adjacent to a residential area or even occupy the ground floor of a residential building. This mixed-use urban arrangement efficiently connects community residents to their daily local destinations. The result is a reduction in the need for automobile use and an allowance for the introduction of multiple mobility options, including walking, biking, a motorized scooter or wheelchair, and of course public transit.

What Is a Neighborhood?
To the general public the definition of a *neighborhood* has evolved over the years. The term is frequently misused to describe where one lives. For example someone

may say, "There are many children in my neighborhood," when they are referring to a subdivision in which they live. Contrary to popular belief, a subdivision is not a neighborhood. A neighborhood is much more than a group of similar-looking housing units.

The definition of a neighborhood includes a variety of characteristics. These include the ability to walk within one-quarter of a mile to a variety of amenities, commercial activity, and public transit. In a properly designed neighborhood, schools and religious facilities are integrated into the residential fabric. Parks, playgrounds, and recreational facilities are nestled among the residential and commercial structures. A neighborhood also includes a variety of residential building types that may include single-family and multifamily structures.

In the book *The New Urbanism: Toward an Architecture of Community*, renowned architects and planners Andres Duany and Elizabeth Plater-Zyberk describe a properly designed neighborhood as having the following characteristics:

> 1) The neighborhood has a center and an edge; 2) The optimal size of a neighborhood is a quarter mile from center to edge; 3) The neighborhood has a balanced mix of activities— dwelling, shopping, working, schooling, worshipping, and recreating; 4) The neighborhood structures, building sites and traffic exist on a fine network of interconnecting streets; 5) The neighborhood gives priority to public space and the appropriate location of civic buildings.[2]

A broad range of housing options can generally be found in urban neighborhoods. Multistory residential buildings and multifamily and single-family homes are often in close proximity. Residential structures are built closer together and close to the street to minimize the space between and to use land more efficiently. Sidewalks are always present and lead to nearby amenities. Streets are wide enough to accommodate automobiles but not unnecessarily wide as to act as a physical barrier.

Commercial amenities are located within one-quarter of a mile of residential housing. Establishments such as markets, retail stores, pharmacies, banks, and restaurants are built directly next to the sidewalk with parking on the street or in the rear of the structure. In addition to being accessible by automobile, commercial establishments in properly built urban neighborhoods are easily and safely accessible by foot, motorized scooter, wheelchair, and public transit.

A common theme found in urban neighborhoods when they are properly designed and built is that of personal mobility choice. By virtue of the compact nature of their physical design and mixed-use zoning characteristics, urban neighborhoods offer convenient mobility options to satisfy daily personal transportation needs. Comprehensive public transit systems that offer options such as streetcars, buses, and subways are embedded into the infrastructure of the neighborhood and complement the freedom of choosing to walk, bike, rollerblade, use a manual wheelchair, use a motorized scooter or power wheelchair, or use an automobile as a driver or passenger.

When living in an urban neighborhood, residents can make use of the variety of convenient mobility options generally available and can often avoid the burden of automobile ownership. Although rider fees for public transit could apply, these are small when compared with the heavy cost of purchasing, maintaining, repairing, licensing, fueling, and insuring an automobile annually. If residents desire automobile ownership or use, they have the option of using it at their discretion.

Because of the compact nature of a properly designed and built urban neighborhood, the opportunities for casual social interaction are far more abundant than in nonurban places. Having people living closer together with all amenities within a 5-minute walk encourages them to get out of their automobiles and use the public sidewalks to accomplish many of their daily tasks. Residents using sidewalks creates a healthier environment. It provides opportunities for unexpected meetings and casual social interaction. This can be of great benefit in helping people feel like they are fully part of their community.

An added public health benefit of built environments that encourage residents to use sidewalks is the increase of physical activity. Residents directly benefit from a lifestyle arrangement that encourages walking to accomplish many daily tasks.

Properly designed urban neighborhoods provide not only greater mobility choice for the individual but also they provide greater independence for young and elderly persons and those with disabilities. By virtue of their built physical environment, these neighborhoods allow individuals to express and maintain a large degree of independence, freedom, and dignity by accomplishing many if not all daily tasks on their own. They can be more fully integrated and feel part of their community just by being out on their own.

CASE STUDIES

In the case studies we will look at three types of living arrangements: suburban, urban, and a combination of the two. We will examine how the design of each type of community can enhance or restrict personal mobility choices, encourage or suppress daily mobility freedom and independence, and how each affects an individual's isolation or integration into a community.

The suburban example is Sterling Heights, Michigan. This community is an example of fully implemented, low-density 1950s planning principles. The urban example is the St. Lawrence neighborhood in Toronto, Ontario, Canada. The St. Lawrence neighborhood is an example of a properly built, traditional mixed-use urban neighborhood. The semiurban example is Birmingham, Michigan, which reflects a combination of single-use and mixed-use planning.

CASE 1: SUBURBAN EXAMPLE

The city of Sterling Heights, Michigan is located a few miles north of Detroit and has a population of approximately 127,000 residents. Led by the industrial giants of the automotive industry in search of cheap land outside Detroit, Sterling Township became home to many new industrial plants during the mid-1950s. New residents followed to the previously rural area, and the township grew until it incorporated as the City of Sterling Heights in 1968.

Sterling Heights is an example of an automobile-centered suburban community that has embraced and fully implemented the 1950s planning concept of single-use zoning. For example residences are separated from commercial areas, and offices are separated from residential and commercial activity. Each use is physically isolated and often located at great distances from the other. In terms of mobility an automobile is generally the sole means for reasonable accessibility to each use.

The community is physically made up of a series of wide perpendicular arterial roads spaced approximately 1 mile apart and forming a 6-mile × 6-mile grid. The arterial roads are six to nine lanes wide and are designed to accommodate large volumes of traffic moving at high speeds. These roads act as dangerous and almost impassible barriers for those not riding in an automobile.

The arterial roads also are wide and visually unappealing, especially to a pedestrian or to anyone not traveling at high speeds inside the comfort of an automobile. This visual unsightliness successfully discourages most pedestrian-based activity. Sidewalks may or may not be present. The idea of traversing vast distances across wide roads and past enormous parking lots to various commercial destinations on foot or in a motorized scooter or wheelchair can be a dismal and even brutal adventure that few choose to undertake.

Within the grid formed by the arterial roads, residential developments have been constructed that have the physical form of a suburban subdivision. These subdivisions consist of homogeneous, low-density housing built far from the street and have an excessive amount of space between them. Once inside the subdivision the only legally permitted use is that of a residential structure. Markets, pharmacies, retail stores, and nonresidential structures are prohibited and must be located outside of the subdivision.

Subdivisions can be large, often containing a vast number of houses, sometimes as many as several hundred. Many subdivisions are without sidewalks, and those that do have them are generally limited to the area inside a specific development or lead only to an arterial road. All daily amenities are inconveniently located outside the subdivision and are generally a great distance from each individual housing unit.

Multifamily condominiums and apartments are also present in the city. However, these also have the physical arrangement of a subdivision and are generally accessible only by automobile from a single access road. These structures are placed far from the street and from each other, and like their single-family subdivision counterparts, they are isolated and separated from all commercial activities and from the rest of the community.

Noticeably lacking in Sterling Heights is the presence of a downtown or any kind of public center where commercial and social activity can take place. Like so much of the suburban United States, all commercial amenities are either located inside a shopping mall or sporadically placed behind large, unsightly parking lots along wide arterial roads. Commercial buildings, such as grocery stores, pharmacies, restaurants, and retail stores, are isolated from area residences; by design, access is made difficult and dangerous without an automobile.

Public transportation options are extremely limited. The regional bus service has several stops within the city. However, these stops are generally inconveniently located and are physically separated from residential subdivisions. Most if not all bus stops would require the use of an automobile to traverse the distance from the bus stop to a typical dwelling. Bus stops also are generally placed along wide arterial roads without the benefit of a transit shelter. This often dangerous and inhospitable situation leaves riders exposed to the elements and standing next to many lanes of high-speed motor vehicle traffic. Not many residents who have a choice dare to venture into such hostile conditions.

Sterling Heights is a community that is designed to restrict mobility choice. To live a reasonable life in this suburb, automobile dependence is mandatory along with all of its associated expenses. Automobile ownership or access to a personal driver or chauffeur service is required to accomplish even the most basic errands. Without automobile access, residents are isolated and are forced to forfeit a great deal of their independence because they have almost no hope of reaching their daily destinations. Residents who are too old or too young and those who have special needs are reduced to the status of second-class citizens.

CASE 2: URBAN EXAMPLE

Founded in 1793, the city of Toronto, Canada has >2.4 million residents. It is located in the southern part of the province of Ontario and sits along the northwestern edge of Lake Ontario. There are many good examples of properly designed urban neighborhoods throughout this city.

One such urban neighborhood is St. Lawrence, which borders the eastern edge of downtown Toronto. The neighborhood is a true mix of uses, including residential, retail, office, recreational, religious, institutional, and transit. Compact and built at high densities, St. Lawrence offers this diverse mix of uses along with every amenity imaginable all within a few square blocks. St. Lawrence gives its residents the power of choice in their daily mobility options and offers ample opportunity for full integration into daily neighborhood life.

Like any properly built higher-density urban neighborhood, buildings in St. Lawrence are built close together and up to the sidewalk. This compact neighborhood design allows amenities to be close and accessible to residences. Many times amenities occupy first-floor retail space below residential units, which further enhances convenience. Street widths tend to be narrower rather than wider, which, along with frequent curb cuts and abundant pedestrian-crossing signals, make them easy to cross.

The streets in St. Lawrence are visually appealing and inviting places. Compact and lined with attractive retail storefronts, restaurants, and cafes, the neighborhood sidewalks act as inviting outdoor spaces that are generally filled with people and activity during most hours of the day.

The St. Lawrence neighborhood offers true convenience in terms of amenities. It offers a fresh food market, a full-service 24-hour grocery store, >100 specialty retail shops, many banks, pharmacies, and numerous restaurants ranging from fine dining to diners and quick carry-outs. St. Lawrence also offers Berczy Park, a quiet, human-scaled green space with a fountain and benches at its center. St. Lawrence is home to several religious institutions and a college and has St. Michael's Hospital at its northern edge. St. Lawrence also is one block away from downtown Toronto and all of the amenities that it has to offer.

At the heart of the St. Lawrence neighborhood is the St. Lawrence Market. Established in 1807, this wonderful amenity occupies a renovated historic building and offers >50 food vendors, including those selling fresh meat, fish, poultry, bread, baked goods, and many specialty food items. Physically located at the center of the neighborhood, residents are never more than just a few blocks away from its offerings.

Having the opportunity to casually meet people in the neighborhood where one resides is an important factor in residents feeling that they are a part of the community. When visiting St. Lawrence, one finds people of all ages and social and income classes. One is likely to find high-paid professionals, retired senior citizens, and young families all living in the same building or on the same block. The sidewalks, parks, markets, and cafes provide ample opportunities for social interaction.

Exiting the front door of their home St. Lawrence residents have convenient access to numerous transportation options all within a short distance. Residents have many choices on how to get to and from their desired destinations to meet their daily needs. Residents who are too young to drive or who have special needs and are unable to drive have the freedom and independence to accomplish their daily trips without a private driver or chauffeur service.

Because the neighborhood has been designed and built in a proper urban fashion, there are many transportation options available besides the automobile. When in the St. Lawrence area one finds most people getting to and from their neighborhood destinations by walking, biking, or using a motorized scooter or wheelchair.

For those who wish to travel to destinations outside the neighborhood, St. Lawrence is well served by the Toronto Transit Commission (TTC). Streetcars run directly through the neighborhood along King Street, Queen Street, and Church Street with stops every couple of blocks. The TTA subway also has a station at King/Yonge Streets at the eastern edge of the neighborhood. Nearby subway stops at Union Station and Queen/Yonge Streets are just two blocks outside the neighborhood. Besides offering a subway stop, Union Station is a hub for the GO Train, which provides regional rail service to points outside of Toronto, and VIA Rail, which provides national rail service to cities and towns throughout Canada.

Close and easily accessible amenities are one of the many advantages of living in the St. Lawrence neighborhood. Having a diverse and abundant variety of amenities and transportation options steps from the front door of neighborhood residences is a neighborhood asset that adds a great deal of convenience, independence, and quality to the lives of the locals.

CASE 3: SEMIURBAN EXAMPLE

Birmingham, Michigan, a northern suburb of Detroit, was founded in 1819 and has approximately 20,000 residents. As a commercial hub for a farming community, for many years the town provided services and products for neighboring rural residents. Its location along the Native American Saginaw Trail (later to be named Woodward Avenue) allowed it to become a population center and a resting point for northern Michigan travelers who moved to and from Detroit.

Birmingham is an example of a small city that historically functioned as an independent population center and over time became engulfed in the suburban expansion of a nearby major metropolis. Most large North American cities have numerous historic small towns, such as Birmingham, that are now part of the suburban landscape. The key difference between these historic suburban communities and the majority of suburbia is that they were initially planned and partially built before the rise and entrenchment of automobile-centric community planning.

The historic centers of these communities generally were planned and built using traditional town planning methods that used a compact, pedestrian-oriented design and permitted mixed-use building opportunities. The initial result was the creation of a small-scale, walkable community that offered residences and commercial establishments in close proximity to each other.

However, as these communities developed over time, especially those that experienced growth from the 1950s through the 1980s, many have adopted suburban characteristics in their newer areas. These areas tend to be farthest from the historic center and characterized by single-use zoning and automobile-centric planning. Although they may contain some urban characteristics, these outer neighborhoods generally lack many of the necessary ingredients of a properly designed and built urban neighborhood.

As with many of these older historic communities, Birmingham has two distinct areas in its built environment. The first and most prominent is its historic center, which has a variety of mixed-use buildings and adjacent multifamily and single-family residences that have been constructed in a proper urban fashion. As the city grew in the latter half of the past century, its newer, outer neighborhoods were planned and built primarily using single-use zoning and are auto-centric in nature.

In more recent years there has been a refocus on Birmingham's historic center. New high-density housing, shops, entertainment centers, and grocery stores along with a wide variety of other amenities have been added or upgraded in its town center. Improved sidewalks, signage, and streetscaping have made its built environment more convenient and user friendly. Residents who live in this part of the city or on the adjacent streets have benefited greatly from these improvements.

Birmingham incorporates numerous housing types in and around its historic center. These include mostly single-family houses in several neighborhoods that surround the downtown, along with higher-density housing closer to and at the center of town. The single-family homes range in size from small cottages to large mansions and range from one to three stories in height. In the historic center of town there are a variety of multifamily housing developments. Row houses and townhouses line several streets adjacent to the downtown commercial district. These structures are similar to single-family houses except that they are connected together.

Apartment buildings are also part of the residential mix in downtown Birmingham. These types of buildings can be condominiums or rental units and provide a higher level of residential density than the townhouse option. Many are zoned for mixed uses and offer first-floor professional or commercial establishments that are a great convenience to residents. Ranging in size from just a few units on two floors to >100 hundred units on 15 floors, these residential buildings create a housing option centered directly in downtown Birmingham and provide effortless pedestrian access to the variety of amenities that exist nearby.

The downtown or commercial center of Birmingham provides most of the conveniences and amenities of a large city district. Within easy walking distances of thousands of residential housing units are a wide variety of food, clothing, and entertainment establishments that are connected with an extensive and convenient network of sidewalks. Restaurants, retail stores, grocery stores, movie theaters, pharmacies, coffee shops, and many other examples are part of the amenity mix that makes this community fundamentally usable and accessible on many levels.

Recreationally the downtown is intertwined with parks and wooded paths that have the ability to present the feeling of being far removed from the city while being only a short distance away. The central green space, Shain Park, is located at the center of town and is the primary civic space adjacent to the city library, city hall, and the entire commercial shopping district.

Public transportation options are limited but available. With bus stops at several points along the community's main street, the transit options are used primarily for riders' travel to other communities in the region.

Overall in terms of mobility, the primary attribute that makes Birmingham an attractive and practical place to live is that when living near or at its center, it offers a way of life that fully incorporates a viable alternative to driving. The physical structure of its compact historic center and adjacent neighborhoods has placed most daily needs within a comfortable distance of residences. Convenient interconnectivity between residents and their daily needs is its key mobility component. The community has been designed so that residents are directly connected to a wide variety of amenities by a comprehensive, attractive, and well-maintained network of sidewalks. The sidewalks, with frequent curb cuts and ample crossing signals, conveniently permit walking, biking, or use by a motorized scooter or wheelchair. An automobile may still be used; however, it can often be used at one's discretion.

SUMMARY

In summary, what alternatives are there to driving? The answer to this question is that it depends primarily on where you live. Some communities offer choice and with it, a certain level of mobility freedom and independence, whereas other communities restrict choice and mandate a singular and often expensive mobility option.

A suburban, subdivision-based lifestyle offers few mobility options beyond driving (or riding in) an automobile. The built environment in these areas is designed in such a way that automobile ownership, a private driver, or chauffeur service is required to maintain a basic level of mobility freedom. When living in a properly designed and built urban environment, residents have many mobility options. These include the automobile, a private driver, or chauffeur service as in suburban living arrangements, but also an intricate and inviting network of sidewalks and the close proximity of amenities and public transit that permit walking and biking along with the use of motorized scooters and power and manual wheelchairs.

When presented with a choice on where to live, it is always better to consider a community that offers a variety of community mobility options, where an automobile can be owned or used at one's discretion, and where daily amenities can be readily accessed.

REFERENCES

1. National Highway Transportation and Safety Administration
2. Duany A, Plater-Zyberk E: The neighborhood, the district and the corridor. In Katz P: *The new urbanism: toward an architecture of community*, New York, 1994, McGraw-Hill, pp. xvii-xx.

Part VI

PROFESSIONAL ETHICS AND EVIDENCE-BASED DRIVER REHABILITATION PRACTICE

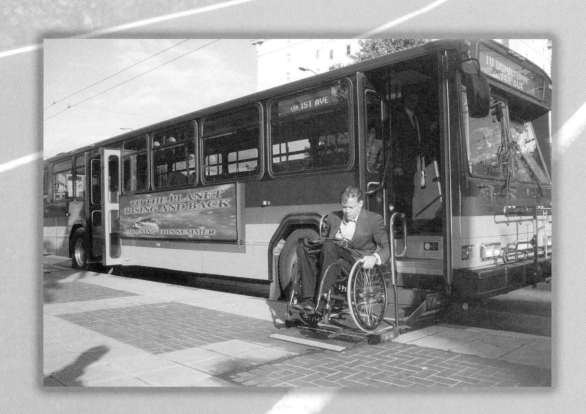

Chapter 23

LEGAL AND PROFESSIONAL ETHICS IN DRIVER REHABILITATION

Janie B. Scott

KEY TERMS

- Professional ethics
- Codes of ethics
- Blood alcohol concentration (BAC)
- Motor Vehicle Administration (MVA)
- National Highway Traffic Safety Administration (NHTSA)
- Medical advisory board (MAB)
- Instrumental activities of daily living (IADL)
- Ethics
- Occupational engagement

CHAPTER OBJECTIVES

After completing this chapter, the reader will be able to do the following:

- Know how many states have different license renewal regulations based on age.
- Know what the state requirements are for physicians and health care professionals to report when they have seen/evaluated/treated someone with a specific medical condition.
- Understand the consequences for not reporting someone.
- Understand what ethical issues and dilemmas driver rehabilitation specialists (DRSs) face.

The purpose of this chapter is to examine some of the legal and ethical issues related to driving and driver rehabilitation. It is not intended to provide the reader with legal advice; rather, it is meant to guide the understanding of legal and ethical issues as they are related to this specialized practice area. Occupational therapists and driver educators specializing in driver rehabilitation, occupational therapy (OT) generalists, and other professional caregivers that provide services to people with disabilities and/or aging-related concerns must possess an understanding of aging, disability, and chronic illness. Additionally, professionals should also recognize and address the psychosocial factors associated with a client's responses to learning that his or her driving has been limited, curtailed, or ended altogether.[1]

So what do ethics have to do with driving? State laws and regulations establish behavioral expectations for professional caregivers and generally provide consequences if those expectations are not met. *Professional ethics* are principles and values articulated by a profession to guide the ethical behavior of practitioners (i.e., clinicians, educators, and researchers) and students. *Codes of ethics* are developed to inform internal and external audiences about the values and beliefs that a particular constituency is expected to emulate. The difference between legal and ethical issues related to this area of practice will be explored throughout this chapter. The driver rehabilitation specialist (DRS), OT student, and OT practitioner (occupational therapist or OT assistant clinician, educator, or researcher) have an obligation to the profession and their clients to know, understand, and apply the legal and ethical principles to their study and practice. When ethical issues are raised in this chapter, reference may be made to the American Occupational Therapy Association's (AOTA) *Occupational Therapy Code of Ethics*, Association for Driver Rehabilitation Specialists (ADED) *Code of Ethics*, or both. Both documents are located in

Appendix C. The intent of identifying specific sections of one or more of the codes is to increase the readers' familiarity with the codes and their application to specific situations.

As you review the content and data in this chapter, keep in mind that drivers and potential drivers of all ages and differing abilities are included implicitly and explicitly. More materials are available that consider issues related to the older driver. Younger persons who have never been issued licenses and have a developmental or acquired disability or individuals who once possessed a driver's license and were injured or disabled are also included in this discussion of legal and ethical issues related to driving and driver rehabilitation. We will briefly review how attitudes toward drinking and driving, *blood alcohol concentration (BAC)* levels, and how substance use and BAC differ among people of different ages and racial and ethnic groups. The purpose of including this information is to underscore the practitioner's need to become knowledgeable about the social and cultural contexts to which each individual client belongs.[2] People's backgrounds, knowledge, and experiences frame their beliefs and value systems. Professionals cannot provide services to individuals without giving recognition to the contextual fabric of their daily lives.

According to the American Medical Association (AMA) and state agencies who issue driver's licenses, a wide range of diagnoses or conditions may affect an individual's ability to drive a motor vehicle safely (Box 23-1). Not all states require a physician, the driver, or someone else (e.g., family members/caregivers, DRS, and health care professionals) to report to the *Motor Vehicle Administration (MVA)* when an individual has a new occurrence or exacerbation of one of these health conditions. It is interesting to note that the majority of these health conditions are seen more frequently among older adults than younger people.

Although "occupational therapist" is frequently identified throughout this chapter, it is not intended to exclude the important role that the OT assistant may play in this practice arena. Rather it is an attempt to reduce redundancy. OT practitioners have a responsibility to adhere to their state regulations governing scope of practice and supervision requirements. The occupational therapist and the OT assistant must also understand conditions for reimbursement by third-party payers. Additionally, other professionals specializing in driver rehabilitation, such as driver educators, can benefit greatly from recognizing and subscribing to the AOTA's *Code of Ethics* whenever possible. The Association for Driver Rehabilitation Specialists (ADED) also has published the *ADED Code of Ethics* that all DRSs, irrespective of professional background and training, should be familiar with as well.

> AOTA's Occupational Therapy Code of Ethics (AOTA Code)
>
> Principle 4. E: Occupational therapy practitioners shall protect service recipients by ensuring that duties assumed by or assigned to other occupational therapy personnel match credentials, qualifications, experience, and scope of practice.
>
> Principle 4. F: Occupational therapy practitioners shall provide appropriate supervision to individuals for whom the practitioners have supervisory responsibility in accordance with Association policies, local, state and federal laws, and institutional values.[3]

DEMOGRAPHICS

United States Census data reflect the anticipated increase in the percentage of older adults between 2000 and 2050. The age group 85+ is the only category where growth is anticipated. Slight declines are expected to occur in all other groupings by 2050. For example, ". . . the United States' older population is growing nearly twice as fast as the total population. . . . these license-holders will drive more miles than older drivers do today."[4] Also of interest are the anticipated changes in racial and ethnic populations (Tables 23-1 and 23-2). The percentage of individuals who identify themselves as solely white is anticipated to decline compared with the rest of the U.S. population. Increases are expected among people in other racial and ethnic groups. Languages other than English spoken at home for individuals age 5 years and older in 2000 were 17.9%. OT managers and other service providers should plan for the effects of these changing demographics. Providers of driver rehabilitation services will need to respond with greater cultural sensitivity, including building bilingual pools of staff as the consumer

BOX 23-1	**Conditions That May Affect Ability to Drive**

Alzheimer's disease
Type II diabetes mellitus
Hypertension
Dementia
Visual deficits
Arthritis
Psychiatric disorders (e.g., depression, schizophrenia, affective disorder, and so forth)
Cerebrovascular accident (Stroke)
Congestive heart failure (CHF)
Syncope and vertigo
Substance abuse
Seizure
Delirium

Table 23-1 Projected Population of the United States, by Age: 2000 to 2050

Age	2000	2010	2020	2030	2040	2050
0-4	6.8%	6.9%	6.8%	6.7%	6.7%	6.7%
5-19	21.7%	20.0%	19.6%	19.5%	19.2%	19.3%
20-44	36.9%	33.8%	32.3%	31.6%	31.0%	31.2%
45-64	22.1%	26.2%	24.9%	22.6%	22.6%	22.2%
65-84	10.9%	11.0%	14.1%	17.0%	16.5%	15.7%
85+	1.5%	2.0%	2.2%	2.6%	3.9%	5.0%

In thousands. As of July 1. Resident Population.

From United States Census Bureau: *United States interim projections by age, sex, race, and Hispanic origin, 2004,* *http://www.census.gov/opc/www/usinterimproj/* Internet release date: March 18, 2004.

Table 23-2 Projected Population Change in the United States, by Race and Hispanic Origin: 2000 to 2050

Percent of Total Population	2000	2010	2020	2030	2040	2050
White alone	81.0	79.3	77.6	75.8	73.9	72.1
Black alone	12.7	13.1	13.5	13.9	14.3	14.6
Asian alone	3.8	4.6	5.4	6.2	7.1	8.0
All other races*	2.5	3.0	3.5	4.1	4.7	5.3

*Includes American Indian and Alaska Native alone, Native Hawaiian and Other Pacific Islander alone, and Two or More Races. As of July 1. Resident population.

From United States Census Bureau: *United States interim projections by age, sex, race, and Hispanic origin, 2004,* *http://www.census.gov/opc/www/usinterimproj/* Internet release date: March 18, 2004.

demands increase. Older drivers will not be the only group who want and need to drive. In 2000, the U.S. Census Bureau reported that 17.4% of the population age 5 and older had disabilities.[5] The Bureau of Transportation Statistics (BTS) estimated that between 1 and 2.3 million households own at least one vehicle modified for a person with a disability.[6] With continued improvements in technology, babies born prematurely, adolescents and adults who sustain traumatic injuries, and people with chronic conditions are more likely to live longer and healthier lives.

The implication for providers of driver evaluation and rehabilitation services is that the demand for services will continue to increase. For the foreseeable future, driving is expected to be viewed as a continuing right of passage and a priority for people of all ages regardless of their functional abilities. The field of OT is in the unique position to anticipate, plan for, and deliver services to this ever-growing and diverse population. AOTA, ADED, *National Highway Traffic Safety Administration (NHTSA)*, and the AMA recognize that occupational therapists have the skills to deliver driver evaluation and rehabilitation services. OT practitioners need to stay alert to the changing demographics and the changes in the laws and reporting requirements to meet both the consumer demands and professional and legal requirements of today and tomorrow.

United States Census data (Tables 23-1 and 23-2) place in context the anticipated growth in the U.S. population from 2000 to 2050 by age group. The segment of the population anticipated to grow in numbers is that of individuals age 85 and older.

The high rate of fatalities among older drivers is not only due to the seriousness of the crashes. The frailty and complex medical conditions of older drivers and their older passengers are significant contributing factors as well.

> Relatively few deaths of older people (1 percent or fewer) involve motor vehicles. . . . However, increasingly these older drivers are keeping their licenses longer and driving more miles than ever before. . . . Seventy-nine percent of deaths in 2002 motor vehicle crashes involving older people were passenger vehicle occupants, and 16 percent were pedestrians. . . . People 65 years and older represented 16 percent of the driving age population in 2002 and were involved in 15 percent of fatal motor vehicle crashes. By 2030, older people are expected to represent 25 percent of the driving age population and 25 percent of fatal crash involvements.[7]

Many sources (NHTSA, Insurance Information Institute [III], etc.) have discussed a tendency for older drivers to self-regulate their driving in response to their recognition of decreased functional capacity and performance. However, when you consider the number of crashes this population is involved in and the consequent result in fatalities, perhaps leaving it up to the individual to self-regulate is not enough. "Today, older adults constitute about 13 percent of the population but represent 16 percent of all traffic deaths."[8] Questions to ask may include, "At what point does the driver begin to self-regulate? Is there a precipitating event (e.g., a crash)?" Older drivers and others whose driving skills may be declining need easy access to a range of driving services and transportation options that help unsafe drivers recognize sooner the decline in skills and danger posed to the community. However, mandating driver screenings based on age rather than functional capacity poses a political challenge and ethical dilemmas.

CHANGING DEMOGRAPHICS

The growing elderly population and the need for older adults to stay in the workforce means that alternative transportation options must be available. Public transportation may be limited or nonexistent in suburban and rural areas. Driving is important for more than just driving to work. The ability to drive provides the individual with opportunities to engage in chosen occupations, shopping, socialization, recreation, and seeking medical care. These are activities important to daily life, health, and quality of life.

"At all ages, males have much higher motor vehicle death rates per 100,000 people compared with females. By age 85 and older, the rate is three times as high among men as among women."[7] A study conducted by Siren, Heikkinen, and Hakamies-Bloomqvist[9] revealed that women have a greater tendency to walk or use other modes of transportation compared with men. Women also drive shorter distances than their male counterparts, reducing the potential for crashes, injury, and death.

DRIVING BEHAVIORS AND ATTITUDES

A Gallup survey[10] studied drinking and driving behaviors and attitudes among racial and ethnic groups. More than half of the survey respondents supported increasing the penalties for people who drink and drive. Groups that advocate for public safety would receive community support. If these survey results are accurate, the public is ready to support BAC levels of 0.08 or less. "Only seven percent of fatally injured drivers 65 years and older had a BAC of 0.08 or greater, compared with over 30 percent among drivers younger than 65."[7] (See Table 23-3 for percentages of drivers killed by age group whose BAC was higher than 0.08.)

The following information will provide you with a basic understanding of some of the attitudes and behaviors captured in a study sponsored by NHTSA and carried out by the Gallup Organization.[10] The data summarized below represent 10,453 respondents age 16-64.

- About 26% of persons age 16-64 have driven a motor vehicle within two hours of consuming alcoholic beverages in the previous year. These persons are referred to as "drinker-drivers" throughout this report. Males are two and one-half times as likely to have driven within two hours of drinking as are females (37% compared to 15%). Non-Hispanic Whites are the most likely to be drinker-drivers (28%), while Asians are the least likely to have driven within two hours of alcohol consumption (13%)[10] (p. i).

- One in ten persons age 16 to 64 has ridden with a driver they thought might have consumed too much alcohol to drive safely in the previous year. One in three of these riders decided that their drivers were unsafe *before* they were riding in the vehicle, but still

Table 23-3 Percentage of Drivers Killed with BAC ≥0.08, 2002

Age	Rate
16-24	34
25-64	38
65+	7

From Insurance Institute for Highway Safety: *Fatality facts, older people 2002*, Arlington, VA, 2003, *www.highwaysafety.org*. Retrieved March 15, 2005.

rode with them. Persons of American Indian/Eskimo and Hispanic descent are almost twice as likely to have ridden with a driver who may have consumed too much alcohol to drive safely[10] (p. ii). When an occupational therapist or OT assistant discovers that their client has been injured as a result of being a passenger of a "drinker-driver," strategies can be offered to assist the client to identify alternatives to riding in a car with someone who has had too much to drink; for example, assign a designated driver, call a taxi, take the keys away, delay his or her departure, avoid going out with that driver if alcohol will be served, and so forth.

DRINKING AND DRIVING AS A PUBLIC SAFETY ISSUE

The public sees drinking and driving as a public safety issue. Health care providers, including OT practitioners, have the opportunity to inquire about these behaviors in their screenings and assessments. When a problem is recognized, education and referrals to substance abuse programs can be provided as a part of the OT generalist's and/or DRS's intervention or recommendations.

"Two-thirds of this age 16 to 64 believes that they themselves should not drive after consuming more than two alcoholic beverages within two hours"[10] (p. ii). The people surveyed underestimated the number of drinks that could be assumed within a two hour limit to achieve the legal limits for blood alcohol concentration (BAC) levels. "The average 170 pound male would be at about a 0.03 BAC after consuming two drinks within two hours"[10] (p. 28).

More than 80% of people in the 16-64 age group have heard of BAC levels. "Non-Hispanic White persons of drinking age are significantly more likely to be aware of BAC levels than other racial groups, with 89% awareness. Less than three fourths of those in other racial groups have heard of BAC levels"[10] (p. 54).

Drinking and driving and other risky behaviors are less likely to be a contributor to crashes among older adults than other age groups.

Occupational therapists, OT assistants, and others may encounter individuals with a variety of substance abuse problems in their daily practice. Individuals receiving OT may present a need for these services in a mental health clinic, while receiving treatment for a hand injury, or while participating in a work rehabilitation program. One of the underlying causes necessitating OT intervention may be abuse of alcohol, illegal drugs, or prescription medications. Practitioners have the opportunity to have an effect on substance abuse behaviors, particularly those related to driving and the potential of the individuals to injure themselves or others due to their substance abuse. Health care professionals have an obligation to understand some of the attitudes and behaviors of those served. Education can become a part of the treatment through an education and prevention approach.

The *February 2004 Hot Topic on Older Drivers* listed the following Key Facts that are relevant to this discussion.
- "In 2002, older people (70 and older) made up 12 percent of all traffic fatalities, 12 percent of vehicle occupant fatalities and 17 percent of pedestrian fatalities, according to NHTSA.
- In 2002, 81 percent of fatal accidents involving older drivers happened during the day. Seventy-five percent involved another vehicle.*
- According to the Insurance Institute for Highway Safety, about half of fatal crashes in 2002 involving drivers 80 years and older occurred at intersections and involved more than one vehicle. This compares with 24 percent among drivers up to age 65."[11]

*Author comment: we frequently hear about those who self-regulate and only drive during the day. These data suggest that this strategy is ineffective.

Wang's review of scientific literature on crash data concluded that "Currently, motor vehicle crashes are the number one cause of injury-related deaths in the 65-74 age group"[4] (p. 9). Crash-related injuries and deaths for individuals in this age group are often associated with medical conditions that impair motor function and cognition. Regardless of the individual's age, the driver rehabilitation professional has an obligation to understand the relationship between the medical condition as well as side effects of medications and psychosocial state relative to driving performance. There is no question of the driving rehabilitation professional's responsibility to evaluate the skills of older drivers and those with disabilities. Society will benefit in terms of lives saved, injuries prevented, and property protected. There is also a need to educate passengers about seat belt use and other safety tips in their roles as passengers. Pedestrian safety issues should become a priority for occupational therapists and OT assistants working in rehabilitation and community practices as well as professionals specializing in driver rehabilitation.

CURRENT LAWS

State Drivers License Renewal Laws Including Requirements for Older Drivers, as of February 2004 (see Appendix A), provides a state-by-state view of requirements for retesting for license renewals for people of all ages, age at which states require older drivers to pass tests, the states in which doctors are required to report medical conditions, and the age at which mail renewals are no longer allowed. Consistency in reporting requirements among states does not exist.

Table 23-4 is an overview of licensing and reporting requirements (see Appendix A). Bioptic telescopes are permitted in over 70% of states. However, the user must comply with certain established conditions, for example, daylight driving only. (See Chapters 6 and 12 for more information on driving with bioptic lenses.) Restricted licenses are common in most states and serve to place limits or special requirements on the driver, including the number of miles driven, the use of sensory aids, or specialized equipment. Fifty-one percent of states have some degree of an age-restricted renewal procedure. Typical requirements expect the licensee of a certain age to renew in person and have a vision screening. Only 14 states require physician reporting, while the majority, greater than 70%, encourage physicians and others to report people with specific health conditions. (Note: Encouragement is not interpreted as a legal obligation to report individuals who meet specific criteria.)

Laws and regulations governing driving change and differ among states. DRSs have a legal and ethical duty to be aware of and adhere to all laws and regulations governing this practice area. OT and other professional practitioners are expected to maintain their knowledge of current legislation and apply those changes to their practice. Compliance with state and federal regulations is an expectation articulated in AOTA Code, Principle 5A. (See Appendix C for more information.)

Occupational therapists who evaluate and make recommendations regarding an individual's ability to drive safely need to be aware of state licensing requirements and reporting laws. Current information about individual state reporting requirements may be found at one of these web sites or by contacting your state MVA directly:
- AMA's Older Drivers Project: http://www.ama-assn.org/go/olderdrivers
- National Highway Traffic Safety Administration. State reporting practices. http://www.nhtsa.gov/people/injury/olddrive/FamilynFriends/state.htm

LEGAL ISSUES

When researching legal issues related to driving, it is fairly easy to find written material about the older driver and methods to institute separate driver renewal procedures based on age. This meets with controversy; some people suggest that it would be discrimination to support the establishment of laws or regulations that focus only on one age group or one segment of the population. Researchers from TransAnalytics, LLC, under the auspices of an NHTSA grant, produced *Model Driver Screening and Evaluation Program, Final Technical Report. Volume 1: Project Summary and Model Program Recommendations.* The NHTSA study engaged the American Association for Motor Vehicle Administrators (AAMVA) to survey their 60 member jurisdictions where they confronted the question of mandatory driver screenings.

Table 23-5 reflects the question posed with the three options and responses from the 60 jurisdictions surveyed. Only six jurisdictions supported the statement, "all drivers over a specified age, who apply for license renewal," should have a driver screening. Twenty-eight (the majority) of jurisdictions indicated support when responding to, "only a 'high risk' subgroup of drivers, likely to include a disproportionate share of older persons, who are brought to the DMV's attention through various referral mechanisms," should be screened. Finally, 26 jurisdictions indicated support for "both of these sets of drivers." It is obvious that different opinions exist. If response "c" is examined closely, a significant percentage of respondents would support both new and expanded driver screening procedures for all drivers over a specified age that apply for license renewal and

Table 23-4 State Licensing and Reporting Requirements: Summary

Response	Number of States
ARE BIOPTIC TELESCOPES ALLOWED?[1]	
Unknown	1
No	14
Yes	36
ARE RESTRICTED LICENSES ALLOWED?[2]	
None	4
Available	47
ARE THERE AGE-BASED RENEWAL PROCEDURES?[3]	
No	25
Yes	26
IS THERE PHYSICIAN/MEDICAL REPORTING?[4]	
Self-reporting	3
May report/encouraged	35
Yes, required	14

1. The majority of states allowing bioptic telescopes did so with conditions. Some of the conditions included for use when driving, daylight driving only, road test required.
2. Examples of conditions imposed on restricted licenses: daylight only, corrective lenses, no highway or interstate driving, external mirrors, special equipment/controls, hearing aids, mileage restrictions.
3. At certain ages, mail renewals are no longer accepted, renewal cycles decrease, vision testing required at time of renewal, physician states the individual is medically fit.
4. A few states specified certain conditions that would necessitate a physician's referral: lapses of consciousness, Alzheimer's disease, seizure disorders. 32 states accept information from other sources, which may include occupational therapists.
From Wang CC, Kosinski CJ, Schwartzberg JG, et al: *Physician's guide to assessing and counseling older drivers,* Washington, DC, 2003, National Highway Traffic Safety Administration.

include the "high risk" subgroup of drivers. This is closer to being age-neutral; however, it is likely to include a disproportionate share of older persons, who are brought to the DMV's attention through various referral mechanisms. If legislated in these 26 jurisdictions, all drivers over a certain age applying for license renewal would be rescreened. Individuals identified as high-risk drivers by physicians, police, family members, or other sources would be screened at the time of license renewal, or at

the time of identification. Age discrimination will be discussed further, later in this chapter.

LEGAL AND REGULATORY TRENDS

A National Driver Register (NDR) captures reports from state MVAs about individuals who have had their licenses suspended, revoked, or denied. Hypothetically, if you or the client's physician reported an individual as

Table 23-5 **Survey of State Licensing Officials**

(a) *All* Drivers Over a Specified Age Who Apply for License Renewal	(b) Only a "High Risk" Subgroup of Drivers, Likely to Include a Disproportionate Share of Older Persons, Who are Brought to the DMV's Attention Through Various Referral Mechanisms	(c) Both of These Sets of Drivers?
Arkansas	Alaska	Alabama
Connecticut	Alberta	British Columbia
Florida	Arizona	Colorado
Kansas	California	Delaware
Maine	Kentucky	Hawaii
Quebec	Louisiana	Idaho
	Manitoba	Illinois
	Massachusetts	Indiana
	Michigan	Iowa
	Minnesota	Maryland
	Missouri	Nebraska
	Montana	New Brunswick
	Nevada	New Hampshire
	New York	New Jersey
	North Dakota	Newfoundland & Labrador
	Nova Scotia	North Carolina
	Oklahoma	Northwest Territories
	Pennsylvania	Ohio
	Prince Edward Island	Ontario
	Rhode Island	Oregon
	Saskatchewan	South Carolina
	Texas	South Dakota
	Utah	Tennessee
	Virginia	Vermont
	Washington (State)	Washington, DC
	West Virginia	Yukon
	Wisconsin	
	Wyoming	

From Staplin L, Lococo KH, Gish KW, et al: *Model Driver Screening and Evaluation Program, Final Technical Report. Volume 1: Project Summary and Model Program Recommendations, Office of Research and Traffic Records,* May 2003, National Highway Traffic Safety Administration.

being unable to drive safely, this information could be referred to a *medical advisory board (MAB)*. If the MAB determines, after investigation, that an individual is no longer competent to drive and this is communicated to the MVA, the MVA may report this to the NDR. The data that the NDR receives vary among states. An individual may contact their local MVA and submit an inquiry to see if they are listed in this database. Likewise an employer or federal transportation agency may learn if someone has been reported to this database. If state-by-state reporting of impaired drivers is more consistently mandated and enforced, the NDR's potential to serve as a major data repository would greatly increase.

DRIVER SCREENING CRITERIA

Research by Staplin et al[12] was motivated by a need to update the AAMVA's driver screening criteria, particularly in anticipation of the growing number of older adults who will be driving in 2000 and beyond. Their hope was to determine a way to screen individuals based on a concept of fitness to drive. The data gathered during this Maryland survey involved MVA sites and community senior centers. Researchers concluded that some action must occur to help keep seniors driving safely for longer periods.

> In a broader sense, this research reinforces the notion that functional screening to assure the 'driving health' of older persons is rightfully viewed in the context of injury prevention. As such, its potential benefits to individuals and to society are profound, *if* integrated with education and counseling to improve awareness about the risks associated with functional loss, referrals for remediation of functional loss whenever possible, and connection to alternative transportation resources to preserve – instead of penalizing – the independent mobility of affected drivers.[12] (p. 2)

Individuals and agencies who consider the fiscal implications associated with mandatory driver screenings often anticipate high costs. Staplin's project also considered cost. Overall the costs per driver were anticipated to be $5.00 or less. If one thinks in terms of cost benefits, the following factors should be considered: cost of screening, rehabilitation, and adaptive equipment, against the costs incurred to persons and property when crashes occur. If at-risk drivers are identified early enough and remediation or revocation of driving privileges occurs, there are potentially great savings to the client and to society. Although cost versus benefit analyses do not drive ethics, the potential benefits to society can be compelling.

THE PHYSICIAN'S ROLE

A growing number of physicians believe they have a role and responsibility to discuss driving health and safety with their patients. The AMA, with the support of NHTSA, created the *Physician's Guide to Assessing and Counseling Older Drivers*, which includes guidance to physicians on screening patients whose conditions may negatively affect their ability to drive safely (Appendix I). The *Guide* also reminds physicians of their duty to report drivers determined to be unsafe to the state MVA, and can be instructive to other driver rehabilitation specialists as well. Portions of the *Physician's Guide* are presented in Appendices A, F, H, and I. The complete *Physician's Guide* in PDF format is available on the book's supplemental CD-ROM (*The Adapted Driving Decision Guide*) as well.

LAWS, REGULATIONS, AND GUIDELINES: APPLICATION TO DAILY LIFE AND PRACTICE

It can be challenging to review laws, regulations, and guidelines and discern how they apply to daily life and practice. Box 23-2 contains an interview with elder-law attorney Leigh H. Bernstein, who agreed to respond to some legal and ethical questions over the telephone. It should be noted that Associate Attorney Bernstein's practice focuses on protection and advocacy for older adults, and that she confronts client and family dilemmas regarding safe driving, public safety, and individual freedoms on a regular basis.

A CLOSER LOOK AT LEGAL AND ETHICAL ISSUES

Personal and professional protection begins when each service provider is well acquainted with the laws, regulations, and ethical duties governing their practice. Review the legal and ethical mandates to identify unsafe/impaired drivers as required by the professional's state and particular professional association. (Refer to Appendix A, the appropriate state's MVA website, the state board that regulates OT practice, ADED, and to AOTA's website for access to this information.)

Driver rehabilitation professionals have a significant responsibility to the individuals they serve and to the community. There is an obligation to ensure that all services provided are competent and adhere to all legal and professional standards. Public safety is at stake. The professionals' responsibility is to *do no harm* (nonmalfeasance). The client, family, doctor, MVA, and community are all stakeholders in the driver rehabilitation professional's duty to uphold that responsibility.

Wang et al asserted that "A background in driver education alone may be insufficient for appropriate evaluation of medically impaired drivers and correct interpretation of the evaluation."[4] When using a commercial driving school instructor for the in-car work,

BOX 23-2	Interview with Elder-law Attorney

Q: If a state recommends/requires physicians, family members or others to report a potentially unsafe driver and they do not and the patient/client crashes and injures self and others, can the individual or family members, or individuals injured sue the physician or occupational therapist for not reporting?

A: Family members (or anyone) can sue anyone at anytime. The suit can be based on the professional's failure to act, which is similar to the duty to rescue someone that is injured. There are almost no regulations that mandate reporting certain conditions to the state MVA. No case law exists where a physician or occupational therapy practitioner is sued. However, some may have been sued and the case settled before going to court.

There was a claim against an insurance agent because the elderly claimant thought that the agent had not advised her properly to carry enough insurance. (The claimant was involved in a crash where significant injuries were involved.) Learning about suits against state MVA examiners (known to occur) is difficult to discover because states are self-insured and the data regarding suits are not captured or disclosed to the public.

Q: If a professional code of ethics includes concepts of beneficence (AOTA Code, Principle 1 A & 1B), nonmalfeasance (AOTA Code, Principle 2A), and confidentiality (AOTA Code, Principle 3E) can the professional be sued if someone was injured even if no law was broken?

A: Although one could be sued for common law negligence, Ms. Bernstein does not see evidence of that occurring. Her opinion was that reporting should be done even if regulations do not require or encourage it due to the professional's obligation to protect the individual and the public from harm. Considering the potential for suits, it is crazy for driver rehabilitation specialists not to make sure that they have proper coverage (malpractice insurance).

[Author comments] Health Information Patient Portability Act (HIPPA) and the codes of ethics emphasis on confidentiality should remind DRSs how to handle information that they may communicate to a third party, like the MVA. Make sure that the client knows reporting requirements before any intervention begins. It would be a good practice to explain privacy rules at the beginning of the relationship and have the client sign a standardized document acknowledging receipt and agreement with this information.

Q: Is there an obligation/duty to more than just the person being evaluated—the family, referring physician, payer, MVA, society?

A: There is an obligation beyond the individual. The client and practitioner need to understand that there is a duty to society based on potential harm. It is the same type of obligation as if a client told the practitioner of their intent to harm themselves or another person. Although physicians in a few states have an obligation to report such instances, it is unclear how many actually comply with the legal and ethical mandate.

Q: Is it discrimination if state regulations only target older adults and/or people with disabilities?

A: Issues related to driving safety are not about age and/or disability discrimination; it is about dysfunction. Critics of legislative efforts need to understand that age and disability can result in changes in functional capacity. Rescreening shouldn't be an insult because changes are a natural part of aging. Public awareness activities would go a long way to dispel negative views of people with disabilities and/or aging-related concerns as well as individuals who rely on formal and informal alternative transportation services. Additionally, there are a variety of laws and regulations which focus on specific age groups, for example, infant hearing screening programs.

the client and referring professional need to understand that the driving school instructor has no medical background or training. If an individual refers a client for these services, the person responsible for generating the referral and the entity he or she works for must recognize the potential liability implications. Let us consider a scenario in which an OT generalist refers a client to a driving school instructor for on-road driver rehabilitation services. An important question that the referring professional should consider before initiating the referral is: "If the commercial driving school instructor makes an uninformed decision because he or she lacks insight into the client's diagnosis (or diagnoses) and its potential effect on the driving task, and that decision results in a client, caregiver, and/or other road users

and pedestrians becoming injured, is the generalist and the organization he or she works for liable?"[13] To be certain, consult with an attorney to help ensure that the professional, the program, the client, the caregiver, and the public at large are adequately protected.

SCREENING HIGH-RISK POPULATIONS FOR DRIVING SAFETY

As was previously stated, if only older adults are screened for their driving safety, and perhaps people with disabilities, there may be a danger that this may be seen as a discriminatory practice. The functional performance of individuals with disabilities may also change with aging, warranting rescreening in accordance with the recommendations proposed for older drivers.

If you do not provide driver screenings to at-risk populations, are you responsible if the driver is engaged in a crash that could have been anticipated? Do occupational therapists have a legal and ethical responsibility to offer screenings to the general public? Relatively few lawsuits have been successfully made against physicians, therapists, or MVA officials when an individual is injured in a crash. (See Box 23-2 for more information on this topic.) DRSs and OT generalists have a legal and ethical obligation to assure that their scope of work is competent and conforms to standards of practice. The professional selects the screening tools, evaluations, and interventions based on client need and the provider's areas of competence. Driver screenings for each individual encountered may not be appropriate. However, if an individual is considered at risk, it is advisable to share those concerns with the client and recommend driver screening by you or a referral source. All recommendations must be documented and include the client's response. A general screening may include a review of driving performance skills, factors that contribute to pedestrian safety, and seat belt use. If safe behaviors are not currently a routine, DRSs should include driving, pedestrian, and seat belt safety into their intervention plans as primary prevention recommendations.

Clinical screenings for all persons include questions about wearing seat belts and whether participation in risky behaviors is likely to occur behind the wheel. It is also important to obtain a perspective of the client's social networks; would the client get in a car as a passenger with someone who is unfit to drive? Remember that 10% of the persons surveyed by Royal[10] had been passengers in vehicles driven by someone whom they perceived had consumed too much alcohol to drive safely. If possible it may be helpful to role play scenarios that equip the individual with strategies on how to deal with these situations.

INFORMED CONSENT

If DRSs practice in a state that has reporting obligations, the client should be informed of their duty to report unfit drivers and under what circumstances. Notification is presented orally and in writing, and signed by the client before any services are initiated. What do DRSs do if the individual refuses to sign? The driving program must anticipate this situation and create a set of policies and procedures to protect the client, practitioner, and institution and/or driver rehabilitation program. Consider developing release of information forms that would articulate legal and ethical obligations to report outcomes of the evaluation to whom and under what circumstances. In states requiring or permitting that outcomes of driver evaluations be shared with the state's MAB or the physician, it is imperative that the client understands the reporting obligations and signs a consent form. Information about which states require, allow, or encourage physicians and others to report unsafe drivers can be found in Appendix A. AOTA's Code addresses the need for patient confidentiality and adherence to laws in Principles 3E and 5A. (See Appendix C for the full text.)

The Health Insurance Portability and Accountability Act of 1996 (HIPAA) must also be taken into account: ". . . the HIPPA *Standards for Privacy of Individually Identifiable Health Information* ("Privacy Rule") permit health care providers to disclose protected health information without individual authorization *as required by law*. It also permits health care providers to disclose protected health information to public health authorities authorized by law to collect or receive such information for preventing or controlling disease, injury, or disability"[4] (p. 70).

If DRSs report their recommendations to the DMV as required by law, it is wise to notify clients in advance and provide the individual with a copy of the submitted report. Sharing information with families can be helpful, but is best done with the consent of the client, especially when the client retains decision-making capacity (AOTA Code, Principle 3E). Accurate documentation is a necessity (AOTA Code, Principle 6C).

APPLICATION OF ETHICS THEORY TO DRIVING AND DRIVER REHABILITATION

What are the ethical responsibilities of the OT assistants and occupational therapists who do not work as DRSs to view driving/mobility as an *instrumental activity of daily living (IADL)*? The AMA, NHTSA, AOTA, ADED, and others recognize the important contributions that OT practitioners contribute to the field of driving. Practitioners at most levels of practice may be delivering a component of service related to this IADL. The occupational therapist working in a school-based practice or community center for individuals with developmental disabilities may think about mobility, and in particular driving, in terms of physical performance and cognitive skills required to retain information and react to environmental changes with efficiency and competence.

Considerations may also extend to the individual's ability to travel safely as a passenger and ability to use public transportation with or without assistance. The clinician working in an acute care, rehabilitation, or mental health setting can incorporate into screening and rehabilitation programs the functional components related to prerequisite skills that are foundational to driving. However, OT generalists should never "fail" a client based on screening criteria alone. The generalist should refer the client to a DRS, who is the only professional capable of providing a comprehensive driver rehabilitation evaluation that incorporates both a thorough clinical evaluation and an on-road evaluation. Similarly, occupational therapists providing in-home rehabilitation services may screen for performance skills related to driving and provide clients with consultation or make a referral as necessary.

One of the things that separate a professional organization from a technical one is the existence of a code of ethics. *Ethics* is one of the components of applied philosophy. A code of ethics establishes principles developed to guide the profession's aspirations and the professional behavior of the organization's members. Codes of ethics typically address concepts of beneficence, nonmaleficence, duties, justice, veracity, and fidelity. The ways these concepts are addressed vary among organizations and professions. Codes of ethics publicly articulate principles and values against which a professional's (and in some environments, a student's) conduct can be measured. The purpose of codes is to guide the behaviors of the profession's members and give the public a measuring stick to evaluate the conduct of an individual or group of individuals. Enforcement procedures are often developed to define the consequences of violations to principles articulated in the code. These procedures establish processes for the review of ethics complaints and recommend specific disciplinary actions, when appropriate.

THE AOTA, ADED, AND NBCOT CODES OF ETHICS

The AOTA and the ADED have codes of ethics that apply to their members. These documents are available for review in the public and members-only sections of each of their web sites, www.aota.org and www.aded.net, respectively. They are also included in this text as Appendix C. The following discussion will draw upon the principles established in these codes. It is important to note that when AOTA members are determined by AOTA's Commission on Standards and Ethics (SEC) to have violated the AOTA *Occupational Therapy Code of Ethics*, some sanctions are communicated privately to the members, while other disciplinary actions are communicated publicly and can ultimately have an effect on the individual's ability to practice OT. ADED does not currently have an ethics committee; however, any com-

plaints received are referred to the Board of Directors for consideration and possible action.

STATE REGULATORY AGENCIES

State boards that regulate the practice of OT incorporate AOTA's Code of Ethics into their practice regulations. State boards regulate the practice of OT and serve to protect the public from practitioners who are not properly licensed or credentialed and do not conform to regulations guiding the practice of OT. Clients, professionals, and the public may submit complaints against a licensed occupational therapist and/or OT assistant that may have violated the state practice act to the board that regulates OT practice. The National Board for Certification in Occupational Therapy (NBCOT) has a Candidate/Certificant Code of Conduct (www.nbcot.org). NBCOT has authority over occupational therapists and OT assistants who hold current NBCOT certification. Their goal is to serve the public interest through their certification process. Additional information about jurisdiction and disciplinary authority is available through these organizations and each state regulatory board.

Ethical principles as cited by AOTA and ADED place the expectation on the practitioner to inform the client fully about the procedures that will be used, anticipated outcomes of the interventions, and any reporting requirements that may exist. This is particularly important, as the outcome of the comprehensive driver rehabilitation evaluation (not the driver screening) may result in the professional's recommendation to the referring physician or to an MAB that the client should be restricted from driving. Providing this information in advance of an intervention allows the client the opportunity to weigh the benefits and consequences of the intervention. The OT generalist and the DRS must respect the individual's right to refuse services, which is part of the client-centered approach. Equally, it is imperative that the client understands the range and scope of the practitioner's confidentiality duties and obligations. (AOTA Code, Principles 3A, B, D, E. ADED Code, Principles A.6.d, B.2.b, B.3. b-c.)

The entire team has a responsibility to clearly explain the scope of the evaluation and training, and the range of potential outcomes (AOTA Code, Principle 3B):

"In situations where clear evidence of substandard driving impairment implies a strong threat to patient and public safety, and where the physician's advice to discontinue driving privileges is ignored, it is desirable and ethical to notify the Department of Motor Vehicles. . . . physicians should disclose and explain to their patients this responsibility to report. . . . physicians should protect patient confidentiality by ensuring that only the minimal amount of information is reported and that reasonable security measures are used in handling that information."[4] (p. 20)

Occupational therapists also have an ethical obligation to respect patient confidentiality (AOTA Code, Principle 3E). The duty also exists to abide by any laws and regulations governing reporting to the state (AOTA Code, Principle 5A). This does not place the DRS in a double bind. The law will take precedence over the Code. An individual can comply with reporting by first making the client aware of the need to do so, and then providing the type and amount of information that is required.

The physician's legal and ethical duties are articulated in the *Physician's Guide to Assessing and Counseling Older Drivers* that was published by the AMA and the NHTSA. The areas identified included the following: protecting the patient, duty to protect, maintaining patient confidentiality, and adhering to state reporting laws. Appendix I has more information on a physician's legal and ethical responsibilities. During the course of this chapter, we will see how these areas are related to OT and the ethical duties outlined in the AOTA *Occupational Therapy Code of Ethics*.

OT generalists would benefit from knowing the red flags that indicate the need to refer a client for a comprehensive driver rehabilitation evaluation; for example, decreased memory, recent stroke or brain injury, confusion, or seizure disorders that do not respond to medication. Policies and procedures written and approved by the hospital or facility administrator, OT manager, DRS, or legal counsel should incorporate legal and ethical duties required by law and standards of practice articulated by AOTA and ADED. These procedures should be reviewed regularly and be a part of the orientation materials for new staff. Procedures developed may address situations in which the client is recommended for a driver evaluation to determine fitness to drive. The program may want to outline when and how to notify the referring physician, the family, or caregivers. The inclusion of documentation requirements and confidentiality guidelines will help the DRS maintain the highest levels of ethical practice.

The U.S. Department of Transportation found that

> . . . older people prefer to drive in a private vehicle as late in life as possible and generally do so safely. . . . older people drive longer than they can walk or use transportation options. . . . those with cognitive deficits and other diminished functional abilities may not recognize their condition and may not properly reduce or cease driving. . . . less than five percent of older people lose their licenses due to action by state licensing authorities."[8] (p. 14)

Health care providers should use this information as a challenge to help identify what performance skills can be improved, and which skills can be identified early as essential for safe driving. Once those critical skills are identified, the driver, caregivers, and others in the support environment need to be educated to help monitor when deficits may be occurring and when it may be advantageous to seek professional services.

EVIDENCE-BASED PRACTICE: A WORTHY GOAL FOR ALL DRIVER REHABILITATION SPECIALISTS

In December 2002, Helen Wood conducted an evidence-based review of the following question: Does public transport training versus no intervention help clients that have sustained traumatic brain injuries (TBIs) or cerebrovascular accidents (CVAs) increase their independence in accessing their local community? According to Wood, ". . . there is no current evidence that transport training whether it is *in vivo*, via classroom teaching, or on an individual basis increases a client's independence in accessing their local community."[15] Incorporation of current evidence into practice is the responsibility of each DRS practitioner. Armed with reliable evidence, the DRS can identify alternative strategies to help clients meet their goals.

Multiple evidence-based research studies and analyses occur in all areas of health care and rehabilitation. Reviews of such data underscore the importance of staying current with research and place responsibility on practitioners to use standardized test measures rather than place undue emphasis on caregiver reporting. This is not to say, however, that family members should be excluded from the evaluation process, as they often contribute useful insight into the client's behavior.

Some of the current research has produced discussions comparing on-road and simulator tests with caregiver reports.[8] Ethical consideration of the testing methods is warranted. The DRS should determine if the testing equipment or environment produces physical discomfort or sickness, whether these tools should be used, and at what cost. One would hope that alternatives to the equipment or environment would be identified that reduce potential harm to the client.

The DRS must recognize his or her obligation to provide a testing environment that conforms to the requirements of the standardized test. Deviations from the standards may affect the outcome of the evaluation. Deviations that do not conform to standards of practice may be considered as ethics violations. See Chapter 24 for more information on evidence-based practice in driver rehabilitation.

MAINTAINING PROFESSIONAL COMPETENCE

Professional ethics require practitioners to ensure that they maintain the highest level of competence. The DRS is expected to take advantage of available education and training. A range of training, continuing education, and mentoring programs are available to professionals in this practice area. Opportunities are readily available, such as the AOTA's web site that features a driver rehabilitation list serve, micro web site that focuses on issues pertaining to elderly drivers, and online asynchronous tutorials. Additionally, AOTA offers an annual conference with some workshops that focus on driver rehabilitation and community mobility. ADED also offers an informational web site, hosts an annual conference, and has initiated a series of four separate workshops conducted throughout the United States on driver rehabilitation topics, including an overview of driver rehabilitation, disabilities, aging, low vision and driving, vehicle modifications, and traffic safety. DRSs and professionals wishing to stay current on issues and expand their knowledge and skills should take advantage of these and other opportunities for professional development (AOTA Code, Principle 4C. ADED Code, Principle C4-5). See Appendix D for more information on continuing professional competency training.

MEDICATIONS AND DRIVING

The *Insurance Information Institute (III) February 2004 report*[11] about older drivers stated that some medications, particularly those that reduce stress, have side effects that are typically most evident during the first week of use. However, drug toxicity can affect cognitive and motor performance at any time. Of course, this is also true for other drivers, including people with disabilities. This underscores the importance for all DRSs working with clients who use medications to understand the benefits, use, history, and side effects for their clients. As we know, a variety of substances (prescribed and illegal) can influence an individual's driving skills regardless of age. Studies have explored knowledge of alcohol use and its effect on driving skills.[10] Overall, people of all ages underestimate the amount of alcohol they can consume and how much consumption influences driving performance. This study also identified differences regarding attitudes and behaviors of different racial/ethnic groups relative to impaired driving and being the passenger in a car with an impaired driver behind the wheel. The occupational therapist has an ethical obligation to understand the behaviors, attitudes, and their social-cultural context and collaboratively provide treatment that incorporates these factors and best practices into the intervention. See Chapter 8 for more information on medications and driving and this chapter for a discussion on alcohol use and driving.

ETHICS AND THE CLINICAL EVALUATION

If the DRS begins an evaluation or recommends one and it is refused, the DRS needs to document the client's refusal to participate, recommendations, and the counseling provided. When a family member is actively involved, share any concerns about the client's resistance to see if alternative approaches can be identified. Perhaps family members can be a part of the team's efforts to encourage the client to have the evaluation, limit driving, or stop driving altogether. It is important to make sure that speaking with the family does not breech the client's right to confidentiality. AOTA's Code, Principle 3D acknowledges the client's right to refuse treatment interventions.

Driving and driver rehabilitation often focus on adults with new occurrences of disability, or whose chronic conditions have worsened. Making services available to all persons regardless of age, race, or socioeconomic status supports the altruistic nature of the AOTA Code of Ethics: "Thus, providing specialized training to safely operate a vehicle or use alternative transportation systems for young adults with a disability is not only a reasonable rehabilitative strategy but also is critical to individuals attaining a sense of self-esteem and independence as contributing members of society"[16] (p. 2).

PUBLIC AWARENESS

Public awareness activities may include DRSs working in collaboration with organizations and agencies concerned about driving and alternative transportation issues. This is an excellent opportunity for individuals with disabilities and older adults to learn about the education, training, and equipment that may allow them to continue to drive safely and access alternative transportation. Practitioners need to continually update their knowledge about the range of equipment and local resources available.

PSYCHIATRIC CONDITIONS, SUBSTANCE ABUSE, AND DRIVING

Discussions of driving issues often focus on issues of physical dysfunction, primarily performance deficits. However, individuals who are substance abusers or who have psychiatric conditions that are not controlled by behavioral approaches, medications (e.g., mood disorders, psychoses), or both may also benefit from a comprehensive driver rehabilitation evaluation. Some questions for consideration are: "Does the client (with one or more of these conditions) have consistent judgment necessary for quick decision making when behind the wheel?" "Is the client subject to impulsive behaviors?" "Does the client have the insight to recognize when his or her condition has begun to deteriorate and will voluntarily limit driving?" DRSs providing services to individuals with these behavioral issues have a responsibility to evaluate the client's safety and make appropriate recommendations.

STOPPING AN EVALUATION THAT IS IN PROGRESS

The driver rehabilitation evaluation should be discontinued when it becomes apparent that an individual's executive function impairment does not enable them to respond to the evaluation.[17] DRSs also have an obligation to use the client's and payer's limited financial resources wisely. It is in the client's best interest to stop the evaluation, rather than evaluating other skills related to driving or engaging in training. It would be misleading to the client and a possible waste of their resources. Similarly, it is not in the clients' best interest to put them in a position to over-learn tests. The client who repeats tests more than once may confound attempts to readminister the same tests in the future; therefore, the DRS should avoid over-testing a client. To illustrate this point, consider a scenario in which the neuropsychologist has recently administered a test that is a standard part of the driver evaluation battery. The DRS should not repeat the same test if there is any possibility that the client's experience may influence test performance and the outcomes data collected. Use available data and seek other assessments that will augment and complement the existing data.[17]

DEVELOPING EVIDENCE-BASED TOOLS

DRSs have the unique opportunity (and responsibility) to participate in research to develop the tools that will reliably predict at-risk drivers and the efficacy of driver rehabilitation interventions. The more evidence that exists to support the assessments and interventions used, the greater the option to build public trust and gain broader payer authorizations; and the individual, community, and service provider benefit from these efforts.

Efforts to contribute to the body of evidence (i.e., knowledge) will reinforce the belief that the procedures used in this practice area are based on the best evidence available. It is also critical and a duty for DRSs to continually update their knowledge and skills to help ensure the highest level of professional competency (AOTA Code, Principles 4B-D). When DRSs learn about a new assessment or treatment strategy, they must check the evidence and become familiar with the

intervention before offering it to clients. Clients are paying for DRSs' services and have the right to expect that service providers are competent in the services they deliver. Find out if the data support compensation strategies over remediation. DRSs have the responsibility to develop competencies before using and introducing new assessments or techniques in evaluation and treatment of clients.

When cognition, and in particular executive function, is impaired, inform the client and family of the associated functional implications and that recovery may take longer. It is important that the DRS deliver verbal and written feedback in a concrete and succinct fashion that the client will understand. It is equally important to teach the caregiver how to be effective when supporting a client and to recognize the necessary precautions (AOTA Code, Principle 3B).

Case Study #1

Paul is an experienced DRS. He has used a battery of assessments that comprise the formal clinical evaluation (versus the informal screening) for the past 2 years. He recently learned about a new version of one of the tools that he used. Paul purchased the new text and materials and plans to replace the old version with the new immediately.

The new version of the test has not been standardized, unlike the old one. Paul thinks that the new version tests a wider variety of skills and appears to be a far better assessment than the previous version. Should he abandon the previous standardized version, and use the new one that is not standardized? What are the consequences to the client if Paul chooses the old version, or the new one?

Codes of ethics emphasize principles of beneficence–to do no harm. Can the client be harmed by Paul's decision? If the client can be harmed, describe the assessment choice likely to produce injury. State regulations and codes of ethics require practitioners to adhere to standards of practice, which includes delivering professional services with competence. Competence is established by mastery over the techniques used. Should Paul use the new and improved tool immediately, because he thinks it is better and more thorough?

Is it the client's right to expect Paul to have the competence and experience to use a new assessment? Paul should explain to the client that he is experienced with the previous standardized version of the assessment in question and has just received a new version that may yield better data to support the client's ability to drive. This process of informed consent would both allow the client to participate in making the decision about which measure to use and reinforce the DRS's commitment to a client-centered approach to driver rehabilitation service delivery (AOTA Code, Principle 3B; ADED Code C.2.c, and C. 4. b).

Cultural Competence

Codes of ethics and federal regulations include use of language that encourages materials and services that are culturally sensitive. Appreciation of the client's and his or her family's culture and beliefs can be valuable in understanding the significance they may place on owning a motor vehicle and maintaining the image and occupation of being a driver. The motor vehicle (object) and role of the driver may be important to the individual and others in the community. When this is true, it is important to recognize and guide the client and his or her support network with strategies that make necessary transitions in a way that supports their new role as passenger and user of alternative transportation versus driver (e.g., remove the car, initiate driving cessation, and explore alternative community mobility options). The car evokes great feelings of pride for many people. The former driver may not want to sell his or her car to a stranger and would interpret it as a great loss. However, if the car is given or sold to a relative and the former driver rides as a passenger to meet some of his or her community mobility needs, it may make the loss less stressful. The DRS and the referring physician can work together in delivering recommendations about restricting or eliminating driving and examining alternative transportation options.

Driving Cessation and the Need for Alternative Transportation

If a DRS determines that a client should no longer drive, the DRS should help the client with that transition by exploring alternative transportation or alternative community mobility services and developing a strategy to help ensure that community mobility remains viable. The DRS must realize that this is an issue that has importance to the individual's psychosocial well-being. The DRS should learn about counseling or support services that may be available during this transition. If it is determined that the individual can no longer drive, there are probably other lifestyle issues that need to be addressed as well. The DRS should investigate whether the reduced ability (or inability) to drive is related to slowed reflexes, poor balance, impaired vision, or a combination of these and other client factors. In these cases, the DRS may want to refer the client to an OT generalist who can look at safety issues in the home. The generalist would examine if the individual is at greater risk for falls and remediation, compensation approaches to ameliorate the problem, or both. If strengthening or mobility solutions are not effective, a DRS can work with the client to determine the need for environmental modifications, including assistive technologies. Remember that occupational therapists and OT assistants treat the whole person in the context of their environment with emphasis on their successful engagement in occupations that are of importance to them. Teach family members how to assist their loved one to get into and out of the vehicle using proper body mechanics and assistive technologies that will reduce the potential risks such as sustaining a back injury or the client falling.

The NHTSA Bureau of Transportation Statistics (BTS) conducted a study in 2002 of individuals with and without disabilities. They created an *Issue Brief* in April 2003 summarizing the survey results. More than 500,000 individuals with disabilities indicated that they never leave their homes because of transportation difficulties (Table 23-6). The implications of the numbers that reflect individuals that are homebound are staggering. Both an individual's quality of life and the nation's economy are negatively affected when there is a loss of a productive worker. As a profession that focuses on *occupational engagement*, there is an ethical responsibility on the part of occupational therapists to help clients as well as their primary and secondary group members (i.e., family and neighbors versus acquaintances and classmates) achieve the level of independence and community involvement that they desire. Advocating for accessible, safe, and cost-effective personal and public transportation is one way to stimulate awareness and positive changes in public policy.

The number of drivers who need vehicle modifications is likely to increase with the growth in the population of people with disabilities, aging-related concerns, or both. Estimates of the number of households that own at least one vehicle modified for a person with a disability range from 1 to 2.3 million households. An exact number is unknown as is the types of adaptive driving equipment used; however, clients will benefit if their providers know about the range of available technology for modified vehicles and alternative transportation services. The DRS must acknowledge the importance of knowing the resources and must be able to initiate appropriate referrals for services and equipment. DRSs have a responsibility to consider the consequences when their clients are no longer able to drive safely, help them identify alternative transportation options, and assist them with developing the skills necessary to access these alternatives. A lack of mobility may lead to isolation and potential physical and emotional deterioration. If the services that the DRS provides do not include community mobility training, a professional and ethical obligation exists to locate providers that do.

Table 23-6 Reasons Expressed by Persons with Disabilities for Never Leaving Home*

Reason	Percent
Don't have a car	45.1
Public transportation availability or cost	31.2
Physical problems due to disability	28.6
Personal problems	26.2

*Percent of total people who said they never leave home due to problems getting transportation that they need (N = 560,823). An individual may have stated more than one reason.

From Bureau of Transportation Statistics: Transportation difficulties keep over half a million disabled at home, *Issue Brief*, April 2003. *http://www.bts.gov/publications/issue_briefs/number_03/html/figure_table.html* Retrieved: June 7, 2004.

Case Study #2

Gerry was 59 years old when he was first diagnosed with Huntington's disease. He was never a particularly good driver; however, lately his wife, Ann, noticed some changes in his driving patterns and skills. Gerry occasionally became confused about how to get to destinations that were previously familiar to him. He would slow or stop the car in the middle of the street and appeared minimally aware of the traffic around him.

Ann tried to explain her concerns about his safety on the road to Gerry, but he now lacked the insight to believe what she told him. Ann tried strategies of hiding the car keys and telling Gerry that his car was broken. These strategies were ineffective and only upset both husband and wife. Gerry's motor performance was deteriorating; the choreic movements were affecting his gait and fine motor coordination. Ann and Gerry's doctor finally convinced Gerry to undergo a comprehensive driver rehabilitation evaluation.

The data gathered and analyzed during Gerry's evaluation resulted in the determination that he was unsafe behind the wheel. He asked the DRS if he could participate in some physical rehabilitation to help retrain his skills and then on-road training if it was necessary. What should the DRS do? Referring to AOTA and ADED's codes of ethics, should Gerry be referred for therapy or training to help him accept his condition? What are the psychosocial and financial implications of agreeing with the client's request? If Gerry and Ann lived in a state that encouraged reporting (by physician, family member, or other source) when someone was deemed no longer able to drive, who should report him to the MVA and why?

ADVOCACY

The AOTA's Code's Principle 1 and 1C address the commitment that the profession has to demonstrate its concern for the well-being of the clients served. One means of accomplishing this is to advocate for the services needed by clients and/or caregivers.[3] Advocacy can take many forms. Advocacy for a client to arrange transportation services to the local mall may involve a telephone call to any number of agencies that provide or identify public and private transportation services, such as the local Senior Information and Assistance office. If few transportation services exist in the client's community, advocacy on behalf of the client may be directed to the local government agencies responsible for funding these services. Successful advocacy efforts often involve collaboration with clients and other service providers. OT generalists, OT assistants, and DRSs are effective members of coalitions, coordinating councils, and advocacy groups. The OT field's advocacy efforts can have an effect across the micro to macro continuum; for example, one individual, a small group, larger constituency group, community, or the broader society can readily benefit directly or indirectly from professional advocacy. Driver rehabilitation team members should also work to help clients and their caregivers identify ways to effectively practice self-advocacy as well. This approach is especially important because clients will not always be engaged in receiving driver rehabilitation and community mobility services.

The AOTA Code clearly indicates the occupational therapist's and OT assistant's responsibility to advocate for their clients. "In addition, as this generation retires from driving, there will be an increased demand for public or private transportation alternatives. . . . To assist this generation in maintaining their independence and aging in place, health services and medical professionals must be prepared and trained today to meet all of the community mobility needs of the future"[16] (p. 2). According to the *Report on Community Mobility/ Driver Safety Intervention as an Area for Specialty Certification*, "A National Highway Traffic Safety Administration (NHTSA) report suggests that family members, friends, and caregivers of older at-risk drivers need information on signs of unsafe driving and its consequences and specific examples of ways in which they and others can intervene, such as taking their family member to a driving evaluation and remediation program or obtaining information on user-friendly, accessible alternative transportation programs (U.S. Department of Transportation, 2001)"[16] (p. 7). People with disabilities could also benefit greatly from these approaches and must not be overlooked in our discourse and professional endeavors meant to ameliorate the negative consequences associated with immobility.

DRSs can help people with disabilities and/or aging-related concerns understand that a driver evaluation can be positive, helping them to remain safer while staying on the road longer. "Educate older people and their caregivers (and others) on how to identify unsafe older drivers and extend safe driving, walking, and use of transit (options). . . . train transportation, health and social service personnel to enable safe mobility and well-being of elderly people"[8] (p. 23). If safe driving is no longer an option, the DRS has an obligation to inform the client of alternate modes of transportation. If alternatives do not exist, the professional has an opportunity to collaborate with agencies and advocate for safe and accessible transportation for people with disabilities and the elderly in their respective communities.

DRSs, clients, and others should become aware of the role that MABs fulfill and that these are not punitive programs. Driver screening programs can confirm an individual's ability to drive or indicate an individual's need to refresh skills, adhere to a restricted license, or discontinue driving altogether. MVAs see a part of their collective role as not only helping to ensure an individual client's safety but the safety of the public at large. They can empower MABs to engage in and support research efforts aimed at developing accurate tools to screen core skills associated with safe driving. OT generalists, OT assistants, and DRSs can become advocates for public safety and injury prevention by their participation in research consortiums or driving and transportation research and planning groups. If state transportation advocates collaborate with their insurance administrations to identify areas in which coverage for driver evaluation and rehabilitation is deficient, the administration may have the authority to take corrective action. DRSs and other health care providers may find ways of contributing data to these insurance reviews and problem solving to ensure that coverage for driving evaluation and training services are available to the driving population who are most at risk.

Although the topic of this chapter addresses driving, pedestrian safety is also an important topic for OT practitioners. Older adults and people with disabilities are likely to cross intersections more slowly than the general population. It is imperative that DRSs provide their clients with strategies for safe street crossing that could lead to reduced injuries and deaths. Older adults who are involved in crashes are more likely to die than other age groups because of their frailty. This is also true for older adults who are hit by vehicles when crossing streets. (See Chapter 19 for more information on traffic safety.)

Individuals with disabilities who are unable to drive or use fixed route transportation services may take advantage of paratransit services. These services provide curb-to-curb or door-to-door assistance; however, these accessible vehicles require reservations sometimes well in advance. Therefore the rider is less able to be spontaneous in their comings and goings throughout the day and especially at night. If the DRS's client is unable to advocate for him or herself, it is an appropriate role for the occupational therapist, OT assistant, and driving rehabilitation professional to work with the client's caregiver to acquire the skills necessary to be an effective advocate.

Active walkers do not have difficulty getting to bus stops and boarding buses and vans. However, people of all ages may have conditions that limit their ability to do this. In these situations, alternate transportation must be identified. Carpools, paratransit services, taxi cabs, and contracted limousine services are potential providers of transportation that would enable the individual to attend school, keep medical appointments, shop for groceries and other personal effects, or pursue leisure interests, such as seeing a first-run movie or theatrical performance. The majority of free or low-cost transportation services are typically available for doctors' appointments or therapy appointments, and by and large are less frequently available in the evenings.

One of the important advocacy goals is to promote a variety of mobility options that are safe, convenient, and affordable. Social marketing strategies are needed to increase the public's willingness to support driver screening programs. This advertising may help to remove the stigmatization of public transport users (which are usually the poor, people with disabilities, and the elderly) and encourage greater use of alternative transportation services. DRSs and other advocates need to educate primary care providers about looking at the decline in functional capacity and its relationship to safe driving. Professionals should present information to state association members at conferences and meetings regarding the relevance of and relationship to this practice area as well as OT practice in the broadest sense. DRSs should join their professional associations to multiply the effect of their advocacy efforts at the intra- and inter-group levels. Often pooling limited financial and human resources by combining efforts to achieve common aims can be extraordinarily effective.

To ensure that transportation services are available to nondrivers, DRSs need to promote the view that transportation is as an essential human service and must be an integral part of the long-term health care system. DRSs and others must become involved in securing Medicare and Medicaid funding for all phases of the comprehensive driver rehabilitation evaluation and training as well as community mobility services for former drivers. This includes responding to calls to action to communicate with legislators to increase funding for driver evaluations and training at the local and national levels. DRSs must engage their clients, caregivers, and other professionals in these advocacy strategies.

Providers of general and specialized OT services have the opportunity to train and educate providers of public and private transportation services in disability awareness and how to assist consumers with special needs. If private, local, and state transportation providers that serve people with disabilities and the elderly do not currently have a disability awareness program for their employees, these providers may welcome the consultation services required to develop one. The occupational therapist can translate knowledge about aging and disabling conditions into sensitive and practical information for drivers, former drivers, and caregivers alike.

Driving is critical to the individual's assessment of their quality of life. Occupational therapists and other senior advocates may identify and join coordinating councils and citizen advocacy groups that are concerned about aging in place and empowering people with disabilities. Consider including employers and the local chambers of commerce as partners in identifying transportation needs and coordinating services. One of the important goals is to help actualize the mission to have transportation seen as an essential human service that must be a part of the long-term health care system.

According to NHTSA,

It is strongly suspected . . . that drivers who do not have alternative transportation continue to drive for longer than they know is safe, simply because they feel they have no choice. Conversely, drivers who have alternative methods of transportation may reduce their driving or cease driving earlier than if those alternatives were not in place. Alternative trans-

portation may increase safety by reducing the numbers and exposure to impaired drivers. Mobility alternative programs differ greatly by locality, and much can be learned by examining existing programs.[18]

Without access to affordable transportation services, people may become homebound. Table 23-6 reflects the percentage of people who do not/cannot leave their homes. It is widely believed that reduction in homebound status decreases isolation, creates opportunities for people to engage in desired occupations, and enhances their quality of living. (See Chapters 1 and 21 for more information on the effect of driving and driving cessation on people with disabilities and/or aging-related concerns.)

DRSs should become involved in their respective communities to help clients and their caregivers plan for a nondriving future. If someone is considering a move to a new home, check out the availability of transportation services as well as the location/proximity of medical, employment, educational, recreational, and leisure opportunities. Encourage individuals that are contending with progressive illnesses to think and plan for their long-term needs. Long-term planning promotes health and reduces the chances of isolation and depression. Encourage individuals with disabilities and elders to participate in their local communities by advocating for the types of transportation services that will meet their long-term community mobility needs.

Case Study #3
Alice just completed an extensive clinical and on-road evaluation of Mr. Smith's driving skills. Mr. Smith has been the primary driver for himself and his group of friends for the past 4 years. He was reluctant to come for the driver evaluation, fearing the outcome of the evaluation process.

Based on his performance, Alice is going to recommend that Mr. Smith restrict his driving and reevaluate his performance again in 6 months to determine whether his restricted driving has been positive or whether additional incidents and caregiver concerns exist. To prepare Mr. Smith and his extended family for the possibility that the temporary restricted driving plan is ineffective, Alice is devising a transition plan for him. Alice received guidance for the appropriate decision to make in this situation from the clinical data collected and from AOTA's and ADED's codes of ethics. Each code speaks to the responsibility of the practitioner to advocate for services that would benefit the client (AOTA Code, Principle 1C, 4G; ADED Code, A.1.d). It is a service to the client and to community safety to help Mr. Smith locate alternate transportation services for himself and his friends. Elimination of transportation services for all involved may lead to social isolation and ultimately a reduction in physical and mental health. If these friends are no longer able to participate in occupations of their choice, their ability to sustain themselves in the community may be jeopardized. Alice or service providers that she locates may teach Mr. Smith about alternate transportation services, their routes, and how to use them. If this service is not available through Alice's place of employment, she can contact Eldercare Locator, the Area Agency on Aging, Citizen Services for Individuals with Disabilities, or the local Center for Independent Living for referrals and assistance.

DEPARTMENTS OF TRANSPORTATION, PROFESSIONAL ORGANIZATIONS, AND KEY EMPLOYERS OF DRSs

OT practitioners have the opportunity to change the availability of, and accessibility to, transportation services. Collaboration with transportation planners will assist them in learning how to be sensitive to the special transportation needs of people with disabilities and/or aging-related concerns. If transportation services feature fixed routes, planners must consider measures to help ensure adequate and appropriate shelter, lighting, seating, and safety. The use of public transportation by individuals unfamiliar with how these systems work requires personal training that covers logistics (where to go, how to get on and off different types of vehicles) and strategies that will increase self-confidence and the feeling of personal safety. Developing client-specific interventions will require an OT needs assessment and task analysis.

When beginning a driver rehabilitation program, it is helpful to anticipate a variety of situations where clients might challenge a DRS's legal and ethical authority to accurately document and report evaluation results that can result in negative consequences such as the state restricting or revoking the client's license. The first step is to review the laws regarding reporting. Develop policies or standards about confidentiality, reporting, involving family members, and so forth. DRSs should think through scenarios where they are challenged by family members or the clients themselves if they report their clients. Be prepared to cite the laws and the legal and ethical responsibilities of the DRS. DRSs should determine in advance what they will do if they discover that an unsafe driver continues to drive against their recommendations. What actions should a DRS take if he or she determines that the client has had his or her license revoked and continues to drive? Under what circumstances will you notify family members or caregivers? When the client was referred by a physician, what information will you convey to the referral source? Understand privacy rules and be prepared to

report information required by law, ethics, or both and limit any information that may be extraneous to the situation. (See Chapter 26 for more information on starting a driver rehabilitation program.)

DRSs have a vital role to play in ensuring public safety. If team members do not have the expertise needed to assess the client's skills and make appropriate recommendations, it is incumbent upon the team to locate a consultant or refer the client to another provider (AOTA Code, Principle 4B, E, G). "Encourage your patients to plan a safety net of transportation options. . ."[16] (p. 27). Work toward a new culture that encourages people nearing retirement to make plans for driving retirement as a part of their life plan. Explore and identify community alternatives to driving. Remember that safe driving is not focused only on older adults; people with disabilities of all ages are part of the focus as well. DRSs should encourage the development of assessment tools and procedures aimed to engage at-risk drivers regardless of their age and/or disability. DRSs must avoid age discrimination and remain vigilant in their efforts to avoid prejudging anyone. However, the professional's duty to prevent injuries extends beyond the client to the community. Therefore, when a DRS is concerned about a client's safety after completing a comprehensive driver rehabilitation evaluation, the DRS has a responsibility to inform the individual of the specific concerns as well as notifying the DMV when state reporting laws apply.

DRSs should contribute to the development of checklists and self-assessment materials to help clients self-evaluate, to help caregivers identify potentially unsafe drivers, and to direct clients and caregivers to local resources and support systems as necessary. Self-assessments that are available to the community may help identify problems with judgment, ability to self-regulate, and any other factor that may impede safe driving before a client's safety and the safety of other road users and pedestrians are compromised. See Chapter 5 and Appendix G for examples of driver self-assessments.

SUMMARY

Population projections for the next several decades estimate a growth in the number of adults living into old age. Additionally, people with disabilities make up the largest minority group, with close to 60 million adults and children in the United States alone as well as approximately 600 million worldwide.[19] DRSs should consider how they can respond to the reality that the two largest segments of the population in the United States present a growing need for access to efficacious and cost-effective driver rehabilitation and community mobility services and equipment. OT practitioners can seize the opportunity to expand their presence in this practice area to enable people of all ages and abilities to begin, resume, or continue driving, or to help them access alternative community transportation services that will enable them to continue engaging in the meaningful occupations of their choosing. Developing this large pool of qualified practitioners will require strategies that include recruitment into the profession, developing educational programming, and specialty certification to reach the needs of students, entry-level practitioners, and those who already have experience in this dynamic practice area. The responsibility to become involved and obtain the knowledge and skills necessary extends to educators, practitioners, and researchers alike. The OT field's involvement in research is critical to support the examination and standardization of research tools, as well as outcome studies that examine the various interventions employed by DRSs to evaluate, educate, and train clients. Meeting the future demands for these services from individuals with disabilities and older adults will be our collective challenge. Student recruitment, increasing the availability of continuing and specialty education, and public awareness activities are needed and must have the involvement of all stakeholders—providers and individuals who will need and demand these services.

Travel within and between communities expands the notion of a DRS's role in driving and community mobility. If community members never drive motor vehicles, or lose the ability to drive safely, they will inevitably require transportation alternatives to help them remain fully engaged in their communities. Without advocacy for community transportation systems, nondrivers are likely to become socially isolated, and that will negatively influence their health, productivity, and wellness. OT generalists, OT assistants, students, and DRSs have an opportunity and ethical responsibility to advocate for driver rehabilitation and community mobility services that are often needed by clients and caregivers. Effective advocacy must occur at the local, state, national, and international levels across the micro to macro continuum, including individuals, small primary groups, larger constituency groups, institutions, agencies, and governmental bodies, to name a few. DRSs will play an ever-increasing role in assisting their clients and caregivers to face and overcome these and other unforeseen challenges within the evolving field of driver rehabilitation and community mobility.

REFERENCES

1. Personal notes from the Driving Expert Panel Meeting, March 19-20, 2004, American Occupational Therapy Association, Bethesda, Maryland.
2. American Occupational Therapy Association: Occupational therapy practice framework: domain and process, *Am J Occup Ther* 56:609-640, 2002.
3. American Occupational Therapy Association: Occupational therapy code of ethics (2000), *Am J Occup Ther* 54:614-616, 2000.
4. Wang CC, Kosinski CJ, Schwartzberg JG, et al: *Physician's guide to assessing and counseling older drivers*, Washington, DC, 2003, National Highway Traffic Safety Administration.
5. United States Census Bureau: *US Interim Projections Age, Race, Ethnicity and Hispanic Origin*, 2004, http://www.census.gov/opc/www/usinterimproj/ Internet Release Date: March 18, 2004.
6. Dalrymple G: Personal communication, June 7, 2004.
7. Insurance Institute for Highway Safety: *Fatality facts, older people 2002*, Arlington, VA, 2003, www.highwaysafety.org. Retrieved December 1, 2003.
8. United States Department of Transportation: *Safe mobility for a maturing society: challenges and opportunities*, Washington, DC, November 2003, The Department.
9. Siren A, Heikkinen S, Hakamies-Blomqvist L: *Older female road users: a review*, 2001, Swedish National Road and Transport Research Institute.
10. Royal D: *Racial and ethnic group comparisons national surveys of drinking and driving – attitudes and behavior – 1993, 1995, and 1997. Volume 1: Findings*, Washington, DC, August 2000, The Gallup Organization, United States Department of Transportation, National Highway Traffic Safety Administration.
11. Insurance Information Institute: *State driver's license renewal laws including requirements for older drivers*, as of February 2004, http://www.iii.org/media/hottopics/insurance/olderdrivers/ Retrieved March 15, 2004.
12. Staplin L, Lococo KH, Gish KW, et al: *Model driver screening and evaluation program, final technical report, Volume 1: Project summary and model program recommendations*, Office of Research and Traffic Records, May 2003, National Highway Traffic Safety Administration.
13. Pierce S: Personal e-mail, 12/4/2003.
14. Reference deleted in pages.
15. Wood H: *Does public transport training versus no intervention help clients with TBI/CVA increase their independence in accessing their local community?* December 2002, http://www.otcats.com/topics/h_wood.pdf
16. Wheatley C, Barnhart P, Davis ES, et al: *Report on community mobility/driver safety intervention as an area for specialty certification*, Rockville, MD, 2004, American Occupational Therapy Association.
17. Schold-Davis E, Wheatley C: *The impact of executive deficits on driving: why would his driving make me so nervous?* AOTA Annual Conference, May 23, 2004.
18. National Highway Traffic Safety Administration, http://www.nhtsa.gov/people/injury/olddrive/OlderRoa/problem_state.htm#04. June 24, 2002.
19. United States Census Bureau, 2000: Retrieved from www.ican.com on October 1, 2004. *Association for Driver Rehabilitation Specialists. (2003) Code of Ethics: http://www.aded.net/files/public/CodeofEthics.doc. Retrieved June 1, 2004.*

Chapter 24

RESEARCH AND EVIDENCE-BASED PRACTICE IN DRIVER REHABILITATION

Franklin Stein

KEY TERMS

- Research model
- Problem-oriented research
- Socratic method
- Quantitative research
- Qualitative research
- Experimental research
- Independent variable
- Dependent variable
- Random assignment
- Researcher bias
- Placebo effect
- Methodological research
- Evaluation research
- Survey research

CHAPTER OBJECTIVES

After completing this chapter, the reader should be able to do the following:

- Understand the importance of research in driver rehabilitation.
- Understand the steps in the research process.
- Understand the differences between and uses of quantitative and qualitative research.
- Describe the different models of research.

The history of driver rehabilitation (and more recently community mobility) coincides with the invention of the automobile around the beginning of the twentieth century. As a means of personal transportation, the automobile symbolized independence and freedom for anyone who possessed the resources to purchase one. The design of the automobile was an outgrowth of the industrial revolution and built upon the success of the railroad during the nineteenth century as a means of transporting people and goods. The automobile enabled an individual to travel independently or with family members or friends. It represented personal autonomy, as did riding a horse or bicycle.

However, the automobile itself as a complex machine raised many issues since it challenged the skill of the driver and created unknown safety problems for the driver, passengers, pedestrians, and other people using various other means of transportation. Society, too, had to accommodate the automobile by creating new highways and roads, designing signs and light signals for controlling traffic, developing rules for driving, and testing the competence of the driver and inspecting the safety of the automobile. In addition, and for the automobile to be an effective means of transportation, the mechanisms of driving had to be made more convenient for drivers. Thus, while the average car was designed for the individual of average height and weight, it was nonetheless designed as ergonomically as possible so that individuals could climb into the seat and sit down with relative ease and comfort. Shock absorbers or struts had to be constructed in the automobile so that the car could travel comfortably on rough roads or over pasturelands. Headlights were designed for night driving, brakes helped to ensure safety in stopping, and tires were designed to withstand punctures from stones or metal objects that were common obstacles during the early days of driving. Engines were built to be able to power the automobile to climb hilly terrain and reach a speed that was not only faster than walking but safe for the traffic patterns and conditions of the roads.

PEOPLE WITH DISABILITIES AND DRIVING

Individuals with disabilities required a variety of accommodations in the design of the automobile to compensate for loss of physical function. Driver rehabilitation began as soon as the automobile was adapted for the individual with a disability to drive a car safely. Research to develop special equipment for the automobile was initiated to enable the driver with a disability to operate a car. The first adaptations involved hand controls to operate the vehicle so that individuals with spinal cord injuries and lower extremity amputations could still operate the gas, brake, clutch, and other necessary driving controls. Methodological research[1] was initiated to discover materials, gadgets, and devices that could be placed in an automobile and be attached to the pedals. These were probably the first research studies into driver rehabilitation.

Later, researchers[2] focused on the driver to determine how individuals with disabilities could be retrained to drive safely. Driver rehabilitation has undergone an evolutionary process. While only automobiles were custom designed for individuals with disabilities in decades past, now a wide array of motor vehicles can be modified to allow wheelchair users and others with disabilities to not only access vehicles using hydraulic ramps or lifts that are operated by a switch, but operate all of the other operational vehicle controls as well. All of these adaptations and engineering designs are the result of research and application in the field. Current research now focuses on evaluating the effectiveness of driver rehabilitation programs for individuals with specific disabilities; for example, recovery from a stroke[3]; having an orthopedic condition,[4] visual problems,[5] Alzheimer's Disease[6]; psychosocial diagnosis[7]; or loss of function due to age.[8] Other areas of research have applied computer technology (i.e., virtual reality experiments for persons with driving phobias).[9]

Studies and public policy developed momentum during the 1950s and 1960s. Issues of focal interest included the relationship of the environment to driving performance and consideration of the safety of drivers with disabilities in such areas as use of seat belts, air bags, and visibility of signs. Highway surfaces that enhance traction in extreme weather conditions and the design of rest areas off the highway that have wheelchair-accessible facilities and reserved parking spaces for individuals with disabilities are two further examples of how research particularly benefited persons with disabilities. Hence, research in driver rehabilitation is an outgrowth of society's need to protect the public from the potential dangers of driving and to protect the rights of individuals with disabilities to have the opportunity to drive.

DEFINITION OF RESEARCH AND ITS APPLICATION TO DRIVER REHABILITATION

What is research and how does it relate to driver rehabilitation? "Research is a systematic and objective investigation as carried out by identifying a problem, stating a hypothesis or guiding question, and collecting primary data"[10] (p. 2). How can research be applied to driver rehabilitation? The three major areas of practice in driver rehabilitation include the following: (1) assessing whether the individual with a disability can drive safely, (2) training the individual to be an effective and safe driver, and (3) designing adaptive devices in motor vehicles to compensate for the individual's loss of function.

These three major areas of practice have generated a number of research studies. For example, in a clinical study exploring the driving skills of individuals with neurological symptoms, Schanke, Osten, and Pedersen[11] from Norway examined the cognitive abilities of individuals who had traumatic brain injuries and their ability to drive. They found that individuals with cognitive deficits could be evaluated through a multimodal approach that included medical, neuropsychological, and on-road evaluations in determining their capacity to drive. Driving simulators in the laboratory have also been used increasingly in research studies to determine the individual's ability to drive. Kotterba, Orth, Eren, et al[12] compared the driving performances of individuals with multiple sclerosis using a driver simulator. They found the driving simulator to be a valuable tool in evaluating driver performance. Lee, Cameron, and Lee[13] compared the effectiveness of the driving simulator with an on-the-road driving evaluation in a group of 129 older drivers. They found that the driving simulator had good validity in measuring driver performance. Virtual reality driving assessment is the newest method in assessing driver performance. Wald and Liu[14] assessed the driving performances of individuals with brain injury. They concluded that virtual reality is a valid method in assessing driver performance. These four studies show the progress based on research in assessing driver performance by starting with on-the-road tests, continuing with driver simulators in the laboratory, and finally using virtual reality assessment.

How does the researcher select a relevant topic for research? In general the *research model* is based on the scientific method, taking into consideration the identification of a significant problem, a relevant literature review, statement of a hypothesis or guiding question, method to test the hypothesis, collection of pertinent data, analysis of results, a conclusion, and recommendations for further research. The results of a research study always have a history or building block that comes before the study and a lead-in to future studies. Research is an evolving process that generates further research.

STEPS IN THE RESEARCH PROCESS

The first step in any research project is to formulate a research question. This involves brainstorming a topic. *Problem-oriented research* is a process of selecting significant issues in a field. For example, contemporary issues in driver rehabilitation generate studies that could involve assessment of an individual's ability to drive, designing powered controls in automobiles that require minimal muscle strength or use of controls for amputees, training requirements for driver evaluators, reliability and validity of driving simulators, evaluating the effectiveness of visual retraining methods, the impact of prescription drugs on driving ability, psychosocial factors and their impact on driving, aging and driving, and cognitive decline and driving. These are just some of the many significant problems in our society that are related to driver rehabilitation.

The second step in the research of driver rehabilitation is to narrow the topic to a significant problem that can be feasibly investigated and will add to the knowledge base. For example, a researcher of driver rehabilitation may be interested in devising a test that can evaluate the driving skills of individuals diagnosed with cognitive disabilities. Is this a significant topic? The initial reaction is that it seems like a reasonable topic. However, the researcher would need to narrow the investigation by a *Socratic method* of internal dialogue or by presenting his or her ideas in a scientific colloquium. A Socratic method applies a question and answer dialogue to clarify an issue. Questions to be raised, for example, are as follows:

1. What type of assessment is being planned to evaluate an individual with a disability (e.g., a paper and pencil test, driving simulator, or virtual reality test)?
2. What are other tests that are currently being used to measure the driving performance of individuals with cognitive disabilities?
3. What is the significance of the problem? For example, approximately how many individuals in the United States have cognitive disabilities and are driving?

Feedback from colleagues will sharpen the objectives of the research and clarify any questions of significance.

The third step for the researcher is to justify the research from the perspective of potential benefits to society and to individuals with disabilities. By citing epidemiological statistics and the possible impact of the results of the study on driver rehabilitation, the researcher provides strong evidence in justifying the investigation. For example, in a study that proposes to focus on drivers with cognitive impairment and their ability to return to safe driving after experiencing a stroke or TBI, etc, epidemiological statistics on the initial incidence of a disease and prevalence of the pertinent cognitive disabilities would be a valuable addition to the proposal. In Canada it is estimated that about 11% of individuals who are driving have a disability.[15] If these figures are extrapolated to the United States with an adult population of about 220 million, over 2.5 million people who are driving have a disability. This is a significant population.

The fourth step in the research process is to do an extensive review of the literature. This requires that a researcher identify and critically review the most salient research in the area of interest. A conceptual review of the literature[10] includes a step-by-step search. There are literally thousands of scientific journals that are potential sources of information for driver rehabilitation. How does the investigator systematically locate the research studies that are relevant? The steps are outlined in Box 24-1.

The first step in locating relevant research studies is to identify key words in the research, such as driver rehabilitation, evaluation of driving performance, car hand controls, driving simulator, fitness for automobile driving, older driver, driving cessation, driving and dementia, etc. The key words can be used in searching databases such as MEDLINE or CINAHL. Pubmed (http://www.ncbi.nlm.nih.gov/entrez/query.fcgi) is a good Internet source for locating research studies in the MEDLINE database. While medical databases are important sources of information, researchers must remember that one's study purpose and the specific aims of the study directly guide the search for appropriate literature. For example, if the purpose of a study is to understand the psychological impact of driving

BOX 24-1	Steps in Locating Relevant Research Studies

Identify key words in the research.
Locate a secondary source.
Initiate a search for additional perspectives.
Locate recent studies.

cessation, or alternatively, the meaning of personal mobility in individual lives, then the researcher might examine more appropriate databases like PsycINFO and SociologicalAbstracts. The second step is to locate a secondary source on the topic that can give an overall view of the subject. For example, if a researcher is interested in the topic of the driving skills of individuals with age-related macular degeneration, then the researcher would search the library for up-to-date books on the subject of macular degeneration and books related to the topic.

Initiating an Internet search for additional and more diverse perspectives on the topic by using the key words identified earlier (e.g., driver rehabilitation and macular degeneration) is the third step in locating relevant studies. Pubmed.com is one source of data that can be accessed on the web. Pubmed is the text-based search and retrieval system derived from the National Center for Biotechnology Information (NCBI) for the major databases. NCBI includes the MEDLARS database from the National Library of Medicine and the database from the National Institutes of Health. Some of the journals related to research on driver rehabilitation that are in the Pubmed system include those listed in Box 24-2. These journals represent only a portion of the database that is of interest to researchers. However, the novice researcher should be aware that Pubmed.com and MEDLINE abstract virtually the same information. These are simply two different methods to obtain this information. Also, these databases have limitations. For example, they tend not to include studies and reports produced by government agencies, research companies, commercial businesses, or industry. Thus, very current and valuable information will be missed without attention to other sources. For example, reports of consumer opinions about older drivers could be found on the AARP web site, information about the impact of seat belt legislation on traffic fatalities may only be released on the web sites of individual state governments, and crash test data may only be available from research institutes

directly. These online sources of information should not be overlooked.

The fourth step is to locate recent studies on driver rehabilitation that are not in the computer databases. The investigator should also consider contacting researchers who have published studies about driver rehabilitation. In using the Pubmed.com database or, increasingly today, even a quick Google.com search, the investigator can locate prominent investigators. Often the web page includes the researcher's e-mail address so they can be contacted directly. As mentioned above, the investigator can also use the Internet to identify previous and ongoing research by contacting agencies that publish or sponsor research in areas that are related to driver rehabilitation. Several major sponsoring agencies are described in Table 24-1. The investigator can also go to a research library and browse the stacks of recent journals that relate to driver rehabilitation to identify relevant studies.

The next step is for the researcher to compile and organize the studies located into categories of theoretical articles, descriptive studies of treatment programs, and research studies that produce original data. It is important for the researcher to carefully organize the studies in a data file that can be easily retrieved. The file should contain the citation and abstract of each study in American Psychological Association format. The file can be organized into primary data research coming from journal articles, dissertations and conference proceedings, review articles that are secondary sources, position papers, and textbooks.

The researcher is now ready to critically evaluate the validity of the content of the study, research article, or review paper of interest. In research articles, the researcher examines the research methodology, including the definition of the sample and main study groups and key variables. The researcher must also critically evaluate the appropriateness of the measures to the study purpose and ensure that the authors selected a design capable of yielding meaningful study results. This is a critical part of the literature review and increases the researcher's confidence that the study findings are valid and useful. The literature review is the sum of the studies located, the analysis of the methodologies, and the summary of the findings.

QUANTITATIVE AND QUALITATIVE RESEARCH MODELS

In order to conduct and use research in driver rehabilitation (and community mobility), it is important to understand both quantitative and qualitative approaches to research. *Quantitative research* is a hypothesis-driven approach to research in which the investigator attempts

---

BOX 24-2 | Sample of Journals That Can Be Found on the Pubmed System

Archives of Physical Medicine and Rehabilitation
Journal of Head Trauma Rehabilitation
Journal of the American Optometric Association
Human Factors
Archives of Ophthalmology
American Journal of Occupational Therapy
Occupational Therapy International
Bulletin of Prosthetic Research

Table 24-1 Major Sponsoring Agencies of Research in Driver Rehabilitation and Safety

Agency Research	URL	Description	Examples of Current Research
The Centre for Transportation Research and Innovation for People (TRIP)	www.tcd.ie/Transport_Research_Centre/	Takes a multidisciplinary approach to research transportation issues, including safety and environmental impact	
University of North Carolina Highway Safety Research Center	www.hsrc.unc.edu/	Emphasizes highway safety	Staplin, Lococo, Byington, et al[16]
United States National Highway Traffic Safety Administration	www-nrd.nhtsa.dot.gov/	Focuses on reducing and preventing motor vehicle injuries and fatalities	
United States Transportation Research Board	www.ntsb.gov/	Keeps statistics on accidents in the U.S. Advises the federal government	
Karolinska Institute, Traffic Medicine Centre, Sweden	info.ki.se/cnsf/geri/tmc/	Concerned with older drivers	Johansson, Lundberg[17] Hakamies-Blomqvist, Johansson, Lundberg[18] Johansson, Bronge, Persson, et al[19] Lundberg, Johansson, and the consensus group[20] Johansson, Bogdanovic, Kalimo, et al[21]
Federal Office of Road Safety	www.irc.uwa.edu.au/research/	Covers road injury prevention, including a database	Ryan, Legge, Rosman[22] Lee, Lee, Cameron, et al[23]
Insurance Institute for Highway Safety	www.hwysafety.org	Research is focused on testing vehicles and identifying design flaws	
National Highway Traffic Safety Administration	www.nhtsa.dot.gov/nhtsa/	Regulates vehicle adaptive equipment	National Highway Traffic Safety Administration[24]
Driver Competency Assessment (DCA)	www.dca.ca/	Offers driving assessments	
National Center for Injury Prevention and Control	www.cdc.gov/ncipc/factsheets/older.htm	Accumulates research studies on the older driver and injury statistics	Stevens, Hasbrouck, Durant, et al[25] National Highway Traffic Safety Administration[26]

to control one or more variables in an objective way so that an outcome can be reliably predicted. Thus, quantitative research focuses on measuring and counting facts and the relationships among variables, and seeks to describe observations through statistical analysis of data. It includes experimental and nonexperimental research and descriptive research (research that attempts to describe the characteristics of a sample or population). *Qualitative research* differs in purpose and practice. Qualitative research is interested in the experiences, interpretations, impressions, or motivations of an individual or individuals, and seeks to describe how people view things and why. It relates to beliefs, attitudes, and changing behavior. In contrast to quantitative research, qualitative research is more interpretative in orientation. It should be recognized, however, that there are many different types of quantitative and qualitative research (Table 24-2). Each type of research brings with it a different disciplinary tradition and tends to rely on different research methods (e.g., indepth interviews, standardized scales, structured questionnaires, participant-observation, focus groups, etc.) as well.

One useful way to distinguish the two approaches is to focus on the study question itself and ask which methodological approach—quantitative or qualitative—can best answer the study question. The primary strength of quantitative research is its ability to control study conditions. This approach starts with a defined and clearly stated hypothesis that does not change during the experiment. In qualitative research, either study questions or a hypothesis provide the starting point for a study, and rather than controlling predetermined variables, qualitative research seeks to understand the multifaceted and complex nature of human experience from the perspective of the subjects of study themselves. Drawing on cultural theory, qualitative research assumes that experiences of life vary significantly and that one cannot interpret the nature of those experiences by mechanically assigning subjects to groups, such as African-American or White, male or female, young or old, paraplegic or tetraplegic, wheelchair user or person using a cane. Although such categories may be relevant to some degree, qualitative research recognizes that understanding the experiences of members of these groups and how the experiences form and change are of greatest importance to really understanding any social phenomenon.

As implied above, different methodological approaches to research and a wide variety of data collection methods are used in research. Some examples of driver rehabilitation research using different methodologies and approaches are described below. As you read through these examples you can see that the purpose of each kind of research dictates a specific approach to the selection of research methods and tools.

EXPERIMENTAL RESEARCH

The classic example of quantitative research is *experimental research*. In this example the researcher tries to control variables and extraneous factors by identifying independent and dependent variables and reducing the effects of extraneous factors. The independent variable is the treatment or intervention applied by the investigator, and the dependent variable is the desired measurable outcome. Extraneous variables are conditions or factors that could potentially affect the results, such as age, intelligence, gender, and degree of disability. For example, Mazer et al[27] are interested in comparing two

Table 24-2 Examples of Research Models

Research Model	Examples
Quantitative	Case-control studies Cross-sectional surveys Case studies Randomized controlled trials
Qualitative	Ethnography Phenomenology Discourse analysis Case studies Life histories Grounded theory

methods to teach visual training (*independent variables*). In this study two independent variables were identified and compared; that is, the Useful Field of View (UFOV) was compared with a traditional visuoperception treatment program to determine which one is more effective in improving driving skills of individuals with visual impairments.

Before a study takes place, the investigator operationally defines the independent variables in enough detail so that other investigators who may desire to corroborate the results can replicate the study. The experimental researcher also operationally defines the *dependent variable*, which is the targeted or desired outcome of the research.

In the Mazer et al[27] study, investigators measured the outcome with three procedures: (1) on-road driving evaluation, (2) perception tests, and (3) a test of attention. In general the dependent variable is operationally defined by a procedure or standardized test that can be easily replicated. The reliability and validity of the outcome measures are reported by the investigator in order to validate the consistency and accuracy of the results. Another important characteristic of experimental design is randomization of participants into treatment groups. In the Mazer et al[27] study, 97 participants that had experienced a stroke were randomly assigned to the two interventions. *Random assignment* means that every participant has an equal chance of being assigned to an intervention. This can be done by assigning numbers to each participant and randomly selecting a number and by so doing, assign the individual to the group. Randomized control eliminates experimenter bias that could occur if the researcher "stacks the deck" by arbitrarily assigning participants to specific interventions and by so doing distorts the results. The random assignment method insures that the groups are equal in such factors as age, intelligence, or severity of illness. Randomization eliminates or reduces the effects of extraneous or systematic variables that could potentially affect the results. The important aspect of experimental research is to eliminate or reduce variables that influence the results.

Administrative or *researcher bias* can occur if the investigator is biased toward one intervention, such as hypothesizing that an automobile simulator is more effective than a controlled on-the-road test in evaluating driver performance. In this hypothetical example the investigator would employ two independent workers with equal skills and education to carry out the interventions and to test the outcome of the study. In experimental research it is necessary to control for the Hawthorne Effect, which is due to the attention and time that a group receives during an experiment. For example, if a researcher spends 30 minutes each day implementing an intervention, then the same amount of time and attention should be given to the comparative or control group. The *placebo effect* can also distort results if the participants in a study believe that the intervention received is effective as compared with a control group that does not believe that the intervention received is effective. To control for the placebo effect, it is important for the investigator to equally motivate each group as well as provide equal time and attention.

METHODOLOGICAL RESEARCH

The invention or the design of a device or instrument to improve a driver's performance is the result of *methodological research*. In this model the researcher objectively tests the reliability and validity of the instrument. Hand devices are typically used to operate the gas pedal, brake, horn, and dimmer switch in a motor vehicle. For example an investigator may be interested in developing a ring that has a hook at the end, to attach to the steering wheel for individuals with an upper limb prosthesis. The investigator should consider a number of variables in designing an effective device that can be adapted for an individual who uses an upper limb hook prosthesis. The device should be easy to install on a standard car and to remove when necessary. It should be attached securely on the steering wheel with little or no chance of failure in operating the device. The material for the ring should be durable and hold up to continuous use over a long period of time. The device should be easy to maneuver and should take limited muscle exertion. Researchers inventing new devices for driver rehabilitation explore a number of areas in detail before the device is put on the market. The steps in carrying out methodological research (Box 24-3) are outlined below.

In the first step of methodological research, the researcher states the purpose of the research (e.g., to design a hand control assistive aid for individuals with spinal cord injury). The purpose of the study should be stated clearly and the end product should be clearly portrayed, such as in a drawing.

The next step is for the researcher to do a quick literature search that may include the Internet, using key words such as hand controls and driving aids. For example, a Google.com search would assist the researcher to locate assistive devices that are currently on the market.

BOX 24-3	Steps in Carrying Out Methodological Research

State purpose.
Do literature search.
Set up laboratory or research environment.

One of the first web sites that the driver rehabilitation researcher should consult is the ADED web site. The Association for Driver Rehabilitation Specialists (ADED) (http://www.driver-ed.org) was established in 1977 to support professionals working in the field of driver education, driver training, and transportation equipment modifications for persons with disabilities. The Association publishes fact sheets that are especially helpful for the beginning researcher on disabilities such as spinal cord injury, multiple sclerosis, cerebral palsy, traumatic brain injury, and arthritis. The ADED web site includes a search menu that is helpful in locating studies that relate to driver rehabilitation and equipment adaptations for cars. Another useful web site is Midwest Mobility (http://www.midwestmobility.com). Midwest Mobility is a distributor of driver aids for individuals with spinal cord injuries and arthritis, and for amputees. This distributor lists Braun, EMC, Howell Ventures, MPS, and Wells-Engberg as manufacturers of steering devices and hand controls for individuals with disabilities. Another company identified from our example Google.com search was Access Mobility Systems, which offers many types of assistive driving devices, including hand controls and pedal extensions for brake and throttle, extensions for steering control, voice recognition, vehicle switches, and touch pad controls. The researcher can accumulate a list of a number of companies that distribute and manufacture hand devices for driving that are suited for individuals with disabilities.

One important concern that arises is in regard to the quality of the device and the group of individuals for whom this device is most useful. How does the investigator design a research study to construct and evaluate an assistive device?

Transport Canada (http://www.tc.gc.ca/tdc/menu.htm) is a valuable source of data for the researcher in evaluating driver controls. Recently a study on left-foot gas pedals for individuals with disabilities was designed in Nova Scotia to evaluate the ergonomic and technical factors. The investigators conducted the study by developing a database of descriptive studies of left-foot gas pedals and related accident reports in using this device. In laboratory studies they investigated the engineering analysis of the design of the device, ergonomic and kinesiology study in using the device, and a task analysis. The researchers concluded that industry-wide guidelines should be used in the design of custom-made left-foot gas pedals.

The next step of methodological research is to set up a laboratory or research environment to objectively study the design of the device, instrument, or hardware. The purposes of the device are operationalized so they can be measured. For example, if the main purpose of the device is to increase the driving perform-

ance of an individual with an amputation, then a driving simulator could be used to measure the outcome. Ku, Jang, Lee, et al[28] developed a virtual driving simulator for individuals with spinal cord injuries:

> The simulator is composed of an actual car, a beam projector, and a large screen. For the interface of our driving simulator, an actual car was adapted and then connected to a computer. We equipped the car with hand control driving devices especially adapted for spinal injury patients. A beam projector was used so that the subjects could see the virtual scene on a large screen set up in front of them. (p. 151)

In the research, the investigators compared the driving performances of individuals without disabilities (control group) with individuals who had spinal cord injuries (experimental group). The control group used standard car equipment for controlling speed and braking while the experimental group used hand controls to operate the gas pedal and brakes. The investigators measured driver performance (outcome) in the virtual reality driver simulator by evaluating appropriate speed, steering stability, ability to keep within the centerline, ability to obey traffic signals, and performance in driving on straight and curved roads. The results indicated that there was no significant difference between the two groups on driver performance. They concluded that the virtual reality driving simulator would be useful in improving the confidence and skill of individuals with spinal cord injuries.

Methodological research can be an ongoing endeavor that provides feedback to the investigator on the usefulness of a device. Research and development are important departments in industry and manufacturing that innovate and change products continuously. Almost every product on the market, such as home appliances, cars, computers, cameras, and cell phones, is the result of ongoing methodological research that includes innovation, design, analysis, application, and redesign.

EVALUATION RESEARCH

Evaluation research as applied to driver rehabilitation is defined as the systematic analysis of a program or organization that provides services to individuals with disabilities. In evaluation research, the purposes are clearly stated, such as certification of a program, evaluation of the effectiveness of the program, justification for expanding services, or receiving external funding, or conversely, providing data to close a program. In general, evaluation research provides objective data that are used for decision making. The Joint Commission on Accreditation of Healthcare Organizations (JCAHO) and the Commission on Accreditation of Rehabilitation Facilities (CARF) are examples of agencies that apply evaluation research in assessing the quality of a program. The steps in evaluation research are outlined here.

The first step of evaluation research is to state the purposes of the evaluations. These can include measuring the outcomes of the driver rehabilitation program, measuring direct and indirect costs of the program, measuring proposed extension of services to other geographical areas, and justifying grant application for external funding of the program.

The next step is to organize an evaluation research team that has the expertise to assess a driver rehabilitation program. Each member of the evaluation team should have a specific area of expertise, such as (1) an occupational therapist who is an expert in on-site driver training, (2) a specialist in evaluating an individual's driving performance through on-road evaluations or simulation, (3) a specialist in vehicle modification, (4) a seating specialist, (5) an administrator of a driver rehabilitation program who is familiar with budgets and personnel issues, and (6) a physician who refers clients for driver rehabilitation. The evaluation research team collects objective data that serve as the results of the study.

The third step is to collect descriptive data. This includes the following: history of the driver rehabilitation program; flow chart of administrative responsibilities and algorithm describing how a client is referred to the program and receives specific assessments and driver training; pictorial description of the physical facilities, including equipment used in assessment and training such as simulators, vans for wheelchair users, and adaptations for vehicle modification; personnel backgrounds and credentials; job descriptions of rehabilitation personnel; rehabilitation services offered; discharge policies and follow-up services provided for clients; statistical data regarding the number of clients served daily, weekly, monthly, and yearly; and schedule of costs for each client and how the program is funded, including local, state, and federal funds, as well as co-payments and grants. Follow-up referrals for vendors providing vehicle modifications, vehicle inspections, and vehicle maintenance are also needed.

Description of outcome measures used to evaluate the effectiveness of the driver rehabilitation program is the fourth step. This can include the client's increased performance in driving, follow-up data on car accidents, driving infractions, driving frequency, ability to use vehicle adaptations, and confidence in driving.

The fifth step in evaluation research is to interview on-site the staff of the driver rehabilitation program involved in assessment of driver performance, vehicle modification, and driver retraining, as well as administrative personnel and clients in the driver rehabilitation program. It is also helpful to interview clients who have completed the program to gain insights from the consumer perspective. This is the opportunity for the evaluation research team to obtain first-hand information regarding the program. Questions posed to the staff members should be well thought through and allow the respondents opportunities to explore issues in depth. For example, the evaluation team may be interested in how staff members make decisions regarding a rehabilitant's readiness to drive. How are the decisions made and what follow-up data are collected to insure that the client is making good progress as a driver?

After the data are collected, the evaluation team synthesizes the descriptive information that was obtained in statistical reports, observations regarding the physical plant, and interviews from staff and clients. This section of the evaluation is an objective reporting of the data collected.

The interpretation and discussion of the data are listed in a separate section, where the evaluation team analyzes the program data based on comparative programs. Standards for performance outcome are examined and applied in evaluating the merits and deficiencies of the program. The findings from research studies related to driver rehabilitation are cited to support points made in the interpretation.

The final section of the evaluation research report includes the summary of the report, conclusions of the study, and recommendations for changes and support for decisions. This section is sometimes referred to as the "executive summary" of the evaluation research report. Using an evaluation research model, does the description provide enough information to determine the quality of the program? What other information should be provided to make an informed opinion about this program? From a consumer's perspective, is the description of the program positive and attractive?

SURVEY RESEARCH

In general, *survey research* is defined as the objective gathering of characteristics, attitudes, and opinions of a targeted population. Survey research as applied to driver rehabilitation includes gathering of data on individuals with disabilities regarding their frequency of driving per week, their main purposes of using a motor vehicle, accidents they may have incurred over a year, consumer evaluations of adaptations used in a motor vehicle, and their attitudes toward driving with a disability.

The survey serves as the research tool. As such, the survey should be reliable and valid; in other words, the questions asked should be clearly stated and directly related to the content of the survey. Extraneous questions should be avoided. For example, in a survey of drivers with a neurological disease, questions regarding the driving abilities and physical and psychological capacities seem appropriate in a survey that seeks information on how a neurological disease affects driving performance. Questions about where the subjects went to high school or about the subject's cultural values may be perceived as extraneous by the subject. Each question on the survey should be carefully thought through and have a rationale for its inclusion in the survey. The length of the survey and the time it takes to complete will affect the survey's validity. Most surveys should be short and not take longer than 10 minutes to complete to avoid subject fatigue and lack of interest. The survey should be written so that subjects with an eighth grade education will understand the wording. Mail surveys usually have a response rate of less than 50%. To increase the response rate, the survey researcher could include a self-addressed, stamped envelope or other incentive. Telephone surveys are cost effective and do have a good response rate if the survey just takes a few minutes to complete. Surveys conducted through e-mail can be cost effective and can also have a good response rate if there is an incentive for the subject to complete the survey and the subjects' anonymity is preserved. Indepth, one-on-one survey interviews are helpful in obtaining qualitative information. The information obtained through personal interviews can be extremely valuable, but these interviews require that the interviewer be knowledgeable about interviewing as well as objective in the listening process. There are pros and cons of all types of survey methodologies. The researcher has to determine the best method for collecting data within a time frame and the finances allocated to carry out the survey.

The reliability of the survey should be pilot tested before applying it to a sample of subjects. The steps involved in survey research include the design of the questionnaire based on the purposes of the survey and the form in which it is presented. Survey questions could be open ended; for example, "What are the problems in driving that have occurred because of your disability?" The survey questions can be posed as an incomplete sentence: "The most difficult time to drive is? (e.g., during inclement weather). Another form for a survey question is the multiple forced-choice item, such as the following: "From the list below, select the item that most applies to you: 1. I feel very comfortable when driving in heavy traffic; 2. I feel comfortable when driving in heavy traffic; 3. I don't feel comfortable when driving in heavy traffic; 4. I feel uncomfortable when driving in heavy traffic; 5. I feel very uncomfortable when driving in heavy traffic." The next step in establishing the reliability and validity of the survey is to have a group of experts in driver rehabilitation and experts in research design critique the survey. The panel of experts evaluates the survey by commenting on the content and clarity of each item. After the survey is revised based on the comments of the experts, the survey researcher then pilot-tests the survey with a small group of subjects to screen out ambiguous items. The individual evaluating the survey in a pilot study

provides feedback regarding the length of the survey and ambiguity of any questions, and perhaps recommends that an item be eliminated or a new item be added. The survey is again revised and is now ready to be used in a research project.

The next important phase of survey research is to select a representative sample. A representative sample should reflect the demographics of the population, including age, gender, geographical distribution, severity of disability, and any other variable that could possibly influence the results. Randomization and random samples are used in obtaining a representative sample. A random sample assumes that every individual in the population has an equal chance of being selected for the study. Tables of random numbers are used to assign potential subjects with an equal opportunity of being selected for the study. Stratified samples are also used in selecting portions of a population for study, such as all men or individuals living in a specific geographical area or individuals with 5/6 cervical spinal cord injuries.

Surveys are frequently used to gauge a population's attitudes toward a controversial subject, such as allowing individuals who have a diagnosis of schizophrenia to obtain a driver's license. For example, in Utah, a study was undertaken to determine the effect of a psychiatric or emotional condition on driving.[29] Through a survey of public records, the researchers obtained and examined the records of individuals with psychosocial disabilities. The data collected included information regarding traffic violations; accidents were separated by fault and no-fault of the driver. The data obtained were compared with public data from so-called unrestricted drivers (drivers without a disability or restriction on driving due to a disability). The information obtained in this study came mostly from public records. In this example the survey relied on the accuracy of the public records. Is this a reliable and valid method to obtain data? On the basis of the results reported in the study,[29] it appears that individuals with a psychosocial disability did not have significantly higher rates of traffic citations or accidents as compared with a sample of individuals without restrictions or disabilities. This study illustrates the use of survey data in comparing the driving performances of a group of individuals with disabilities with a "normal group."

In another survey DeCarlo et al[30] applied a standardized questionnaire to a randomized group of 126 elderly individuals with a diagnosis of maculopathy. The questionnaire was administered through telephone interviews. The participants were selected from a list of individuals who had attended a low vision rehabilitation clinic in the last year. Of the 126 individuals contacted, 30 of the individuals reported that they were continuing to drive. The researchers found that the drivers reported driving an average of 4 days a week for approximately 10 miles. About 50% of the drivers in general avoided situations that would make them vulnerable to accidents such as rain, heavy traffic, driving during the evening, and driving on interstate highways.

SUMMARY

Research is an important part of driver rehabilitation and community mobility. The research conducted today leads to improvements in mobility for disabled and older drivers in the future. Several different research models can be employed; the researcher must choose the best one to fit the scope and needs of his or her study.

REFERENCES

1. Reger SI, McGloin AT, Law, DF, et al: Aid for training and evaluating of handicapped drivers, *Bull Prosthetic Research* 10:35-39, 1981.
2. Haslegrave CM: Driving for handicapped people, *Int Disabil Stud* 13(4):111-120, 1991.
3. Akinwuntan AE, DeWeerdt W, Feys H, et al: Reliability of a road test after stroke, *Arch Phys Med Rehabil* 84(12):1792-1796, 2003.
4. Egol KA, Sheikhazadeh A, Mogatederi S, et al: Lower-extremity function for driving an automobile after operative treatment of ankle fracture, *J Bone Joint Surg Am* 85(7):1185-1189, 2003.
5. Keeffe JE, Jin CF, Weih LM, et al: Vision impairment and older drivers: who's driving? *Br J Ophthalmol* 86(10):1118-1121, 2002.
6. Fox GK, Bowden SC, Bashford GM, et al: Alzheimer's disease and driving: prediction and assessment of driving performance, *J Am Geriatr Soc* 45:949-953, 1997.
7. Hauri-Bionda R, Bar W, Friedrich-Koch A: Driving fitness/driving capacity of patients treated with methadone, *Schweiz Med Wochenschr* 10:1538-1547, 1998.
8. Stutts JC, Wilkins JW: On-road driving evaluations: a potential tool for helping older adults drive safely longer, *J Safety Res* 34:431-439, 2003.
9. Wald J, Taylor S: Preliminary research on the efficacy of virtual reality exposure therapy to treat driving phobia, *Cyberpsychol Behav* 6:459-465, 2003.
10. Stein F, Cutler S: *Clinical research in occupational therapy*, ed 4, San Diego, 2000, Singular/Thomson.
11. Schanke AK Osten PE, Hofft E, et al: Assessment of cognitive ability to drive after brain injury, *Tidsskrift for den Norske laegeforening* 119:954-958, 1999.
12. Kotterba S, Orth M, Eren E, et al: Assessment of driving performance in patients with relapsing-remitting multiple sclerosis by a driving simulator, *Euro Neurol* 50(3):160-164, 2003.
13. Lee HC, Cameron D, Lee AH: Assessing the driving performances of older adult drivers: on-road versus simulated driving, *Accid Anal Prev* 35(5):797-803, 2003.
14. Wald J, Liu L: Psychometric properties of the driVR: a virtual reality driving assessment, *Stud Health Technol Inform* 81:564-566, 2001.
15. Transport Canada: The potential of intelligent transportation systems to increase accessibility to transport for elderly and disabled people (TP 12926E). Accessed 2/17/05 through the web: *www.tc.gc.ca/tdc/summary/12900/12926e.htm*
16. Staplin L, Lococo K, Byington S, et al: *Guidelines and recommendations to accommodate older drivers and pedestrians*, Report No FHWA-RD-01-051, McLean, VA, 2001, Federal Highway Administration.
17. Johansson K, Lundberg C, editors: *Aging and driving. Effects of aging, diseases and drugs on sensory functions, perception, and cognition, in relation to driving ability*, Proceedings, Stockholm, 1994, Karolinska Institute.
18. Hakamies-Blomqvist L, Johansson K, Lundberg C: Medical screening of older drivers as a traffic safety measure—a comparative Finnish-Swedish evaluation study, *J Am Geriatr Soc* 44:650-653, 1996.
19. Johansson K, Bronge L, Persson A, et al: Can a physician recognize an older driver with increased crash risk potential? *J Am Geriatr Soc* 44:1198-1204, 1996.
20. Lundberg C, Johansson K, and the consensus group: Dementia and driving. An attempt at consensus, *Alzheimer's Dis Assoc Disord* 11(1):28-37, 1997.
21. Johansson K, Bogdanovic N, Kalimo H, et al: Alzheimer's disease and apolipoprotein E e4-allele in older drivers who died in automobile accidents, *Lancet* 349:1143-1144, 1997.
22. Ryan GA, Legge M, Rosman D: Age related changes in drivers' crash risk and crash type, *Accid Anal Prev* 30(3):379-387, 1998.
23. Lee HC, Lee AH, Cameron D, et al: Using a driving simulator to identify older drivers at inflated risk of motor vehicle crashes, *J Safety Res* 34(4):453-459, 2003.
24. National Highway Traffic Safety Administration, Bureau of Transportation Statistics: *Common vehicle modifications for persons with disabilities*, September 2002, *www.nhtsa.dot.gov/cars/rules/adaptive/ BTSRN/ResearchNote0209.html* accessed July 20, 2004.
25. Stevens JA, Hasbrouck L, Durant TM, et al: Surveillance for injuries and violence among older adults, *MMWR Surveillance Summaries* 48 (SS-8):27-50, 1999.
26. National Highway Traffic Safety Administration, Department of Transportation (US): *Traffic safety facts 2002: older population*, Washington, DC, 2003, NHTSA, [cited 2003 December 10]. Available from: URL: *http://www-nrd.nhtsa.dot.gov/pdf/nrd-30/ NCSA/TSF2002/2002oldfacts.pdf.*
27. Mazer et al: Effectiveness of a visual attention retraining program on the driving performance of clients with stroke, *Arch Phys Med Rehabil* 84(4):541-550, 2003.
28. Ku JH, Jang DP, Lee BS, et al: Development and validation of virtual driving simulator for the spinal injury patient, *Cyberpsychol Behav* 5:151-156, 2002.
29. Diller E, Cook L, Leonard D, et al: *Evaluating drivers licensed with medical conditions in Utah, 1992-1996*, U.S.DOT/NHTSA Pub No. DOT HS 809 023, Washington, DC, 1999.

Chapter 25

EMERGENT FUNCTIONAL BRAIN IMAGING AND DRIVER REHABILITATION*

Richard J. Genik II • Li Hsieh • Christopher C. Green

KEY TERMS

- Functional neuroimaging
- Gray matter
- White matter
- Neural correlates
- Baseline
- Behavior
- Brain network

CHAPTER OBJECTIVES

After completing this chapter, the reader will be able to do the following:

- Be knowledgeable about the current state-of-the-art technology in neuroimaging.
- Understand the various imaging modalities and how they work.
- Learn about the application of these imaging techniques in evaluation of driving performance for clients with brain injuries during the rehabilitation process.
- Recognize the importance in developing a new perspective for driver rehabilitation in convergence between advanced technology and rehabilitation approaches.

*This work is supported in part by General Motors Foundation and National Defense University.

NEXT GENERATION IMAGING IN DRIVER REHABILITATION

Functional imaging of the brain is the most important emergent medical technology for those studying rehabilitation involving restoration or reassignment of neural activity. The methodology, detailed in this chapter, makes use of a way to actually watch people think and observe how cognition, workload, and emotionality relate to each other. The research world is currently evaluating clinical techniques that allow real-time monitoring of the brain activity during the recovery process, especially after closed-head or traumatic brain injury (TBI).[1-3] This chapter is intended to assist the driver rehabilitation specialist (DRS) by giving an overview of the current state-of-the-art methodologies in neuroimaging for specialists who will soon be testing this technology. Also, we look forward to where the field is going in the next decade, and detail how this evolving technology will serve patients and clients. Extensive references are included for those interested in further literature reviews or comprehensive physics and engineering explanations of the various technologies beyond the brief treatment presented here. Our aim is to enable the DRS to unlock the "person in the brain" to promote an optimal level of recovery and functioning in a variety of contexts including driving and community mobility.

FROM BASICS TO DRIVING

Functional neuroimaging is the study of brain activity related to a specific internal or external function such as finger tapping, where one may expect to observe activity in the areas of the motor cortex, or passive visual stimulation, where one may expect to observe activity in the primary visual cortex. The entire central nervous system is constantly active with many functions occurring simultaneously, even when a person is at rest.

Gray matter is the brain tissue where thinking takes place, and *white matter* serves to transmit signals between clumps of gray matter. Determining the exact areas of gray matter activity associated with a function, called the *neural correlates* for that function, is accomplished by taking a measurement during performance of a function and comparing it with a measurement used as a control, called the *baseline*. In a simple example, the brain is monitored while the subject taps his index finger against his thumb for a specified time interval, called the "stimulus interval," and then remains still for an equal period of time, called the "baseline interval." The stimulus-baseline pairs are repeated several times to obtain a stable average, and the difference between the two averages reveals the neural correlates of finger tapping.

The stimulus design in the previous example is known as "boxcar" or "block" design. This design contrasts with an event-related design, in which stimuli are presented or tasks are performed at irregular intervals (Figure 25-1). The averaging of the data is more involved in event-related designs, although the result is the same: a mean measurement for each functional state, in which the difference reveals the neural correlates.

In general, mean measurements are not single images. The precise nature of the mean measurement depends on the modality used in a given complete experimental setup, or paradigm. Stimulus and baseline intervals in a boxcar design are nearly always set equal, and the period is often called the "Inter-Stimulus Interval," or ISI. The various technologies, detailed in the next section, all result in differential maps showing the areas of neural activity determined by the specific modality.

Complex functionality includes multiple task-induced and stimuli-induced neural responses. A complex functionality that is repeatable because it is instinctual or learned is termed a *behavior*. Complex behaviors can include a compilation of neural correlates called a *brain network*, and several brain networks may be involved in behaviors such as driving. It should be noted that the definitions are not universal due to ongoing evolution of the field and nonstandardization; paradigm, for example, is also sometimes used as shorthand for stimulus paradigm, the time course of all sensory stimuli within an experiment. Additionally, the terms "brain network" or "neural system" are preferred instead of "neural network" for a set of neural correlates; a neural network is previously defined as a statistical data classification technique, and this technique is used in neuroimaging.

Until recently the areas of the brain that were essential for fitness to drive could only be inferred from neuropsychological test performances through correlation with actual on-road driving ability.[4,5] With the advent of new neuroimaging technology, observation and analysis of the actual neural correlates and brain networks that subserve driving are possible.[6,7] Additionally, patterns of activation that serve as compensatory mechanisms for driving for brain injury survivors can be examined. Understanding the complexity of driving behavior as it pertains to neural activation could revolutionize the way driving ability is conceptualized and assessed, as well as guide the development of new technologies for driver rehabilitation.

The methodology used to generate neural correlates specific to a function is a far cry from reading minds, as some of the more hyperbolic literature sometimes implies. Neuroimaging tools are presented here that provide complementary pieces that strengthen the broader evaluation and rehabilitation puzzle outlined by the other chapters in this text.

TBI FOLLOWING AUTOMOTIVE ACCIDENTS

Safe operation of a motor vehicle requires a complex interaction of motor skills and perceptual and cognitive abilities. Survivors of TBI typically are permitted to resume driving a motor vehicle without medicolegal consideration; however, brain damage can substantially compromise fitness to drive.[5,8,9] Research suggests that 40% to 60% of individuals resume driving after brain injury, yet nearly two thirds of these individuals do not receive a formal evaluation for driving competency.[5,10-13] Not all licensed clients with acquired brain damage drive, and literature on disability and driving strongly indicates that handicaps per se are not related to increased rates of motor vehicle crashes or traffic violations. In fact some researchers propose that

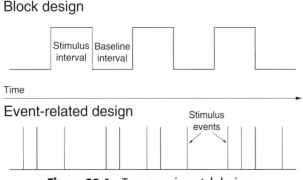

Figure 25-1 Two experimental designs.

persons with disabilities are highly motivated to be good drivers.[12]

Many clients with TBIs who resume driving, however, have residual deficits that impair their driving performance.[14] Despite the number of people who survive brain injuries and resume driving, little is known about the actual effect of the neurological insult on neural activation and driving ability. The most common type of neurological insult secondary to motor vehicle accidents is diffuse axonal injury (DAI), which occurs after subcortical white matter tracks are stretched and pulled to the extent that significant permanent damage occurs. This type of injury most commonly results in slowed information processing speed and decreased cognitive flexibility as information transfer between gray matter areas is partially interrupted or requires rerouting around damaged white matter pathways.[15] Speed and flexibility of cognitive processes are essential factors in safe driving, and neuroimaging allows both qualities to be benchmarked and tracked during rehabilitation.

TRANSMISSION-RELATED INJURY OR INTERRUPTION

In addition to direct neural injury, functional impairment can be caused by injury or interruption of brain signals during transmission to the extremities either through spinal cord injury (SCI) or traumatic amputation (TA) of the extremity itself. Current research in neuroimaging involves developing techniques to image the spinal cord to determine the quantitative extent to which transmitted neural signals propagate.[16-18] If successful, this will allow localization of signal losses using an orthogonal measure for visualization of the physical injury. Additionally, a new measure to accurately track progression of spinal cord rehabilitation will be available. It has also been proposed to use real-time neuroimaging feedback to assist in training TA clients to use artificial limbs that are controlled via neural transmission through existing circuitry. The hope is that extensive and detailed multi-modal feedback training with neuroprosthetics will allow extended function for very complex behaviors such as driving and reduce the need for vehicle modifications (i.e., structural changes to the vehicle, adapted driving aids, or both).

GROWTH IN THE REHABILITATION TEAM

Neuroimaging technology will continue to develop over the next decade. The process of moving leading-edge research from clinical evaluation to routine technical task will echo in an evolution of the rehabilitation team. It is likely that in the next few years, world-class rehabilitation teams will temporarily add a couple of members. A PhD cognitive neuroscientist will be required to develop experimental paradigms to test and track a client's progress. A PhD physicist specializing in experimental design, familiar with the basic principles and operation of all of the modalities in use and trained in data postprocessing techniques, will be required to set up and check system integration from stimulus delivery to response logging, to image processing and quality control. Such multidisciplinary supervisors will develop the training program for research assistants and courses for postgraduate training programs. By the end of this decade the clinical rehabilitation team will likely include only a single person with a postgraduate education and training in medical physics with a specialty in functional neuroimaging.

The DRS participating in testing and evaluation of neuroimaging during this development phase will require general knowledge of the techniques to be employed. This is the subject of the next section.

RELEVANT TECHNOLOGIES IN NEUROIMAGING FOR REHABILITATION

Several modalities are currently available to produce images of differential function states. Detailed here are the techniques associated with electroencephalography (EEG), magnetoencephalography, magnetic resonance imaging (MRI), and near-infrared spectrometry. The goal of this tutorial is to allow the DRS to understand the how, what, and why of each modality rather than serve as a comprehensive training manual, since such training is specific to equipment and manufacturer, and scanning techniques are likely to evolve within the useful life of this text. Additional functional techniques exist that exploit contrast and tracing agents alone, namely positron emission tomography (PET) and single photon emission computed tomography (SPECT), and in conjunction with x-rays, namely computed tomography (CT or "CAT") and angiography; however, all four of these modalities require exposing the patient to ionizing radiation, and although minimal risk is assumed per scan, they are not ideal for the multiple measurements required during a comprehensive rehabilitation program in which longitudinal scans track progress.

ELECTROENCEPHALOGRAPHY

Neuronal activity and transmission of signals between neurons is accomplished through biochemical reactions that have the net effect of movement of ions in solution. The ionic charges do not exist in a vacuum, and the motion of these charged particles affects the surrounding tissues by disturbing nearby bound electrons much as the motion of a speedboat on a lake creates a wake of diffuse eddies and currents in the surrounding water. These currents in turn create their own induced currents, and so on, until finally these internal electrical disturbances appear on the surface of the skin and can be measured via noninvasive surface electrodes. The original movement of charge is termed the "primary current," and the sympathetic movements are called "volume currents." The electrical response on the skin is, for all practical purposes, simultaneous with the neuronal firings and therefore an accurate temporal measure of activity. However, the deeper the origin of activity, the weaker and more diffuse the signal at the skin, so acceptable spatial accuracy is limited to cortical activity in most cases. The measurement of these currents, detected as a time-dependent voltage difference between two points, is the basis of EEG.

Electrical signals from the brain typically result in voltage differences at the skin of a few to tens of microvolts (mV). Electrodes are placed on the scalp at equidistant points between fixed landmarks on the head and are specified for their lobule location and distance from center. Voltage differences measured between the electrodes, and a reference value, determine the signal for a given channel. The reference value is set using one of three different schemes, called "derivations." In common derivation, all electrode signals are measured against a single standard such as the ear electrodes; A1, A2, or A1 connected to A2 are typically used. The average reference derivation takes the arithmetic mean of all electrodes, and each channel is measured against the instantaneous result. The bipolar derivation measures the difference between adjacent electrodes, usually starting in the front (F3-C3, C3-P3, etc.). The standard 21-channel configuration is shown in Figure 25-2. An extended standard placement and nomenclature exists for up to 74-channel electrode configurations, and proposed standards are being considered for up to as many as 300 channels.

EEG signals are classically traced out on a multichannel chart recorder, where the deflection of each pen is proportional to the measured instantaneous voltage in that channel; this type of recording device is generally called a "polygraph." The vast majority of brain activity produces alternating electrical signals with frequencies less than 30 Hz. Additionally, signals are classified by frequency, with beta activity greater than 13 Hz, alpha activity between 8 and 13 Hz, theta activity between 4 and 7 Hz, and delta activity less than 4 Hz. Normal adults who are awake with their eyes open will exhibit beta and alpha activity. Drowsy adults may exhibit theta activity, while delta is normally only seen in deep sleep.

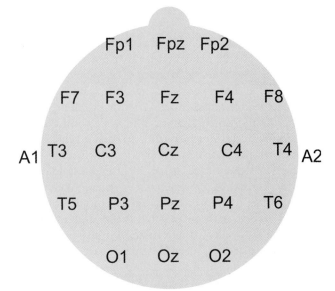

Figure 25-2 Standard 21-channel 10/20 electrode configuration, for 10% to 20% distribution along anatomical markers. *Fp*, Frontal pole; *F*, frontal; *C*, central; *T*, temporal; *P*, parietal; *O*, occipital; *A*, ear references. *z*, for "zero" to avoid confusion with *O*, indicates midline, with odd numbers on the left, and even numbers to the right.

Alpha and beta signals should be observed around the frontal and temporal lobules and on the occipital lobule near the visual cortex during driving behavior. Signals may be quantified by fixing a reference of alpha and beta strength in mV and extent in number of electrodes above a threshold of activity during a visual fixation and standard motor exercise. The absolute value of a reference may be used for general tracking of improvement during rehabilitation, and relative performance during the driving behavior can be used to track multi-task execution progress.

Event related potentials (ERPs) may be observed as single or multiple deflections of channels between 0.1 and 30 Hz, depending on the nature of the stimulus, and occurring at a set time lag after a stimulus event. A stimulus is repeated several times and the signals are averaged to obtain a stable result that is above the inherent noise.[19,20]

MAGNETOENCEPHALOGRAPHY

Primary currents produce sympathetic volume currents via an electrical interaction between the various charged participants. Both primary and volume currents also produce magnetic fields. The strength of these magnetic fields is inherently small, screened by tissue interactions, and weakens with distance. Although unlike measuring potential differences at the scalp, which requires solid and stable electrical contact between the electrodes and the skin, measuring the magnetic field only requires a sensor close to the skin because the magnetic field propagates in free space. The challenge in quantifying the magnetic field changes from neural activity is finding a device that is sensitive enough to detect changes on the order of 100 femtoTesla (fT), where one fT is one thousandth of one millionth of one millionth of a Tesla (10^{-15} T). By comparison, the magnetic field of the Earth at the surface is measured in tens of microTesla, about one hundred million times stronger. The sensor that performs this difficult job is a small loop of special wire cooled to a temperature near −454° F by bathing it in liquid helium. This superconducting quantum interference device (SQUID) measures the time-varying magnetic field at a point near the scalp, and an array of SQUIDs mounted inside a cryogenic helmet constitute the detection apparatus of a magnetoencephalogram (MEG) (Figure 25-3). A MEG specifically designed for detection of brain activity is also called a "neuromagnetometer."

Interpretation of MEG measurements is slightly less challenging than EEG. Both modalities can be thought of as measuring a two-dimensional shadow and then trying to determine the set of three-dimensional objects that likely produced the shadow, without knowing the number or location of objects and illuminating light sources. Using the previous metaphor, the challenge of interpretation is like measuring the waves breaking on the shoreline and trying to determine the number and location of watercraft responsible. In EEG, cortical primary currents will partially mask propagation of gyral and subcortical-induced volume currents, though not completely; therefore, a given cortical activation pattern can be mimicked by a greater amount of gyral activation. Although the overall field strength is smaller, the measured magnetic field depends on the direction of the current that produced it: cortical surface primary currents parallel to the scalp produce good signal, while gyral activations, where the primary currents flow perpendicular to the scalp, are not well detected with commercially available hardware. The masking of subcortical currents is less with magnetic fields and still leads to multiple activation patterns that can produce the same field map, although with gyral activation nearly excluded, localization is easier. Fortunately, for the purposes of driver rehabilitation, we concentrate on qualitative existence of activation in functional paradigms and relative quantitative improvement in signal strength within and between modalities.

A final important point about MEG is that because of the sensitivity of the instrument, measurements must take place in a shielded room. Combined with the extent of the cryogenics required to keep the SQUIDs cold and precision instrumentation to read the minute induced electrical signals, MEG systems cost between ten and one hundred times that of an EEG system.[19,21,22]

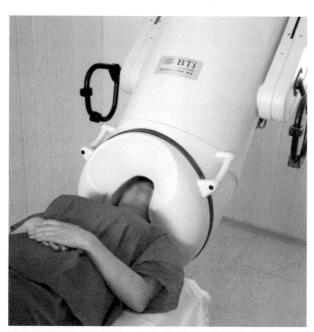

Figure 25-3 Example of a 148-channel MEG. The sensors are located near the scalp, while the associated electronics are further up. The bulk of the cylinder above the head is cryogenics. (Courtesy Henry Ford Hospital, Detroit, Mich.)

FUNCTIONAL MAGNETIC RESONANCE IMAGING

The concepts that make MRI a powerful tool are easy to explain. Radiofrequency (RF) energy that is about the same as found in FM-band is transmitted while the subject is in a strong static magnetic field (the MRI magnet). The static field orients a small (but measurable) number of the hydrogen nuclei (single protons) in the brain in a parallel direction. The applied RF field flips the orientation (because the selected frequency exactly matches the resonant frequency of the spinning hydrogen protons and transfers energy to them) and the RF is then turned off. As the protons relax from this excited state and realign, energy is given up, and the same antenna-system (oriented in three dimensions) that sent the RF now measures the relaxation energy as it returns. Mathematical processing of the directions, timing, and amount of RF that returns all create a picture. The picture is exact, and there is no better way to noninvasively visualize the anatomy of the brain than this technology.

Comprehensive physics and engineering details are best left to another venue; besides, the majority of these details are not important to the DRS. There are, however, a couple of concepts worth noting so that the terminology used makes sense.

On top of the static field is added a smaller time-varying magnetic field called the "gradient field." This varying field changes the characteristics of the returned energy based on the spatial location of tissue in a known manner. Furthermore, energy characteristics returned are different depending on whether a given proton is part of a water or lipid molecule, and whether surrounding molecules have significant magnetic properties; for example, iron atoms in deoxygenated blood molecules (deoxyhemoglobin) exhibit paramagnetic properties seen in bulk iron and distort the local magnetic field enough to cause a few percent reduction in the amplitude of the returned RF signal from neighboring water molecules. Combining the spatial and tissue composition information, a three-dimensional picture is reconstructed.

The gradient fields are produced via electromagnets in the form of coils mounted on the inside bore of an MRI scanner. The gradient control system switches the field around in a preplanned manner, called the "sequence," to maximize signal for the specific effect under study. This rapid changing of electrical current magnitude and direction in the gradient coils produces the noise heard during image acquisition.

Every tissue containing hydrogen has associated magnetic properties that determine two half-life time constants. T1, typically measured in seconds, describes how fast the average molecule in a tissue returns input RF energy by relaxing and realigning its spin to the static field. T2, typically measured in tens of milliseconds, describes how long spins within a tissue stay aligned to one another as they are relaxing. Standard MR sequences concentrate on a measurement of either T1 or T2. More precisely, the sequence produces a contrast image based on weighting each three dimensional pixel, called a voxel, by an amount proportional to T1, T2, or whichever physical property the sequence was designed to measure.

It is very important to remember that even when the gradient system is deactivated and the machine is not making any noise, the large static field is still present in the scan room; the typical signage reads "WARNING: THE MAGNET IS ALWAYS ON." The static field itself is safe for living tissue, but ferromagnetic objects can become dangerous projectiles around the magnet. No objects attracted to magnetic fields should ever be brought into the scan room. In addition, the MR field will erase all information from credit cards and magnetic ID badges, so leave these objects outside of the magnet room when assisting in these scans.

BOLD Imaging

The most important functional technique currently in widespread use is called "blood oxygen level dependent" (BOLD) imaging. Localized neural activity consumes oxygen. The body responds to this increased local depletion by increased blood flow and blood volume to areas in need. The net effect of this reaction is to increase the ratio of oxy- to deoxyhemoglobin in the draining venules and veins surrounding the area of activation. Since oxyhemoglobin is diamagnetic (the iron atoms are "rusted") and deoxyhemoglobin is paramagnetic, this change in local magnetic susceptibility can be seen in sequences that mainly contrast T2. The time course characterizing this change in blood ratio is called the hemodynamic response function (hrf), and it typically peaks at t = 3 to 9 seconds (where t = 0 seconds at neuronal firing), subsides at t = 8 to 12 seconds, and returns to baseline at t = 12 to 20 seconds. The peak signal strength is typically 1% to 5% of the total MR signal (depending on the static field strength, with higher fields producing a larger change), so like EEG and MEG, many repetitions are required to obtain a good average above inherent noise.

BOLD measurements are most often acquired using echo-planar imaging (EPI). These sequences are currently capable of producing a moderate resolution whole brain image in less than 2 seconds. This sampling frequency allows several points during hrf evolution to be measured at each repetition. This technique is most often called BOLD-EPI.

Susceptibility Weighted Imaging (SWI)

Susceptibility weighted imaging (SWI) is a new proprietary technique using venous deoxyhemoglobin content as an indicator of neuronal injury. Currently undergoing clinical evaluation, it is expected to prove superior to traditional gradient-echo techniques in evaluating DAI because it images gray-white matter boundaries at unprecedented resolution (1 mm × 1 mm or better) and allows for visualization of the venous side of the injury. SWI partial-brain imaging requires several tens of seconds and therefore is primarily used in structural tracking; however, initial clinical evaluation using SWI in functional paradigms is ongoing.

Diffusion Weighted Imaging (DWI)

Diffusion weighted imaging (DWI) is a routine technique available in the traditional T1 and T2 applied sequences. It is an excellent method for gauging the age and the characterization of hemorrhage and infarction in brain injury. Additional postacquisition calculations allow for an "apparent diffusion coefficient" (ADC) to be obtained of the areas of injury.

Application of this technique to TBI and other brain pathologies is in the early stages of clinical evaluation.

Diffusion Tensor Imaging (DTI)

Diffusion tensor imaging (DTI) is a postacquisition data processing technique for images that have recorded water diffusion. Under clinical evaluation by teams across the country, DTI takes advantage of axonal structural anisotropy. In an isotropic environment such as a spherical bottle of water, a sequence measuring diffusion along the Z direction will yield identical results to one measuring along the X direction. In a confined tube such as an axon of white matter, however, maximum signal will be obtained when the sequence acquisition direction is along the axonal axis. Using a mathematical technique to combine 6 or 12 axis of acquisition, it is possible to reconstruct active white matter tracks in the brain. This advanced technique is applicable to diagnosing track disruption seen in DAI, resulting in a greater understanding of the pervasiveness of typical white matter damage, how it might affect driver performance, and allowance of another window to track rehabilitation progress. DTI sequences require several minutes of acquisition time and are currently exclusively under investigation in nonfunctional scans for anatomical evaluation; however, the very nature of the sequence does reveal dynamic functionality of white matter.

Standard Anatomical Imaging and Coregistration

Routine high-resolution sequences such as FLASH or MPRAGE are used in creating standard three-dimensional T1-weighted images. These images, besides their clinical usefulness in demarcating gray and white matter areas of the brain, are important for something called "coregistration." Individual normal brains contain the same areas around the same structures; the visual cortex is always located between these fissures, the right-hand motor operation is performed on this gyrus, etc. And even though brain anatomical structure is well known, there are small individual differences in size and location, as well as normal variations in assigned functionality. These individualities require recognition in any quantitative evaluation: if the peak of right side visual activation in an EEG study is stronger in electrode O1 for one subject versus T3 for another, it is because (1) the electrodes were misplaced, (2) there is a normal deviation between the location of the visual cortex relative to skull landmarks used to place the electrodes, or (3) one of the subjects has injured his or her visual cortex and an adjacent area in the brain has adapted and assumed control of that function. The last of these options is the entire reason for performing neuroimaging during rehabilitation, but the first two should be accounted for before assuming the third.

There exist a few standard human brain anatomical T1 MRI. MNI305 and the newer ICBM152 are standards that constitute the mean of 305 and 152 subject pools, respectively. One can use mathematical techniques to warp, say, subject EPI onto the standard brain. This warping of one image onto another is called "coregistration." More important to individual subjects during rehabilitation, though, is coregistering EPI, DWI, or DTI with a subject's own high-resolution T1 image (SWI is already high-resolution). Also, standard techniques are emerging to automatically coregister EEG and MEG sensor locations either by anatomical landmarks visible on the whole head image, or by manually marking the head with a drop of vitamin E or similar lipid that will show up very bright on a T1 image. Vitamin E pills are routinely taped to the right side of subject's foreheads for a similar reason as taping a metal "R" on an x-ray film.[23]

NEAR INFRARED SPECTROSCOPY (NIRS)

Near infrared spectroscopy (NIRS) is a very new technique that is beginning to be used in clinical evaluation. This technique relies on the BOLD effect just like BOLD-EPI but instead of exploiting the magnetic susceptibility difference, it exploits a chemical difference between oxy- and deoxyhemoglobin, namely the different optical absorption spectra: one appears bright red and the other slightly bluish. This difference in color is also present at near infrared wavelengths. In a similar light-penetrating fashion to shining a flashlight completely through one's hand, NIRS shines two wavelengths of light into the skull and records the reflection showing peaks at oxy- and deoxyhemoglobin (Figure 25-4). Each sensor requires a wide area to be illuminated to collect enough signal, and spatial

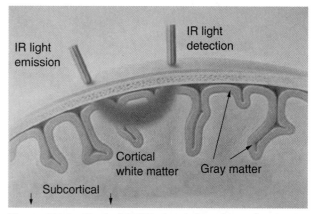

Figure 25-4 Cortical BOLD signal detection using NIRS. Infrared light shone through the skull is reflected differently depending on the time-dependent concentrations of oxyhemoglobin and deoxyhemoglobin.

resolution is measured in tens of mms, about a factor of 10 larger than conventional functional magnetic resonance imaging (fMRI) and comparable with the cost advantage. Current commercial production includes 48-channel systems with the sensors embedded in a flexible skull cap similar to large channel EEG. The illumination sources and sensors can be the ends of optical fibers and are theoretically MR compatible.[24]

MULTI-MODAL STUDIES

Tremendous promise is already evident when combining two or more functional techniques. MRI and NIRS measure the BOLD signal and thus share a common temporal resolution. MRI is the gold standard for spatial resolution. EEG and MEG directly measure neural activity and have similar temporal resolution that is superior to BOLD, where the signal itself is an indirect measure of brain activation.

In additional to using a three-dimensional anatomical MRI as the benchmark for coregistration, one can theoretically combine functional MR with NIRS for simultaneous measurement of the BOLD signal. Once calibrated against three-dimensional BOLD-EPI images, longitudinal scans to track progress can be done with the significantly cheaper NIRS system. Moreover, because of the decreased spatial resolution in NIRS, the subject may move about with the optical sensor array attached to the head, versus fMRI where the subject must maintain a millimeter or better constant cranial position. Furthermore, simulation and training equipment for use outside of the magnetic environment provides greater flexibility for rehabilitation programs. For example, the MR-compatible visual stimulation system alone requires capital and maintenance outlay close to that of an entire NIRS scanner.

BOLD imaging isn't a panacea for rehabilitation; the imaging technique itself assumes normal oxygen usage and hemodynamic response, and TBI or other maladies that may bring a client to a DRS can reduce, alter, or completely interrupt this cycle. Fortunately, it is a fact that if neurons are firing under conscious control, then an EEG can detect it. Using a commercially available EEG, the DRS can pinpoint generally where activation should be occurring, and the team neuroscientist can manually adjust the postacquisition data analysis to compensate for an altered hemodynamic response. Moreover, it is likely in the next 10 years that a combined clinical paradigm of EEG and BOLD-EPI and/or NIRS will constitute a standardized spatio-temporal diagnostic technique.[19,21,25-27]

MRI scanners generate mT gradient fields, and this is a billion times stronger than fields measured by SQUIDs in neuromagnetometers. Although it is theoretically possible to compensate for the known gradient fields generated by the MR control system, the MR electronics are not designed to control the field to the accuracy that would be required; this would be similar in magnitude to trying to measure the width of a human hair using the bumper of an automobile and reading the change on the odometer. The same stimulus paradigm can be presented in both machines separately and the results combined offline. In this case it is important to note that timing on the MR is more critical than usual; whereas a BOLD-EPI time-series can possess a timing error of a couple of hundred ms and not produce much difference in the mean parametric map, MEG signals only last a few hundred ms at most, and therefore the combined analysis is quite a bit trickier. By the end of the decade, this problem should be resolved through automation; in the mean time, the DRS should be aware of this possible confound. The same timing consideration applies to combining MRI and EEG.

Comparisons between activation measurements using MEG and EEG are still in clinical evaluations.[19] MEG should prove to be a more repeatable technique for longitudinal comparisons. Given that the sensor array is not distorted by variances in skull shape, the lower sensitivity to gyral and subcortical activations may prove useful for certain rehabilitation tasks, and it is certainly more comfortable for the subject to avoid a shampoo with conductive goo; however, it has yet to be shown that these advantages are significant enough to justify a factor of 20 difference in expenditures. The authors' prediction is that in the next 10 years, MEG will have an essential but limited role in world-class rehabilitation centers and/or multi-laboratory collaborations.

Combination of all four techniques is possible. The postprocessing of quad-modal hybrid data presents a challenge to current clinical researchers. Rehabilitation specialists should see combination tools and complete analyses packages of clinical quality appearing in about 5 years, around the time that neuroimaging itself will become leading-edge practice throughout all rehabilitation programs.

NEW TECHNOLOGY IN DRIVING STUDIES: USE OF A SIMULATED DRIVING ENVIRONMENT

Assessment of driving safety using a simulator offers the advantage of presenting challenging scenarios that could not be replicated on a standardized basis in a real-life, on-road driving evaluation. As such, the use of simulators is gaining interest as a means for both driving assessment and intervention. Several studies support the ecological validity of simulators in the assessment of fitness to drive. A Doron Precision System's simulator showed a strong validity in predicting satisfactory road performance among adults with stroke and adolescents with disabilities. Similarly, a study of persons with HIV indicated that both the simulator and neuropsychological tests predicted significant variance in on-road conditions.[28-30] See Chapter 10 for more information on driving simulators.

Important to note for functional imaging is that a complete cockpit and driver interface simulation is not required in all instances. For normal adults, any learned complex behavior can be elicited through the introduction of a critical mass of sensory cues. The required cues are different for different individuals because some put their brain in driving mode as soon as they enter the passenger compartment. In a real-world setting, this can lead to the behavioral phenomena of back-seat driving, although not all passenger commentary on driver performance should be considered an involuntary expression of mind-on-the-drive. Furthermore, some individual tasks within the driving behavior can be studied outside of a complete simulation. Hand responses to lights, for example, exercise neural correlates of visual event detection and subsequent motor activation, which are both integral parts of the driving behavior. Early studies show that the same activation patterns elicited in the simple task are components of similar tasks in more complex assignments. Eliciting the driving behavior and examining neural correlates are the topics of the next section.

THE ROLE OF REHABILITATION

Simulated driving and studies of the neural correlates of detection and response tasks are detailed below in the context of normal adult driving behavior. Understanding of what is normal is essential when defining rehabilitation goals. We explore studies of normal behavior to serve as a reference since expertise in the topic is sparsely distributed. Finally, we present a typical and also a detailed clinical study and include their motivational contexts, even if not directly related to rehabilitation, to emphasize the interdisciplinary nature of all work in the neuroimaging field.

Pre-Injury Data

In addition to knowledge of what is considered nominal neural activation in functional driving evaluation, any information collected from a subject prior to an injury can be useful in evaluating the extent of injury and individualizing a rehabilitation program. This will likely be part of general behavioral screening, but there are functional neuroimaging-specific data that can be

useful. We limit our discussion here to the modalities detailed above, and moreover exclusively discuss digital retrieval of images; we save a discussion of analog films for a future specialized venue, other than to say that a re-read of previous images has likely provided any useful information to clinical specialists prior to entering driver rehabilitation.

Digital imaging in medicine started the process of standardization in 1983; 10 years later a completed draft standard was published, and 10 years after that, the standardization process has started to deliver on the promise of picture archiving and retrieval in a multi-vendor environment. Most major manufacturers of imaging devices still internally use a proprietary image format and storage model; however, all of them currently archive their images to the Digital Image and Communications in Medicine (DICOM) standard. Retrieval of old clinical exam data is accomplished through one of several commercial DICOM conversion tools widely available for MRI and CT scans, with additional DICOM modalities to become available in the next few years. EEG, MEG, and NIRS are not currently included as part of the DICOM strategic vision, although they can be incorporated under the waveform information object standard and likely will have a standard in the next decade. It should finally be noted that the DICOM strategy includes cross-modality data combinations, which will provide standardized combination interfaces in the next decade.

In addition to software retrieval and interpretation issues, most digital information (the so-called raw scan data), if retained at all, is likely stored on media for which there may be an issue to find hardware to read. In almost all cases, the medical record gatekeeper should be able to provide the digital information in a readable format. Media hardware storage is also part of DICOM.

Going forward, more instances will be seen where a readily available MRI can be found for a given patient, although it will likely just be an anatomical exam. Old MRI scans will be of lower resolution than available today; nonetheless, they may contain limited useful information for rehabilitation purposes. Specifically, if on a modern three-dimensional MRI some structural deficit is found that could have been caused by the current injury, an old MRI may prove that the defect was present prior to loss of function. Even in the case that the defect cannot be visualized on the old scan, with access to the digital data it is possible to determine whether the old scan is consistent or not with the new scan, and such reinterpretation tools will be widely available in the next decade (driven by nascent SCI research). Information from an old MRI re-read is important to include on the rehabilitation chart for clients undergoing a program that includes functional neuroimaging, even if the results were inconclusive.

In the event a patient may have undergone a previous EEG exam, functional data from a strobe exam to elicit a visual response may have been recorded. The standard strobe exam should be repeated in this case to look for changes that may be injury related. In cases without strobe data where the original EEG interpretation (and possible re-read executed before a driver rehabilitation program) shows normal activity, no additional information is of use for functional neuroimaging. Abnormal activity in the previous exam is important to note in the rehabilitation chart.

It is unlikely in the next 10 years that many driver rehabilitation clients will have prior MEG or NIRS scan data available.

The complete functional neuroimaging suite of scans can be executed by examining only the preinjury functional information gleaned from a standard subject interview. Preinjury data are useful, but they are not required.

EMERGENCE OF MULTI-LABORATORY COLLABORATIONS

Construction of a complete standard behavioral rehabilitation center can require capital outlays in the range of a few million dollars; a state-of-the-art neuroimaging center including the capability to perform every scanning procedure described in this chapter will require upwards of $10,000,000 for equipment and specialized infrastructure alone. This capitalization requirement alone necessitates the collaboration of multiple clinical centers in the next decade to perform the full range of subject evaluation and tracking.

FUNCTIONAL IMAGING OF SIMULATED DRIVING

An essential issue for human factor research is to examine and evaluate the design of human machine interfaces for the safe and efficient operation of complex equipment under multi-tasking conditions. Multi-tasking is required for both primary driving (steering, braking, navigation) and secondary tasks (e.g., a cell phone conversation).[6,7,31,32] Evaluating neural activity as a function of task load is an important tracking element in a program of rehabilitation.

Task load and overload has proven a challenging question through use of standard behavioral techniques on normal adults. The ways in which in-vehicle devices and external events influence mind-on-the-drive are currently under investigation, and little is known about functioning at the neuronal level during distraction of a performance task resulting from multi-tasking. For example, self-reports of situational awareness assume drivers are aware they are distracted, which may not always be the case.

Eye movement analysis is a useful indicator of driver cognition, but it may not detect cases in which drivers look right at something and do not see it, an effect called "looked-but-did-not-see," or "cognitive blindness."[33,34] Measuring driver reaction times and miss rates to unexpected events in on-road testing is useful, but there can be large variability and low repeatability because of the need to keep the events random and unexpected. Response time measurements are purely behavioral, and do not elucidate underlying neural mechanisms.[7,35]

The ability to noninvasively examine the effects of dual-task states on driving performance has not been attempted until now. Direct measurement of the underlying neural mechanisms for event detection and response during multi-tasking might prove effective in improving designs to optimize driver attention to the roadway when performing secondary tasks in the vehicle. One of the goals of direct measurement is to determine exactly how and why the performance of secondary tasks such as answering a phone and conversing using a hands-free telematics system can affect primary driving. With the power of these neuroimaging systems, we can better understand the fundamental mechanisms underlying the multi-tasking driving behavior. Subsequently, such knowledge is critical to the design of safe and effective telecommunications systems for the driver. Without the fundamental nature of driver distraction, a telematics or navigation system cannot be designed to reduce driver distraction.

A current project at the Transportation Imaging Laboratory (TIL) at Wayne State University (WSU; Detroit, MI) attempts to directly measure mind-on-the-drive through use of safe and noninvasive fMRI and MEG. This study provided an opportunity for one of the first attempts to directly and objectively measure and understand mind-on-the-drive in a driving-like scenario with current technology. The scientific goal of this study was to determine the underlying cognitive mechanisms that might underlie mind-off-road; that is, to determine the neural basis of mental attention shifts that underlie driver errors, or driver distraction. Results from pilot studies are encouraging. By improving understanding of the fundamental mechanisms underlying driver inattention, time and expense will likely be saved in designing in-vehicle systems to optimize mind-on-the-drive.[32]

CASE STUDY: MEG NEUROIMAGING STUDY ON DRIVING PERFORMANCE FOR NORMAL ADULTS

With the superb temporal and moderate spatial resolution for functional brain mapping, MEG allowed the research team at WSU to explore the neural mechanisms underlying driving distraction while the subjects are engaged in event-detection tasks during a driving paradigm. Subjects viewed a real-world driving video and responded (with a foot pedal) to red light stimuli (events) presented either centrally or peripherally on the driving scene. A 148-channel whole head Neuromagnetometer (4 Dimensional Neuroimaging) was used to measure magnetic fields in 5 individuals between 30 and 55 years of age (4 females; 1 male) who all possessed a current driver's license and signed an informed consent form approved by the Henry Ford Hospital (HFH) Internal Review Board.

Each subject lay comfortably (in the supine position) on a bed inside a magnetically shielded room, with the driving scene in front of him or her. Standard automatic probe position routine was applied to locate the subject's head relative to the location of the neuromagnetometer detector coils.[36] The neuromagnetometer helmet containing the detector array was placed around the subject's head in close proximity to the skull surface. A mirror system was used to enable the subject to view the projected driving video. The subject was asked to lie as still as possible without excessive eye blinks and body movements during data collection. Multiple data collection sessions were conducted; each lasted 4 minutes. Each subject was monitored by video camera and two-way audio speaker system during the time he or she was in the shielded room. All MEG data were band-pass filtered from 0.1 Hz to 100 Hz, and digitally sampled at 508.63 Hz.

The driving scene simulated the actual images seen while driving. Subjects viewed a real-world driving video and responded by pushing a foot pedal with their right foot every time to a red LED light up (stimuli events) presented either centrally or peripherally on the driving scene. MEG data were back averaged on the foot pedal response. The foot pedal response turned off the light and produced a visual evoked response, followed by an auditory response to the sound of the foot pedal being pressed down. About 40 red light stimuli were presented in each scanning session (Figure 25-5). Cortical activation between 0 ms and 650 ms was analyzed to determine the latency and source of neuronal activity of attention processes.[37,38]

In order to do the functional brain mapping of the driving distraction, it is necessary to correlate MEG areas of cortical activity with specific anatomical structures. Each subject's MRI was co-registered into each subject's head digitization points collected at the beginning of the MEG study.[36] The techniques for co-registration of MEG and MRI are well established and used in all HFH clinical MEG studies. This allows precise correspondence between anatomical structures and MEG areas of cortical activation. The MRI scan was performed on a 3-Tesla GE whole body MRI scanner.

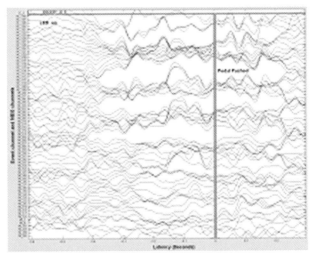

Figure 25-5 Averaged evoked MEG data. Bold trace shows averaged lights on and foot pedal response to 40 events.

This volumetric scan was a three-dimensional inversion recovery spoiled gradient echo sequence with TE:4.5 ms, TI:300 ms, and TR:10.4 ms, and the imaging matrix was 256 × 256 × 200 voxels (Figure 25-6).

MEG data were averaged during certain periods of time relative to the onset of the foot pedal. The red light was on 580 ms before the foot pedal onset, which evoked occipital cortex activity. This visual activation was followed by activation associated with attention and decision making in the superior frontal gyrus and anterior cingulate gyrus (t=−470 ms). Motor activity (t=−270 ms) in the precentral gyrus corresponding to foot and leg control was followed by foot pedal response pad

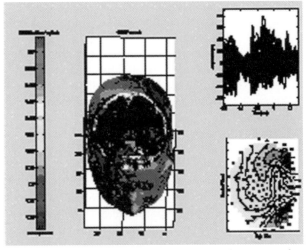

Figure 25-6 MR-FOCUSS localization results averaged over 900 ms. MEG graph in upper right corner displays all 148 MEG channels with significant events marked. Contour plot in lower right corner depicts average magnetic field pattern.

(t=0). This action turned off the light and produced a visual evoked response (t = 95 ms) in the occipital cortex and a bilateral auditory response (t = 111 ms) in the auditory cortex. The superb temporal resolution of MEG enabled us to determine the following sequential cortical activations. Occipital activation was seen with the light on and the light off. Prefrontal and anterior cingulate gyrus activation was shown right after the light came on, which is likely to be associated with attention and decision making in response to the red light detection task. Motor cortex activation was detected during eyeball movement (light on) and foot movement. These were brief intervals and correlated well with known locations for visual and specific motor cortex locations. Frontal-parietal networks were dominant during the driving task. Our findings suggest that driving tasks recruit neural systems for visual-motor multi-modal processing and integration. Therefore, the application of event-related MEG in investigating neural processing during simulated driving tasks is quite promising.

DETAILED CLINICAL RESEARCH EXAMPLE: NEURAL CORRELATES OF DRIVING IN A SAMPLE OF TBI SURVIVORS USING REAL-TIME fMRI

Resumption of driving is a critical issue for many brain injury survivors, yet the cognitive and perceptual processes involved in driving are not well understood. Many studies have attempted to operationalize the cognitive and perceptual abilities that predict fitness to drive, but traditional driving measures do not provide any information about the neural correlates that subserve driving, nor do they expose the driver to standardized driving scenarios that are specifically designed to engage aspects of cognition that are considered important in safe driving.

We have examined neural activation and driving performance in a sample of TBI survivors using real-time fMRI and comparing performance indices with those obtained on a driving simulator that is commonly used in the assessment of driving ability.

A driving paradigm developed and validated by General Motors and adapted for the fMRI magnet has been used to examine the effects of various aspects of brain injury on driving ability. The fMRI methodology used in this study incorporates BOLD, SWI, DWI, and DTI technology. To our knowledge, the application of these technologies to examine the relationship between driving ability and brain injury is unprecedented.

Normal Adults

In the control group, we used event-related functional MRI in a driving simulation to identify the neural sys-

tems engaged in the driving task. Our hypotheses included (1) a large frontal-parietal functional network for detection of tasks during driving, (2) brain activation patterns modulated by multi-tasking experiences, (3) different brain activation for various workloads, and (4) various stages and networks for multi-tasking and executive functions.

Testing our hypotheses involved identifying neural systems engaged in multi-tasking during simulated driving. We also analyzed the differences in activated brain systems based on the demands of the simulated driving tasks by using both block and event-related analyses. We developed a testable paradigm for evaluation of the detection of distraction during a driving task, and measured the brain activation changes in the prefrontal and parietal areas in response to different workload and networks of multi-tasking and executive functions.

The noninvasive MRI methodology provides us a chance to look into an individual's brain activation while the individual engages in a cognitive task. This method allows us to scan normal healthy children and adults, and also the clients with brain damage or neurological disease. In our study, 6 normal adults (3 males; 3 females) participated in our MRI driving study. All of them provided a written informed consent form approved by the WSU Internal Review Board. Subjects were all right-handed and were within the age range of 22 to 27 years.

Each subject was asked to perform three tasks during the MRI scanning session. The first task was the Central Event Detection Task (CEDT). In this task, the subject was presented with a pair of liquid crystal display (LCD) goggles through which he or she could see a red light at the bottom of a screen with a dark background. The subject was to detect and respond to each red light stimulus by pressing a push button with the right index finger. The second task was the Simulated Driving. In this task, the subject was presented a driving video through the LCD goggles. The subject was to actively attend to the driving video. The third task combined simulated driving with the CEDT. The red light stimuli were presented at random intervals throughout all conditions. A 40-second block was use for each experimental condition followed by a 40-second rest period to allow the brain activation to return to baseline. During this rest baseline, the subject was presented with a white crosshair at the center of the screen to provide a visual fixation point. A boxcar design was used for each 5-minute scanning session with alternating 40-second periods between the active condition and the fixation condition (Figure 25-7). Each scanning series contains only one experimental task with 4 blocks of the 40-second experimental period. The task, which required red light event detec-

Boxcar analysis scheme

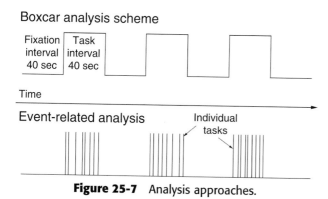

Figure 25-7 Analysis approaches.

tion, contained 7 red light events in a pseudo-random order in each 40-second experimental period. Both the brain activations and behavioral responses (including the correction rate and reaction time) of each individual were collected during the MRI driving task.

Scanning was conducted using the 1.5 T Siemens Sonata at the MR Research Center at Wayne State University. The MRI scans included anatomical and functional imaging sequences. The parameters for the anatomical imaging sequence were T1-weighted axial three-dimensional volume acquired, TR = 11.5 ms, TE = 3.9 ms, flip angle = 15°, number of slices = 104 slices, slice thickness = 1.25 mm, matrix size = 256 × 256 pixels. The parameters for the functional imaging sequence were: T2*-weighted images (EPI), TR = 2s, TE = 40 ms, FA = 90 degrees, number of slices = 22, matrix size = 64 × 64 pixels, FOV = 400 mm, slice thickness = 6.0 mm with 10% gap, voxel size = 6.25 × 6.25 × 6.6 mm, number of TRs = 180.

Regarding imaging data preprocessing and statistical analysis, the Statistical Parameter Mapping (SPM99) and Brain Voyager were used. The preprocessing steps included slice time correction, normalization individual brain, scaling to Talairach space, phase and three-dimensional motion correction, high pass temporal filtered at 3 cycles per run, and 6 mm spatial smoothing. The statistical analysis was performed according to a boxcar design with alternating 40-second periods of the driving task and the rest baseline condition. An alternative event-related analysis was also performed, which was used specifically to time lock the subject's responses according to the red light events.

According to the boxcar analysis, healthy subjects showed a large frontal-parietal network that was particularly strong in the frontal, parietal, occipital, and thalamus regions while engaging the CEDT during the driving scene, in comparison with the simulated driving task while viewing the driving scene. These results strongly suggested the subjects' involvement in coordinating visual attention, attention control, stimulus pro-

cessing, response selection, and motor execution, and provides convincing evidence that a learned executive-function-controlled behavior, the driving behavior, was successfully elicited in the limited simulation presented during the experiment. Brain activations in the simulated driving task by viewing the driving scene alone involved significant increase in the left precentral gyrus, left superior parietal lobule, left supramarginal gyrus, left inferior frontal gyrus, visual cortex, cerebellum, anterior cingulate gyrus, and basal ganglia. Activation of these brain regions suggested a greater role for motor coordination and control, vigilance, preparatory motor processes, and the regulation of the temporal aspects of specific motor responses, again strong evidence of evoked driving behavior even absent the response task.

The event-related analysis provides a close-up window to look at the brain activity with a fine-grain and more precise perspective. In the red light detection task alone, increased brain activations of the left precentral gyrus, left superior parietal lobe, left inferior frontal gyrus, and cingulate gyrus were recruited for focus attention, stimulus processing, response decision making, and motor execution (Figure 25-8). The simulated driving analysis with CEDT shows similar brain networks as the boxcar analysis, in comparison with the fixation condition and with the simulated driving alone (Figures 25-9 and 25-10). Such a consistent finding provides logical validation for the cognitive neuroscience network for driving behavior, as well as for the application of the functional MRI methodology in the investigation of a high-level, multi-tasking activity such as driving.

Traumatic Brain Injury (TBI) Clients

We performed the same driving tasks with 2 clients who sustained TBIs. SWI images indicated some vascular and tissue damages in the clients' brains (Figure 25-11) that cannot be seen in the regular anatomical MRI scans nor in the functional MRI scans.

The TBI clients' performance in reaction time and correction rate during the driving tasks were worse than the healthy controls. The Event Related fMRI Analysis indicated that TBI-001 showed limited activations in the left inferior frontal gyrus, left precentral gyrus, and anterior cingulate gyrus in the comparison between the CEDT during simulated driving and fixation condition (threshold of t = 3.2, p < 0.0016) (Figure 25-12). In contrast, TBI-002 showed a little more activation in the left inferior frontal gyrus, left precentral gyrus, anterior cingulate gyrus, and bilateral superior parietal regions.

The difference in brain activation between clients and normal control is as expected. The TBI clients' brain activation patterns were less consistent and more

Average across six subjects

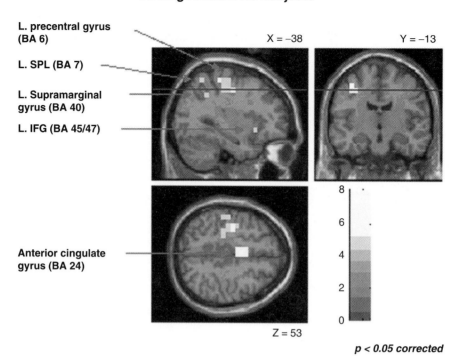

Figure 25-8   CEDT versus fixation: event related.

Average across six subjects

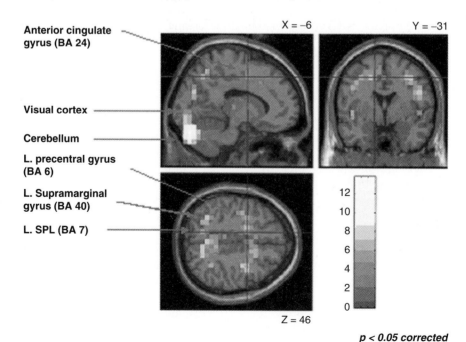

Figure 25-9   Simulated driving with CEDT versus fixation: event related.

Average across four subjects

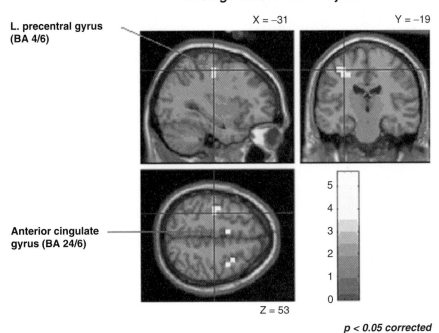

L. precentral gyrus (BA 4/6)

Anterior cingulate gyrus (BA 24/6)

X = –31

Y = –19

Z = 53

p < 0.05 corrected

Figure 25-10 Simulated driving with CEDT versus simulated driving: event related.

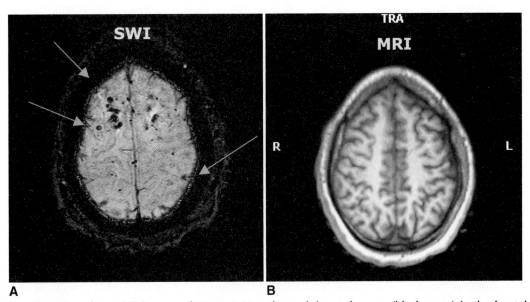

A

B

Figure 25-11 SWI **(A)** and MRI **(B)** images of TBI-001: Vascular and tissue damage (black spots) in the frontal and temporal regions.

Continued

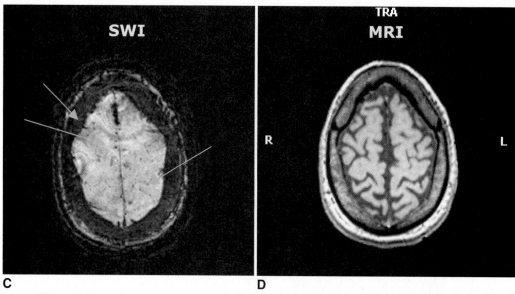

Figure 25-11 cont'd SWI **(C)** and MRI **(D)** images of TBI-002: Vascular and tissue damage (black spots) in the brain regions.

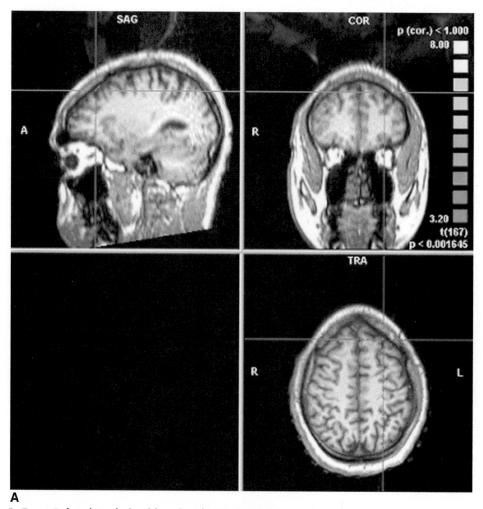

Figure 25-12 A, Event Related Analysis of functional MRI (fMRI) image of TBI-001 between the Central Event Detection Task (CEDT) during simulated driving and fixation baseline (threshold of t=3.2, p<0.0016): brain activations in the left inferior frontal gyrus, left precentral gyrus, and anterior cingulate gyrus.

Continued

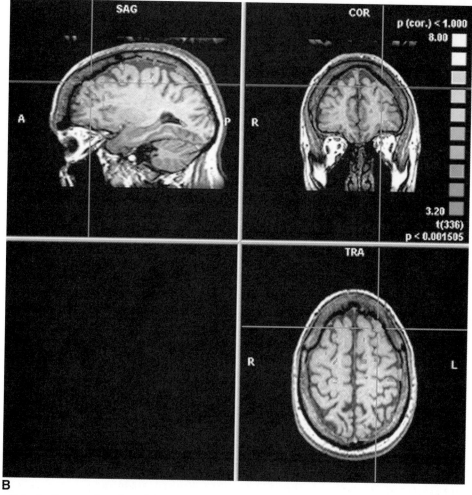

Figure 25-12 cont'd **B,** Event Related Analysis of fMRI image of TBI-002 in the comparison between the CEDT during simulated driving and fixation baseline (threshold of t=3.2, p<0.0015): brain activations in the left inferior frontal gyrus, left precentral gyrus, anterior cingulate gyrus, and bilateral superior parietal regions.

scattered in comparison with the normal controls. Furthermore, even within the client group, there are different brain activation patterns between these two clients, which is positively associated with their differences in the SWI images; that is, the TBI-001 with more vascular and tissue damage showed less and limited brain activations, whereas the TBI-002 with less brain damage showed a bit more activation in the areas similar to normal controls.

The combination of various functional neuroimaging techniques (such as fMRI and MEG) together with SWI has shown to be a powerful, well-rounded diagnostic tool to help us better understand both normal and pathological neural networks involved in complex multi-task behavior such as driving. With these advanced neuroimaging and analysis techniques, researchers are able to investigate a complicated research area such as driving and develop a potential

evaluation and treatment battery that is complementary to the traditional methodology.

SUMMARY

Presented here has been a brief review of the noninvasive neuroimaging technologies in use today and that likely will be included as a future component in a comprehensive driver rehabilitation program. The information in this review included an introduction to the developing terminology, the basics of functional imaging and its application to driver rehabilitation, an overview of the biophysical principles underlying each modality, and a detailed clinical research example. Combining the research of neurosurgery, psychiatry and behavior, and neurology forms a new synergy to allow the DRS to provide the best program possible to unlock full potential recovery. The current data accumulation from clients with TBIs and SCIs will allow advances applicable to all areas. When politics or payment schedules are conflicting with rehabilitation goals because no external progress has been seen, imaging can decide whether improvement has occurred and whether rehabilitation should continue.

Our emergent vision is that the next decade starts now. Every new clinical research result is useful to evaluate eventual applications of neuroimaging technology. The path forward will be a leap, not a walk, as technology is moving faster than our vision. The question is no longer whether neuroimaging will be useful for rehabilitation, but how soon research funding will appear to help produce concrete results and usable paradigms for clinical application.

REFERENCES

1. Hillary FG, Steffener J, Biswal BB, et al: Functional magnetic resonance imaging technology and traumatic brain injury rehabilitation: guidelines for methodological and conceptual pitfalls, *J Head Trauma Rehabil* 17(5):411-430, 2002.
2. Lew HL, Lee EH, Pan SS, et al: Electrophysiologic abnormalities of auditory and visual information processing in patients with traumatic brain injury, *Am J Phys Med Rehabil* 83(6):428-433, 2004.
3. Muller SV, von Schweder AJ, Frank B, et al: The effects of proprioceptive stimulation on cognitive processes in patients after traumatic brain injury, *Arch Phys Med Rehabil* 83(1):115-121, 2002.
4. Akinwuntan AE, DeWeerdt W, Feys H, et al: Reliability of a road test after stroke, *Arch Phys Med Rehabil* 84(12):1792-1796, 2003.
5. Brouwer WH, Zomeren AHv, Wolffelaar PCv: Traffic behavior after severe traumatic brain injury. In Deelman BG, Saan RJ, Zomeren AHv, Editors: *Traumatic brain injury: clinical, social, and rehabilitational aspects*, Rockland, Mass, 1990, Swets & Zeitlinger.
6. Graydon FX, Young RA, Benton MD, et al: Visual event detection during simulated driving: identifying the neural correlates with functional neuroimaging, *Transportation Res Traffic Transport Psychol*, in press.
7. Walter H, Vetter SC, Grothe J, et al: The neural correlates of driving, *Neuroreport* 12(8):1763-1767, 2001.
8. Coleman RD, Rapport LJ, Ergh TC, et al: Predictors of driving outcome after traumatic brain injury, *Arch Phys Med Rehabil* 83(10):1415-1422, 2002.
9. Galski T, Bruno RL, Ehle HT: Driving after cerebral damage: a model with implications for evaluation, *Am J Occup Ther* 46(4):324-332, 1992.
10. Fisk GD, Schneider JJ, Novack TA: Driving following traumatic brain injury: prevalence, exposure, advice and evaluations, *Brain Inj* 12(8):683-695, 1998.
11. Priddy DA, Johnson P, Lam CS: Driving after a severe head injury, *Brain Inj* 4(3):267-272, 1990.
12. Shore D, Gurgold G, Robbins S: Handicapped driving: an overview of assessment and training, *Arch Phys Med Rehabil* 61:481, 1980.
13. van Zomeren AH, Brouwer WH, Minderhoud JM: Acquired brain damage and driving: a review, *Arch Phys Med Rehabil* 68(10):697-705, 1987.
14. Voller B, Auff E, Schnider P, et al: To do or not to do? Magnetic resonance imaging in mild traumatic brain injury, *Brain Inj* 15(2):107-115, 2001.
15. Stokx LC, Gaillard AW: Task and driving performance of patients with a severe concussion of the brain, *J Clin Exp Neuropsychol* 8(4):421-436, 1986.
16. Guye M, Parker GJ, Symms M, et al: Combined functional MRI and tractography to demonstrate the connectivity of the human primary motor cortex in vivo, *Neuroimage* 19(4):1349-1360, 2003.
17. Matsuyama Y, Kawakami N, Yanase M, et al: Cervical myelopathy due to OPLL: clinical evaluation by MRI and intraoperative spinal sonography, *J Spinal Disord Tech* 17(5):401-404, 2004.
18. Toosy AT, Werring DJ, Orrell RW, et al: Diffusion tensor imaging detects corticospinal tract involvement at multiple levels in amyotrophic lateral sclerosis, *J Neurol Neurosurg Psychiatry* 74(9):1250-1257, 2003.
19. Barkley GL, Baumgartner C: MEG and EEG in epilepsy, *J Clin Neurophysiol* 20(3):163-178, 2003.
20. Michel CM, Murray MM, Lantz G, et al: EEG source imaging, *Clin Neurophysiol* 115(10):2195-2222, 2004.
21. Lutkenhoner B: Magnetoencephalography and its Achilles' heel, *J Physiol Paris* 97(4-6):641-658, 2003.
22. Wheless JW, Castillo E, Maggio V, et al: Magnetoencephalography (MEG) and magnetic source imaging (MSI), *Neurologist* 10(3):138-153, 2004.
23. Jezzard P, Matthews PM, Smith SM, editors: *Functional MRI: an introduction to methods*, New York, 2003, Oxford University Press.
24. Ferrari M, Mottola L, Quaresima V: Principles, techniques, and limitations of near infrared spectroscopy, *Can J Appl Physiol* 29(4):463-487, 2004.
25. He B, Lian J: High-resolution spatio-temporal functional neuroimaging of brain activity, *Crit Rev Biomed Eng* 30(4-6):283-306, 2002.
26. Krakow K, Baxendale SA, Maguire EA, et al: Fixation-off sensitivity as a model of continuous epileptiform discharges: electroencephalographic, neuropsychological and functional MRI findings, *Epilepsy Res* 42(1):1-6, 2000.
27. Voller B, Benke T, Benedetto K, et al: Neuropsychological, MRI and EEG findings after very mild traumatic brain injury, *Brain Inj* 13(10):821-827, 1999.
28. Cimolino N, Balkovec D: The contribution of a driving simulator in the driving evaluation of stroke and disabled adolescent clients, *Can J Occup Ther* 55:119-125, 1988.
29. Galski T, Bruno RL, Ehle HT: Prediction of behind-the-wheel driving performance in patients with cerebral brain damage: a discriminant function analysis, *Am J Occup Ther* 47(5):391-396, 1993.
30. Lundqvist A, Gerdle B, Rönnberg J: Neuropsychological aspects of driving after a stroke in the simulator and on the road, *Appl Cogn Psychol* 14(2):135-150, 2000.
31. Just MA, Carpenter PA, Keller TA, et al: Interdependence of nonoverlapping cortical systems in dual cognitive tasks, *Neuroimage* 14(2):417-426, 2001.

32. Young RA, Hsieh L, Graydon FX, et al: Mind-on-the-drive: real-time functional neuroimaging of cognitive brain mechanisms underlying driver performance and distraction, *Proceedings of the Society of Automotive Engineering*, in press, 2005.

33. Angell LS, Young RA, Hankey JM, et al: *An evaluation of alternative methods for assessing driver workload in the early development of in-vehicle information systems*, SAE Government/Industry Meeting Washington D.C., May 13-15, 2002, Society of Automotive Engineers.

34. Young RA, Angell LS: *The dimensions of driver performance during secondary tasks.* Paper presented at International Driving Symposium on Human Factors in Driver Assessment, Training, and Vehicle Design, Park City, Utah, University of Iowa, July 2003.

35. Farber E, Blanco M, Foley JP, et al: *Surrogate measures of visual demand while driving.* Paper presented at The XIVth Triennial Congress of the International Ergonomics Association and Human Factors and Ergonomics Society's 44th Annual Meeting, San Diego, July 30-August 4, 2000.

36. Bowyer SM, Moran JE, Mason KM, et al: MEG Validation Parameters for Clinical Evaluation of Interictal Epileptic Activity, *J Clin Neurophysiol* 20(2):87-93, 2003.

37. Bowyer SM, Moran JE, Mason KM, et al: MEG localization of language-specific cortex utilizing MR-FOCUSS, *Neurology* 62(12):2247-2255, 2004.

38. Moran JE, Bowyer SM, Tepley N: Multi-Resolution FOCUSS source imaging of MEG Data, *Biomedizinische Technik* 46:112-114, 2001.

Part VII

PROGRAM AND PROFESSIONAL DEVELOPMENT IN A RAPIDLY EVOLVING FIELD

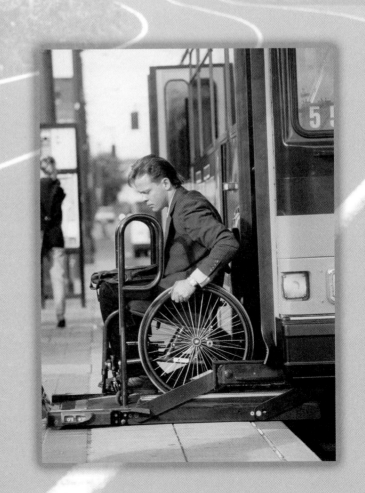

Chapter 26

DEVELOPING A DRIVER REHABILITATION PROGRAM

Thomas D. Kalina • Elizabeth L. Green

KEY TERMS

• Credentialing

CHAPTER OBJECTIVES

After completing this chapter, the reader will be able to do the following:

• Identify key aspects of a program business plan.
• Describe several program delivery models.
• Understand the critical importance of proper staffing.
• Identify program implementation steps.
• Appreciate the liability considerations when operating a driver rehabilitation program.

Cars were in their infancy when people started modifying them to accommodate disabilities. Quentin Coley lost both his arms in a 1905 train accident. His strong desire for community mobility led him to modify one of the first Ford Model Ts in Dallas, Texas. He used a special ring to enable himself to drive with his prosthetic arm. His primary problem was applying the gas, as the first Model Ts used a hand gas feed on the steering wheel. He adapted the car with what might have been the first foot-operated accelerator. He lectured all across America and drove well past his 90th birthday.[1]

The desire to drive today is even stronger as we have become dependent on the automobile for most of our community mobility needs. Driver rehabilitation has progressed from a few creative individuals inventing devices to a profession comprised of a whole team of professionals who provide a constellation of driver rehabilitation services. Advanced evaluation and training programs target complex challenges that are often associated with the client's diagnosis or diagnoses as well as diminished function because of the aging process. Manufacturers, distributors, and mobility equipment dealers are providing new and innovative adapted driving products and techniques to modify vehicles of all shapes and sizes. Programs now benefit clients with a wide variety of conditions, many of whom require specialized clinical and on-road evaluations and training regimens. Many of the clients served today do not require vehicle adaptations but instead need an objective evaluation of driving ability and a comprehensive strategy to address their need for alternative transportation if it is determined that they are not a candidate for driving.

The demand for driver rehabilitation and alternative community mobility services is expected to increase significantly as the population ages within the United States. Development of effective driver rehabilitation programs will be essential in meeting this growing demand. This chapter provides guidelines for establishing a driver rehabilitation program. It is primarily geared toward a hospital or community-based facility that is considering offering driver rehabilitation services; however, it is extremely important that driver rehabilitation programs also adopt a strategy to address their clients' alternative transportation needs as well.

Those considering developing a business plan and starting a driver rehabilitation program must remember that research, specialized training, and careful planning are critical components required to help ensure a successful program. Many of the topics covered in this chapter will be helpful for a driver rehabilitation specialist (DRS) in private practice who is relatively new to the field (e.g., working as a DRS for less than 1 to 2 years); however, most DRSs have had many years of experience in driver rehabilitation before attempting to start their own private practices.

DEVELOPING A BUSINESS PLAN

The DRS needs to be aware of many factors before starting a private practice. These include performing a needs assessment, identifying referral sources, identifying reimbursement sources, and surveying the competition.

NEEDS ASSESSMENT

Who are the likely customers for a driver rehabilitation program? The first step in exploring the potential for a program is determining the demand for the intended services to the prospective clients in a particular geographic area. Potential clients could include anyone with a physical, mental, or cognitive disability. Adaptations including structural modifications to vehicles and adaptive driving aids can make driving accessible to persons with disabilities, aging-related challenges, or both and may be as simple as a steering knob or as complex as a joystick driving system. Clients with learning disabilities may not require adaptive controls or structural vehicle modifications but may need special instructions to develop safe driving skills and habits or to identify and use alternative transportation available in their communities. Concerns about older drivers will continue to grow as the population ages, creating an increasing demand for services. Clients, young and old, that cannot drive could benefit from a community mobility or alternative transportation evaluation to help them explore alternatives to driving, such as paratransit, a passenger van, or mass transit, to name a few.

Public health statistics that reflect morbidity rates (i.e., incidence of various diagnostic groups) within a particular geographic area where a DRS will potentially be providing driver rehabilitation and community mobility services are available from local or regional planning agencies. Understanding population demographics including health-related statistics is one step that will help the entrepreneurial-minded DRS to begin gauging the potential demand for services. Careful consideration should also be given to factoring in the needs of prospective clients who will not be driving as well as the needs of their caregivers. If a hospital is developing a program, its marketing staff will have this information as well. Some of the more common diagnostic groups of experienced drivers needing driver rehabilitation services include dementia, stroke, multiple sclerosis (MS), spinal cord injury (SCI), amputation, acquired brain injury (ABI), Parkinson's disease (PD), and hand injuries. Tracking admissions into the hospital and its affiliates (e.g., outpatient centers) and estimating how many clients may require assistance in returning to driving, using alternative transportation, or both can help the DRS predict the demand from the hospital's current admissions. For a program to be financially successful it will likely need to recruit clients from outside the system. This is especially true of new drivers with conditions that could affect safe driving (e.g., cerebral palsy, spina bifida, short stature, and learning disabilities).

Many common health conditions are frequently seen in the older population; thus, the percentage of people in the service area over 65 years of age is another important indicator of the potential demand for services. Undoubtedly, the demand for driver rehabilitation and alternatives to driving that enable dependable community mobility services will increase significantly in the next 15 to 20 years, as people that comprise the baby boomer generation reach retirement age. This age group is heavily dependent upon the automobile and is expected to seek services that address driver rehabilitation and perhaps alternatives to driving that enable community mobility should they experience a disability that affects their ability to drive or get around their communities by other means. Their adult-age children are likely to be concerned about their elderly parents' safety and may depend on a driving program to provide an objective evaluation, effective education and training, or strategies to contend with driving cessation.

REFERRAL SOURCES

A program must draw from many referral sources to be successful. The Commission for Accreditation of Rehabilitation Facilities (CARF) requires a rehabilitation facility to provide driver rehabilitation services either directly or through a referral to a qualified provider in the area.[1a] Identifying potential referral sources is an important step in designing a program that will remain viable in the long run. A comprehensive list of referral sources identifies those physicians, other health care providers, and agencies in the community. Providing these prospective customers with educational in-services can increase awareness about driver rehabilitation generally and the DRS's program specifically. Typical community referral sources to consider when marketing and building a program are discussed below.

Physicians

Physicians are the first-line referral source. Some states require physicians to refer clients with certain medical conditions such as seizures and dementia that impair driving performance. Physicians are encouraged by the American Medical Association (AMA) to perform a driver screening and make appropriate referrals for those clients who have medical, cognitive, or psychomotor deficits that may interfere with driving. (See the AMA's *Physician's Guide to Assessing and Counseling Older Drivers.*) Drivers and their families often ask physicians whether they should continue, resume, or stop driving. State Division of Motor Vehicles (DMV) personnel often request medical reports from physicians during an investigation to determine a client's eligibility to drive. Primary care physicians, psychiatrists, internal medicine specialists, and general practitioners follow drivers over time. These physicians are good resources for building a driver evaluation program's referral base. Other physicians that may address a client's driving status include neurologists, neurosurgeons, orthopedic surgeons, and ophthalmologists among others.

Social Workers

The social worker or case manager is concerned with the resources a person has after being diagnosed with a disability, illness, or functional decline due to an injury, illness, the aging process, or any combination of these and other factors; therefore, they are an excellent referral source as well as important members of the driver rehabilitation team.

State Division of Motor Vehicles (DMV) Personnel

The DMV determines whether a driver is legally eligible to operate a motor vehicle. A driver with questionable abilities may be enrolled in the DMV medical review program. Each state has its own criteria and regulations governing the use of medical review programs. It is important for a driving program to be included on the DMV resource list once the program is open for business.

Self-Referrals

Individual drivers may request a driver rehabilitation evaluation, community mobility evaluation, or both. Offering educational opportunities to the general public can increase awareness of factors that limit or interfere with driving and community mobility skills. For instance, offering a workshop or speaking at a group's meeting such as the AARP, stroke survivor club, and arthritis support group can generate referrals as clients and caregivers learn about the resources that are available to them.

Family Members

Parents of children with disabilities, children of older adults contending with dementia, and spouses of individuals who are dealing with the effects of strokes, ABIs, and other debilitating conditions are an important link to connecting community safety with personal independence. Providing educational in-services to caregiver

support groups, attending health fairs, and focusing direct marketing on caregivers and spouses are important steps in identifying and gathering referral sources.

Parish Nurses

Working through local churches, some programs employ parish nurses who offer preventive health care and education to church members. They address the mental, physical, and spiritual well-being of the church's members as well as provide a link between parishioners and their primary care physicians. A parish nurse, in this capacity, may refer drivers and passengers to a driver rehabilitation and community mobility program.

Workers' Compensation Agency Personnel

The workers' compensation insurance company personnel are charged with assisting employees who have been injured at work in regaining health and wellness so that they may resume gainful employment as soon as it is possible. Losing the ability to drive due to a work-related injury or illness may prolong this process. The workers' compensation case manager may authorize payment of driver evaluation and training (i.e., rehabilitation) in an effort to assist the employee with a quick resumption of work duties.

State Vocational Rehabilitation Services Personnel

When illness or injury precludes an individual from returning to work, vocational rehabilitation serves as a community resource for provision of services, training, and adaptive equipment to facilitate the resumption of self-care and vocational activities. Vocational Rehabilitation (VR) often uses the expertise of a DRS to provide comprehensive driver rehabilitation services to help ensure that a client begins or resumes driving so that he or she can commute to and from work or an education or training program. The DRS should develop a contract with his or her state's VR agency; this should be viewed as a high priority when establishing a program.

State Independent Living Rehabilitation Services Personnel

Independent Living Rehabilitation (ILR) is charged with assisting persons unable to work because of their age, health status, or both. The goal of ILR counselors is to help their clients achieve their highest level of independence. Referring their clients to a driver rehabilitation program will assist the clients in moving toward achieving this goal.

Allied Health Professionals

Rehabilitation therapists, including occupational (OTs), physical therapists (PTs), and speech and language pathologists (SLPs), have the most direct and consistent access to clients who can benefit from driver rehabilitation and community mobility services; needless to say, these professionals are a valuable resource for prospective referrals. Provision of departmental in-services and workshops will increase awareness and knowledge of driver rehabilitation and community mobility needs of, and services for, clients and their caregivers.

REIMBURSEMENT

Next to the quality of the professional services provided, reimbursement is the most important factor in determining whether a program will ultimately survive. The primary sources of funding for driver rehabilitation services are clients who can afford to pay for services "out of pocket" (i.e., self-pay), state VR agencies, and workers' compensation agencies. Basic medical insurance coverage (e.g., HMOs, Blue Cross and Blue Shield, Medicaid, and Medicare) have typically not covered driver rehabilitation or community mobility services because driving is not always considered a medical necessity. With a vigilant effort, some programs have been successful in obtaining coverage from some insurance carriers including Medicare on a case by case basis. For some programs, the provision of occupational therapy services can be billed and paid for by major medical insurance entities. It is important for a new program to have in place a pre-certification system to determine whether the prospective client's insurance will cover the cost of the evaluation, training, or both before services are rendered.

Medicare pays for the provision of general occupational therapy services. It will be the responsibility of the service provider to check with their Medicare Fiscal Intermediary to determine the correct billing code to use for a driver rehabilitation evaluation, community mobility evaluation, or both as well as on-road training and whether or not Medicare will authorize payment of such services. This knowledge will be vital information to include in the program's business plan. The service provider will need to determine if the Medicare reimbursement rate will be sufficient to cover the cost of the services rendered in the program. Many programs typically require clients to self-pay (sometimes prior to providing the service); thus, the program avoids the complications associated with preauthorizing payments, handling Medicare claims, appealing insurance denials, and jumping through the various "hoops" that the many third-party payers demand.

COMPETITION SURVEY

Identifying competitors is an essential part of the needs assessment. It is essential to investigate what services are currently being provided in the program's service area. If there are no programs, the DRS should consider why one has not been developed to date. The possible factors such as low population or reimbursement constraints will help the DRS to assess whether a program's viability will be feasible. Urban areas can usually support a driver rehabilitation program simply because of the high numbers of people with disabilities, aging-related challenges, or both. Developing a program in a rural area will likely have less demand for its services. Other factors make a rural-based program less attractive including the increased time it would take clients to travel to and from a rural-based facility or the increased overhead (i.e., time and money) if the DRS travels to his or her clients' homes.

If there is a driving program in the DRS's area, he or she should determine the level of service and evaluate if a new program can meet an unfilled need, either geographically or in the type of services provided. For example the existing program may serve only VR clients thus leaving an opening for the growing demand for older driver evaluations. If the other program does not have a van, there may be opportunities to serve clients that require specialized evaluations and training in an adapted full-sized van or minivan. It is important to keep in mind that few people will require a van equipped with advanced adapted driving controls and extensive vehicle modifications. To illustrate this point consider one program that started in the early 1980s that was eager to meet the demands of people with any type of disability. The program purchased a van equipped for persons diagnosed with tetraplegia (quadriplegia), a van for persons diagnosed with paraplegia, and a car. The DRS soon realized that maintaining two vans was not cost-effective because most of their clients needed a car versus a van. In addition there was another van program in their area. In the final analysis, they could have seen more clients had they purchased two cars and only one van.

PROGRAM DELIVERY MODELS

There are several different delivery models, each with various advantages and disadvantages: clinical evaluations only, clinical and simulator assessments, and clinical evaluations and in-vehicle evaluations. See also Chapters 1 and 4 for more information about program delivery models.

CLINICAL EVALUATIONS ONLY

A clinical evaluation or screening program is designed to provide information to help guide clients and physicians on how to address issues pertaining to a return to driving or alternatives to driving that enable community mobility, such as identifying and using alternative transportation. Predriver clinical evaluations consist of obtaining the client's medical and driving history, thorough visual assessment, physical evaluation (e.g., range of motion, strength, coordination, sensation, sitting balance, transfers, and mobility status), reaction time test, visual-perceptual assessments, and cognitive assessments (e.g., memory, traffic sign recognition, attention).

Sprigle et al[2] found that most of the practitioners conducting driving evaluations were OTs. Driving requires the synthesis of many skill areas in a fast-moving, risk-filled environment; thus, the information that is derived from evaluating a client in a clinical setting should rarely, if ever, be used to make a final judgment about his or her driving readiness. On-road driving behavior is the most critical factor in assessing driver safety, but this key performance variable cannot be tested in a clinical or community setting while the client and DRS are sitting at a table. For example an OT would likely not judge kitchen safety by performing only a vision assessment. The client's task performance must be observed while he or she is in the kitchen to truly assess kitchen safety.

Screening a client in a clinic or some other setting is useful for ruling out driving for individuals with significant impairments (e.g., field cuts or severe physical or perceptual limitations); however, the vast majority of people referred will require an in-vehicle evaluation while on the road and behind the wheel of a motor vehicle. To create a predriving clinical evaluation–only program that is worthwhile, the clients should subsequently be referred to a program that conducts on-road evaluations. It is important to work with an established program to help ensure that clients will accept the results of the initial clinical evaluation, thereby preventing duplication of testing services. To understand how clinical performance relates to actual driving skills, the therapist conducting the evaluations in a predriving clinical evaluation–only program should try to observe as many on-road evaluations as possible.

CLINICAL AND SIMULATOR ASSESSMENTS

Advantages of incorporating a driving simulator into the evaluation and training services include the ability to assess client responses to challenging stimuli (e.g., inclement weather, animate and inanimate obstacles, night driving) and practice with adapted driving aids in a low-risk virtual environment prior to getting behind the wheel and hitting the road. Simulators are ideally suited for airline pilots, shuttle crews, and police officers because the ability to repeatedly practice high-risk skills is safe and cost-effective. However, persons with disabilities also can benefit from accessing and utilizing driving simulators for remediation and training of driving skills in a controlled environment.

Determining whether or not the benefits that a simulator provides for driver evaluation, training, and research justify the cost is debatable. It is important to note that researchers differ in their opinions about whether or not simulators reliably predict driving behavior and performance in real driving situations. Failing a simulator test, the client may rightly react by saying, "You didn't test me in a real car!" From a cost standpoint, an effective simulator usually costs more than a car and it will require devoted floor space. In a self-pay environment, clients may be unwilling to pay for several lessons on a simulator. If a program is struggling to choose between a car and a simulator, the most cost-effective way to meet the client's needs is most likely a car. (See Chapter 10 for more details regarding driving simulators.)

CLINICAL EVALUATIONS AND IN-VEHICLE EVALUATIONS

Providing both the predriving clinical evaluation and in-vehicle or on-road evaluation allows a program to offer comprehensive driver rehabilitation evaluations and the ability to follow-up with on-road driver training services. The clinical evaluation will likely be conducted by an OT that specializes in driver rehabilitation services. There are several ways to provide the in-vehicle evaluation, depending on the anticipated customer volumes.[3] If the business plan shows a need for the service but the client volumes initially are low, contracting with a local driving school to provide some of the on-road training can reduce the program's start-up costs. It is important to collaborate with a driver educator who can provide on-road training with sensitivity and objectivity. It is recommended that the OT working as a DRS ride in the back seat of the training vehicle and the driver educator ride in the front passenger seat during a client's first and last on-road training sessions.[1a] The OT who is a DRS and providing the clinical evaluations and the driver educator will need to agree on optimal methods of communication, case documentation style and format, and how to handle disagreements regarding driver and/or community mobility recommendations.

When working with a contracted driving school, communication with the client can be compromised because several people that work in different locations are involved in the evaluation process, training process, or both. The health care organization (e.g., hospital) should also carefully look at existing and potential liability issues. What is the hospital's liability if the contracted school makes a mistake? Again, it is ideal to have the OT working as a DRS observe the on-road evaluation and training from the back seat.

If the volume of clients served is sufficient, the most efficient, comprehensive, and potential cost-effective program would be one that offers both clinical and on-road evaluations. A driver educator could be hired full-time or part-time to work collaboratively with an OT who is working as a DRS and may have voluntarily become a certified driver rehabilitation specialist (CDRS), a licensed driving instructor, or both. State laws vary regarding the licensing requirements for driving instructors; therefore, the therapist-as-instructor option may not be possible.

Consider the following issues:
- Does your state regulate driver instructors that work with adults?
- Does your state keep a list of accepted driver rehabilitation programs? If so, what are the state's requirements for a program to be listed and remain in good standing?

A committed therapist working as a DRS should be willing to take the academic courses required to become a driving instructor.

Conducting both the clinical evaluation and on-road evaluation sessions allows a client to benefit from "one-stop-shopping" and have the evaluation potentially completed in 1 visit. The continuity of having the same person present during both portions of the overall comprehensive driving evaluation will benefit the client when establishing rapport as well. It will also help the evaluator get a more complete picture of the client.

PROFILE OF THE DRIVER REHABILITATION SPECIALIST (DRS)

The field of driver rehabilitation (and more recently alternative community mobility) is rapidly expanding, and working in the capacity of a DRS is a rewarding and exciting career. The nature of the profession is also one in which risk and liability are important factors to consider. Working with a client in a vehicle is inherently more risky than the activities occurring in the average therapy clinical or community setting. The DRS often works independently, and the decisions he or she makes have a direct effect on a client's safety, independence, and well-being. OTs working as DRSs are held accountable to standards from the American Occupational Therapy Association (AOTA). (See Chapter 23 and appendixes C, D, and I for more information on professional ethics and standards of prac-

tice.) Skills DRSs bring to their jobs will affect their performance, influence their decision-making, increase or decrease their risk level, and have an effect on their ability to communicate with their clients. This section discusses the basic profile of a DRS; Box 26-1 details the occupational outlook.

SPECIALIZED TRAINING

The DRS is a professional who has received specialized training in this area of practice. Professionals who become DRSs are generally OTs or driver educators; however, PTs, SLPs, state certified driver instructors, and others are entering the field as well. DRSs must remain in good standing with their respective profession's state and national licensure and/or registry. Because driver rehabilitation (and now we are also including community mobility) is a specialty, the type, amount, and sophistication of structural vehicle modifications and adapted driving equipment are constantly changing; therefore, continuing education is a necessity. The Association of Driver Rehabilitation Specialists (ADED) offers voluntary professional certification for eligible candidates. The AOTA's Representative Assembly (RA) also recently voted to support the development of a certificate in driver rehabilitation, community mobility, or both that will be granted by the AOTA. Contact the AOTA (www.aota.org) for more information.

SKILLED OBSERVATION

A great majority of information about the client is obtained by honing decision-making skills that require skilled and knowledgeable observation. Simply escorting a client to the office can yield important information about their ability to follow verbal and/or written directions, their sense of space and topographic orientation in the hallway, and visual perceptual skills, including the ability to scan the environment to identify the office door, for example. Additionally a client's speed of gait, evidence of gait disturbance, upper body function, and use of adaptive mobility equipment can also be observed during the few minutes that transpire after meeting a client face-to-face. Observation during the clinical evaluation can inform the evaluator about the client's interaction skills, ability to follow instructions, ability to focus on a particular task, attention to details, temperament, and how he or she handles stressful situations. When evaluating the client on the road and behind the wheel of a motor vehicle, the DRS will find the previously observed behaviors to be valuable information. By the time the on-road evaluation takes place, the DRS will have an idea of how the client follows instructions, handles stress, solves problems, and attends to the

BOX 26-1   Driver Rehabilitation Specialist Job Analysis

The U.S. Department of Labor *Occupational Outlook Handbook (OOH)* provides detailed career information and identifies what a particular job entails and the training and experience necessary, and provides information on salary and job outlook. Because there is not a specific listing for driver rehabilitation specialists in the OOH, it served as the model for this analysis in order to provide consistent basic information about the specialty.

SIGNIFICANT POINTS

The driver rehabilitation specialist (DRS) is a licensed/ registered professional with at least a 2-year degree in the following: kinesiology, occupational therapy, physical therapy, speech and language pathology, or state-approved driver instructor or driver education teacher.

Although DRS certification is available and recommended, it may not be a requirement for provision of services in all states. Refer to the Association of Driver Rehabilitation Specialists (ADED) for current certification requirements (www.aded.net).

NATURE OF THE WORK

Using a combination of clinical assessments and skilled, functional observations, a DRS helps to determine a client's fitness for driving after being challenged by disease, traumatic injury, chronic disability, or normal changes associated with aging. The DRS provides on-road evaluations to help clients resume safe and competent motor vehicle operation. The DRS not only evaluates whether a client is capable of driving, but determines whether adaptive equipment or adapted driving behaviors are indicated for competent motor vehicle operation. The DRS will also determine the amount, frequency, and duration of training required to improve a driver's skills with newly learned behaviors or prescribed adapted driving equipment.

The DRS assists clients in performing all necessary tasks for motor vehicle operation including motor vehicle selection, adaptive driving equipment prescription, vehicle structural modifications for accessibility, and basic vehicle operation skills. A DRS may provide classroom education as part of a driver rehabilitation program as well as behind-the-wheel driver training. Home exercise programming may be provided to improve flexibility, coordination, or strength for improvement in vehicle control skills. Independent study may also be directed in order to facilitate learning and improvement in the client's awareness and understanding of motor vehicle law, vehicle operation, and defensive driving strategies.

For those with functional limitations, the DRS may prescribe adapted driving equipment and training for vehicle operation competence. For example a driver with paraplegia will be educated and trained to efficiently and safely transfer into and out of the motor vehicle, load and stow the wheelchair, position the seat, use hand controls for gas and brake operation, and interface with a steering device for adapted steering. For those with age-related limitations, the DRS may teach adapted driving habits, select and instruct in alternate driving routes, recommend driv-

ing restrictions, and assist the driver and his or her family in identifying alternative transportation resources in the face of impending driving retirement or cessation.

Recording testing results, skilled observations, and findings is an important part of any driver evaluation or rehabilitation program. Accurate, objective, and timely records are essential for evaluating clients, communicating progress, reporting status, and for billing purposes. Reports are generally shared with referring physicians, third party payers, the client, and other pertinent agencies working with the client.

WORKING CONDITIONS

DRSs will work in a combination of a clinical setting and an in-vehicle setting. The clinical setting can be based in a hospital outpatient therapy area, free-standing outpatient therapy clinic, private practice office, or in a university therapy clinic setting. The in-vehicle services are provided in a motor vehicle that has been purchased by the program and is outfitted with various types of adaptive driving equipment used for evaluation and rehabilitation purposes. Some driver evaluation programs offer the clinical evaluation and either refer the driver to another facility for the on-road evaluation or will contract with a driving school to provide these services. Most DRSs work a 40-hour work week on a typical Monday through Friday schedule. Some facilities offer extended, evening, or weekend hours to accommodate their clientele. DRSs often perform driver evaluation and rehabilitation work as part of their traditional occupational therapy services, administrative duties, teaching commitments, or a combination of these and other duties.

A clinical evaluation setting will use a number of standardized tests to assess cognitive, psychological, and psychomotor function. Testing equipment for vision screening and reaction time is also used. The driver evaluation vehicle is another piece of equipment used by the DRS. The vehicle is generally a four-door vehicle equipped with automatic transmission and various adaptive driving equipment used for evaluation and training purposes. The vehicle is also outfitted with dual control brakes that the DRS will operate from the front passenger's seat while on the road with a client. Some facilities also use an adapted van for evaluation and training of persons requiring more advanced or highly technical driving equipment due to severity of functional loss. The majority of adapted driving equipment used for evaluation is removable and adjustable, and the DRS will be responsible for installing and adjusting the equipment per individual client needs.

The job can be tiring, as the DRS will be required to physically assist with client transfers, install and adjust necessary driving equipment, and remain alert during on-road evaluation and training sessions. A fair amount of time is spent on nonbillable activities as well as fielding questions by clients, their families, and caregivers. Regular marketing and program promotion is an essential part of the job.

Continued

| BOX 26-1 | Driver Rehabilitation Specialist Job Analysis–cont'd |

EMPLOYMENT

The primary employers of DRSs are outpatient hospital programs, university clinical research programs, and state rehabilitation programs. Some DRSs are self-employed in private practice. Clients are referred by physicians, state DMV medical review programs, state rehabilitation programs, other health care professionals, and by clients themselves and their family members.

The Association of Driver Rehabilitation Specialists (ADED) is an organization devoted to the ongoing education of driver rehabilitation specialists and offers a certification program for individuals seeking professional credentialing and ongoing education in the field. As of December 1, 2003, ADED listed 305 current Certified Driver Rehabilitation Specialists (CDRSs). The American Occupational Therapy Association (AOTA) has listed driver rehabilitation as one of their top ten emerging practice areas. This practice area has been identified for a growth area within occupational therapy in response to the growing elder population.

TRAINING, ADVANCEMENT, AND OTHER QUALIFICATIONS

Model practices were defined in a document co-created by the National Mobility Equipment Dealers Association (NMEDA) and ADED. The "Model Practices for Driver Rehabilitation for Individuals with Disabilities" was designed for distribution to all state Vocational Rehabilitation agencies to promote "safety, quality, and consistency in the provision of driver rehabilitation and vehicle modification services to consumers with disabilities."[4] NMEDA and ADED intended for the document to be used to promote the creation of new driver rehabilitation and vehicle modification programs, as well as assisting with the expansion of existing programs and services. According to this document, requirements for DRSs were identified as such:

- All DRSs must have a bachelor's degree, operate under a professional license, and have a minimum of 3 years of qualifying experience. Or a practitioner may have an associate's degree and 6 years of full-time experience in driver rehabilitation.
- DRSs must be able to provide documentation of a minimum of 3 years of full-time experience providing driver rehabilitation services to individuals with disabilities.

ADED offers certification in the field of driver rehabilitation in order to protect the public by "Providing measurement of a standard of current knowledge desirable for individuals practicing driver rehabilitation; encouraging individual growth and study, thereby promoting professionalism among driver rehabilitation specialists; formally recognizing driver rehabilitation specialists who fulfill the requirement for certification."[5] Refer to current guidelines from ADED for certification criteria.

The AOTA offers continuing education in the field of driver rehabilitation evaluation. Driver evaluation workshops (that now emphasize the importance of including community mobility as part of the overall services offered) can be attended at AOTA's annual conference. Also, an online course entitled *Older Driver Screening and Evaluation: The Forgotten IADL* was designed for all occupational therapists at the intermediate professional level interested in working with the elderly. ADED offers an annual conference featuring workshops for the new, intermediate, and advanced level professionals involved in the provision of driver rehabilitation services.

Professionals interested in specializing in driver rehabilitation services need patience, compassion, strong verbal and written communication skills, and the ability to quickly build rapport and gain the trust of their clients. The DRS is exposed to dangerous situations every time he or she is in a vehicle with a client, which makes the ability to think quickly, plan ahead, anticipate a client's actions or reactions, and remain calm under pressure important attributes. Strong teaching and coaching skills are also required.

JOB OUTLOOK

As the population ages, the need to address older driver safety increases. The older population is growing nearly twice as fast as the total U.S. population, and the fatality rates for drivers 85 and older are 9 times higher than the rate for drivers 25 to 69 years old.[6] There is an obvious need for emerging practice areas to address the issue of older driver safety and prevention of automobile accidents that result in injuries, damaged property, and/or death. The DRS will also be involved in addressing the mobility needs of the disabled population, regardless of age.

EARNINGS

The majority of professionals providing driver rehabilitation services are occupational therapists; the following earnings data are provided using information from the U.S. Department of Labor *Occupational Outlook Handbook*. The median annual earnings for an occupational therapist (O*NET 29-1122.00) in 2000 was $49,450, and those individuals falling around the fiftieth percentile (i.e., midrange) earned between $40,460 and $57,890.[7] The majority of OTs providing driver rehabilitation services are based in hospitals and offices. The OOH lists the hospital medical OT salary for 2000 at $50,430 while the average salary for those OTs employed to work in offices owned by other health care professionals, such as physicians or physical therapists, is $49,520. A number of OTs are providing driver rehabilitation services through their own private practices; salary information for this group is unavailable.

surrounding environment inside and outside of the vehicle. This information can be used to prevent dangerous on-road situations and requires the DRS to constantly apply an identification, prediction, decision, and plan-of-action sequence simultaneously while observing both the client and internal and external driving environments. Skilled, honed, and accurate observation skills are necessary for quick responses and the highest level of safety during on-road evaluation and training sessions. See Chapters 12 and 13 for more information on on-road evaluation and on-road training.

COMMUNICATION SKILLS

The ability to communicate is important to the DRS on several levels. First, body language is present upon the first meeting with the client and can affect the rapport-building process. The DRS should project a sense of hospitality, trustworthiness, empathy, and competence. These traits can be projected either positively or negatively the moment that the client first meets the DRS. Secondly, verbal communication skills used to glean information, provide instruction, and reassure the client are also important factors that will affect the evaluation process. While in the vehicle, the DRS must be able to provide clear and precise driving instructions, put the client at ease, and verbally control the vehicle operator's actions in the face of impending traffic or roadway hazards. Strong teaching and coaching skills are valuable assets to any DRS in helping put clients at ease, making instruction understandable, and maintaining a controlled situation. Developing good rapport with the client is important, because communication during the in-vehicle evaluation is important for safety. In many instances, hazardous driving situations can be avoided by a simple word or gesture by the DRS. If the DRS has not taken the time to gain rapport and instill trust in the client, the DRS will not have much control over the vehicle or the driver. Safety is the most important factor in any comprehensive driver rehabilitation evaluation. Without a strong relationship that reflects good rapport and trust between the DRS and client as well as the ability to reduce driver anxiety, the risk of collision increases.

The DRS also must be skilled at communicating results that may be viewed as undesirable, too. When a client does not pass a driver evaluation, the DRS has the responsibility to share this information with the driver and in some circumstances his or her family. Basic independence is tied closely with the ability to drive, and learning that one is no longer safe to drive can be devastating news. Clients react very differently to the news; they can be reticent, angry, defiant, tearful, or even hostile. The DRS must have many communication tools in order to convey this news delicately yet forthrightly and in a way that the client can fully comprehend. One must

give concrete, objective information along with the more subjective impressions to support the recommendations. See Chapters 7 and 21 and Appendix H for more information on neuropsychology and driving, driving cessation, and counseling clients no longer fit to drive.

OBJECTIVITY AND CONSISTENCY

Valid evaluations of driving ability require that the client and the referral source obtain accurate and sound recommendations. A part of a DRS's recommendation comes from a "gut feeling" or intuition that answers the question, "Would I let this person drive my child to school, or my elderly parent to the doctor's office?" Although subjective information may guide the DRS in making a decision, it will simply not be valid information for an investigation, inquiry, or ethical probe. Therefore, solid decisions must be based on objective (and usually quantifiable) data, sound medical knowledge, and research that adhere to the scientific method. (See Chapter 24 for more information on research and evidence-based practice in driver rehabilitation.) The DRS is held responsible by professional ethics to treat each client consistently, objectively, and fairly. The DRS's reports should follow a consistent format that provides the same level of detailed information, including recommendations that are grounded in their professional observations, thorough analysis of assessment data, and expectations related to current and future driving performance. See Chapter 23 to explore legal and professional ethics in driver rehabilitation.

EVALUATION SKILLS

The careful selection and application of evaluation assessment tools is a critical job task and is generally guided by the program's evaluation protocol and the client's diagnosis or disability. Choosing valid, pertinent, and logical evaluation tools will give the DRS information that he or she can use to support his or her recommendations. Using unnecessary or unproven testing tools does not add to the validity of the evaluation or the credibility of the data collected and adds to the overall time and expense. Making sense of the observed information, clinical testing, and on-road performance is the artistry and skill set of the DRS. The DRS must draw logical and objective conclusions in order to provide the client and referral source with appropriate recommendations that will lead to desired outcomes.

CRITICAL THINKING

While there are many definitions of critical thinking, the basic premise is that critical thinkers draw conclusions and make judgments and decisions based on the contextual information they are processing. Critical thinkers also make judgments and observations about their own thinking processes, analyzing how they came to certain conclusions and definitions. Critical thinkers are flexible with their thoughts and able to adjust their conclusions based on new information while continuously seeking new sources of information. Box 26-2 identifies the characteristics of critical thinkers.

Putting education, observation, evaluation, and assessment together while making sound judgments and projecting empathy and trustworthiness toward the client is a talent that may not be available to every OT generalist, driver educator, or other professional wishing to become a DRS. There is an art to simultaneously shouldering the combined responsibilities of evaluator, instructor, advocate, and resource provider. The talent lies in the clinician's ability to see the big picture, predict client's actions and reactions, determine the most appropriate driving situation for the client, and communicate this information. Driver evaluation and rehabilitation can be the most dangerous and simultaneously rewarding specialty area within rehabilitation that a health care professional or driver educator can be engaged in. The added talents of being able to remain calm in a crisis, choosing when to let a client make a driving error, and when to step in as well as deciding when to provide verbal feedback (irrespective of whether it is viewed by the client as positive or

negative) are also part of the art of driver rehabilitation services offered by a DRS working in a respectable and legitimate program.

COSTS OF STARTING A PROGRAM

Start-up and operating costs are the main costs associated with starting a program.

START-UP COSTS

The cost of setting up a program will greatly depend on the program's delivery model. One essential cost of developing a program is the staff time required to conduct a feasibility study. Funds must also be committed to train the therapist and/or instructor. Specialty coursework or hiring a consultant is highly recommended, because the DRS in training will not have had this specialty training in school. *Credentialing* is important in this field, too. More extensive education and training lends credibility and fosters respect for the professional in question by consumers and colleagues alike as well as promoting the notion that the professional is well qualified to provide driver rehabilitation services. Education and training coupled with experience also help prepare professionals planning to sit for the CDRS exam offered annually by ADED.

Clinical equipment start-up costs are negligible unless the program plans to use a simulator or other specialized assessment tool(s). Obtaining and equipping a vehicle will be the biggest up-front expense. Leasing a car has pros and cons. With a lease, there will be less up-front costs, and trading in a vehicle in a few years will help the program stay current with equipment and vehicle options. The downside to a vehicle lease is the expense of equipping a different vehicle every few years. The cost to properly configure and equip a training vehicle can range from $3000 to $5000. Obtaining a donated vehicle and adapted driving equipment will result in a significant cost savings. When obtaining a donated vehicle, be sure that the car meets programmatic needs. It could be frustrating to accept a free car from a local dealer only to find that it cannot be equipped properly or that it lacks the minimal safety features, such as driver-side and passenger-side airbags. Equipment manufacturers may donate equipment, as it certainly helps them to have clients evaluated and trained with their equipment.

VR agencies can be an important source for start-up funding. Having an effective driver rehabilitation and community mobility program in the area can make a significant difference in the employability of clients with disabilities. This assistance may be critical if the program hopes to obtain an expensive evaluation van.

BOX 26-2	**Characteristics of a Critical Thinker**

- Asks pertinent questions
- Assesses statements and arguments
- Is able to admit a lack of understanding or information
- Has a sense of curiosity
- Is interested in finding new solutions
- Is able to clearly define a set of criteria for analyzing ideas
- Is willing to examine beliefs, assumptions, and opinions and weigh them against facts
- Listens carefully to others and is able to give feedback
- Sees that critical thinking is a lifelong process of self-assessment
- Suspends judgment until all facts have been gathered and considered
- Looks for evidence to support assumptions and beliefs
- Is able to adjust opinions when new facts are found
- Looks for proof
- Examines problems closely
- Is able to reject information that is incorrect or irrelevant[8]

OPERATIONAL COSTS

Staff salaries will be the largest continuous operating expense. Driving programs are typically expensive to operate due to the large amount of time required for nonbillable services (e.g., phone calls, documentation, consultations, vehicle modification research, and marketing). Time is spent talking to potential clients and referral sources that may never result in them coming to the program for services. Programs will become a public resource and the staff will need time to answer many phone inquiries about issues pertaining to driver rehabilitation and community mobility. Other expenses include fuel, vehicle maintenance, marketing, support staff, insurance, and typical office operation costs. The physical space required depends on whether the program needs to have a devoted space. A full-time program will require office space, storage, and perhaps room for a simulator. If only a few evaluations are conducted each week, using a private room for the clinical evaluations may suffice.

Driving programs will never generate the revenue generated by the typical therapy department because of the one-on-one nature of the evaluations and training. Unlike the services provided by the OT generalist, who may lead several groups of clients each day, performing group treatment to cut expenses is not feasible for the therapist working as a DRS. The program's profitability may largely depend on the amount of indirect hospital costs attributed to the program as well as grant funding. To avoid revenue loss for the health care facility that hosts a driver rehabilitation program, the program should aim to meet at least its direct costs. If a program is losing money, this loss should be balanced with the overall value to the clients and the community, the public relations benefits, and crossover referrals to other therapies and health-related services.

PROGRAM IMPLEMENTATION

Program implementation involves many factors, including creating a mission statement, developing a policy, finding referrals, documenting, reporting impairments, using clinical screening tools, choosing a driver evaluation and training automobile, and developing marketing strategies. Correctly implementing these factors can help the DRS create a successful private practice.

MISSION STATEMENT

A mission statement will guide the program and help succinctly explain the program to others. Developing a mission statement will help the program define its purpose and set a general course over the following 3 to 5 years or longer. The mission statement will likely change over time as the program grows and changes to meet the changing needs of its customers. The following provides components of a mission statement that is typical of many driving programs throughout the United States:

- Enable individuals to achieve their fullest potential through safe driving, community mobility, or both
- Clarify driving ability for individuals with questionable driving skills
- Serve as a public resource for issues related to driving and persons with disabilities, aging-related challenges, or both

POLICY DEVELOPMENT

Policies and procedures are essential tools that guide health care services, particularly the high-risk practice area of driver rehabilitation. These policies can be cited in a court of law, so it is prudent to be certain that these important documents have administrative approval and do not increase the organization's or program's liability. Possible topics include referral method, admissions requirements, evaluation and training protocols, policies for writing adapted equipment prescriptions, and how and when to report clients unfit for driving to state licensing departments.

REFERRALS

Most programs will require a physician's referral, especially if an OT working as a DRS is conducting the evaluation. Driving instructors may not be required by law to have a physician's prescription, but it is a good idea to obtain one anyway for issues requiring medical follow-up. A basic prescription pad referral stating "Driver Rehab" is usually not adequate, especially if you do not have access to the full medical history. An easy-to-complete referral form that gathers the basic medical history could be faxed to the physician. The form should include information on diagnosis or diagnoses, onset, prognosis, past medical history, visual limitations, seizure history, cardiac and orthopedic precautions, and medications.

DOCUMENTATION

The protocols and documentation for the evaluations and lessons will serve as the road map for how the program operates. (See Chapters 6, 9, 12, 13, 14 and 15 as well as Appendix A for more information on areas that should be addressed in a comprehensive driver rehabilitation evaluation and training regimen and how to document the results.) How the information is documented may depend on the amount of clerical and computer support available. A checklist is an easy format to complete, but it may not provide the necessary detailed description of the client's performance that is required in all cases. Documentation should be thorough, so the DRS and others privy to the client's information can understand what happened during the evaluation as needed; for example, a court case could surface years after the evaluation, and well-documented evaluations are critical to minimize liability. Pierce[1a] recommends that documentation should be written as if a lawyer will be scrutinizing the details. With computerized documentation, the information is entered into a database and linked to an evaluation form that is generated as an electronic or hard copy report with speed and efficiency. The data are also available for program evaluation and research purposes.

A detailed adapted equipment prescription is usually written after the client has passed the state license coding requirements and is then "legal" to drive with or without structural vehicle modifications, adaptive driving aids, or both. The prescription should be complete and include key information that the client will need to procure the adaptive driving aids and/or vehicle modifications regardless of the funding source, because modifications the client wants or needs are not always reimbursed by his or her funding source or sources.

REPORTING IMPAIRMENTS

Additional policies and procedures should address the following questions: What will be your policy if a client fails the program and driving is not recommended? Does the DMV require a report? The AMA recommends that physicians report clients with significant risk, regardless of the state reporting requirements.[9] Who should report, the driving program or the referring physician? These difficult issues should be addressed with the assistance of legal counsel. (These questions are discussed in further detail in Chapters 12 and 23 as well as appendices A and I.) Additionally information can be found in Antrim and Engum,[10] Jacobs,[11] and Annas.[12]

CLINICAL ASSESSMENT TOOLS

Many of the tools required to conduct clinical assessments used to evaluate clients may already be available in the hospital's occupational therapy department. Visual assessment protocols and devices may include some type of automated vision tester that can measure a variety of visual functions. A basic wall chart can yield good information on basic visual acuity and allows the examiner to observe the client's eyes during the assessment. A contrast sensitivity chart may be a specific expense, as the occupational therapy clinic many not have one. Wands for assessing saccades and visual field cuts are important.

Other basic devices include perceptual tests, a brake reaction time tester, goniometer, and eye patches.

More complex and expensive assessment tools, such as simulators, the Useful Field of View (UFOV), and Dynavision are also available and can be useful if you have time to perform these tasks during your initial clinical evaluation. These tools provide a valid way to assess the client's status; however, they may be difficult to administer if the predriving clinical evaluation is limited to 1 hour in duration.

CHOOSING A DRIVER EVALUATION AND TRAINING VEHICLE

Finding one evaluation vehicle that will meet all the needs of a program may be difficult due to competing demands. For instance, if the DRS chooses a two-door car for ease of transfers, he or she may have to give up the ability to see and access the gas pedal from the instructor's side if the vehicle has a center console. What is best for the client's eventual needs may not be best for the driver evaluation and training program, as the program must meet the needs of a large and diverse group of clients. Use the following list to evaluate the vehicle under consideration for acquisition for a driving program:

- Good visibility in the front and rear of the vehicle for both the driver and the instructor (i.e., DRS)
- Adequate accessibility to the gas pedal for the instructor (rules out center consoles)
- Power adjustable driver's seat
- Adequate room to install a left foot gas pedal to the left of the brake
- Column-mounted gear shift
- Easy-to-read dashboard instrumentation (especially the gear indicator)
- Split bench seats
- Large side-view mirrors

When the choices are narrowed to one or two cars, consult a vendor to see if installing the desired hand controls is feasible. Wrap-around dashboards may not allow for the installation of some hand controls. Access the ADED web site bulletin board to see what vehicles other programs are considering or go to the AOTA micro site dedicated to providing information about the elderly and driving issues for more information. Advice from other programs is very helpful, but it is important for each program to conduct their own research when assessing the potential needs of their current and prospective customers. Gathering this information will also help guide clients when they ask for advice on vehicle selection.

Equipping an Evaluation Vehicle
Equipping the vehicle with adaptations is a critical step when developing a driver rehabilitation program, because the equipment (and how it is installed) will

typically dictate what type of clients you can serve and how well you can serve them. To reduce client anxiety and maximize safety, most of the equipment should be removable, as many clients may not need adapted equipment. Older clients especially are often confused by unfamiliar devices and may inadvertently select the wrong device. Adjusting to a new vehicle is difficult enough; adding distractions could become dangerous. Clients are also prone to blaming the extra equipment if they perform poorly and fail their driving evaluation; they may have a valid point.

Table 26-1 is a listing of equipment that might be included in an evaluation automobile. (See also Chapters 5 and 11 for a detailed description of these devices.) It is critical to find a mobility equipment dealer or vehicle modifier that has the ability to install mountings that enable quick release of the hand controls. If set up correctly, it is possible for the DRS to install the controls in less than 5 minutes and remove them from the vehicle in less than 1 minute and without the use of tools. This flexibility allows the DRS and client to experiment with different equipment during the evaluation to quickly determine the best device. Be certain to complete a thorough review of the vehicle

before leaving the vehicle modifier's shop; the DRS should know how to install and adjust all the adapted driving controls.

Choosing a Driver Evaluation and Training Van

If the program's business plan includes evaluations of clients driving adapted vans, the first decision is deciding what type of van would best serve your clients' needs. A full-sized van will likely be the best choice if the program can only afford one van, because a greater range of clients could be evaluated as a result of height restrictions in a minivan. If the client wants a minivan, but was trained in a full-sized van, it is important to observe the person in a minivan prior to writing the final prescription to be certain that difficulties making the transition are kept to a minimum. Table 26-2 lists guidelines of what might be included in an evaluation van. It is important to emphasize that van modifications are complex and require careful research and planning. The information listed is only meant as a guideline when considering options. (See Chapter 11 for a more complete description of how the modifications are performed.) As mentioned above in the car section, the devices

---

Table 26-1 Listing of Possible Equipment for an Evaluation Vehicle

Who Uses It	Possible Equipment
Driver	Left foot gas pedal (quick release)
	Variety of hand controls, on right and left (push-pull, push-right angle, sure grip on left)
	Steering devices (knob, post, tri-pin, quad or C cuff, V-grip)
	Right turn signal extension
	Left gear shift extension
	Hand parking brake
	Removable chest strap is required for clients with reduced trunk stability
	Cushions to help shorter drivers gain better visibility
	Pedal extensions (small extensions, to extensive extensions for very short clients)
	Air bag on-off switch (used when working with short clients)
	Removable pedal shield that covers the gas pedal (used when working with hand controls or a left foot gas pedal to minimize risk and allow for comfortable right foot placement)
	Remote placement of turn signals, horn, high beams, wiper for the occasional client that may not be able to access the standard car controls
Instructor	Training brake
	Rear view mirror
	Eye-check mirror to monitor the client's eye movements
	Horn switch
	Brake light/turn signal light indicator on the dash for monitoring simultaneous gassing/braking and incorrect turn signals

Table 26-2   Listing of Possible Equipment for a Full-Sized Evaluation Van

Van Component	Equipment
Entry System	The floor should be lowered by 6 inches with a 3-inch removable spacer in the driver's compartment Raised roof Raised door Powered side-entry doors Fully automatic lift on the side of the vehicle Magnetic entry in side rear reflector Inside lift control on console Primary controls (removable so van can be customized to each client) Servo hand control (i.e., right or left mount) with interface devices; for example, tri-pin steering device, amputee ring, spinner knob, and glove. MPD 3700 right and left hand controls Push right angle hand control (left and right), with regular handle, offset handle and quad handle Sure-grip hand control on the left Push-pull hand control on right and left Extended steering column Adapted steering wheel (Note: options include horizontal steering system with 7" wheel and factory size wheel, digital steering systems, and other specialty systems) Variable effort steering system (i.e., zero, reduced, or standard effort steering) Back-up steering system Steering devices (e.g., post, knob, tri-pin, palm grip, V-grip) Variable effort brakes Electronic gear selector
Secondary Controls	Remote secondary controls, including turn signals, wipers, horn, high beam for elbow activation (variable mounting on right and left) Voice scan or voice-activated system for secondary controls Electric parking brake Quad extensions on dash controls
Console (central location)	Ignition/starter Gear selector Headlights/low beams 4-way flasher Wiper/washer control Electric parking brake Windows Lift controls Entry door controls Small console on the *left* for ignition and shifter if the client will be using the hand control on the *right* Hand control on the right
Seating	Removable 6-way captain's chair (to be installed in either the driver's position or in rear of the van, useful as a seat when the van is moving) Flexible seat belt/shoulder belt system for wheelchair drivers Retractable manual lockdown system for clients driving from their power wheelchairs as well as those individuals who will be riding as passengers while remaining in their wheelchairs in the rear of the vehicle. Both positions must include seat and shoulder belts that can be adjusted for an appropriate fit.

These modifications are for a Ford E-350 XLT van, cargo doors, with trailer towing package.
Refer to Table 26-1 for recommended equipment for the instructor.

should be removable and easily adjusted to meet the needs of a variety of clients.

PROGRAM EVALUATION

Measuring outcomes in a driver rehabilitation program can be difficult because there is not one set of measures of success that is recognized by the professional community or the general public. Additionally goals differ for each client and cannot always be generalized from one individual to another, even when they are presenting the same diagnosis and similar deficits. For example a successful outcome may well be that for one client he or she returns to safe driving, versus another client who failed the evaluation, is unsafe, and is no longer driving, thus reducing the risk for other roadway users.

Client satisfaction surveys may also yield skewed outcome data because the clients that do not pass the comprehensive driver rehabilitation evaluation may express displeasure with the program. Other methods may be required to evaluate the program's effectiveness. Outcome studies and surveys of clients receiving training will monitor the effectiveness of the training sessions and may yield estimates of the average number of lessons a diagnostic group may require. Surveying training clients after discharge will determine if they were pleased with the training and equipment installation and how the adaptive equipment performed over time. Funding and referral sources could be surveyed to see if the program is meeting their needs. Frequently clients referred to a driver rehabilitation program do not always follow through with obtaining an evaluation; tracking nonmaterialized referrals might help to begin shedding light on the reasons they did not participate. Marketing efforts can be evaluated by tracking referral and funding sources. Did the mass mailing generate additional referrals? Has the payer mix changed over time? Targeted program evaluation methods will help the program evolve to meet the current and future needs of the clients and referral sources.

MARKETING STRATEGIES

A key aspect of program implementation is a targeted marketing campaign. Marketing should start internally at a facility and expand to the larger institution, health system, and community only after the problems have been worked out of the new program.[13] Once the DRS is ready to advertise to the public, an extensive marketing plan should be developed to reach key referral sources.

Promotional materials will be essential for speaking engagements, mailings, and public exhibits. A general brochure could be complemented by specialty handouts developed by the program, ADED, and AOTA, or a professional graphic designer. Interesting profiles of successful clients will generate newspaper articles that can be reprinted for distribution long after the initial article appears. A program should develop a marketing folder with key information (e.g., promotional materials, referral forms, and state law information) to send to a referral source that wants to know more about the program.

Media presentations (e.g., slide shows, videos, PowerPoint presentations) would show how the program operates and allow people to view how the equipment works. A PowerPoint presentation could be geared to a variety of referral sources and customized to fit the particular needs of each group. The presentation disk, or perhaps a video in a variety of formats (e.g., CD-ROM, VHS, DVD), could be left for review after the in-service has concluded. Local and/or national television exposure is often possible due to the nature of the issues addressed, especially those that pertain to older drivers. Make sure local television, radio, and newspaper reporters are aware of the special services provided by the program.

Marketing is also critical for both new and established programs. The rapid turnover in the health care field may result in a nearby hospital not realizing the DRS down the street has opened a driver rehabilitation program, even though the DRS gave a stimulating in-service there 2 years ago. Keep track of all referral sources in a database and send out occasional letters, broadcast faxes, or e-mail communiqués to alert them to any new major developments. The public relations benefits of the program are one of its greatest assets. Promoting the program will give the hospital a reputation as a provider of comprehensive care. Providing these special services (e.g., driver rehabilitation and community mobility presentations) can help differentiate one facility or program as superior over others that otherwise provide similar services in a highly competitive health care environment.

ENTREPRENEURIAL OPPORTUNITIES

Experienced DRSs have begun to open private practices in this specialized field. Someone interested in opening a driver rehabilitation practice would have to follow most of the basic steps outlined in this chapter, but it is likely that the DRS will have a good understanding of the market environment in their location due to their experience and established professional network. The DRS will have to decide how to set up the business (e.g., sole proprietorship, S-corporation, limited liability corporation) and will likely need legal as well as accounting and tax advice from a certified public accountant on how to formally set up the business. A physical store front (i.e., as opposed to, or in addition to, a web site) may be required in some states, or the DRS may be able to work out of a home office. If the clients are met at their homes, the DRS will have to possess a thorough knowledge of the area to select appropriate evaluation and training routes. Hiring staff to perform office functions or on-road services will add to the capacity, but also to the complexity of the overall operation. It will be especially important to have the proper insurance to protect the DRS and the business from liability in this high-risk practice area.

LIABILITY AND LEGAL ISSUES

When designing and operating a driver rehabilitation program, professionals are held to standards imposed by state and federal laws as well as professional organizations, including AOTA and ADED. A program must ensure that it will meet all state requirements for conducting a driving school. The program must also be certain that laws pertaining to professional licensure, certification, and/or registration are not being violated. For example, can a driver evaluator with no formal education that addressed medically related topics perform a visual perception evaluation? Conversely, can an OT provide behind-the-wheel instruction to a client who is under the age of 18 without the proper credentials? These and other questions must be addressed to help ensure that each client receives the best possible care and the professional does not needlessly put himself or herself and the business at risk.

Besides meeting the basic requirements for licensure, certification, and/or registration, the DRS must be concerned with the implications of the decisions rendered after an evaluation. When considering whether a driver is safe to resume or to begin independent driving, it is suggested that the practitioner be comfortable with the answers to the following questions:

- Can or should this client resume driving a vehicle?
- What are my obligations and responsibilities in this matter?
- If the client is not ready to resume or initiate independent driving, what alternatives can I help the client identify and safely use to help ensure engagement in his or her community?

Responsibility is shared among many parties when considering driving recommendations. The client has the civic and ethical responsibility to be concerned for the general public, namely pedestrians and other roadway users. In many states it is mandatory that clients report to their state DMV if they had an illness or injury that interferes with their ability to operate motor vehicles. Few states require physicians or health care professionals to notify licensing authorities of any medical conditions that jeopardize the safety of the driver, the

community, or both. Regardless of state guidelines and legislature, the AMA Recommendations on Impaired Drivers[9] places an ethical responsibility on the physician to report unsafe drivers and explore options to ensure community mobility and improve safety. (See Chapters 21 and 23 for a discussion on driving cessation and professional and legal ethics and Appendix A for a listing of state driver licensing requirements and reporting laws.)

Driving is of course a privilege and not a right, and the driver has the responsibility to cease driving if there is a question about his or her safety while on the road and behind the wheel of a motor vehicle. It can be deemed negligent if a DRS does not alert either the physician or the state DMV of unsafe drivers if they have knowledge that they could be harmful to themselves or others. The physician, under guidelines and a code of ethics, has responsibility to protect clients and the public. The driver rehabilitation program has a responsibility to ensure that its DRSs abide by all state and federal laws and act ethically and responsibly as well as protect the general public by ensuring that the care clients receive is from qualified, trained professionals. The state DMV has the responsibility and legal authority to determine driving capacity and licensure. Questions to ask pertaining to liability and ethics include the following:

- What is the role of the physician in regard to medical concerns and an individual's ability to drive safely?
- Does the physician or health provider have immunity if they report clients that they feel are at risk?
- Are individuals required to report changes in their physical status, mental status, or both only when renewing their licenses?
- How does the DRS's state address loss of consciousness, seizures, visual impairment, and other factors that can affect driving?
- What restrictions can be placed on an individual's license, and what is the process for putting those restrictions on the license?

SUMMARY

Because driving is a high-risk instrumental activity of daily living, driver rehabilitation is a high-risk profession. The many legal, ethical, and logistical considerations that must be considered before starting a program may deter many well-intentioned health care professionals. The demand for ongoing education, training, and research as well as the requirement to maintain awareness of emerging technology may also be perceived as a barrier for many professionals attempting to balance not only responsibilities to a driver rehabilitation program, but other duties contained within their broader job descriptions. Regardless of these obstacles, the population is aging and the elderly as well as people with physical disabilities, cognitive disabilities, or both are beginning to expect equal access to a full and robust social life. Finally America's dependence on the automobile has facilitated the need for comprehensive driver rehabilitation and community mobility programs that are essential for any community.

A driver rehabilitation program serves to improve and enhance independence, increase public safety, and provide clients with options for dependable, affordable, and accessible alternatives to driving that enable community mobility. The profession of driver rehabilitation is more than a job; it is a calling for many specialists throughout North America and the world. These individuals often see themselves as the catalysts for positive change and a means by which clients can experience real empowerment. For those individuals wanting to advance their careers by seeking additional education that values evidence-based practice so as to provide competent driver rehabilitation services, the rewards are numerous. The profession is not for every health care professional or driver educator, but for those that meet the criteria and standards it can be an enjoyable and rewarding career. For the older driver that needs driver refreshment training, the driver with a disability that benefits from adapted driving equipment, or the new driver that requires specialized and intensive driver education, driver rehabilitation is a valuable asset to the client in particular and the broader community in general.

REFERENCES

1. Quentin Corley, Los Angeles Times, April 14, 1918 and Interview with author, March 19, 1936.
1a. Pierce S: Legal considerations for a driver rehabilitation program, *Phys Disabil Special Interest Section Newsletter* 16(1):1-4, 1993.
2. Sprigle S, Morris BO, Nowachek G, et al: Assessment of the evaluation procedures of drivers with disabilities, *Occup Ther J Res* 15(3):147-164, 1995.
3. Erisman CL: (1987). Disabled drivers program: in house versus contract service, *Phys Disabil Special Interest Section Newsletter* 10(4):2, 1987.
4. National Mobility Equipment Dealers Association, Association for Driver Rehabilitation Specialists: *Model practices for driver rehabilitation for individuals with disabilities,* May 2002, *http://www.driver-ed.org/i4a/pages/index.cfm?pageid=198.*
5. *Certification,* The Association for Driver Rehabilitation Specialists, http://www.driver-ed.org/i4a/pages/index.cfm?pageid=120. Accessed February 28, 2005.
6. Traffic Safety Facts: *Older population,* U.S. Department of Transportation, National Highway Traffic Safety Administration, March 16, 2004, *http://www-fars.nhtsa.dot.gov/pubs/7.pdf.7.*
7. Bureau of Labor Statistics, U.S. Department of Labor: *Occupational outlook handbook, 2004-05 Edition,* Occupational Therapists, March 18, 2004, http://www.bls.gov/oco/ocos078.htm.
8. Ferrett S: *Peak performance: success in college and beyond,* New York, 1997, McGraw-Hill.
9. AMA Policy # E-2.24: *Impaired drivers and their physicians,* June 2000. Retrieved July 13, 2004, http://www.ama-assn.org/apps/pf_new/pf_online?f_n=browse&doc=policyfiles/HnE/E-2.24.HTM.
10. Antrim JM, Engum ES: The driving dilemma and the law: patients' striving for independence vs. public safety, *Cognitive Rehabil* 7(2):16-19, 1989.
11. Jacobs S: Reporting the handicapped driver, *Arch Phys Med Rehabil* 59:387-390, 1978.
12. Annas GJ: Confidentiality and the public: when must the physician warn others of the potential dangerousness of his patient's condition? *Orthopedic Review* 4(5):55-57, 1975.
13. Kalina TD: Expanding opportunities: marketing your driving program, *Phys Disabil Special Interest Section Newsletter* 16(1):6-7, 1993.

Glossary

Accommodation: The focusing of the lens of the eye in response to the distance of an object from the viewer.

Acquired brain disorder: Any medical event or pathological process that causes damage to the brain resulting in neuropsychological impairment (e.g., traumatic brain injury, stroke, or dementia).

Activities of daily living (ADL): Activities in daily life on which hinge the client's emotional well-being and sense of self (e.g., self-care, work, and leisure).

Adaptations: Changes or additions that allow vehicle access to drivers and passengers with physical disabilities, aging-related concerns, or both.

Adapted vehicles: Vehicles whose design and structure are such that the additions and adaptations necessary for people with disabilities have been applied after-market.

Advocacy: The role taken on by the DRS when the driver is vulnerable to factors beyond his or her control, and where the DRS is able to influence the outcome. Examples may include licensing, parking, and access to certain services and benefits, such as funding and alternative community mobility.

Ancillary team members: Other health care professionals who help ensure that clients achieve their driver rehabilitation goals, community mobility goals, or both (e.g., primary care physicians, psychologists, registered nurses).

Anthropometrics: The study of human physical dimensions.

Anthropomorphic test drivers (ATD): Otherwise known as crash test dummies, these data-collecting devices, along with sophisticated computer models, both of which simulate human response and injury during a vehicle crash, are used to gauge human impact response and injury tolerance during a variety of crash scenarios.

Assistive technology: Devices that aid a person in his or her daily life as necessary (e.g., canes, wheelchairs, adaptive driving aids).

Attention: A hierarchical concept that captures many different aspects of cognition, including the ability to focus for short or long periods on a single stimulus (i.e., simple or sustained attention) and the ability to attend to multiple pieces of information simultaneously (i.e., complex or divided attention).

Attentional resources: The cognitive functions and behaviors available to the client at any given time to adjust his or her level of concentration to the appropriate area of concern.

Baseline: A measurement used by those administering various tests as a manner of gauging a client's performance. A baseline is usually determined by the results of the same tests by those without impairments.

Behavior: A complex functionality that is repeatable because it is instinctual or learned.

Bioptics: Optical devices used to accommodate persons granted restricted low vision driving privileges.

Blood alcohol concentration (BAC): The concentration of alcohol in a person's blood stream at a given moment in time.

Brain network: A grouping of neural correlates that may all function together to perform a particular task.

Central field of view: The portion of the field of view seen by the macula.

Certified driver rehabilitation specialists (CDRS): Professionals who have completed certification requirements set forth by the Association for Driver Rehabilitation Specialists (ADED).

Chunking: The merging of two or more codes into larger units (such as multiple symbol signs, interstate route numbers and shields, color coding, and so forth), minimizing reaction time.

Client-centered approach (or client-centered model): An approach to treatment whereby the DRS includes the client in every part of the evaluation and treatment program, including the decision of what plan of action to choose.

Clinical: The practice of administering tests and examinations in an occupational therapy clinic. The term is used to differentiate this evaluation method from the on-road (i.e., behind-the-wheel) evaluation.

Clinical reasoning: A method of reasoning founded upon evidence-based practice, and deduction and research skills.

Code of ethics: A set of rules developed to inform internal and external audiences about the values and beliefs that a particular constituency is expected to emulate. They publicly articulate principles and values against which a professional's (and in some environments, a student's) conduct can be measured.

Coding: The observation, reading, and comprehension of written or displayed information. Examples include stop lights, yield signs, and hand signals from traffic police.

Community mobility: The ability of members of a community to use dependable, cost-effective, and accessible alternatives to driving for travelling over distances less than 500 miles within a specific geographic area. Community mobility (or alternative community mobility) is synonymous with alternative transportation.

Compensation: Changes made to various processes to aid the client in achieving goals as determined by his or her abilities or potential for recovery.

Compensatory techniques: Techniques used by clients to aid in daily activities. These devices (physical or not) help the client compensate for disabilities, aging-related challenges, or both.

Competencies: Underlying capacities and attributes within a number of different categories.

Computerized graphic imagery (CGI): A design technique used in computerized driving simulations to allow the driver and the driving environment to interact.

Construct validity: Qualities in a test that require it be run in such a manner as to properly measure that which is being tested.

Content validity: Secondary to construct validity, it requires that the test incorporate a representative sample of performance components for each construct to be assessed.

Contrast sensitivity: The ability of the eye to detect various shades of gray or color shades (i.e., nuances).

Credentialing: The official academic background or professional foundation that lends credibility to the DRS. Appropriate and valid credentials help to reassure the client and the public at-large that the specialist has the proper education, training, and in some cases experience to evaluate and treat clients. Credentials also promote trust and respect of professionals within the field of driver rehabilitation and related fields.

Criterion validity: The measurement and comparison of a client's performance against both the performances of unimpaired subjects, and also against the performance of other similarly impaired drivers.

Cultural lag: The amount of time it takes for a given industry to respond to the unforeseen negative consequences that impact consumers of new technology.

Current procedural terminology (CPT) codes: CPT codes may be used by physicians and non-physicians who are state licensed to perform and bill for the services rendered.

Dark adaptation: The accommodation of the eyes in response to a change in the environment's lighting conditions from bright to dark.

Dependent variable: The treatment or intervention applied by the investigator.

Divided attention: The performance or mental processing of two or more stimuli simultaneously.

Documentation: Writing down a client's status once an evaluation has been completed or how treatment has impacted the client's performance outcomes (e.g., ability to resume safe motor vehicle operation, access alternatives to driving that enables community mobility, or both).

Driving cessation plan: A plan created by the driver rehabilitation specialist along with the client if he or she is not able to drive a motor vehicle. The creation of this plan is based on the client's current status or anticipated prognosis determined by the professional driver rehabilitation team members.

Driver readiness: The level of preparedness of a prospective driver as determined by the DRS.

Driver rehabilitation evaluations: A series of tests or assessments conducted by DRSs with the aim of determining their clients' driver-readiness. The clinical evaluation and the on-road evaluation comprise a comprehensive driver rehabilitation evaluation.

Driver rehabilitation specialist (DRS): An occupational therapist, other health care professional, driver educator, or other professional who is recognized as competent to perform clinical and on-road driver rehabilitation evaluations, as well as design and implement on-road training regimens.

Driver remediation plan: A plan created by the DRS and client when that client does not successfully pass the on-road driver evaluation. Remediation plans include steps meant to help a client improve his or her overall functional abilities related to the driving task and prepare him or her to retake any portion of the comprehensive driver rehabilitation evaluation.

Driver underload: A period of time when the level of a driver's concentration may drop due to a reduced number of stimuli, such as when driving for long periods of time at a constant speed can create a false sense of security.

Driving cessation: Usually following driving reduction, the complete elimination of driving from the client's activities.

Driving fitness: The suitability of the client for safe driving.

Driving reduction: The lessening of the amount of driving done by a client.

Driving simulation: A system that mimics the sensation and experience of driving in a virtual environment.

Drug: Any natural or synthetic substance that when taken into the body results in a change in medical, behavioral, or perceptual states for either medically therapeutic or non-medical purposes.

Dynamic visual acuity: The ability of the client to see details in certain objects when the object, the viewer, or both are moving.

Efficient mobility: The ability for a person or group of people to move between two points quickly and without great diversion (e.g., an ambulance driver responding to a motor vehicle collision or firefighters to a building fire).

Employment plan: A plan created by the client and the vocational rehabilitation counselor that outlines the development of job skills (e.g., the pursuit of education) as an avenue toward gainful employment, and obtaining job training in preparation for employment.

Ergonomic design: A design method meant to create products and environments that optimize comfort, functionality, and safety for the majority of people.

Ethics: A set of principles established by professional organizations, institutions, or groups to guide their members' professional conduct, such as treating clients with respect and demonstrating appropriate bedside manners for the betterment of both the client and the organization. These principles also aid in standardizing evaluation and treatment protocols for any client in the care of a member.

Evaluation research: As applied to driver rehabilitation, this research model is defined as the systematic analysis of a program or organization that provides services to individuals with disabilities, aging-related concerns, or both.

Evaluation vehicle: The vehicle in which the on-road or behind-the-wheel evaluation will take place.

Evidence-based practice: A means of providing driver rehabilitation services where the client's course of treatment is evidence-based. An evidence-based practitioner will design efficacious treatment based on sound theory and proven methods usually reported in scholarly publications and often reported at professional conferences.

Executive function: The ability to coordinate multiple areas of the brain to achieve a desired outcome, such as solving novel problems, changing actions based on previous behavior, developing strategies, and sequencing a series of complex tasks.

Executive functioning: A level of brain function reserved for upper levels of thought rather than physical movement or emotion.

Executive functions: The upper mental abilities of a client, such as with divided attention and problem solving.

Experimental research: A means of investigating a given hypothesis through scientific trials. The aim of experimental research is to eliminate or reduce variables that influence the results.

Face validity: A test that appears to have validity and, after measuring the test against specific measures of validity, may or may not be valid.

Federal Motor Vehicle Safety Standards (FMVSS): A set of standards set forth by the federal government that requires vehicles to have manufacturer-installed restraint systems which comply with minimum crashworthiness and occupant-protection design and performance requirements.

Field of view (FOV): The portion of the viewing area that can be perceived by the client without turning the head, irrespective of acuity. The field of view has natural limitations defined by the eyebrows and cheekbone structure as well as the shape and size of the nose. The "out the windshield" view that is seen by the driver and measured in numbers of degrees.

Functional assessment: A test to determine if the client has factors such as the strength, range of motion, and balance to safely operate a motor vehicle, as well as the ability to successfully transfer into and out of the vehicle and stow an ambulation aid or wheelchair as necessary.

Functional classification: The assignment to a class of related drugs according to its intended effect.

Functional deficits: Impairments that impact a client's ability to perform tasks associated with driving, community mobility, or both.

Functional neuroimaging: The study of brain activity related to a specific internal or external function in a specific area of the brain, depending on what type of stimulus is being used.

Gray matter: The tissue in the brain dedicated to thinking.

Housing density: The amount of residential dwellings per acre. Suburban housing tends to be at very low densities, sometimes as low as one residential unit per acre.

Independent variable: The desired measurable outcome.

Instrumental activities of daily living (IADL): Activities in daily life that improve the quality of life of a patient, but aren't critical to a patient's emotional well-being and sense of self.

Intelligent transport systems (ITS): Those systems designed to aid the driver with real-time information about the road ahead, the vehicle, or outside conditions. These systems may be in or out of the vehicle, such as radio traffic reports or in-vehicle mapping systems.

Interface: The primary information source for a given system; for example, the speedometer conveys information about the vehicle's current speed.

International Classification of Functioning, Disability, and Health (ICF): Created by the World Health Organization, the ICF provides a standard lexicon for describing interrelationships between health, disability, functioning, and other related issues such as driving.

In-vehicle demonstration: The explanation and orientation of the client by the DRS to all of the recommended vehicle modifications and how they function.

In-vehicle intelligent transport systems (IITS): Systems in a vehicle designed to aid the driver in traversing the roadways safely. An example of an IITS is the cruise-control system.

Kinesthetic awareness: Being aware that one's extremity or extremities are moving, and in which direction.

Language functioning: An individual's ability to communicate by comprehending verbal information (in an auditory or written form) and respond to such information through the use of verbal or nonverbal communication.

Loading device: Those products used to lift and transport unoccupied wheelchairs or motorized scooters. These can be used to compensate for a lack of strength but this may still not be useful if the client does not have the coordination skill to operate switches or attach the loading device to the mobility aid.

Make inoperative prohibition: The ban on alterations to given parts in vehicles based on safety concerns of the manufacturer. Dealers must have an understanding of the Federal/Canadian Motor Vehicle Safety Standards (FMVSS/CMVSS), and whenever vehicles are being altered, mobility equipment dealers are expected to be knowledgeable of any applicable standards or guidelines that might be impacted by such modifications.

Managed care: A general term for several types of health insurance plans. Managed care plans are created with incentives for enrollees to purchase services within established networks. The types of managed care plans include preferred provider organizations (PPOs) and health maintenance organizations (HMOs), both generally offered through employer group insurance plans. CHAMPUS, Medicare, and Medicaid are government-funded programs.

Mapped simulation: An approach used in creating CGI driving simulations in which roads can be driven at will as opposed to staying on a predetermined route.

Mass automobility: The ability of a large number of people to move about through the use of an individual means of transportation. It did not come to dominate the American transportation system until the 1950s, when the decline in mass transit systems across the country made automobile ownership more of a necessity.

Mass transit: A means of transportation offered to the public as an alternative to a private vehicle. Mass transit choices (i.e., subways, commuter railroads, buses, and trolleys) are important only in a few large cities in North America, though Americans prefer airplanes for travel of more than 500 miles.

Medical Advisory Board (MAB): The state-level government entity that works with the Motor Vehicle Administration or Department of Motor Vehicles to review cases in which a driver has or had a disability or condition that would prevent the operation of a motor vehicle without some type of aid or vehicle modification.

Memory functioning: The ability to perform each of the following three stages and the degree to which they can be performed: encoding (the ability to acquire new information), consolidation (the transformation of new information to permanent storage), and retrieval (the ability to recall learned material).

Methodological research: A model of research in which the researcher objectively tests the reliability and validity of the instrument.

Mixed-use zoning: The designation given to an area whose buildings may have a variety of uses. Traditionally found in urban settings, this type of zoning allows for workplaces and homes to be side-by-side, across the street, or even in the same building.

Mobility device: A manual or power wheelchair, scooter, or ambulation aid that facilitates indoor and outdoor personal mobility.

Motion perception: The ability to perceive changes in spatial location of anything in the visual field.

Motor Vehicle Administration (MVA): The state-level government entity dedicated to the registration, licensing, testing, and supervision of drivers and their vehicles. Known in most states as the Department of Motor Vehicles or DMV.

National Highway Traffic Safety Administration (NHTSA): A government entity dedicated to the reduction and prevention of traffic accidents.

National Mobility Equipment Dealers Association (NMEDA): Founded in 1988, NMEDA is primarily composed of dealer members; however, the association has manufacturers as a secondary membership as well. Professional members make up a third component of the membership, which include DRSs, rehabilitation engineers, vehicle modification inspectors, state and federal government employees with a role in the industry, and others.

Negative transfer: The extent to which previously learned skills may interfere with the acquisition of new skills in relation to a condition or disability.

Neighborhood: The definition of a neighborhood includes a variety of characteristics. These include the ability to walk within a quarter mile to a variety of amenities, commercial activity, and public transit.

Neural correlates: A general term referring to areas of the brain dedicated to specific functions.

Occupational engagement: The ability of a client to interact physically with the surrounding environment. Can be associated with leisure activities, but in self-care and work activities as well.

Occupational therapy driving specialists: Those professionals who have specialized in driver rehabilitation services and are working as DRSs.

Occupational therapy generalists: Occupational therapists who have not specialized in any particular area or areas of practice.

Off-road assessment: Conducted by the DRS to determine the abilities of the driver in several areas before starting an on-road evaluation. The abilities being tested include, but are not limited to, the following: the client's ability to safely transfer into and out of the driver's position, the need for adaptive driving equipment, the client's brake reaction time, and the effects on the client of vehicle dynamics. If individuals will be using adaptive driving equipment for the first time or they are inexperienced drivers, the initial driving assessment could occur in an off-road area to optimize safety.

On-road evaluation: An evaluation conducted by the DRS to determine the abilities of the driver in

several areas in order to make appropriate recommendations pertaining to an individual's driving status.

Operational behavior: First of three hierarchal levels of driving performance and behavior, it is concerned with routine vehicle maneuvering at the level of vehicle control operations. It is generally at the skill-based level (in the Skills-Rules-Knowledge hierarchy), except for novice drivers.

Orientation and mobility specialist: Someone who provides instruction to individuals with varying degrees of vision loss on specific techniques, strategies, and modifications necessary to help ensure safe and efficient mobility in a wide variety of environments.

Original equipment manufacturer (OEM): A term referring to the companies that design and produce commercially available stock or off-the-shelf products.

Peripheral vision: The portion of the field of view along the outer limits of the entire field.

Pharmacodynamics: The study of the biochemical and physiologic effects of drugs and their mechanism of action. A drug's actions may be structurally specific or nonspecific.

Pharmacokinetics: The study of a particular drug's concentration levels and effect on body systems as it passes through the body during the absorption, distribution, metabolism, and excretion phases.

Pharmacology: The study of the preparation, properties, uses, and actions of drugs. The DRS should be familiar with how medications work in the body, how they are named, how they are classified, and how they can impact driving performance.

PIEV time: Standing for Perception, Intellection, Emotion, and Volition, PIEV time is the total time from seeing and becoming aware of some kind of internal or external stimulus or stimuli to actually executing a response.

Placebo effect: The adoption of traits thought to be connected to the process of the experiment. For example, clients in a medication experiment may take on side effects, treatment results, or both even though they are not taking the actual medication, but rather a placebo.

Predictive validity: A test has predictive validity when it is indicative of how the client will perform in a novel situation.

Predriving evaluation: The process of investigating discrete fundamental performance areas that are considered to be critical to the task of operating a motor vehicle, otherwise known as the clinical evaluation. DRSs meet with clients to assess several factors involved with driving including visual acuity, visual perception, hearing, range of motion, functional strength and endurance, sensation, reaction time, transfers, cognition, and the driver's overall knowledge of the rules of the road. The comprehensive driver rehabilitation evaluation report should provide summaries of each one of these areas.

Predriving screen: A diagnostic given to clients to determine whether there is a need to initiate a referral for a driver rehabilitation evaluation by a DRS. Occupational therapy generalists may perform a screen during an ADL or IADL evaluation and refer their clients to an occupational therapist specializing in driver rehabilitation.

Primary safety: The risk factor for involvement in a motor vehicle crash.

Primary team members: Those members of the driver rehabilitation program who provide key driver rehabilitation services irrespective of the program's service delivery model, team structure, or service offerings.

Problem-oriented research: Research directed at resolving or investigating issues that are relevant to a specific field.

Processing speed: The latency in verbal or motor responses to a stimulus. Although impairments in processing speed often accompany attentional deficits, a deficit in either of these domains individually may be problematic in the context of driving resumption.

Professional ethics: Principles and values articulated by a profession to guide the ethical behavior of practitioners (i.e., clinicians, educators, and researchers) and students.

Programmed observations: A predetermined set of driving skills that, if not successfully accomplished, will indicate deficiencies in the driver's skill level.

Proprioception: The knowledge of the position of an extremity in space.

Ptosis: The covering of the upper portion of the cornea. With the eyes open, the upper lids should be even with the superior margin.

Pure risk: Situations that require a driver's assessment of risk may be classified as a pure or a speculative risk assessment. A pure risk exists when there is a chance of loss but no chance of gain.

Qualitative research: A type of research interested in the experiences, interpretations, impressions, or motivations of an individual or individuals, and seeks to describe how people view things and why. It relates to beliefs, attitudes, and changing behavior. In contrast to quantitative research, qualitative research is more interpretative in its orientation.

Quantitative research: A hypothesis-driven approach to research where the investigator attempts to control one or more variables in an objective way so that an outcome can be reliability predicted. Thus, quantitative research focuses on measuring and counting facts and the relationships among variables, and seeks to describe observations through statistical analysis of data.

Random assignment: A situation established during an experiment in which every participant has an equal chance of being assigned to a given circumstance.

Reaction time: The more common term for PIEV time; the total time from seeing and becoming aware of some kind of internal or external stimuli to actually executing a response.

Recreational activities: Those activities outside of the workplace that allow us to relax and experience a satisfying lifestyle.

Reliability: The quality of a test given when a sustained effort from the test subject results in the same test result.

Remediation: Remedial interventions are those intended to improve driving performance by enhancing one or more of the driver's basic capacities, associated functional abilities, or more general behavioral characteristics. In driver rehabilitation, remediation commonly focuses on musculoskeletal, sensory, or cognitive abilities, or socio-cultural characteristics such as habits, values, or behavioral roles.

Remediation program: A course of action determined by the DRS to help the client develop the necessary client factors such as strength or cognitive skills to meet predetermined goals, such as passing a standard license test.

Research model: In general the research model is based on the scientific method. It takes into consideration the identification of a significant problem, a relevant literature review, statement of a hypothesis or guiding question, a method to test the hypothesis, collection of pertinent data, analysis of results, conclusion, and recommendations for further research.

Researcher bias: The potential inclination of the investigator of one outcome over another. Researcher bias has the potential to influence the results of an experiment, thereby negating the outcome, correct or not.

Risk: In general terms, risk is usually defined as the product of the probability of a particular negative consequence, multiplied by the severity of that consequence.

Risk assessment: The continuous gauging of possible consequences of actions a driver may take when selecting his or her speed and route while driving.

Route-based simulation: An approach used in creating CGI driving simulations in which a predetermined route is driven. In those route-based simulations, regardless of whether a driver turns or fails to turn at an intersection, the roadway that is displayed is the same as originally planned.

Scanning: The ability of the eyes to search within the field of view to locate an object.

Scotomas: Damaged areas of the macula that result in distorted, hazy, or blank areas in the visual field.

Seating components: Devices that aid trunk, pelvic, and extremity positioning. Lower extremity positioning components include lateral thigh supports, abductor pommels, pivot pads, angle adjustable footplates, and toe or ankle straps. Upper limb positioning options include arm troughs, lap trays, and wrist or forearm straps, to name a few.

Seating specialist: A health care professional whose role is to choose and modify the primary mobility device to allow the client the greatest level of independence and safety in all daily living activities but especially personal mobility and perhaps the ability to perform pressure relief. This includes personal mobility within both living spaces and the community.

Secondary safety: The systems put in place to reduce injury to the driver and passengers during a motor vehicle crash.

Selective attention: The ability of the client to direct attention to certain stimuli while ignoring others.

Service delivery model: A generic plan of action, which may be tailored to the individual's needs, which serves as a starting point for the DRS as a way of establishing how to best serve the needs of the client.

Shared potential benefits: A term referring to the possible benefit common to one group of people.

Side effects: The unintended effects of a drug on a client. These results may be harmful (e.g., high blood pressure), or helpful (e.g., relaxation).

Sight: The information gathered by the photoreceptor cells of the retina and the resulting nerve impulses transmitted by the optic neural pathway.

Simulator sickness: The generic experience of feeling sick as a result of exposure to computer-generated stimuli, which includes visual and vestibular symptoms that resemble motion sickness.

Single-use zoning: The separation of structures in a given area for one specific use.

Socratic method: A method of teaching or problem-solving in which a question and answer dialogue occurs.

Space perception: The ability to perceive the relative distances of objects and the absolute distance from an object to observer.

Spatial cognition: The ability of the client to take into consideration the placement and direction of certain objects in the visual field.

Speculative risk: Speculative risk exists when there is a chance of gain as well as a chance of loss. Nondriving examples of speculative risk include casino gambling, horse racing, and various lotteries.

Static visual acuity: The ability of the client to see details in certain objects when neither the object nor the viewer is moving.

Strategic behavior: Third of three hierarchal levels of driving performance and behavior, it is the consideration of goals and more general driving context; for example decisions about whether or not to drive under particular conditions and route planning. It is most commonly considered knowledge-based in the Skills-Rules-Knowledge hierarchy.

Superelevation: The modification in a highway design to work with the laws of mechanics under which a vehicle operates to result in the safest means of travelling on a roadway.

Superelevation at curves: The modification of a roadway in a curved path so that the centrifugal forces at work upon the vehicle do not cause the vehicle to slide off the roadway. This is often achieved by building the road at a set angle that works in direct relation to the speed limit.

Survey research: A model of research in which attitudes, characteristics, and opinions of a targeted population are gathered objectively. Survey research as applied to driver rehabilitation includes gathering of data on individuals with disabilities or aging-related challenges or both regarding their frequency of driving per week, their main purposes of using a motor vehicle, accidents they may have incurred over the previous year, consumer evaluations of adaptations used in a motor vehicle, and their attitudes towards driving with a disability.

Tactical behavior: Second of three hierarchal levels of driving performance and behavior, it is the application of road rules and adaptation to the demands of the immediate road and traffic conditions, including performance of maneuvers such as turning, overtaking and parking; it may be performed at various levels of automatization, but much of it is rule-based for most drivers in the Skills-Rules-Knowledge hierarchy.

Tactical driving: Similar to defensive driving, this method helps to ensure that appropriate decisions are made with sufficient time to avoid potentially hazardous and even deadly situations.

Technology abandonment: The discontinuance of assistive technology devices, usually due to dissatisfaction or disillusion with the utility of the device.

Telematics: Telematics is the general umbrella under which fall all computer and communication-related technologies intended for the vehicle's occupants. These include applications such as voice communications (e.g., cell phones, GM's OnStar), in-vehicle navigation (e.g., BMW's iDrive), crash avoidance, and driver vision enhancement.

Tertiary safety: The systems put in place to minimize the extent of harm by maximizing post-crash support.

Therapeutic use: The intended medical effect of a medication, which is sometimes used to classify a drug (e.g., antibiotics or antidepressants).

Therapeutics: The study of how drugs are used to prevent and treat disease.

Tracking: Scanning plus motion; the ability to find and fixate on an object, and, if it is a moving object such as a vehicle or pedestrian, follow its movement.

Traffic control devices: Devices that are part of the highway infrastructure and assist drivers in understanding the driving environment for safe and efficient operation.

Traffic signals: Devices created and placed to provide regulations, warnings, and guidance information to all road users.

Transit wheelchairs: Wheelchairs equipped with the transit option, known simply as WC/19 wheelchairs.

Universal design: The design of a product whose aim is to improve the lives of people with disabilities and whose design allows for the product's use in a variety of circumstances (a lift that fits into any number of vehicle types, for example).

Validity: The relevance of a given test to the skill, strength, or ability being tested.

Vehicle modifier: Also known as the mobility equipment dealer or vendor, this person plays a primary role in the provision of driver rehabilitation and community mobility services.

Vision: The manner in which the brain converts neural impulses into what we perceive, and interprets this information.

Visual acuity: The ability and degree to which a client can recognize detail at various distances.

Visual field: The portion of the viewing area that can be perceived by the client without turning the head, irrespective of acuity. The field of view has natural limitations defined by the eyebrows and cheekbone structure as well as the shape and size of the nose.

Visual function: The degree to which a client is able to see.

Visuomotor functioning: The ability of a client to drive the vehicle according visuospatial cues (e.g., turning the wheel to follow the road or causing the car to swerve to avoid a pedestrian).

Visuospatial functioning: The ability of a client to recognize cues in the visual field (e.g., recognizing that the road curves to the left or there is a person crossing the street).

Vocational rehabilitation: Vocational rehabilitation (VR) services are often used to assess a client's work-related capacity and to help remove barriers to employment, including assisting a client to secure resources that would enable him or her to drive to and from work.

Wheelchair lift: Interior- or under vehicle–mounted lifts that raise the person and his or her mobility device into a van.

Wheelchair tiedown and occupant restraint system (WTORS): Systems that ensure the safety of those traveling in a vehicle, even if those passengers are in wheelchairs or other mobility devices.

White matter: The tissue in the brain dedicated to transmitting signals between clumps of gray matter.

DOCUMENTATION AND BILLING INFORMATION

Appendix A

STATE DRIVER LICENSING REQUIREMENTS AND REPORTING LAWS*

Each state has its own licensing and license renewal criteria for drivers of private motor vehicles. In addition, certain states require physicians to report unsafe drivers or drivers with specific medical conditions to the driver licensing agency. This appendix contains licensing agency contact information, license requirements and renewal criteria, reporting procedures, and Medical Advisory Board information listed by state. These materials are provided to physicians and other driver rehabilitation professionals as a reference to aid them in discharging their legal and ethical responsibilities. The information in this appendix should not be construed as legal advice nor used to resolve legal problems. If legal advice is required, physicians and other professionals should consult an attorney who is licensed to practice in their state. Information for this appendix was primarily obtained from each state's driver licensing agency and reflects the most current information at the time of publication. Please note that this information is subject to change. When information for this appendix was not available from an individual state's driver licensing agency, the following references were used:

Coley MJ, Coughlin JF: State driving regulations. Adapted from National Academy on an Aging Society. *The Public Policy and Aging Report* 11, 2001.

Epilepsy Foundation: Driver information by state. Available at: http://www.efa.org/answerplace/drivelaw/searchform.cfm. Accessed January 10, 2003.

Insurance Institute for Highway Safety: US driver licensing renewal procedures for older drivers. Available at:

http://www.hwysafety.org/safety_facts/state_laws/older_drivers.htm. Accessed May 12, 2003. Massachusetts Medical Society: *Medical Perspectives on*

Impaired Driving, ed 1. Available at: *www.massmed.org/pages/impaireddrivers.asp*. Accessed May 12, 2003.

National Highway Traffic Safety Administration: State reporting practices.

Available at: *http://www.nhtsa.gov/people/injury/olddrive/FamilynFriends/state.htm*. Accessed May 12, 2003.

Peli E, Peli D: *Driving with confidence: a practical guide to driving with low vision,*. Singapore, 2002, World Scientific Publishing Co. Pte. Ltd.

State and provincial licensing systems: comparative data, Arlington, VA, 1999, American Association of Motor Vehicle Administrators.

Supplemental Technical Notes. In Staplin L, Lococo K, Byington S, Harkey D: *Guidelines and recommendations to accommodate older drivers and pedestrians*, Washington, DC, 2001, Federal Highway Administration.

ALABAMA

Driver Licensing Agency
Alabama Department of Public Safety 334 242-4239

Contact Information
Driver License Division
PO Box 1471
Montgomery, AL 36102-1471
www.dps.state.al.us

Licensing Requirements
Visual Acuity

Each eye with/without correction	20/40
Both eyes with/without correction	20/40

---

*This section has been reprinted with permission from the AMA.

549

If one eye blind—other with/ without correction	20/40
Absolute visual acuity minimum	20/60 in best eye with or without corrective lenses
Are bioptic telescopes allowed?	No

Visual Fields
| Minimum field requirement | 110° both eyes |
| Visual field testing device | Keystone view |

Color Vision Requirement For new and professional drivers only

Restricted Licenses Available

License Renewal Procedures
Standard
Length of license validation	4 years
Renewal options and conditions	In-person
Vision testing required at time of renewal?	No
Written test required?	No
Road test required?	No

Age-based Renewal Procedures No special requirements for age.

Reporting Procedures
Physician/Medical Reporting Physician reporting is encouraged.

Immunity Available

Legal Protection Available

DMV Follow-up Driver notified in writing of referral. For diabetes, seizures, and convulsions, a form is sent to be completed by patient's doctor.

Other Reporting Will accept information from courts, police, other DMVs, family members, and anyone who completes and signs the appropriate forms.

Anonymity Not anonymous or confidential. The client may request a copy of his/her medical records by completing the necessary forms, having them notarized, and paying the proper fee for copying these records.

Medical Advisory Board
Role of the MAB
The MAB assists the Director for Public Safety with the medical aspects of driver licensing. It consists of at least 18 members, with the chairman elected on an annual basis.

MAB Contact Information
The MAB assists the Medical Unit, which may be reached at 334 242-4239.

ALASKA
Driver Licensing Agency
Alaska Department of Motor Vehicles 907 269-5551

Contact Information
3300 B. Fairbanks Street
Anchorage, AK 99503
www.state.ak.us/dmv

Licensing Requirements
Visual Acuity
Each eye with/without correction	20/40
Both eyes with/without correction	20/40
If one eye blind—other with/without correction	20/40
Absolute visual acuity minimum	20/100 needs report from eye specialist. License request determined by discretion.
Are bioptic telescopes allowed?	Only under certain conditions (specifically recommended by physician) with regards to lighting conditions and number of miles to and from specific locations. Physicians must submit a letter stating "with the bioptic telescopes this patient can safely operate a motor vehicle without endangering the public under the following conditions: _____."

Visual Fields
| Minimum field requirement | None |

Color Vision Requirement None

Restricted Licenses Available

License Renewal Procedures
Standard

Length of license validation	5 years
Renewal options and conditions	Mail-in every other cycle
Vision testing required at time of renewal?	Yes, at in-person renewal
Written test required?	No
Road test required?	No

Age-based Renewal Procedures
No renewal by mail for drivers aged 69+.

Reporting Procedures
Physician/Medical Reporting None. However, a licensee should self-report medical conditions that cause loss of consciousness to the DMV.

Immunity None

Legal Protection N/A

DMV Follow-up All medical information submitted to the DMV is reviewed by Department of Public Safety personnel.

Other Reporting Law enforcement officers, other DMVs, and family members may submit information.

Anonymity N/A

Medical Advisory Board
Role of the MAB
Alaska does not retain a medical advisory board.

ARIZONA
Driver Licensing Agency
Arizona Department of Transportation 800 251-5866

Contact Information
Motor Vehicle Division
PO Box 2100
Phoenix, AZ 85001-2100
www.dot.state.az.us/mvd/mvd.htm

Licensing Requirements
Visual Acuity

Each eye with/without correction	20/40
Both eyes with/without correction	20/40
If one eye blind—other with/without correction	20/40
Absolute visual acuity minimum	20/60 in best eye restricted to daytime only
Are bioptic telescopes allowed?	No

Visual Fields

Minimum field requirement	70° E, 35° N
Visual field testing device	Keystone view

Color Vision Requirement For commercial drivers only

Restricted licenses Daylight-only licenses available

License Renewal Procedures
Standard

Length of license validation	12 years
Renewal options and conditions	N/A
Vision testing required at time of renewal?	Yes
Written test required?	No
Road test required?	If recommended by the Medical Review Program.

Age-Based Renewal Procedures
At age 65, reduction of cycle to 5 years. No renewal by mail after age 70.

Reporting Procedures
Physician/Medical Reporting Yes (not specified)

Immunity Available

Legal Protection Reporting immunity is granted.

DMV Follow-up The DMV follows physician recommendations.

Other Reporting Will accept information from courts, police, other DMVs, family members, and other sources.

Anonymity Available

Medical Advisory Board
Role of the MAB
The Medical Review Program staff reviews reports to determine if a licensee requires a re-examination of driving skills, written testing, or medical/psychological evaluation.

MAB Contact Information
Arizona Department of Transportation
Medical Review Program
Mail Drop 818Z
PO Box 2100
Phoenix, AZ 85001
623 925-5795
623 925-9323 fax

ARKANSAS

Driver Licensing Agency
Arkansas Office of Motor Vehicles 501 682-1631

Contact Information
PO Box 3153
Little Rock, AR 72203
www.state.ar.us/dfa/odd/motor_vehicle.html

Licensing Requirements
Visual Acuity

Each/both eyes without correction	20/40
Each/both eyes with correction	20/50
If one eye blind—other without correction	20/40
If one eye blind—other with correction	20/50
Absolute visual acuity minimum	20/40 in better eye for unrestricted license; 20/60 for restricted license
Are bioptic telescopes allowed?	Yes, under certain circumstances: 20/50 through telescope, 20/50 through carrier, minimum field of vision 105°

Visual Fields

Minimum field requirement	105° both eyes
Visual field testing device	Optec screening machine

Color Vision Requirement None

Type of Road Test Standardized

Restricted Licenses Daylight-only licenses available at physicians' recommendation (licensee must meet minimum visual requirements).

License Renewal Procedures
Standard

Length of license validation	4 years
Renewal options and conditions	In-person, by mail only if out of state
Vision testing required at time of renewal?	Yes
Written test required?	No
Road test required?	No

Age-based Renewal Procedures
None

Reporting Procedures
Physician/Medical Reporting Physician reporting is encouraged.

Immunity None

Legal Protection None

DMV Follow-up Medical information is reviewed by the director of Driver Control. An appointment is scheduled within 2 weeks of receipt. At that time, a medical form is given to the licensee for completion by a physician. If the medical exam is favorable, a road test is given.

Other Reporting Will accept information from courts, police, other DMVs, and family members.

Anonymity N/A

Medical Advisory Board
Role of the MAB
Arkansas does not have a medical advisory board. However, unsafe drivers may be referred to Driver Control at:
Arkansas Driver Control
Hearing Officer
Room 1070
1910 W. 7th
Little Rock, AR 72203
501 682-1631

CALIFORNIA

Driver Licensing Agency
California Department of Motor Vehicles 916 657-6550

Contact Information
2415 First Avenue, Mail Station C152
Sacramento, CA 95818-2698
www.dmv.ca.gov

Licensing Requirements
Visual Acuity

Each eye with correction	Screening standard: One eye 20/70 if other is 20/40.
Failure to meet standard results in referral to vision specialist and possible road test.	
Both eyes with correction	20/40 (also a screening standard)
If one eye blind—other with/without correction	20/40 (with road test given unless it is a stable, long-standing condition)
Absolute visual acuity minimum	Better than 20/200, best corrected, in at least one eye. Cannot use bioptic telescopes to meet standard.
Are bioptic telescopes allowed?	Yes, for daylight driving only.

Visual Fields

Minimum field requirement	None

Color Vision Requirement None

Type of Road Test The Driving Performance Evaluation (DPE) is administered for original licensing and for some experienced impaired drivers (e.g., drivers with vision problems). For other experienced impaired drivers (e.g., drivers with cognitive deficits), the Supplemental Driving Performance Evaluation (SDPE) is administered.

Restricted Licenses A variety of restrictions are available—most commonly for corrective lens wearers.

License Renewal Procedures
Standard

Length of license validation	5 years
Renewal options and conditions	In-person or (if applicant qualifies) mail renewal for no more than two license terms in sequence.
Vision testing required at time of renewal?	Yes, at in-person renewal
Written test required?	Yes, at in-person renewal
Road test required?	Only if there is significant evidence of driving impairment.

Age-based Renewal Procedures
No renewal by mail at age 70 and older.

Reporting Procedures
Physician/Medical Reporting Physicians are required to report all patients diagnosed with "disorders characterized by lapses of consciousness." The law specifies that this definition includes Alzheimer's disease "and those related disorders that are severe enough to be likely to impair a person's ability to operate a motor vehicle." Physicians are not required to report unsafe drivers. However, they are authorized to report, given their good faith judgment that it is in the public's interest.

Immunity Yes, if the condition is required to be reported. (A physician who has failed to report such a patient may be held liable for damages.) If the condition is not required to be reported, there is no immunity from liability.

Legal Protection Only if the condition is required by law to be reported.

DMV Follow-up The medical information obtained from the physician is reviewed by DMV hearing officers within the Driver Safety Branch. The driver is re-examined; at the conclusion of the process, the DMV may take no action, impose restrictions, limit license term, order periodic re-examinations, or suspend or revoke the driver's license.

Other Reporting The DMV will accept information from the driver himself or herself, courts, police, other DMVs, family members, and virtually any other source.

Anonymity If so requested, the name of the reporter will not be divulged (unless a court order mandates disclosure).

Medical Advisory Board
Role of the MAB
The MAB gathers specialists for panels on special driving related topics (e.g., vision). These panels develop policy recommendations for the DMV regarding drivers with a particular type of impairment. No recommendations are made regarding individuals as such.

MAB Contact Information
The MAB no longer meets as a group. For further information regarding the role of the MAB, contact:
Post Licensing Policy
California Department of Motor Vehicles
2415 First Avenue, Mail Station C163
Sacramento, CA 95818-2698
916 657-5691

Colorado

Driver Licensing Agency
Colorado Department of Motor Vehicles
303 205-5646

Contact Information
Driver License Administration
1881 Pierce Street, Room 136
Lakewood, CO 80214
www.mv.state.co.us/mv.html

Licensing Requirements
Visual Acuity

Each eye with/without correction	20/40*
Both eyes with/without correction	20/40
If one eye blind—other with/without correction	20/40
Absolute visual acuity minimum	No absolute minimum acuity.
The DMV will license any individual whom a physician/optometrist feels is not a danger.	
Are bioptic telescopes allowed?	Yes

Visual Fields

Minimum field requirement	None**

Color Vision Requirement None

Restricted Licenses Available based on doctor's recommendations

License Renewal Procedures
Standard

Length of license validation	10 years
Renewal options and conditions	If eligible, mail-in every other cycle

Vision testing required at time of renewal?	Yes, at in-person renewal
Written test required?	Only if point accumulation results in suspension
Road test required?	No, unless condition has developed since last renewal that warrants road test.

Age-based License Procedures
At age 61, renewal period is reduced to every 5 years; no renewal by mail at age 66+.

Reporting Procedures
Physician/Medical Reporting Drivers should self-report medical conditions that may cause a lapse of consciousness, seizures, etc. Physicians are encouraged but not required to report patients who have a medical condition that may affect their ability to safely operate a motor vehicle.

Immunity N/A

Legal Protection No civil or criminal action may be brought against a physician or optometrist licensed to practice in Colorado for providing a written medical or optometric opinion.

DMV Follow-up The driver is notified in writing of the referral and undergoes a re-examination. Medical clearance may be required from a physician, and restrictions may be added to the license.

Other Reporting Will accept information from courts, police, other DMVs, and family members.

Anonymity Not anonymous or confidential

Medical Advisory Board
Role of the MAB
Colorado does not currently retain a medical advisory board.

Connecticut

Driver Licensing Agency
Connecticut Department of Motor Vehicles
860 263-5700

Contact Information
60 State Street (within Hartford or outside CT)
Wethersfield, CT 06161-2510
860 842-8222
www.dmvct.org (elsewhere in CT)

---

*Unless the consumer is blind in one eye, individual eye acuity is not normally tested nor is there an individual eye minimum acuity requirement. The DMV is concerned with the acuity of both eyes together, unless the applicant is applying for a Commercial Driver's License.

**Based on discussions with ophthalmologists and optometrists, the DMV does not currently test peripheral vision or color vision as accommodations can be made for these deficiencies. However, testing is performed for phoria.

Licensing Requirements
Visual Acuity

Each eye with/without correction	20/40
Both eyes with/without correction	20/40
If one eye blind—other with/without correction	20/40
Absolute visual acuity minimum	20/70 in better eye for restricted license; some circumstances allow for restricted license at 20/200
Are bioptic telescopes allowed?	No

Visual Fields

Minimum field requirement	100° monocular; 140° binocular
Visual field testing device	Optec 1000

Color Vision Requirement None (only for commercial drivers)

Type of Road Test The general on-the-road skills test is conducted by a DMV instructor or licensing agent.

The test for a "graduated license" is conducted by off-site staff who make an appointment with the applicant at his or her residence and conduct the test in a state-owned, dual-control vehicle. Applicants with specific needs are trained/tested by a Handicapped Driver Training Unit–certified driving instructor.

Restricted License Graduated license considerations include the applicant's health problem/condition, accident record, and driving history. Restrictions include daylight only, corrective lenses required, no highway driving, automatic transmission only, external mirrors required, special controls or equipment, and hearing aid required.

License Renewal Procedures
Standard

Length of license validation	6 years
Renewal options and conditions	In-person at DMV full-service branch, mobile unit scheduled locations, satellite offices, license renewal centers, and authorized AAA offices.
Vision testing required at time of renewal?	No
Written test required?	No

Road test required?	Only for new applicants and for these applicants whose license has been expired for 2 or more years.

Age-based Renewal Procedures
Applicants age 65+ may renew for 2 years. Applicants age 65+ may renew by mail only upon submission of a written application showing hardship, which shall include—but is not limited to—distance of applicant's residence from DMV renewal facility.

Reporting Procedures
Physician/Medical Reporting Section 14-46 states that a "physician may report to the DMV in writing the name, age, and address of any person diagnosed by him to have any chronic health problem which in the physician's judgment will significantly affect the person's ability to safely operate a motor vehicle."

Immunity No civil action may be brought against the commissioner, the department or any of its employees, the board or any of its members, or any physician for providing any reports, records, examinations, opinions, or recommendations. Any person acting in good faith shall be immune from liability.

Legal Protection Only the laws regarding immunity apply.

DMV Follow-up The driver is notified in writing of his or her referral to the MAB. If the MAB requires additional information for review in order to make a recommendation, the driver is requested to file the additional medical information.

Other Reporting State regulations require "reliable information" to be on file for the DMV to initiate a medical review case. This includes a written, signed report from any person in the medical/law enforcement profession or a third-party report on the DMV affidavit, which requires signing in the presence of a notary public.

Anonymity All information on file in a medical review case is classified as "confidential." However, it is subject to release to the person or his or her representative upon written authorization from the person to release the data.

Medical Advisory Board
Role of the MAB
The MAB must be comprised of eight specialties
1. General medicine or surgery
2. Internal medicine

3. Cardiovascular medicine
4. Neurology or neurological surgery
5. Ophthalmology
6. Orthopedic surgery
7. Psychiatry
8. Optometry

The MAB advises the commissioner on health standards relating to safe operation of motor vehicles; recommends procedures and guidelines for licensing individuals with impaired health; assists in developing medically acceptable standardized report forms; recommends training courses for motor vehicle examiners on medical aspects of operator licensure; undertakes any programs/activities the commissioner may request relating to medical aspects of motor vehicle operator licensure; makes recommendations and offers advice on individual health problem cases; and establishes guidelines for dealing with such individual cases.

MAB Contact Information
Connecticut Department of Motor Vehicles
Medical Review Division
60 State Street
Wethersfield, CT 06161-2510
860 263-5223
860 263-5774 fax

DELAWARE
Driver Licensing Agency
Delaware Division of Motor Vehicles 302 744-2500

Contact Information
PO Box 698
Dover, DE 19903
www.delaware.gov/yahoo/DMV

Licensing Requirements
Visual Acuity

Each eye with/without correction	20/40
Both eyes with/without correction	20/40
If one eye blind—other with/without correction	20/40
Absolute visual acuity minimum	20/50 for restricted license; beyond 20/50 driving privileges denied
Are bioptic telescopes allowed?	Yes, on a case-by-case basis with daytime-only restrictions

Visual Fields

Minimum field requirement	None

Color Vision Requirement None

Restricted Licenses Daytime-only licenses available

License Renewal Procedures
Standard

Length of license validation	5 years
Renewal options and conditions	In-person only
Vision testing required at time of renewal?	Yes
Written test required?	No
Road test required?	No

Age-based Renewal Procedures
None

Reporting Procedures
Physician/Medical Reporting Physicians should report patients subject to "losses of consciousness due to disease of the central nervous system." Failure to do so is punishable by a fine of $5.00 to $50.00.

Immunity Available

Legal Protection N/A

DMV Follow-up The driver is notified in writing of the referral, and his or her license is suspended until further examination.

Other Reporting The DMV will accept information from courts, other DMVs, police, and family members.

Anonymity The DMV protects the identity of the reporter.

Medical Advisory Board
Role of the MAB
If the DMV receives conflicting or questionable medical reports, the reports are sent to the MAB. The MAB determines whether the individual is medically safe to operate a motor vehicle.

MAB Contact Information
Contact the MAB through Delaware Health and Social Services at:
1901 N. DuPont Highway
Main Building
New Castle, DE 19720

302 255-9040
302 744-4700
302 255-4429 fax
dhssinfo@state.de.us

DISTRICT OF COLUMBIA

Driver Licensing Agency
District of Columbia Department of Motor Vehicles
202 727-5000

Contact Information
301 C Street, NW
Washington, DC 20001
www.dmv.washingtondc.gov

Licensing Requirements
Visual Acuity

Best eye with/without correction	20/40
Other eye with/without correction	20/70
If one eye blind—other with/without correction	20/40
Absolute visual acuity minimum	20/40; 20/70 in better eye requires 140 E visual field for restricted license.
Are bioptic telescopes allowed?	No

Visual Fields

Minimum field requirement	130° both eyes (may be approved by director at 110°)
Visual field testing device	Confrontation or perimetry

Color Vision Requirement For new drivers only

Restricted Licenses Daytime-only licenses available (acuity must be 20/70 or greater and field of vision 140° or greater).

License Renewal Procedures
Standard

Length of license validation	5 years
Renewal options and conditions	Drivers with a clear driver record and no medical requirements can now renew their license on-line
Vision testing required at time of renewal?	Yes
Written test required?	Yes; however, drivers are allowed a 6-month grace period
Road test required?	Licensees with physical disabilities may require a road test at the time of renewal. Also, senior citizens may be required to take the road test on an observational basis.

Age-based Renewal Procedures
At age 70, the licensee must submit a letter from his or her physician stating that the licensee is medically fit to drive based on vision and physical and mental capabilities.

Reporting Procedures
Physician/Medical Reporting Permitted but not required.

Immunity None

Legal Protection None

DMV Follow-up N/A

Other Reporting Any concerned citizen may report.

Anonymity Reporters are allowed to remain anonymous.

Medical Advisory Board
Role of the MAB
Washington, DC does not currently retain a medical advisory board.

FLORIDA

Driver Licensing Agency
Florida Department of Highway Safety and Motor Vehicles 850 922-9000

Contact Information
Neil Kirkman Building
2900 Apalachee Parkway
Tallahassee, FL 32399-0500
www.hsmv.state.fl.us/html/dlnew.html

Licensing Requirements
Visual Acuity

Each/both eyes without correction	20/40; if 20/50 or less, applicant is referred to eye specialist for possible improvement
Each/both eyes with correction	20/70; worse eye must be better than 20/200

If one eye blind—other with/without correction	20/40
Absolute visual acuity minimum	20/70
Are bioptic telescopes allowed?	No

Visual Fields

Minimum field requirement	130° horizontal
Visual field testing device	None; Goldman by eye specialist if indicated

Color Vision Requirement None

Restricted Licenses Drivers may be licensed to drive with the following restrictions: corrective lenses, outside rearview mirror, business and/or employment purposes only, daylight driving, automatic transmission, power steering, directional signals, grip on steering wheel, hearing aid, seat cushion, hand control or pedal extension, left foot accelerator, probation interlock device, medical alert bracelet, educational purposes, graduated license restrictions, and other restrictions.

License Renewal Procedures
Standard

Length of license validation	4 to 6 years, depending on driving history
Renewal options and conditions	In-person every third cycle
Vision testing required at time of renewal?	At in-person renewal
Written test required?	May be required based on driving history and/or observation of physical or mental impairments
Road test required?	May be required based on observation of physical or mental impairments

Age-based renewal procedures
Effective January 2004, vision testing is required at each renewal for drivers over the age of 79.

Reporting Procedures
Physician/Medical Reporting Any physician, person, or agency having knowledge of a licensed driver's or applicant's mental or physical disability to drive may report the person to the Department of Highway Safety and Motor Vehicles (DHSMV). Forms are available on the DHSMV Web site, as well as at local driver license offices. The Division of Driver Licenses' (DDL)

Medical Review Section provides other forms as the situation requires.

Immunity N/A

Legal Protection The law provides that no report shall be used as evidence in any civil or criminal trial or in any court proceeding.

DMV Follow-up The DHSMV investigates, sanctions actions if needed, and notifies the driver in writing.

Other Reporting The law authorizes any person, physician, or agency to report.

Anonymity Available

Medical Advisory Board
Role of the MAB
The MAB advises the DHSMV on medical criteria and vision standards and makes recommendations on mental and physical qualifications of individual drivers.

MAB Contact Information
Dr. Jack MacDonald, MAB Chairperson
DHSMV/DDL/Driver Improvement Medical Section
2900 Apalachee Parkway
Tallahassee, FL 32399-0570
850 488-8982
850 921-6147 fax

GEORGIA
Driver Licensing Agency
Georgia Department of Motor Vehicle Safety
678 415-8400

Contact Information
PO Box 1456
Atlanta, GA 30371
www.dmvs.ga.gov

Licensing Requirements
Visual Acuity

Each eye with/without correction	20/60
Both eyes with/without correction	20/60
If one eye blind—other with/without correction	20/60
Absolute visual acuity minimum	20/60 in either eye with or without corrective lenses.

Are bioptic telescopes allowed?	Yes, with acuity of 20/60 through telescope and 20/60 through carrier lens. Biopic telescopes are also permitted for best acuity as low as 20/200, with restrictions.

Visual Fields

Minimum field requirement	140° both eyes
Visual field testing device	Juno vision machine

Color Vision Requirement None

Restricted Licenses Available

License Renewal Procedures
Standard

Length of license validation	4 years
Renewal options and conditions	In-person
Vision testing required at time of renewal?	Yes
Written test required?	No
Road test required?	No

Age-based Renewal Procedures
None

Reporting Procedures
Physician/Medical Reporting Physicians should report patients with diagnosed conditions hazardous to driving and/or any handicap that would render the individual incapable of safely operating a motor vehicle.

Immunity None

Legal Protection None

DMV Follow-up Medical evaluation and retest

Other Reporting Will accept information from anyone with knowledge that the driver may be medically or mentally unfit to drive.

Anonymity None

Medical Advisory Board
Role of the MAB
The Medical Advisory Board advises agency personnel on individual medical reports and assists the agency in the decision-making process.

MAB Contact Information
Georgia Department of Motor Vehicle Safety
Medical Unit
PO Box 80447
Conyers, GA 30013

HAWAII
Driver Licensing Agency
Honolulu Division of Motor Vehicles & Licensing
808 532-7730

Contact Information
Drivers License Branch
1199 Dillingham Boulevard, Bay A-101
Honolulu, HI 96817
www.co.honolulu.hi.us/csd

Licensing Requirements
Visual Acuity

Each eye with/without correction	20/40
Both eyes with/without correction	20/40
If one eye blind—other with/without correction	20/40
Absolute visual acuity minimum	20/40 for better eye
Are bioptic telescopes allowed?	Not allowed to meet visual field requirements; however, permitted for use while driving

Visual Fields

Minimum field requirement	70° one eye
Visual field testing device	Eye testing machine or eye specialist certification

Color Vision Requirement None

Restricted Licenses Available

License Renewal Procedures
Standard

Length of license validation	6 years
Renewal options and conditions	In-person or by mail
Vision testing required at time of renewal?	Yes
Written test required?	No
Road test required?	Only if necessary

Age-based Renewal Procedures
Drivers aged 15 to 17 renew every 4 years; drivers aged 18 to 71 renew every 6 years. After age 72, drivers must renew every 2 years.

Reporting Procedures
Physician/Medical Reporting Permitted but not required.

Immunity None

Legal Protection None

DMV Follow-up Driver notified in writing of referral.

Other Reporting Will accept information from courts, police, other DMVs, and family members.

Anonymity N/A

Medical Advisory Board
Role of the MAB
The MAB advises the DMV on medical issues regarding individual drivers. Actions are based on the recommendation of the majority.

MAB Contact Information
For general information, contact the Department of Transportation at 808 692-7656
For case specific information, contact the county of issue at:
Honolulu: 808 532-7730
Hawaii: 808 961-2222
Kauai: 808 241-6550
Maui: 808 270-7363

IDAHO
Driver Licensing Agency
Idaho Transportation Department 208 334-8716

Contact Information
Division of Motor Vehicles, Driver Services
PO Box 7129

Boise, ID 83707
www2.state.id.us/itd/dmv

Licensing Requirements
Visual Acuity

Each eye with/without correction	20/40
Both eyes with/without correction	20/40
If one eye blind—other with/without correction	20/40
Absolute visual acuity minimum	20/40 in better eye for unrestricted license; 20/50 to 20/60 requires annual testing; 20/70 denied license
Are bioptic telescopes allowed?	Yes, if acuity is 20/40 through lens, 20/60 through carrier

Visual Fields

Minimum field requirement	None

Color Vision Requirement None

Restricted Licenses Available

License Renewal Procedures
Standard

Length of license validation	4 years
Renewal options and conditions	Mail-in every other cycle
Vision testing required at time of renewal?	Yes
Written test required?	No
Road test required?	Only if requested by examiner, law enforcement agency, family member, or DMV. An annual road test may be required to coincide with vision or medical retesting requirements.

Age-based Renewal Procedures
After age 69, no renewal by mail.

Reporting Procedures
Physician/Medical Reporting Yes (not specified)

Immunity None

Legal Protection A physician may not be sued for submitting required medical information to the department. Reports received by the Driver's License Advisory Board for the purpose of assisting the department in determining whether a person is qualified to be licensed may not be used as evidence in any civil or criminal trial.

DMV Follow-up License suspended upon referral.

Other Reporting Will accept information from family members, other DMVs, and law enforcement officers.

Anonymity Not anonymous or confidential.

Medical Advisory Board
Role of the MAB
The medical information submitted is initially reviewed by employees within the Driver Support Division who work specifically with medical cases. If there is a question whether to issue a license, the information is reviewed by the Driver's License Advisory Board, which is composed of a small group of representatives and the sheriff.

MAB Contact Information
Vicky Fisher
DLR/Medical Unit Supervisor
208 334-8736
vfisher@itd.state.id.us

ILLINOIS
Driver Licensing Agency
Illinois Office of the Secretary of State

Contact Information
Driver Services Department—Downstate
217 785-0963
2701 S. Dirksen Parkway
Springfield, IL 62723
Driver Services Department—Metro 312 814-2975
17 N. State Street, Suite 1100
Chicago, IL 60602
www.sos.state.il.us/departments/drivers/drivers.html

Licensing Requirements
Visual Acuity

Both eyes without correction	20/40
Both eyes with correction	20/40
If one eye blind—other with/without correction	20/40
Absolute visual acuity minimum	20/40 in better eye for unrestricted license; 20/70 in better eye for daylight-only restrictions.
Are bioptic telescopes allowed?	Yes, if acuity is 20/100 in better eye and 20/40 through bioptic telescope.

Visual Fields

Minimum field requirement	105° one eye, 140° both eyes
Visual field testing device	Stereo Optical testing machine

Color Vision Requirement None

Restricted Licenses Restrictions include daytime-only driving and two outside mirrors on the vehicle.

License Renewal Procedures
Standard

Length of license validation	4 years
Renewal options and conditions	Mail-in every other cycle for drivers with clean records and no medical report
Vision testing required at time of renewal?	At in-person renewal
Written test required?	Every 8 years unless driver has a clean driving record
Road test required?	Only for applicants age 75+

Age-based Renewal Procedures
Drivers age 75+: no renewal by mail; vision test and on-road driving test required at each renewal. Drivers age 81 to 86: renewal every 2 years. Drivers age 87+: renewal every year.

Reporting Procedures
Physician/Medical Reporting Physicians are encouraged to inform patients of their responsibility to notify the Secretary of State of any medical conditions that may cause a loss of consciousness or affect safe operation of a motor vehicle within 10 days of becoming aware of the condition.

Immunity Yes

Legal Protection N/A (Illinois is not a mandatory reporting state.)

DMV Follow-up The driver is notified in writing of the referral and required to submit a medical report.

Determination of further action is based on various scenarios.

Other Reporting Will accept information from courts, other DMVs, law enforcement agencies, members of the Illinois medical advisory board, National Driver Register (NDR), Problem Driver Pointer System, Secretary of State, management employees, Federal Motor Carrier Safety Administration, and driver rehabilitation specialists.

Anonymity Available

Medical Advisory Board
Role of the MAB
The MAB reviews each medical report and determines the status of the licensee's driving privileges. The decision of the MAB is implemented by the Secretary of State.

MAB Contact Information
Supervisor, Medical Review Unit
Office of the Secretary of State
Driver Services Department
2701 S. Dirksen Parkway
Springfield, IL 62723
217 785-3002

INDIANA*
Driver Licensing Agency
Indiana Bureau of Motor Vehicles 317 233-6000 x2

Contact Information
Driver Services
100 N. Senate Avenue, Rm N 405
Indianapolis, IN 46204
www.ai.org/bmv

Licensing Requirements
Visual Acuity

Each eye with/without correction	20/40
Both eyes with/without correction	20/40
If one eye blind—other without correction	20/50
Absolute visual acuity minimum	20/40 in best eye: no restrictions; 20/50 one eye: outside rearview mirror required; 20/50 both eyes: glasses also required; 20/70 both eyes: outside rearview mirror and proof of normal visual fields required, daylight driving only.
Are bioptic telescopes allowed?	Yes, for best acuity as low as 20/200 with some restrictions, if 20/40 can be achieved with telescope.

Visual Fields

Minimum field requirement	70° one eye, 120° both eyes
Visual field testing device	Not specified

Color Vision Requirement Only for commercial and bioptic drivers

Restricted Licenses Daytime-only and required outside rearview mirror licenses available.

License Renewal Procedures
Standard

Length of license validation	4 years
Renewal options and conditions	In-person
Vision testing required at time of renewal?	Yes (acuity and peripheral fields)
Written test required?	N/A
Road test required?	Only for those with 14+ points or three convictions in 12-month period.

Age-based Renewal Procedures
At age 75, renewal cycle is reduced to 3 years.

Reporting Procedures
Physician/Medical Reporting None. However, there is a statute requiring that physicians and others who diagnose, treat, or provide care for handicapped persons report the handicapping condition to the state Board of Health within 60 days.

Immunity None

Legal Protection N/A

DMV Follow-up Driver notified in writing of referral.

Other Reporting Will accept information from courts, police, other DMVs, family members, and other sources.

---

*Information was not available from this state's licensing agency. The information above was gathered from the resources listed at the beginning of this appendix.

Anonymity N/A

Medical Advisory Board
Role of the MAB
The MAB advises the Bureau of Motor Vehicles on medical issues regarding individual drivers. Actions are based on the recommendation of the majority and/or specialist.

Iowa

Driver Licensing Agency
Iowa Motor Vehicle Division 800 532-1121

Contact Information
Park Fair Mall
100 Euclid Avenue
PO Box 9204
Des Moines, IA 50306-9204
515 244-8725
www.dot.state.ia.us/mvd

Licensing Requirements
Visual Acuity

Each eye with/without correction	20/40
Both eyes with/without correction	20/40
If one eye blind—other with/without correction	20/40
Absolute visual acuity minimum	20/50 for daylight driving only; 20/70 in better eye for daylight driving only up to 35 mph; 20/100 requires recommendation from a vision specialist; if worse, recommendation from the MAB is required; absolute minimum is 20/200.
Are bioptic telescopes allowed?	No

Visual Fields

Minimum field requirement	140° both eyes
Outside mirrors required if 70° T + 45° N one eye, 115° both eyes. If less than 95° both eyes and 60° T + 35° N one eye, MAB recommendation required.	

Visual field testing device	Keystone-Optic 100 Vision Tester

Color Vision Requirement None

Type of Road Test Non-fixed course in general traffic

Restricted Licenses
Available

License Renewal Procedures
Standard

Length of license validation	5 years
Renewal options and conditions	In-person, extensions available if out of state for 6 months.
Vision testing required at time of renewal?	Yes
Written test required?	No
Road test required?	If physical or mental conditions are present.

Age-based Renewal Procedures
Persons under the age of 18 or aged 70 and older are issued 2-year licenses.

Reporting Procedures
Physician/Medical Reporting A physician may report to the motor vehicle division "the identity of a person who has been diagnosed as having a physical or mental condition which would render the person physically or mentally incompetent to operate a motor vehicle in a safe manner."

Immunity Available

Legal Protection Under 321.186, "a physician or optometrist making a report shall be immune from any liability, civil or criminal, which might otherwise be incurred or imposed as a result of the report."

DMV Follow-up Driver notified in writing of referral. License suspended upon referral.

Other Reporting Will accept information from courts, other DMVs, police, and family members.

Anonymity Not anonymous or confidential.

Medical Advisory Board
Role of the MAB
The MAB reviews medical/vision reports as requested and makes recommendations regarding the individual's capability to drive safely.

MAB Contact Information
The MAB may be contacted through the Iowa Medical Society at:
Iowa Medical Society
1001 Grand Avenue
West Des Moines, IA 50265-3502
515 223-1401

KANSAS

Driver Licensing Agency
Kansas Division of Motor Vehicles 785 296-3963

Contact Information
Docking State Office Building 785 296-0691 fax
PO Box 2188
Topeka, Kansas 66601-2128
www.accesskansas.org/living/cars-transportation.
  html

Licensing Requirements
Visual Acuity

Each eye with/without correction	20/40
Both eyes with/without correction	20/40
If one eye blind—other with/without correction	20/40
Absolute visual acuity minimum	20/40 in better eye for unrestricted license; 20/60 in better eye requires doctor's report; drivers with 20/60 or worse must demonstrate ability to operate a vehicle and maintain safe driving record for 3 years.
Are bioptic telescopes allowed?	Yes, with eye doctor's report.

Visual Fields

Minimum field requirement	110° with both eyes and 55° monocular

Color Vision Requirement None

Type of Road Test Non-fixed course

Restricted Licenses Up to four restrictions can be added at doctor's/examiner's discretion. These may include corrective lenses required; daylight only; no interstate driving; no driving outside business area; driving within city limits only; mileage restrictions in increments of 5 miles up to 30 miles total; outside mirror required; mechanical aid required; automatic transmission required; prosthetic aid required; and licensed driver in front seat required.

License Renewal Procedures
Standard

Length of license validation	6 years
Renewal options and conditions	In-person
Vision testing required at time of renewal?	Yes
Written test required?	Yes
Road test required?	By examiner challenge, for visual acuity of 20/60 or worse, or at medical doctor's request.

Age-based Renewal Procedures
At age 65, renewal cycle is reduced to 4 years.

Reporting Procedures
Physician/Medical Reporting Statutes specify that physicians are not required to volunteer information to the division or to the medical advisory board concerning the mental or physical condition of any patient.

Legal Protection Patients must sign a form permitting the MD or OD to release information to the DMV. Persons so reporting in good faith are statutorily immunized from civil actions for damages caused by such reporting.

DMV Follow-up Driver is notified in writing of referral.

Other Reporting Will accept information from courts, other DMVs, police, family members, and concerned citizens.

Anonymity Letters of concern must be signed. Applicants may request a copy of the letter.

Medical Advisory Board
Role of the MAB
The MAB assists the Director of Vehicles and Driver Review in interpreting conflicting information and formulating action based on the recommendation of specialists. It also helps determine the driving eligibility of complicated or borderline cases.

MAB Contact Information
Kansas Driver Review
Medical Advisory Board

915 SW Harrison, Room 162
Topeka, KS 66626

KENTUCKY

Driver Licensing Agency
Kentucky Division of Driver Licensing 502 564-6800

Contact Information
501 High Street
Frankfort, KY 40602
www.kytc.state.ky.us/drlic

Licensing Requirements
Visual Acuity

Each eye with/without correction	20/40
Both eyes with/without correction	20/40
If one eye blind—other with/without correction	20/40
Absolute visual acuity minimum	20/200 with corrective lenses
Are bioptic telescopes allowed?	Yes, with acuity of 20/60 or better through telescope and 20/200 through carrier lens

Visual Fields

Minimum field requirement	120° E and 80° N in the same eye
Visual field testing device	N/A

Color Vision Requirement None

Restricted Licenses Available

License Renewal Procedures
Standard

Length of license validation	4 years
Renewal options and conditions	In-person
Vision testing required at time of renewal?	No
Written test required?	No
Road test required?	No

Age-based Renewal Procedures
None

Reporting Procedures
Physician/Medical Reporting Yes (not specified)

Immunity Yes

Legal Protection None

DMV Follow-up Driver is notified in writing of referral to medical advisory board.

Other Reporting Will accept information from courts, other DMVs, family members, and police.

Anonymity None

Medical Advisory Board
Role of the MAB
The medical advisory board identifies drivers with physical or mental impairments that impede their ability to safely operate a motor vehicle.

MAB Contact Information
Lisa Bowling
502 564-6800 x2552
502 564-6145 fax

LOUISIANA

Driver Licensing Agency
Louisiana Office of Motor Vehicles 877 368-5463

Contact Information
PO Box 64886
Baton Rouge, LA 70896
www.expresslane.org

Licensing Requirements
Visual Acuity

Both eyes without correction	20/40
Both eyes with correction	20/40
If one eye blind—other with/without correction	20/40
Absolute visual acuity minimum	20/40 in better eye for unrestricted license; 20/50 to 20/70 in better eye for restricted license; 20/70 to 20/100 in better eye may qualify for a restricted license. If less than 20/100 in better eye, driver is referred to the medical advisory board.
Are bioptic telescopes allowed?	No

Visual Fields

Minimum field requirement	None

Color Vision Requirement None

Restricted Licenses Restrictions include daytime driving only, weather restrictions, radius limitations, and no interstate driving.

License Renewal Procedures
Standard

Length of license validation	4 years
Renewal options and conditions	In-person or by mail every other cycle. Can also be renewed by Internet and interactive voice response unless license has been expired 6 months or more.
Vision testing required at time of renewal?	Yes
Written test required?	If license has been expired 1 year or more.
Road test required?	If license has been expired 2 years or more.

Age-based Renewal Procedures

No renewal by mail for drivers over the age of 70.

Reporting Procedures

Physician/Medical Reporting There is no statutory provision requiring physicians to report patients. However, if a medical report is filed, it must address the medical concern for which it was required; contain the physician's signature, address, and phone number; and be dated within 60 days from the date received by the Department. The physician's opinion of the applicant's ability to safely operate a motor vehicle is desired but not required.

Immunity A physician who provides such information has statutory immunity from civil or criminal liability for damages arising out of an accident.

Legal Protection Louisiana has statutory protection for good faith reporting of unsafe drivers.

DMV Follow-up Driver is notified in writing of referral.

Other Reporting Will accept information from DMV employees or agents in the performance of duties, law enforcement officers, health care providers, or family members.

Anonymity Not anonymous or confidential. However, an order from a court of competent jurisdiction is required before the identity of the reporter can be released.

Medical Advisory Board
Role of the MAB

Medical reports requiring further attention are forwarded to the Data Prep Unit marked Attention: Conviction/Medical Unit. The conviction/medical unit evaluates these reports and may request an evaluation by the MAB. The MAB then recommends actions.

MAINE

Driver Licensing Agency

Maine Bureau of Motor Vehicles 207 624-9000

Contact Information

29 State House Station
101 Hospital Street
Augusta, ME 04333-0029
www.state.me.us/sos/bmv

Licensing Requirements
Visual Acuity

Best eye with/without correction	20/40
If one eye blind—other with/without correction	20/40
Absolute visual acuity minimum	20/70 with restrictions
Are bioptic telescopes allowed?	No

Visual Fields

Minimum field requirement	140° both eyes; 110° for restricted license.
Visual field testing device	Titmus II or Stereo Optical vision screening equipment

Color Vision Requirement None

Restricted Licenses Restrictions include daytime driving only, radius limitations, and special equipment requirements.

License Renewal Procedures
Standard

Length of license validation	6 years

Vision testing required at time of renewal? — Vision tested at age 40, 52, 65, and every 4 years thereafter.

Written test required? No
Road test required? No

Age-based Renewal Procedures
At age 65, the license renewal cycle is reduced to every 4 years.

Reporting Procedures
Physician/Medical Reporting Yes (not specified)

Immunity N/A

Legal Protection A physician acting in good faith is immune from any damages as a result of the filing of a certificate of examination.

DMV Follow-up The DMV will require a medical evaluation form to be completed by a physician at periodic intervals.

Other Reporting Will accept information from courts, other DMVs, police, family members, and other sources.

Anonymity Not anonymous or confidential. The identity of the reporter may be revealed at an administrative hearing if requested.

Medical Advisory Board
Role of the MAB
The Medical Advisory Board reviews the medical information submitted whenever an individual contests an action of the Division of Driver Licenses. Reports received or made by the Board are confidential and may not be disclosed unless the individual gives written permission.

MAB Contact Information
Linda French, RN
Medical Review Coordinator
207 624-9101

MARYLAND
Driver Licensing Agency
Maryland Motor Vehicle Administration 301 729-4550

Contact Information
6601 Ritchie Highway, NE
Glen Burnie, MD 21062
800 950-1682
www.mva.state.md.us

Licensing Requirements
Visual Acuity

Each eye with/without correction — 20/40

Both eyes with/without correction — 20/40

If one eye blind—other with/without correction — 20/40

Absolute visual acuity minimum — 20/70 in better eye for restricted license; 20/70 to 20/100 in better eye requires special permission from medical advisory board.

Are bioptic telescopes allowed? — Yes, with visual acuity of 20/70 through telescope and 20/100 through carrier lens. Restrictions include daytime driving only and required outside mirrors.

Visual Fields

Minimum field requirement — Continuous field of vision at least 140° for unrestricted license; 110° for restricted license.

Visual field testing device — Stereo Optical Optec 1000 vision screener

Color Vision Requirement Only for commercial drivers

Restricted Licenses Restrictions include daytime driving only and required outside mirrors for low vision drivers.

License Renewal Procedures
Standard

Length of license validation — 5 years

Renewal options and conditions — In-person

Vision testing required at time of renewal? — Yes (visual acuity and visual fields)

Written test required? No
Road test required? No

Age-based Renewal Procedures
Medical report required for new drivers age 70 and older.

Reporting Procedures

Physician/Medical Reporting Maryland law provides for the discretionary reporting to the Motor Vehicle Administration of persons who have "disorders characterized by lapses of consciousness."

Immunity N/A

Legal Protection A civil or criminal action may not be brought against any person who makes a report to the Medical Advisory Board and who does not violate any confidential or privileged relationship conferred by law.

DMV Follow-up Driver is notified in writing of referral. License is suspended, and further examination is required.

Other Reporting Will accept information from courts, other DMVs, police, family members, and other sources.

Anonymity Confidentiality available if requested by reporter.

Medical Advisory Board
Role of the MAB
The MAB advises the Motor Vehicle Administration on medical issues regarding individual drivers. Actions are based on the recommendation of the majority and/or specialist.

MAB Contact Information
Ms. Nancy Snowden 410 768-7513

MASSACHUSETTS
Driver Licensing Agency
Massachusetts Registry of Motor Vehicles 617 351-4500

Contact Information
PO Box 199100
Boston, MA 02119-9100
www.state.ma.us/rmv

Licensing Requirements
Visual Acuity

Each eye with/without correction	20/40
Both eyes with/without correction	20/40
Absolute visual acuity minimum	20/40 in better eye for unrestricted license; 20/50 to 20/70 in better eye for daylight-only restriction.
Are bioptic telescopes allowed?	Yes, if peripheral vision is at least 120° and acuity is corrected to 20/40 through the bioptic telescope and 20/100 through the carrier lens. The bioptic lens must meet certain requirements: it must be monocular, fixed focus, no greater than 3× magnification, and must be an "integral part of the lens."

Visual Fields

Minimum field requirement	120°
Visual field testing device	Optec 1000 vision testing machine

Color Vision Requirement Drivers must be able to distinguish red, green, and amber.

Restricted Licenses Daytime-only restrictions available.

License Renewal Procedures
Standard

Length of license validation	5 years
Renewal options and conditions	In-person or via Internet.
Vision testing required at renewal?	Yes
Written test required?	No; however, DMV reviews on a case-by-case basis and will administer a written test if indicated.
Road test required?	No; however, DMV reviews on a case-by-case basis and will administer a road test if indicated.

Age-based Renewal Procedures
None

Reporting Procedures
Physician/Medical Reporting Massachusetts is a self-reporting state. It is the responsibility of the driver to report to the Registry of Motor Vehicles any medical condition that may impair driving ability. However,

physicians are encouraged to report unfit drivers to the Registry of Motor Vehicles.

Immunity N/A

Legal Protection The law does not provide any protection from liability, nor does it promise confidentiality due to the "Public Records" law, which states simply that a driver is entitled to any information upon receipt of written approval.

DMV Follow-up If the report comes from the general public or a family member, it must be in writing and signed. If the report is accepted, the driver is contacted by mail and asked to obtain medical clearance to certify that he or she is safe to drive. If the DMV does not receive a response within 30 days, a second request is mailed. If there is still no response, then the license is revoked. If the report is from a law enforcement officer or physician, it is considered an "immediate threat." The driver is contacted by mail and requested to voluntarily surrender his or her license or submit medical clearance within 10 days. If there is no response, then the license is revoked.

Other Reporting Will accept information from courts, other DMVs, police, family members, and other sources.

Anonymity None

Medical Advisory Board
Role of the MAB
The MAB provides guidance to the Registry of Motor Vehicles when there are medical issues relating to an applicant's eligibility for a learner's permit or driver's license or when an individual's privilege to operate a motor vehicle has been—or is in danger of being—restricted, suspended, or revoked.

MAB Contact Information
Mary Strachan
Massachusetts Registry of Motor Vehicles
Medical Affairs Bureau
PO Box 199100
Boston, MA 02119-9100
617 351-9222
www.state.ma.us/rmv

MICHIGAN
Driver Licensing Agency
Michigan Department of State 517 322-1460

Contact Information
7707 Rickle Road

Lansing, MI 48918
www.michigan.gov/sos

Licensing Requirements
Visual Acuity

Each eye with/without correction	20/40
Both eyes with/without correction	20/40 to and including 20/50
If one eye blind—other with/without correction	20/50
Absolute visual acuity minimum	Minimum of 20/70 in better eye with daylight-only restriction; minimum of 20/60 if progressive abnormalities or disease of the eye exists.
Are bioptic telescopes allowed?	Yes. A road test is required.

Visual Fields

Minimum field requirement	110° to 140° in both eyes; if less than 110° to/including 90°, there are additional conditions and requirements.
Visual field testing device	Not specified

Color Vision Requirement None

Type of Road Test Standardized course and requirements

Restricted Licenses Restrictions are based on review of medical input and re-examination testing. Examples include radius limitations, daylight-only driving, and no expressway driving.

License Renewal Procedures
Standard

Length of license validation	4 years
Renewal options and conditions	Mail-in every other cycle, if free of convictions.
Vision testing required at time of renewal?	Yes
Written test required?	Yes
Road test required?	Yes, if license has been expired more than 4 years.

Age-based Renewal Procedures
No

Reporting Procedures

Physician/Medical Reporting Physicians are encouraged to report unsafe drivers. They may do so by completing a "Request for Driver Evaluation" form (OC-88). This form can be downloaded from the Michigan Department of State Web site.

Immunity None

Legal Protection None

DMV Follow-up The driver is notified in writing of the referral. The notification includes a notice of date, time, and location of driver re-examination, as well as any medical statements to be completed by the driver's doctor.

Other Reporting The Department accepts referrals for re-examination from family, police, public officials, and others who have knowledge of a driver's inability to drive safely or health concerns that may affect his or her driving ability.

Anonymity Reporting is not anonymous. However, the Department will release the name of the reporter only if he or she is a public official (e.g., police, judge, or state employee). The names of non-public official reporters will be released only under court order.

Medical Advisory Board

Role of the MAB
The MAB advises the Department of State on medical issues regarding individual drivers. Actions are based on the recommendation of specialists.

MAB Contact Information
For additional information, contact the Driver Assessment Office at 517 241-6840.

MINNESOTA

Driver Licensing Agency
Minnesota Department of Public Safety 651 296-6911

Contact Information
Driver and Vehicle Services
445 Minnesota Street
St. Paul, MN 55101
www.dps.state.mn.us/dvs

Licensing Requirements
Visual Acuity

Each eye with/without correction	20/40
Both eyes with/without correction	20/40
If one eye blind—other with/without correction	20/40
Absolute visual acuity minimum	20/70 in better eye with speed limitations; 20/80 referred to a driver evaluation unit; 20/100 denied license.
Are bioptic telescopes allowed?	No

Visual Fields

Minimum field requirement	105°

Color Vision Requirement None

Restricted Licenses Restrictions include daytime driving only, area restrictions, speed restrictions, and no freeway driving.

License Renewal Procedures
Standard

Length of license validation	4 years
Renewal options and conditions	In-person
Vision testing required at time of renewal?	Yes
Written test required?	Only if license has been expired for more than 1 year
Road test required?	Only if license has been expired for more than 5 years

Age-based Renewal Procedures
None

Reporting Procedures
Physician/Medical Reporting Physician reporting is encouraged. Physicians may contact the Medical Unit in writing; no specific form is required.

Immunity Yes

Legal Protection Not addressed in driver licensing laws.

DMV Follow-up Driver is notified in writing of referral. License is suspended upon referral, and further examination is conducted.

Other Reporting Will accept information from courts, other DMVs, police, family members, or other sources.

Anonymity Reporting cannot be done anonymously. However, the identity of the reporter will be held confidential unless the court subpoenas records.

Medical Advisory Board
Role of the MAB
The MAB advises the Department of Public Safety on medical issues regarding individual drivers. Actions are based on the recommendation of the majority.

MAB Contact Information
The MAB can be contacted through the Medical Unit at:
Minnesota Department of Public Safety
Medical Unit
445 Minnesota Street, Suite 170
St. Paul, MN 55101-5170
651 296-2021

MISSISSIPPI*

Driver Licensing Agency
Mississippi Department of Public Safety 601 987-1200

Contact Information
Driver Services
1900 E. Woodrow Wilson
Jackson, MS 39216
www.dps.state.ms.us

Licensing Requirements
Visual Acuity

Each eye with/without correction	20/40
Both eyes with/without correction	20/40
Absolute visual acuity minimum	20/70 with daytime-only restriction
Are bioptic telescopes allowed?	Yes, with acuity of 20/50 or better through the telescope and 20/200 through the carrier lens. Also, visual field must be >105°, and the telescope must have magnification no greater than 4×.

Visual Fields

Minimum field requirement	140° both eyes; one eye T 70°, N 35° with two outside mirrors

---

*Information from this state's licensing agency was not available. The information above was gathered from the resources listed at the beginning of this appendix.

Visual field testing device	Not specified

Color Vision Requirement None

Restricted Licenses Available

License Renewal Procedures
Standard

Length of license validation	4 years
Renewal options and conditions	In-person; renewal via Internet permitted every other cycle
Vision testing required at time of renewal?	Yes
Written test required?	N/A
Road test required?	N/A

Age-based Renewal Procedures
None

Reporting Procedures
Physician/Medical Reporting Permitted but not required

Immunity No

Legal Protection N/A

DMV Follow-up N/A

Other Reporting Will accept information from courts, other DMVs, police, and family members.

Anonymity N/A

Medical Advisory Board
Role of the MAB
N/A

MAB Contact Information
N/A

MISSOURI
Driver Licensing Agency
Missouri Department of Revenue 573 751-4600

Contact Information
Division of Motor Vehicle and Driver Licensing
Room 470, Truman Office Building
301 W. High Street
Jefferson City, MO 65105
www.dor.state.mo.us

Licensing Requirements
Visual Acuity

Each eye with/without correction	20/40
Both eyes with/without correction	20/40
If one eye blind—other with/without correction	20/50
Absolute visual acuity minimum	20/160 with restrictions
Are bioptic telescopes allowed?	Not for meeting vision requirements; however, they can be used for skills tests and while driving.

Visual Fields

Minimum field requirement	55° or better in each eye; 85° in one eye only with restrictions.
Visual field testing device	Objective/quantitative

Color Vision Requirement None

Restricted Licenses As long as the client meets the vision requirements, Missouri has restrictions for equipment, speed, radius (location of driving), time of day and/or length of time driving, or any restriction a doctor or examiner recommends.

License Renewal Procedures
Standard

Length of license validation	6 years
Renewal options and conditions	In-person or renewal by mail if out of state.
Vision testing required at time of renewal?	Yes
Written test required?	If license has been expired for more than 6 months (184 days). Also, if an individual is cited, after the review process a written test may be required.
Road test required?	If license has been expired for more than 6 months (184 days). Also, if an individual is cited, after the review process a road test may be required.

Age-based Renewal Procedures
At age 70, renewal cycle is reduced to 3 years.

Reporting Procedures
Physician/Medical Reporting Reporting is not required. However, for any condition that could impair or limit a person's driving ability, physicians may complete and submit a statement (Form 1528, "Physician's Statement"). Form 1528 is available on the Missouri Department of Revenue Web site.

Immunity Yes, an individual is immune from civil liability when a report is made in good faith.

Legal Protection Medical professionals will not be prevented from making a report because of their physician-patient relationship (302.291. Rsmo).

DMV Follow-up Depending on the information received, the DMV may request additional information; add restrictions; require a written exam, skills test, vision exam, or physical exam; or deny the privilege of driving.

Other Reporting Will accept information from courts, DMV clerks, police officers, social workers, and family members within three degrees of consanguinity.

Anonymity Available

Medical Advisory Board
Role of the MAB
The MAB evaluates each case on an individual basis. Action is based on the recommendation of the majority.

MAB Contact Information
Missouri Department of Review
Attention: Medical Review
PO Box 200
Jefferson City, MO 65105-0200
573 751-2730

MONTANA
Driver Licensing Agency
Montana Department of Justice 406 444-1773

Contact Information
Motor Vehicle Division
Scott Hart Building, Second Floor
303 N. Roberts
PO Box 201430
Helena, MT 59620-1430
www.doj.state.mt.us

Licensing Requirements
Visual Acuity

Each eye with/without correction	20/40

Both eyes with/without correction	20/40
If one eye blind—other with/without correction	20/40
Absolute visual acuity minimum	20/70 in better eye with restrictions on daylight and speed; 20/100 in better eye for a possible license with restrictions.
Are bioptic telescopes allowed?	Yes, with acuity of 20/100 or better through carrier lens.

Visual Fields

Minimum field requirement	Only for commercial drivers
Visual field testing device	Optec 1000

Color Vision Requirement Only for commercial drivers

Type of Road Test The road test includes a figure 8; three left and three right turns; two stop signs; driving through an intersection; and parallel parking.

Restricted Licenses Available

License Renewal Procedures
Standard

Length of license validation	8 years. If renewing by mail, a 4-year license is issued, and the next renewal requires a personal appearance by the applicant.
Vision testing required at time of renewal?	Yes
Written test required?	At the discretion of the examiner if safe operation of the motor vehicle is in question.
Road test required?	Same as written requirement.

Age-based Renewal Procedures
Between ages 68 and 74, all issued/renewed licenses expire on the client's 75th birthday. At age 75, renewal cycle is reduced to 4 years.

Reporting Procedures
Physician/Medical Reporting Physicians are encouraged to report.

Immunity There is a statute granting physicians immunity from liability for reporting in good faith any patient whom the physician diagnoses as having a condition that will significantly impair the patient's ability to safely operate a motor vehicle.

Legal Protection N/A

DMV Follow-up N/A

Other Reporting Will accept information from courts, other DMVs, police, family members, and other sources.

Anonymity Not anonymous or confidential. If requested, the state is required to disclose to the driver the name of the reporter.

Medical Advisory Board
Role of the MAB
Montana does not retain a medical advisory board.

NEBRASKA

Driver Licensing Agency
Nebraska Department of Motor Vehicles 402 471-2281

Contact Information
Nebraska State Office Building
301 Centennial Mall South
PO Box 94789
Lincoln, NE 68509-4789
www.dmv.state.ne.us

Licensing Requirements
Visual Acuity

Each eye with/without correction	20/40
Both eyes with/without correction	20/40
If one eye blind—other with/without correction	20/40
Absolute visual acuity minimum	20/70, if the other eye is not blind. Seventeen restrictions are used, depending on vision in each eye.
Are bioptic telescopes allowed?	Yes, with acuity of 20/70 or better through the telescope.

Visual Fields

Minimum field requirement	140° both eyes. If less than 100°, then license denied.
Visual field testing device	Not specified.

Color Vision Requirement Only for commercial drivers.

Type of Road Test The road test includes elements such as emergency stops, right turns, and left turns.

Restricted Licenses Available

License Renewal Procedures
Standard

Length of license validation	5 years
Renewal options and conditions	In-person. Individuals who are out of state during their renewal period may renew via mail.
Vision testing required at time of renewal?	Yes
Written test required?	Only if license has been expired over 1 year or license is suspended, revoked, or cancelled.
Road test required?	Only if license has been expired over 1 year or license is suspended, revoked, or cancelled.

Age-based Renewal Procedures
None

Reporting Procedures
Physician/Medical Reporting Reporting is encouraged but not required.

Immunity No

Legal Protection No

DMV Follow-up The driver is notified by certified mail that he or she must appear for retesting. The driver is also required to submit a vision and medical statement completed by his or her physician(s) within the past 90 days.

Other Reporting Will accept information from law enforcement officers and other concerned parties.

Anonymity Not anonymous. However, the reporter's identity remains confidential unless the driver appeals the denial or cancellation of his or her license in District Court.

Medical Advisory Board
Role of the MAB
The MAB advises the DMV concerning the physical and mental ability of an applicant or holder of an operator's license to operate a motor vehicle.

MAB Contact Information
Sara O'Rourke, Driver's License Administrator
Nebraska Department of Motor Vehicles
301 Centennial Mall South
PO Box 94789
Lincoln, NE 68509
Sorourke@notes.state.ne.us

NEVADA
Driver Licensing Agency
Nevada Department of Motor Vehicles 702 486-4368 (Las Vegas)

Contact Information
555 Wright Way 775 684-4368 (Reno/Sparks/ Carson City, NV 89711 Carson City)
www.dmvnv.com 877 368-7828 (rural Nevada)

Licensing Requirements
Visual Acuity

Each eye with/without correction	20/40
Both eyes with/without correction	20/40
If one eye blind—other with/without correction	20/40
Absolute visual acuity minimum	20/50 (if other eye is no worse than 20/60); daylight driving only.
Are bioptic telescopes allowed?	Yes, with acuity of 20/40 through telescope and 20/120 through carrier lens, and 130 E visual field.

Visual Fields

Minimum field requirement	Binocular 140° for unrestricted license; binocular 110° to 140° for restricted license.
Visual field testing device	Keystone testing equipment and Optec 1000 testing equipment

Color Vision Requirement None

Restricted Licenses Daytime-only license available.

License Renewal Procedures
Standard

Length of license validation	4 years

Renewal options and conditions	Mail-in every other cycle
Vision testing required at time of renewal?	Yes
Written test required?	No, unless license classification has changed.
Road test required?	No, unless license classification has changed.

Age-based Renewal Procedures
At age 70, a vision test and medical report are required for mail-in renewal.

Reporting Procedures
Physician/Medical Reporting Physicians are required to report patients diagnosed with epilepsy, any seizure disorder, or any other disorder characterized by lapse of consciousness.

Immunity Yes

Legal Protection Yes

DMV Follow-up The DMV notifies the driver by mail and may suspend his or her license.

Other Reporting Will accept information from courts, other DMVs, police, and family members.

Anonymity Available

Medical Advisory Board
Role of the MAB
The MAB advises the DMV in the development of medical and health standards for licensure. It also advises the DMV on medical reports submitted regarding the mental or physical condition of individual applicants.

MAB Contact Information
Currently not applicable. The department has the authority to convene a medical advisory board, as stated in Nevada Administrative Code 483.380. However, due to budget constraints, Nevada does not have an advisory board at present.

NEW HAMPSHIRE
Driver Licensing Agency
New Hampshire Department of Safety 603 271-2251

Contact Information
Division of Motor Vehicles
James A. Hayes Building
10 Hazen Drive
Concord, NH 03305-0002
www.state.nh.us/dmv

Licensing Requirements
Visual Acuity

Both eyes with/without correction	20/40
One eye with/without correction	20/30
Absolute visual acuity minimum	20/70, restricted to daytime only
Are bioptic telescopes allowed?	Yes

Visual Fields

Minimum field requirement	None
Visual field testing device	Stereo Optical viewer

Color Vision Requirement None

Restricted Licenses Daytime-only licenses available.

License Renewal Procedures
Standard

Length of license validation	5 years
Renewal options and conditions	N/A
Vision testing required at time of renewal?	Yes
Written test required?	No
Road test required?	No

Age-based Renewal Procedures
At age 75, road test is required with renewal.

Reporting Procedures
Physician/Medical Reporting Physicians are encouraged to report.

Immunity N/A

Legal Protection Not available, as reporting is not a requirement.

DMV Follow-up Full re-examination and, in some cases, an administrative hearing.

Other Reporting Will accept information from courts, other DMVs, police, and family members.

Anonymity Not anonymous or confidential.

Medical Advisory Board
Role of the MAB
New Hampshire does not retain a medical advisory board.

NEW JERSEY

Driver Licensing Agency
New Jersey Motor Vehicle Commission 609 292-6500

Contact Information
PO Box 160
Trenton, NJ 08666
www.state.nj.us/mvs

Licensing Requirements
Visual Acuity

Each eye with/without correction	20/50
Both eyes with/without correction	20/50
If one eye blind—other with/without correction	20/50
Absolute visual acuity minimum	20/50
Are bioptic telescopes allowed?	Yes, with acuity of 20/50 through telescope

Visual Fields

Minimum field requirement	None

Color Vision Requirement Color vision is tested in new drivers, but licenses are not denied based on poor color vision.

Type of Road Test Standardized

Restricted Licenses Available

License Renewal Procedures
Standard

Length of license validation	4 years
Renewal options and conditions	In-person (digitized photos will be implemented in 2003).
Vision testing required at time of renewal?	Periodically
Written test required?	If recommended by examiner.
Road test required?	If recommended by examiner.

Age-based Renewal Procedures
None

Reporting Procedures
Physician/Medical Reporting Physicians are required to report patients who experience recurrent loss of consciousness.

Immunity Yes

Legal Protection No

DMV Follow-up The driver is notified in writing of the referral. There is a scheduled suspension of the license, but the driver may request due process in an administrative court.

Other Reporting Will accept information from police, family, other DMVs, and courts. The letter must be signed.

Anonymity Not available

Medical Advisory Board
Role of the MAB
The Motor Vehicle Commission supplies forms for each type of medical condition that may be a cause for concern. These forms must be completed by the driver's physician. Problem cases are referred to the MAB, which then makes licensing recommendations based on the information provided.

MAB Contact Information
New Jersey Motor Vehicle Commission
Medical Division
PO Box 173
Trenton, NJ 08666
609 292-4035

NEW MEXICO

Driver Licensing Agency
New Mexico Taxation and Revenue Department
888 683-4636

Contact Information
Motor Vehicle Division
PO Box 1028
Joseph Montoya Building
Santa Fe, NM 87504-1028
http://www.state.nm.us

Licensing Requirements
Visual Acuity

Each eye with/without correction	20/40
Both eyes with/without correction	20/40
If one eye blind—other with/without correction	20/40
Absolute visual acuity minimum	20/80 in better eye with restrictions.
Are bioptic telescopes allowed?	No

Visual Fields

Minimum field requirement	120° external and 30° nasal field of one eye
Visual field testing device	Not specified

Color Vision Requirement None

Restricted Licenses Available

License Renewal Procedures
Standard

Length of license validation	4 or 8 years
Vision testing required at time of renewal?	Yes
Written test required?	May be required
Road test required?	May be required

Age-based Renewal Procedures
Drivers may not apply for 8-year renewal if they will turn 75 during the last 4 years of the 8-year period. At age 75, the renewal interval decreases to 1 year.

Reporting Procedures
Physician/Medical Reporting Yes (not specified)

Immunity Yes

Legal Protection Yes

DMV Follow-up
Driver is informed by mail that his or her license will be cancelled in 30 days unless he or she submits a medical report stating that he or she is medically fit to drive. If a report is not submitted, the license will be cancelled.

Other Reporting Will accept information from courts, other DMVs, police, and family members.

Anonymity Not anonymous or confidential.

Medical Advisory Board
Role of the MAB
The MAB reviews the periodic medical updates that are required for drivers with specific medical conditions (e.g., epilepsy, diabetes, and certain heart conditions). The DMV learns of these conditions through questions asked on the application.

MAB Contact Information
New Mexico Taxation and Revenue Department
Motor Vehicle Division
Driver Services
PO Box 1028
Joseph Montoya Building
Santa Fe, NM 87504-1028
505 827-2241

NEW YORK

Driver Licensing Agency
New York State Department of Motor Vehicles
212 645-5550

Contact Information
6 Empire State Plaza (New York City metropolitan area)
Albany, NY 12228
800 342-5368
www.nydmv.state.ny.us (area codes 516, 631, 845, 914)
800 225-5368 (all other area codes)
518 473-5595 (outside the state)

Licensing Requirements
Visual Acuity

Each eye with/without correction	20/40
Both eyes with/without correction	20/40
If one eye blind—other with/without correction	20/40
Absolute visual acuity minimum	For applicants with visual acuity less than 20/40 but not less than 20/70, Form MV-80L can be completed and submitted for licensing consideration.
Are bioptic telescopes allowed?	Yes. Applicants with 20/80 to 20/100 best-corrected acuity require minimum 140° E horizontal visual fields plus

20/40 acuity through bioptic telescope lens.

Visual Fields

Minimum field requirement	140° E horizontal visual fields
Visual field testing device	Not specified

Color Vision Requirement None

Restricted Licenses Restrictions include daytime driving only, limited radius from home, and annual renewal.

License Renewal Procedures

Standard

Length of license validation	8 years
Renewal options and conditions	In-person or mail-in.
Vision testing required at time of renewal?	Yes. Clients must pass a vision test at the DMV office or submit Form MV-619.
Written test required?	No
Road test required?	No

Age-based Renewal Procedures
None

Reporting Procedures

Physician/Medical Reporting Permitted but not required.

Immunity No

Legal Protection N/A

DMV Follow-up If a physician reports a condition that can affect the driving skills of a patient, the DMV may suspend the driver's license until a physician provides certification that the condition has been treated or controlled and no longer affects driving skills. If the DMV receives a report from a source that is not a physician, the DMV considers each case individually.

Other Reporting Will accept information from courts, other DMVs, police, family members, and other sources. Letters must be signed.

Anonymity Not anonymous. Also, if a person in a professional or official position (i.e., physician) reports, the DMV will disclose the identity of the reporter; however, if the reporter does not fall under this category, the identity of the reporter is protected under the Freedom of Information Law.

Medical Advisory Board

Role of the MAB

The MAB advises the commissioner on medical criteria and vision standards for the licensing of drivers.

MAB Contact Information
New York State Department of Motor Vehicles
Medical Review Unit
Room 220
6 Empire State Plaza
Albany, NY 12228-0220

NORTH CAROLINA

Driver Licensing Agency
North Carolina Department of Transportation
919 715-7000

Contact Information
Division of Motor Vehicles
1100 New Bern Avenue
Raleigh, NC 27697
www.dmv.dot.state.nc.us

Licensing Requirements

Visual Acuity

Each/both eyes without correction	20/40
Each/both eyes with correction	20/50
If one eye blind—other with/without correction	20/30 or better
Absolute visual acuity minimum	20/100; 20/70 if one eye is blind
Are bioptic telescopes allowed?	No. However, the applicant can initiate a medical appeal process if so desired.

Visual Fields

Minimum field requirement	60° in one eye
Visual field testing device	Keystone; Stereo Optec 1000

Color Vision Requirement None

Road Test Standardized road test; certain tasks must be completed to pass.

Restricted Licenses Restrictions include daytime driving only, speed restrictions, and no interstate driving.

License Renewal Procedures
Standard

Length of license validation	5 years
Renewal options and conditions	In-person
Vision testing required at time of renewal?	Yes
Written test required?	Yes
Road test required?	No

Age-based Renewal Procedures
Drivers age 60 and older are not required to parallel park on their road test.

Reporting Procedures
Physician/Medical Reporting Physicians are encouraged to report unsafe drivers.

Immunity North Carolina statutes protect the physician who reports an unsafe driver.

Legal Protection No

DMV Follow-up Driver is notified in writing of referral.

Other Reporting Will accept information from courts, other DMVs, police, family members, and other sources. Letters must be signed.

Anonymity Not anonymous or confidential. The driver may request a copy of his or her records.

Medical Advisory Board
Role of the MAB
The MAB reviews all medical information that is submitted to the DMV and determines what action should be taken. These actions can be appealed.

MAB Contact Information
North Carolina Division of Motor Vehicles
Medical Review Unit
3112 Mail Service Center
Raleigh, NC 27697
919 861-3809
Fax: 919 733-9569

NORTH DAKOTA

Driver Licensing Agency
North Dakota Department of Transportation
701 328-2600

Contact Information
Drivers License and Traffic Safety Division
608 East Boulevard
Bismarck, ND 58505-0700
www.state.nd.us/dot

Licensing Requirements
Visual Acuity

Each eye with/without correction	20/40
Both eyes with/without correction	20/40
If one eye blind—other with/without correction	20/40
Absolute visual acuity minimum	20/80 in better eye if 20/100 in other eye
Are bioptic telescopes allowed?	Yes, if client has 20/130 acuity through the carrier lens, 20/40 through the telescope, and full peripheral fields.

Visual Fields

Minimum field requirement	105° with both eyes
Visual field testing device	Optec 1000 vision tester

Color Vision Requirement None

Restricted Licenses Restrictions include daytime driving only (pending a sight-related road test) and area and distance restrictions.

License Renewal Procedures
Standard

Length of license validation	4 years
Vision testing required at time of renewal?	Yes
Written test required?	No
Road test required?	No

Age-based Renewal Procedures
None

Reporting Procedures
Physician/Medical Reporting Physicians are permitted by law to report to the Drivers License and Traffic Safety Division in writing the name, date of birth, and address of any patient over the age of 14 whom they have reasonable cause to believe is incapable, due to physical or mental reason, of safely operating a motor vehicle.

Immunity Physicians who in good faith make a report, give an opinion, make a recommendation, or participate in any proceeding pursuant to this law are immune from liability.

Legal Protection Available. North Dakota Century Code addresses medical advice provided by physicians.

DMV Follow-up Vision and/or medical reports may be required.

Other Reporting Will accept information from courts, other DMVs, police, and family members.

Anonymity Not available.

Medical Advisory Board
Role of the MAB
The MAB participates in drafting administrative rules for licensing standards.

MAB Contact Information
Ileen Schwengler
Drivers License and Traffic Safety Division
701 328-2070

OHIO
Driver Licensing Agency
Ohio Department of Public Safety 614 752-7500

Contact Information
Bureau of Motor Vehicles
PO Box 16520
Columbus, OH 43216-6520
www.state.oh.us/odps

Licensing Requirements
Visual Acuity

Each eye with/without correction	20/40
Both eyes with/without correction	20/40
If one eye blind—other with/without correction	20/30
Absolute visual acuity minimum	20/70 in better eye with restrictions.
Are bioptic telescopes allowed?	Yes, if client has 20/70 acuity through telescope and 20/200 acuity through carrier lens.

Visual Fields

Minimum field requirement	Each eye must have 70° temporal reading.
Visual field testing device	Keystone Vision II

Color Vision Requirement There is a requirement (not specified).

Type of Road Test Standardized course

Restricted Licenses There are various restrictions, including daytime driving only for persons with vision in both eyes who have a visual acuity between 20/50 and 20/70; daytime driving only for persons with vision in one eye only who have a visual acuity between 20/40 and 20/60; right or left outside mirror required for persons who are blind in one eye but have 70° temporal and 45° nasal peripheral vision in the other eye. Persons with certain medical or physical conditions may be required to furnish periodic medical statements or take periodic driver's license examinations.

License Renewal Procedures
Standard

Length of license validation	4 years
Renewal options and conditions	In-person. Clients may renew by mail only if they are out of state.
Vision testing required at time of renewal?	Yes
Written test required?	No
Road test required?	No

Age-based Renewal Procedures
None

Reporting Procedures
Physician/Medical Reporting Ohio will accept and act on information submitted by a physician regarding an unsafe driver. The physician must agree to be a source of information and allow the Bureau of Motor Vehicles to divulge this information to the driver.

Immunity No

Legal Protection No

DMV Follow-up A letter is sent requiring the driver to submit a medical statement and/or take a driver's license examination. The driver is given 30 days to comply.

Other Reporting Will accept information from courts, law enforcement agencies, hospitals, rehabilitation facilities, family, and friends.

Anonymity Not anonymous or confidential.

Medical Advisory Board
Role of the MAB
Ohio does not have a medical advisory board. The Bureau of Motor Vehicles contacts a medical consultant for assistance with difficult cases or for policy-making assistance.

OKLAHOMA
Driver Licensing Agency
Oklahoma Department of Public Safety 405 425-2059

Contact Information
Driver License Services
PO Box 11415
Oklahoma City, OK 73136-0415
www.dps.state.ok.us

Licensing Requirements
Visual Acuity

Each eye with/without correction	20/60
Both eyes with/without correction	20/60
If one eye blind—other with/without correction	20/50
Absolute visual acuity minimum	20/100 in better eye with restrictions.
Are bioptic telescopes allowed?	No. Laws do not allow for consideration of licensing or restrictions.

Visual Fields

Minimum field requirement	70° in the horizontal meridian with both eyes together.
Visual field testing device	Not specified.

Color Vision Requirement None

Type of Road Test Non-fixed course.

Restricted Licenses Restrictions are based on physician recommendations and can include daylight driving only, speed limitations, or local driving only.

License Renewal Procedures
Standard

Length of license validation	4 years
Renewal options and conditions	In-person
Vision testing required at time of renewal?	No

Written test required?	No
Road test required?	No

Age-based Renewal Procedures
None

Reporting Procedures
Physician/Medical Reporting Physicians are permitted to report to the Department of Public Safety any patient whom they have reasonable cause to believe is incapable of safely operating a motor vehicle.

Immunity Any physician reporting in good faith and without malicious intent shall have immunity from civil liability that might otherwise be incurred.

Legal Protection By statute the physician has full immunity.

DMV Follow-up The driver is notified in writing of the referral and required to appear for an interview at the Department. The Department also requires a current medical evaluation from a qualified practitioner.

Other Reporting Will accept information from any verifiable source with direct knowledge of the medical condition that would render a driver unsafe.

Anonymity Not available.

Medical Advisory Board
Role of the MAB
The MAB advises the Department of Public Safety on medical issues regarding individual drivers. Actions are based on the recommendation of the majority and/or specialist.

MAB Contact Information
Oklahoma Department of Public Safety
Executive Medical Secretary
PO Box 11415
Oklahoma City, OK 73136-0415
Attn: Mike Bailey

OREGON
Driver Licensing Agency
Oregon Department of Transportation 503 945-5000

Contact Information
Driver and Motor Vehicle Services
1905 Lana Avenue NE
Salem, OR 97314
www.odot.state.or.us/dmv

Licensing Requirements
Visual Acuity

Each eye with/without correction	20/40
Both eyes with/without correction	20/40
If one eye blind—other with/without correction	20/40
Absolute visual acuity minimum	20/70 in better eye with restrictions.
Are bioptic telescopes allowed?	Bioptic telescopic lenses are not permitted to meet acuity standards; however, they may be used while driving. The client must pass the vision test with the carrier lens only.

Visual Fields

Minimum field requirement	110° in horizontal plane (one or both eyes).
Visual field testing device	Both Keystone driver vision screening system and OPTEC vision screening instruments are used.

Color Vision Requirement None

Type of Road Test Standardized course.

Restricted Licenses Daytime driving only for visual acuity between 20/40 and 20/70.

License Renewal Procedures
Standard

Length of license validation	8 years
Renewal options and conditions	Mail-in every other cycle.
Vision testing required at time of renewal?	Only after age 50.
Written test required?	No
Road test required?	No

Age-based Renewal Procedures

After age 50, vision screening is required every 8 years.

Reporting Procedures

Physician/Medical Reporting Oregon is in the process of phasing in a statewide mandatory medical impairment-based reporting system. Physicians and health care providers meeting the definition of "primary care provider" are required to report persons presenting functional and/or cognitive impairments that are severe and cannot be corrected/controlled by surgery, medication, therapy, driving devices, or techniques. The state also has a voluntary reporting system that can be utilized by doctors, law enforcement officers, family, and friends who have concerns about an individual's ability to safely operate a motor vehicle. Reports submitted under the voluntary system may be based on a medical condition or on unsafe driving behaviors exhibited by the individual.

Immunity Under the mandatory reporting system, primary care providers are exempt from liability for reporting.

Legal Protection Under the mandatory reporting system, the law provides the primary care provider with legal protection for breaking the patient's confidentiality.

DMV Follow-up In most cases, the driving privileges of individuals reported under the mandatory system are immediately suspended. An individual may request the opportunity to demonstrate the ability to safely operate a motor vehicle via knowledge and driving tests. For cognitive impairments (and for specific functional impairments), a medical file and driving record are sent to the State Health Office for determination of whether the individual is safe to drive at the current point in time.

Other Reporting Under the voluntary system, the DMVS will accept information from courts, other DMVs, law enforcement officers, physicians, family members, and other sources.

Anonymity Reporting is not anonymous. Under the mandatory system, only the medical information being reported is confidential. Under the voluntary system, the DMVS will make every attempt to hold the reporter's name confidential if requested.

Medical Advisory Board
Role of the MAB

Oregon does not retain a medical advisory board. The State Health Office reviews medical cases and makes licensing decisions by reviewing an individual's medical condition and ability to drive.

MAB Contact Information

For more information regarding the review of medical cases, contact:

Oregon Driver and Motor Vehicle Services
Driver Programs Section

Attn: Melody Sheffield
1905 Lana Avenue NE
Salem, OR 97314
503 945-5520

PENNSYLVANIA

Driver Licensing Agency
Pennsylvania Department of Transportation
800 932-4600 (within state)

Contact Information
Driver and Vehicle Services 717 391-6190 (out of state)
1101 S. Front Street
Harrisburg, PA 17104-2516
www.dot.state.pa.us

Licensing Requirements
Visual Acuity

Each eye with/without correction	20/40
Both eyes with/without correction	20/40
If one eye blind—other with/without correction	20/40
Absolute visual acuity minimum	20/40 in better eye for unrestricted license; up to 20/100 binocular vision for a restricted license.
Are bioptic telescopes allowed?	Not permitted for meeting acuity standards; however, they are permitted for driving. Must have acuity of 20/100 or better with carrier lens only.

Visual Fields

Minimum field requirement	120° both eyes
Visual field testing device	PENNDOT does not regulate the kind of testing device used.

Color Vision Requirement None

Type of Road Test A standardized road test, similar to those used for the first-time permit application drivers.

Restricted Licenses Restrictions are related to vision and include daytime driving only, area restrictions, dual mirrors, and class restrictions.

License Renewal Procedures
Standard

Length of license validation	4 years
Renewal options and conditions	Internet, mail, in-person
Vision testing required at time of renewal?	No
Written test required?	No
Road test required?	No

Age-based Renewal Procedures
Drivers aged 65+ renew every 2 years. Drivers aged 45+ are requested to submit a physical and vision exam report prior to renewing (through a random mailing of 1,650 per month).

Reporting Procedures
Physician/Medical Reporting "All physicians and other persons authorized to diagnose or treat disorders and disabilities defined by the Medical Advisory Board shall report to PENNDOT in writing the full name, DOB, and address of every person 15 years of age and older, diagnosed as having any specified disorder or disability within 10 days." Physicians must report neuromuscular conditions (e.g., Parkinson's), neuropsychiatric conditions (e.g., Alzheimer's dementia), cardiovascular, cerebrovascular, convulsive, and other conditions that may impair driving ability.

Immunity "No civil or criminal action may be brought against any person or agency for providing the information required under this system."

Legal Protection Available

DMV Follow-up PENNDOT sends the appropriate correspondence to the driver asking him or her to submit the necessary forms and examination reports.

Other Reporting Will accept information from courts, other DMVs, police, emergency personnel, family members, neighbors, and caregivers. Reports must be signed in order to confirm reporter facts.

Anonymity Reporting is not anonymous, but the identity of the reporter will be protected.

Medical Advisory Board
Role of the MAB
The MAB advises PENNDOT and reviews regulations proposed by PENNDOT concerning physical and mental criteria (including vision standards) relating to the licensing of drivers. The MAB meets once every 2 years or as needed.

Rhode Island*

Driver Licensing Agency
Rhode Island Division of Motor Vehicles 401 588-3020

Contact Information
286 Main Street
Pawtucket, RI 02860
www.dmv.state.ri.us

Licensing Requirements
Visual Acuity

Each eye with/without correction	20/40
Both eyes with/without correction	20/40
If one eye blind—other with/without correction	20/40
Absolute visual acuity minimum	20/40 in better eye
Are bioptic telescopes allowed?	Unknown. (However, bioptic telescopes are mentioned in regulations.)

Visual Fields

Minimum field requirement	Unknown

Color Vision Requirement None

Restricted Licenses Not available

License Renewal Procedures
Standard

Length of license validation	5 years
Renewal options and conditions	Unknown
Vision testing required at time of renewal?	Yes
Written test required?	No
Road test required?	No

Age-based renewal procedures
At age 70, the renewal cycle is reduced to 2 years.

Reporting Procedures
Physician/Medical Reporting Any physician who diagnoses a physical or mental condition that, in the physician's judgment, will significantly impair the person's ability to safely operate a motor vehicle may voluntarily report the person's name and other information relevant to the condition to the medical advisory board within the Registry of Motor Vehicles.

Immunity Any physician reporting in good faith and exercising due care shall have immunity from any liability, civil or criminal. No cause of action may be brought against any physician for not making a report.

Legal Protection N/A

DMV Follow-up Driver is notified in writing of referral.

Other Reporting Will accept information from courts, other DMVs, police, and family members.

Anonymity N/A

Medical Advisory Board
Role of the MAB
The MAB advises the Division of Motor Vehicles on medical issues regarding individual drivers. Actions are based on the recommendation of the majority.

South Carolina

Driver Licensing Agency
South Carolina Department of Public Safety 803 737-4000

Contact Information
Department of Motor Vehicles
PO Box 1993
Blythewood, SC 29016
www.scdps.org

Licensing Requirements
Visual Acuity

Each eye with/without correction	20/40
Both eyes with/without correction	20/40
If one eye blind—other without correction	20/40
If one eye blind—other with correction	20/40; must have outside mirror.
Absolute visual acuity minimum	20/40 in better eye for unrestricted license; 20/70 in better eye if other eye is 20/200 or

---

*Information from this state's licensing agency was not available. The information above was gathered from the resources listed at the beginning of this appendix.

better; 20/40 in better eye if other eye is worse than 20/200.

Are bioptic telescopes allowed?	Not permitted for meeting acuity standards; however, they are permitted for driving.

Visual Fields

Minimum field requirement	If total angle <140°, the individual is referred to the MAB.
Visual field testing device	Not specified.

Color Vision Requirement None

Restricted Licenses Restrictions include mandatory corrective lens, mandatory outside mirrors, daylight driving only, neighborhood driving only, and speed and time restrictions.

License Renewal Procedures
Standard

Length of license validation	5 years
Renewal options and conditions	In-person. Renewal by mail is permitted if there have been no violations in the past 2 years, and no suspensions, revocations, or cancellations.
Vision testing required at time of renewal?	Yes
Written test required?	Only if the client has 5+ points on his or her record or if there appears to be a need.
Road test required?	Only if there appears to be a need.

Age-based Renewal Procedures
None

Reporting Procedures
Physician/Medical Reporting Permitted but not required.

Immunity No

Legal Protection N/A

DMV Follow-up License is suspended upon referral, and further examination is conducted.

Other Reporting Will accept information from courts, other DMVs, and police.

Anonymity N/A

Medical Advisory Board
Role of the MAB
The MAB determines the mental or physical fitness of license applicants through a medical evaluation process and makes recommendations to the department's director or designee on the handling of impaired drivers.

MAB Contact Information
South Carolina Driver Improvement Office
PO Box 1498
Columbia, SC 29216

SOUTH DAKOTA
Driver licensing agency
South Dakota Department of Public Safety
800 952-3696 (within state)

Contact Information
Office of Driver Licensing 605 773-6883 (out of state)
118 W. Capitol Avenue
Pierre, SD 57501
www.state.sd.us/dcr/dl/sddriver.htm

Licensing Requirements
Visual Acuity

Each eye with/without correction	20/50
Both eyes with/without correction	20/40
If one eye blind—other with/without correction	20/40
Absolute visual acuity minimum	20/40 in better eye for unrestricted license; 20/60 in better eye with restrictions.
Are bioptic telescopes allowed?	Yes, driver must pass a skills test.

Visual Fields

Minimum field requirement	None

Color Vision Requirement None

Type of Road Test Standardized course.

Restricted Licenses Restrictions include daylight driving only, mandatory outside rearview mirrors, mandatory corrective lenses, and driving limited to 50-mile radius from home or to the neighborhood.

License Renewal Procedures
Standard

Length of license validation	5 years
Renewal options and conditions	In-person; renewal by mail for military and military dependents only.
Vision testing required at time of renewal?	Yes
Written test required?	No
Road test required?	No

Age-based Renewal Procedures
None

Reporting Procedures
Physician/Medical Reporting Physicians may report unsafe drivers if they so choose by submitting a "Request Re-Evaluation" form. The form can be found on the Office of Driver Licensing Web site.

Immunity No

DMV Follow-up An appointment is scheduled, and the driver is notified to appear for an interview. A written test and road test may be required.

Other Reporting Will accept information from courts, other DMVs, police, family members, and other sources.

Anonymity Not available.

Medical Advisory Board
Role of the MAB
South Dakota does not have a medical advisory board. Medical information is reviewed by Department of Commerce & Regulation personnel. If the Department has good cause to believe that a licensed operator is not qualified to be licensed, it may upon written notice of at least 5 days require him or her to submit to an examination or interview. The Department shall take appropriate action, which may include suspending or revoking the license, permitting the individual to retain his or her license, or issuing a license subject to restrictions.

TENNESSEE
Driver Licensing Agency
Tennessee Department of Safety 615 741-3954

Contact Information
Motor Vehicle Services
1150 Foster Avenue
Nashville, TN 37249
www.state.tn.us/safety

Licensing Requirements
Visual Acuity

Each eye with/without correction	20/40
Both eyes with/without correction	20/40
If one eye blind—other with/without correction	20/40
Absolute visual acuity minimum	20/40 in better eye with/without correction for unrestricted license; minimum 20/60 in each/both eyes with restrictions.
Are bioptic telescopes allowed?	Yes, provided that acuity is 20/200 in better eye through the carrier lens, 20/60 through the telescope, visual field is 150° or greater, and the telescope magnification is no greater than 4×.

Visual Fields

Minimum field requirement	For professional drivers only.
Visual field testing device	Stereo Optec

Color Vision Requirement Only for commercial drivers.

Type of Road Test Standardized course with specific requirements.

Restricted Licenses Restrictions include area limitations.

License Renewal Procedures
Standard

Length of license validation	5 years
Renewal options and conditions	In-person; mail and Internet renewal are permitted every other cycle.
Vision testing required at time of renewal?	No
Written test required?	No
Road test required?	No

Age-based Renewal Procedures
None

Reporting Procedures

Physician/Medical Reporting Permitted but not required.

Immunity Yes

Legal Protection No

DMV Follow-up Driver is notified in writing of referral.

Other Reporting Will accept information from courts, other DMVs, police, family members, and other sources.

Anonymity Not available

Medical Advisory Board

Role of the MAB
The MAB is composed of volunteer physicians, who review medical reports and make recommendations. Actions are based upon the recommendation of the majority.

MAB Contact Information
Contact the MAB through the Driver Improvement Office at 615 251-5193.

TEXAS

Driver Licensing Agency
Texas Department of Public Safety 512 424-2967

Contact Information

Driver License Division
PO Box 4087
Austin, TX 78773-0001
512 424-2602
www.txdps.state.tx.us

Licensing Requirements
Visual Acuity

Each/both eyes without correction	20/40
Each/both eyes with correction	20/50
If one eye blind—other without correction	20/25 with eye specialist statement.
If one eye blind—other with correction	20/50 with eye specialist statement.
Absolute visual acuity minimum	20/40 in better eye for unrestricted license;

	20/70 in better eye with restrictions.
Are bioptic telescopes allowed?	Yes, provided that the client has acuity of 20/40 through the telescope and passes the road test.

Visual Fields

Minimum field requirement	None

Color Vision Requirement There is a requirement for all new drivers (not specified).

Type of Road Test Standardized course

Restricted Licenses Restrictions are based on medical advice and may include daytime driving only where the speed limit <45 mph and no expressway driving.

License Renewal Procedures
Standard

Length of license validation	6 years
Renewal options and conditions	In-person; if the client is eligible, renewal by Internet, telephone, or mail is also available.
Vision testing required at time of renewal?	At in-person renewal.
Written test required?	No
Road test required?	No

Age-based Renewal Procedures
None

Reporting Procedures

Physician/Medical Reporting Any physician licensed to practice medicine in the state of Texas may inform the Department of Public Safety. This release of information is an exception to the patient-physician privilege. There is no special reporting form; a letter from the physician will suffice.

Immunity Yes

Legal Protection Yes

DMV Follow-up The driver is notified in writing of the referral and required to provide medical information from his or her personal physician.

Other Reporting Will accept information from courts, other DMVs, police, family members, and other sources.

Anonymity Not anonymous or confidential. However, an attempt is made to protect the identity of the reporter. If the client requests an administrative hearing, the identity of the reporter may be revealed at that time.

Medical Advisory Board
Role of the MAB
The MAB advises the Department of Public Safety on medical issues regarding individual drivers. The Department bases its actions on the recommendation of the physician who reviews the case.

MAB Contact Information
Texas Department of Public Safety
Medical Advisory Board
PO Box 4087
Austin, TX 78773
512 424-2344

UTAH
Driver Licensing Agency
Utah Department of Public Safety 801 965-4437

Contact Information
Driver License Division
PO Box 30560
Salt Lake City, UT 84130-0560
www.driverlicense.utah.gov

Licensing Requirements
Visual Acuity

Each eye with/without correction	20/40
Both eyes with/without correction	20/40
If one eye blind—other with/without correction	20/40
Absolute visual acuity minimum	20/100 in better eye with restrictions.
Are bioptic telescopes allowed?	No

Visual Fields

Minimum field requirement	120° horizontal and 20° vertical for an unrestricted license; 90° horizontal with restrictions.
Visual field testing device	Stereo Optical (DMV 2000)

Color Vision Requirement None

Restricted Licenses Restrictions include daytime driving only where the speed limit <45 mph and radius limitations.

License Renewal Procedures
Standard

Length of license validation	5 years
Renewal options and conditions	In-person; mail-in every other cycle if no suspensions, revocations, convictions, and not more than four violations.
Vision testing required at time of renewal?	Only for clients aged 65 and older.
Written test required?	No
Road test required?	No, unless examiner feels the applicant's ability to drive is in question.

Age-based Renewal Procedures
Vision testing required at license renewal for clients aged 65 and older.

Reporting Procedures
Physician/Medical Reporting Permitted but not required.

Immunity Any physician or person who becomes aware of a physical, mental, or emotional impairment that appears to present an imminent threat to driving safety and reports this information to the Department of Public Safety in good faith shall have immunity from any damages claimed as a result of so doing.

Legal Protection No

DMV Follow-up Driver is notified in writing of referral. License is suspended upon referral.

Other Reporting Will accept information from courts, other DMVs, police, family members, and other sources.

Anonymity Not anonymous or confidential.

Medical Advisory Board
Role of the MAB
The MAB advises the Director of the Driver License Division and recommends written guidelines and standards for determining the physical, mental, and emotional capabilities appropriate to various types of driving in an effort to minimize the conflict between the individual's desire to drive and the community's desire for safety.

MAB contact information
Dana H. Clarke
Chair, Utah Medical Advisory Board
PO Box 30560
University of Utah Hospital
Salt Lake City, UT 84130-0560

Kurt Stromberg
Executive Committee Program Coordinator, Utah
Driver License Division
Research Park
615 Arapeen Drive, #100
801 965-3819
801 965-4084 fax
Salt Lake City, UT 84108
Kstromberg@utah.gov

VERMONT

Driver Licensing Agency
Vermont Agency of Transportation 802 828-2000

Contact Information
Department of Motor Vehicles
120 State Street
Montpelier, VT 05603-0001
www.aot.state.vt.us

Licensing Requirements
Visual Acuity

Each eye with/without correction	20/40
Both eyes with/without correction	20/40
If one eye blind—other with/without correction	20/40
Absolute visual acuity minimum	20/40 in better eye.
Are bioptic telescopes allowed?	Yes, with a daytime driving–only restriction and vehicle weight restriction (10,000 lbs.). Also, the client must pass a road test.

Visual Fields

Minimum field requirement	Each eye 60°; 60° external and 60° nasal for one eye only.
Visual field testing device	Not specified.

Color Vision Requirement None

Restricted Licenses There are restrictions for clients who wear glasses or contact lenses and for those who utilize biopic telescopes.

License Renewal Procedures
Standard

Length of license validation	2 to 4 years
Renewal options and conditions	By mail and in-person.
Vision testing required at time of renewal?	No
Written test required?	No
Road test required?	No

Age-based Renewal Procedures
None

Reporting Procedures
Physician/Medical Reporting Physicians may provide information to the DMV only with the permission of the patient.

Immunity No

Legal Protection No

DMV Follow-up Driver is notified of the referral by mail.

Other Reporting Will accept information from courts, other DMVs, police, concerned citizens, or family members. The letter must be signed.

Anonymity Not anonymous or confidential. However, the reporter's identity is held confidential until a hearing is requested by the client.

Medical Advisory Board
Role of the MAB
Vermont no longer retains a medical advisory board.

VIRGINIA

Driver Licensing Agency
Virginia Department of Motor Vehicles
866 368-5463

Contact Information
PO Box 27412
Richmond, VA 23269
www.dmv.state.va.us

Licensing Requirements
Visual Acuity

Each eye with/without correction	20/40
Both eyes with/without correction	20/40

If one eye blind—other with/without correction	20/40
Absolute visual acuity minimum	20/40 in better eye for unrestricted license; 20/70 in better eye with daylight-only restriction; 20/200 in better eye with other restrictions.
Are bioptic telescopes allowed?	Yes, provided that acuity is 20/200 through carrier lens and 20/70 through telescope. A test is required.

Visual Fields

Minimum field requirement	100° monocular and binocular; 70° monocular and binocular with daylight-only restriction.
Visual field testing device	Stereo Optical/Titmus 10 mm W @ 333 mm.

Color Vision Requirement None

Type of Road Test A behind-the-wheel test is administered with the DMV examiner instructing and evaluating the person on specific driving maneuvers.

Restricted Licenses Restrictions may be based on road test performance, medical conditions, violation of probation, or court convictions. The restrictions include mandatory corrective lenses, hand controls, radius limitations, daylight driving only, mandatory ignition interlock device, and driving only to and from work/school.

License Renewal Procedures
Standard

Length of license validation	5 years
Renewal options and conditions	Customers may use an alternative method of renewing their driver's license every other cycle unless their license has been suspended or revoked, they have two or more violations, there is a DMV medical review indicator on the license, or they fail the vision test. Alternative methods include mail-in, Internet, touch-tone telephone, fax, and ExtraTeller.
Vision testing required at time of renewal?	Yes
Written test required?	If the customer has had two or more violations in the past 5 years.
Road test required?	No

Age-based Renewal Procedures
None

Reporting Procedures
Physician/Medical Reporting Physicians are not required to report unsafe drivers. However, for physicians who do report unsafe drivers, laws have been enacted to prohibit release of the physician's name as the source of the report.

Immunity No

Legal Protection Virginia code β 54.1-2966.1 states that if a physician reports a patient to the DMV, it shall not constitute a violation of the doctor-patient relationship unless the physician has acted with malice.

DMV Follow-up Drivers are notified in writing that the DMV has initiated a medical review and advised of the medical review requirements. Drivers are also advised of any restrictions or suspension imposed as a result of the review.

Other Reporting The DMV relies upon information from courts, other DMVs, law enforcement officers, physicians, and other medical professionals, relatives, and concerned citizens to help identify drivers who may be impaired.

Anonymity Not anonymous. Virginia law provides confidentiality, but only for relatives and physicians.

Medical Advisory Board
Role of the MAB
The MAB enables the DMV to monitor drivers throughout the state who may have physical or mental problems. The MAB assists the Commissioner with the development of medical and health standards for use in the issuance of driver's licenses. The MAB helps the DMV avoid the issuance of licenses to persons suffering from any physical or mental disability or disease that will prevent their exercising reasonable and ordinary control over a motor vehicle while driving it on highways. The MAB reviews the more complex cases,

including those referred for administrative hearings, and provides recommendations for medical review action.

MAB Contact Information
Ms. Jacquelin C. Branche, RN
Virginia Department of Motor Vehicles
Medical Review Services
PO Box 27412
Richmond, VA 23269
804 367-0531
804 367-1604 fax
Dmvj3b@dmv.state.va.us

WASHINGTON

Driver Licensing Agency
Washington Department of Licensing 360 902-3600

Contact Information
Driver Services
1125 Washington Street SE
PO Box 9020
Olympia, WA 98507-9020
www.dol.wa.gov

Licensing Requirements
Visual Acuity

Each eye with/without correction	20/40
Both eyes with/without correction	20/40
If one eye blind—other with/without correction	20/40
Absolute visual acuity minimum	20/40 in better eye for unrestricted license; 20/70 in better eye with restrictions.
Are bioptic telescopes allowed?	Yes; training and testing are required.
Visual fields	110° in horizontal meridian, binocular and monocular.
Visual field testing device	Optec 1000; Keystone Telebinocular; Keystone DVSII

Color Vision Requirement There is a requirement for new and professional drivers (not specified).

Type of Road Test Standardized scoring using approved test routes at each licensing office.

Restricted Licenses Restricted licenses may be issued depending on the circumstances. Corrective lenses may

be required to meet the minimum acuity, and the client may be restricted to daytime driving only based on an eye care practitioner's report or after failing a night-time driving test. If needed to compensate for visual or physical impairment, there may be equipment restrictions, route or distance restrictions, or geographic area limits.

License Renewal Procedures
Standard

Length of license validation	5 years
Renewal options and conditions	In-state renewals are in-person only. If out of state, the applicant can renew by mail once.
Vision testing required at time of renewal?	Yes
Written test required?	Only if warranted by results of vision, health, or medical screening.
Road test required?	Only if warranted by results of vision, health, or medical screening.

Age-based Renewal Procedures
None

Reporting Procedures
Physician/Medical Reporting Permitted but not required.

Immunity No

Legal Protection No

DMV Follow-up The DMV sends a letter to the driver with information detailing due process and action following any failure to respond.

Other Reporting Will accept information from courts, other DMVs, police, family members, and other competent sources. If in doubt, the reporting party may be required to establish his or her firsthand knowledge and standing for making a report.

Anonymity Not anonymous or confidential.

Medical Advisory Board
Role of the MAB
Washington does not retain a medical advisory board.

West Virginia

Driver Licensing Agency
West Virginia Department of Transportation
800 642-9066 (within state)

Contact Information
Division of Motor Vehicles 304 558-3900 (out of state)
Building 3, Room 113
1800 Kanawha Boulevard, East
Charleston, WV 25317
www.wvdot.com

Licensing Requirements
Visual Acuity

Both eyes with/without correction	20/40
If one eye blind—other with/without correction	20/40
Absolute visual acuity minimum	20/60 in better eye; if less, the client must submit a report from an optometrist or ophthalmologist declaring the client's ability to drive safely.
Are bioptic telescopes allowed?	No

Visual Fields

Minimum field requirement	None

Color Vision Requirement None

Type of Road Test Standard road skills exam.

Restricted Licenses Not available

License Renewal Procedures
Standard

Length of license validation	5 years. Under the "Drive for Five" program, all driver's licenses expire in the client's birth month at an age divisible by five (e.g., 25, 30, 35, and so on).
Renewal options and conditions	In-person
Vision testing required at time of renewal?	No

Written test required?	No
Road test required?	No

Age-based Renewal Procedures
None

Reporting Procedures
Physician/Medical Reporting Physicians are permitted and encouraged to report.

Immunity No

Legal Protection No

DMV Follow-up A medical report is sent to the driver, to be completed by his or her physician. If the driver fails to comply, then the driver's license is immediately revoked.

Other Reporting Will accept information from law enforcement officers and family members.

Anonymity Not anonymous or confidential.

Medical Advisory Board
Role of the MAB
The MAB reviews medical cases and advises the Division on how the driver's medical condition may affect his or her ability to drive safely. If the MAB concludes that the driver is unsafe, it may recommend to the Commissioner of Motor Vehicles that the license be revoked. The Commissioner then makes the final licensing decision.

MAB Contact Information
Joetta Gore 304 558-0238

Wisconsin

Driver Licensing Agency
Wisconsin Department of Transportation
608 266-2353

Contact Information
Bureau of Driver Services
Hill Farms State Transportation Building
4802 Sheboygan Avenue
PO Box 7910
Madison, WI 53707-7910
www.dot.wisconsin.gov

Licensing Requirements
Visual Acuity

Each eye with/without correction	20/40

If one eye blind—other with/without correction	20/40
Absolute visual acuity minimum	20/100 in better eye with or without correction.
Are bioptic telescopes allowed?	Not for meeting vision standards, but can be used in driving.

Visual Fields

Minimum field requirement	70° in better eye for regular unrestricted license.
Visual field testing device	Stereo Optical machine

Color Vision Requirement Only for commercial drivers.

Type of Road Test Knowledge and sign tests are administered prior to the road test. The limited area test is on a non-fixed course, but is otherwise standardized.

Restricted Licenses Restrictions can be recommended by a physician or vision specialist or determined by the road test. Restrictions include daytime driving only, radius limitations, and/or freeway restrictions.

License Renewal Procedures
Standard

Length of license validation	8 years
Renewal options and conditions	In-person; by mail if client is out of state.
Vision testing required at time of renewal?	Yes
Written test required?	Determined by DOT, vision specialist, or physician.
Road test required?	Determined by DOT, vision specialist, or physician.

Age-based Renewal Procedures
None

Reporting Procedures
Physician/Medical Reporting Physicians are encouraged though not required to report. They can report by submitting form MV3141 ("Driver Condition or Behavior Report") or a letter on letterhead stationary. Form MV3141 is available on the DOT Web site.

Immunity Yes

Legal Protection Yes

DMV Follow-up Driver is notified in writing of requirement(s). Depending on requirement(s), he or she is given 15, 30, or 60 days to comply. If driver does not comply within the time period given, the driver's license is cancelled. Driver is notified in writing of cancellation.

Other Reporting Will accept information from courts, other DMVs, police, family members, and other sources.

Anonymity Not anonymous or confidential. (Wisconsin has an Open Records Law.) However, individuals can submit "Pledge of Confidentiality" form MV3454 with form MV3141. Form MV3454 is available on the DOT Web site.

Medical Advisory Board
Role of the MAB
The MAB advises the Bureau of Driver Services on medical issues regarding individual drivers. Wisconsin has two types of MAB:
1. By-Mail Board: Paper file is mailed to three physicians specialists (i.e., neurologist, endocrinologist, and ophthalmologist) for recommendations based on the client's medical condition(s).
2. In-Person Board: The client has an interview with three physicians (psychiatrist, neurologist, and internist).

Actions are based on the recommendation of the majority, the client's driving record, medical information provided by the client's physician, and, if appropriate, driving examination results.

WYOMING
Driver Licensing Agency
Wyoming Department of Transportation 307 777-4800

Contact Information
Driver Services
5300 Bishop Boulevard
Cheyenne, WY 82009-3340
307 777-4810
www.dot.state.wy.us

Licensing Requirements
Visual Acuity

Each eye with/without correction	20/40
Both eyes with/without correction	20/40
If one eye blind—other with/without correction	20/40

Absolute visual acuity minimum	20/100 in better eye with restrictions.
Are bioptic telescopes allowed?	Yes, provided that acuity is 20/100 or better through both carrier lenses. There is a distance restriction for at least 1 year.

Visual Fields

Minimum field requirement	120° binocular for new, renewal, and professional drivers.
Visual field testing device	Keystone machine

Color Vision Requirement None

Restricted Licenses Restrictions include daytime driving only and weather and distance restrictions.

License Renewal Procedures
Standard

Length of license validation	4 years
Renewal options and conditions	In-person; mail-in every other cycle.
Vision testing required at time of renewal?	Yes
Written test required?	No
Road test required?	Only if warranted by vision statement from physician or examiner.

Age-based Renewal Procedures
None

Reporting Procedures
Physician/Medical Reporting Physician reporting is encouraged, though not required.

Immunity Physicians providing information concerning a patient's ability to drive safely are immune from liability for their opinions and recommendations.

Legal Protection N/A

DMV Follow-up If necessary, the DOT obtains additional information from the physician through completion of a Driver Medical Evaluation form.

Other Reporting Will accept information from courts, other DMVs, police, and family members.

Anonymity N/A

Medical Advisory Board
Role of the MAB
Wyoming does not retain a medical advisory board.

CPT CODES

The following Current Procedural Terminology (CPT) codes can be used for driver assessment and counseling, when applicable. These codes were taken from *Current Procedural Terminology (CPT)*. 4th ed., Professional ed. Chicago, IL: American Medical Association; 2003.

When selecting the appropriate CPT codes for driver assessment and counseling, first determine the primary reason for your patient's office visit, as you would normally. The services described in this Guide will most often fall under Evaluation and Management (E/M) services. Next, select the appropriate E/M category/ subcategory. If you choose to apply codes from the Preventive Medicine Services category, consult Table 1 for the appropriate codes. If any additional services are provided over and above the E/M services, codes from Table 2 may be additionally reported.

Table 1   Evaluation and Management—Preventive Medicine Services

If the primary reason for your patient's visit falls under the E/M category of Preventive Medicine Services, choose one of the following codes:

99386 40-64 years **99387** 65 years and older	**New Patient, Initial Comprehensive Preventive Medicine** Evaluation and management of an individual including an age and gender appropriate history, examination, counseling/anticipatory guidance/risk factor reduction interventions, and the ordering of appropriate immunizations(s), laboratory/diagnostic procedures. *These codes can be used for a complete Preventive Medicine history and physical exam for a new patient (or one who has not been seen in three or more years), which may include assessment and counseling on driver safety. If significant driver assessment and counseling take place during the office visit, Modifier-25 may be added to the codes above.*
99396 40-64 years **99397** 65 years and older	**Established Patient, Periodic Comprehensive Preventive Medicine** Reevaluation and management of an individual including an age and gender appropriate history, examination, counseling/anticipatory guidance/risk factor reduction interventions, and the ordering of appropriate immunization(s), laboratory/diagnostic procedures. *Codes from the Preventative Medicine Services 99386-99387 and 99396-99397 can only be reported once per year. If driver assessment and counseling take place during the office visit, Modifier-25 may be added to the codes above.*

Modifier-25 is appended to the office/outpatient service code to indicate that a significant, separately identifiable E/M service was provided by the same physician on the same day as the preventive medicine service.

99401 Approximately 15 minutes **99402** Approximately 30 minutes **99403** Approximately 45 minutes **99404** Approximately 60 minutes	**Counseling and/or Risk Factor Reduction Intervention** Preventive medicine counseling and risk factor reduction interventions provided as a separate encounter will vary with age and should address such issues as family problems, diet and exercise, substance abuse, sexual practices, injury prevention, dental health, and diagnostic and laboratory test results available at the time of the encounter. (These codes are not to be used to report counseling and risk factor reduction interventions provided to patients with symptoms or established illness.) These are time-based codes, to be reported based upon the amount of time spent counseling the patient. *Driver safety or driving retirement counseling fall under the category of injury prevention. Please note that for driving retirement counseling, a copy of the follow-up letter to your patient can be included in the patient's chart as additional documentation.*

Table 2 Additional Codes

The codes below can be used for administration of ADReS. If you complete the entire assessment, you can include codes 99420, 95831, and either 99172 or 99173. The ADReS Score Sheet can serve as the report.

99420	**Administration and Interpretation of Health Risk Assessment Instrument**
95831	**Muscle and Range of Motion Testing** Muscle testing, manual (separate procedure) with report; extremity (excluding hand) or trunk.
99172	**Visual Function Screening** Automated or semi-automated bilateral quantitative determination of visual acuity, ocular alignment, color vision by pseudoisochromatic plates, and field of vision (may include all or some screening of the determination(s) for contrast sensitivity, vision under glare).
99173	**Screening Test of Visual Acuity, quantitative, bilateral** The screening used must employ graduated visual acuity stimuli that allow a quantitative estimate of visual acuity (e.g., Snellen chart).

PROFESSIONAL ETHICS, CONTINUING COMPETENCE, AND ORGANIZATIONS

Appendix C

CODES OF ETHICS AND STANDARDS OF PRACTICE*†

INTRODUCTION

The Association for Driver Rehabilitation Specialists (ADED) is a professional organization whose members are dedicated to enhancing the lives of individuals with disabilities and impairments by providing services that assist such individuals in the attainment of skills that enable safe and independent driving and transportation through the use of adapted vehicles and adaptive driving equipment.

Membership in ADED commits members to follow the *Code of Ethics* and comply with the *Standards of Practice*. Driver rehabilitation specialists possessing the CDRS (Certified Driver Rehabilitation Specialist) certification are likewise committed to such compliance.

The ADED Code of Ethics is a set of principles set forth to guide the professional conduct of driver rehabilitation specialists. The *Standards of Practice* defines the minimum requirements that govern professional behaviors in the provision of driver rehabilitation services. Establishment of the *Code of Ethics* and *Standards of Practice* demonstrates ADED's commitment to fostering excellence in the field of driver rehabilitation.

---

*Effective Date: 8/1/03.

†This section has been reprinted with permission from ADED and AOTA.

ADED CODE OF ETHICS

CONTENTS

PRINCIPLE A: Demonstrating Concern for the Well-being of Clients Served
PRINCIPLE B: Respecting the Rights of Clients Served
PRINCIPLE C: Fostering Excellence in the Field of Driver Rehabilitation by Achieving and Maintaining a High Standard of Competence
PRINCIPLE D: Complying with Laws and Association Precepts Governing the Driver Rehabilitation Profession
PRINCIPLE E: Providing Accurate Information Regarding Driver Rehabilitation Services
PRINCIPLE F: Treating Colleagues and Other Professionals with Fairness, Discretion, and Integrity
PRINCIPLE G: Promoting a Greater Understanding of Driver Rehabilitation Issues by Others in Rehabilitation, Health Care, and Education, and by Seeking Public Awareness through Communication about Such Issues

PRINCIPLES REVIEWED

Principle A: Demonstrating Concern for the Well-being of Clients Served
A.   1.   Client Welfare
    a.   Primary Obligation. The primary obligation of the driver rehabilitation specialist is to promote the welfare of clients. A client is defined as an individual with a disability or impairment

who is receiving services from a driver rehabilitation specialist.

b. Safety. Driver rehabilitation specialists ensure the physical safety of clients by ensuring that all equipment used in the provision of services is in proper working order, is utilized in an appropriate manner, and in an appropriate setting.

c. Impairment. When the potential exists for the personal problems of the driver rehabilitation specialist to cause harm to a client, themselves, or others, the driver rehabilitation specialist refrains from offering services in the affected areas of practice until the situation has been rectified. Such problems may include physical illness, emotional issues, and psychological impairments.

d. Family and Caregiver Involvement. Driver rehabilitation specialists foster family and caregiver understanding and enlist family and caregiver involvement when appropriate.

A. 2. Provider Objectivity
a. Personal Needs. Driver rehabilitation specialists avoid situations and refrain from actions that meet their personal needs at the expense of client needs.

b. Personal Bias. Driver rehabilitation specialists avoid imposing their own values, beliefs, and attitudes upon clients.

c. Judgment and Objectivity. Driver rehabilitation specialists avoid situations, activities, and relationships that interfere with professional judgment and objectivity.

A. 3. Appropriate Relationships
a. Non-exploitation. Driver rehabilitation specialists are aware of the issues of influence and dependency within the client relationship and do not exploit the client's trust.

b. Sexual Intimacy. Driver rehabilitation specialists do not engage in any type of sexual intimacies with clients.

c. Sexual Harassment. Driver rehabilitation specialists do not engage in sexual harassment. Sexual harassment may include unwelcome or unwanted sexual advances, requests for sexual favors, and other verbal or physical conduct of a sexual nature.

A. 4. Fees for Service
a. Establishing Fees. Driver rehabilitation specialists establish fees that are fair, reasonable, equitable, and commensurate with the services to be performed.

b. Advance Understanding. Fees and methods of payment and collection for non-payment are clearly explained to clients in advance of services rendered.

A. 5. Avoidance, Termination, and Referral
a. Refusal of a Potential Client. If the driver rehabilitation specialist determines that he or she would/could not be of professional assistance to a potential client, the relationship should be avoided, and the client should be referred to an appropriate resource if possible.

b. Appropriate Termination. The driver rehabilitation specialist terminates services if the services are no longer required, the client can no longer benefit from services, the driver rehabilitation specialist has reached the limit of his or her competency with respect to the service being provided, the driver rehabilitation specialist has experienced an impairment that would interfere with the safe provision of services, for non-payment of fees, or when institutional or legal limits do not allow provision of further services. The client should be referred to an appropriate resource if feasible.

A. 6. Client Records
a. Appropriate Records. The driver rehabilitation specialist maintains appropriate and necessary records reflecting accurate, objective information.

b. Confidentiality of Records. The driver rehabilitation specialist ensures confidentiality of records in all mediums with respect to maintenance, storage, handling, and destruction.

c. Client Access. The driver rehabilitation specialist provides adequate access for clients to their records.

d. Informed Consent. The driver rehabilitation specialist obtains informed written consent from clients to disclose or transfer records to legitimate third parties. The driver rehabilitation specialist understands that informed consent does not waive confidentiality.

Principle B: Respecting the Rights of Clients Served

B. 1. Respecting Diversity
a. Nondiscrimination. Driver rehabilitation specialists do not engage in discrimination on the basis of sex, age, color, natural origin, race, religious beliefs, or type of disability.

b. Cultural Diversity. Driver rehabilitation specialists actively attempt to understand the culturally diverse backgrounds of their clients as they impact driver rehabilitation services.

B. 2. Right to Information and Self-determination
a. Self-determination. Driver rehabilitation specialists involve clients in the determination of goals and priorities.

b. Disclosure to Clients. Prior to assessment, the driver rehabilitation specialist informs the client of the purposes, goals, potential outcomes, techniques, procedures, limitations, potential risks, and benefits of services. The driver rehabilitation specialist discloses the limitations of confidentiality, including those resulting from the use of computer technology and the transmission of electronic communication. Also disclosed are the consequences of refusal of services. The driver rehabilitation specialist takes steps to ensure client understanding and informed consent.

B. 3. Right to Privacy

   a. Respecting and Guarding Privacy. The driver rehabilitation specialist respects the client's right to privacy and the confidential nature of client information. The driver rehabilitation specialist takes steps to avoid illegal, unnecessary, and inadvertent disclosure of confidential information. This includes guarding the safety and security of confidential records, regardless of medium.

   b. Client Waiver. The right to privacy may be waived by the client, a legal guardian, or by a legally appointed representative.

   c. Essential Disclosure. When driver rehabilitation specialists are compelled to disclose confidential information without a client waiver, such as in a court-ordered disclosure, only essential information is disclosed. If feasible, the client should be informed prior to such disclosure.

   d. Associates. Driver rehabilitation specialists make every effort to ensure that all associates, including co-workers, volunteers, and contractors, maintain privacy and confidentiality.

Principle C: Fostering Excellence in the Field of Driver Rehabilitation by Achieving and Maintaining a High Standard of Competence

C. 1. Code and Standards

   a. *Code of Ethics.* The driver rehabilitation specialist has the responsibility to become familiar with, develop an understanding of, and follow the ADED *Code of Ethics.*

   b. *Standards of Practice.* The driver rehabilitation specialist has the responsibility to become familiar with, develop an understanding of, and follow the ADED *Standards of Practice.*

C. 2. Professional Competence

   a. Boundaries of Competence. Driver rehabilitation specialists practice only within their areas of expertise as defined by the boundaries of their competence. These boundaries are determined by their education, training, professional experience, and professional credentials.

   b. Diverse Populations. Driver rehabilitation specialists will endeavor to gain personal awareness, knowledge, sensitivity, and skills needed to provide services to a diverse client population.

   c. New Specializations. Driver rehabilitation specialists provide services in specialized areas new to them only after obtaining the appropriate education and training necessary to develop the skills required to provide such new services. During the skill development phase, driver rehabilitation specialists make provisions for ensuring the quality of service provision as well as protecting client safety and the safety of others.

   d. Employment Assignments. Driver rehabilitation specialists only accept employment, assignments, cases, and referrals for which they are qualified by education, training, professional experience, and professional credentials. Driver rehabilitation specialists hire for driver rehabilitation positions, make assignments to, provide client cases to, and make referrals only to individuals who are qualified and competent.

   e. Continuing Education. Driver rehabilitation specialists pursue continuing education to maintain an awareness of current information pertinent to their areas of specialization and to maintain competence in the skills they utilize in service provision.

C. 3. Public Responsibility

   a. Unjustifiable Gains. Driver rehabilitation specialists do not use their professional positions to obtain unearned, unfair, or unjustified gains.

   b. Conflicts of Interest. Driver rehabilitation specialists do not knowingly place themselves in positions that would constitute conflicts of interest. If it becomes apparent that such a situation exists, the driver rehabilitation specialist takes appropriate steps to rectify the situation, such as removing oneself from the situation or full disclosure of the conflict of interest.

   c. Dishonesty. Driver rehabilitation specialists do not engage in any act or omission of a dishonest, deceitful, or fraudulent nature in the conduct of their professional activities.

C. 4. Assessment Techniques

   a. Development. Driver rehabilitation specialists hold paramount the welfare of clients in the development and dissemination of clinical and driver assessment techniques. Steps are taken to ensure the appropriate utilization of such techniques as well as the appropriate interpretation of results.

b. Utilization. Driver rehabilitation specialists use only assessment techniques that they are qualified and competent to use. They do not misuse assessment results or interpretations.

c. Client's Right to Know. The driver rehabilitation specialist respects the client's right to know the results of an assessment and to be informed of the basis for interpretation and recommendations.

C. 5. Teaching and Training Programs

a. Teacher/Trainer Role. Driver rehabilitation specialists who are functioning as teachers or trainers are qualified and competent as driver rehabilitation practitioners and teachers/trainers. They are knowledgeable regarding applicable legal and ethical matters. They conduct education and training programs in an ethical manner consistent with the ADED *Code of Ethics* and *Standards of Practice*. They maintain appropriate relationship boundaries with students and trainees and do not subject them to discrimination or sexual harassment.

b. Acknowledgments. Driver rehabilitation specialists give credit to students and trainees for their contributions to research, development of assessment techniques, and publications.

c. Endorsement. Driver rehabilitation specialists provide endorsements for certification, licensure, employment, or completion of an academic or training program only to students and trainees who are qualified to receive such endorsements.

d. Responsibility for Client Welfare. Driver rehabilitation specialists who supervise services provided by students or trainees are responsible for ensuring that such services are provided in a professional manner, respect clients' rights, and demonstrate concern for the welfare of the client.

C. 6. Resolving Ethical Issues

a. Knowledge of Standards. Driver rehabilitation specialists are responsible for knowing and understanding the ADED *Code of Ethics* and *Standards of Practice*.

b. Seeking Clarification. A driver rehabilitation specialist should seek advice if there is uncertainty as to whether or not a particular behavior constitutes a violation of the ADED *Code of Ethics* and *Standards of Practice*.

c. Employment Conflicts. If acting on behalf of an employer appears to place the driver rehabilitation specialist in violation of the ADED *Code of Ethics* and *Standards of Practice*, the

driver rehabilitation specialist should seek immediate advice.

Principle D: Complying with Laws and Association Precepts Governing the Driver Rehabilitation Profession

D. 1. Legal Standards

a. Responsibility. Driver rehabilitation specialists have the responsibility to obey the laws and statutes of the legal jurisdictions in which they practice.

b. Legal versus Ethical. If obeying the laws or statutes of the legal jurisdictions in which the driver rehabilitation specialist practices places the driver rehabilitation specialist in conflict with the ADED *Code of Ethics* and *Standards of Practice*, the driver rehabilitation specialist should seek immediate advice.

c. Legal Limitations. Driver rehabilitation specialists are familiar with and observe the legal limitations of the services they offer to clients.

D. 2. Client Records. Driver rehabilitation specialists maintain appropriate records as necessitated by law, statute, regulations, and institutional requirements. Records will be maintained for at least the number of years consistent with jurisdictional requirements and are destroyed in a manner ensuring confidentiality.

Principle E: Providing Accurate Information Regarding Driver Rehabilitation Services

E. 1. Advertising Practices—Restrictions. Driver rehabilitation specialists advertise their services to the public only in an accurate, honest, straightforward manner. They advertise only services that they are qualified and competent to provide.

E. 2. Credentials

a. Stated Credentials. Driver rehabilitation specialists claim only professional credentials possessed including degrees and training programs that have been completed and certifications and licenses obtained. Driver rehabilitation specialists take steps to correct any known misrepresentation or misinterpretation of their credentials by others.

b. Credential Usage. Driver rehabilitation specialists use their credentials only in manners consistent with the guidelines established by the issuing bodies.

c. Misrepresentation. Driver rehabilitation specialists do not misrepresent their credentials by identifying them in a fraudulent or deceptive manner. They do not attribute more to their credentials than the credentials actually represent. They do not claim or imply that other driver rehabilitation specialists are not qualified to provide driver rehabilitation services solely because they do not possess certain credentials.

E. 3. Reporting—Reports to Third Parties. Driver rehabilitation specialists provide to appropriate third parties reports that are objective, accurate, and honest with respect to their actions, assessments, interpretation, and recommendations.

Principle F: Treating Colleagues and Other Professionals with Fairness, Discretion, and Integrity

F. 1. Responsibility to Other Professionals
   a. Disparaging Comments. Driver rehabilitation specialists do not disparage or discredit other professionals with respect to competency or quality of services.
   b. Personal Public Statements. When making personal statements in a public context, driver rehabilitation specialists take steps to ensure that the audience knows that they are speaking only from their personal perspective and that they are not speaking on behalf of all such professionals, the ADED, or the profession.
   c. Confidentiality. Driver rehabilitation specialists take steps to safeguard confidential information about colleagues and staff.
   d. Accurate Representation. Driver rehabilitation specialists accurately represent the qualifications, views, contributions, and findings of colleagues.

Principle G: Promoting a Greater Understanding of Driver Rehabilitation Issues by Others in Rehabilitation, Health Care, and Education and Seeking Public Awareness through Communication about Such Issues

G. 1. Professional Association Involvement—Participation. Driver rehabilitation specialists actively participate in local, state, and national associations that foster the development and improvement of driver rehabilitation.
G. 2. Public Responsibility
   a. Media Presentations. When driver rehabilitation specialists provide information via any public medium or format, they take steps to ensure that the information is accurate, consistent with current literature and practice, and in line with the ADED *Code of Ethics* and *Standards of Practice*.
   b. Personal Public Statements. When making personal statements in a public context, driver rehabilitation specialists take steps to ensure

that the audience knows that they are speaking only from their personal perspective and that they are not speaking on behalf of all driver rehabilitation specialists, the ADED, or the profession.

ADED STANDARDS OF PRACTICE

The ADED *Standards of Practice* delineate the minimum requirements governing professional behavior for driver rehabilitation specialists. As such, these requirements represent standards by which driver rehabilitation specialists must abide. Failure to do so constitutes unethical behavior. For clarification, corresponding sections of the ADED *Code of Ethics* are cited.

CONTENTS

PRINCIPLE A: Demonstrating Concern for the Well-being of Clients Served
PRINCIPLE B: Respecting the Rights of Clients Served
PRINCIPLE C: Fostering Excellence in the Field of Driver Rehabilitation by Achieving and Maintaining a High Standard of Competence
PRINCIPLE D: Complying with Laws and Association Precepts Governing the Driver Rehabilitation Profession
PRINCIPLE E: Providing Accurate Information Regarding Driver Rehabilitation Services
PRINCIPLE F: Treating Colleagues and Other Professionals with Fairness, Discretion, and Integrity
PRINCIPLE G: Promoting a Greater Understanding of Driver Rehabilitation Issues by Others in Rehabilitation, Health Care, and Education, and by Seeking Public Awareness through Communication about Such Issues

PRINCIPLES REVIEWED

Principle A: Demonstrating Concern for the Well-being of Clients Served
Standard A-1: Safety
      Driver rehabilitation specialists must take steps to ensure the physical safety of clients by ensuring that all equipment used during service provision is in proper working order, is utilized in an appropriate manner, and in an appropriate setting. (See A.1.b)

Standard A-2: Impairment
Driver rehabilitation specialists must refrain from offering professional services when their personal problems or impairments are likely to harm a client, themselves, or others. (See A.1.c)

Standard A-3: Non-exploitation
Driver rehabilitation specialists must avoid dual relationships and must not exploit clients. (See A.3.a)

Standard A-4: Sexual Intimacy
Driver rehabilitation specialists must avoid dual relationships and must not engage in any type of sexual intimacies with their clients. (See A.3.b)

Standard A-5: Sexual Harassment
Driver rehabilitation specialists do not engage in dual relationships and do not engage in sexual harassment. (See A.3.c)

Standard A-6: Establishing Fees
Driver rehabilitation specialists must establish fees that are fair, reasonable, equitable, and commensurate with services to be performed. (See A.4.a)

Standard A-7: Advance Understanding of Fees
Driver rehabilitation specialists must explain to clients in advance of services their fee structures, methods of payment, and methods of collection and consequences for non-payment. (See A.4.b)

Standard A-8: Inability to Assist Clients
Driver rehabilitation specialists must terminate professional relationships and refer clients to appropriate resources if feasible when unable to be of professional assistance. (See A.5.a and b)

Standard A-9: Appropriate Records
Driver rehabilitation specialists must maintain appropriate client records reflecting accurate, objective information. (See A.6.a)

Standard A-10: Confidentiality of Records
Driver rehabilitation specialists must take steps to ensure the confidentiality of client records in all media. (See A.6.b)

Standard A-11: Client Access to Records
Driver rehabilitation specialists must provide access for clients to their records. (See A.6.c)

Standard A-12: Informed Consent
Driver rehabilitation specialists must obtain informed written consent from clients to disclose or transfer records. (See A.6.d)

Principle B: Respecting the Rights of Clients Served

Standard B-1: Nondiscrimination
Driver rehabilitation specialists must not discriminate against clients. (See B.1.a)

Standard B-2: Disclosure to Clients
Driver rehabilitation specialists must fully inform clients about all aspects and limitations of service provision prior to rendering services and take steps to ensure client understanding. (See B.2.b)

Standard B-3: Right to Privacy
Driver rehabilitation specialists must take steps to avoid illegal, unnecessary, and inadvertent disclosure of confidential information, including guarding the safety and security of confidential records, regardless of medium. (See B.3.a)

Standard B-4: Essential Disclosure of Confidential Information
Driver rehabilitation specialists must only disclose information that is essential to the situation when compelled to disclose confidential information without a client waiver, such as in a court-ordered disclosure. (See B.3.c)

Standard B-5: Confidentiality Requirements for Associates
Driver rehabilitation specialists must take steps to ensure that all associates, including co-workers, volunteers, and contractors, maintain privacy and confidentiality of client services and records. (See B.3.d)

Principle C: Fostering Excellence in the Field of Driver Rehabilitation by Achieving and Maintaining a High Standard of Competence

Standard C-1: ADED *Code of Ethics* and *Standards of Practice*
Driver rehabilitation specialists must adhere to the ADED *Code of Ethics* and *Standards of Practice*. (See C.1.a and b)

Standard C-2: Boundaries of Competence
Driver rehabilitation specialists must only practice within their boundaries of competence. (See C.2.a)

Standard C-3: New Specializations
Driver rehabilitation specialists must obtain the appropriate education and

training before offering services in areas of specialization new to them. (See C.2.c)

Standard C-4: Qualified for Service Provision
Driver rehabilitation specialists must only accept employment, assignments, cases, and referrals for which they are qualified and must only hire, make assignments to, provide client cases to, and make referrals to individuals who are qualified and competent. (See C.2.d)

Standard C-5: Continuing Education
Driver rehabilitation specialists must pursue continuing education to maintain professional competence. (See C.2.e)

Standard C-6: Unjustified Gains
Driver rehabilitation specialists must not use their professional positions to obtain unearned, unfair, or unjustified gains. (See C.3.a)

Standard C-7: Conflicts of Interest
Driver rehabilitation specialists must avoid conflicts of interest. (See C.3.b)

Standard C-8: Dishonesty
Driver rehabilitation specialists must not engage in any act or omission of a dishonest, deceitful, or fraudulent nature in the conduct of their professional duties. (See C.3.c)

Standard C-9: Development of Assessment Techniques
Driver rehabilitation specialists must take steps to guard the welfare of clients when developing assessment techniques. (See C.4.a)

Standard C-10: Utilization of Assessment Techniques
Driver rehabilitation specialists must use only assessment techniques that they are qualified and competent to use. (See C.4.b)

Standard C-11: Client's Right to Know
Driver rehabilitation specialists must inform the client of assessment results, interpretations, and recommendations. (See C.4.c)

Standard C-12: Teacher/Trainer Role
Driver rehabilitation specialists who are functioning as teachers or trainers must be competent as driver rehabilitation practitioners and teachers/trainers, must be knowledgeable regarding applicable legal/ethical matters, must maintain appropriate relationship boundaries, must not discriminate, and must not engage in sexual harassment. (See C.5.a)

Standard C-13: Acknowledgments
Driver rehabilitation specialists must give appropriate acknowledgments for contributions. (See C.5.b)

Standard C-14: Endorsements
Driver rehabilitation specialists must give only appropriate warranted endorsements. (See C.5.c)

Standard C-15: Responsibility for Client Welfare
Driver rehabilitation specialists who supervise students or trainees maintain responsibility for client welfare and must take steps to ensure such welfare. (See C.5.d)

Standard C-16: Knowledge of Standards
Driver rehabilitation specialists must know and understand the ADED *Code of Ethics* and *Standards of Practice*.

Standard C-17: Employment Conflicts
Driver rehabilitation specialists must seek immediate advice if acting on behalf of an employer who appears to place the driver rehabilitation specialist in violation of the ADED *Code of Ethics* and *Standards of Practice*.

Principle D: Complying with Laws and Association Precepts Governing the Driver Rehabilitation Profession

Standard D-1: Responsibility for Complying with Laws and Statutes
Driver rehabilitation specialists must obey the laws and statutes of the legal jurisdictions in which they practice. (See D.1.a)

Standard D-2: Legal Limitations of Services
Driver rehabilitation specialists must be familiar with and observe the legal limitations of the services they offer. (See D.1.c)

Standard D-3: Retention of Client Records
Driver rehabilitation specialists must maintain client records in a safe, secure, confidential manner for at least the number of years consistent with jurisdictional requirements. (See D.2.a)

Principle E: Providing Accurate Information Regarding Driver Rehabilitation Services

Standard E-1: Advertising Restrictions
Driver rehabilitation specialists must only advertise to the public services that they are qualified and competent to perform and must do so only in an

accurate, honest, straightforward manner. (See E.1.a)

Standard E-2: Stated Credentials

Driver rehabilitation specialists must claim only professional credentials possessed, including degrees and training programs completed and certifications and licenses obtained, and must not misrepresent their credentials or attribute more to them than they actually represent. (See E.2.a. and c)

Standard E-3: Reports to Third Parties

Driver rehabilitation specialists must only provide to appropriate third parties reports that are objective, accurate, and honest with respect to their actions, assessments, interpretations, and recommendations. (See E.3.a)

Principle F: Treating Colleagues and Other Professionals with Fairness, Discretion, and Integrity

Standard F-1: Personal Public Statements

Driver rehabilitation specialists must, when making personal statements in a public context, take steps to ensure that the audience knows that they are speaking only from their personal perspectives and that they are not speaking on behalf of all such professionals, the ADED, or the profession. (See F.1.b)

Standard F-2: Confidentiality

Driver rehabilitation specialists must take steps to safeguard confidential information about colleagues and staff. (See F.1.c)

Standard F-3: Accurate Representation

Driver rehabilitation specialists must accurately represent the qualifications, views, contributions, and findings of colleagues. (See F.1.d)

Principle G: Promoting a Greater Understanding of Driver Rehabilitation Issues by Others in Rehabilitation, Health Care, and Education and Seeking Public Awareness through Communication about Such Issues

Standard G-1: Media Presentations

Driver rehabilitation specialists must, when providing information via any public medium, take steps to ensure that the information is accurate, current, and not misleading in any way. (See G.2.a)

Standard G-2: Personal Public Statements

Driver rehabilitation specialists, when making personal statements in a public context, must take steps to ensure that the audience knows that they are speaking only from their personal perspective and that they are not speaking on behalf of all driver rehabilitation specialists, the ADED, or the profession.

SECTION II

American Occupational Therapy Association (AOTA) Code of Ethics (2000)

PREAMBLE

The American Occupational Therapy Association's *Code of Ethics* is a public statement of the common set of values and principles used to promote and maintain high standards of behavior in occupational therapy. The American Occupational Therapy Association and its members are committed to furthering the ability of individuals, groups, and systems to function within their total environment. To this end, occupational therapy personnel (including all staff and personnel who work and assist in providing occupational therapy services, e.g., aides, orderlies, secretaries, and technicians) have a responsibility to provide services to recipients in any stage of health and illness who are individuals, research participants, institutions and businesses, other professionals and colleagues, students, and the general public.

The *Occupational Therapy Code of Ethics* is a set of principles that applies to occupational therapy personnel at all levels. These principles to which occupational therapists and occupational therapy assistants aspire are part of a lifelong effort to act in an ethical manner. The various roles of practitioner (occupational therapist and occupational therapy assistant), educator, fieldwork educator, clinical supervisor, manager, administrator, consultant, fieldwork coordinator, faculty program director, researcher/scholar, private practice owner, entrepreneur, and student are assumed.

Any action in violation of the spirit and purpose of this *Code* shall be considered unethical. To ensure compliance with the *Code*, the Commission on Standards and Ethics (SEC) establishes and maintains the enforcement procedures. Acceptance of membership in the American Occupational Therapy Association commits members to adherence to the *Code of Ethics* and its enforcement procedures. The Code of Ethics, Core Values and Attitudes of Occupational Therapy Practice (AOTA, 1993) and the Guidelines to the Occupational

Therapy Code of Ethics (AOTA, 1998) are aspirational documents designed to be used together to guide occupational therapy personnel.

Principle 1. Occupational therapy personnel shall demonstrate a concern for the well-being of the recipients of their services. (beneficence)

A. Occupational therapy personnel shall provide services in a fair and equitable manner. They shall recognize and appreciate the cultural components of economics, geography, race, ethnicity, religious and political factors, marital status, sexual orientation, and disability of all recipients of their services.

B. Occupational therapy practitioners shall strive to ensure that fees are fair and reasonable and commensurate with services performed. When occupational therapy practitioners set fees, they shall set fees considering institutional, local, state, and federal requirements, and with due regard for the service recipient's ability to pay.

C. Occupational therapy personnel shall make every effort to advocate for recipients to obtain needed services through available means.

Principle 2. Occupational therapy personnel shall take reasonable precautions to avoid imposing or inflicting harm upon the recipient of services or to his or her property. (nonmaleficence)

A. Occupational therapy personnel shall maintain relationships that do not exploit the recipient of services sexually, physically, emotionally, financially, socially, or in any other manner.

B. Occupational therapy practitioners shall avoid relationships or activities that interfere with professional judgment and objectivity.

Principle 3. Occupational therapy personnel shall respect the recipient and/or his or her surrogate(s) as well as the recipient's rights. (autonomy, privacy, confidentiality)

A. Occupational therapy practitioners shall collaborate with service recipients or their surrogate(s) in setting goals and priorities throughout the intervention process.

B. Occupational therapy practitioners shall fully inform the service recipients of the nature, risks, and potential outcomes of any interventions.

C. Occupational therapy practitioners shall obtain informed consent from participants involved in research activities and indicate that they have fully informed and advised the participants of potential risks and outcomes. Occupational therapy practitioners shall endeavor to ensure that the participant(s) comprehend these risks and outcomes.

D. Occupational therapy personnel shall respect the individual's right to refuse professional services or involvement in research or educational activities.

E. Occupational therapy personnel shall protect all privileged confidential forms of written, verbal, and electronic communication gained from educational, practice, research, and investigational activities unless otherwise mandated by local, state, or federal regulations.

Principle 4. Occupational therapy personnel shall achieve and continually maintain high standards of competence. (duties)

A. Occupational therapy practitioners shall hold the appropriate national and state credentials for the services they provide.

B. Occupational therapy practitioners shall use procedures that conform to the standards of practice and other appropriate AOTA documents relevant to practice.

C. Occupational therapy practitioners shall take responsibility for maintaining and documenting competence by participating in professional development and educational activities.

D. Occupational therapy practitioners shall critically examine and keep current with emerging knowledge relevant to their practice so they may perform their duties on the basis of accurate information.

E. Occupational therapy practitioners shall protect service recipients by ensuring that duties assumed by or assigned to other occupational therapy personnel match credentials, qualifications, experience, and scope of practice.

F. Occupational therapy practitioners shall provide appropriate supervision to individuals for whom the practitioners have supervisory responsibility in accordance with Association policies, local, state and federal laws, and institutional values.

G. Occupational therapy practitioners shall refer to or consult with other service providers whenever such a referral or consultation would be helpful to the care of the recipient of service. The referral or consultation process should be done in collaboration with the recipient of service.

Principle 5. Occupational therapy personnel shall comply with laws and Association policies guiding the profession of occupational therapy. (justice)

A. Occupational therapy personnel shall familiarize themselves with and seek to understand and abide by applicable Association policies; local, state, and federal laws; and institutional rules.

B. Occupational therapy practitioners shall remain abreast of revisions in those laws and Association policies that apply to the profession of occupational therapy and shall inform employers, employees, and colleagues of those changes.

C. Occupational therapy practitioners shall require those they supervise in occupational therapy–related activities to adhere to the *Code of Ethics.*

D. Occupational therapy practitioners shall take reasonable steps to ensure employers are aware of occupational therapy's ethical obligations, as set forth in this *Code of Ethics,* and of the implications of those obligations for occupational therapy practice, education, and research.

E. Occupational therapy practitioners shall record and report in an accurate and timely manner all information related to professional activities.

Principle 6. Occupational therapy personnel shall provide accurate information about occupational therapy services. (veracity)

A. Occupational therapy personnel shall accurately represent their credentials, qualifications, education, experience, training, and competence. This is of particular importance for those to whom occupational therapy personnel provide their services or with whom occupational therapy practitioners have a professional relationship.

B. Occupational therapy personnel shall disclose any professional, personal, financial, business, or volunteer affiliations that may pose a conflict of interest to those with whom they may establish a professional, contractual, or other working relationship.

C. Occupational therapy personnel shall refrain from using or participating in the use of any form of communication that contains false, fraudulent, deceptive, or unfair statements or claims.

D. Occupational therapy practitioners shall accept the responsibility for their professional actions that reduce the public's trust in occupational therapy services and those who perform those services.

Principle 7. Occupational therapy personnel shall treat colleagues and other professionals with fairness, discretion, and integrity. (fidelity)

A. Occupational therapy personnel shall preserve, respect, and safeguard confidential information about colleagues and staff, unless otherwise mandated by national, state, or local laws.

B. Occupational therapy practitioners shall accurately represent the qualifications, views, contributions, and findings of colleagues.

C. Occupational therapy personnel shall take adequate measures to discourage, prevent, expose, and correct any breaches of the *Code of Ethics* and report any breaches of the *Code of Ethics* to the appropriate authority.

D. Occupational therapy personnel shall familiarize themselves with established policies and procedures for handling concerns about this *Code of Ethics,* including familiarity with national, state, local, district, and territorial procedures for handling ethics complaints. These include policies and procedures created by the American Occupational Therapy Association, licensing and regulatory bodies, employers, agencies, certification boards, and other organizations that have jurisdiction over occupational therapy practice.

REFERENCES

American Occupational Therapy Association: Core values and attitudes of occupational therapy practice, *Am J Occup Ther* 47:1085-1086, 1993.

American Occupational Therapy Association: Guidelines to the occupational therapy code of ethics, *Am J Occup Ther* 52:881-884, 1998.

AUTHORS

The Commission on Standards and Ethics (SEC):

Barbara L. Kornblau, JD, OTR, FAOTA, Chairperson
Melba Arnold, MS, OTR/L
Nancy Nashiro, PhD, OTR, FAOTA
Diane Hill, COTA/L, AP
Deborah Y. Slater, MS, OTR/L
John Morris, PhD
Linda Withers, CNHA, FACHCA
Penny Kyler, MA, OTR/L, FAOTA, Staff Liaison
for
The Commission on Standards and Ethics
Barbara L. Kornblau, JD, OTR, FAOTA, Chairperson

Adopted by the Representative Assembly 2000M15
Note: This document replaces the 1994 document, Occupational Therapy Code of Ethics (*Am J Occup Ther* 48:1037-1038).

Previously published and copyrighted in 2000 by the American Occupational Therapy Association in the *American Journal of Occupational Therapy* 54:614-616.

CONTINUING COMPETENCE IN DRIVER REHABILITATION

Joseph M. Pellerito, Jr. • *Cynthia J. Burt*

Competence is a major determinant of a professional's effectiveness when providing clients driver rehabilitation and community mobility services. Driver rehabilitation specialists (DRSs) must conform to various clinical, nonclinical, and interpersonal standards that provide a foundation on which efficacious and evidence-based practice can emerge. Being able to measure competence is essential for determining the ability and readiness of DRSs to provide quality services to the general public. In the final analysis, however, it is an ethical responsibility for every DRS to stay abreast of leading-edge assessment and treatment strategies, as well as modification procedures and adapted driving equipment that are supported in the professional literature. For more information on professional ethics and driver rehabilitation, see Chapter 23.

There are numerous ways to define competence generally, as well as within the context of professional driver rehabilitation and community mobility service delivery. For example the *Merriam-Webster Dictionary* defines the word competent as, "proper or rightly pertinent, having requisite or adequate ability or qualities, legally qualified or adequate having the capacity to function or develop in a particular way." The U.S. Agency for International Development described competence as encompassing knowledge, skills, abilities, and traits.[1] It is gained in the health care professions through preservice education, in-service training, and work experience. Finally the PEW Commission's Interprofessional Workgroup on Health Professions Regulation defines professional competence as the application of knowledge and skills in interpersonal relations, decision making, and physical performance consistent with the professional's practice role and public health welfare and safety considerations.[2]

Although competence is a precursor to doing a job correctly, measuring performance is also crucial to determining whether providers are actually applying their knowledge in a professional and competent manner. Providers can possess knowledge but not demonstrate adequate skills because of individual factors; for example, DRSs have different abilities, training, experience, goals, values, and inertia. There are also important external factors that impact skill level and performance; for example, administrators who demonstrate a strong commitment for continuing education in terms of approving release time and funding, access to state-of-the-art equipment, and organizational support that fosters a culture that values continuing education.

Continuing education and training is the link that facilitates continuing competence as well as efficacious and evidence-based practice. In many professions the requisites for measuring competence change over time as various factors reshape the scope of practice and as individual practitioners specialize in any given area of practice.[3] Continuing competence, therefore, is the ongoing application and integration of knowledge and critical thinking, as well as interpersonal and psychomotor skills essential for safe and effective service delivery. Of course, service delivery is also impacted by other factors as well, such as the particular field or profession under consideration and its unique professional culture; the roles and responsibilities a professional assumes within the program and organization he or she is working for; the physical environment (e.g., condition of the client's vehicle, topography, weather patterns, transportation infrastructure, and so forth); and, perhaps most important, the knowledge and insight clients and caregivers bring to the table when articulating their needs and expectations to the DRS and other driver rehabilitation team members.

The indicators of continuing competence change over time as various factors reshape the scope and expand the boundaries of any professional practice. Continuing competence involves the satisfactory demonstration of observable and quantifiable behaviors, as well as the acquisition of concepts pertaining to driver rehabilitation; for example, assessment, planning, analysis, modification of the intervention, supervision, research and scholarship, service, and education. Interpersonal and behavioral characteristics of continuing competence include safe, efficient, and effective service delivery; time management; adherence to recognized standards and ethical codes of practice; and responsibility for professional growth and development on an ongoing basis.[4] Allied health professionals have long debated the best ways to assess continuing competence. This task is especially important in professions that subscribe to rapidly changing evaluation and intervention strategies, as well as rely on leading edge technology such as driver rehabilitation. Hinojosa et al[5] asserted that "Rapid changes in technology and difficulty inherent in managing a great amount of information place all of us in danger of becoming incompetent." To stay current, DRSs must keep up with advances in driver assessment and rehabilitation, general physical medicine and rehabilitation, driver education, wheeled mobility and seating, pharmacology, adapted driving aids, vehicle modifications, reimbursement, the automotive and traffic safety industries, and local and national traffic laws. In addition to the diverse knowledge base that DRSs must continually cultivate and expand, they often practice under the oversight of more than one professional organization. An occupational therapist who specializes in driver rehabilitation, for example, could be certified as an occupational therapy generalist or occupational therapy assistant by the National Board for the Certification of Occupational Therapists (NBCOT); be an active member of the American Occupational Therapy Association (AOTA); be a member of, and certified by, the Association for Driver Rehabilitation Specialists (ADED); and be registered or licensed by his or her state licensing or registration agency/authority. Additionally the professional in this example could also maintain licensure as a driving instructor and have completed the academic coursework to become certified as a driver educator. Needless to say, each of these organizations has its own criteria for ensuring that its respective members/stakeholders maintain a prescribed level of continuing competence with voluntary or compulsory compliance expected. No wonder the public (not to mention much of the professional community) is often confused or unaware of the best avenues for seeking out effective driver rehabilitation professional services. Until there is greater collaboration between these organizations, adhering to expectations for continuing competence, professional ethics, and standards of practice that each entity promotes will continue to be a moving target for DRSs and potentially confusing to the general public.

Individuals in the United States and other places around the world who desire a foundation as an occupational therapy generalist before becoming DRSs must demonstrate entry-level competence in occupational therapy practice. Competence is usually recognized after the prospective occupational therapy generalist has graduated from an occupational therapy program that is accredited by the Accreditation Council for Occupational Therapy Education (ACOTE), which is affiliated with AOTA. The education also includes an internship (i.e., fieldwork experience) and an entry-level examination for certification leading to licensure or registration. The most effective methods for ensuring continued competence once a graduate enters the field of driver rehabilitation have long been debated. Periodic reexamination was deemed costly and not well received by members in good standing within various professional organizations. An alternative approach to periodic reexamination was participation in continuing education. Many licensure and regulatory agencies began calling for mandatory continuing education for certification and licensure renewal. This approach has become somewhat controversial because there has been little research to support the relationship between continuing education and competence; however, it is expected that continuing education and training will remain the preferred method to foster continuing competence.

In July 2003 the Federation of Associations of Regulatory Boards (FARB) held a national summit to develop strategies for ensuring that health care professionals remain competent throughout their careers. The organizations that participated included the AOTA, NBCOT, American Physical Therapy Association (APTA), and many others. The summit's overall objective was to identify a set of programs that will help assure the public of continuing education and training of health care professionals to help ensure an ongoing and acceptable level of professional competence. One of their discussions focused on determining which competency assessment mechanism should be relied on. The panel believed that testing is the easiest and most reliable but not always the most appropriate choice. They discussed peer review as the single best approach because it included actual observation of performance, but they believed it was too costly and difficult to ensure reliability and validity because reviewers are influenced by their own subjective perceptions and interpersonal relationships to some extent. They also discussed portfolio and self-assessment tools that have some peer review elements and concluded that irrespective of the method, measuring competence must focus on the practitioner's current performance. The precise methods of competency assessment are less important than the outcomes gathered as the result of an effective evaluation of a practitioner's knowledge, skills, attitudes, and other important aspects of performance.[6]

The AOTA, NBCOT, and ADED have implemented continued competency plans and recertification requirements based on the need for ongoing professional development. AOTA's self-initiated plan focuses on therapists exploring their specific professional responsibilities, performing a self-assessment, identifying professional development needs in light of AOTA's Standards of Continuing Competence (Box D-1), developing a plan for continuing competence, implementing the plan, documenting continuing competence and changing performance outcomes, implementing changes, and demonstrating competence on an ongoing basis. The AOTA has proposed that triggers such as changes in reimbursement, entering a new

practice area, practicing in isolation, licensure requirements, intrinsic motivations, personal goals, and employer mandates be the impetus for practitioners to examine their professional competence.[5]

The NBCOT has a mandatory plan for recertification that requires a requisite number of professional development units (PDUs) during a predetermined certification period. They also provide a self-assessment tool that is initiated by professional transitions or triggers as well. NBCOT has identified 30 professional development activities and has assigned a PDU value for each activity. The activities include continuing education, volunteer service, attaining specialty certification, making professional presentations, publication, mentoring, reflective practice with an advanced colleague, guest lecturing, reading of peer-reviewed material, providing professional in-service training or instruction, presenting to local organizations, manuscript review, academic coursework, professional study groups, research, fellowship training, independent study, and development of instructional materials. Random samples of practitioners who are renewing their certification are audited for compliance.[7]

ADED also has its own mandatory requirements for recertification that require certified driver rehabilitation specialists (CDRSs) to accumulate a specific number of points for specific professional activities during the previous certification period. Professional activities are assigned a point value and include approved workshops, lectures and seminars, academic course completion, publishing, development of instructional materials, and presenting at ADED's annual conference.

Standards of practice and codes of ethics are the basis for competencies for which practitioners are held accountable. Any DRS with a professional background in occupational therapy must meet the Standards of Practice and adhere to the Code of Ethics for both the AOTA and ADED. The Code of Ethics and Standards of Practice in both organizations closely parallel one another and do not impose additional burden to the practitioner to meet the standards of both organizations. Using AOTA's Professional Development Tool or NBCOT Self-Assessment Resource Tool can assist DRSs in developing a personal continuing competency plan based on their practice needs and allow for meeting the initial certification or recertification criteria for the DRS.

Individuals providing driver rehabilitation services can and should draw from a wide variety of arenas when developing a personal continuing competency plan. From the medical arena, the practitioner may gain understanding of how impairments, conditions, disabilities, medications, and therapeutic interventions and equipment may affect prerequisite skills that are necessary for safe driving. From the driver education arena,

BOX D-1	**Standards for Continuing Competence for Occupational Therapy Practitioners**

- Knowledge—The occupational therapy practitioner shall demonstrate understanding and comprehension of the information required for the multiple roles he or she assumes.
- Critical reasoning—The occupational therapy practitioner shall employ reasoning processes to make sound judgments and decisions within the context of his or her role.
- Interpersonal abilities—The occupational therapy practitioner shall develop and maintain professional relationships with others within the context of his or her role.
- Performance skills—The occupational therapy practitioner shall demonstrate the expertise, proficiencies, and abilities to competently fulfill his or her role.
- Ethical reasoning—The occupational therapy practitioner shall identify, analyze, and clarify ethical issues or dilemmas in order to make responsible decisions within the changing context of his or her roles.

Data from American Occupational Therapy Association: Standards for continuing competence, *Am J Occup Ther* 5(6):599-600, 1999.

the practitioner may gain knowledge in the area of teaching individuals the rules of the road (e.g., traffic laws) and actual driving skills, as well as vehicle control strategies. From the vehicle modification arena, the practitioner can gain knowledge about vehicle modification options and procedures, as well as adaptive driving equipment. From the traffic safety arena, the practitioner may gain knowledge about vehicle safety, older driver safety, and roadway design that fosters the health, safety, and well-being of all road users. Finally the automotive industry can contribute to the practitioner's competence by providing knowledge in the area of individual vehicle specifications, features, and universal design. For more information on universal design, see Chapter 16.

Irrespective of the assessment tool or tools that a practitioner chooses to use with the aim of fostering continued competence, the assessment methods should include self-reflection of one's strengths and weaknesses, as well as peer review and external evaluation of the individual's scope of practice, the community's needs, and identified triggers. When practitioners base their continuing competence plans on these factors, they will be individually tailored to meet the needs of the practitioner, which will inevitably benefit his or her clients and the wider community.

REFERENCES

1. Kak N, Burkhalter B, Cooper MA: *Measuring the competence of healthcare providers* (Issue Paper No. 2), 2001, US Agency for International Development.
2. Gragnola CM, Stone E: *Considering the future of health care workforce regulation,* San Francisco, 1997, UCSF Center for the Health Professions.
3. Pew Health Professions Commission: 1995
4. Mayhan YD, Holm MB, Fawcett L, editors, and the National Commission on Continued Competency in Occupational Therapy: *Continued competency in occupational therapy: recommendations to the profession and key stakeholders,* Gaithersburg, MD, 1999, National Board for Certification in Occupational Therapy.
5. Hinojosa J, et al: Standards for continuing competence for occupational therapy practitioners, *OT Practice* 5(20), 2000.
6. Federation of Associations of Regulatory Boards: *Demonstrating continuing professional competence: A national summit to develop strategies for assuring that health care professionals remain competent throughout their careers,* (Meeting report), San Francisco, California, 2003.
7. The National Board for Certification in Occupational Therapy, Inc. (NBCOT) Retrieved April 25, 2005 from http://www.nbcot.org.

ADED YESTERDAY, TODAY, AND TOMORROW

SECTION I

The Past and Present

Deena Garrison Jones

Reading through the chapters in this book, one will discover that the primary aim of any reputable driver rehabilitation program is to empower clients to be competent and responsible drivers as well as proficient consumers of alternative transportation and the ubiquitous transportation infrastructure (e.g., gas stations, freeway rest areas, roads, and bridges) that supports our global car culture. The rationale that supports this aim presumes that driver rehabilitation specialists (DRSs) will provide their clients with more than performing predriving clinical and on-road evaluations or teaching them how to use adaptive driving equipment during an on-road training session. The DRS performing the predriving and on-road evaluations must be familiar with the unique issues that are presented by people with disabilities, the elderly, and their caregivers. In other words, the DRS must possess a keen understanding of the associated conditions, impairments, and disabilities that can preclude people from driving and accessing alternative transportation. Specialists must also be cognizant of the special needs that caregivers often present as well as the evaluation and training processes required to assess existing and develop future skills necessary for successful driver rehabilitation and community mobility outcomes.

Initially hospitals and private facilities could not find instructors for their clients who were in need of driver rehabilitation and alternative community mobility services. So where are the specialists who follow all applicable federal, state, and local laws and policies while providing driver rehabilitation services for people with disabilities, aging-related challenges, or both? By and large, they are members of the Association for Driver Rehabilitation Specialists (ADED) who have become certified driver rehabilitation specialists (CDRSs). CDRSs have diverse professional backgrounds and experience in rehabilitation, education, or some other healthcare–related field. Most CDRSs have a background in occupational therapy; however, CDRSs may also be educated and trained, for example, as physical therapists, pharmacists, and driver educators. The occupational therapist presents an ideal professional foundation that readily complements the skills required to provide driver rehabilitation services. Occupational therapists subscribe to a client-centered approach and view each client holistically; that is, a client is not seen narrowly as simply a diagnosis, but broadly as a human being who has psychosocial, cognitive, biological, spiritual, and emotional needs and wants. Some models of practice include teaming an occupational therapist with another member of the driver rehabilitation team such as a driver educator who may lack the medical training but possesses complementary skills developed over years of experience.

THE EARLY YEARS

Prior to the development of driver rehabilitation as a recognized field comprising highly skilled practitioners, commercial driving instructors who lacked formal medical training taught people with disabilities how to drive. As the need for driver rehabilitation services intensified and driving tasks along with technological solutions became more complex, certified classroom driver educators and on-road driving instructors worked with occupational therapists, physical therapists, and kinesiotherapists to try and understand how disabilities impacted driving outcomes in an effort to better serve their clients. Soon a handful of occupational therapists from different parts of the country wanted to provide specialized driver rehabilitation services and began evaluating their clients' driving potential clinically. It was not long before therapists realized that the clinical evaluation provided only a part of the total picture, and eventually on-road driving performance was being formally evaluated.

ADED was formed in 1977 because of this early collaboration between professionals who possessed different backgrounds and levels of experience. They shared one important thing in common—the desire to provide efficacious driver rehabilitation services to people with disabilities (the elderly were served later as the population demographics changed over time). During an interview with Jerry Bouman, the second president of ADED, he vividly recalled the first ADED meeting:

> We met in Detroit, Michigan with 30 other people from 10 different states. The Rehabilitation Institute, represented by Gary Gurgold, OTR and Scott Robins, OTR hosted the meeting. The organization was primarily started to foster support of one another in the work that we were doing. Prior to the beginning of ADED, it always felt like each of us was on our own. It gave all of us a tremendous boost in confidence to find so many other people who shared similar experiences, doubts, and concerns.[1]

The type of organizational structure, official name, and selection of the first group of officers to lead the newly formed organization were determined by this early group of pioneers at the first meeting.

THE MANUFACTURERS' PERSPECTIVE

Keeping drivers and passengers safe often requires the use of modified vehicles and adaptive driving equipment, especially for people with disabilities. ADED encourages the development of aftermarket adaptive driving equipment to maximize driving and passenger options for people with disabilities, the elderly, and their caregivers. Freedom of movement within one's community is an essential part of an active life. There are many aftermarket vendors that design and manufacture customized driving controls that keep people actively involved in the world around them.[2] Numerous manufacturers of driver rehabilitation products have been involved with ADED:

> As a manufacturer, we are able to introduce our innovations and new products to the ADED membership and reach a larger and more informed audience. The scope of the audience has increased, our products receive greater visibility and use in the marketplace, and the ultimate goal of freedom for the individual is accomplished. Without ADED members, the ability to communicate with the consumer to keep them abreast of new product developments would be greatly diminished.[2]

As early as 1952, the Drive-Master Company designed a push-pull hand control that has naturally led to the mass production of other mobility products. Peter Ruprecht of Drive-Master, recipient of the 1998 ADED Research and Applied Engineering Award, did not remember when he first got involved with ADED, but he recalled building evaluator vans for numerous specialty driving schools. Peter recalled some of the founding members of ADED with whom he has worked, such as Jiri C. Sipajlo, Ed Colvert, Carmella Strano, Mike Shipp, Paul St. Pierre, and Lola Hershberger. Peter also remembered one particular inventive evaluator who drove his vehicle to the vendor's shop:

> . . . to demonstrate what the evaluator had done with a coat hanger operating some OEM (original equipment manufacturer) piece of equipment. The evaluator wanted the vendor to duplicate his coat hanger adaptation so that the client could drive his or her own vehicle. It was a riot and I wish we had pictures of some of his crazy gadgets! People would call and describe an item or some driving task they needed to perform; most of the time we would design and fabricate the product for them and for the next person that needed the same or similar product. This is how the industry got going, but the industry has greatly advanced so that clients, vendors, and evaluators have choices with adaptive equipment.[3]

Back in the early 1980s, Drive-Master designed and manufactured smaller steering wheels, reduced-effort braking, horizontal steering, power pans, and other products that enabled wheelchair users to get behind the wheel and drive. "Everyone was always calling to find out how to get an adapted vehicle, buy parts to build one themselves, or how to perform an evaluation using the custom-made products."[3]

ADED's leadership recognized early on that the field of driver rehabilitation (and later alternative community mobility) for people with disabilities and others needed to include professionals who specialized in equipment fabrication and modification. ADED changed its name from the Association of Driver Educators of the Disabled and became incorporated as the Association for Driver Rehabilitation Specialists in 1997 in order to better reflect the diversity of its members; however, they kept the ADED acronym because of its brand identity and name recognition. ADED has evolved over the years to become an international, nonprofit association that is dedicated to enhancing the lives of individuals with disabilities, the elderly, and their caregivers by providing services that assist people in attaining the skills that are required to operate motor vehicles safely and efficiently for as long as possible.[4]

ADED is the premier professional association that represents the men and women working within this highly specialized area of practice, and the association works to support its members working in the field. The organization addresses the professional needs of its members by providing educational resources including timely information on its web site, hosting an annual educational conference, managing the CDRS credentialing process, and providing ongoing education and training sessions throughout the United States.

ADED AWARDS

Among the many highlights of the annual ADED conferences has been the presentation of awards including the Lifetime Honorary Member Award, the Achievement Award, the Distinguished Service Award, the Scholar Award, the Research and Applied Engineering Award, the Commercial Service Award, the Virginia Anderson Award, and the Exemplary Award. The ADED awards offer an historical view of the industry as well. The names on the perpetual plaques include founding members, industry giants, and people who are respected for their work in advancing the field of driver rehabilitation.[5]

ADED worked collaboratively with members of its sister organization, the National Mobility Equipment Dealers Association (NMEDA), to foster the highest quality of services and compliance with safety standards for equipment development and prescription. There is a synergy that occurred when the driver educators, clinicians, vendors, and manufacturers work together, "learning from each other to provide better services to our clients by combining all of the talents that each professional brings to the table."[1]

THE EVOLUTION OF ADED

ADED continued to grow, and local ADED chapters were established throughout the United States. ADED's Certificate of Professional Recognition began in 1988 and led to the development of the certification examination process by 1992. The CDRS exam was developed in 1995, which continues to be offered for professionals seeking to obtain the CDRS credential.

The ADED certification exam is an entry-level exam and helps define the minimum knowledge that an entry-level practitioner must possess, which has helped to ensure specialists possess basic core knowledge and experience. The CDRS credential signifies that an individual is competent to "plan, develop, coordinate, and implement driver rehabilitation services for people with disabilities."[4] The purpose of the ADED certification process is to protect the public by providing a program that defines the standard of practice and current knowledge required of individuals practicing driver rehabilitation; encouraging individual growth and study; promoting professionalism and ethical behavior among its members; and formally recognizing DRSs who not only fulfill the requirement for certification but are rewarded for exceptional service, teaching, or research.[4] Members of ADED commit to follow the Code of Ethics and comply with their Standards of Practice. CDRSs are likewise committed to such compliance. Standards of Practice set forth the minimal requirements that govern professional behavior in the provision of driver rehabilitation services. The ADED Code of Ethics is a set of principles to guide the professional conduct of the CDRS.

Quality driver rehabilitation services can only be achieved when standards are adopted and the proper oversight is in place. ADED is in the process of developing a Best Practices publication that will be used by its members. ADED leadership will use competency-based criteria and specific methodology for evaluating the CDRS's knowledge and competency in relation to these standards. The creation of the Best Practices will help foster uniform driver rehabilitation services across the membership. ADED will require its members to adhere to the forthcoming Best Practices in order to satisfy demands of the health care industry that expects that any professional group develop and adhere to accepted standards of practice. These Best Practices will provide a risk management framework for the CDRS as well.

Newcomers to the organization often share a perspective that supports the notion that ADED is a place to learn and share information while gaining *support and understanding* from the experienced members within the organization:

> I had my first exposure to people with disabilities in my driving school business. I was always trying to find a way to give people more mobility. I realized there were a considerable amount of safety issues associated with teaching people to drive, so I developed an instructor's brake that has superior braking power, greater comfort, and a safety-lock pin to disable the primary brake pedal. I then got involved with ADED because as I see it, ADED members are the guardians who help to ensure that people with disabilities receive every opportunity to gain independence, yet at the same time, filter out those individuals who are not capable of operating a motor vehicle safely.[6]

Clients have also benefited from the services ADED offers:

> I feel safer knowing that ADED exists to serve both clients and manufacturers for specialized driving adaptations. I hope that they continue their work and receive support from the manufacturers and clinicians alike. However, as ADED pushes for more stringent testing, evaluation protocols, and training for the clients, I am afraid that the cost of driving equipment will grow too high for people with disabilities to be able to pay for such services. I hope that this is a factor that ADED considers as it lobbies for changes in the laws.[7]

ADED understands that many clients have limited financial resources and are often on fixed incomes. ADED members work closely with traditional (e.g., workers' compensation, vocational rehabilitation services, auto insurance companies, philanthropic organizations, and religious institutions) and nontraditional (e.g., Kiwanis Club, Optimist Club, churches, synagogues, and mosques) funding sources, and clients. Automotive manufacturers such as General Motors, Ford, Toyota, and Daimler Chrysler have also created rebate programs that provide reimbursement of a portion of the cost of aftermarket adaptive equipment.

ALLIANCES

ADED has formed alliances with the Society of Automotive Engineers (SAE), NMEDA, the American Occupational Therapy Association (AOTA), the American Driver and Traffic Safety Association (ADTSA), the American Kinesiotherapy Association, the Driving School Association of America (DSAA), AAA Foundation for Traffic Safety, American Association of State Highway and Transportation Officials, American Association of Motor Vehicle Administrators (AAMVA), Canadian Association of Road Safety Professionals, Disabled Drivers Motor Club-UK, Rehabilitation Engineering and Assistive Technology Society of North America (RESNA), and Neuro-Optometric Rehabilitation Association (NORA).

A GROWING ORGANIZATION

The industry has grown including the relationships with OEMs, regulatory agencies, and the consumers through an exponential increase in the sales of adapted vehicles. The role of the CDRS is changing in order to keep up with the changing population demographics, technology advancements, and the expectation that they will provide services that address community mobility, driving cessation, and alternative transportation. ADED is at a critical juncture in its development

and place within the driver rehabilitation and community mobility industry. The evolution of the automotive adaptive equipment industry over the past three decades has changed the disability equipment market. As Tom Egan stated:

> We are literally riding the crest of a demographic wave with no end in sight. The number of vehicles modified annually is in the tens of thousands. At last count, over 400,000 vehicles that were modified with adaptive equipment were on the road. People who are 50-years-old and older represent the fastest-growing demographic group in the US. Currently there are more than 76 million people age 50 and over in North America. By 2020, this number is expected to increase 36 percent to 116 million or one in three Americans. There are currently 58 million people with disabilities, over 2 million of them in wheelchairs. The so-called 'third' age, ages 50-75, is upon us. Demographic forces and the inevitable results of a maturing industry have combined to take our industry to the next level of attractiveness from a business perspective.[8]

For ADED and the CDRS this means more clients and the need for greater accountability.

ADED is becoming a more recognizable name to many prospective clients. As clients have begun to assert their rights thanks to organizations and companies such as the AARP and iCan!, Inc., their attitudes are reflected in their buying patterns and what they expect from their driver rehabilitation evaluations. Irrespective of whether clients come to the driver evaluator wanting specific adaptive driving equipment without knowing whether or not the equipment will work for them, or they have no idea of what might be available that could help them either drive or identify reliable alternative transportation, CDRSs will continue to provide the answers. ADED and its members will also continue to play a key role in helping to ensure that helpful and accurate information about driver rehabilitation and community mobility will be disseminated to automotive dealers, OEMs, adaptive driving equipment vendors, health care professionals, law enforcement personnel, prospective and actual clients, and the public at large.[4]

SECTION II

The Future

Chad Strowmatt • Lori Benner

The future of driver rehabilitation should continue to be bright for many compelling reasons. First, as the population ages, there is an increasing demand for driver rehabilitation and alternative community mobility services that address the unique needs of the elderly and their concerned family members. Second, people with disabilities will continue to require the expertise offered by DRSs to help ensure that driving can be a viable goal after an injury or illness. Finally, community mobility services, namely, alternative transportation and driving cessation intervention, have created a new and dynamic service area for the driver rehabilitation team.

The training of, and collaboration between, professionals in the field ultimately benefit the clients served. Today and in the future, DRSs will be involved in professional activities that often impact an individual's quality of life; those activities include predriving and on-road evaluations, on-road training, vehicle acquisition and modification, automotive design, communication with officials in state and federal government agencies to advocate for favorable laws that improve reimbursement for services and equipment, and promoting the importance of driver rehabilitation services to the general public and potential referral sources such as case managers and physicians.

ADED will continue to provide its members with an organization that has been, and will continue to be, actively involved in education and training in response to the rapidly evolving field of driver rehabilitation. The organization's Mission Statement reflects this commitment:

> The Association of Driver Educators for the Disabled (ADED) is devoted primarily to the support of professionals working in the field of driver education and transportation equipment modification for persons with disabilities. The Association provides key components of education and information dissemination. ADED's functional services will be accomplished through educational conferences, professional development programs, research support, legislative efforts, and encouraging equipment development to maximize transportation options for persons with disabilities.[4]

What distinguishes ADED from other organizations is its focus on promoting an interdisciplinary approach to providing evaluation and training, which results in safe, cost-effective, and helpful options for adapted driving, alternative transportation, or both for the clients served. The members of ADED also believe that collaboration between various disciplines promotes innovative solutions to complex challenges that impair personal mobility. Occupational therapists, driver educators, other allied health professionals, engineers, rehabilitation specialists, vocational rehabilitation counselors, manufacturers, vendors, and others work together for the health, safety, and well-being of the clients and caregivers receiving services.

ADED will also continue to host yearly conferences with opportunities for continuing education and networking between its members and other attendees. The current focus of ADED is on recruiting new DRSs to meet an expanding demand for services by providing education on driver rehabilitation to professionals new to, or considering entering, the field. ADED is also committed to providing continuing education to DRSs with experience in the field. The organization is currently organizing educational courses that will reflect a core curriculum that covers the many facets of driving and driver rehabilitation. The curriculum is expected to be influenced by community needs, innovations in vehicle design, and the implementation of legislation at the state and federal levels. It is also anticipated there will be a growing need for specialization within the field to address the increasing demand for high-tech driving systems as well as services that address issues impacting the innovative solutions to the unique challenges of an aging population within the United States.

The clients served by DRSs will continue to request information about their fitness to drive, the medical implications of their condition on the tasks associated with driving, and the most reasonable solution to promote safe and efficient driving, alternative community mobility, or both. The baby boomer generation is fast approaching the age range that can result in declining health status that negatively affects driving fitness. A special challenge presented by many people within this cohort is their belief that they should be able to continue to live very active lives, including driving as their primary means for community mobility, irrespective of their functional capacity. The number of Americans aged 65 years and older is expected to double from 35 million today to 70 million by 2030, when there will be 60 million licensed drivers aged 70 and older.[9] The organization's mission, therefore, is to meet that demand and provide the highest quality services to balance the independence of the driver with the safety and well-being of all roadway users.

There are approximately 300 individuals in the world today who have voluntarily earned the CDRS designation. Historically CDRSs have most likely worked in rehabilitation facilities located in urban areas. However, CDRSs and DRSs are increasingly practicing in private practice settings and programs within small community-based hospitals. These isolated practice arenas make interdisciplinary collaboration and sharing of leading-edge information that support evidence-based practice a real challenge. In addition traditional in-house continuing education is less available for professionals working in specialized practice areas.

ADED is sponsoring course offerings to help the entry-level DRS gain the basic information needed to begin providing efficacious driver rehabilitation services. The organization's goal is to train individuals on the fundamentals of driver rehabilitation as well as the impact that medical conditions, low vision, and aging have on the driving task. Additionally courses enable the participants to explore the vehicle modification process, driver education strategies, and important issues pertaining to traffic safety. As the curriculum is developed through regional training centers, ADED's certification program will promote evidence-based practice and gain credibility in the professional community. For the experienced DRS, the long-term goal is to develop endorsements for each of the specialty areas in which DRSs consistently practice.

As a not-for-profit 501 (c-3) organization, ADED is also applying for grant funding to provide educational opportunities to promote evidence-based practice guidelines and research, as well as publish a journal for DRSs. ADED is working closely with NMEDA to improve the overall quality of the recommendations DRSs formulate and document in order to help ensure that clients receive the appropriate equipment to compensate for functional impairment. NMEDA has a quality assurance program (QAP) to help modification businesses achieve a well-defined level of professional services to meet the needs of their customers. It must be stressed that the integration of the driver rehabilitation professional with the actual installer of adaptive equipment is critical to the success and safety of our clients. Relatively speaking, ADED and NMEDA are in their infancy and must be able to adapt to the changing world in which we operate. Our clientele is living longer, surviving more serious accidents, and living with more serious medical conditions. In addition the cost of service delivery is rising. The costs of gasoline, auto insurance, and adaptive equipment are all rising at a remarkable rate. The importance of providing clients with a comprehensive driver rehabilitation evaluation, a complete and satisfactory installation of assistive devices, a final client-vehicle fitting, on-road training, and maintenance of these devices is part of the DRS's knowledge base.

AOTA has begun to work with the National Highway Traffic Safety Administration (NHTSA) to address the need for expanding the numbers of DRSs committed to address the driver rehabilitation and alternative community mobility needs of an aging baby boomer population within the United States. The first initiative is to increase occupational therapists' awareness of their ideal position to address the driving task within the activities of daily living (ADL) framework. AOTA has classified driving as an instrumental activity of daily living (IADL). IADL are often complex activities that individuals choose to engage in within various environmental contexts.[10] Driver rehabilitation is a growing niche service area.[10]

Occupational therapists generally provide driving services to older clients on one of three levels. At the first level, therapists in a wide range of clinical and community settings may evaluate clients and refer them to programs that provide driving assessments or guide access to community resources that offer alternative community mobility programs. At the second level, occupational therapists with some specialized training in driver rehabilitation help older drivers, as well as younger clients, to incorporate goals specifically related to driving and community mobility into their rehabilitation program to strengthen subskills in preparation for resuming driving, if at all possible. Therefore occupational therapists can assist older drivers on some level. However, only occupational therapists who specialize in driver rehabilitation can actually perform a comprehensive driver rehabilitation evaluation including conducting predriving clinical evaluations and on-road evaluations and training. These services comprise the third level of service delivery.[10] An aging population coupled with the limited number of professionals practicing in the field makes the initiative by the AOTA an important development. Professionals must start addressing community mobility as a daily activity for all clients served and not forget the specialized subset of skills required to do an on-road evaluation to keep both the client and DRS safe. Furthermore most DRSs believe that it is inappropriate to render an opinion on an individual's ability or inability to drive without completing a comprehensive driver rehabilitation evaluation that includes the on-road evaluation. While there have been efforts to correlate performance on clinical testing and simulator usage with successful on-road performance, the correlation has not been strong enough to draw conclusions about "passing or failing" a client without first completing the on-road evaluation.

Clearly the need for more professionals in the field is strong, and it is unclear if just one profession such as occupational therapy can produce sufficient numbers of DRSs to meet the expanding need for driver rehabilitation services. The interdisciplinary model is another model that is evolving in an effort to meet the demand; however, occupational therapists engaged in this specialized practice area will play a key role here as well. ADED will continue to promote this exciting and rewarding field to a variety of professionals, including occupational therapists, driver educators, and other allied health professionals, versus making it exclusive to a single or select number of professions.

Lobbying the health insurance industry to facilitate its understanding of the importance of driver evaluation and rehabilitation is critical to the future of the profession. The most obvious benefit of driver evaluation services for the aging population is in accident prevention. Many elderly drivers modify their driving practices as they age and through the help of programs, such as AARP's 55 Alive, recognize their declining reaction times, visual skills, and physical fitness for driving. However, there are many individuals who need a more structured approach for evaluating their fitness to drive, as they are not always willing or able to recognize their deficits. Some states require that physicians report at-risk drivers; however, physicians often need the assistance from a DRS to make an accurate assessment. Funding of evaluation services for the aging driver and remediation of remediable deficits will save millions in health care dollars spent as a result of injuries and fatalities due to unsafe drivers. The response of Medicare intermediaries to the request of payment for driver rehabilitation services has been inconsistent. While some occupational therapists have been successful in getting Medicare to pay for these services, there has been no clear avenue for other professionals to approach Medicare, and many Medicare intermediaries do not recognize driver rehabilitation services as a Medicare-eligible service. See Chapter 15 for more information on funding.

The American Medical Association (AMA) has written a position paper regarding the older driver and driver rehabilitation services. This may help to promote the need for driver evaluation and rehabilitation funding and to recognize driving as a health care issue. NHTSA is also working closely with a variety of groups to meet the needs of all drivers.

For those with a disability, no matter what the age, the eventual funding of driver rehabilitation services within the medical model will promote wellness, a return to work, and meaningful life and socialization opportunities, which will decrease costs associated with the negative consequences of lacking mobility such as unemployment and depression.

Historically health insurance policies have not recognized the therapeutic value of driver rehabilitation within the medical model. Despite groups such as the Commission on Accrediting Rehabilitation Facilities (CARF) and the Joint Commission for the Accreditation of Hospital Organizations (JCAHO) that require rehabilitation and hospital facilities to provide their patients and clients with access to driver rehabilitation professionals and services, the health care funding industry, such as Medicare and Medicaid, has not fully funded these types of services. Vocational rehabilitation programs within state governments, workers' compensation, and auto insurance have traditionally been the primary funding sources for the services of driver rehabilitation professionals and for the high cost of adaptive equipment and its installation. However, frequently the need for a vocational goal prohibits clients from being eligible for vocational rehabilitation services. In many states, the role of the DRS within the vocational rehabilitation model will be an important

one. Controlling the costs associated with driver rehabilitation services, improving the quality of services, and reducing technology abandonment and other negative consequences that result from providing clients with prescriptions that do not reflect evidence-based practice will benefit the entire driver rehabilitation industry, and especially the client.

The auto industry has been steadily developing vehicles that are safer and more user-friendly. Having better lines of sight, better fitting seats, speed-sensitive steering, adjustable foot pedals, more advanced crash-avoidance equipment options, and advanced crash-protection devices is helping to expand the role of the DRS who considers these and other critical applications of technology that help the clients served.

Historically, educating professionals in driver education and traffic safety has been conducted within teacher certification programs in colleges and universities. However, their mission was to prepare teachers to educate first-time teenage and adult drivers. These programs were generally directed at teachers or DRSs who wanted additional education in how to prepare students to engage in this important life activity. However, over the past 15 to 20 years, these programs have declined, and more and more driving instructors are being trained within satellite programs that are shorter in duration than the traditional certification programs. ADED will have to help educate DRSs and CDRSs who want to increase their knowledge in the field of driver rehabilitation. DRSs working in the field of driver rehabilitation and alternative community mobility will continue to be responsible for training first-time drivers who have medical conditions from birth, such as cerebral palsy, spina bifida, neuromuscular diseases, and orthopedic conditions. ADED's involvement in the education and training of driver rehabilitation professionals should continue to increase the number of certified professionals from its current level of more than 300 to numbers that can better meet the growing demand for these services.

REFERENCES

1. Bauman J: Personal correspondence, March 31, 2004.
2. Schultz B: Personal correspondence, March 30, 2004.
3. Repurecht P: Personal correspondence, March 31, 2004.
4. Association for Driver Rehabilitation Specialist: 1997. Available at: http://www.aded.org. Accessed March 23, 2004.
5. Lillie S: ADED Awards, *News Brake* 27:10-11, 2002.
6. Trikilas S: Personal correspondence, April 4, 2004.
7. Connor D: Personal correspondence, March 31, 2004.

8. Egan T: *Megatrends for mobility: does history repeat itself?* Paper presented at the Annual National Mobility Dealers Association Conference, Dallas, February 2004.

9. U.S. Department of Transportation: *Safe mobility for a maturing society: challenges and opportunities,* Washington, DC, 2003, U.S. Department of Transportation.

10. American Occupational Therapy Association OT Practice: *Driver rehabilitation, a growing niche,* May 10, 2004.

EDUCATIONAL MATERIALS, COMMUNITY MOBILITY, AND DRIVING CESSATION

EDUCATIONAL MATERIALS FOR CLIENTS AND CAREGIVERS*

PATIENT, FAMILY, AND CAREGIVER RESOURCE SHEETS

The materials in this appendix are handouts for patients, their family members, and caregivers. We encourage physicians and driver rehabilitation specialists (DRSs) to make copies of these handouts and use them when discussing driving issues. These handouts were designed to be user-friendly and simple to read. All patient education materials were written at or below a sixth grade reading level, and all family and caregiver materials were written at a seventh grade reading level. Listed below are additional resources and references for the materials in this appendix:

At the crossroads—a guide to Alzheimer's disease, dementia, and driving, Hartford, CT, 2000, The Hartford.
Creating mobility choices: the older driver skills assessment and resource guide, Washington, DC, 1998, American Association of Retired Persons.
Drivers 55 plus: check your own performance, Washington, DC, 1994, AAA Foundation for Traffic Safety.
Driving safely as you get older: a personal guide, Harrisburg, PA, 1999, Pennsylvania Department of Transportation.
Driving safely while aging gracefully, Washington, DC, 1999, USAA Educational Foundation.
Family conversations that help parents stay independent, Washington, DC, 2001, American Association of Retired Persons.
How to help an older driver: a guide for planning safe transportation, Washington, DC, 2000, AAA Foundation for Traffic Safety.

---

*Portions of this section have been reprinted with permission from the AMA.

LePore PR: *When you are concerned—a handbook for families, friends and caregivers worried about the safety of an aging driver*, Albany, NY, 2000, New York State Office for the Aging.
Older drivers on the go: making decisions they can live with, *UMTRI Research Review* 32:1-5, 2001.
Family and friends concerned about an older driver, Washington, DC, 2001, National Highway Traffic Safety Administration.

AM I A SAFE DRIVER?

Check the box if the statement applies to you.
☐ I get lost while driving.
☐ My friends and family members say they are worried about my driving.
☐ Other cars seem to appear out of nowhere.
☐ I have trouble seeing signs in time to respond to them.
☐ Other drivers drive too fast.
☐ Other drivers often honk at me.
☐ Driving stresses me out.
☐ After driving, I feel tired.
☐ I have had more "near misses" lately.
☐ Busy intersections bother me.
☐ Left-hand turns make me nervous.
☐ The glare from oncoming headlights bothers me.
☐ My medication makes me dizzy or drowsy.
☐ I have trouble turning the steering wheel.
☐ I have trouble pushing down on the gas pedal or brakes.
☐ I have trouble looking over my shoulder when I back up.
☐ I have been stopped by the police for my driving recently.

☐ People will no longer accept rides from me.

☐ I don't like to drive at night.

☐ I have more trouble parking lately.

If you have checked any of the boxes, your safety may be at risk when you drive. Talk to your doctor or DRS about ways to improve your safety when you drive.

Tip #1: Take care of your health. Visit your doctor regularly. Ask about tests and immunizations that are right for your age group. Eat a healthy diet. Your diet should be low in fat and high in fiber.

• Eat plenty of vegetables, fruits, beans, and whole grains.

• Eat low fat proteins in the form of lean red meat, poultry, and fish.

• Get enough calcium by drinking low fat milk and eating low fat yogurt and cheese.

• Eat a variety of foods to get enough vitamins and minerals in your diet.

• Drink lots of water.

Exercise to stay fit. Be active every day at your own level of comfort.

• Walk, dance, or swim to improve your endurance.

• Work out with weights to increase your strength.

• Stretch to maintain your flexibility.

Don't drink too much alcohol. People over the age of 65 should try not to have more than one drink per day. (A drink is one glass of wine, one bottle of beer, or one shot of liquor.) And remember: never drink alcohol with your medicines!

Don't use tobacco in any form. This means cigarettes, cigars, pipes, chew, or snuff. If you need help quitting, talk to your doctor.

Tip #2: Keep yourself safe. Make your home a safe place.

• Keep your home, walkways, and stairways well lit and uncluttered.

• Keep a fire extinguisher and smoke detectors in your home. Make sure the batteries in your smoke detectors work.

• Adjust the thermostat on your hot water tank so that you don't burn yourself with hot water.

Prevent falls.

• Make sure all throw rugs have nonslip backs so they don't throw you!

• Slip-proof your bathtub with a rubber mat.

Stay safe in the car.

• Wear your safety belt—and wear it correctly. (It should go over your shoulder and across your lap.)

• Never drink and drive!

• Don't drive when you are angry, upset, sleepy, or ill.

• If you have concerns about your driving safety, talk to your doctor.

SUCCESSFUL AGING TIPS

Tip #3: Take care of your emotional health. Keep in touch with family and friends.

It's important to maintain your social life! Exercise your mind. Keep your mind active by reading books, doing crossword puzzles, and taking classes.

Stay involved. Join community activities or volunteer projects. Somebody needs what you can offer!

Keep a positive attitude!

• Focus on the good things in your life, and don't dwell on the bad.

• Do the things that make you happy.

• If you've been feeling sad lately or no longer enjoy the things you used to, ask your doctor for help.

Tip #4: Plan for your future. Keep track of your money. Even if someone else is helping you manage your bank accounts and investments, stay informed.

Know your own health. This is important for receiving good medical care.

• Know what medical conditions you have.

• Know the names of your medicines and how to take them.

• Make a list of your medical conditions, medicines, drug allergies (if any), and the names of your doctors. Keep this list in your wallet.

Make your health care wishes known to your family and doctors.

• Consider filling out an advance directives form (i.e., living will). This form lets you state your health care choices or name someone to make these choices for you.

• Give your family and doctors a copy. This way, they have a written record of your choices in case you are unable to tell them yourself.

• If you need help with your advance directives, talk to your doctor.

Create a transportation plan.

If you don't drive, know how to get around.

• Ask family and friends if they would be willing to give you a ride.

• Find out about buses, trains, and shuttles in your area.

• If you need help finding a ride, contact your local Area Agency on Aging.

Patient and Caregiver Educational Materials
Tip #1: Drive with care.

Always—

• Plan your trips ahead of time. Decide what time to leave and which roads to take. Try to avoid heavy traffic, poor weather, and high-speed areas.

- Wear your safety belt—and wear it correctly. (It should go over your shoulder and across your lap.)
- Drive at the speed limit. It's unsafe to drive too fast or too slow.
- Be alert! Pay attention to traffic at all times.
- Keep enough distance between you and the car in front of you.
- Be extra careful at intersections. Use your turn signals and remember to look around you for people and other cars.
- Check your blind spot when changing lanes or backing up.
- Be extra careful at train tracks. Remember to look both ways for trains.
- When you take a new medicine, ask your doctor or pharmacist about side effects. Many medicines may affect your driving even when you feel fine. If your medicine makes you dizzy or drowsy, talk to your doctor to find out ways to take your medicine so it doesn't affect your driving.

Never—
- Never drink and drive.
- Never drive when you feel angry or tired. If you start to feel tired, stop your car somewhere safe. Take a break until you feel more alert.
- Never eat, drink, or use a cell phone while driving.

If—
- If you don't see well in the dark, try not to drive at night or during storms.
- If you have trouble making left turns at an intersection, make three right turns instead of one left turn.
- If you can, avoid driving in bad weather, such as during rain, sleet, or snow.

Tip #2: Take care of your car.
- Make sure you have plenty of gas in your car.
- Have your car tuned up regularly.
- Keep your windshields and mirrors clean.
- Keep a cloth in your car for cleaning windows.
- Replace your windshield wiper blades when they become worn out.
- Consider using Rain-X or a similar product to keep your windows clear.
- If you are shopping for a new car, look for a car with power steering and automatic transmission.

Tip #3: Know where you can find a ride. How do you get around when your car is in the shop? If you don't know the answer to this question, it's time for you to put together a "transportation plan." A transportation plan is a list of all the ways that you can get around. Use this list when your car is in the shop or when you don't feel safe driving.

Your transportation plan might include:
- Rides from friends and family
- Taxi
- Bus or train
- Senior shuttle

If you need help creating a transportation plan, your doctor can get you started.

Tip #4: Take a driver safety class. To learn how to drive more safely, try taking a class. In a driver safety class, the instructor teaches you skills that you can use when you are driving. To find a class near you, call one of the following programs:

AARP 55 ALIVE Driver Safety Program
1 888 227-7669
AAA Safe Driving for Mature Operators Program
Call your local AAA club to find a class near you.
National Safety Council Defensive Driving Course
1 800 621-7619
Driving School Association of the Americas, Inc.
1 800 270-3722

These classes usually last several hours. They don't cost much—some are even free. As an added bonus, you might receive a discount on your auto insurance after taking one of these classes. Talk to your insurance company to see if it offers a discount.

As experienced drivers grow older, changes in their vision, attention, and physical abilities may cause them to drive less safely than they used to. Sometimes these changes happen so slowly that the drivers are not even aware that their driving safety is at risk. If you have questions about a loved one's driving safety, here's what you can do to help him or her stay safe AND mobile.

Is your loved one a safe driver?

If you have the chance, go for a ride with your loved one. Look for the following warning signs in his or her driving:
- Forgets to buckle up
- Does not obey stop signs or traffic lights
- Fails to yield the right of way
- Drives too slowly or too quickly
- Often gets lost, even on familiar routes
- Stops at a green light or at the wrong time
- Doesn't seem to notice other cars, people walking, or bike riders on the road
- Doesn't stay in his or her lane
- Is honked at or passed often
- Reacts slowly to driving situations
- Makes poor driving decisions

Other signs of unsafe driving include:
- Recent near misses or fender benders
- Recent tickets for moving violations

- Comments from passengers about close calls, near misses, or the driver not seeing other vehicles
- Recent increase in the car insurance premium

Riding with or following this person every once in a while is one way to keep track of his or her driving. Another way is to talk to this person's spouse or friends.

If you are concerned about your loved one's driving, what can you do?

Talk to your loved one. Say that you are concerned about his or her driving safety. Does he or she share your concern?

- Don't bring up your concerns in the car. It's dangerous to distract the driver! Wait until you have his or her full attention.
- Explain why you are concerned. Give specific reasons—for example, recent fender benders, getting lost, or running stop signs.
- Realize that your loved one may become upset or defensive. After all, driving is important for independence and self-esteem.
- If your loved one doesn't want to talk about driving at this time, bring it up again later.

Your continued concern and support may help him or her feel more comfortable with this topic.

- Be a good listener. Take your loved one's concerns seriously.

HOW TO HELP THE OLDER DRIVER

Help make plans for transportation. When your loved one is ready to talk about his or her driving safety, you can work together to create plans for future safety.

- Make a formal agreement about driving. In this agreement, your loved one chooses a person to tell him or her when it is no longer safe to drive. This person then agrees to help your loved one make the transition to driving retirement. You can find a sample agreement in *At the Crossroads: A Guide to Alzheimer's Disease, Dementia & Driving*. Order a free copy by writing to:

At the Crossroads Booklet, the Hartford, 200 Executive Boulevard, Southington, CT 06489.

- Help create a transportation plan. Your loved one may rely less on driving if he or she has other ways to get around.

Encourage a visit to the doctor. The doctor can check your loved one's medical history, list of medicines, and current health to see if any of these may be affecting his or her driving safety. The doctor can also provide treatment to help improve driving safety.

Encourage your loved one to take a driving test.

A driver rehabilitation specialist (DRS) can assess your loved one's driving safety through an office exam and driving test. The DRS can also teach special techniques or suggest special equipment to help him or her drive more safely. (To find a DRS in your area, ask your doc-

tor for a referral or contact the Association for Driver Rehabilitation Specialists [ADED]. Contact information for ADED is listed on the following page.) If a DRS is not available in your area, contact a local driving school or your state's Department of Motor Vehicles to see if they can do a driving test.

How to help when your loved one retires from driving. At some point, your loved one may need to stop driving for his or her own safety and the safety of others on the road. You and your loved one may come to this decision yourselves, or at the recommendation of the doctor, DRS, driving instructor, or Department of Motor Vehicles. When someone close to you retires from driving, there are several things you can do to make this easier for him or her:

- Create a transportation plan. It's often easier for people to give up driving if they have other ways to get around. Help your loved one create a list of "tried-and-true" ride options. This list can include:
  - The names and phone numbers of friends and relatives who are willing to give rides, with the days and times they are available.
  - The phone number of a local cab company.
  - Which bus or train to take to get to a specific place. Try riding with your loved one the first time to help him or her feel more comfortable.
  - The phone number for a shuttle service. Call the community center and regional transit authority to see if they offer a door-to-door shuttle service for older passengers.
  - The names and phone numbers of volunteer drivers. Call the community center, church, or synagogue to see if they have a volunteer driver program.
  - If you need help finding other ride options, contact the Area Agency on Aging. (The contact information is on the next page.)

If your loved one can't go shopping, help him or her shop from home. Arrange for medicines and groceries to be delivered. Explore on-line ordering or subscribe to catalogs and "go shopping" at home. See which services make house calls—local hairdressers or barbers may be able to stop by for a home visit.

Encourage social activities. Visits with friends, time spent at the senior center, and volunteer work are important for one's health and well-being. When creating a transportation plan, don't forget to include rides to social activities. It's especially important for your loved one to maintain social ties and keep spirits high during this time of adjustment.

Be there for your loved one. Let your loved one know that he or she has your support. Offer help willingly and be a good listener. This is an emotionally difficult time, and it's important to show that you care.

Where can I get more help?
Contact the following organizations if you need more help assessing your loved one's driving safety or creating a transportation plan.

American Automobile Association (AAA) Foundation for Traffic Safety
1 800 993-7222
www.aaafoundation.org
Call the toll-free number or visit the Web site to order free booklets on how to help an older driver.

American Association of Retired Persons (AARP)
55 ALIVE Driver Safety Program
1 888 227-7669
www.aarp.org/drive
Visit the Web site to find safe driving tips, information on aging and driving, and details about the 55 ALIVE Driver Safety Program—a classroom course for drivers age 50 and older.

In this course, participants review driving skills and learn tips to help them drive more safely.

Call the toll-free number or visit the Web site above to find a class in your loved one's area.

Area Agency on Aging (AAA)
Eldercare Locator: 1 800 677-1116
www.aoa.gov
The local Area Agency on Aging can connect your loved one to services in the area, including ride programs, Meals-on-Wheels, home health services, and more. Call the Eldercare Locator or visit the Web site above to find the phone number for your loved one's local Area Agency on Aging.

Association for Driver Rehabilitation Specialists (ADED)
1 800 290-2344
www.driver-ed.org or www.aded.net
Call the toll-free number or visit the Web site to find a DRS in your loved one's area.

Easter Seals
1 312 726-7200
Easter Seals' *Caregiver Transportation Toolkit* includes a video, booklet, and list of helpful products and resources for family caregivers and volunteer drivers. To order the toolkit, call the number above or write to: Easter Seals National Headquarters, 230 Monroe Street, Suite 1800, Chicago, IL 60606.

National Association of Private Geriatric Care Managers (NAPGCM)
1 520 881-8008
www.caremanager.org
A geriatric care manager can help older persons and their families arrange long-term care, including transportation services. Call the phone number or visit the Web site above to find a geriatric care manager in your loved one's area.

National Association of Social Workers (NASW)
www.socialworkers.org
A social worker can counsel your loved one, assess social and emotional needs, and assist in locating and coordinating transportation and community services. To find a qualified clinical social worker in your loved one's area, search the NASW Register of Clinical Social Workers.

Who doesn't drive?
If you don't drive, you're in good company. Many people stop driving because of the hassle and expense of auto insurance, car maintenance, and gasoline. Other people stop driving because they feel unsafe on the road. Some people never learned how to drive in the first place! Although most Americans use their cars to get around, many people get by just fine without one. In this sheet, we suggest ways to get by without driving.

Where can you find a ride?
Here are some ways to get a ride. See which ones work best for you.
- Ask a friend or relative for a ride. Offer to pay for the gasoline.
- Take public transportation. Can a train or bus take you where you need to go? Call your regional transit authority and ask for directions.
- Take a taxicab. To cut down on costs, try sharing a cab with friends. Also, find out if your community offers discounted fares for seniors.
- Ride a Senior Transit Shuttle. Call your community center or local Area Agency on Aging (AAA) to see if your neighborhood has a shuttle service.
- Ask about volunteer drivers. Call your community center, church, or synagogue to see if it has a volunteer driver program.
- Ride a Medi-car. If you need a ride to your doctor's office, call your local Area Agency on Aging to see if a Medi-car can take you there.

If you can't go out to get something, have it come to you.

Many stores will deliver their products straight to your door.
- Have your groceries delivered. Many stores deliver for free or for a low fee. You can also ask your family, friends, or volunteers from your local community center, church, or synagogue if they can pick up your groceries for you.
- Order your medicines by mail. Not only is this more convenient—it's often less expensive, too. Order only from pharmacies that you know and trust.
- Have your meals delivered to you. Many restaurants will deliver meals for free or for a low fee. Also, you may be eligible for Meals-on-Wheels, a program that delivers hot meals at a low cost. Call your local Area

Agency on Aging for more information about Meals-on-Wheels.

- Shop from catalogs. You can buy almost everything you need from catalogs: clothing, pet food, toiletries, gifts, and more! Many catalogs are now also available on the Internet.

GETTING BY WITHOUT DRIVING

Where can you find more information about services in your area?
The following agencies can provide you with information to get you started:
Area Agency on Aging (AAA)
Eldercare Locator
1 800 677-1116

Call this toll-free number and ask for the phone number of your local Area Agency on Aging (AAA). Your local AAA can tell you more about ride options, Meals-on-Wheels, and senior recreation centers in your area.
National Institute on Aging (NIA)
Resource Directory for Older People
1 800 222-2225

Call this toll-free number and ask the National Institute on Aging (NIA) to send you its Resource Directory for Older People. This 111-page directory lists organizations that provide services for older people.

Put it all together.

Fill out the table below with names and phone numbers of services in your area. Keep this information handy by placing it next to your phone or posting it on your refrigerator.

Service Phone Numbers

Name of Company	Phone Number	Contact Name

Physician's guide to assessing and counseling older drivers,
American Medical Association/National Highway Traffic Safety Administration/U.S. Department of Transportation, June 2003.

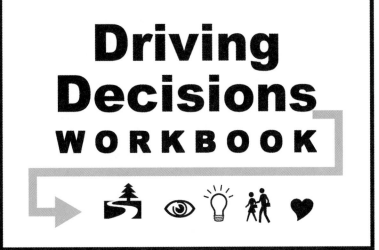

UMTRI-2000-14

MARCH 2000

This work was sponsored by General Motors Corporation pursuant to an agreement between General Motors and the United States Department of Transportation. The opinions, findings, and conclusions expressed in this document are those of the authors and not necessarily those of General Motors Corporation or the United States Department of Transportation.

ACKNOWLEDGMENTS

We acknowledge several individuals who were essential to the completion of this work. Lidia Kostyniuk, Fredrick Streff, and Patricia Waller contributed valuable input into development of a framework for thinking about older-driver issues. Neil Alexander, Jesse Blatt, Lawrence Decina, Allen Dobbs, Sally Guthrie, Regula Herzog, Paula Kartje, Lawrence Lonero, Richard Marottoli, Cynthia Owsley, Donald Reinfurt, Sandra Rosenbloom, Kenneth Stack, Jane Stutts, and Jean Wilkins contributed important feedback on development of the workbook itself. Tiffany Fordyce, Jonathon Vivoda, and Jennifer Zakrajsek assisting in pilot testing and validation of the workbook. Finally, we acknowledge the support of the University of Michigan Claude D. Pepper Older Americans Independence Center (NIA Grant #AG08808) for providing lists of potential subjects for the pilot testing and validation of the workbook.

David W. Eby
Lisa J. Molnar
Jean T. Shope

Social and Behavioral Analysis Division
University of Michigan
Transportation Research Institute

Driving Decisions WORKBOOK

David W. Eby

Lisa J. Molnar

Jean T. Shope

Driving Decisions Workbook

All of us need to be able to get around. Getting around is important not only for running errands, going to appointments, and getting to work, but in order to visit with friends and family, to have fun, and to just get out of the house. Most of us prefer to get around by driving a car. Some of us, however, may have changes in our abilities, such as seeing, that make it more difficult to drive safely. Some changes occur with age and happen so slowly over time that we may not even have noticed them. In order to make good decisions about driving, it is important to know as much as possible about any changes in ability we've had, how these changes might be related to safe driving, and what we can do about them.

This workbook will help you learn about age-related changes in abilities and habits that could affect safe driving. After you respond to questions about yourself, feedback is provided about what various changes may mean for driving and what you can do to increase safety.

The workbook contains five sections—each has to do with an area that affects safe driving. Each section should take 5-10 minutes to read and complete. Within each section, there are questions on different topics. For each question, please circle the answer that best describes your situation. Arrows connect certain answers to feedback—information about various problems and suggestions to deal with those problems.

Regardless of your answers, you may want to read all of the feedback to learn more about what various changes could mean for your driving in the future. Or, you may be thinking of other people who may have had these changes. Knowing more about age-related changes that can affect driving helps us to anticipate situations and plan ahead for them.

You can go through the workbook by yourself, with a friend, or with your family. Everyone can benefit from knowing more about how to keep driving safely.

The five sections in this workbook include:

 On the Road

◉ **Seeing**

💡 **Thinking**

🧍🧍 **Getting Around**

♥ **Health**

ON THE ROAD

Questions:

How stressful for you is <u>driving in unfamiliar areas</u> during the daytime?

Not at all   Not very   Somewhat   Very

How much difficulty do you have following directions or a map in <u>unfamiliar areas</u>?

None   A little   Some   A lot

Do you avoid driving to new places far away from home?

No   Yes

Feedback:

Driving in unfamiliar areas may be a problem for you. Certain types of driving errors are more likely on unfamiliar than familiar routes, including stopping over the limit lines, driving too slowly, and turning too wide or too short.

► Plan your trip ahead of time and write down driving instructions.

► Do a trial run with a passenger before your actual trip.

► Choose left-turn locations where traffic signals have arrows.

► Ask someone to ride with you to read a map or street signs.

► Be prepared for an emergency by thinking of potential problems. Take along emergency signs and phone numbers.

► Reduce distractions in your car (for example, don't smoke, eat, talk on phone, put on makeup, shave, watch scenery, or daydream).

ON THE ROAD 1

Questions:

How stressful for you is <u>driving at night</u>?

Not at all   Not very   Somewhat   Very

During <u>night driving</u>, do you think that most other drivers on the road are driving too fast?

No   Yes

During <u>night driving</u>, how much difficulty do you have reading well-lit signs?

None   A little   Some   A lot

During <u>night driving</u>, how much difficulty do you have seeing because of oncoming headlights, even when they are properly dimmed?

None   A little   Some   A lot

During <u>night driving</u> in the <u>past year</u>, how many traffic tickets or warnings have you had?

None   One   Two or more

During <u>night driving</u> in the <u>past year</u>, how many times have you almost or actually been in a traffic accident?

None   One   Two or more

In the past year, has a friend, relative, or doctor expressed concern about your driving at <u>night</u>?

No   Yes

Feedback:

Night driving may be a problem for you. This could be from a decline in vision over time. More information on vision loss is given in the section on "seeing."

► Before starting out, give your eyes at least 5 minutes to adjust to the darkness.

► Avoid wearing tinted glasses or sunglasses.

► Make sure that your car's windshield, windows, mirrors, and headlights are clean.

► Always dim your headlights for oncoming cars.

► Try to drive on well-lit streets—the more light there is, the easier it is to read signs, and the less headlight glare there is.

► Consider getting an eye exam.

► If you must go out at night, make sure to drive more cautiously.

► Reduce the amount of night driving you do, or stop altogether.

ON THE ROAD 2

Questions:

Feedback:

How stressful for you is <u>driving in bad weather</u> (such as rain, snow, or fog)?

    Not at all   *Not very*   *Somewhat*   *Very*

How much does rain on the windshield bother you?

    None   *A little*   *Some*   *A lot*

While <u>driving in bad weather</u> in the <u>past year</u>, how many times have you almost or actually been in a traffic accident?

    None   *One*   *Two or more*

In the past year, has a friend, relative, or doctor expressed concern about your driving in bad weather?

    No   *Yes*

Driving in bad weather may be a problem for you. Bad weather can affect your ability to see well and drive safely.

▶ Choose your driving conditions wisely. Avoid driving in bad weather by checking weather conditions before you start out.

▶ Make sure you are well stocked with food and other household necessities so that you don't have to go out in bad weather.

▶ If you must drive in bad weather, turn on your lights regardless of the time of day.

▶ Make sure that your car's windshield, windows, mirrors, and headlights are clean.

▶ Check your brakes before starting out to make sure they're working.

▶ Increase your "cushion of safety" by allowing more distance between you and the car in front of you. While stopped in traffic, you should be able to see the tires of the car in front of you.

▶ Be alert to changing road conditions.

▶ If weather becomes bad, park well off the road and wait—if you are on the freeway, get off at an exit before finding a safe place to park.

▶ Slow down in anticipation of slippery spots.

 ON THE ROAD 3

Questions:

Feedback:

How stressful for you is <u>driving in heavy traffic</u>?

    Not at all   *Not very*   *Somewhat*   *Very*

How much difficulty do you have pulling out into a busy street or freeway?

    None   *A little*   *Some*   *A lot*

How often do other cars proceed when you feel you have the right of way at intersections with stop signs?

    Never   *Rarely*   *Sometimes*   *Often*

How often do other drivers honk at you?

    Never   *Rarely*   *Sometimes*   *Often*

While <u>driving in heavy traffic</u> in the <u>past year</u>, how many traffic tickets or warnings have you had?

    None   *One*   *Two or more*

While <u>driving in heavy traffic</u> in the <u>past year</u>, how many times have you almost or actually been in a traffic accident?

    None   *One*   *Two or more*

In the past year, has a friend, relative, or doctor expressed concern about your driving in <u>heavy traffic</u>?

    No   *Yes*

Driving in heavy traffic may be a problem for you. This may be due to changes in your vision, your thinking, or your movement abilities. These changes are discussed in sections on "seeing," "thinking," and "getting around." Together, these changes may reduce your ability to react quickly and safely to the demands of driving in heavy traffic.

Studies show that intersections that cause trouble for older drivers are those with right-of-way and left-turn decisions. Drivers may have trouble using information from several sources at once, anticipating what others may do, paying attention to traffic signs and signals, and being aware of their own position in traffic.

▶ Avoid driving in congested, fast-moving traffic.

▶ Find out before you leave home about road closings and construction (through radio, newspapers, TV).

▶ Plan your routes in advance to reduce the number of left turns you must make.

▶ Increase your cushion of safety by allowing more distance between your car and the car in front of you.

▶ Stay current on rules of the road and become familiar with new lane markings and traffic signals and signs.

▶ Let other drivers and pedestrians know your intentions by positioning your car in the proper lane and signaling.

▶ Check all your mirrors often—we tend to focus on what's ahead, but traffic comes from many directions.

▶ Consider taking a driving refresher course. You may want to contact your AARP or AAA office or Area Agency on Aging to find out more about such courses.

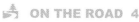 ON THE ROAD 4

Questions:

In the past year, have you dozed or "nodded off" for a moment while driving?

No   *Yes*

In the past year, have you had to open the window, play the radio, or have a passenger talk with you in order to stay alert while driving?

No   *Yes*

How stressful for you is driving long distances?

Not at all   *Not very*   *Somewhat*   *Very*

▶ **Feedback:**

You may get overly tired while driving. Older drivers are especially prone to "highway hypnosis" with increased blinking, dozing off, lapses in time not remembered, voices and sounds that seem far away or louder than normal, and your car slowing down without your awareness that you let up on the gas.

▶ Start out well rested—don't drive if you are tired or sleepy.

▶ Pace yourself—take a break every 1-2 hours on long trips.

▶ Get out of the car and stretch or walk on breaks.

▶ Drink plenty of water.

▶ Increase your strength and flexibility by exercise to help prevent tiredness.

▶ Ask someone else to drive when tired.

▶ Remember that most methods people use to stay awake while driving only work for a short period of time, and sometimes not at all.

ON THE ROAD 5

Questions:

Overall, how stressful for you is driving?

Not at all   *Not very*   *Somewhat*   *Very*

How much difficulty do you have backing up?

None   *A little*   *Some*   *A lot*

How much difficulty do you have making right turns?

None   *A little*   *Some*   *A lot*

How much difficulty do you have making left turns across traffic?

None   *A little*   *Some*   *A lot*

How often do you find yourself disoriented while driving?

Never   *Rarely*   *Sometimes*   *Often*

▶ **Feedback:**

You could be having a general problem with your driving. Here are some things you can do:

▶ Plan your route before you start, so you can focus your effort on driving, rather than finding your way.

▶ Adjust mirrors and seat before starting.

▶ Always check your mirrors and blind spots, and signal well before making a lane change.

▶ Stay informed of changes in highway regulations, traffic signals, and symbols.

▶ Consider taking a driving refresher course. Contact your AARP or AAA office or Area Agency on Aging to find out more about such courses.

▶ Consider having a medical, vision, or driving check-up.

▶ When driving an unfamiliar car, take time to locate all controls before you start out.

▶ Travel when there is little traffic, such as during the middle of the day.

▶ Avoid left turns, if possible. This can be done by planning your travel routes in advance.

▶ Reduce distractions while driving, such as listening to the radio, talking with a passenger, or sightseeing.

▶ Gather information on local alternatives to driving such as public transportation, taxi services, or senior ride programs, and try them out.

ON THE ROAD 6

Questions:

In the past year, have you noticed that someone preferred to ride with someone else or drive, rather than ride with you driving?

No   *Yes*

In the past year, has a friend or family member refused to ride with you because of your driving?

No   *Yes*

In the past year, has a friend, relative, or doctor expressed concern about your driving?

No   *Yes*

Feedback:

Relatives, friends, and doctors can be a valuable and objective source of information about your driving. Research shows that many older drivers expect their family and friends to discuss driving problems with them, but such conversations can be difficult. Family and friends may try to share their concerns about driving but some older drivers may resist hearing those concerns.

▶ Ask a trusted person to honestly tell you how safely they think you drive.

▶ If others express concern, you might consider reducing or stopping your driving.

▶ Consider taking a driving refresher course. Contact your AARP or AAA office or Area Agency on Aging to find out more about such courses.

▶ Consider having an evaluation of your driving done. Ask your local driving schools, doctor, or Area Agency on Aging to find our where you might get an evaluation done.

ON THE ROAD 7

Questions:

How many times have you almost or actually been in a traffic accident in the past year?

None   *One*   *Two or more*

How many traffic tickets or warnings have you had in the past year?

None   *One*   *Two or more*

Feedback:

Drivers who have almost or actually been in traffic accidents are more likely to have an accident in the future, regardless of whether or not they were at fault. If you have come close to being in an accident, think about how you might have prevented the situation. Could you have reacted differently? Did you fail to see something? Why was the other car honking at you?

Tickets can also be an early warning sign of driving problems. Some drivers are aware of their limits and cope with them. Others, however, overestimate their abilities. The most frequent problems of older drivers include failure to observe signs and signals, careless crossing of intersections, failure to yield, changing lanes without regard for others, improper backing, and driving too slowly. Inattention and having too much information to handle at once seem to be the root of most of these conditions.

▶ Consider taking a driving refresher course. Contact your AARP or AAA office or Area Agency on Aging to find out more about such courses.

▶ Consider having a private evaluation of your driving done. Ask your local driving schools, doctor, or Area Agency on Aging to find out where you might get an evaluation done.

ON THE ROAD 8

SEEING

In answering these questions, assume that you are wearing glasses or contact lenses if you normally do.

Questions:

Would you say your eyesight now using both eyes (with glasses or contact lenses, if you wear them) is:

Excellent　　*Good*　　*Fair*　　*Poor*

How much do you worry about how well you see now?

Not at all　　*A little*　　*Some*　　*A lot*

Has a doctor ever told you that you are blind in one eye?

No　　*Yes*

Feedback:

You may have a vision problem. As we age, we experience declines in our vision. There are several types of vision declines that could increase the chance of being in an accident. These declines relate to our ability to read traffic signs, recover our focus at night, quickly detect brake lights, and correctly judge the speed and location of other cars around us. While some vision problems are not correctable, many problems can be corrected under a doctor's care.

▶ It is important to get regular eye exams.

▶ Let the eye doctor know about any changes in your vision.

SEEING 1

Questions:

How much difficulty do you have seeing due to the glare from your windshield when the sun is low in the sky?

None　　*A little*　　*Some*　　*A lot*

When driving at night, how much are you bothered by the properly dimmed headlights of oncoming cars?

Not at all　　*A little*　　*Some*　　*A lot*

How much difficulty do you have seeing something when lights are being reflected from it (for example, watching television when the room lights are shining on the screen)?

None　　*A little*　　*Some*　　*A lot*

Feedback:

You may have difficulty with "glare recovery." As we age, our eyes become more sensitive to glare, making it more difficult to see while driving at night. Studies show that older people need a lot more time than younger people to see properly after lights are shined into their eyes. Some drivers try to solve this problem by wearing sunglasses at night, but that actually makes it more difficult to see at night and makes for a more dangerous driver.

▶ It is important to have regular eye exams.

▶ Let the eye doctor know about any problems you may be having with glare recovery.

▶ Try to avoid driving at night.

▶ Avoid looking directly into the headlights of other cars on the road.

▶ Try to drive on well-lit streets—the more light there is, the less headlight glare there is.

SEEING 2

Questions:

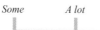**Feedback:**

How much difficulty do you have reading ordinary newspaper print?

None   *A little*   *Some*   *A lot*

How much difficulty do you have reading small print in a telephone book, on a medicine bottle, or on a map?

None   *A little*   *Some*   *A lot*

When driving at night, does your instrument panel seem blurry or out-of-focus even though it is bright enough?

No   *Yes*

You may be having a problem with near-vision; that is, the ability to see things clearly that are close. As we age, our ability to see details, such as printed words or the car's instrument panel, may decline. Problems with near-vision can also be caused by cataracts which often can be treated successfully.

Because glasses or contact lenses may help you see better, it is important to:

▶ Get regular eye exams.

▶ Tell the eye doctor about any changes in your near-vision.

SEEING 3

Questions:

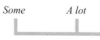**Feedback:**

When you are not moving, how much difficulty do you have reading a sign or recognizing a picture because it is moving (such as an advertisement on a passing bus or truck)?

None   *A little*   *Some*   *A lot*

How much difficulty do you have, because of your eyesight, recognizing people across a room?

None   *A little*   *Some*   *A lot*

Do you need to squint in order to see things far away or to watch television?

No   *Yes*

You may be having a problem with far-vision; that is, the ability to see things clearly that are far away. In driving, problems with far-vision may make it difficult to read road signs and see lines painted on the road. Studies show that problems with far-vision increase with age and can increase our chance of being in an accident. Problems with far-vision can also be made worse by cataracts which can often be treated successfully.

Because glasses or contact lenses may help you see better, it is important to:

▶ Get regular eye exams.

▶ Tell your eye doctor of any changes in your far-vision.

SEEING 4

Questions:

How often when you are driving and looking straight ahead, do other vehicles seem to come into your peripheral or side vision unexpectedly?

Never   Rarely   Sometimes   Often

When merging into traffic, how often are you "surprised" by a vehicle that you didn't notice until it was quite close to you?

Never   Rarely   Sometimes   Often

While looking ahead, whether driving or not, how much difficulty do you have noticing things off to the side?

None   A little   Some   A lot

Feedback:

You may have reduced peripheral or side vision, the ability to see off to the sides without moving our head or eyes. The larger our side vision, the more we can see without moving our head or eyes. Research shows that as we age, our side vision decreases. Studies also show that decreased side vision can increase a person's chance of being in an accident. Decreased side vision makes it harder to see cars and people off to the side, making it difficult to react in time to avoid a problem.

Things you can do that may help you partly overcome a problem with reduced side vision include:

▶ Move your head and eyes to the sides occasionally as you drive.

▶ Adjust the existing mirrors on your car to increase your range of vision.

▶ Use special mirrors that increase your range of vision.

👁 SEEING 5

Questions:

How much difficulty do you have indoors seeing when the lights are dim (for example, reading a menu in a dimly lit restaurant)?

None   A little   Some   A lot

How much difficulty do you have at night keeping your car's instrument panel in focus because it is just too dim?

None   A little   Some   A lot

How much difficulty do you have seeing the taillights of other vehicles because they are not bright enough?

None   A little   Some   A lot

Feedback:

You may have decreased sensitivity to light. Sensitivity to light has to do with our ability to see things when the light is dim, such as at night. Studies show that sensitivity decreases with age—the older we are the more light we need to see things and the longer it takes for our eyes to adjust to changes in lighting conditions. Decreased sensitivity might make it more difficult to drive at night and, therefore, less safe.

▶ It is important to notice changes in your sensitivity to light.

▶ Get regular eye exams.

▶ Try to avoid driving at night.

▶ Increase the brightness of your car's instrument panel if it can be adjusted.

▶ If you must drive at night, drive more cautiously.

▶ Try to drive on well-lit streets—the more light there is, the better you will be able to see.

▶ Make sure your windshield, lights, and mirrors are clean.

👁 SEEING 6

Questions:

How much difficulty do you have judging your speed without looking at the speedometer?

 None *A little*   *Some*   *A lot*

How much difficulty do you have judging distances for parking?

 None *A little*   *Some*   *A lot*

How much difficulty do you have judging how fast you are approaching a stopped vehicle?

 None *A little*   *Some*   *A lot*

Feedback:

You may be having a problem with depth perception—our ability to accurately judge the distance between other objects and us. In driving, we use depth perception to merge with and to cross traffic, as well as for parking. Studies show that these abilities may decline with age—older drivers perceive distance less accurately than younger drivers do.

▶ It is important to be aware of changes in your vision.

▶ Have your eyes checked by your eye doctor regularly.

▶ Allow more distance between your car and the car in front of you.

▶ Pay attention to cars braking far ahead of you—not just the car immediately in front of you—so you are more ready to stop.

                                        👁 SEEING 7

THINKING

Questions:

In general, how much difficulty do you have carrying on a conversation and listening to the radio or television at the same time?

 None *A little*   *Some*   *A lot*

While you are driving, how much difficulty do you have also talking with passengers?

 None *A little*   *Some*   *A lot*

While you are driving, how much difficulty do you have also changing the radio station?

 None *A little*   *Some*   *A lot*

Feedback:

You may be having a problem with "divided attention"—the ability to do two things at once, such as keeping track of your driving speed and what other cars are doing at the same time. Research shows that tasks requiring divided attention, such as driving, become harder as we age. In normal driving, we must divide our attention among several things. The task becomes more difficult when there are distractions, either in the car (a radio or passenger) or outside (bad weather).

▶ Keep your eyes on the road while you are driving.

▶ Reduce distractions inside your car, such as talking with passengers, trying to read a road map, changing radio stations, or talking on the phone.

▶ Drive when there are fewer distractions outside (such as bad weather or heavy traffic).

▶ Plan your trip in advance.

▶ Have a passenger help you find your way.

▶ Avoid driving in unfamiliar areas.

▶ Avoid busy traffic situations.

                                        💡 THINKING 1

Questions:

How much difficulty do you have finding something on a crowded shelf?

None　　*A little*　　*Some*　　*A lot*

How much difficulty do you have carrying on a conversation when there is noise in the background (such as other people talking)?

None　　*A little*　　*Some*　　*A lot*

How much difficulty do you have finding a certain sign among many other signs (for example, finding a restaurant sign on a street with many other signs)?

None　　*A little*　　*Some*　　*A lot*

Feedback:

You may be having a problem with "selective attention"—the ability to ignore what is **not** important while focusing on what **is** important. In driving, this means our ability to quickly direct attention to the most important events. Studies show that selective attention abilities are poorer among older than younger adults, and that as selective attention abilities decline, the chance of being in an accident increases. Many problems for older drivers involve not seeing or correctly understanding road signs, as well as failing to yield the right-of-way. These problems come from not paying attention to the right things in the driving situation.

▶ Avoid driving where there are many signs.

▶ Plan your trip in advance.

▶ Have a passenger help you find your way.

▶ Avoid driving in unfamiliar areas.

▶ Avoid busy traffic situations.

 THINKING 2

Questions:

How much difficulty do you have understanding people who speak quickly?

None　　*A little*　　*Some*　　*A lot*

How often do you have to slow down to read unfamiliar road signs?

Never　　*Rarely*　　*Sometimes*　　*Often*

How often are you uncomfortable because traffic seems to be moving too quickly?

Never　　*Rarely*　　*Sometimes*　　*Often*

Feedback:

The speed of your thinking and decision making may have decreased. Research shows that this speed declines with age. This change can lead to slow or hesitant driving, unexpected lane changes, and slowed reactions to driving situations. All of these things combine to increase the chance of being in a traffic accident.

▶ Plan your trip in advance.

▶ Avoid busy traffic situations.

▶ Take routes that are less crowded.

▶ Avoid areas where drivers tend to drive very fast.

▶ Consider asking your doctor about checking your "*cognition*" (that is, your thinking).

THINKING 3

Questions:

In the past year, how often have you missed an appointment because you forgot about it?

    Never   *Rarely*   *Sometimes*   *Often*

In the past year, how often have you had difficulty finding your car in a parking lot?

    Never   *Rarely*   *Sometimes*   *Often*

In the past year, how often have you had difficulty finding your way home from a familiar place (such as the grocery store)?

    Never   *Rarely*   *Sometimes*   *Often*

Feedback:

You may be having a problem with your memory. Memory helps us use a familiar traffic route and remember the rules for safe driving behavior. Our memory is also important in problem solving and decision making. Studies show that some older adults have difficulty recalling things when they want to remember them. Even otherwise healthy older drivers may have trouble remembering what to do in certain driving situations or recalling driving rules or laws. This problem increases the chance of being in a traffic accident and should be taken seriously.

▶ You may want to ask your doctor about checking your memory.

▶ Consider taking a driving refresher course. Contact your AARP or AAA office or Area Agency on Aging to find out more about such courses.

▶ Plan your trip ahead and write down the route.

▶ Drive the route ahead of time to become familiar with it.

▶ Look up information that you are having trouble remembering. This will help you remember it in the future.

 THINKING 4

 # GETTING AROUND

Questions:

How much pain, stiffness, or weakness do you have in your hips, knees, ankles, or feet?

    None   *A little*   *Some*   *A lot*

How much difficulty do you have getting in and out of a car?

    None   *A little*   *Some*   *A lot*

How much difficulty do you have turning your head to back up or to check for traffic?

    None   *A little*   *Some*   *A lot*

Feedback:

You may have decreased flexibility—how far we can move a joint or stretch a muscle. As we age, our flexibility can be reduced, making it harder to do certain driving tasks. Decreased neck flexibility makes it hard to turn our heads leading to difficulty backing up, checking for traffic at intersections, and changing lanes. Discomfort in joints can slow reaction time and reduce our ability to turn the steering wheel or step on the brake. Fortunately, studies show that flexibility can often be improved through exercise and stretching.

▶ Check with your doctor or senior center about programs in your area that might help you improve your flexibility.

▶ Avoid long periods of driving without a stretch break.

▶ Avoid driving when muscle or joint pain is intense.

▶ Avoid driving when muscles are stiff.

▶ Fit your car with special mirrors.

▶ Begin a fitness program. It's never too late to start.

Questions:

How much difficulty do you have opening and closing doors in public buildings?

None   *A little*   *Some*   *A lot*

How much difficulty do you have holding the steering wheel firmly?

None   *A little*   *Some*   *A lot*

How much difficulty do you have pressing the brake pedal?

None   *A little*   *Some*   *A lot*

Feedback:

You may have decreased muscle strength. Lack of strength in our arms or legs may interfere with our ability to accelerate, brake, or steer while driving. Studies suggest that we can improve our strength through exercise.

▶ Check with your doctor or senior center to find out about programs in your area that might help you to improve your strength.

▶ Check into fitting your car with devices that help people drive who have reduced strength.

▶ If your car does not have power steering or brakes, consider buying a car with those features.

▶ Begin a fitness program. It's never too late to start.

 GETTING AROUND 2

Questions:

Can you quickly put your foot on the brake pedal?

Yes   *No*

Do you feel that your reactions are quick enough to handle a dangerous driving situation?

Yes   *No*

Could you swerve suddenly if necessary to avoid an unexpected hazard?

Yes   *No*

Feedback:

Your ability to quickly react to things may be reduced. In order to react quickly to something we must 1) see what the problem is, 2) decide what to do, and 3) do something. Slowed reaction times can occur because one or more of these three steps has slowed down. Research shows that as we age, our reaction time slows, particularly in situations that require us to respond to more than one thing at once.

▶ Because slowed reaction time may result from certain age-related medical conditions, it is important to get regular physical exams.

▶ Ask your doctor to check your reaction time.

▶ Try to avoid heavy traffic situations.

▶ Plan your trip in advance.

 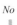 GETTING AROUND 3

HEALTH

Questions:

How much difficulty would you have walking a half mile without help if you had to?

    None   *A little*   *Some*   *A lot*

How much difficulty would you have climbing two flights of stairs without help if you had to?

    None   *A little*   *Some*   *A lot*

In general, would you say that your physical fitness is:

    Excellent   *Good*   *Fair*   *Poor*

Feedback:

Your overall physical fitness affects your ability to function on a day-to-day basis. Problems with daily physical functioning may precede problems in other areas, such as driving. Overall functioning is also important because older drivers may have several minor physical or medical problems, each of which taken separately may not affect their driving ability very much, but when taken together, could make driving dangerous.

▶ You have far more control over your personal fitness and health than you might think. Begin a fitness program. It is never too late to start.

▶ What you eat, how much you exercise, regular visits to the doctor, and following your doctor's advice can help you stay healthy and keep driving safely.

♥ HEALTH 1

Question:

Has a doctor ever told you that you have diabetes or high blood sugar?

    No   *Yes*

Feedback:

Diabetes can interfere with your ability to drive safely. In diabetes, blood sugar can be high, which is treated by insulin and other medications, as well as diet and exercise. People treated for diabetes are at risk for low blood sugar, which can result from a change in their medication, unexpected effort, irregular meals, or other factors. Low blood sugar can lead to impaired judgement or loss of consciousness, causing a driver to lose control of the car.

▶ It is important to talk with your doctor about any symptoms you are experiencing that might be related to your diabetes.

▶ Follow your doctor's advice about driving restrictions.

♥ HEALTH 2

Questions:

Has a doctor ever told you that you had a stroke?

   No   *Yes*

Do you have paralysis, weakness, or mental difficulties due to stroke?

   No   *Yes*

Feedback:

A stroke can interfere with the ability to drive safely because of partial or complete paralysis, weakness, or mental difficulties.

▶ If you have had a stroke, it is important that you undergo a thorough assessment by a doctor to determine if you should be driving and under what conditions.

▶ Remember that impaired consciousness or decreased awareness, or confusion or dizziness, can make driving unsafe.

▶ Muscle strength and coordination are needed to control the car safely. A loss of control of the limbs caused by paralysis may not necessarily prevent you from driving safely, but vehicle controls may need to be adapted.

♥ HEALTH 3

Question:

Has a doctor ever told you that you have Parkinson's Disease?

   No   *Yes*

Feedback:

Symptoms of Parkinson's include tremors, slowness of movement, and rigidity that can interfere with the ability to drive safely. These symptoms can greatly prolong reaction times so that a driver may be unable to respond quickly enough to changing conditions.

▶ It is important for you to be aware of changes in your symptoms.

▶ Report any changes to your doctor.

▶ Monitor with your doctor your ability to drive.

♥ HEALTH 4

Questions:

Has a doctor ever told you that you have seizure disorder or syncope?

    No   *Yes*

In the past two years, have you had a blackout, fainting spell, or seizure?

    No   *Yes*

Both seizure disorders and syncope involve a sudden loss of consciousness, a serious concern for driving safely. Studies show that, overall, drivers with seizure disorders have an increased risk of traffic accidents and injury. Every state in the US has some type of driving restriction for drivers with seizure disorder.

▶ If you have had a sudden loss of consciousness such as a blackout, fainting spell, or seizure, it is important that you see your doctor.

▶ If you have a seizure disorder, your doctor will need to figure out what type of seizures you have and what the best treatment should be.

▶ If you are having syncope, your doctor will need to assess all of your symptoms to determine whether you can drive safely.

Questions:

▶**Feedback:**

How often do you have difficulty staying awake when you want to?

    Never   *Rarely*   *Sometimes*   *Often*

At night, how often do you have difficulty falling asleep or staying asleep?

    Never   *Rarely*   *Sometimes*   *Often*

Has anyone ever told you that you snore loudly?

    No   *Yes*

In the past two years, have you ever fallen asleep while driving?

    No   *Yes*

Has a doctor ever told you that you have sleep apnea or narcolepsy?

    No   *Yes*

Sleep apnea and narcolepsy can interfere with the ability to drive safely. Sleep apnea involves the relaxation of the muscles of the throat during sleep, causing breathing to stop. Such sleep disturbances lead to excessive daytime sleepiness and the possibility of suddenly falling asleep without warning. People with sleep apnea syndrome have an increased risk of traffic accidents.

Narcolepsy also results in excessive sleepiness. While some people with narcolepsy are able to force themselves to stay awake through strong motivation and various measures (for example, open windows or cold air), they can be subject to sleep attacks without warning, placing them at high risk for traffic accidents. Medications used to treat narcolepsy may impair driving.

▶ Accurate diagnosis and treatment of sleep apnea and narcolepsy is essential, and requires overnight sleep assessment.

▶ Driving restrictions may be necessary.

▶ Remember that most methods people use to stay awake while driving only work for a short period of time, and sometimes not at all.

Questions:

Has a doctor ever told you that you have dementia or Alzheimer's disease?

No   *Yes*

Feedback:

Dementia and Alzheimer's disease seriously interfere with short-term memory and clear judgments that are essential to minute-to-minute driving decisions.

▶ It is important that you have your doctor evaluate your mental and physical health regularly.

▶ Always follow your doctor's orders regarding driving.

▶ Drive when traffic is less stressful and avoid difficult road conditions.

▶ Keep your driving trips short and direct.

▶ Do not drive too fast or too slow.

▶ Drive defensively—anticipate situations.

▶ Use family, friends, and neighbors as important resources for feedback about your driving.

▶ You should not drive at all if significant memory loss, disorientation or cognitive impairment exists. If you are unsure, you should have a driving evaluation with regular follow-ups.

 HEALTH 7

Question:

Do you take any medications for your heart or high blood pressure (other than aspirin)?

No   *Yes*

Feedback:

Some heart and blood pressure medications can cause dizziness, drowsiness, or mood changes that could affect your driving ability.

▶ Make sure to read medication labels and follow directions carefully.

▶ It is important to check with your doctor or pharmacist about the possible side effects of the drug(s) you are taking, especially effects that could impair driving abilities.

▶ Also ask what, if anything, you can do to counter side effects that affect driving.

▶ Consider checking with your doctor about changing the time you take your medication so that it does not interfere with driving.

▶ Never stop your medication or change the dosage without checking with your doctor.

♥ HEALTH 8

Questions:

Do you ever take any medications for anxiety (such as Valium, Xanax, Klonapin, Ativan, etc.)?

No   *Yes*

Do you ever take any medications to help you sleep (such as Halcion, ProSom, Ambien, etc.)?

No   *Yes*

Feedback:

Studies suggest that drugs for anxiety or sleep problems increase the risk of traffic accidents. In addition, the interactions between some of these drugs and alcohol can be dangerous.

▶ Make sure to read medication labels and follow directions carefully.

▶ It is important to check with your doctor or pharmacist about the possible side effects of the drug(s) you are taking, especially effects that could impair driving abilities.

▶ Also ask what, if anything, you can do to counter side effects that affect driving.

▶ Consider checking with your doctor about changing the time you take your medication so that it does not interfere with driving.

▶ Never stop your medication or change the dosage without checking with your doctor.

♥ HEALTH 9

Question:

Do you ever take any medications for depression (such as Prozac, Pamelor, Elavil, Zoloft, etc.)?

No   *Yes*

Feedback:

Drugs for depression can lead to problems with attention, memory, and motor coordination. While there are differences among these drugs, studies show that in general, they impair driving performance and increase the risk of traffic accidents. This risk appears to increase as the dosage of medication increases.

▶ Make sure to read medication labels and follow directions carefully.

▶ It is important to check with your doctor or pharmacist about the possible side effects of the drug(s) you are taking, especially effects that could impair driving abilities.

▶ Also ask what, if anything, you can do to counter side effects that affect driving.

▶ Consider checking with your doctor about changing the time you take your medication so that it does not interfere with driving.

▶ Never stop your medication or change the dosage without checking with your doctor.

♥ HEALTH 10

Question:

Do you ever take any medications for allergies or allergic symptoms?

  No   *Yes*

Feedback:

Older antihistamines are well known to cause drowsiness and impair driving ability. Newer antihistamines should be used in preference.

▶ It is important to check with your doctor or pharmacist to see what type of antihistamine you are taking.

▶ Make sure to read medication labels and follow directions carefully.

▶ It is important to check with your doctor or pharmacist about the possible side effects of the drug(s) you are taking, especially effects that could impair driving abilities.

▶ Also ask what, if anything, you can do to counter side effects that affect driving.

▶ Consider checking with your doctor about changing the time you take your medication so that it does not interfere with driving.

▶ Never stop your medication or change the dosage without checking with your doctor.

♥ HEALTH 11

Questions:

Do you ever take any prescription medications for pain, such as codeine?

  No   *Yes*

Feedback:

Pain medications are widely used among older adults. Studies show that use of these may interfere with your ability to drive safely.

▶ Make sure to read medication labels and follow directions carefully.

▶ It is important to check with your doctor or pharmacist about the possible side effects of the drug(s) you are taking, especially effects that could impair driving abilities.

▶ Also ask what, if anything, you can do to counter side effects that affect driving.

▶ Consider checking with your doctor about changing the time you take your medication so that it does not interfere with driving.

▶ Never stop your medication or change the dosage without checking with your doctor.

♥ HEALTH 12

Question:

Feedback:

How many different prescription drugs do you take?

None   *One*   *Two or more*

As we age, our body chemistry changes and drugs have stronger effects than when we were younger. We also tend to take more medications. In high doses, or when combined, drugs can impair the skills and reflexes of otherwise good drivers. Many drugs can cause drowsiness, affect vision, and have other side effects that are serious hazards on the road but may go unnoticed. They may even impair our ability to decide whether we can drive safely.

▶ Make sure to read medication labels and follow directions carefully.

▶ Check with your doctor or pharmacist about the possible side effects of the drugs you are taking, especially effects that could impair driving abilities.

▶ Also ask what, if anything, you can do to counter side effects that affect driving.

▶ Closely monitor your reactions and report them to your doctor or pharmacist.

▶ Take medicine only in prescribed amounts at the proper times.

▶ Consider checking with your doctor about changing the time you take your medication so that it does not interfere with driving.

▶ Never stop your medication or change the dosage without checking with your doctor.

▶ Do not drive when using prescription drugs that make you sleepy or affect your ability to drive.

♥ HEALTH 13

Questions:

Feedback:

Do you ever take over-the-counter medications for sleep, pain, or allergies?

No   *Yes*

Do you ever take any dietary or herbal supplements (such as St. John's Wort, Kava Kava, Valerian root, etc.)?

No   *Yes*

Not only do medications affect the way your body functions, but dietary and herbal supplements also do, and could lead to dangerous interactions. Your driving abilities could be affected.

▶ Make sure all of your doctors know about all the medications or supplements you are taking. Bring all your medications and supplements with you when you see your doctor.

▶ Ask your doctor or pharmacist to check for dangerous interactions.

▶ Make sure to read medication and supplement labels and follow directions carefully.

▶ Check with your doctor or pharmacist about the possible side effects of the medications or supplements you are taking, especially effects that could impair driving abilities.

▶ Also ask what, if anything, you can do to counter side effects that affect driving.

▶ Consider checking with your doctor about changing the time you take your medication so that it does not interfere with driving.

▶ Never stop your medication or change the dosage without checking with your doctor.

♥ HEALTH 14

Questions:

Do you drink alcoholic beverages?

    No   *Yes*

Feedback:

Another drug that you may not think of as a drug, is alcohol. Alcohol has a powerful effect on our bodies, both physical and psychological. Alcohol is the single most important factor in fatal traffic accidents.

▶ As we age, our bodies handle alcohol differently, so we should drink less.

▶ Never drive after drinking. Make arrangements for someone else to drive if you know you will be drinking.

▶ It's important to avoid alcohol when taking medications. With few exceptions, combining alcohol and other drugs decreases driving abilities, and in some cases, can cause coma or death.

♥ HEALTH 15

Questions and Answers

 I am a good driver but what can I do to be even safer on the road?

 Even safe drivers can do things to help prevent accidents. If you don't already do them, here are several things you can do to be safer on the road:

→ Make sure your car is in good working order.

→ Always use your safety belt.

→ Try to drive during the safest times, such as during the middle of the day.

→ Take a refresher driving course. Cars, roads, and traffic laws keep on changing. A refresher course is a good way to stay up with those changes. Contact your *American Association of Retired Persons* (AARP) or *American Automobile Association* (AAA) office or *Area Agency on Aging* to find out more about such courses.

→ Continue to monitor your driving abilities with this workbook or testing given by a doctor or organization.

→ Do not drive after drinking alcohol, when you are tired, or when you are not confident of your driving.

Some of my answers in the workbook led to the suggestion that I have a doctor's check up. How can I be sure that the doctor understands my concerns and addresses my needs?

Doctor offices are very busy and it can sometimes seem as if doctors do not have enough time to talk with you about your concerns. Here are some suggestions for making sure that your concerns are addressed:

→ Think about your relationship with your doctor as a partnership— your job is to actively ask questions and raise concerns. Your doctor's job is to help meet your needs.

→ Write down and prioritize your questions and concerns (including medication issues) before your visit and bring them with you.

→ Understand your insurance benefits—know, in general, what services are covered.

→ Consider bringing another person with you to help listen, remember information, and be sure your concerns are addressed.

→ Bring up your most important questions and concerns first.

→ Be honest with your doctor so he or she can best help you. Remember that the information you share is confidential.

→ Make sure your doctor knows that you drive.

→ Take notes to refer to later. Ask your doctor to write down information for you.

→ Find out how to contact your doctor if you have further questions, are having problems, or your treatment is not working.

Q and A 2

  I've thought about having an evaluation of my driving done, but I worry that my license might be taken away. What should I do?

There are places where you can have your driving evaluated without the results being reported to the driver licensing agency. Contact a local driving school, geriatric center, *Area Agency on Aging*, or *AARP* or *AAA* office to find out about where you can have your driving evaluated in your area.

→ Be open and honest with yourself about the results.

→ If the evaluation shows that you are having driving problems, you should consider how you can change your driving to be most safe. The person giving you the evaluation should be able to give you suggestions.

→ Keep in mind that there may be many ways for you to adapt or reduce your driving so that you can drive safely and keep your license.

→ Remember, too, that one day you may have to stop driving completely in order to protect yourself and others from serious injury.

Q and A 3

If I decide to reduce or stop my driving, how can I still get around?

Options for getting around will vary depending on where you live, where you need to go, and how well you can walk. Consider contacting a local *Area Agency on Aging* or AARP office about transportation options in your area. Here's what may be available and a brief description of each:

→ *Buses, trains, and subways*: Each of these run on a set route with a set schedule and specific stops. These options require you to walk to and from stops. They are usually low cost and schedules and routes can be obtained by contacting the agency that runs the service.

→ *Taxis and dial-a-ride*: These provide transportation from one place, such as your home, to another place, such as the store, and can include just you or other riders. Typically, you call the company that runs the service and tell them where you want to go and they come and pick you up and take you there for a fee. There is little walking involved. You may have a short wait to be picked up.

→ *Community transportation*: Some communities have organizations that have set up programs to provide transportation for specific groups such as seniors. These programs are usually responsive to the needs of their riders. Check to see if your community provides such transportation.

→ *Family, friends, and neighbors*: If you have family, friends, or neighbors nearby, they may be able to help out with transportation. Although you may not like to ask for a ride, you can do your part by paying for gas, lunch, or returning a different favor.

→ *Walking and bicycles*: Depending on your health, you may be able to meet some of your needs through walking or riding a bicycle/tricycle. This option has the added benefit of helping you maintain your fitness.

Q and A 4

My abilities and driving seem okay right now, but that could change. What can I do to make sure I have my transportation needs met in the future?

In the same way that we plan for retirement, we should plan for meeting our future transportation needs. As we get older, we begin to reduce our driving, such as at nighttime, and some of us stop driving altogether. Here are some things to think about to help you plan for a future where your transportation needs are safely met:

→ Continue to be aware of and check your driving abilities, since they can change quickly. This workbook can help you. Any ability that you think may be declining should be assessed by a doctor or other qualified person.

→ Stay in practice, even if your spouse or someone else prefers to do the driving right now. Keeping up your driving skills will help you drive safely in the future when you may need to drive more.

→ When deciding about where to live, think about how you could get around if you were unable to or chose not to drive yourself. For example, would there be other transportation options such as buses or taxis available at night or in bad weather? Would family or friends be close by to help out?

→ Begin riding the bus, taxi, subway, or train every now and then, so that you become familiar with these options for getting around in case you need them in the future.

Q and A 5

I know someone whose driving has become worse. What can I do to help that person?

If you know someone who is having problems with driving, let the person know you are concerned. Talking with someone about his or her unsafe driving may not be easy but it can provide important information for the person. Here are some ways you can help:

→ Give the person a copy of this workbook. Let him or her work through it alone or offer to help.

→ Talk with the person's spouse or friends about whether they have noticed unsafe driving. Discuss with them how to approach the driver.

→ Offer to provide occasional transportation.

→ If you are concerned about someone who is a family member, talk with his or her doctor to see if the doctor will bring up driving during their next visit.

→ Help the person begin to plan for reducing driving.

Appendix *H*

COUNSELING THE PATIENT WHO IS NO LONGER SAFE TO DRIVE*

Mr. Phillips returns for follow-up after undergoing driver assessment and rehabilitation. From the driver rehabilitation specialist (DRS) report, you know that his DRS has helped fit his car with a steering wheel spinner knob to compensate for decreased hand grip and a wide-angle rearview mirror to compensate for decreased neck rotation. Mr. Phillips has successfully undergone training with these adaptive devices and now states that he is driving more confidently with them. You counsel him on the Tips for Safe Driving and Successful Aging Tips, advise him to continue exercising, and encourage him to start planning alternative transportation options.

You continue to provide care for Mr. Phillips' chronic conditions and follow up on his driving safety. Three years later, Mr. Phillips' functional abilities have declined to the extent that you believe it is no longer safe for him to drive. You also feel that further driver rehabilitation is unlikely to improve his driving safety. Mr. Phillips has decreased his driving over the years, and you tell him that it is now time for him to retire from driving. Mr. Phillips replies, "We've talked about this before, and I figured it was coming sooner or later." He feels that rides from family, friends, and the senior citizen shuttle in his community will be adequate for his transportation needs, and he plans to give his car to his granddaughter.

One week after this visit, you see a new patient. Mrs. Allen is a 76-year-old widow who has not seen a doctor in the past 5 years despite urging by her daughter, who accompanies her to the clinic today. She presents with a sore throat, fever, and chills. Mrs. Allen is unable to provide you with any history, and she has trouble following instructions throughout the clinic visit. Your rapid strep test confirms strep throat, and you prescribe antibiotics and ask her to return in one week for follow-up and a full

physical exam. You are concerned about her cognitive state, and wonder if it is due to the infection. You confirm that Mrs. Allen's daughter drove her to the clinic, and you ask Mrs. Allen to refrain from driving until you see her for follow-up.

Two days later, you receive a phone call from Mrs. Allen's daughter. The daughter reports an improvement in her mother's symptoms, but now wishes to speak to you about her mother's mental decline. She reports that her mother, who lives alone, is having increasing difficulty dressing herself, performing personal hygiene tasks, and completing household chores. She is particularly concerned about her mother's daily trips to the grocery store 2 miles away. Mrs. Allen has gotten lost on these trips and—according to the store manager—has handled money incorrectly. Dents and scratches have appeared on the car without explanation. Mrs. Allen's daughter has asked her mother to stop driving, but Mrs. Allen responds with anger and resistance each time. The daughter would like to know how to manage her mother's long-term safety and health, and—most urgently—how to address the driving issue. What do you tell her?

For many, driving is a source of independence and self-esteem. When an individual retires from driving, he or she not only loses a form of transportation but also all the emotional and social benefits derived from driving.

For various reasons, physicians may be reluctant to discuss driving retirement with their patients. Physicians may fear delivering bad news or depriving the patient of mobility and all its benefits. Physicians may avoid discussions of driving altogether because they believe that a patient will not heed their advice.

These concerns are all valid. However, physicians have a responsibility to protect their patients' safety through assessment of driving-related functions, exploration

*Reprinted with permission from the American Medical Association.

655

of medical and rehabilitation options to maintain their patients' driving safety, and—when all other options have been exhausted—recommendations of driving restriction or driving retirement. Physicians are influential in a patient's decision to stop driving; in fact, advice from a doctor is one of the most frequently cited reasons that a patient retires from driving.[1]

In this appendix, we discuss the key steps in counseling a patient on driving retirement and provide strategies for managing challenging cases.

HOW DO YOU RECOMMEND DRIVING RETIREMENT TO YOUR PATIENT?

If you must recommend driving retirement to your patient, there are several things you can do to make this conversation more comfortable for both of you. First, use the term *driving retirement* to help normalize the experience. After all, retirement is generally considered a more natural and positive life experience than "quitting" or "giving up." Second, involve your patient in the decision-making process by openly discussing why his or her driving safety is at risk and addressing his or her needs and concerns. Third, acknowledge that safe mobility is a priority by encouraging your patient to develop a list of alternative transportation options.

When discussing driving retirement with your patient, you may find it helpful to follow these four steps.

EXPLAIN TO YOUR PATIENT WHY IT IS IMPORTANT TO RETIRE FROM DRIVING

If your patient has undergone Assessment of Driving-Related Skills (ADReS) or assessment by a DRS, explain the results of the assessment in simple language. Clearly explain what the results tell you about his or her level of function, and then explain why this function is important for driving. State the potential risks of driving, and end with the recommendation that your patient retire from driving.

For example, you could say to Mr. Phillips:

> "Mr. Phillips, the results of your eye exam show that your vision isn't as good as it used to be. Good vision is important for driving, because you need to be able to see the road, other cars, pedestrians, and traffic signs. With your vision, I'm concerned that you'll get into a car crash. For your own safety and the safety of others, it's time for you to retire from driving."

This recommendation may upset or anger your patient. Let him or her know that this is normal, and that you understand his or her reaction.

While you should be sensitive to the practical and emotional implications of driving retirement, it is also necessary for you to be firm with your recommendation. At this time, it is best to avoid engaging in disputes or long explanations. Rather, you should focus on making certain your patient understands your recommendation and understands that this recommendation was made for his or her safety.

DISCUSS TRANSPORTATION OPTIONS

Now that you have recommended driving retirement, the next step is to explore alternative transportation options with your patient. Encourage your patient to maintain his or her mobility by creating a transportation plan—a list of alternatives to driving.

You can begin discussing transportation options by asking the following questions:

- How do you usually get around when your car is in the shop?
- Do these get you everywhere you need to go?
- Have you ever thought about how you would get around if you couldn't drive?

Discuss whether these options can fulfill all of your patient's transportation needs, and suggest other options for your patient to consider. (A list of alternatives to driving can be found in Box H-1.) Address any barriers your patient identifies, including financial constraints, limited service and destinations, reluctance to depend on family and friends for rides, and challenging physical requirements for accessibility (e.g., unsheltered bus stops and steep bus stairs).

Help your patient choose the most feasible transportation options. In developing a transportation plan, recommend to your patient that he or she contact the local Area Agency on Aging (AAA) for information about local resources such as taxis, public transportation, and senior-specific transportation services.

Remind your patient to plan for transportation to social services because it is important—especially at this time—for him or her to maintain a strong social support system.

BOX H-1	Alternatives to Driving

- Walking
- Public transportation
- Rides from family and friends
- Cabs
- Paratransit services
- Community transportation services
- Hospital shuttles
- Medi-car
- Delivery services and house calls
- Volunteer drivers (through the church, synagogue, or community center)

In addition to exploring transportation options, your patient should also consider how to eliminate unnecessary trips by combining activities and utilizing delivery and house-call services. For example, your patient can reduce the number of trips needed by scheduling all appointments in the same area for the same day or arranging to have groceries or medications delivered.

Encourage your patient to involve family members in the creation of a transportation plan. With your patient's permission, contact family members and encourage them to offer rides and help formulate a weekly schedule for running errands. They can also arrange for the delivery of groceries, newspapers, medications, and other necessities and services. (See Box H-2 for more tips.)

REINFORCE DRIVING CESSATION

Because your patient may initially offer resistance or fail to comprehend your recommendation for driving retirement, it is important to reinforce this recommendation at the current and future office visits.

To reinforce this recommendation:
- Ask your patient if he or she has any questions regarding the assessment or your recommendation. Reassure your patient that you are available to answer questions and provide further assistance.
- Ask your patient to repeat back to you why he or she must not drive. Emphasize that this recommendation is for personal safety and the safety of others on the road.
- A prescription with the words "Do Not Drive" may help your patient understand that your recommendation constitutes "official" medical advice. (See Box H-3 for other reinforcement tips.)
- If your state has a reporting law, discuss this with your patient before submitting the required report.

(A discussion of the legal and ethical role of the physician and a state-by-state list of reporting laws can be found in Appendices I and A, respectively.)
- Send your patient a follow-up letter (see Figure H-1 for a sample letter). This letter should be written in language that is easy to understand and should emphasize your concern for his or her safety and well-being. Send copies to the patient and—with his or her permission—to concerned family members, and keep another copy in the patient's chart as documentation.
- Ask your patient to return to your office in 1 month for follow-up.

FOLLOW UP WITH YOUR PATIENT

At your patient's 1-month follow-up appointment, you should:
- Ask your patient if he or she has successfully developed and utilized a transportation plan.
- If indicated, assess your patient for signs of isolation and depression.

You can begin the discussion by asking your patient how he or she got to the appointment that day. For example, you could say to Mr. Phillips:

Physician: Good morning, Mr. Phillips. It's good to see you again. Did you have any problems getting to the office today?
Mr. Phillips: No, not at all.
Physician: How did you get here today?
Mr. Phillips: My son dropped me off. We've worked out a schedule so that he and his wife can give me rides to all my appointments.
Physician: That's wonderful! Aside from these rides, have you found any other ways to get around?

During the office visit, remember to be alert to signs of depression, neglect, and isolation. Driving cessation

---

BOX H-2	Tips for Involving the Family

- Encourage family members to promote the health and safety of their loved one by supporting your recommendations and assisting in the creation of a transportation plan.
- Encourage questions regarding patient care.
- If a third party accompanies your patient into the examination room, involve all parties in the discussion. Take care not to ignore your patient.
- Provide resources to the family.
- Refer the family to the National Family Caregivers Association (NFCA) at 800 896-3650 or www.nfcacares.org to find resources and tips on caring for their loved one.
- Be alert to signs of caregiver burnout.

BOX H-3	Tips to Reinforce Driving Cessation

Tip 1: Give the patient a prescription on which you have written, "Do Not Drive." This aids as a visual reminder for your patient and also emphasizes the strength of your message.
Tip 2: Remind your patient that this recommendation is for his or her safety and for the safety of other road users.
Tip 3: Ask the patient how he or she would feel if he or she got into a crash and injured someone else.
Tip 4: Use economic arguments. Point out the rising price of gas and oil, the expense of car maintenance (tires, tune-ups, insurance), registration/license fees, financing expenses, and the depreciation of car value.
Tip 5: Have a plan in place that involves family member support for alternative transportation.

July 1, 2003

Clayton Phillips
123 Lincoln Lane
Sunnydale, XX 55555

Dear Mr. Phillips:

I am writing to follow up on your clinic visit on June 20, 2003. During the visit, we talked about yor safety when you drive a car. I tested your vision (eyes), strength, movement, and thinking skills, and asked you about your health problems and medicines. Because your vision, strength and movement might make you drive unsafely, I recommended that you retire from driving.

I know that driving is important to you, and I know that it is hard to give up driving. Still, your safety is more important than driving. To help you get around, you can ask for rides from your son and your friends. You can also use the senior bus in your neighborhood. The Patient Resource Sheet (enclosed) has some other ideas that we talked about. As we agreed, I am also sending a copy of these materials to your son so that the two of you can read them together.

I want to make sure you can still do your chores, visit your friends, and go other places without a car. It is important for you to maintain your lifestyle. Please see me again in one month—we will talk about how this is working for you.

As we discussed, the state of _____ requires me to refer unsafe drivers to the Department of Motor Vehicles (DMV). Because I am required by law to do this, I have sent a report to the _____ DMV. The DMV will send you a letter in a few weeks to discuss your driver's license.

Please call my office if you have any questions. I look forward to seeing you next month.

Sincerely,

Your Physician

Enc: Patient Resource Sheet
cc: Your son

* Note that this sample letter has been written at a 5th grade reading level, as measured by the SMOG Readability Formula.

Figure H-1 Sample follow-up letter from the physician to the client that reiterates the recommendation that the client cease driving.

has been associated with an increase in depressive symptoms in the elderly.[2,3] In addition to direct effects on the patient's well-being, depressive symptoms have been linked to physical decline and mortality in the elderly.[4] Ask your patient how he or she is managing without driving, and assess for depression (see Box H-4) and neglect (see Box H-5) as indicated. Educate family members and caregivers about signs of depression, and encourage them to contact you if they have concerns about their loved one's well-being.

Continue to assess and manage your patient's functional impairments and the underlying disorders. If they improve to the extent that your patient is safe to drive again, discuss this with your patient and help him or her develop a plan for a safe return to driving. This can include a driver evaluation performed by a DRS and limiting driving to familiar, uncongested areas until the patient regains his or her confidence.

SITUATIONS THAT REQUIRE ADDITIONAL COUNSELING

It may be necessary to provide additional counseling to encourage driving retirement or to help your patient cope with this loss. In this section, we discuss situations that require additional counseling and offer recommendations for the management of these situations.

BOX H-4	**Questions to Assess for Depression**

- How has your mood been lately?
- Have you noticed any changes in appetite?
- Have you noticed any changes in sleeping habits?
- Have you noticed feeling particularly tired or anxious lately?
- Have you been taking part in and enjoying your usual activities?[5]

BOX H-5	**Signs of Neglect or Self-Neglect**

- Patient has an injury that has not been properly treated
- Symptoms of dehydration and/or malnourishment without illness-related cause
- Weight loss
- Soiled clothing
- Evidence of inadequate or inappropriate administration of medications

---

SITUATION 1: THE RESISTANT PATIENT

If your patient is belligerent or refuses to retire from driving, it is important for you to understand why. Knowing this will help you address your patient's concerns.

In the care of your patient, you may find it helpful to:
- Let your patient know that you are listening.

Use empathetic statements when addressing your patient's concerns. Remind your patient that you are an advocate for his or her safety and health.

For example, you could say to your patient:

> **Physician:** Mr. Adams, it worries me that you drove yourself to the appointment today. At our last visit, we talked about why it was no longer safe for you to drive, and I recommended that you retire from driving. Can you tell me why you're still driving?
>
> **Mr. Adams:** Well, Doctor, I don't understand it. My driving is just fine. Frankly, I don't think you have the right to tell me not to drive.
>
> **Physician:** I know this is a frustrating situation for you. I also know that it's not easy for you to retire from driving, but I still think it's best for your safety and health. As your doctor, your safety and health are my concern. I want to make sure we understand each other, and I'd like to help you as much as possible. Can you tell me some of your concerns about retiring from driving?

- Have the patient define when he or she feels a person would be unsafe to drive.

This may help your patient become involved in the decision to retire from driving, and help you assess his or her judgment and insight.

> **Physician:** Mr. Adams, when do you think it's best for a person to retire from driving?
>
> **Mr. Adams:** Well, when they're running red lights and getting into crashes, I guess.
>
> **Physician:** Do you know anyone who drives like this?
>
> **Mr. Adams:** A friend of mine doesn't drive too well. He drives all over the road and runs red lights. I don't want to get into the car with him anymore because I don't trust his driving.
>
> **Physician:** That sounds like a scary situation for your friend and for other people on the road. I think it's time for him to retire from driving. Do you think it's a good idea for people to retire from driving when they're a danger to themselves and others?

Many older drivers are able to identify peers whose driving they consider unsafe, yet may not have the insight to make similar observations about their own driving. By asking your patient about friends whose driving is unsafe and why he or she considers their driving unsafe, your patient may be able to recognize similarities in his or her own driving performance.

Assure your patient that he or she will not be alone in driving retirement. After all, many people make the decision when safety becomes a concern. Encourage your patient to seek a second opinion if he or she feels that additional consultation is necessary.
- Have your patient identify support systems.

Ask your patient to list friends and relatives who have retired from driving and ways that they have continued to remain active and mobile. Also, your patient can list family members, neighbors, religious groups, and other support groups that are able and willing to help with transportation decisions. Remind your patient to plan for transportation to social activities so that he or she can maintain a social life.

• Help your patient view the positives.

Often, discussions of driving retirement tend to focus on the negative aspects, such as "losing independence" or "giving up freedom." Help your patient view the positives by pointing out that this is a positive step towards his or her safety and the safety of other road users. Mention the benefits of not owning a car and of utilizing community services (such as decreased costs and the potential to meet new people).

• Refer your patient to a social worker.

Your patient may need additional help securing resources and transitioning to a life without driving. Social workers can provide counseling to patients and their families, assess your patient's psychosocial needs, assist in locating and coordinating community services and transportation, and enable your patient to maintain safety, independence, and a high quality of life. The National Association of Social Workers Register of Clinical Social Workers is a valuable resource for locating a social worker in your area who has met national verified professional standards for education, experience, and supervision. You can access the Register or place an order online at www.socialworkers.org.

SITUATION 2: YOUR PATIENT PRESENTS WITH SYMPTOMS OF DEPRESSION

Driving cessation has been associated with an increase in depressive symptoms.[2,3] This can result from a combination of factors, including social isolation, feelings of loss, and perceived poor health status. If your patient presents with signs or symptoms of depression, assess further by asking specific questions (see Box H-4).

Talk to your patient and appropriate family members about the symptoms of depression and available options. These can include referral to a mental health professional for full assessment and treatment or direct referral for individual therapy, group therapy, or social/recreational activities. Acknowledge that your patient has suffered a loss and that this is a difficult time for him or her. Let your patient know that these feelings are normal.

SITUATION 3: YOUR PATIENT LACKS DECISION-MAKING CAPACITY

If your patient presents with significant cognitive impairment, lacks insight and decision-making capacity,

or both, it is imperative that you employ the aid of the appointed guardian or caregiver to help the patient comply with your recommendation of driving retirement. Let family and caregivers know that they play a crucial role in helping the patient find safer alternatives to driving.

If necessary, an expert evaluation can be used to appoint a legal guardian for the patient. In turn, the guardian may forfeit the patient's car and license on behalf of the safety of the patient. These actions should be used when needed, but only as a last resort.

SITUATION 4: YOUR PATIENT SHOWS SIGNS OF SELF-NEGLECT OR NEGLECT

At times, a patient may not be able to secure resources for himself or herself and may lack support from family, friends, or the appointed caregiver. If you suspect that your patient does not have the capacity to care for himself or herself—or that family and caregivers lack the ability to adequately care for your patient—be alert to signs of self-neglect and neglect (see Box H-5).

Self-neglect is defined as the failure to provide for one's own essential needs, while neglect is the failure of a caregiver to fulfill his or her caregiving responsibilities due to willful neglect or an inability arising from disability, stress, ignorance, lack of maturity, or lack of resources. If you identify signs of neglect or self-neglect, notify the Adult Protective Services (APS). APS will investigate and confirm cases of neglect and self-neglect and arrange for services such as case planning, monitoring, and evaluation and medical, social, economic, legal, housing, law enforcement, and other emergency or supportive services. To obtain contact information for your state APS office, call the Eldercare Locator at 1 800 677-1116.

REFERENCES

1. Persson D: The elderly driver: deciding when to stop, *Gerontologist* 33:88-91, 1993.
2. Marottoli RA, Mendes de Leon C, Glass TA, et al: Driving cessation and increased depressive symptoms: prospective evidence from the New Haven EPESE, *J Am Geriatr Soc* 45:202-210, 1997.
3. Fonda SJ, Wallace RB, Herzog AR: Changes in driving patterns and worsening depressive symptoms among older adults, *J Gerontol* 56:S343-351, 2001.
4. Berkman LF, Berkman CS, Kasl S, et al: Depressive symptoms in relation to physical health and functioning in the elderly, *Am J Epidemiol* 124:372-388, 1986.
5. American Psychiatric Association: *Diagnostic and statistical manual of mental disorders,* ed 4, text revision, Washington DC, 2000, American Psychiatric Association.

LEGAL AND ETHICAL RESPONSIBILITIES OF THE PHYSICIAN*†

Appendix I

Upon further evaluation of Mrs. Allen, you diagnose her with Alzheimer's disease. It is readily apparent that her condition has progressed to the extent that she is no longer safe to drive and that rehabilitation is not likely to improve her driving safety. You tell Mrs. Allen that she must retire from driving for her own safety and the safety of others on the road. You also explain that the state reporting law requires you to report her to the DMV. Initially, Mrs. Allen does not comprehend, but when you specifically tell her that she can no longer drive herself to the grocery store every day, she becomes agitated and screams, "I hate you!" and "I'm going to sue you!" The daughter understands your decision to report Mrs. Allen to the DMV, but is now concerned that she will encounter legal problems if her mother attempts to drive without a license. She asks if it is absolutely necessary for you to report her mother. What do you say?

Driving is a difficult topic to address, particularly when there is the risk of damaging the patient-physician relationship, violating patient confidentiality, and potentially losing patients. To complicate matters, many physicians are uncertain of their legal responsibility, if any, to report unsafe drivers to their state Department of Motor Vehicles (DMV).[1,2] As a result, physicians are often faced with a dilemma: should they report the unsafe driver to the state DMV at the expense of breaching confidentiality and potentially damaging the patient-physician relationship or should they forego reporting and risk being liable for any future patient or third-party injuries? This appendix will help clarify your legal and ethical responsibilities. In particular, we will discuss the duties of the physician, offer recommendations on how to balance these duties, and provide strategies for putting them into practice. To aid you in navigating legal terminology and concepts, we have assembled a list of definitions (Box I-1). Because reporting laws vary by state, Appendix A lists a state-by-state reference list of reporting laws, licensing requirements, license renewal information, and DMV contact information.

THE PHYSICIAN'S LEGAL AND ETHICAL DUTIES

Current legal and ethical debates highlight duties of the physician that are relevant to the issue of driving. These include protecting the patient, protecting public safety, maintaining patient confidentiality, and adhering to state reporting laws.

PROTECTING THE PATIENT

Protecting the patient's physical and mental health is considered the physician's primary responsibility. This includes not only treatment and prevention of illness but also caring for the patient's safety. With regards to driving, physicians should advise and counsel their patients about medical conditions and possible medication side effects that may impair their ability to drive safely. Case law illustrates that failure to advise the patient about such medical conditions and medication side effects is considered negligent behavior.[3-5]

DUTY TO PROTECT: PROTECTING PUBLIC SAFETY

In addition to caring for their patients' health, physicians may, in certain circumstances and jurisdictions,

---

*Please note that this Appendix is provided for informational purposes only. It is not intended to constitute legal advice. If legal advice is required, the services of a competent professional should be sought.

†This section has been reprinted with the permission of the American Medical Association.

661

BOX I-1	Common Terminology

Mandatory Medical Reporting Laws: In some states, physicians are required to report patients who have specific medical conditions (e.g., epilepsy, dementia) to their state Department of Motor Vehicles (DMV). These states generally provide specific guidelines and forms that can be obtained through the DMV.

Physician Reporting Laws: Other states require physicians to report "unsafe" drivers to their state DMV, with varying guidelines for defining "unsafe." The physician may need to provide (a) the patient's diagnosis and (b) any evidence of a functional impairment that can affect driving (e.g., results of neurological testing) to prove that the patient is an unsafe driver.

Physician Liability: Case law illustrates situations in which the physician was held liable for civil damages caused by his or her patient's car crash when there was a clear failure to report an at-risk driver to the DMV prior to the incident.

Immunity for Reporting: Several states exempt physicians from liability for civil damages brought by the patient if the physician reported the patient to the DMV beforehand.

Anonymity and Legal Protection: Several states offer anonymous reporting and/or legal protection against civil actions for damages caused by reporting in good faith. Many states will maintain the confidentiality of the reporter, unless otherwise required by a court order.

Duty to Protect: Case law in certain jurisdictions demonstrates that physicians have a legal duty to warn the public of danger their patients may cause, especially in the case of identifiable third parties. With respect to driving, mandatory reporting laws and physician reporting laws provide physicians with guidance regarding their duty to protect.

Renewal Procedures: License renewal procedures vary by state. Some states have age-based renewal procedures; that is, at a given age, the state may reduce the time interval between license renewal, restrict license renewal by mail, require specific vision, traffic law, and sign knowledge testing, and/or require on-road testing. Very few states require a physician's report for license renewal.

Restricted Driver's License: Some states offer the restricted license as an alternative to revoking a driver's license. Typical restrictions include prohibiting night driving, restricting driving to a certain radius, requiring adaptive devices, and shortening the renewal interval.

Medical Advisory Boards: Medical Advisory Boards (MABs) generally consist of local physicians who work in conjunction with the DMV to determine whether mental or physical conditions may affect an individual's ability to drive safely. MABs vary between states in size, role, and level of involvement.

Driver Rehabilitation Programs: These programs, run by driver rehabilitation specialists (DRSs), help identify at-risk drivers and improve driver safety through adaptive devices and techniques. Clients typically receive a clinical evaluation, driving evaluation, and—if necessary—vehicle modifications and training.

---

have some responsibility for protecting the safety of the public.[*,6,7] With regards to driving, legal precedents demonstrate that in some cases, physicians can be held liable for their patient's car crash and for third-party injuries caused by their patient. Several cases have found physicians liable for third-party injuries because they failed to advise their patients about medication side effects,[3,4,6,7] medical conditions,[5,8-10] and medical apparati[11] that may impair driving performance.

Maintaining Patient Confidentiality

Confidentiality is defined as the physician's ethical obligation to keep information about the patient and his or her care unavailable to those—including the

---

* It should be noted that the Tarasoff ruling per se, upon which the principles of "Duty to Warn" and "Duty to Protect" are based, originally applied only in the state of California and now applies only in certain jurisdictions. The U.S. Supreme Court has not heard a case involving these principles. Many states have adopted statutes to help clarify steps that are considered reasonable when a physician is presented with someone making a threat of harm to a third party.

---

patient's family, the patient's attorney, and the government—who do not have the authorization to receive this information.[12,13] Confidentiality is crucial within the physician-patient relationship because it encourages the free exchange of information, allowing the patient to describe symptoms for diagnosis and treatment.[14] Without confidence in the confidentiality of their care, individuals may be less likely to seek treatment, disclose information for effective treatment, or trust the health care professional. There are several exceptions to maintaining confidentiality. Information may be released if the patient gives his or her consent. Also, information may be released without patient authorization in order to comply with various reporting statutes (such as child abuse reporting statutes) and court orders.

Many physicians are reluctant to report impaired drivers to the DMV for fear of jeopardizing the patient-physician relationship,[15] breaching patient confidentiality, and—more recently—violating the Health Insurance Portability and Accountability Act of 1996 (HIPAA). However, while some courts have previously held the health care system liable for breaching confidentiality,[15] physicians generally enjoy immunity for complying with mandatory reporting statutes in good faith.[12] Some states specifically protect health care professionals from liability for reporting unsafe drivers in good faith. Furthermore, the HIPAA *Standards for Privacy of Individually Identifiable Health Information* ("Privacy Rule") permit health care providers to disclose protected health information without individual authorization *as required by law.* It also permits health care providers to disclose protected health information to public health authorities authorized by law to collect or receive such information for preventing or controlling disease, injury, or disability.

ADHERING TO STATE REPORTING LAWS

Physicians must know and comply with their state's reporting laws. Because each state has its own reporting laws, we have provided a state-by-state reference list in Appendix A. Please note that in states where there are no laws authorizing physicians to report patients to the DMV, physicians must have patient consent in order to disclose medical information. In these states, physicians who disclose medical information without patient consent may be held liable for breach of confidentiality. Nonetheless, this should not dissuade physicians from reporting when it is necessary and justified, as reporting may provide protection from liability for future civil damages.

PUTTING IT ALL TOGETHER

With these competing legal and ethical duties, how can you fulfill them while legally protecting yourself? In this section, we provide recommendations for achieving this balance.

COUNSEL YOUR PATIENT

Patients should be advised of medical conditions, procedures, and medications that may impair driving performance. (A reference list of medical conditions and medications that may impair driving performance, with recommendations for each one, can be found in Chapter 9.)

RECOMMEND DRIVING CESSATION AS NEEDED

As discussed in the previous chapters, you should recommend that a patient retire from driving if you believe that the patient's driving is unsafe and cannot be made safe by any available medical treatment, adaptive device, or adaptive technique. As always, base your clinical judgment on the patient's function rather than age, race, or gender.[16]

KNOW AND COMPLY WITH YOUR STATE'S REPORTING LAWS

You must know and comply with your state's reporting laws. If you fail to follow these laws, you may be liable for patient and third-party injuries. If your state has a mandatory medical reporting law, report the required medical condition(s) using the DMV's official form. If your state has a physician reporting law, submit your report using the DMV's official form and/or any other reporting guidelines. If the DMV's guidelines do not state what patient information must be reported, provide only the minimum of information required to support your case.

REDUCE THE IMPACT OF BREACHING PATIENT CONFIDENTIALITY

In adhering to your state's reporting laws, you may find it necessary to breach your patient's confidentiality. However, you can do several things to reduce the impact of breaching confidentiality on the patient-physician relationship. Before reporting your patient to the DMV, tell your patient what you are about to do. Explain that it is your legal responsibility to refer him or her to the state DMV, and describe what kind of follow-up he or she can expect from the DMV.

Assure your patient that out of respect for his or her privacy, you will disclose only the minimum of information required and hold all other information confidential. Even in states that offer anonymous reporting, it is a good idea to be open with your patients. When submitting your report, provide only the information required. Consider giving your patient a copy of his or her report. By providing your patients with as much information as possible, you can involve them in the process and give them a greater sense of control. Before contacting your patient's family members and caregivers, request the patient's permission to speak with these parties. If your patient maintains decision-making capacity and denies permission for you to speak with these parties, you must respect the patient's wishes.

DOCUMENT THOROUGHLY

Through documentation, you provide evidence of your efforts to assess and maintain your patient's driving safety. In the event of a patient or third-party crash injury, thorough documentation may protect you against a lawsuit. To protect yourself legally, you should document your efforts, conversations, recommendations, and any referrals for further testing in the patient's chart.[17] In other words, you should document all the steps of PPODS (see Chapter 1) that you have performed, including the following:

- Any direct observations of functional deficits, red flags, or crash-related injuries that lead you to believe that your patient may be at risk for medically impaired driving.
- Any counseling specific to driving (e.g., documenting that the patient is aware of the warning signs of hypoglycemia and its effects on driving performance).
- Formal assessment of your patient's function (e.g., documenting that the patient has undergone Assessment of Driving-Related Skills [ADReS] and including the ADReS scoring sheet in the chart).
- Any medical interventions and referrals you have made to improve the patient's function and any repeat testing to measure improvement.
- A copy of the driver rehabilitation specialist (DRS) report, if the patient has undergone driver assessment and/or rehabilitation.
- Your recommendation that the patient continues driving or ceases driving.
- If you recommend that the patient cease driving, include a summary of your interventions (e.g., "discussed driving retirement with patient and sent letter to reinforce recommendation," "discussed transportation options and gave copy of *Getting By Without Driving*," "contacted family members with patient's permission," and "reported patient to DMV with patient's knowledge"). Include copies of any written correspondence in the chart.
- Follow-up for degree of success in utilizing alternative transportation options and any signs of social isolation and depression. Document any further interventions, including referral to a social worker, geriatric care manager, or mental health professional.

ADDITIONAL LEGAL AND ETHICAL CONCERNS

What should you do if you find yourself in a particularly challenging situation? In this section, we offer recommendations for several potential situations:

Situation 1: *My patient threatens to sue me if I report him or her to the DMV.*
A patient's threat to sue should by no means influence you against complying with your state's reporting laws. If a patient threatens to sue, there are several steps you can take to protect yourself in the event of a lawsuit:
- Know if your state has passed legislation specifically protecting health care professionals against liability for reporting unsafe drivers in good faith.
- Even if your state has not passed such legislation, physicians generally run little risk of liability for following mandatory reporting statutes in good faith.[12] Consult your attorney or malpractice insurance carrier to determine your degree of risk.
- Make certain you have clearly documented your reasons for believing that the patient is an unsafe driver. Be aware that physician-patient privilege does not prevent you from reporting your patient to the DMV. Physician-patient privilege, which is defined as the patient's right to prevent disclosure of any communication between the physician and patient by the physician, does not apply in cases of required reporting.

Situation 2: *Should I report an unsafe driver even if my state does not have any reporting laws?*
In this situation, the physician's first priority is to ensure that the unsafe driver does not drive. If this can be accomplished without having the patient's license revoked, then there may be no need to report the patient to the DMV. However, if your patient refuses to stop driving despite your best efforts, then you must consider which is more likely to cause the greatest amount of harm: breaching the patient's confidentiality versus allowing the patient to potentially injure himself or herself and third parties in a motor vehicle crash. According to AMA Ethical Opinion E-2.24, "in situations where clear evidence of substantial driving impairment implies a strong threat to patient and public safety, and where the physician's advice to discontinue driving privileges is ignored, it is desirable and ethical to notify the Department of Motor Vehicles." Before reporting your patient, you may address the risk of liability for breaching patient confidentiality by following the steps listed under Situation 1.

Situation 3: *My patient has had his or her license suspended by the DMV for unsafe driving, but I am aware that he or she continues to drive.*
This patient is clearly violating the law, and several questions are raised: Is the physician responsible for upholding the law at the expense of breaching patient confidentiality? Since the license has been revoked by the DMV, is the driving safety of the patient now in the care of the DMV, the physician, or both?
   There are several steps you can take in this situation:
- Ask your patient why he or she continues to drive. Address the specific causes brought up by your patient (see Appendix H for recommendations). With your patient's permission, the family should be involved in finding solutions.
- Ask your patient if he or she understands that he or she is breaking the law. Reiterate your concerns about

the patient's safety, and ask how he or she would feel about causing a crash and potentially being injured or injuring someone else. Discuss the financial and legal consequences of being involved in a crash without a license or auto insurance.

- If your patient is cognitively impaired and lacks insight into this problem, the issue must be discussed with the individual who holds decision-making authority for the patient and with any other caregivers. These parties should understand their responsibility to prevent the patient from driving.

- If your patient continues to drive and your state has a physician reporting law, adhere to the law by reporting your patient as an unsafe driver (even if you have already done so previously, resulting in the revocation of your patient's license). If your state does not have a physician reporting law, base your decision to report as in Situation 2. The DMV, as the agency that grants and revokes the driver's license, will follow up appropriately.

Situation 4: *My patient threatens to find a new doctor if I report him or her to the DMV.*
This situation, while unfortunate, should not prevent you from adhering to your state's reporting laws. As a physician, it is your responsibility to care for your patients' health and safety, regardless of such threats. There are several strategies that may help you diffuse this situation:

- Reiterate the process and information used to support your recommendation that the patient retire from driving.

- Reiterate your concern for the safety of your patient, his or her passengers, and those sharing the road.

- Remind your patient that you try to provide the best possible care for his or her health and safety. State that driving safety is as much a part of patient care as encouraging patients to wear a safety belt, keep a smoke detector in the home, floss their teeth, and have regular physical check-ups.

- Encourage your patient to seek a second opinion. The patient may see a DRS if he or she has not already done so, or consult another physician.

- If your state DMV follows up on physician reports with driver retesting, inform the patient that just as it

is your responsibility to report him or her to the DMV, it is the patient's responsibility to prove his or her driving safety to the DMV. Emphasize that the DMV makes the final decision, and that only the DMV can revoke the license. Remind your patient that you have done everything medically possible to help him or her pass the driver test.

- As always, maintain your professional behavior even if your patient ultimately makes the decision to seek a new physician.

REFERENCES

1. Kelly R, Warke T, Steele I: Medical restrictions to driving: the awareness of patients and doctors, *Postgrad Med J* 75:537-539, 1999.
2. Miller D, Morley J: Attitudes of physicians toward elderly drivers and driving policy, *J Am Geriatr Soc* 40:722-724, 1993.
3. *Gooden v Tips*, 651 SW 2d 364 (Tex Ct App 1983).
4. *Wilschinsky v Medina*, 108 NM 511 (NM 1989).
5. *Freese v Lemmon*, 210 NW 2d 576, 577-578, 580 (Iowa 1973).
6. *Kaiser v Suburban Transportation System*, 65 Wash 2d 461, 398 P.2d 14 (Wash 1965).
7. *Duvall v Goldin*, 362 NW 2d 275 (Mich App 1984).
8. *Calwell v Hassan*, 260 Kan 769, 770, 925 P.2d 422 (Kan 1996).
9. *Myers v Quesenberry*, 144 Cal App 3d 888, 894, 193 Cal Rptr 733, 743 (1983).
10. *Schuster v Alternberg*, 424 NW 2d 159 (Wis 1988).
11. *Joy v Eastern Maine Medical Center*, 529 A2d 1364 (Me 1987).
12. Duckwork K, Kahn M: Interface with the legal system. In Tasman A, Kay J, Lieberman JA, et al, editors: *Psychiatry*, Philadelphia, 1997, WB Saunders, pp 1803-1821.
13. Justice J: Patient confidentiality and pharmacy practice, *The Consult Pharmacist* 12, 1997.
14. Retchin SM, Anapolle J: An overview of the older driver, *Clin Geriatr Med* 9:279-296, 1993.
15. Tripodis VL: Licensing policies for older drivers: balancing public safety with individual mobility, *Boston College Law Rev* 38 B.C.L. Rev 1051, 1997.
16. Equal Protection Clause of the Fourteenth Amendment to the United States Constitution.
17. Carr DB: The older adult driver, *Am Fam Physician* 61:141-148, 2000.

INDEX

G

Gadget Matrix, 17
Gasoline-powered automobiles and technical improvements, 26
Gasoline-powered vehicles dominate market, 25
Gastrointestinal disorders, drugs that treat, 194
Goals and related characteristics, client, 299-300
Golf carts, 422
Gray matter, 500
GRIMPS (Gross Impairments Screening), 106
Groups, IITS issues relevant to different client, 383-385
Guide, Adapted Driving Decision, 77-102
  client-centered approach, 78-80
  driver readiness, 81-87
  driver rehabilitation, 80
  driver rehabilitation services, 78-80
  driver rehabilitation team members and services, 81
  driving cessation, 98-101
  driving controls, 94-98
  enhanced quality of life, 80
  evaluating driver rehabilitation programs, 81
  key driver rehabilitation services, 80-81
  navigating guide, 78
  technology discontinuance, 80
  vehicle selection, 87-94
Guidelines, laws, regulations and, 473

H

Hand controls, 249
Handles, push, 206-207
Hazardous activity, driving as a, 8-9
Hazards, 400
  driver expectancy and, 398-404
    driver information, 398-404
    expectancy, 399
    hazards, 400
    information handling, 399
    memory, 399
    priority of information, 399-400
    reaction time, 399
    sight distance, 400-401
    specific information display techniques, 401
    visually displayed information, 398-399
  highway factors that constitute, 398-404
    driver information, 398-404
    expectancy, 399
    hazards, 400
    information handling, 399
    memory, 399
    priority of information, 399-400
    reaction time, 399
    sight distance, 400-401

Hazards *(Continued)*
    specific information display techniques, 401
    visually displayed information, 398-399
Health care plans and reimbursement, 336-337
Health care reimbursement, issues in, 337-342
  claims appeal process, 341-342
  covered services and exclusions, 338-340
  documentation, 338
  medical necessity, 340
  out-of-network providers, 340
Health issues, hearing loss interactions and other, 152-153
Healthy, older drivers, 173
Hearing
  optimizing driver's, 151-152
  review of, 146-150
    causes of hearing loss, 146-147
    cochlear implants, 147
    coping with hearing loss, 148
    frequency of hearing loss, 147-148
    general effects of hearing loss, 148
    hearing impairment and increased crash risk, 149-150
    impact of hearing loss on communication, 148
    impact of hearing loss on driving, 148-149
    treatment of hearing loss, 147
Hearing, clinical evaluation of, 146-153
  review of hearing, 146-150
Hearing impairment and increased crash risk, 149-150
Hearing impairments, on-road evaluation and clients with, 285-292
  alternatives to speech in vehicles, 287-288
  case study, 291
  communication methods used in dynamic driving environments, 289
  communication strategies that work best for client, 286
  compensation strategies for hearing loss, 288-289
  difficulties experienced while driving, 285
  environment that facilitates new learning, 285-288
  implementing on-road evaluation, 289-290
  licensing issues, 290
  lip or speech reading and sign language, 287
  open approach to issue of hearing loss, 286
  optimizing communication process, 285-288
  self-regulation of driving, 290-291

Hearing loss
  causes of, 146-147
  compensation strategies for, 288-289
  coping with, 148
  frequency of, 147-148
  general effects of, 148
  impact on communication, 148
  impact on driving, 148-149
  interactions and other health issues, 152-153
  off-road assessment for, 150-153
  open approach to issue of, 286
  treatment of, 147
Heart disease, 426
Henry, Ford, 38-39
High-risk populations, screening for driving safety, 474-475
Highway. *See* Road; Roadway
Highway-driver-vehicle relationship, 392-397
Highway factors that constitute hazards, 398-404
Highway infrastructure, 404-413
  cross slopes, 405
  design elements of roadways, 405-413
  lane widths, 404-405
  shoulders, 405
  sidewalks and curbs, 405
Highway signage, consistency of, 404
Highways, improved roads and, 27
Highways in America, proliferation of, 43
History
  medication, 196
  ocular, 136-139
HMOs (health maintenance organizations), 337
Hoist lifts, 94
Horizontal alignment, 405-406
Horseless carriages, 25
Hospital model, acute care, 67
Housing density, 456
Human as processor of information, 14-15
Hybrid engines, 24-25

I

IADL (instrumental activity of daily living), 47, 104, 475
ICF (International Classification of Functioning, Disability, and Health), 8
IITS to meet individual needs, choosing correct, 385-386
  compensation versus remediation, 385-386
  ITS and future challenges, 386-387
  maintenance of IITS, 386
  trialing and training needs, 386
IITSs (in-vehicle intelligent transport systems), 373
  analyzing demands of, 377-381
  interface design, 374-377